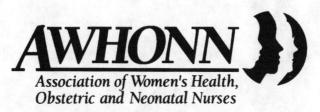

Perinatal Nursing

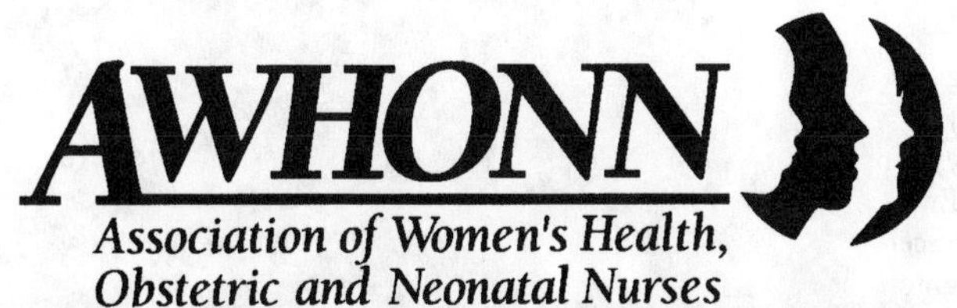

Perinatal Nursing

Second Edition

Kathleen Rice Simpson, PhD, RNC, FAAN
Perinatal Clinical Nurse Specialist
St. John's Mercy Medical Center
St. Louis, Missouri

Patricia A. Creehan, MS, MA, RNC, ACCE
Perinatal Clinical Nurse Specialist
Palos Community Hospital
Palos Heights, Illinois

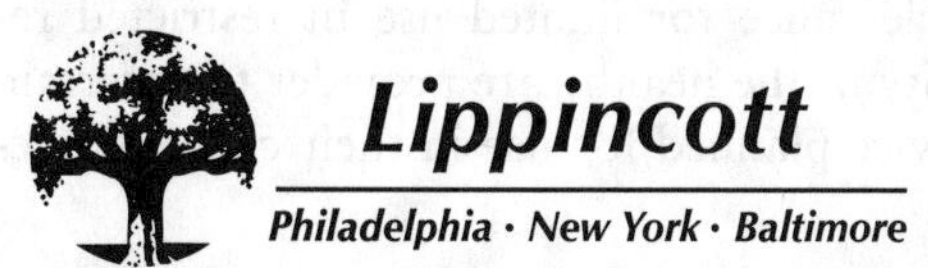

Acquisitions Editor: Jennifer E. Brogan
Assistant Editor: Susan Barta Rainey
Senior Project Editor: Sandra Cherrey Scheinin
Senior Production Manager: Helen Ewan
Production Coordinator: Michael Carcel
Design Coordinator: Brett MacNaughton
Manufacturing Manager: William Alberti
Indexer: Nancy Newman
Interior Design: Joan Wendt
Cover Design: Melissa Walter
Compositor: Pine Tree Composition
Printer: Victor Graphics

2nd Edition

9 8 7 6 5 4 3

Library of Congress Cataloging-in-Publication Data
Simpson, Kathleen Rice.
Perinatal nursing / Kathleen Rice Simpson, Patricia A. Creehan.--2nd ed.
p. cm.
At head of title: AWHONN, Association of Women's Health, Obstetric and Neonatal Nurses.
Includes bibliographical references and index.
ISBN 0-7817-2510-0 (alk. paper)
1. Maternity nursing. I. Creehan, Patricia A. II. Association of Women's Health, Obstetric and Neonatal Nurses. III. Title.
RG951 .A985 2001
610.73'678--dc21 00-067266

Care has been taken to confirm the accuracy of the information presented and to describe generally accepted practices. However, the authors, editors, and publisher are not responsible for errors or omissions or for any consequences from application of the information in this book and make no warranty, express or implied, with respect to the contents of the publication.

The authors, editors and publisher have exerted every effort to ensure that drug selection and dosage set forth in this text are in accordance with current recommendations and practice at the time of publication. However, in view of ongoing research, changes in government regulations, and the constant flow of information relating to drug therapy and drug reactions, the reader is urged to check the package insert for each drug for any change in indications and dosage and for added warnings and precautions. This is particularly important when the recommended agent is a new or infrequently employed drug.

Some drugs and medical devices presented in this publication have Food and Drug Administration (FDA) clearance for limited use in restricted research settings. It is the responsibility of the health care provider to ascertain the FDA status of each drug or device planned for use in their clinical practice.

To

the perinatal nurses at St. John's Mercy Medical Center in St. Louis, Missouri and Palos Community Hospital in Palos Heights, Illinois

and

my parents William and Dorothy, my husband Dan, and my children Daniel, Kate, Michael, John, and Elizabeth

KRS

my parents Raymond and Ruth

PAC

CONTRIBUTORS

Debbie Fraser Askin, MN, RNC
Assistant Professor, Faculty of Nursing
Neonatal Nurse Practitioner
University of Manitoba
Winnipeg, Manitoba, Canada
CHAPTER 14: Newborn Adaptation to Extrauterine Life

Mary Lee Barron, MSN, RN-CS, FNP
Instructor, Family Nurse Practitioner Program
St. Louis University School of Nursing
St. Louis, Missouri
CHAPTER 7: Antenatal Care

Lynn Clark Callister, PhD, RN
Associate Dean and Associate Professor
Brigham Young University
Provo, Utah
CHAPTER 4: Integrating Cultural Beliefs and Practices Into the Care of Childbearing Women

Bonnie Flood Chez, MSN, RNC
Perinatal Clinical Nurse Specialist Consultant
President, Nursing Education Resources
Tampa, Florida
CHAPTER 2: Professional and Legal Issues

Patricia A. Creehan, MS, MA, RNC, ACCE
Perinatal Clinical Nurse Specialist
Palos Community Hospital
Palos Heights, Illinois
CHAPTER 11: Pain Relief and Comfort Measures During Labor
CHAPTER 15: Newborn Physical Assessment
CHAPTER 16: Newborn Nutrition

Nancy Friest Dahlberg, MS, RNC
Clinical Nurse Manger
Minnesota OB Homecare
Allina Health System
Minneapolis, Minnesota
CHAPTER 19: Postpartum Home Care

Joan Drukker Dauphinee, MS, RNC
Staff Nurse
UPMC Shadyside Hospital
LDRP Unit
Pittsburgh, Pennsylvania
CHAPTER 8: High-Risk Pregnancy—Multiple Gestation

Jeanne Watson Driscoll, RN, MS, CS
Clinical Nurse Specialist
Principal
Hestia Institute: Center for Women and Families
Wellesley, Massachusetts
CHAPTER 6: Psychosocial Adaptation to Pregnancy and Postpartum

Margaret Comerford Freda, EdD, RN, CHES, FAAN
Associate Professor, Department of Obstetrics and Gynecology and Women's Health
Albert Einstein College of Medicine
Montefiore Medical Center
Bronx, New York
Editor, *MCN: The American Journal of Maternal Child Nursing*
CHAPTER 8: High-Risk Pregnancy—Preterm Labor and Birth

Dotti C. James, PhD, RN
Assistant Professor, Perinatal Nursing
St. Louis University School of Nursing
St. Louis, Missouri
CHAPTER 12: Postpartum Care

Jo M. Kendrick, MSN, RNC, OGNP
Obstetrics and Gynecology Nurse Practitioner
University of Tennessee
Medical Center at Knoxville
Department of Obstetrics and Gynecology
Knoxville, Tennessee
CHAPTER 8: High-Risk Pregnancy—Diabetes
CHAPTER 9: Labor and Birth

Ann Blystad Keppler, MN, RN
Clinical Nurse Specialist, Family Maternity Center
Coordinator, Postpartum Care Center Clinic
Coordinator, Parent Education
Evergreen Hospital Medical Center
Kirkland, Washington
Clinical Faculty
School of Nursing
University of Washington
Seattle, Washington
CHAPTER 18: Discharge Planning

Tekoa L. King, CNM, MPH
Nurse–Midwife
Associate Clinical Professor
Department of Obstetrics and Gynecology
School of Medicine
University of California San Francisco
San Francisco, California
CHAPTER 10: Fetal Assessment During Labor

G. Eric Knox, MD
Director of Patient Safety
Children's Hospitals and Clinics
The Twin Cities of Minneapolis and St. Paul
Professor of Obstetrics and Gynecology
University of Minnesota Medical School
Minneapolis, Minnesota
CHAPTER 3: Perinatal Teamwork: Turning Rhetoric Into Reality

Karren Kowalski, PhD, RN, FAAN
Consultant
Kowalski & Associates
Denver, Colorado
CHAPTER 13: Perinatal Loss and Bereavement

Cynthia F. Krening, MS, RNC
Perinatal Clinical Nurse Specialist
Family Birthplace
Presbyterian/St. Luke's Medical Center
Denver, Colorado
CHAPTER 8: High-Risk Pregnancy—Pulmonary Complications

Carol Jean Luppi, BSN, RNC
Clinical Educator
Co-Chair Critical Care Obstetric Nursing Team
Center for Labor and Birth
Brigham and Women's Hospital
Boston, Massachusetts
CHAPTER 5: Physiologic Changes of Pregnancy
CHAPTER 8: High-Risk Pregnancy—Cardiac Disease

Patricia L. Nash, MSN, RNC, NNP
Neonatal Nurse Practitioner Staff Member
NICU Staff Educator
Cardinal Glennon Children's Hospital
St. Louis, Missouri
CHAPTER 17: Common Neonatal Complications

Judith H. Poole, PHD, RNC
Perinatal Outreach Education Coordinator
Department of Obstetrics and Gynecology
Carolinas Medical Center
Charlotte, North Carolina
CHAPTER 8: High-Risk Pregnancy—Hypertensive Disorders

Ann Ropp, MS, RN
Vice President
Women's and Children's Services
St. Luke's Shawnee Mission Health System
Kansas City, Missouri
CHAPTER 1: Managing the Quality of Care

Kathleen Rice Simpson, PhD, RNC, FAAN
Perinatal Clinical Nurse Specialist
St. John's Mercy Medical Center
St. Louis, Missouri
CHAPTER 1: Managing the Quality of Care
CHAPTER 2: Professional and Legal Issues
CHAPTER 3: Perinatal Teamwork: Turning Rhetoric Into Reality
CHAPTER 9: Labor and Birth
CHAPTER 10: Fetal Assessment During Labor
CHAPTER 18: Discharge Planning

Mary Ellen Burke Sosa, MS, RNC
Clinical Teaching Associate
Brown University School of Medicine
Clinical Nurse Specialist
Women and Infants Hospital
Providence, Rhode Island
CHAPTER 8: High-Risk Pregnancy—Bleeding and Maternal Transfer

Kathleen Thorman, PhD, RN, BSN, MA
Administrator, Women and Children
St. John's Mercy Medical Center
St. Louis, Missouri
CHAPTER 1: Managing the Quality of Care

Marsha Walker, RN, IBCLC
Lactation Consultant
Weston, Massachusetts
CHAPTER 16: Newborn Nutrition

REVIEWERS

Debbie Fraser Askin, MN, RNC
Assistant Professor, Faculty of Nursing
Neonatal Nurse Practitioner
University of Manitoba
Winnipeg, Manitoba, Canada

Jana Atterbury, MSN, RNC
Maternal Child Clinical Nurse Specialist
Lake Forest Hospital
Lake Forest, Illinois

Susan Bakewell-Sachs, PhD, RN, APN, C
Associate Professor of Nursing
Coordinator of Family Nurse Practitioner Program
The College of New Jersey School of Nursing
Ewing, New Jersey
Pediatric Nurse Practitioner
The Children's Hospital of Philadelphia
Philadelphia, Pennsylvania

Cheryl Tatano Beck, DNSc, CNM, FAAN
Professor
School of Nursing
University of Connecticut
Storrs, Connecticut

Monica C. Berry, RN, JD, LLM, FASHRM
Senior Risk Consultant
Healthcare Consulting Services
St. Paul Companies, Inc.
Deerfield, Illinois

Susan Blackburn, PhD, RN,C, FAAN
Professor, Department of Family and Child Nursing
University of Washington
Seattle, Washington

Debbie Bocar, MS, MEd, RN, IBCLC
Lactation Consultant
Oklahoma City, Oklahoma

Barbara Buchko, MSN, RN
Clinical Nurse Specialist
Department of Nursing
Women and Children Service Line
York Hospital
York, Pennsylvania

Jennifer W. Burton, MSN, RNC, PNNP
Perinatal Nurse Practitioner
Maternal Child Nursing
Rush-Presbyterian-St. Luke's Medical Center
Chicago, Illinois

Sandra K. Cesario, PhD, RNC
Clinical Assistant Professor
College of Nursing
University of Oklahoma
Claremore, Oklahoma

Octavio Chirino, MD, FACOG
Chairman, Department of Obstetrics and Gynecology
St. John's Mercy Medical Center
St. Louis, Missouri

Phyllis Portnoy Cohen, RNC, MS
Clinical Nurse Specialist, Perinatal Outreach
Division of Obstetrics and Gynecology
Long Island Jewish Medical Center
New Hyde Park, New York

Paul Craig, RN, JD
Risk Manager
St. Francis Memorial Hospital
San Francisco, California

Marie A. Cueman, MS, RN, CNAA
President
Cueman Associates, Consulting Firm
Faculty
Fairleigh Dickinson University
Hackensack, New Jersey

Cindy Curtis, RN, IBCLC
Registered Nurse, Maternal and Child Health
Director of Lactation Center
Culpeper Memorial Hospital
Culpeper, Virginia

Kit S. Devine, ARNP, MSN
Women's Health Nurse Practitioner and Practice Site Manager
Fertility and Endocrine Associates
Louisville, Kentucky
Adjunct Faculty
Bellarmine College
Louisville, Kentucky

Susan M. Ellerbee, PhD, RNC, IBCLC
Associate Professor
University of Oklahoma College of Nursing
Lactation Consultant
University Hospital
Oklahoma City, Oklahoma

Nannette Libertore Gillette, MSN, RN, IBCLC
Clinical Director
Birth Center and Perinatal Special Care Unit
MultiCare Health System
Tacoma, Washington

Linda Goodwin, MEd, RNC
Manager, Family Birthplace & Family Beginnings
Group Health Hospitals
Seattle and Redmond, Washington

Cecile Graf, MSN, RNC
Perinatal Outreach Educator
Nebraska Methodist Hospital
Omaha, Nebraska

Linda K. Grossglauser, MSN, NNP, RNC
Neonatal Nurse Practitioner
St. John's Mercy Medical Center
St. Louis, Missouri

Ellen Hodnett, PhD, RN
Professor in Perinatal Nursing Research
University of Toronto
School of Nursing
Toronto, Ontario, Canada

Maureen Kelley, PhD, CNM, FACNM
Associate Clinical Professor
Director, Nurse Midwifery Education Program
Nell Hodgson Woodruff School of Nursing
Emory University
Atlanta, Georgia

Tekoa King, CNM, MPH
Nurse–Midwife
Associate Clinical Professor
Department of Obstetrics and Gynecology
School of Medicine
University of California, San Francisco
San Francisco, California

G. Eric Knox, MD
Director of Patient Safety
Children's Hospitals and Clinics
The Twin Cities of Minneapolis and St. Paul
Professor of Obstetrics and Gynecology
University of Minnesota Medical School
Minneapolis, Minnesota

Linda Koehl, MS, RNC
Education/Quality Coordinator
Department of Women and Children
Rush-Presbyterian-St. Luke's Medical Center
Chicago, Illinois

Susan Leavitt, BSN, RN
Director, Maternity Center
Elliot Hospital
Manchester, New Hampshire

Patricia McCartney, PhD, RN
Clinical Assistant Professor
School of Nursing
State University of New York
University at Buffalo
Staff Nurse, Labor and Delivery
Children's Hospital of Buffalo
Buffalo, New York

Mary Lou Moore, PhD, RNC, FACCE, FAAN
Associate Professor, Obstetrics and Gynecology
Wake Forest University School of Medicine
Winston-Salem, North Carolina

Merry-K. Moos, MPH, RN, FNP
Research Associate Professor
University of North Carolina
Division of Maternal and Fetal Medicine
Department of Obstetrics and Gynecology
Chapel Hill, North Carolina

Elizabeth Peter, PhD, RN
Assistant Professor
Faculty of Nursing and Joint Center for Bioethics at the University of Toronto
Toronto, Ontario
Canada

Mary Elizabeth Philips, MSN, RN
Nurse Manager, LDR Unit
St. John's Mercy Medical Center
St. Louis, Missouri

Martina Letko Porter, MS, MBA, RNC
Principal and Consultant
Letko Porter Group
Alexandria, Virginia

Nancy O'Brien-Abel, MN, RNC
Perinatal Clinical Nurse Specialist/Clinical Faculty
Department of Obstetrics and Gynecology
University of Washington School of Medicine
Seattle, Washington

Deborah A. Raines, PhD, RNC
Associate Professor
Virginia Commonwealth University
Richmond, Virginia

Joyce Roberts, PhD, CNM
Professor, Nurse-Midwifery and Women's Health Graduate Program
Ohio State University
Columbus, Ohio

Catherine Rommal, BS, RNC, FASHRM
Manager, Education Services and Product Development
Healthcare Professional Liability Division
Farmers Insurance
Los Angeles, California

Patricia M. Sauer, MSN, RNC
Clinical Nurse Specialist
Labor and Delivery and High-Risk Obstetrics
Northside Hospital
Atlanta, Georgia

Erna Snelgrove-Clarke, MN, RN, IBCLC
Nursing Research Associate
Maternal, Newborn and Women's Health
Nursing Research Department
IWK Grace Health Centre
Halifax, Nova Scotia, Canada

Mary Ellen Burke Sosa, MS, RNC
Clinical Teaching Associate
Brown University School of Medicine
Clinical Nurse Specialist
Women and Infants Hospital
Providence, Rhode Island

Anne Simmonds Spence, BScN, LCCE, CD (DONA)
Faculty, The Michener Institute for Health Sciences
President, The Childbirth Network, Inc.
Consultant, University of Toronto
Maternal and Infant Reproductive Health Unit
Toronto, Ontario, Canada

Ellen Tappero, MN, RNC, NNP
Executive Editor, *Neonatal Network: The Journal of Neonatal Nursing*
Neonatal Nurse Practitioner
Exempla Lutheran Medical Center
Wheat Ridge, Colorado

Keiko L. Torgerson, BSN, MSM, RNC
Operations Officer, 81st Aerospace Medicine Squadron
Keesler Medical Center
Keesler Air Force Base, Mississippi

Carol Trotter, PhD, RNC, NNP
Neonatal Nurse Practitioner
St. John's Mercy Medical Center
St. Louis, Missouri
Adjunct Clinical Associate Professor
Coordinator of Neonatal Nurse Practitioner Option
University of Missouri—St. Louis
Barnes College of Nursing
St. Louis, Missouri

Sara Rice Wheeler, DNS, RNCS, LCPC
Clinical Instructor, Maternal Child Health
University of Illinois at Chicago
College of Nursing
Urbana Regional Campus
Urbana Illinois

Lenore R. Williams, MSN, RN, CNS
Director, Professional Nurse Associates
Health Design Plus
Hudson, Ohio

Sue A. Woodson, CNM, RNC, MSN
Nurse–Midwife
University of Virginia
Charlottesville, Virginia

FOREWORD

Nursing practice is continually being redefined in response to an explosion of knowledge and advances in technologic applications in healthcare. Nursing research has emerged as a significant force in shaping nursing practice in the 21st century, and will continue to provide numerous opportunities for the exploration of important questions relevant to the practice arena. Concurrently, major shifts in the healthcare delivery system have had an impact on nursing practice, including an emphasis on health promotion and risk reduction, growth in community-based care, cost containment, and an unprecedented increase in managed care and highly integrated care systems.

This book provides a comprehensive review of perinatal nursing practice and presents an evidence-based approach to nursing care for mothers, their newborns, and families. The publication of this second edition is particularly important, considering the constant pressures to reduce cost in the clinical setting while promoting quality outcomes. Nurses find themselves in a day-to-day struggle as they attempt to balance quality patient care with fewer resources than ever before. Fewer nurses are caring for more patients than a decade ago. We are facing a nationwide shortage of professional registered nurses in general, as well as a decrease in the numbers of nurses in specialty practice. While the emphasis on cost containment is likely to continue as policy makers debate the relative merits of various health delivery systems, nurses will maintain a leadership role in refocusing the discussion to quality patient outcomes. The integration of the best evidence into clinical practice many times results in significant cost savings while promoting the best possible outcomes for mothers and babies. Adoption of a philosophy of care by all perinatal healthcare providers acknowledging that pregnancy, labor, and birth are normal processes and that unnecessary interventions add risk of iatrogenic injuries and more costs of care, would go a long way toward improving perinatal practice. This book provides a foundation for providing care that is based on the best available evidence.

Specific nursing issues that arise from the rapid pace of change in the healthcare system include the following:

- The need for a highly skilled, well-prepared, and competent nursing workforce that possesses the knowledge base needed to deliver care to women and newborns.
- The importance of the unique relationship between the perinatal nurse and childbearing women and their families.
- The continuing need for health teaching and support for the mother, newborn, and family as a cornerstone of nursing responsibilities.
- Changes in the practice settings.
- An increased awareness by consumers about preventable adverse outcomes in the healthcare setting and pressures to reduce errors by healthcare providers.
- An emphasis on individualization of care considering the sociocultural diversity of the population.

AWHONN is pleased to present this valuable resource as a tool for continued intellectual and professional growth of perinatal nurses. Through the promotion of excellence in nursing practice, the association's mission of improving the healthcare outcomes of women and newborns is realized. It is my hope that you will use this book often and share the information with your colleagues in the practice arena.

Martha G. Lavender, RN, MSN, DSN
2001 President, AWHONN

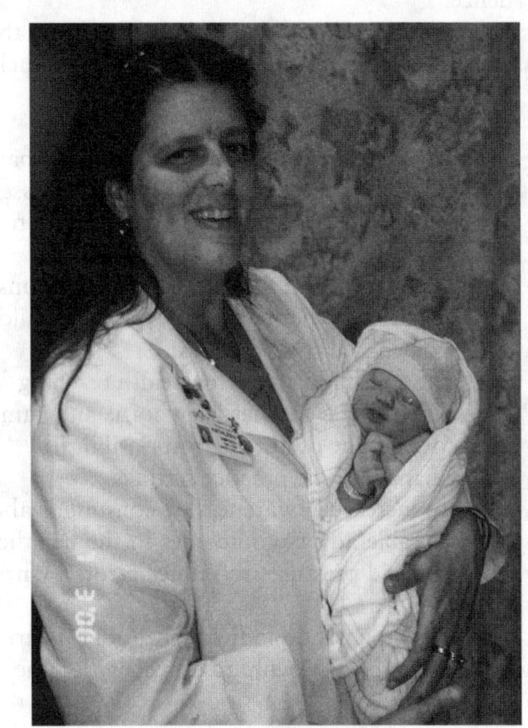

Kathleen Simpson

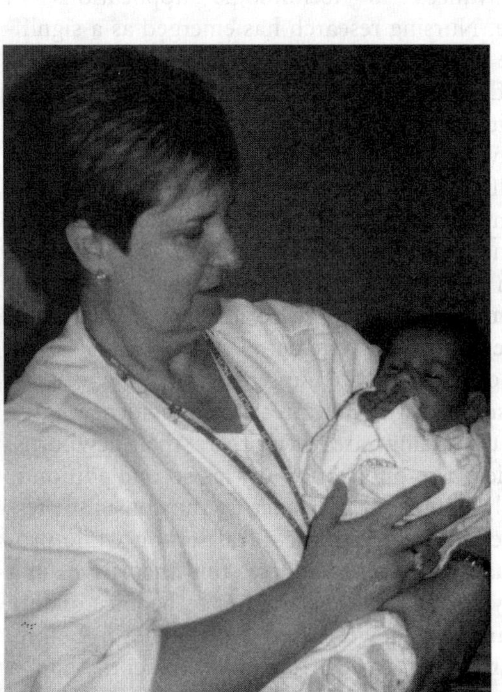

Patricia Creehan

INTRODUCTION

The goal of this text is to provide perinatal nurses with the knowledge and evidence to promote the best possible outcomes for mothers and babies. There have been significant advances in the practice of perinatal nursing since publication of the first edition of *AWHONN's Perinatal Nursing*. We have made every attempt to provide the best evidence and latest standards for all areas of clinical practice. Two new chapters have been added: *Perinatal Teamwork: Turning Rhetoric Into Reality* and *Integrating Cultural Beliefs and Practices Into The Care Of Childbearing Women.* Working together with physician and midwife colleagues to provide care collaboratively to childbearing women, is critical to our success as perinatal healthcare providers. A thorough knowledge and understanding of cultural practices and beliefs of all childbearing women is essential to provide comprehensive perinatal nursing care. Increasingly women with complications of pregnancy are cared for in community hospitals. Thus, we expanded the chapter on perinatal complications to include multiple gestation, diabetes, cardiac disease, and pulmonary complications, in addition to the existing content on bleeding, preterm labor, and hypertensive disorders of pregnancy. We provided practical strategies to decrease risk of adverse outcomes and promote evidence-based care. An item bank has been added to facilitate use of the text as a resource for orientation and continuing education.

This text reflects the philosophy that pregnancy, labor, and birth are natural processes for most women. Healthy women do well with minimal selected interventions within the context of a well-designed safety net (ie, the ability to intervene when necessary in a clinically timely manner). It is important to remember that unnecessary interventions introduce the risk of iatrogenic maternal–fetal injuries. We have attempted to present pregnancy, labor, and birth as healthy life events rather than medical events. However, effective strategies for providing nursing care to mothers and babies when complications do arise are also covered.

As perinatal nurses we must critically examine the continued medicalization of the childbirth process. As technologic advances are introduced, high-tech, low-touch care is in danger of becoming the norm. The best hope for advocating for safe and effective perinatal nursing care is a firm commitment to providing care based on the combined weight of available evidence. This commitment involves making an effort to become educated about how to critique research and apply the evidence to everyday clinical practice. Knowledge is power. This power is within all perinatal nurses who arm themselves with the skills required to have clinical discussions with physician colleagues and hospital administrators based on evidence, and thus become true partners in determining the best practices for caring for mothers and babies.

Over the past five years many readers have given us helpful suggestions for additions and revisions. We were fortunate to have expert nurse, physician, and midwife colleagues collaborate with us as contributors and reviewers. We invited a physician colleague as a contributor to give us another perspective on effective perinatal teamwork. The collective work of all of these individuals served to make this edition a valuable resource for practicing perinatal nurses. We sincerely hope our fellow AWHONN members and all perinatal nurses will find this text practical and useful in the clinical setting.

Kathleen Rice Simpson, PHD, RNC, FAAN
Patricia A. Creehan, MS, MA, RNC, ACCE

ACKNOWLEDGMENTS

The authors gratefully acknowledge Jennifer Brogan, Director of Clinical Practice, and Susan Barta Rainey, Assistant Editor, at Lippincott Williams & Wilkins for their advice, patience, editorial assistance, and enthusiasm. We would also like to acknowledge Saundra Brenner, Jennifer Platt, Mayris Woods, Kathy Alsup, and Gretchen Dalzell, who are medical librarians at Saint John's Mercy Medical Center in St. Louis, MO, and Karen Sullivan, medical librarian at Palos Community Hospital in Palos Heights, IL, who spent many hours locating resources and checking references. We also thank David Becker, medical photographer at St. John's Mercy Medical Center, for his expertise in photographing fetal monitoring strips and the cover photo.

CONTENTS

PART 1
Foundations for Practice 1

CHAPTER 1
MANAGING THE QUALITY OF CARE 1

Economics of Healthcare in the United States 2
Challenges Facing Nurse Managers of Perinatal Services 4
Summary 18

CHAPTER 2
PROFESSIONAL AND LEGAL ISSUES 21

Professional Issues 22
Legal Issues 29
Summary 47
Appendix 2A Framework for Root Cause Analysis in Response to a Sentinel Event 50

CHAPTER 3
PERINATAL TEAMWORK: TURNING RHETORIC INTO REALITY 53

Why Teams? 53
Why Not Teams? 54
Team Members Changing Perceptions of Each Other: Good News and a Further Foundation for Building Effective Perinatal Teams 58
What is a Team? 58
Healthcare Under Pressure: Resulting Stress Makes Teamwork Difficult 59
Team-Based Perinatal Care: Self-Assessment 59
Challenges and Opportunities with Perinatal Teamwork 65
Potential Benefits of Perinatal Teamwork 65
Summary 66

CHAPTER 4
INTEGRATING CULTURAL BELIEFS AND PRACTICES INTO THE CARE OF CHILDBEARING WOMEN 68

Cultural Frameworks 69
Childbearing and the Meaning of Birth 71
Practices Associated With Childbearing 72
Gender Roles 72
Experiences of Pain 73
Major Cultural Groups in the United States 73
Nontraditional Cultural Groups 80
Biologic and Physiologic Variations Between Groups 81
Barriers to Integrating Culture into Nursing Care 82
Techniques to Integrate Culture into Nursing Care 84
Long-Term Strategies 88
Summary 89
Appendix 4A Culture Care Resources 94

PART 2
Antepartum 95

CHAPTER 5
PHYSIOLOGIC CHANGES OF PREGNANCY 96

Reproductive Hormonal Changes During Pregnancy 96
Cardiovascular System 98

Respiratory System 101
Renal System 103
Gastrointestinal System 105
Metabolic Changes 107
Endocrine System 108
Neurologic System 109
Integumentary System 109
Musculoskeletal System 110
Reproductive System 110
Host Defense and Immunity 111
Summary 112

CHAPTER 6
PSYCHOSOCIAL ADAPTATION TO PREGNANCY AND POSTPARTUM 115

Aspects of Psychosocial Nursing Care 115
Adaptations During Pregnancy 117
Adaptations During Labor and Birth 120
Adaptations in the Postpartum Period 121
Summary 124

CHAPTER 7
ANTENATAL CARE..................... 125

Birth in the United States 125
Access to Prenatal Care 127
Effects of Prenatal Care on Birth Outcome 129
Prenatal Risk Assessment 130
Fetal Development 147
Fetal Surveillance 147
Plan for Nursing Care and Intervention 154
Collaborative Management and Follow-up 154
Summary 158
Appendix 7A Perinatal Substance Abuse Assessment Guide 161
Appendix 7B Abuse Assessment 164
Appendix 7C Immunization During Pregnancy 166

CHAPTER 8
HIGH-RISK PREGNANCY 173

Hypertensive Disorders 173
Bleeding 190
Preterm Labor and Birth 207
Diabetes 219
Cardiac Disease 235
Pulmonary Complications 243
Multiple Gestation 253
Maternal Transfer 274
Summary 276
Appendix 8A Guidelines for Home Care Management of Selected High-Risk Pregnancy Conditions 292

PART 3
Intrapartum 297

CHAPTER 9
LABOR AND BIRTH 298

Overview of Labor and Birth 298
Emotional Support During Labor and Birth 328
Clinical Interventions for Laboring Women in Labor 329
Cesarean Birth 350
Summary 358
Appendix 9A Admission Assessment 366
Appendix 9B Labor Flow Sheet 369
Appendix 9C Cervical Ripening and Induction of Labor Analysis 376

CHAPTER 10
FETAL ASSESSMENT DURING LABOR 378

Historic Perspectives 378
Definitions and Appropriate Terms Describing Fetal Heart Rate Patterns 379
Techniques of Fetal Heart Rate Monitoring 380
Physiologic Basis for Fetal Heart Rate Monitoring 383
Characteristics of the Normal Fetal Heart Rate 390
Interventions for Nonreassuring Fetal Heart Rate Patterns 391
Fetal Heart Rate Patterns 392
Assessment of Pattern Evolution 402
Ancillary Tests of Fetal Well-Being 405
Nursing Assessment and Management Strategies 409

Ongoing Issues Related to the Use of Fetal Heart Rate Monitoring During Labor 411
Summary 412

CHAPTER 11
PAIN RELIEF AND COMFORT MEASURES DURING LABOR 417

Physiologic Basis for Labor Pain 417
Physiologic Responses to Pain 418
Psychosocial Factors Influencing Pain Perception 418
Nonpharmacologic Pain Management Strategies 423
Pharmacologic Pain Management Strategies 432
Summary 442

PART 4
Postpartum 445

CHAPTER 12
POSTPARTUM CARE 446

Anatomic and Physiologic Changes During the Postpartum Period 446
Postpartum Nursing Care 452
Complications During the Postpartum Period 455
Individualizing Care for Women with Special Needs 463
Postpartum Learning Needs Assessment and Education 464
Selected Postpartum Teaching Topics 465
Women's Perspectives on the Transition to Parenthood 468
Family Transition to Parenthood 468
Summary 470
Appendix 12A Daily Postpartum Assessments and Interventions 473

CHAPTER 13
PERINATAL LOSS AND BEREAVEMENT 476

The Phenomenology of Loss 476
Psychological Perspective of Grief 480
Sociologic Perspective of Bereavement 483
Spiritual Perspective of Bereavement 484
Ontologic Perspective of Bereavement 485
Nursing Management 485
Healing the Healer 490
Summary 490

PART 5
The Newborn 493

CHAPTER 14
NEWBORN ADAPTATION TO EXTRAUTERINE LIFE............... 494

Influence of Maternal History 494
Physiologic Changes During Transition 494
Stabilization and Resuscitation of the Newborn 502
Initial Assessment of the Newborn 502
Procedures Performed in the Birthing Room 506
Promoting Family–Newborn Attachment 508
Exposure to Group B Beta-Hemolytic Streptococcus 508
Hepatitis B Vaccine 510
Summary 511

CHAPTER 15
NEWBORN PHYSICAL ASSESSMENT ... 513

Gestational Age Assessment 513
Integument Assessment 514
Head Assessment 517
Eye Assessment 520
Ear Assessment 521
Nose Assessmnt 523
Mouth Assessment 524
Neck Assessment 524
Chest and Lung Assessment 525
Cardiovascular SystemAssessment 528
Abdominal Assessment 530
Genitourinary System Assessment 532
Musculoskeletal System Assessment 534
Neurologic Assessment 539
Summary 541
Appendix 15A Characteristics of Infant State 543
Appendix 15B Characteristics of the Ballard Gestation Age Assessment Tool 546
Appendix 15C Developmental Reflexes 548

CHAPTER 16
NEWBORN NUTRITION 550

Incidence of Breast-Feeding 550
Physiology of Milk Production 551
Biospecificity of Human Milk 553
Breast-Feeding Process 554
Breast-Feeding Management 557
Potential Breast-Feeding Problems 561
Medications and Breast-Feeding 568
Formula Feeding 568
Lactation Suppression 571
Summary 571

CHAPTER 17
COMMON NEONATAL COMPLICATIONS 575

Respiratory Distress 575
Congenital Heart Disease 579
Hypoglycemia 582
Hyperbilirubinemia 584
Neonatal Sepsis 587
Neonatal Abstinence Syndrome 591
Transport and Return Transport 596
Summary 596
Appendix 17A Algorithm for Management of Hyperbilirubinemia in the Healthy Term Infant 599
Appendix B Loyola University Perinata Network: Acutely Ill Neonatal Transport Collaborative Carepath 603
Appendix C Loyola University Perinatal Network: Neonatal Return Collaborative Carepath 606

PART 6
The Transition from Hospital to Home 610

CHAPTER 18
DISCHARGE PLANNING 610

Current Issues 611
Prenatal Patient Database 612
Prenatal Classes 612
Educational Methods and Materials 618
Family Preference Plan 618
Learning-Needs Assessment 620
Case Management 623
Role of the Staff Nurse 625
Care Paths 626
Postdischarge Follow-up 627
Program Evaluation 630
Summary 631
Appendix 18A Pregnancy, Having a Baby, and Parenting Pathway 633

CHAPTER 19
POSTPARTUM HOME CARE 643

Review of the Literature 643
Models of Services 645
Essential Components of Quality Perinatal Home Care Services 646
Nursing Assessments 649
Nursing Interventions 651
Outcome Monitoring and Quality Care 651
Nurse Providers of Perinatal Home Care 652
Summary 653
Appendix 19A Home Care Assessment Form 656
Appendix 19B Telephone Assessment Form 658
Appendix 19C Maternal Assessment Form 660
Appendix 19D Infant Assessment Form 662
Appendix 19E Patient Satisfaction Form 664

APPENDIX A Item Bank Questions and Answer Key 667

INDEX.................................. 707

PART 1

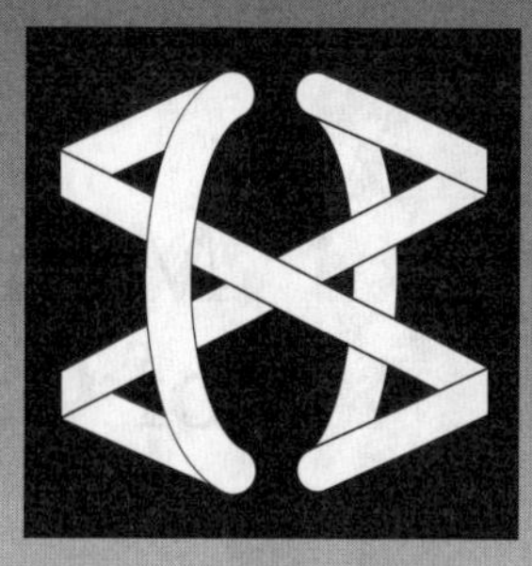

FOUNDATIONS FOR PRACTICE

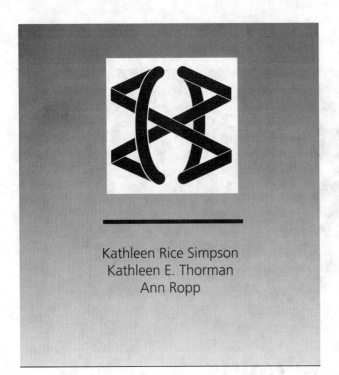

Kathleen Rice Simpson
Kathleen E. Thorman
Ann Ropp

CHAPTER 1

Managing the Quality of Care

Multiple factors influence the ability to consistently provide quality care and achieve the best possible outcomes for mothers and babies. Perinatal nurse managers face distinct challenges in the new century. The nurse manager must operate within fiscal restraints based on projected volume of births and other perinatal services, continually decreasing reimbursement rates and the margins needed to meet institutional targets for financial viability. Attempting to comply with professional standards and guidelines from organizations such as the Joint Commission on Accreditation of Healthcare Organizations (JCAHO) (2000), the Association of Women's Health, Obstetric and Neonatal Nurses (AWHONN), the American College of Obstetricians and Gynecologists (AGOG), and federal and state regulations requires significant time as well as financial and staff resources. Recruiting and retaining competent nurses has become especially challenging as the population of nurses in the United States ages, and because there are fewer applicants and graduates of nursing programs. Specialty areas of nursing practice such as perinatal nursing have been affected by this shortage in most areas of the country. Staff morale is at risk because of chronic understaffing and nurses caring for more patients than in the past. Maintaining high levels of patient satisfaction is challenging when care is provided by nurses who feel overworked, underpaid, and undervalued in the current environment. Physician satisfaction is a key factor in retaining physicians on staff who bring their patients to the institution for revenue-generating care and treatment. Working with physician colleagues who are feeling the pressure of demands for efficiency by third-party payers and hospital administrators can strain existing relationships. Achieving quality clinical outcomes within the context of these multiple challenges remains a top priority for perinatal nurse managers. To survive today, perinatal nurse managers must do much more than manage. They must be inspirational leaders, mentors, facilitators, mediators, visionaries, risk takers, strategists, and financial experts.

ECONOMICS OF HEALTHCARE IN THE UNITED STATES

Healthcare costs in the United States exceeded 1 trillion dollars in 1997, or more than $4,090 per person, a substantial increase since 1993, when total costs were $910 billion and per person costs were $3,300 (Beil, 1999; Freies et al., 1993). In 1997, healthcare costs accounted for 13.5% of the gross domestic product (GDP) (Beil, 1999). Most healthcare economists think this figure will continue to grow in the next decade, rising by at least 1% higher than the GDP. Some predict an increase in U.S. healthcare costs to $2.1 trillion dollars by 2007 (Coile, 1999). This prediction depends in part on the probability that the impact managed care has made on costs has been fully realized and that normal inflationary factors will contribute to higher costs. Managed care enrollment has maximized at 85% of the potential population. Other factors influencing the probable doubling of the nation's healthcare costs in the next decade are the growing population of older Americans, greater life expectancies, increased consumer demand, and rising costs of pharmaceuticals and other innovations in medical technology (Coile, 1999).

Administrative costs as a percentage of total hospital costs have risen steadily over the last decade (Woolhandler & Himmelstein, 1997). Administrative costs and overall costs of care were significantly higher in for-profit hospitals compared with private not-for-profit hospitals (Woolhandler & Himmelstein, 1997). Despite early promise, many managed care plans have not been financially successful. Health maintenance organizations (HMOs) in the United States collectively lost $490 million dollars in 1998, and 56% of HMOs did not make a profit in 1998 (Weiss, 1999). This is a real issue for tax payers and healthcare consumers because HMOs may attempt to drop Medicaid or Medicare patients and patients with significant health problems. The burden of care for the sickest Americans may fall to the federal, state, and local governments (Weiss, 1999).

The government's share of healthcare costs has increased significantly over the past decade. In 1990, healthcare spending by federal, state, and local governments accounted for about 40% of the nation's total healthcare bill, but by 1997, this percentage had risen to 46% of the total, an estimated $507 billion dollars. In contrast, private resources funded 54% of healthcare costs ($585 billion) in 1997, a decrease from 60% in 1990. Although there have been efforts to shift costs to the private sector, the U.S. government's share has continued to rise since 1965, when Medicare and Medicaid programs were enacted (Iglehart, 1999).

The United States spends far more GDP dollars on healthcare than other industrialized nations, but available data do not suggest our system provides better care or has better patient outcomes. Infant mortality rates are frequently used as quality indicators of national healthcare services. Despite spending billions on prenatal care, preterm birth prevention programs, and high-tech neonatal services, the United States consistently ranks unfavorably compared with other developed countries, and the preterm birth rate is the highest since 1970 (11.6% versus 7.0%), when these data began to be systematically collected (Ventura, Martin, Curtin, Mathews, & Park, 2000).

These dollars are not dispersed equally across populations. Access to care continues to be a problem for many in the United States. The number of Americans without health insurance has increased by 10.1 million since 1989 (Carrasquillo, Himmelstein, Woolhandler, & Bor, 1999). According to the latest data, approximately 43.4 million Americans (including 11 million children) are uninsured (U.S. Census Bureau, 1998). This figure represents more than 16% of the population and is at the highest level in more than a decade (Iglehart, 1999). Young adults between the ages of 18 and 24 are the age group most likely to be without healthcare insurance. When census data are evaluated by ethnic groups status, African Americans and Hispanics are the largest uninsured population. Thirty-eight percent of African Americans and 34% of Hispanics have no healthcare coverage, a significant difference compared with only 12% of non-Hispanic whites who are without insurance (U.S. Census Bureau, 1998). Approximately 45 million Americans have incomes under the poverty level, and another 45 million have such small incomes that they are considered the working poor (U.S. Census Bureau, 1998). One third of those under the poverty level are uninsured despite Medicaid programs, as are one third of the working poor. Despite economic prosperity, the numbers and rates of uninsured Americans continue to rise, underscoring the need for fundamental changes in the country's healthcare delivery system. Although there is virtually universal agreement that some changes are needed, there has been no consensus among various stakeholders about the exact nature and scope of these changes.

The number of births in 1999 (the latest year for which data are available) totaled 3,957,829, a 1% increase over 1998 (Martin et al., 1999). Although most of the data for natality statistics are underreported on certificates of live birth, there are enough data to suggest that costly interventions during labor and birth are rising steadily. At least 35% of women receive oxytocin during labor, 85% use continuous electronic fetal monitoring, and 66% have an epidural catheter placed for labor analgesia (Curtin & Park, 1999). The rate of vacuum-assisted births has increased 77% since 1989 (Curtin & Park, 1999). The cesarean birth rate rose 4% from 21.2% in 1988 to 22% in 1999, reversing a previous 7-year downward trend (Curtin & Martin, 1999).

The most common reason for admission to U.S. hospitals is childbirth (Agency for Health Care Policy and Research [AHCPR], 1999). In 1980, length of stay (LOS) for vaginal birth averaged 3.2 days but had dropped to 1.7 days by 1995 (Curtin & Park, 1999). In 1998, average LOS for vaginal birth increased to 2.1 days (AHCPR, 1999). This increase is related to state laws passed in 1995 and 1996 and the federal law (Newborns' and Mothers' Health Protection Act of 1996) that took effect in 1997 and 1998, requiring insurance companies to pay for a 48-hour LOS for vaginal birth. The cost of an extra inpatient day per mother and baby is approximately $1,400 (Raube & Merrell, 1999). Considerable controversy exists about whether an increase in LOS from 1 to 2 days after vaginal birth decreases the risk of neonatal readmission (Behram, Moschler, Sayegh,

Garguillo, & Mann, 1998; Braveman, Egerter, Pearl, Marchi, & Miller, 1995; Lock & Ray, 1999; Maisels & Kring, 1998; Mandle, Brennan, Wise, Tronick, & Homer, 1997). Approximately 2% of newborns in the United States are readmitted during the first 2 weeks of life (Raube & Merrell, 1999). Even if an additional inpatient day prevented all neonatal readmissions, the cost of care for mothers and babies increases by 18% when mothers choose to stay 2 days instead of 1 day after vaginal birth (Raube and Merrell, 1999). Newborns with complications of low birth weight had an average LOS of 23 days (AHCPR, 1999).

Financial Implications for Perinatal Care

Financial crises in U.S. hospitals are commonplace. Individual hospitals are reporting bankruptcy, while profits from the healthcare industry are at an all-time high (Holzemer, 1996). Hospitals that have not changed traditional methods of operation are generating insufficient income to cover expenses. Mergers and consolidations of competitors have resulted in fewer choices for childbearing women and have resulted in decreased services in many of the surviving hospitals (Holzemer, 1996). Since January 1, 1999, the Balanced Budget Act of 1997 has had serious and far-reaching effects on U.S. hospitals. Changes in the methods for calculating Medicare and Medicaid reimbursement have had substantial negative effects on the financial status of all hospitals but have been particularly difficult for teaching hospitals. Many teaching hospitals have reported losses in the millions of dollars. These losses are significant for perinatal nurses, because teaching hospitals are traditionally referral centers for women with complications of pregnancy and for preterm and medically fragile newborns. Socially and financially disadvantaged pregnant women, who tend to be uninsured, underinsured, or Medicaid recipients, have a higher risk of preterm birth and other complications of pregnancy. Quality care for these women and newborns is at risk if teaching hospitals continue to suffer major economic losses. Hospitals may be unable or unwilling to continue the level of services ordinarily provided for the pregnant women they serve. Vital programs such prenatal education and lactation support services that are historically not sources of revenue may have to be discontinued. Economic pressures are compelling perinatal nurse managers to develop new ways of coping with the challenges of balancing cost and quality.

CHALLENGES FACING NURSE MANAGERS OF PERINATAL SERVICES

Cost Containment Versus Cost Consciousness

The financial stability of healthcare institutions hinges on their ability to consistently provide high-quality care in a cost-effective manner. Previous reimbursement structures did not provide incentives to evaluate costs. The traditional fee-for-service insurance plans paid 100% of billed charges. Nurses were rarely involved in the evaluation of patient care in terms of cost (Simpson, 1993). The days of 100% reimbursement are gone and not likely to return. Approximately 85% of patients with private healthcare are enrolled in managed care programs. Managed care has forced institutions to evaluate the cost implications of doing business as usual.

Perinatal unit financial and human resource allocation are under intense scrutiny. Although the fundamental goals of any healthcare institution are to maximize health and conserve resources, as nurse managers know, these goals often appear to be in conflict (Gardner, 1998). When pressures to meet "the bottom line" increase, cost containment is sometimes the only framework for evaluating clinical practices, products, and services. Nurse managers are frequently challenged by financial goals with time lines and targets, and disregard that practice changes based on cost data alone can be short-sighted and potentially contribute to adverse maternal-fetal outcomes (Simpson & Knox, 1999). A more realistic approach, based on sound scientific data and professional standards, must be used to determine which practices can be eliminated or modified and which practices are critical to support the best possible outcomes for mothers and babies.

Knowledgeable nurse managers must advocate for a clinically appropriate plan for fiscal prudence, but to create maximum leverage for change, it is critical to understand the differences between the philosophies of cost containment and cost consciousness in managing expenses. "Cost containment is an attempt to decrease or contain costs by whatever means necessary to meet preset financial targets" (Simpson & Knox, 1999, p. 123). In a clinical environment where cost containment is the priority, costs are the only variable used to plan perinatal care and services. The real impact of cost containment can be known only in retrospect. "Cost consciousness is a philosophy for allocation of human resources based on a careful review of existing research, including analysis of risks and benefits as well as long-term patient implications" (Simpson & Knox, 1999, p. 123). This data-driven process, prospectively applied as well as concurrently analyzed, uses multiple data sources as the foundation for planning perinatal care and services. Using the cost consciousness philosophy, costs are only one variable in the entire patient quality–patient safety equation. Although cost containment is primarily focused on the financial bottom line, cost consciousness is a data-driven approach to financial resource allocation that includes a clinical and organizational perspective. Cost consciousness uses scientific knowledge, standards, and guidelines from professional organizations and the consensus of perinatal providers as a means of eliminating costly routine and unnecessary practices not found to be efficacious in the delivery of appropriate perinatal care (Simpson & Knox, 1999). Cost consciousness is a key component of evidence-based care. An evidence-based approach can eliminate waste and ensure that best practices are continued and that perinatal care professionals have the resources to continue to provide the kind of care that can contribute to the best possible outcomes for mothers and babies (Simpson & Knox, 1999).

Perinatal nurse managers must be assertive in developing successful strategies to promote evidence-based care to avoid being victims of an administrative decision related to cost containment. However, this professional assertiveness cannot work if perinatal nurse managers operate in isolation. Collaboration with key physician leaders is imperative. Sometimes, cost-cutting plans can adversely affect patient safety, and risk managers can be valuable allies to assist with a data-driven presentation to administrators about the institution's professional liability risks. Together, armed with data about the latest evidence and standards, nurse and physician leaders can present a credible alternative approach to managing unit resources within realistic budget targets. First-line perinatal managers have the most knowledge about the impact of cost reduction initiatives on patient care outcomes, but they must have the ability to convey that knowledge to upper-level administrators in an effective, compelling way. The increased emphasis on cost of care and its relationship to quality of care is a reality. This is an opportunity for perinatal nurses and nurse managers to take a leadership role by active participation in the process, with retention of high-quality patient-care delivery systems as the ultimate goal.

Integrating Evidence into Routine Clinical Practice

Although nurse managers are responsible for ensuring that practices on their unit are cost-effective and based on current research and science, this is often much easier said than done. Much of contemporary perinatal practice is based on ritual, myth, and "the way we've always done it" (Simpson & Knox, 1999) (Display 1–1). "The way we've always done it" may be comfortable for many providers, and the process of changing the status quo can be challenging and time consuming for nurse managers. There is a growing body of evidence about the pros and cons of various perinatal practices that can be used to advocate for safe and effective care. However, without a thorough research-based knowledge of all the practices that together constitute perinatal care, it is difficult for nurse managers to determine which practices are critical to maintain the best possible outcomes for mothers and babies (Simpson, 1999). Important aspects of creating a clinical culture that supports evidence-based perina-

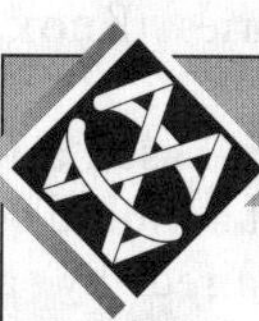

DISPLAY 1–1

Common Rituals in Perinatal Practice

- Documentation systems that require multiple entries for the same patient data
- Routine admission laboratory blood work for healthy women with prenatal records
- Routine discharge laboratory blood work for women who had a normal birth experience
- Routine screening of healthy newborns using blood pressure assessment, hematocrit, and glucose testing
- Strict bed rest therapy as a preterm birth prevention strategy
- Home uterine activity monitoring as a preterm birth prevention strategy
- Continuous electronic fetal monitoring
- Confining women in labor to bed
- Women in labor allowed no oral intake (ie, NPO)
- Use of automatic blood pressure devices during labor
- Arbitrary time frames for length of the second stage of labor
- Nurse or physician coached, closed-glottis pushing during the second stage of labor
- Routine episiotomy
- Restrictive visiting policies
- Restrictive videotaping and camera use during labor and birth

Adapted from Simpson, K.R., & Knox, G.E. (1999). Strategies for developing an evidence-based approach to perinatal care. *MCN The American Journal of Maternal Child Nursing, 24* (3), 122–132.

tal care include true collaboration and healthy communication between physicians and nurses, careful review of pertinent guidelines and standards from professional organizations and regulatory agencies (and the resource implications that are imbedded within them), and a thorough understanding of available clinical research and support from all parties (including senior hospital administrators) for this rigorous approach (Simpson & Knox, 1999).

As evidence is critically evaluated, an essential principle about childbirth emerges: pregnancy, labor, and birth are natural, and most interventions are unnecessary. Generally, providing perinatal care based on the premise that birth is a natural process requiring minimal selected interventions results in the highest-quality, low-cost care (Simpson & Knox, 1999). Unnecessary interventions add to costs of care and can lead to iatrogenic maternal or fetal injuries (Knox, Simpson, & Garite, 1999).

The first step in developing an evidence-based approach to perinatal care is establishment of a multidisciplinary practice committee jointly chaired by a physician and nurse who are recognized by their peers for their clinical expertise and have the ability to influence positive change (Simpson, 1999). Nurses in administrative roles often are not clinical experts. It is an unrealistic expectation that administrative leaders possess clinical expertise for all areas of practice. The nurse manager may not always be the ideal candidate to act as co-chair of the practice committee. This role can be delegated to a senior staff nurse, clinical educator, or clinical nurse specialist, but as the unit leader, the nurse manager needs to ensure that the practice committee nurse co-chair has administrative support to promote and uphold implementation of committee initiatives. Membership should include perinatal service administrators, managers, advanced practice nurses, staff nurses, and physician representatives from perinatal, neonatal, and anesthesia medicine. Providers from other disciplines and departments such as pharmacy, social services, grief support, lactation services, and risk management can be added as ad hoc members, encouraged to attend and required to participate if issues involving their departments are under consideration (Simpson & Knox, 1999).

A perinatal practice committee has two purposes: to establish the basis for and define current institutional practices and to redefine practices accordingly as knowledge, professional guidelines, or regulatory requirements change (Simpson & Knox, 1999). This formal committee structure works best when the committee has been empowered to develop unit polices and protocols and make decisions about practice changes based on a review of appropriate literature and standards. In the initial stages of committee work, it may be helpful to ask an expert on evaluating and critiquing research to provide education to the group so that all members are at the same level of knowledge about this critical process (Simpson & Knox, 1999). Multiple sources of data can be used to develop evidence-based practices (Display 1–2). Institutional access to the Internet can facilitate obtaining data rapidly (Drake, 1999). For the committee to work effectively, there needs to be consensus among committee members that no practice will be approved that is inconsistent with available evidence, standards, and guidelines from professional organizations. This evidence, standards, and guidelines framework can avoid lengthy discussions about practices that are not in the best interests of patients and that could increase institutional liability should litigation result from an adverse outcome. Development of a unit philosophy or purpose statements that designate mothers and babies as the focus of care is helpful for guiding the objectives of the practice committee (see Chapter 3, Display 3–3). When current or proposed practice protocols are reviewed, the process can be discussed within the framework of what is best for the patients. Acknowledge that the best approach for patients may sometimes be inconvenient for providers and could result in slightly higher costs.

Commitment to practice based on evidence and standards is an ongoing process that requires more professional energy than the usual methods of implementing and evaluating changes in patient care (Simpson & Knox, 1999). In some unit cultures, it may be unusual for physicians and nurses to jointly evaluate current literature and standards as the basis of practice protocol development. Many institutions have separate nurse and physician committee structures that develop policies, but this type of committee structure is outdated and inefficient. Parallel committees contribute to professional coexistence rather than professional cohesiveness and collaboration. Physicians and nurses are members of the same team providing care and should work on this process together. Changes in practice cannot occur without respectful collaborative discussions with physician colleagues (Simpson, 1999). Significant changes in unit operations and culture do not occur overnight, and professional relationships that involve trust and mutual respect evolve progressively and are based on many interactions (Simpson & Knox, 1999). Developing an environment in which evidence-based care is jointly promoted and implemented may take months or years. However, the desired outcome will occur only if proactive steps are started. Nurse managers are the unit leaders and must act as the catalyst to move forward.

The nurse manager, in collaboration with the chairman of the department of obstetrics and gynecology

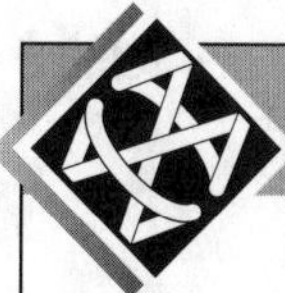

DISPLAY 1–2

Suggested Internet Resources for Developing Evidence-Based Practices

Association of Women's Health, Obstetric and Neonatal Nurses *(http://www.awhonn.org)*
American College of Obstetricians and Gynecologists *(http://www.acog.org)*
American Academy of Pediatrics *(http://www.aap.org)*
American College of Nurse Midwives *(http://www.acmn.org)*
American Nurses Association *(http://www.ana.org)*
American Association of Critical Care Nurses *(http://www.aacn.org)*
Association of periOperative Registered Nurses *(http://www.aorn.org)*
American Society of Perianesthesia Nurses *(http://www.aspan.org)*
American Society of Anesthesiologists *(http://www.asahq.org)*
National Association of Neonatal Nurses *(http://www.nann.org)*
Joint Commission on Accreditation of Healthcare Organizations *(http://www.jcaho.org)*
Agency for Health Quality and Research *(http://www.ahqr.gov)*
Centers for Disease Control and Prevention *(http://www.cdc.gov)*
CenterWatch Clinical Trials Listing Service *(http://www.centerwatch.com/MAIN.HTM)*
United States Food and Drug Administration *(http://www.fda.gov)*
March of Dimes *(http://www.modimes.org)*
Cochrane Database of Systematic Reviews *(http://www.cochrane.com)*
United States Preventive Services Task Force *(http://www.uspstf.gov)*
National Guideline Clearinghouse *(http://www.guildline.gov)*
Best Practices Network *(http://www.best4health.org)*

Adapted from Simpson, K.R., & Knox, G.E. (1999). Strategies for developing an evidence-based approach to perinatal care. *MCN The American Journal of Maternal Child Nursing, 24*(3), 122–132.

(or any other physician in a leadership role), can initially develop strategies to motivate the other members of the perinatal team. After key members have been recruited and agree to participate, the practice committee can begin to designate its scope and purpose. The best approach to early protocol development is to start with less controversial practices for which there is substantial evidence and standards and guidelines from professional organizations such as prevention of early onset group B streptococcal disease in the newborn, cervical ripening, induction of labor, and interventions for nonreassuring fetal heart rate patterns during labor. After these protocols are developed based on existing professional standards and guidelines and the committee is successful with implementation, practices that have conflicting or less rigorous data support can be evaluated. As the process evolves, nurse managers and physicians must take the leadership role in keeping the commitment to evidence-based care on track. The committee leaders must continually challenge the group to give up routine practices that are not beneficial to maternal-fetal outcomes. After the committee has developed a collaborative relationship, has achieved success in implementing several evidence-based protocols, and members are comfortable with open interaction, a frank discussion about practices that are based on provider convenience rather than solid data about enhancing patient outcomes is required. A unit philosophy that supports the patient as the focus of perinatal care can be helpful in guiding this discussion.

Although a collaborative approach to clinical decision-making based on evidence and standards may not come about as quickly as desired, the ongoing investment in time and energy to become oriented to the process and make it successful is worthwhile. The main advantages of an evidence-based approach to perinatal care are care practices can be defended as budgets become more restricted; establishment of true collaborative relationships between nurse and physician colleagues can have a positive spillover effect on clinical operations and therefore on patient safety; assurance to the public and purchasers of services that practices are clinically sound, consistent with scientific data and on existing professional standards of care; and a reduction in risk of professional liability (Simpson & Knox, 1999).

Regulatory Agencies and Professional Standards

Multiple professional organizations promulgate standards and guidelines for practice that have implications for perinatal care providers (Display 1–3).

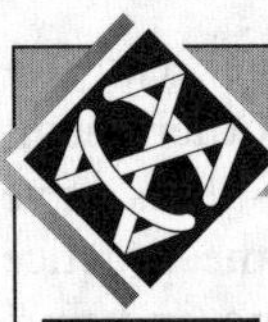

DISPLAY 1–3

Professional Organizations with National Standards Related to Perinatal Nursing Practice

Association of Women's Health, Obstetric, and Neonatal Nurses (AWHONN)
American Nurses Association (ANA)
American Association of Critical Care Nurses (AACN)
American College of Obstetricians and Gynecologists (ACOG)
American Academy of Pediatrics (AAP)
American Society of PeriAnesthesia Nurses (ASPAN)
American Society of Anesthesiologists (ASA)
Association of periOperative Registered Nurses (AORN)
National Association of Neonatal Nurses (NANN)

Local, state, and federal regulations and statutes are additional sources of standards that must be met by institutions providing perinatal services. The nurse manager must be aware of the standards and develop strategies to ensure that unit practices meet these criteria. This is especially challenging because they are continually changing and may have different interpretations by hospital administrators, nurses, physicians, and consumers. One way for nurse managers to keep abreast of current standards and guidelines published by professional organizations is institutional financial support for membership in these organizations. Clinical educators and clinical nurse specialists can assist the nurse manager by providing information about trends in perinatal care and implications for practice. The quality department in each institution should have a systematic process to inform nurse managers as local, state, and federal regulations and JCAHO standards are issued or revised.

Outcome Monitoring

Outcome monitoring is not new to the nursing profession. One of the earliest proponents of outcome evaluation was Florence Nightingale, who used morbidity and mortality statistics to demonstrate effects of substandard care during the Crimean War. Although current methods of data collection and analysis are much more sophisticated, the goals remain the same: measurement and evaluation of patient outcomes related to the nursing care provided.

Identifying Nurse-Sensitive Outcomes

Defining and measuring quality nursing care can be a complex process because providers, consumers, and third-party payers have various expectations and definitions of what constitutes quality. Quality of care, or the clinical aspects of care delivered, is frequently measured by patient outcomes, quality improvement processes, and clinical indicators. Quality of service, or the manner in which patient care is delivered, is typically measured by patient satisfaction surveys (Crain, 1993). Both aspects of quality are equally important and play a key role in evaluating total effectiveness of perinatal care delivery systems. Frequently, quality of service is the single factor used by patients to judge the overall quality of care received (Crain, 1993). Patients consider quality of service to include the characteristics of their experience of care beyond the expected technical competence in diagnostic and therapeutic procedures (Kenagy, Berwick, & Shore, 1999). Patients may not feel qualified to judge technical quality, and they assess their healthcare by other dimensions that reflect factors they value such as timeliness of care and provider empathy and kindness. Service characteristics are an important determinant of patient loyalty in an increasingly competitive market (Kenagy et al., 1999). Quality care, as documented by clinical outcomes and costs, is used by third-party payers to select institutional providers for healthcare plan members, and by regulatory agencies and accrediting bodies in the review process.

When analyzing quality indicators for nursing care, an important consideration is identification of nurse-sensitive outcome measures. Most measures that are analyzed are not directly linked to the nurse's ability to influence outcomes, but rather are related to multiple other factors including patients, physicians, allied health professionals, and hospital operations, policies, and clinical protocols. The role the patient plays in implementing recommendations from nurses and other healthcare providers is sometimes underestimated. Patients often have more direct control over outcomes than any single healthcare team member. Outcomes directly depend on the knowledge, skills, abilities, efforts, and motivations of the patient (Pierce, 1997). A significant portion of nursing activities are directly related to carrying out physician orders or following established hospital policies and protocols. Dependent nursing functions include implementation of medical orders and medical treatments; independent functions include assessment, decision making, interventions, and follow-up; and interdependent functions include activities that nurses engage in that partially or completely depend on functions of other healthcare providers, such as promoting continuity and coordinating care (Irvine, Sidani, & Hall, 1998). Determining which outcomes nurses may be held accountable for requires differentiating the impact of dependent, independent, and interdependent nursing activities (Irvine et al., 1998).

Outcomes of healthcare are generally categorized as patient-focused, provider-focused, and organization-focused measures (Jennings, Staggers, & Brosch, 1999). Nurse-sensitive outcomes are a key component of patient-focused outcome measurement. Nurse-sensitive outcome measures have been identified by the American Nurses Association (ANA, 1997) and the Institute of Medicine (Wunderlich, Sloan, & Davis, 1996). These outcome measures include nursing skill mix, costs of nursing care, educational preparation of nursing staff, and nursing satisfaction with their professional role. The process of delivering nursing care includes assessment, care planning, and care implementation such as physical care, counseling, education, and documentation (Pierce, 1997). Patient satisfaction is an essential indicator for evaluation of the implications and quality of nursing care delivered. In perinatal services, nurse-sensitive outcomes may include supportive care during labor and birth; patient knowledge of labor and birth; postpartum care and newborn care; successful pain management during labor, birth, and the postpartum period; and overall satisfaction with the childbirth process.

Impact of Downsizing, Re-engineering, and Decreased Resources on Patient Outcomes

The restructuring and downsizing of nursing services that occurred in many healthcare institutions during the 1990s dismantled nursing leadership and diminished nursing influence at the healthcare decision-making table (Shamian, 2000). Fewer nurses in leadership positions in hospitals resulted in fewer nurses to advocate for a sensible approach to cost-saving measures that included the potential impact on quality nursing care delivery and, ultimately, patient outcomes. Financial healthcare consulting teams that did not include nurses actively involved in clinical care were hired by many hospitals with the goal of decreasing the financial bottom line. Professional registered nurses make up two thirds of the inpatient workforce and were the target of cost-cutting strategies (Knox, Kelley, Simpson, Carrier, & Berry, 1999). As a result, nursing staff and management positions were eliminated, resulting in fewer nurses caring for more patients, the addition of unlicensed assistive personnel, and several units consolidated under one nurse manager.

Analysis of outcomes of nursing care must include consideration of available resources and operational processes. A skill mix with high numbers of unlicensed assistive personnel, chronic understaffing, and lack of available equipment, space, and ancillary services make nursing care delivery challenging in many institutions. Nurses report dissatisfaction working with unlicensed assistive personnel and their ability to perform delegated tasks and communicate pertinent information (Barter, McLaughlin, & Thomas, 1997). Adding unlicensed assistive personnel to the skill mix does not provide more time for professional nursing activities, because with this care model, more patients are assigned per nurse, and nurses remain responsible for delegated tasks (Barter et al., 1997; Ventura, 1999). Downsizing and re-engineering initiatives that have been implemented in an effort to decrease costs and increase productivity have had a significant impact on the ability of nurses to provide consistent quality care (Knox et al., 1999). Nurses who are continually forced to "do more with less" struggle with how to provide quality care that leads to appropriate patient outcomes.

These cost containment strategies have the potential for unplanned detrimental effects on patient satisfaction, nursing satisfaction, and clinical outcomes of care (Knox et al., 1999). Excellent nursing care directly depends on committed and supported nurses (Kenagy et al., 1999). No matter how effective the existing process of nursing care, it is the nurses who are providing the care that make the difference. Nurses who are continually lacking the resources to do their best are at risk for poor morale and dissatisfaction with their professional role (Ventura, 1999). This is an important issue because nursing satisfaction often mirrors patient satisfaction (Kenagy et al., 1999). Unhappy, disgruntled nurses struggling with limited resources and too many patients produce unhappy, disgruntled patients, whereas nurses who are supported by an environment and infrastructure designed to make them successful produce loyal, happy patients who tell others about their high level of satisfaction (Kenagy et al., 1999). Nurse managers must ensure that the hospital's allocation of resources for perinatal services are adequate to enhance the ability of perinatal nurses to provide quality care for mothers and babies. Managers must make sure that their voices are heard by upper-level administrators who may not fully understand the implications for patient care and safety when personnel cuts are being considered. This includes decreases in staff nurse positions and others in supportive roles such as assistant nurse managers, nurse educators, clinicians, and clinical nurse specialists. When budgets are tight, usually the first to go are nurses who are responsible for nursing education and competence validation and for ensuring that clinical practices and policies are based on the latest evidence and standards. Nursing management positions are also cut, resulting in consolidation of units and the surviving nurse manager being responsible for more nurses than can be adequately supervised, mentored, and nurtured (Simpson, 2000). The ability to follow up on clinical issues, hold nursing staff accountable for nursing practice, and promote professional development is severely compromised. Ample data in the literature support an argument that fewer nurses caring for more patients leads to increased patient morbidity and adverse outcomes and decreased satisfaction of nurses and their patients (Blegen, Goode, & Reed, 1998; Bond, Raehl, Pitterle, & Franke, 1999; Kovner & Gergen, 1998; Lichtig, Knauf, & Milholland, 1999). These researchers found that a higher proportion of registered nurses caring for patients was consistently related to lower adverse outcome rates, shorter lengths of stay, and lower nurse-sensitive patient morbidities (Blegan et al., 1998; Bond et al., 1999; Kovner & Gergen, 1998; Lichtg et al., 1999). The nurse manager can use these data to argue that any plans for downsizing, re-engineering, or restructuring of the clinical workforce should be evaluated in the context of the potential impact on quality care. Although decreasing the proportion of registered nurses may appear be a cost-saving measure initially, as patient morbidities and adverse outcomes increase over time and patient and nursing satisfaction decrease, there may be significant unplanned negative financial implications.

Identifying Realistic Goals for Outcomes of Perinatal Nursing Care

An analysis of patient care delivery methods must include well-defined criteria for quality care and desired patient outcomes. Definitions of quality outcomes based on current lengths of stay must be developed by individual institutions. Clinical pathways and clinical algorithms are useful in defining quality parameters if clear expectations are listed with specific outcome criteria. Variances can be tracked and strategies to improve outcomes continually redesigned.

Institutional definitions and evaluations of quality outcomes must incorporate professional standards of care and JCAHO clinical indicators. The ultimate success of new strategies for care that is high quality and cost effective is related to the ability to gain support from key persons in administrative, nursing, medical, and allied health disciplines within the institution. A multidisciplinary approach and follow through is essential. After quality outcomes and goals are clearly defined and agreed on by all members of the healthcare team, the processes to achieve those goals and indicators to track ongoing results can be developed.

Although LOSs have stabilized, the challenge to set realistic patient care outcomes continues. Even though there are anecdotal reports of problems related to "early discharge," there is no definitive scientific evidence that mandated LOS is superior to an appropriate LOS that is determined by the woman and her physician or certified nurse midwife when the LOS is determined by valid clinical criteria. Adding 24 hours to the inpatient stay for healthy mothers and babies has not been shown to be clinically beneficial for postpartum care outcomes. For example, the challenge of how much information can be provided to and absorbed by new parents in a day or two during the postpartum period remains, whether mothers and babies stay for 1 or 2 days. Classic research by Rubin (1961) has suggested that women may not be able to assimilate parenting information in the immediate postpartum period. However, in the inpatient setting, perinatal nurses have limited hours to try to present this important content. During the inpatient postpartum period, new mothers are often too fatigued to learn new information. The inpatient postpartum stay often consists of juggling newborn feeding schedules, visitors, congratulatory telephone calls, technical aspects of care, and other hospital routines. The new mother may be exhausted from these activities and have limited time to recover from labor and birth, let alone assimilate important information about postpartum self-care and newborn care. Innovative programs to identify women early in pregnancy and encourage participation in parenting classes during the prenatal period have been developed to meet those learning needs in other ways. Surveys to elicit parent preferences for specific teaching needs during hospitalization have been used with success in some perinatal units. Core content can be defined by perinatal nurses to provide for all women after birth (ie, safety issues and self-care needs). Women then select other parenting information as needed, resulting in individualized care and avoidance of repetitive or previously mastered material. Differences in parity, experience, and support systems available affect individual learning needs. Booklets and videotapes may be given to parents to use at home. Parent "warmlines" are useful to answer questions after discharge.

Physiologic determinants of outcomes also must be adjusted based on LOS. Bowel and bladder function, lochia characteristics, perineal healing, lactation, and involution processes are not at the same levels 1 to 2 days after birth as 3 to 4 days postpartum. Realistic, attainable goals must be identified for each physiologic care parameter, and plans to achieve those goals clearly outlined. Each perinatal center must develop strategies to meet the needs of the specific population served. Some methods of evaluation of the success of these strategies are patient-satisfaction surveys and tracking perinatal readmissions and calls to the mother–baby unit and primary care providers about postpartum and newborn care issues.

Benchmarking

Benchmarking in healthcare is the continuous process of evaluating one hospital's performance against the performance of hospitals that are recognized as representing best practices in a specific area. The goal is to promote successful operations so that an organization not only survives, but thrives in a competitive market. Measures typically used in benchmarking are financial, operational, clinical, and quality, but much of the emphasis is on financial data. In a national benchmarking project to identify the top 100 hospitals in the United States, standards by which hospitals were judged included three categories: financial management, operations, and clinical practices (Morrissey, 1998). Financial management measures were expense per adjusted discharge, cash-flow margins, and asset-turnover ratio. Operations measured were average LOS, proportion of outpatient revenues, and index of total facility occupancy. Clinical practices were evaluated by calculating risk-adjusted mortality and risk-adjusted complications. When evaluating perinatal services, measures used included hours worked per birth, indirect costs for patients who do not give birth, full-time equivalents per birth, cesarean birth rates, vaginal birth after previous cesarean birth rates, and hours per patient for postpartum women and newborns.

Advantages of benchmarking include the ability to learn from other hospitals that have been successful and use that information to implement practices that have been shown to improve performance. The free flow of ideas and sharing of information that occurs as a result of benchmarking can be a vital component of quality improvement processes. Typically, hospitals use benchmark data from other hospitals that are similar in size and scope of clinical services. Although this facilitates accurate comparisons, there are potential negative ramifications for this approach if used exclusively. If the other hospitals in the benchmarking data set are matched exactly, it is possible that their clinical processes are very similar, and there is a risk that hospitals could be benchmarking against mediocrity (Lau, 1996). Best practices are often found in other types of organizations and can be adapted to meet individual needs to improve operations. One of the concerns about benchmarking when data from dissimilar hospitals are used to measure performance is that it is inappropriate to "compare apples with oranges." An alternative way of approaching this type of comparison is to consider that they are both "fruit." Even though hospitals may not be very similar, there are data about practices and processes that can be valuable in seeking improvement in overall performance (Lau, 1996). Avoid the mindset "but we are different," and use the data to consider changes in clinical practice and operations that may improve quality.

Many hospitals participate in benchmarking consortia, but other sources of benchmarking data can be used. The Best Practice Network, sponsored by various professional organizations is one source of benchmarking data that provides useful information on multiple clinical and operational topics. Benchmarking can be accomplished within a healthcare system or by developing informal relationships with key professionals in other hospitals outside the system. Several steps are essential in benchmarking: determine which factors are critical to the success of the organization in the marketplace, identify hospitals that have been successful in these areas, and obtain information about how they have been able to achieve that success. Relationships between nurse managers developed through membership in professional nursing organizations may facilitate obtaining data from hospitals in competing healthcare systems that would otherwise be unavailable for benchmarking purposes. Sharing and obtaining information about best practices and implementing changes based on quality performance measures, is a significant role of the perinatal nurse manager and contributes to the potential for success in meeting the ongoing challenges of balancing cost of care with quality of care.

Accreditation and Certification of Healthcare Organizations

The mission of JCAHO is to improve the quality of care provided to the public through the provision of healthcare accreditation and related services that support performance improvement in healthcare institutions (JCAHO, 2000). This organization was founded in 1951 by the American College of Surgeons, the American College of Physicians, the American Hospital Association, the American Medical Association, and the Canadian Medical Association to create an independent not-for-profit association whose primary purpose was to provide voluntary accreditation. In 1965, Congress passed the Medicare Act with a provision that hospitals accredited by JCAHO were deemed to be in compliance with most of the Medicare Conditions of Participation for hospitals. With this legislation, JCAHO accreditation became a de facto requirement for most hospitals to participate in Medicare and Medicaid, but there was still allowance for hospitals to be certified by state agencies to receive federal and state funding for services provided. About 80% of the 6,200 hospitals participating in Medicare are accredited by JCAHO, and about 20% of hospitals nationwide are certified by state agencies (Office of Inspector General [OIG], 1999). Without federal and state reimbursement for services, most hospitals would not be financially viable, and the accreditation or certification process is therefore an important component of institutional strategies and goals for quality performance.

The scope and character of the JCAHO accreditation process have evolved over the years. JCAHO has made a number of changes in their survey process, including a current promotion of a strong emphasis on enhancing organizational performance to improve patient outcomes. Continuously monitoring, analyzing, and improving performance of clinical and other processes are essential requirements (JCAHO, 2000). JCAHO instituted the sentinel event policy in 1998 to encourage self-reporting of medical errors to learn about the relative frequencies and underlying causes of sentinel events, share lessons learned with other healthcare organizations, and reduce the risk of future sentinel events. Chapter 2 describes the JCAHO sentinel event policy.

In 2000, JCAHO approved four focus areas for the initial development of core sets of performance measures for which there is good evidence of effectiveness and benefit to improved patient outcomes. According to JCAHO (2000), a core measure is a standardized quantitative measurement tool that has precisely defined specifications (including risk adjust methods where appropriate) and a standardized data collection process. These core performance measures were identified by expert panels in a process that designated priority areas based on conditions, procedures, and functions that have significant potential to lead to improvement in healthcare: high volume, high risk, high cost, and significant stakeholder interest (JCAHO, 2000). Based on the core measures, JCAHO can expect institutions to examine opportunities for improvement and demonstrate quantitative improvements in performance through appropriate data analysis and clinical or management actions (JCAHO, 2000). The core measurement set applicable to perinatal care is Pregnancy and Related Conditions. Within this performance set are patients at 24 through 34 weeks' gestation who received antenatal steroids before birth, vaginal birth after previous cesarean birth, vaginal births with third- or fourth-degree lacerations, and neonatal mortality. Although JCAHO maintains it does not use these data to directly decide on accreditation, the intent is to use core performance measures as a significant part of the accreditation process and to allow comparisons of performance among hospitals (JCAHO, 2000). Future core measures under consideration are presence of a prenatal record at time of admission, episiotomy rate, indication for or rate of elective labor induction, primary cesarean birth rate, attempted (unsuccessful) vaginal birth after cesarean birth, neonatal transfer to a perinatal center, and maternal transfer to a perinatal center (JCAHO, 2000).

In 1999, the Department of Health and Human Services' Office of Inspector General issued a report citing major deficiencies in the external oversight system intended to make sure the nation's hospitals are safe, and recommended specific strategies for change (OIG, 1999). Some of the deficiencies noted were the inability of JCAHO to detect substandard patterns of care or individual practitioners with questionable skills, the limited time JCAHO surveyors were on site, when JCAHO surveyors were not briefed on a hospital's background and prior safety record before they visited, and when hospitals were allowed to select the medical records that were examined by the surveyors (OIG, 1999). The OIG report recommended that the Health Care Financing Administration (HCFA) take a more active role in ensuring that state agencies and JCAHO conduct meaningful and timely surveys of hospitals, including more unannounced surveys, more random selection of records during the review process, and more rigorous evaluation of hospitals' continuous quality improvement efforts and efforts to increase public disclosure of the performance of hospitals by posting detailed information on the Internet (OIG, 1999). According to the OIG, in the past, JCAHO has been too collegial in relationships with hospitals and has not been holding hospitals accountable for all clinical practices and compliance with standards of accreditation. Hospitals that are certified by state agencies have less external oversight than those accredited by JCAHO. The percent of non–JCAHO-accredited hospitals not surveyed within the 3-year industry standard increased from 28% in 1995 to 50% in 1997, including some hospitals in rural areas that have gone as long as 8 years without a survey (OIG, 1999). The OIG mandated that HCFA insure JCAHO and state agencies appropriately survey participating hospitals and make the information accessible to the public. In response to the OIG report,

JCAHO changed the format for unannounced surveys. Random surveys are done at approximately 5% of all JCAHO-accredited hospitals. With the new format, hospitals no longer receive advance notice of the random, unannounced survey, and these surveys are conducted 9 to 30 months after a scheduled survey. It is unclear whether this new program of unannounced surveys can improve quality of care and enhance patient outcomes, but perinatal nurse managers must be continually vigilant in promoting compliance with the standards of state agencies and JCAHO, so that an unannounced survey does not result in significant negative findings that could affect certification or accreditation status.

Service Excellence

Patient Satisfaction

Nurse managers have direct control over the type and quality of the nursing care that is provided on their units. Definitions of quality care are derived from established guidelines and standards of care and often are measured in terms of clinical and financial outcomes. However, it is not enough to provide excellent quality perinatal nursing care if childbearing women and their families do not perceive it as such (Howard, 1999). A key element is understanding patient expectations of care, because patients often describe quality care in terms different from those used by healthcare providers (Kenagy et al., 1999). Although technical aspects of care are critically important in successful patient outcomes, psychosocial aspects of care may be what patients remember most when asked to rate satisfaction with nursing services. Listening to concerns, providing information, spending time, caring, maintaining empathetic attitudes, having respect for privacy, and not keeping the patient waiting are issues patients feel are elements of quality nursing care (Geary, Fanagan, & Boylan, 1997). Women desire as much control as possible over the childbirth experience (Graham et al., 1999; McCrea & Wright, 1999). A shared decision-making model in which patients actively participate in decisions about their care following provision of adequate information by nurses and physicians has a positive affect on patient satisfaction (Frosch & Kaplan, 1999). Patients' expectations of quality also include a nurse-patient relationship based on mutual trust and respect (Hegedus, 1999).

Family-centered prenatal care contributes to increased personal satisfaction from the childbirth experience, greater self-confidence in caring for the newborn, and a closer relationship with the newborn. A woman's confidence and ability to give birth are enhanced or diminished by every person who provides care and by the environment in which she gives birth (Coalition for Improving Maternity Services [CIMS], 1996). Rooming-in positively affects satisfaction related to increased support and information provided by perinatal nurses and a more individualized approach to care (McKay & Phillips, 1984). The evolution from restrictive visiting policies to open units has allowed family members and friends meaningful participation in the celebration of the birth of the new baby and enhanced patient satisfaction. Women who perceive nurses as answering their questions, providing personalized care, maintaining their personal privacy, and providing information in preparation for discharge have increased satisfaction with perinatal nursing services (Alexander, Sandridge, & Moore, 1993; CIMS, 1996; Copeland & Douglas, 1999; Hegedus, 1999). Principles of the Mother-Friendly Childbirth Initiative (CIMS, 1996) can be used to promote perinatal services that can enhance patient satisfaction. An Internet source (*http://www.healthy.net/cims*) provides more information.

Patient expectations for excellent service and quality nursing care include many factors, some of which the nurse manager may not be able to control. Patients may associate quality nursing care with hospital services that are not within the domain of nursing practice. In competitive markets, where patients have the ability to choose the hospital in which to give birth from among several competing hospitals and healthcare systems, factors such as the design, newness, and beauty of the birthing suites; waiting times for elective induction of labor; availability of private rooms for postpartum care; general hospital visiting policies; parking; and safety can make the difference in hospital selection. Nursing practices and unit operations that require enormous energy on the part of the perinatal nurse manager, such as following accepted standards and guidelines for care from professional organizations; local, state, and federal regulations; and ensuring that care providers are competent, are basic expectations of childbearing women and their families. Patients expect the care delivered to be safe. They expect to be given the right medications on time in the correct dosage and by the correct route. They expect to be treated with dignity and respect. They expect care providers to be empathetic to their concerns, knowledgeable about their clinical condition, and competent in their professional roles. They expect their family members and friends to be welcomed as participants in the childbirth process. They expect their babies to be identified properly, to be protected from abduction, and to be given to the right mother. They expect to be given adequate and accurate information about how to care for themselves and their babies when they go home. They expect their rooms to be clean, good-tasting food to be served hot or cold as appropriate, and calls for assistance to be answered quickly. When these expectations are not met, patients may feel their basic trust in the nurses and the hospital has been violated (Kenagy et al., 1999). Patients rarely blame their physicians for lapses in hospital services. Perinatal nurse managers should consider that a high level of patient satisfaction may hinge on the hospital's ability to go above and beyond these basic expectations. In addition to data collected from formal patient satisfaction surveys, unsolicited calls and letters from patients provide valuable insights into patient expectations for quality care.

Nursing care is an important determinant of overall patient satisfaction with hospitalization (Finkelstein, Harper, & Rosenthal, 1999; Hegedus, 1999). Satisfaction with nursing care is a crucial patient outcome associated with new and return business (Kenagy et al., 1999). A satisfied patient typically relates a positive experience to only one or two others, whereas a dissatisfied patient shares a negative experience with at least 10 others (Masters & Masters, 1993). Childbearing women and families' intention to return to the institution for future health needs, as well as new patients attracted by the positive experiences of former patients, are critical to the economic well-being of healthcare institutions (Kenagy et al., 1999). Women make most family healthcare decisions and, if satisfied with their childbirth experience, continue to use that healthcare institution for future family healthcare needs (Triolo, 1987). Healthcare institutions must develop systems to determine patients' perceptions of quality nursing care and continually monitor patient satisfaction with these expectations. If a patient indicates dissatisfaction with a component of care, timely investigation and a follow-up discussion with the those involved can assist in developing strategies for improvement (Dasu & Rao, 1999).

One way for perinatal centers to gain insight into patients' expectations and perceptions of quality nursing care is to hold focus groups for women who have used the institution during childbirth. Valuable information solicited from previous patients can be useful in improving content validity of tools developed to measure patient satisfaction. Few questionnaires designed to measure patient satisfaction with sufficient validity and reliability have been reported in the literature, although work toward this goal is evolving (Alexander et al., 1993; Carey & Seibert, 1993; Finkelstein et al., 1999; Hegedus, 1999). Instrument design in this area remains a challenge for institutions and nurse researchers because satisfaction with nursing care is a multidimensional concept. Central to this concept is incorporation of nurses' relationships with patients into the satisfaction model (Copelan & Douglas, 1999; Hegedus, 1999).

During the mid-1990s, many perinatal centers redesigned the physical space in their perinatal units because third-party payer reimbursements were based on a 24-hour LOS for vaginal birth and 48- to 72-hour LOS for cesarean birth. These new designs resulted in conversion to labor-delivery-recovery postpartum rooms (LDRPs) and decreased numbers of nursery and postpartum beds. Perinatal nurse managers struggled with how to meet the multiple needs of patients in an abbreviated time frame and developed strategies to overcome the limitations imposed by the short LOS. The recent increase in the postpartum LOS that occurred after consumer outcries resulted in legislative mandates to allow childbearing women to stay at least 2 days after birth. These changes have had dramatic consequences for managers of perinatal services, who now find themselves trying to handle increased patient census within the physical layout designed for 24-hour LOS for vaginal births and 48- to 72-hour LOS for cesarean births of the mid-1990s. Most women prefer a private room during the postpartum period and are dissatisfied when they have preregistered for these accommodations but they are not available during their inpatient stay. The need for yet another physical redesign to add more LDRPs or postpartum and nursery beds is influencing current costs of perinatal care and presents a significant challenge to patient satisfaction for nurse managers.

JCAHO (2000) requires organizations to collect satisfaction data from patients. Data may be collected through satisfaction surveys, regularly scheduled meetings held with patients and families or focus groups. Patient-satisfaction instruments that are reliable and valid are increasingly important. Perinatal centers desiring to maintain or increase their market share of births need to be active participants in this process. The gap between care perinatal nurses provide and care desired by childbearing women can be minimized through the use of well-designed patient-satisfaction surveys (Alexander et al., 1993; Finkestein et al., 1999; Young, Minnick, & Marcantonio, 1996). In addition to collecting patient-satisfaction data, there must be a method of reporting this information to providers and consumers. Results can be used to heighten nurses' awareness of patient-satisfaction issues and modify practice to reflect the patient's expectations of quality nursing care. Staff nurse involvement in the process of collecting and analyzing survey data can lead to more commitment to improving patient satisfaction outcomes.

Patient Rights

Consumer advocacy groups and legislators have promoted patient rights in recent years. JCAHO has been actively involved in developing accreditation standards that reflect increased awareness of the relationship between patient rights and quality care. In July 1999, the HCFA of the U.S. Department of Health and Human Services (DHHS) published new patient rights rules as part of the Medicare and Medicaid Programs Hospital Conditions of Participation. The rules set forth six standards that are designed to ensure minimum protection of each patient's physical and emotional health and safety. A summary of the patient rights follows (42 CFR Part 482, July 1999).

Standard A: Notice of Rights

A hospital must inform each patient, or when appropriate, the patient's representative (as allowed under state law), of the patient's rights in advance of furnishing or discontinuing patient care whenever possible. The hospital must establish a process for prompt resolution of patient grievances and must inform a patient who to contact to file a grievance. The hospital's governing body must approve and be responsible for the effective operation of the grievance process and must review and resolve grievances, unless it delegates the responsibility in writing to a grievance committee. The grievance process must include a mechanism for timely referral of patient concerns regarding quality of care or premature discharge to the appropriate use and quality-control peer-review organization.

Standard B: Exercise of Rights

The patient has the right to participate in the development and implementation of his or her plan of care. The patient or his or her representative (as allowed under state law) has the right to make informed decisions regarding his or her care. The patient's rights include being informed of his or her health status, being involved in care planning and treatment, and being able to request or refuse treatment. This right must not be construed as a mechanism to demand the provision of treatment or services not deemed medically unnecessary or inappropriate. The patient has the right to formulate advance directives and to have the hospital comply with these directives, in accordance with federal law. The patient has the right to have a family member or representative of his or her choice and his or her own physician notified promptly of his or her admission to the hospital.

Standard C: Privacy and Safety

The patient has the right to personal privacy, the right to receive care in a safe setting, and the right to be free from all forms of abuse or harassment.

Standard D: Confidentiality of Patient Records

The patient has the right to confidentiality of his or her clinical records. The patient has the right to access information contained in his or her clinical records within a reasonable time frame. The hospital must not frustrate the legitimate efforts of individuals to gain access to their own records and must actively seek to meet these requests as quickly as its record keeping system permits.

Standard E: Restraint for Acute Medical and Surgical Care

The patient has the right to be free from restraints of any form that are not medically necessary or are being used as a means of coercion, discipline, convenience, or retaliation by staff. A restraint can be used only if needed to improve the patient's well-being and less restrictive interventions have been determined to be ineffective.

Standard F: Seclusion and Restraint for Behavior Management

The patient has the right to be free from restraints of any form that are not medically necessary or are being used as a means of coercion, discipline, convenience, or retaliation by staff. Seclusion or a restraint can be used only in emergency situations, if needed, to ensure the patient's physical safety if less restrictive interventions have been determined to be ineffective.

There are many conditions and limitations to the use of seclusion and restraints contained the language of the Conditions of Participation. A detailed list and full discussion are provided in *Patient Rights: Medicare and Medicaid Conditions of Participation* (42 CFR Part 482, 1999). The Patient Rights have implications for perinatal services. Perinatal nurse managers must be familiar with these rules and ensure that unit practices are consistent with the six standards.

Although the Patient Rights is mandated as part of the Medicare and Medicaid Programs, Conditions of Participation, other groups have promoted patient rights specifically for perinatal services. The Maternity Center Association (MCA, 1998) has developed the *Statement of the Rights of Childbearing Women.*

Adopting all or part of the Rights of Childbearing Women can contribute to service excellence and patient satisfaction. Selected key points of the *Statement of the Rights of Childbearing Women* (MCA, 1998) are included in Display 1–4.

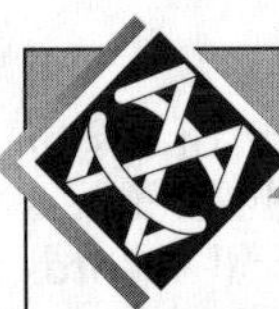

DISPLAY 1–4

Key Points of the *Statement of the Rights of Childbearing Women*

- Every woman has the right to receive care that is consistent with the best available current scientific evidence on its effectiveness.
- Every woman has the right to be fully informed about the benefits, risks, and costs of the procedures, drugs, tests, and treatments considered for use during her pregnancy, labor, birth, and postpartum periods, or for use by her child, and the right to informed consent or refusal.
- Every woman has the right to complete information about her pregnancy, including unrestricted access to her clinical record and any needed help with interpreting its contents.
- Every woman has the right to maternity care that is appropriate to her cultural and religious background.
- Every woman has the right to maternity care that identifies and addresses social and behavioral factors that put her or her baby at increased risk of harm.
- Every woman has the right to receive continuous social, emotional, and physical support throughout labor and birth from a professional who has knowledge of labor support. She also has the right to have a companion or companions of her choice present throughout labor and birth.
- Every woman has the right to choose from a variety of natural and pharmacologic methods to control and relieve the pain of labor. She has the right to change her mind at any time during pregnancy and labor and to make new choices.
- Every woman has the right to decide collaboratively with her caregivers when she and her baby will leave the birth site for home, based on their individual conditions and circumstances.

Maternity Center Association. (1998). *Statement of the rights of childbearing women.* New York, NY: Author.

More information and the complete set of the Rights of Childbearing Women can be obtained by contacting the Maternity Center Association (*http://www.maternity.org*). The MCA has publications suitable for patient education materials, including *Your Guide to Safe and Effective Care During Labor and Birth*. The World Health Organization (WHO, 1996) also has developed a patient education resource that women may find helpful in planning for labor and birth, *Care in Normal Birth: A Practical Guide*. Review of these materials can assist perinatal nurse managers in planning care that meets the needs of childbearing women and enhances their satisfaction during the inpatient stay.

Professional Nursing Personnel Issues

Nurse managers absolutely depend on staff nurses to implement established nursing protocols and provide quality nursing care. However, attracting and retaining excellent staff nurses is increasingly challenging. Experienced nurses have a wide range of alternatives to the inpatient setting, including ambulatory care, homecare, telephone triage, independent practice, managed care firms, pharmaceutical companies, research, teaching, information technology companies, healthcare policy, and private industry. The lack of qualified applicants for specialty nursing practice roles has caused some nurse managers to consider hiring new graduates for positions in units not traditionally open to new nurses, such as labor and delivery (Phillips & Szymanowski, 1999). However, adequate numbers of new graduates may not be available to fill the gap. According to the American Association of Colleges of Nursing (AACN, 2000), nursing school enrollments fell by 4.6% in 1999 compared with 1998. This decline is the fifth consecutive drop in enrollments since 1995 (AACN, 2000). Some nursing schools reported intentional decreases in enrollment because of shortages in qualified nurse educators. The average age of registered nurses is 44 years, representing an increase from 40 years in 1980 (AACN, 2000). Consequently, many nurses will be retiring in the next 10 to 15 years. Nursing schools and hospitals must collaborate to avoid a more significant nursing shortage in the next few years. Internships for new graduates and fellowship programs that provide support for the transition from student to professional registered nurse have been shown to work well for some institutions in recruiting and retaining new nurses. Nursing schools that offered nontraditional flexible approaches to education such as more convenient regional education sites and use of the Internet and other distance learning technologies reported increases in enrollment (AACN, 2000).

The impact of a shortage of experienced nurses combined with the implications of cutting nursing positions during the widespread downsizing and re-engineering initiatives of the 1990s have resulted in nurses who feel chronically overworked and stressed (Leveck & Jones, 1996; Shamian, 2000; Ventura, 1999). In one survey, inpatient nurses reported that short staffing has had serious consequences, including increasing the risk of adverse patient outcomes and forcing them to provide care with which they were not personally satisfied (Ventura, 1999). Changes in the cause of short staffing that have occurred since the mid-1990s are evident in the survey results. When the survey was conducted in 1998, nurses reported short staffing resulted from their institutions cutting nursing positions in an effort to decrease costs. In the latest survey, nurses reported that short staffing was related to a shortage of nurses to fill available positions (Ventura, 1999). In a survey conducted in Minnesota and commissioned by the Minnesota Nurses' Association (MNA), nurses reported being short staffed 72% of the time, primarily in specialty units, emergency departments, and perioperative services (Diemert, 1999). According to the MNA survey, nurses are concerned that compromises in patient care result from inadequate staffing; lack of supportive working environments for nurses affects the quality of patient care; description and documentation of staffing variables limits determining appropriate staffing at the unit level; and maintaining professional nursing practice standards is difficult in situations where staffing is considered inadequate (Diemert, 1999). Survey respondents gave examples of what they considered to be compromises in patient care. Seventy percent of nurses who completed the survey indicated that assessment, observation, and monitoring of patients were not done as scheduled (Diemert, 1999). Other examples with the potential to compromise patient outcomes included basic hygiene, feeding, toileting, positioning, and walking not done on time or at all; medications (including intravenous fluids) and other medical orders not administered on time or at all; communication such as emotional support or teaching with patients and families not done; and special procedures, treatments, and laboratory tests not done on time or at all (Diemert, 1999).

Minnesota nurses reported dissatisfaction with nurse managers who have had their scope of responsibility expanded, resulting in less time to be available to staff nurses and for mentoring new nurses (Diemert, 1999). These results are similar to those of Sochalski and colleagues (1998), who found that nurses trusted their nurse managers less than their nursing peers and thought the lack of nurturing and support by their nurse managers caused them to feel abandoned (Sochalski et al., 1998). In contrast, nurses who thought their nurse managers had ready access to resources, information, support, and opportunity believed that their nurse managers were more likely to share their power with the staff nurses they supervise (McDermott, Laschinger, & Shamian, 1996). These results are not surprising to nurse managers who have been trying to do their best with limited resources. However, for nurse managers of specialty units, the shortage of nurse candidates to fill available positions does not seem likely to be resolved in the near future.

Although there is no immediate solution to the shortage of experienced nurses, it is important for nurse managers to appreciate the impact of chronic understaffing on the nurses they supervise. Working every shift without enough nurses to adequately care for patients results in nursing fatigue, burnout, and job-related stress. Sochalski and coworkers (1998) found that nurses' emotional exhaustion exceeds the norms of other employee groups. In addition to emotional exhaustion, the personal health condition of nurses is poor compared with other employee groups (Sochalski et al., 1998). Nurses are devoted to improving the health status of their patients, but their own health status has suffered as a result of job-related stress during the years of chronic understaffing (Shamian, 2000). Increased nursing stress has been found to be a significant predictor of the quality of care and adverse patient outcomes (Dugan et al., 1996; Leveck and Jones, 1996). Quality of work life has an impact on the quality of care delivered (Shogren & Calkins, 1995). Quality of work life for nurses can be evaluated by examining work-related staff illnesses and injury rates, turnover or vacancy rates, use of supplemental staffing, flexibility of human resource policies and benefit packages, and levels of nurse satisfaction (Shogren & Calkins, 1995). When nurses continually feel that they are unable to deliver the quality of care they feel is in the best interests of their patients, satisfaction with the professional role is diminished, and they are likely to seek other opportunities for employment (Levek & Jones, 1996; Seago, 1996; Ventura, 1999).

Nurses new to the profession are different than nurses of the past. Thirty-four percent of the total workforce in the United States is composed of Generation X workers, who were born between 1961 and 1981 (Phillips, 2000). These nurses do not enter the work setting with the intention of long tenure in one institution. Their philosophy is "work to live" rather than "live to work" (Bradford & Raines, 1992). Retaining a Generation X nurse requires strategies that are different from those used for Baby Boomers, many of whom started their first job with the unspoken goal of remaining with the same institution indefinitely

(Phillips, 2000). Generation X nurses require a reason to stay rather than a reason to go, and retention strategies must be adapted to meet their specific needs. Successful strategies include providing career planning, opportunities for advancement, tuition reimbursement, frequent positive feedback on job performance, and continued challenges in the clinical setting (Phillips, 2000). Generation X nurses thrive on being able to exercise their creative abilities to solve complex clinical problems. Unlike their Baby Boomer counterparts, Generation X nurses are comfortable with change and use of computer technology (Phillips, 2000). When significant changes are needed in unit operations or new technology such as computer documentation systems and e-mail communication is being introduced, Generation X nurses may be the first to adapt and embrace these changes. Nurse managers can use the talents and enthusiasm of this generation to assist with the diffusion of innovations. The shrinking pool of qualified applicants for available nursing positions should be a catalyst for nurse managers to create and foster a workplace that highlights the needs and work ethic of Generation X nurses and provides incentives to for them stay (Phillips, 2000).

Although there are significant challenges for nurse managers in recruiting and retaining excellent staff nurses, some strategies have been effective. Hospitals that report fewer problems with recruitment, retention, and absenteeism have models of care that promote clinical decision-making by nurses and empowerment of nursing staff (McDermott et al., 1996; Seago, 1996). There is a strong association between nurses who feel empowered and their loyalty and commitment to the institution (Shamian, 2000). Promoting clinical decision-making and empowering nurses are strategies that any nurse manager can use and that do not require additional financial and human resources. These strategies may require a change in management or leadership style, but they are worth the effort if excellent nurses are committed to remaining with the institution. Nurses who perceive that they have access to resources, information, opportunities for career advancement, and support for their work are more likely to remain in their positions (Shamian, 2000). Professional and career development opportunities are key factors in retaining qualified, committed nurses (American Organization of Nurse Executives [AONE], 1999). Professional and career development opportunities need not mean promotion from the staff nurse position. Career development can include providing continuing education programs and encouragement to seek additional education by taking advantage of the existing hospital tuition reimbursement program. Nurses who feel they are respected and valued by their nurse managers have greater commitment to their current roles (Sochalski et al., 1998). A small amount of time invested in complimenting staff nurses for a job well done and acknowledging their daily contributions can result in a positive relationship between the nurse manager and staff nurses and commitment to their position. Quality of life issues are high priorities for nurses. Hospitals that promote balanced life and family-friendly work environments are more likely to recruit and retain excellent nurses (AONE, 1999). Flexibility and innovation are the keys to developing scheduling plans that promote quality of life.

Although nurse managers cannot solve all recruitment and retention issues because of factors outside their control in the present healthcare environment, these suggestions, based on evidence from surveys of nurses, can assist in promoting loyalty and commitment to the institution. The costs of recruiting and orienting a new nurse for a specialty unit can be significant (Phillips & Szymanowski, 1999). Nurse managers must develop effective strategies to retain excellent nurses to support quality patient outcomes.

SUMMARY

Balancing the cost-quality equation continues to be one of the biggest challenges for perinatal nurse managers. For institutions providing perinatal services to survive, financially sound and proactive measures that continually monitor quality care and patient outcomes are critical. Determining patient expectations of care and improving satisfaction with nursing care delivery are essential. Promoting nursing satisfaction is key, because nursing satisfaction is directly related to patient satisfaction and to the nurse's commitment and loyalty to the institution. Perinatal nurse managers have an opportunity to take a leadership role in ensuring that financial solutions to clinical situations have a quality-care focus that do not overlook existing evidence and standards of care. A cost-conscious approach to perinatal care ensures that cost is not the single variable in determining quality and increases the likelihood that mothers and babies are provided safe care by competent care providers.

REFERENCES

Alexander, L., Sandridge, J., & Moore, L. (1993). Patient satisfaction: An outcome measure for maternity services. *Journal of Perinatal and Neonatal Nursing, 7*(2), 28–39.

Agency for Healthcare Policy and Research (1999). *Hospital inpatient statistics*. Silver Springs, MD: AHCPR Publications Clearinghouse.

American Association of Colleges of Nursing (2000). *1999–2000 Enrollment and graduations in baccalaureate and graduate programs in nursing*. Washington, DC: Author.

American Nurses Association. (1997). *Implementing nursing's report card: A study of RN staffing, length of stay and patient outcomes*. Washington, DC: Author.

American Organization of Nurse Executives. (1999). *Alert on staffing*. Chicago, IL: Author.

Barter, M., McLaughlin, F. E., & Thomas, S. A. (1997). Registered nurse role changes and satisfaction with unlicensed assistive personnel. *Journal of Nursing Administration, 27*(1), 29–38.

Behram, S., Moschler, E. F., Sayegh, S. K., Garguillo, F. P., & Mann, W. J. (1998). Implementation of early discharges after uncomplicated vaginal deliveries: Maternal and infant complications. *Southern Medical Journal, 91*(6), 541–545.

Beil, C. W. (1999). By the numbers: Healthcare vital statistics. *Modern Healthcare, 29*(Suppl), 4–15.

Blegen, M. A., Goode, C. J., & Reed, L. (1998). Nurse staffing and patient outcomes. *Nursing Research, 47*(1), 43–50.

Bond, C. A., Raehl, C. L., Pitterle, M. E, & Franke, T. (1999). Health care professional staffing, hospital characteristics, and hospital mortality rates. *Pharmacotherapy, 19*(2), 130–138.

Bradford, L. J., & Raines, C. (1992). *Twenty-something: Managing and motivating today's new workforce*. New York: Master Media.

Braveman, P., Egerter, S., Pearl, M., Marchi, K., & Miller, C. (1995). Problems associated with early discharge of newborn infants: Early discharge of newborns and mothers: A critical review of the literature. *Pediatrics, 96*(4, Pt. 1), 716–726.

Carey, R. G., & Seibert, J. H. (1993). A patient survey system to measure quality improvement: Questionnaire reliability and validity. *Medical Care, 31*(9), 834–845.

Carrasquillo, O., Himmelstein, D. U., Woolhandler, S., & Bor, D. H. (1999). Going bare: Trends in health insurance coverage 1989 through 1996. *American Journal of Public Health, 89*(1), 3–42.

Coalition for Improving Maternity Services. (1996). *The mother-friendly childbirth initiative: The first consensus initiative of the coalition for improving maternity services*. Washington, DC: Author.

Coile, R. C. (1999). Top 10 health care trends for 1999. *Russ Coile's Health Trends, 11*(3), 1, 4–13.

Copeland, D. B., & Douglas, D. (1999). Communication strategies for the intrapartum nurse. *Journal of Obstetric, Gynecologic and Neonatal Nursing, 28*(6), 579–586.

Crain, C. A. (1993). Service excellence. *Nursing matters*. St. Louis, MO: St. John's Mercy Medical Center.

Curtin, S. C. & Martin, J. A. (2000). Births: Preliminary data for 1999. *National Vital Statistics Reports, 48*(14), 1–21.

Curtin, S. C., & Park, M. M. (1999). Trends in the attendant, place and timing of births, and in the use of obstetric interventions: United States, 1989–97. *National Vital Statistics Reports, 47*(27), 1–13.

Dasu, S., & Rao, J. (1999). Nature and determinants of customer expectations of service recovery in health care. *Quality Management in Health Care, 7*(4), 32–50.

Diemert, C. (1999). Concern for care. St. Paul, MN: Minnesota Nurses Association.

Drake, E. (1999). Internet technology: resources for perinatal nurses. *Journal of Obstetric, Gynecologic, and Neonatal Nurses, 28*(1) 15–21.

Dugan, J., Lauer, E., Bouquot, Z., Dutro, B. K., Smith, M., & Widmeyer, G. (1996). Stressful nurses: The effect on patient outcomes. *Journal of Nursing Care Quality, 10*(3), 46–58.

Finkelstein, B. S, Harper, D. L., & Rosenthal, G. E. (1999). Patient assessments of hospital maternity care: A useful tool for consumers? *Health Services Research, 34*(2), 623–640.

Fries, J. F., Koop, C. E., Beadle, C. E., Cooper, P. P., England, M. J., Greaves, R. F., Sokolov, J. J., & Wright, D. (1993). Reducing health care costs by reducing the need and demand for medical services: The health project consortium. *New England Journal of Medicine, 329*(5), 321–325.

Frosch, D. L., & Kaplan, R. M. (1999). Shared decision making in clinical medicine: Past research and future directions. *American Journal of Preventive Medicine, 17*(4), 285–294.

Gardner, M. (1998). Cost analysis in obstetrics and gynecology. *Clinical Obstetrics and Gynecology, 41*(2), 296–306.

Geary, M., Fanagan, M., & Boylan, P. (1997). Maternal satisfaction with management in labour and preferences for mode of delivery. *Journal of Perinatal Medicine, 25*(5), 433–439.

Graham, W. J., Hundley, V., McCheyene, A. L., Hall, M. H., Gurney, E., & Milne, J. (1999). An investigation of women's involvement in the decision to deliver by caesarean section. *British Journal of Obstetrics and Gynaecology, 106*(3), 213–220.

Hegedus, K. S. (1999). Providers' and consumers' perspective of nurses' caring behaviours. *Journal of Advanced Nursing, 30*(5), 1090–1096.

Holzemer, W. L. (1996). The impact of multiskilling on quality of care. *International Nursing Review, 43*(1), 21–25.

Howard, J. (1999). Hospital customer service in a changing healthcare world: Does it matter? *Journal of Healthcare Management, 44*(4), 312–325.

Iglehart, J. K. (1999). The American health care system: Expenditures. *New England Journal of Medicine, 340*(1), 70–76.

Irvine, D., Sindani, S., & Hall, L. M. (1998). Finding value in nursing care: A framework for quality improvement and clinical evaluation. *Nursing Economics, 16*(3), 110–116, 131.

Jennings, B. M., Staggers, N., & Brosch, L. R. (1999). A classification scheme for outcome indicators. *Image, Journal of Nursing Scholarship, 31*(4), 381–388.

Joint Commission on Accreditation of Healthcare Organizations. (2000). *Hospital Accreditation Comprehension Manual for Hospitals* Oakbrook Terrace, IL: JCAHO.

Kenagy, J. W., Berwick, D. M., & Shore, M. F. (1999). Service quality in health care. *Journal of the American Medical Association, 281*(7), 661–665.

Knox, G. E., Kelley, M., Simpson, K. R., Carrier, L., & Berry, D. (1999). Downsizing, reengineering and patient safety: Numbers, newness and resultant risk. *Journal of Healthcare Risk Management, 19*(4), 18–25.

Knox, G. E., Simpson, K. R., & Garite, T. J. (1999). High reliability perinatal units: An approach to the prevention of patient injury and medical malpractice claims. *Journal of Healthcare Risk Management, 19*(2), 27–35.

Kovner, C., & Gergen, P. J. (1998). Nurse staffing levels and adverse events following surgery in U. S. hospitals. *Image, Journal of Nursing Scholarship, 30*(4), 315–321.

Lau, S. (1996). *Benchmarking: A workbook for healthcare materials management professionals*. Chicago, IL: American Hospital Association.

Leveck, M. L., & Jones, C. B. (1996). The nursing practice environment, staff retention, and quality of care. *Research in Nursing and Health, 19*(4), 331–343.

Lichtig, L. K., Knauf, R. A., & Milholland, D. K. (1999). Some impacts of nursing on acute care hospital outcomes. *Journal of Nursing Administration, 29*(2), 25–33.

Lock, M., & Ray, J. G. (1999). Higher neonatal morbidity after routine early hospital discharge: Are we sending newborns home too early? *Canadian Medical Association Journal, 161*(3), 249–253.

Maisels, M.J., & Kring, E. (1998). Length of stay, jaundice, and hospital readmission. *Pediatrics, 101*(6), 995–998.

Mandl, K. D., Brennan, T. A., Wise, P. H., Tronick, E. Z., & Homer, C. J. (1997). *Archives of Pediatric Adolescent Medicine, 151*(9), 915–921.

Masters, M. L., & Masters, R. J. (1993). Building TQM into nursing management. *Nursing Economics, 11*(5), 274–278.

Maternity Center Association. (1998). *Statement of the rights of childbearing women*. New York, NY: Author.

McCrea, B. H., & Wright, M E. (1999). Satisfaction in childbirth and perceptions of personal control in pain relief during labour. *Journal of Advanced Nursing, 29*(4), 877–874.

McKay, S., & Phillips, C. (1984). *Family centered maternity care: Implementation strategies*. Rockville, MD: Aspen Publishing.

McDermott, K., Laschinger, H. K. S., & Shamian, J. (1996). Work empowerment and organizational commitment. *Nursing Management, 27*(5), 44–47.

Morrissey, J. (1998). All benchmarked out: Even the top 100 hospitals can't find many more ways to be more productive. *Modern Healthcare, 28*(49), 38–46.

Office of Inspector General. (1999). *Inspector general calls for improved oversight of hospitals*. Washington, DC: Office of Inspector General.

Patient Rights: Medicare and Medicaid Conditions of Participation. *Final Rule*. 42, CFR, part 482 (1999).

Phillips, M. E., & Szymanowski, M. (1999). Should a year on a medical surgical unit be a prerequisite for new graduates who want to be labor and delivery nurses? *MCN, The American Journal of Maternal Child Nursing, 24*(6), 278–279.

Phillips, M. E. (2000). *Generation X: Workplace redesign*. Unpublished paper, Graduate Nursing Program, Barnes College of Nursing at the University of Missouri, St. Louis.

Pierce, S. F. (1997). Nurse-sensitive health care outcomes in acute care settings: An integrative analysis of the literature. *Journal of Nursing Care Quality, 11*(4), 60–72.

Raube, K., & Merrell, K. (1999). Maternal minimum-stay legislation: Cost and policy implications. *American Journal of Public Health, 89*(6), 922–923.

Rubin, R. (1961) Puerperal change. *Nursing Outlook 9*, 753-755.

Seago, J. A. (1996). Work group culture, stress and hostility: Correlations with organizational outcomes. *Journal of Nursing Administration, 26*(6), 39–47.

Shamian, J. (2000). Re-energizing hospital care. *Reflections on Nursing Leadership, 26*(1), 24–26.

Shogren, B., & Calkins, A. (1995). *Minnesota Nurses' Association research project on occupational injury/illness in Minnesota between 1990–1994*. St. Paul, MN: Minnesota Nurses' Association.

Simpson, K. R. (1993). Meeting the challenge of the 1990s: Strategies to provide quality perinatal services in an era of decreasing reimbursement. *Journal of Perinatal and Neonatal Nursing, 7(2)*, 1–9.

Simpson, K. R. (1999). Routine care during labor and birth: Is this really how we want to practice perinatal nursing or are we ready to advocate for childbearing women and insist on evidence-based care? *Mother Baby Journal, 4*(4), 5–7.

Simpson, K. R., & Knox, G. E. (1999). Strategies for developing an evidence-based approach to perinatal care. *MCN The American Journal of Maternal Child Nursing, 24*(3), 122–132.

Simpson, K. R. (2000). Creating a culture of safety: A shared responsibility. *MCN, The American Journal of Maternal Child Nursing, 25*(2), 61.

Sochalski, J., Aiken, L. H., Shamian, J., Muller-Mundt, G., Hunt, J. M., Giovannetti, P., & Clarke, H. F. (1998). Building multidisciplinary research. *Reflections, 24*(3), 20–23.

Triolo, P. K. (1987). Marketing women's health care. *Journal of Nursing Administration, 17*(11), 9–15.

United States Census Bureau. (1998). *United States Census Report*. Washington, DC: Author.

Ventura, S. J., Martin, J. A., Curtin, S. C., Mathews, T. J. & Park, M. M. (2000). Births: Final data for 1998. *National Vital Statistics Reports, 48*(3), 1–100.

Ventura, M. J. (1999). Staffing issues. *RN, 62*(2), 26–30.

Weiss Ratings Incorporated. (1999). *HMOs continue to lose money*. Washington, DC: Author.

Woolhandler, S., & Himmelstein, D. U. (1997). Costs of care and administration at for-profit and other hospitals in the United States. *New England Journal of Medicine, 336*(11), 769–774.

World Health Organization. (1996). *Care in normal birth: A practical guide*. Geneva, Switzerland: Author.

Wunderlich, G. S., Sloan, F. A., & Davis, C. K. (1996). *Nursing staff in hospitals and nursing homes: Is it adequate?* Washington, DC: National Academy Press.

Young, W. B., Minnick, A. F., & Marcantonio, R. (1996). How wide is the gap in defining quality care? Comparisons of patient and nurse perceptions of important aspects of patient care. *Journal of Nursing Administration, 26*(5), 15–20.

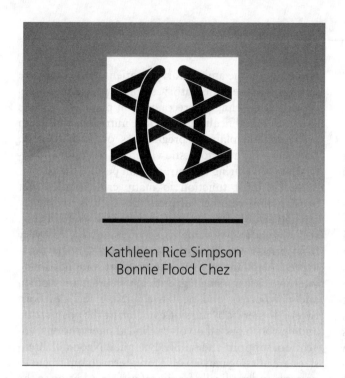

Kathleen Rice Simpson
Bonnie Flood Chez

CHAPTER 2

Professional and Legal Issues

Service to humanity was the primary mission of the first women who chose nursing as a profession, just as it is for the women and men who enter nursing today. When Florence Nightingale founded the modern nursing profession in the 1850s, she was motivated by courage, compassion, and the desire to make a difference. These goals and ambitions remain the foundation for contemporary professional nursing practice. She and her fellow nursing pioneers went to the Crimean War zone armed with practice guidelines and protocols, with the belief that research-based interventions provided with a systematic approach to specific clinical situations could improve patient outcomes, increase trauma survival rates, and address the psychosocial needs of injured soldiers.

Nightingale's success with the injured and sick soldiers during the Crimean War solidified her role in founding the profession of nursing as it is known today (Donahue, 1996). After the war, she returned to England to continue the tasks of educating nurses and developing practice guidelines and quality improvement measures. The Standard Nomenclature of Diseases and the Model Hospital Statistical Form developed by Nightingale facilitated data collection about best practices and provided the basis for her arguments to improve patient care. She was able to show that care provided by competent, devoted nurses who had received adequate education, affected inpatient morbidity and mortality rates. Developing programs for nursing education and classification of diseases linked with specific evidence-based nursing interventions were among her greater contributions. These activities helped to identify nursing practice as a separate but collaborative healthcare profession. Nightingale was the first nurse to demonstrate what modern nurses know today: careful analysis of rigorously collected data presented by those who are passionate about patient welfare is what is needed to make a positive difference for mothers and babies.

A century and a half after Nightingale's heroic efforts during the Crimean War and her contributions to establishing nursing as a profession, public esteem and trust in nurses are at very high levels. A Harris (1999) poll revealed that 92% of the general public trust information about healthcare provided by nurses. Eighty-five percent of Americans indicated they would be pleased if their sons or daughters became nurses. In a Gallup poll (1999), nurses were ranked number one in honesty and ethics by the American public. Of the 45 professions and occupations considered by survey respondents, nurses received the highest scores (73% ranked nurses' honesty and ethics very high or high, compared with pharmacists at 69% and physicians at 57%).

Over the years, various regulatory agencies, federal and state legislatures, accrediting bodies, and professional organizations have developed practice guidelines and standards for education, licensure, credentialing, and certification for nurses. The intention is to provide for the public welfare, assuring patients and their family members that nursing care will be given by competent nursing professionals. As the body of medical and nursing knowledge has expanded, the subspecialty of perinatal nursing has emerged, benefitting from an increased research database and improved technologies. This chapter provides an overview of professional and legal issues related to perinatal nursing practice in this new century.

PROFESSIONAL ISSUES

Perinatal Nursing Practice

Every day, more than 11,000 babies are born to women in approximately 6,000 hospitals in the United States (Ventura, Martin, Curtin, Mathews, & Park, 2000). These mothers and babies are cared for during pregnancy, labor, birth, and the postpartum period by perinatal nurses dedicated to providing a safe and therapeutic environment to promote the best possible outcomes for their patients. According to the *Standards and Guidelines for Professional Nursing Practice in the Care of Women and Newborns* from the Association of Women's Health, Obstetric and Neonatal Nurses (AWHONN), "Nursing care of women and newborns is centered on the principle of treating the patient as a whole being within the context of the family and community. This type of care requires the integration of substantial knowledge, the ability to recognize and use new scientific information, and use of a complex set of communication and organization skills" (AWHONN, 1998b, p. ix). Perinatal nursing is unique among nursing specialties because nurses caring for pregnant women always have a minimum nurse to patient ratio of 1:2. Any medication, therapy, or intervention for pregnant women affects two individuals, each with potentially different outcomes (Poole, 1992). Like the mother, the fetus is a distinct patient, requiring assessments, interventions, evaluation, and medical record documentation of the nursing care provided (Simpson, 1997a). Providing care for two patients, including one that cannot be directly observed is a challenge that requires nurses with refined critical thinking and priority setting skills (Phillips & Szymanowski, 1999).

As a specialty area of professional practice, perinatal nursing offers a wide diversity of clinical opportunities. Nursing care during labor and birth offers the opportunity for autonomy, clinical action, and quick decision-making that is not usually experienced by nurses in other specialty areas. Few professional experiences are more rewarding than attending the birth of a healthy newborn and sharing the joy with the new mother and her family. There is nothing to compare with emerging from a potentially disastrous clinical situation, such as a prolapsed umbilical cord, abruptio placenta, shoulder dystocia, or severely depressed newborn at birth, with a healthy mother and baby. However, there is much more to perinatal nursing than intrapartum care.

Perinatal nurses practice in a wide variety of clinical settings and have the opportunity to use all of the knowledge and skills learned during undergraduate nursing education. Preconception, prenatal, labor, birth, and postpartum care is provided over the telephone and in the ambulatory, inpatient, and home care settings. In the ambulatory setting, perinatal nurses provide counseling in preconception planning, genetic issues, prenatal health promotion, nutrition, childbirth preparedness, planned pregnancies or birth control, grief support, and domestic violence screening and interventions. During the intrapartum period, the perinatal nurse must function in many critical roles that overlap those of other subspecialties such as emergency nursing (eg, obstetric triage), perioperative nursing (eg, cesarean birth), postanesthesia nursing (eg, recovery from birth-related anesthesia), medical-surgical nursing (eg, pregnant women with medical complications), intensive care nursing (eg, critically ill pregnant women and newborns), and pediatric nursing (eg, newborn care). Mother-baby nursing care during the postpartum and newborn period involves clinical interventions, education, support, and family dynamics. Neonatal intensive care nursing may involve long-term commitment to preterm and medically fragile infants. In addition to the clinical component of care, families in the neonatal intensive care unit depend on neonatal nurses for support and critical information to successfully manage the crisis of having a critically ill infant. No other specialty in nursing offers a wider range of activities and opportunities to make a difference in the lives of women, newborns, and their families. Perinatal nursing is focused on supporting families and creating our future. Although approximately 4% of registered nurses in the United States are male (Geolot, 1999), perinatal nursing remains predominantly a specialty of nurses who are women. This woman-to-woman connection is very powerful for perinatal nurses and childbearing women.

Licensure

Nursing licensure in the United States is governed by nurse practice acts enacted by state legislatures. The legal basis for licensure is government's power to protect the public's health, safety, and welfare. Licensure sets the standards for entry into practice, defines a scope of practice, and allows for disciplinary action. Each state has a requirement that all persons functioning in the role of a registered nurse be licensed by that state. Although there have been efforts by the National Council of State Boards of Nursing to develop an interstate compact for mutual recognition of state licensure, several controversial issues are associated with this initiative, including licensure in the state of residence rather than in the state of practice, potential for multiple claims of jurisdiction to discipline nurses, inadequate protection of consumers, and different licensing for basic and advanced practice nurses (AWHONN, 1999). The interstate compact as proposed has not become a reality. However, it is possible that a revised interstate compact for mutual recognition of state licensure may result in consensus and approval by various stakeholders in the next few years.

State boards of nursing develop nurse practice acts, defining the practice of nursing for individual states. Nurses should be aware of the specific wording of the nurse practice acts of their respective states, because the definition of nursing and scope of practice can vary from state to state. For example, some nurse practice acts prohibit nurses from inserting intrauterine pressure catheters during labor, and others have strict guidelines for the role of the nurse during epidural anesthesia for women in labor. Nurse practice acts may include specific criteria about delegation and supervision of unlicensed assistive personnel (UAPs). Nurse practice acts also allow an administrative body, usually the State Board of Nursing, to impose various disciplinary actions if the conduct of the nurse violates a provision of the act that threatens the health and safety of a citizen (Rostant, 1999). Grounds for discipline include fraud and deceit, criminal acts, substance abuse, mental incompetence, unprofessional conduct, incompetence due to negligence, and inability to practice nursing with reasonable skill and safety (Booth & Caruth, 1998). In addition to granting licensure, state boards have the power to deny, revoke, or suspend the license of a registered nurse. Most states have statutes that identify when malpractice has occurred and outline the burden of proof that is required in a malpractice case (Rostant, 1999). Educational criteria identify individuals qualified to write national licensure examinations.

Standardization of licensure examinations has improved the quality of this process and facilitated licensure reciprocity between states. Development of the National Council of State Boards Licensing Examination (NCLEX) with standard minimum passing scores ensures that nurses practicing in all areas of the country have met the same stringent educational and examination criteria before entering into clinical practice.

Licensure also takes into account the two distinct yet overlapping roles of nurses in perinatal nursing: the specialty nurse and the advanced practice nurse (ie, clinical nurse specialists, nurse practitioners, certified nurse midwives, and certified registered nurse anesthetists who specialize in perinatal services). Each of these roles begins with basic nursing education and progresses with specialized education. Nurses who choose to practice in a particular clinical specialty may seek certification to validate their special knowledge. In 1993, the National Council of State Boards of Nursing (NCSBN) defined advanced practice nurses as nurses in advanced clinical practice who possess a graduate degree with a major in nursing or "concentration in an advanced nursing practice category, which includes didactic and clinical components, advanced knowledge in nursing theory, physical and psychosocial assessment, appropriate interventions, and management of healthcare" (NCSBN, 1993, p. 3).

A graduate degree for advanced practice nurses has been recommended by various professional nursing organizations, but this requirement is not yet mandated by most state boards of nursing. A graduate degree is likely to be a requirement for advanced practice nurses in the future. Certification for advanced practice nurses is required by most state boards of nursing. For some advanced practice roles, such as perinatal nurse practitioners and perinatal clinical nurse specialists, there is no certification process available. Advanced practice nurses integrate education, research, management, leadership, and consultation into their clinical role and function in collegial relationships with nursing peers, physicians, and others who influence the health environment (Hagedorn & Gardner, 1999).

Certification

Certification is a process by which a nongovernmental agency or association certifies that an individual licensed to practice a profession has met certain predetermined standards specified by that profession for a specialty practice (ANA, 1979). More than 350,000 nurses in the United States and Canada hold professional certification (Cary, 2000). The certification process provides tangible recognition of an individual registered nurse's professional achievement in a defined functional or clinical area of nursing (American Nurses Credentialing Center [ANCC], 2000). Certification gives the obstetric, gynecologic, or neonatal nurse an additional credential that attests to his or her attainment of special knowledge in a specific area beyond the basic nursing degree (National Certification Corporation for the Obstetric, Gynecologic, and Neonatal Nursing Specialties [NCC], 2000). The certification process helps maintain and promote quality nursing care that benefits individual nurses, the nursing profession, and the public (NCC, 2000). A survey commissioned by ANCC in 1999 found that 87% of consumers would be more confident if they knew their nurse was a certified specialist. Although each specialty group has its own objectives for certification, the following goals usually are included:

- Assessment of special knowledge
- Promotion of excellence in practice
- Encouragement of professional growth
- Standardization of qualifications necessary for specialty practice

- Advancement of specialty knowledge and standards

A study funded by ANCC (Cary, 2000) found many positive aspects of specialty certification. Approximately 19,500 certified nurses representing more than 50 different certification credentials participated in the survey. Certified nurses reported feeling more confident in their ability to detect early signs and symptoms of complications in their patients and to initiate early and prompt interventions for such complications (Cary, 2000). Certified nurses felt that certification enabled them to experience fewer adverse events and errors in patient care than before they were certified (Cary, 2000). One possible explanation for these findings is that nurses who seek certification are more motivated to achieve high levels of performance and professionalism. Voluntary certification involves an initial commitment to review the literature pertinent to their specialty area of practice to prepare for examination and ongoing commitment to keep abreast of current developments because of continuing education and practice requirements for certification maintenance. Certification may be a marker for excellence in nursing practice. Other important results of this study include certified nurses who report more personal growth and job satisfaction and fewer disciplinary events and work-related injuries than their colleagues (Cary, 2000). Certified nurses reported salary increases, advancements, and bonuses as a result of certification (Cary, 2000). Clearly, certified nurses feel there is value in holding certification.

Perinatal nurses have many avenues available for seeking certification. Some examples of nationally recognized certification programs are included in Display 2–1. Some healthcare institutions have developed credentialing or certification programs for their own employees that are specific to an area of practice, such as mother–baby nursing; labor, delivery, and recovery (LDR) nursing; labor, delivery, recovery, and postpartum (LDRP) nursing; electronic fetal monitoring (EFM); childbirth education; lactation consulting; and grief counseling. These programs may be a requirement for employment and are generally nontransferable to other institutions.

Certification is available from professional organizations for specific areas of perinatal nursing practice. NCC offers certifications in six nursing practice specialties and certificates of added qualification for four subspecialties. The NCC certification process for Neonatal Nurse Practitioners (NNP) and Women's Health Care Nurse Practitioners (WHNP) is considered entry into practice criteria in many states. Lamaze International offers certification as a Lamaze certified childbirth educator (LCCE), the International Board of Lactation Consultant Examiners offers certification as a lactation consultant (IBCLC), and the Doulas of North America (DONA) provides course work and examination leading to certification as a professional labor support provider (LSP).

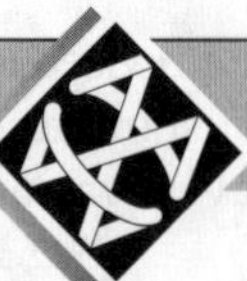

DISPLAY 2–1

Certification Resource Sites for Perinatal Nurses

Academy of Certified Birth Educators and Labor Support Professionals
http://www.acbe.com

American Association of Critical Care Nurses (AACN)
http://www.certcorp.org

American Association of Legal Nurse Consultants (AALNC)
http://www.aalnc.org

American College of Nurse Midwives (ACNM)
http://www.acnm.org

American Nurses Credentialing Center (ANCC)
http://www.ana.org

International Board of Lactation Consultant Examiners (IBLCE)
http://www.nursingcenter.com

International Childbirth Education Association (ICEA)
http://www.icea.org

Lamaze Childbirth Educator Certification (LCEC), formerly ACCE-APSO Lamaze Certified Childbirth Educator
http://www.lamaze-childbirth.com

National Certification Corporation for the Obstetric, Gynecologic, and Neonatal Nursing Specialties (NCC)
http://www.nccnet.org

The fees, prerequisites, certification examinations, and continuing education requirements for certification and recertification depend on the certifying body. Generally, a specific number of clinical hours in the specialty practice area and designated years of experience are examination prerequisites, although sometimes, as in the case of certification examinations given by ANCC, academic preparation at the baccalaureate level is required. Some certification companies require nurses to complete a company-sponsored course as well. Most certification processes involve a written examination. Recertification usually requires continued practice in the specialty area, continuing education hours or reexamination, and an additional maintenance fee. Some certifying agencies recertify by examination only.

Issues Related to Certification

The many options for certification within the perinatal nursing specialty can cause confusion for nurses desiring a credential to validate and document their level of knowledge and expertise in a specific area of practice, and confusion for consumers who may be at a loss to understand the meaning of those additional initials following the registered nurse's name. Controversy continues concerning nonnursing bodies providing certification for nurses and offering the same certification to nurses and other healthcare providers. Questions related to the validity and reliability of items used in these various certification examinations have not been adequately addressed. National recognition and acceptance of the certification credential may be limited if it is obtained through a company or institution that is not sponsored or endorsed by a national professional organization. Certification processes developed by an individual or small group of individuals may merely reflect regional practice. These individuals may lack experience in item writing and examination development and may not have the personnel or financial resources for adequate psychometric evaluation of results. The best approach is to select a certification process that has been determined to be psychometrically sound and legally defensible. An additional quality indicator is accreditation by the National Commission for Certifying Agencies (NCCA) or recognition by the American Board of Nursing Specialties (ABNS).

Because considerable time and expense is involved in the certification and recertification process, including the examination fees, preparation for the examination, and continuing education requirements, the importance of these issues should not be minimized (Simpson, 1990). Display 2–2 contains general questions that may be useful to the candidate for certification. After careful analysis, nurses should choose the program that best meets their needs and resources, while recognizing the program's strengths and weaknesses (Nichols, 1993).

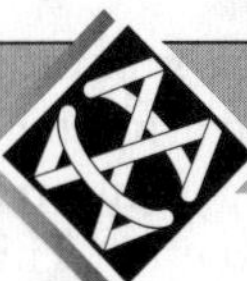

DISPLAY 2–2

Suggestions for Evaluating Certification Programs

- Who is the sponsoring organization of the certification program?
- What is the program's philosophy of certification? How is certification defined by the organization?
- What are the entry requirements?
- What are the objectives of the program?
- How much time does the certification program take?
- How long has the certification program been established?
- How many nurses have been certified by the organization since the program began?
- Is the same certification offered to healthcare providers or educators who are not nurses?
- If a course is required, what does the curriculum include? How many hours of continuing education are given? What organization approves the continuing education?
- Can the educational portion be taken for college credit?
- Who are the faculty, and what are their credentials?
- Is the content outline of the examination available to the candidates?
- Are recognized review courses offered?
- Who provides the review courses?
- What materials are needed to prepare for examination?
- Is there a method for determining validity and reliability of test items?
- What is the mechanism for psychometric evaluation of examination results?
- Who is responsible for item development and what are their credentials?
- What is the reputation of the certification program among the healthcare and nursing community?
- Is the certification credential recognized nationally? Internationally?

Adapted from Nichols F.H. (1993). Issues in perinatal education. *AWHONN'S Clinical Issues in Perinatal and Women's Health Nursing, 4* (1), 55–59.

Educational Preparation for Entry into Professional Nursing Practice

One of the most significant barriers for advancing the professional and economic status of nursing today is the issue of educational criteria for entry into professional nursing practice. There are three common ways to become a registered professional nurse: a diploma from a 2- or 3-year hospital-based school of nursing, a 2-year associate's degree from a community college, and a 4-year baccalaureate degree. Other nontraditional programs allow nonnurses to enter a master's degree in nursing program and become a registered nurse and a nurse practitioner concurrently. This multi-avenue process is confusing to other healthcare providers and consumers and is a hindrance to obtaining adequate financial reimbursement. If an educational program were designed now for a profession that deals with life and death every day, it is unlikely that this profession in the 21st century would have individuals with the same title and license, regardless of whether they have no college education, some college education, a baccalaureate degree, or graduate degree (Freda, 1999). Unfortunately, according to the latest data, 59% of registered professional nurses in the United States do not hold a 4-year college degree (Geolot, 1999). Because nurses are the poorest prepared educationally of all healthcare professionals, they are also the lowest paid and the least respected (Christman, 1998). Pay equity and professional respect are important issues to all nurses.

As the science that is the basis of nursing practice is changing, nursing practice is changing, and these changes are occurring rapidly in a system that is demanding an evaluation of the outcomes of care (Gennaro & Lewis, 2000). Without a baccalaureate degree, how can nurses be expected to review the literature, interpret standards and guidelines, accurately evaluate evidence, and determine best practices based on science rather than on tradition (Gennaro & Lewis, 2000)? In response to evolving changes in the healthcare system and requirements for interpretation and application of scientific knowledge, other healthcare professions have increased the level of education required for their members (Gennaro & Lewis, 2000). There is no other group of healthcare providers that nurses interact with professionally without requirements for at least a 4-year college degree.

Collaboration and mutual respect between physicians and nurses depend on an adequate level of education for nurses who want to be partners in care (Simpson & Knox, 2000). As the nursing profession attempts to develop a collaborative, interdependent relationship with the medical profession and leave the outdated hierarchical, dependent relationship behind, baccalaureate education for nurses becomes essential. According to a 1999 Harris poll, 76% of Americans believe nurses should have at least a 4-year college education. As a profession, we have been struggling with this issue for too long. A date should be set for requiring a baccalaureate degree, current registered nurses should be grandfathered in, and we should look to the future of the profession (Freda, 1999). It is time that we move forward united in providing consumers with the care they deserve, delivered by professionals who have been adequately educated to provide that care (Gennaro & Lewis, 2000). A more detailed discussion of this topic and the impact on teamwork between perinatal care providers is discussed in Chapter 3.

Competence Validation

Healthcare institutions need to maintain a focus on quality outcomes while complying with guidelines and standards from multiple professional organizations and regulatory agencies. The Joint Commission on Accreditation of Healthcare Organizations (JCAHO, 2000) has published standards for nursing orientation, continuing education, competence assessment, and ongoing collection of aggregate data to identify and respond to nursing staff's learning needs. Institutions must identify areas of core competence that are specific to each nursing unit and develop processes to validate nurses' level of competence. Validation only on the basis of skill checklists is not enough to meet this standard. A system to validate the knowledge base that is required for clinical practice must also be developed and implemented. Completion of written self-assessment tools, computer-simulated examinations, oral or written case presentations, peer and manager reviews, and medical record audits examining individual practice are commonly used methods of validating areas of core competence. The critical issue is to incorporate the expected skills verification and the requisite knowledge-based evaluation into the competence validation process. Most current methods of competence validation fall far short of achieving this goal. Traditional written tests may be useful in determining whether the nurse has the appropriate knowledge about a specific clinical practice area but provide little or no information about technical expertise. Possession of a thorough knowledge base does not necessarily mean that the nurse has the ability to translate that knowledge into safe clinical practice (Afriat, Simpson, Chez, & Miller, 1994). It is important to go beyond evaluating core knowledge. The ability to use that knowledge must also be considered as part of the overall competence validation process (AWHONN, 1998a). Traditional skills checklists are commonly used to document clinical expertise, but this method gives no indication about whether the technically expert nurse has the ability to think critically and consider the implications of the clinical intervention. Verification of clinical skills is only one component of the competence validation process.

Competence validation and documentation of that process should be done at the completion of the unit orientation, at specific time intervals during the first year, and on an annual basis thereafter. Nurses who are expected to provide care in areas that deliver services secondary to their primary area of expertise must also meet minimum competence requirements in those areas (JCAHO, 2000). This standard is especially important for perinatal nurses who may be routinely expected to provide care for a variety of patients of different acuity levels in multiple settings, including women during the antepartum, intrapartum, and postpartum periods, and infants in the newborn nursery, intermediate care nursery, and neonatal intensive care nursery. Perinatal units can refer to the *Standards and Guidelines for Professional Nursing Practice in the Care of Women and Newborns* (AWHONN, 1998b) and the *Comprehensive Accreditation Manual for Hospitals* (JCAHO, 2000) for lists of nursing practices that may reflect the expected practice in each institution. *AWHONN's Competence Validation for Perinatal Care Providers* (Simpson & Creehan, 1998) includes multiple tools to assist perinatal nurses with this process.

A more complex issue is whether competent nurses consistently use their knowledge and clinical skills over time and for each patient interaction. Multiple factors, including nurse-to-patient staffing ratios, unit operations, fatigue, interpersonal stress, and interactions with other care providers, influence the ability of competent nurses to provide safe and effective perinatal care on a routine basis (Buerhaus, 1999; Jones et al., 1988). No one method can address all of the issues involved in competence validation, nor can one method ensure that the competent nurse will provide safe and effective care in every interaction, but some methods work better than others (Simpson, 2001). If the goal of competence validation is to enhance the likelihood that nurses will provide safe and effective care to all women and babies during each clinical interaction, use of a process that includes a well-designed medical record audit tool may be one of the best approaches (Simpson, 1998a).

Medical Record Audits

Medical record audits are particularly helpful with validation of competence related to intrapartum nursing but can also be adapted to antepartum or mother–baby nursing. An audit of the medical record provides substantial data about requisite knowledge and clinical skills for each area of specialty practice. This method is comprehensive and objective, avoiding the observer bias inherent in the skills checklist approach. The process can be incorporated into the unit's annual competence validation program for all nurses and allows identification of nurses who could benefit from additional education and clinical practice experience. Ideally, nurses who are identified as deficient in some areas and therefore receive more education and follow-up, will provide better care. If clinical practice does not improve, this process provides objective, supportive information for appropriate disciplinary action. Feedback to nurses based on audits can heighten awareness about the importance of accurate medical record documentation. Improvements in documentation and clinical practice can decrease professional and institutional liability (Rommal, 1996). Overall accuracy; consistency with established institutional policies and procedures, standards, and guidelines from professional organizations; legibility; and clinical practice issues can be evaluated during the intrapartum, immediate postpartum, and newborn periods, using selected parameters from the criteria included in Display 2–3.

A full discussion of how to design, implement, and evaluate the medical record audit process, including a sample medical record audit tool, is discussed in the chapter in *AWHONN's Competence Validation for Perinatal Care Providers* (Simpson & Creehan, 1998), "Using Guidelines and Standards from Professional Organizations as a Framework for Competence Validation" (Simpson, 1998b).

Continuing Education

The dynamic nature of perinatal nursing practice makes it imperative that nurses keep abreast of advancements in knowledge and new technologies. Fewer financial resources for nursing education are available than in the past in most institutional budgets. However, there remains a joint responsibility between professional nurses and their employers to ensure that nurses have current knowledge so clinical practice can be based on the latest evidence. Perinatal nurses are responsible for obtaining new knowledge and maintaining competence in their practice. They must have an awareness of changing practices and professional and ethical issues, seek new knowledge and clinical skills by attending in-service education and professional continuing education programs, be cognizant of pertinent research data and professional literature, and incorporate newly acquired knowledge and skills into practice (AWHONN, 1998b).

Subscribing to professional nursing journals, attending continuing education offerings, and belonging to professional nursing organizations are methods to obtain knowledge of new practice guidelines and research in the field. Journal clubs, organized by nurses in specialty practice areas, that meet on a regular basis to review the latest articles in perinatal nursing and medical journals are one way to ensure currency in

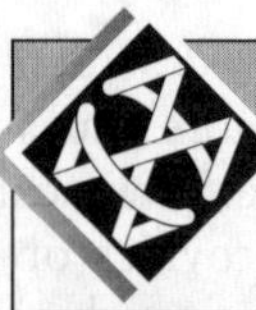

DISPLAY 2-3

Suggested Components of a Medical Record Audit

- Are the nurses' notes legible?
- Are the times noted on the Admission Assessment, Labor Progress Chart, and the initial electronic fetal monitoring (EFM) strip consistent with each other within a reasonable time frame?
- Is there documentation of notification of the physician of admission within the time frame outlined in the policies and procedures?
- Is fetal well-being established before ambulation?
- Does the EFM fetal heart rate (FHR) baseline match the FHR baseline noted on the Labor Progress Chart?
- Does the EFM FHR baseline variability match the FHR baseline variability noted on the Labor Progress Chart?
- If there is evidence of decreased FHR variability, is it noted on the Labor Progress Chart?
- If there is evidence of decreased FHR variability, are appropriate nursing interventions charted on the Labor Progress Chart?
- If there are FHR decelerations on the EFM strip, are they correctly noted on the Labor Progress Chart?
- Are appropriate nursing interventions charted on the Labor Progress Chart during nonreassuring FHR patterns?
- Is there documentation of physician notification on the Labor Progress Chart during nonreassuring FHR patterns?
- If there are FHR accelerations noted on the Labor Progress Chart, are they on the EFM strip?
- Are maternal assessments noted on the Labor Progress Chart according to policy?
- If there is evidence of a nonreassuring FHR pattern, is oxytocin dosage increased?
- If there is evidence of a nonreassuring FHR pattern, is oxytocin dosage decreased or discontinued?
- If there is evidence of uterine hyperstimulation, are appropriate nursing interventions charted on the Labor Progress Chart?
- If there is evidence of adequate labor, is oxytocin dosage increased?
- If there is evidence of uterine hyperstimulation, is oxytocin dosage increased?
- Does the frequency of uterine contractions on the EFM strip match what is noted on the Labor Progress Chart?
- Is the uterine activity monitor (external tocodynamometer or intrauterine pressure catheter) adjusted to maintain an accurate baseline?
- Are oxytocin dosage increases charted when there is an inaccurate uterine baseline tracing or an uninterpretable FHR tracing?
- Are medications given when there is an uninterpretable FHR tracing before administration?
- Does documentation continue during the second stage of labor?
- Are women in the second stage of labor encouraged to push with contractions when the FHR is nonreassuring (ie, variable FHR decelerations occur with each contraction)?
- If the FHR is nonreassuring during the second stage of labor, is oxytocin discontinued?
- Does the time of birth match the end of the EFM strip?
- If the woman had regional analgesia or anesthesia, is a qualified anesthesia provider involved in the decision to discharge from the postanesthetic care unit (PACU).
- If the woman had regional analgesia or anesthesia, is the discharge from PACU care scoring evaluation documented?
- Are maternal assessments documented during the immediate postpartum period every 15 minutes for the first hour?
- Are newborn assessments documented during the transition to extrauterine life at least every 30 minutes until the newborn's condition has been stable for 2 hours?

practice. Publication processes often delay the dissemination of articles and research reports by a year or longer, and "current" articles usually report studies that were completed during the previous year. Innovative programs are available to provide current information such as computer-assisted instructional programs (CAIs), video tape series, and teleconferences. Institutions can purchase these resources as one approach to offer quality programs to a large number of nurses at a relatively low cost per staff member. CAIs, video tapes, and textbooks can become part of a unit's lending library, allowing staff members to borrow resources for home use at their convenience. Continuing education may also be obtained through self-study programs, journal articles, and Internet sites. A variety of perinatal and neonatal nursing educational resources are available through AWHONN, NCC, Lippincott Williams & Wilkins, and the March of Dimes.

Attendance at perinatal nursing conferences and workshops is a common method of assimilating new information. Not only is the course content useful to practice, but conference attendance provides opportunities to discuss clinical and operational issues with professional colleagues from other institutions and other areas of the country. Regional differences in practice can be identified, and those differences that may be an improvement for individual institutions may be promoted and implemented as a result of national conference participation. Some institutions elect to bring a nurse speaker on site for the benefit of all staff rather than send several nurses to a national perinatal conference as a more cost-effective method of providing continuing education. There are merits to this approach, but collaboration and sharing with colleagues from other areas of the country is limited. Informal telephone networks with nursing colleagues and subscription to professional discussion lists through the Internet can be used to overcome this limitation.

LEGAL ISSUES

Nursing Accountability and Responsibility

The perinatal nurse is responsible for decisions and actions within the domain of nursing practice (American Nurses Association [ANA], 1998). There are several important aspects of this responsibility:

- Promotion of a safe and therapeutic environment for the recipients and providers of nursing care
- Accurate and truthful description of nursing care provided
- Acquisition of specialized knowledge and skills and ongoing continuing education to provide specialized care
- Demonstration and validation of competence in nursing practice

Nurses are directly accountable to the public for their practice and are answerable for actions in the provision of patient care (ANA, 1998). The authority for the practice of nursing is based on a social contract that acknowledges professional rights and responsibilities as well as mechanisms for public accountability. Standards provide a means by which a profession clearly describes the focus of its activities, the recipients of service, and the responsibilities for which its practitioners are accountable (ANA, 1998). The ANA's (1998) *Standards of Clinical Nursing Practice* outlines the expectations of the full professional role within which all nurses must practice, and AWHONN's (1998b) *Standards and Guidelines for Professional Nursing Practice in the Care of Women and Newborns* outlines the additional expectations of the professional role of the perinatal nurse. Professional accountability is closely linked to the concept of legal accountability. Legal accountability is defined in part by nurse practice acts, parameters of professional practice established by professional organizations, institutional standards, and legislative changes that affect practice and policies, procedures, and protocols within the practice environment. In nursing malpractice cases, the particular application of legal accountability is usually established by expert witness testimony.

In addition to the legal injunction that all nursing actions be performed in a safe and effective manner, the courts have upheld the nurses' affirmative duty to protect patients from harm. The basis for affirmative duty actions can be found in states' nurse practice acts, the *ANA Code of Ethics* (1985), and standards for professional conduct that are published by professional organizations. The courts recognize nurses as professionals who possess the specialized knowledge and skills required to act interdependently as a collaborative member of a team of caregivers; dependently, carrying out the prescribed healthcare regimen of the primary care provider; and independently as an individual professional on behalf of patients. To do so, perinatal nurses must be cognizant of institutional policies, procedures, and protocols. Perinatal nurses must have a knowledge of physician-prescribed medical and surgical interventions, drug actions and interactions, normal and abnormal laboratory values, and physical examination and assessment skills (Poole, 1992). Competence in a variety of technical skills and critical thinking are requisite. Keen assessment skills and the ability to intervene quickly and accurately are particularly important during emergent situations.

Ethical decision-making is also an inherent part of perinatal nursing practice. Frequently, dilemmas involve one or more of the following: cost-containment issues that may jeopardize patient welfare; end-of-life care; informed consent; incompetent, unethical, or illegal practices of colleagues; and access to care (Chally & Loriz, 1998). Nurses must differentiate decisions that are in the province of the individual nurse from those that require consultation or collaboration with other members of the healthcare team. In addition to the *ANA Code for Nurses* (1985), which provides guidance in the ethics of nursing practice, institutional ethics committees offer assistance in clarifying ethical principles involved and recommending the most ethical courses of action.

Issues Related to Working with Unlicensed Assistive Personnel

The nursing profession determines the scope of nursing practice and defines and supervises the education, training, and use of UAPs involved in providing direct patient care (ANA, 1996). UAPs can contribute as members of the healthcare team under the direction of the professional registered nurse, but the registered nurse is ultimately responsible for the coordination and delivery of nursing care to women and newborns (AWHONN, 1998). The role of the UAP is to assist, not replace, the professional registered nurse (ANA, 1996; AWHONN, 1997, 1998). Certain nursing functions are solely within the scope of nursing practice, and oversight of the activities of the UAP is integral and necessary to implementation of UAP roles (ANA, 1996; Rhodes, 1997).

The AWHONN (1997) position statements, *The Role of Unlicensed Assistive Personnel in the Nursing Care for Women and Newborns* and *Registered Professional Nurses and Unlicensed Assistive Personnel* (ANA, 1996), provide a framework for determining which tasks may be appropriate for delegation in selected clinical situations and examples of nursing care activities for women and newborns that cannot be delegated based on that framework. Review of these publications before development and implementation of a patient care model using UAPs is essential.

The nursing process is traditionally described as including four essential components: assessment, planning, implementation, and evaluation. It is not appropriate to delegate nursing activities that comprise the core of the nursing process and that require specialized knowledge, judgment, competence, and skill (ANA, 1996). In selecting certain aspects of nursing care that can be delegated to UAPs, it is critical to consider whether the tasks meet these exclusion criteria. The delegated task must be a subcomponent of the total nursing process. The registered professional nurse is accountable when delegating nursing tasks and supervising UAPs who carry out those nursing tasks. It is generally agreed that the registered nurse remains legally responsible for the nursing activities delegated to the UAP, although individual state laws may vary (ANA, 1996).

A review of NCSBN (1995) definitions is useful in understanding the role of the registered professional nurse when working with UAPs. *Delegation* is transferring to a competent individual the authority to perform a selected nursing task in selected situations (NCSBN, 1995). Delegation passes on the responsibility for task performance but not the accountability for the outcome of the task (ANA, 1996). *Accountability* is being responsible and answerable for actions and inactions of self or others in the context of delegation (NCSBN, 1995). *Supervision* is the provision of guidance or direction, evaluation, and follow-up by the registered professional nurse for accomplishment of a nursing task delegated to UAPs (NCSBN, 1995).

Patient assessment is a professional nursing responsibility and cannot be delegated to UAPs (JCAHO, 1997). Confusion seems to exist about the difference between collecting data and assessment. *Data* are uninterpreted observations or facts reported to the registered professional nurse (JCAHO, 1997). *Assessment* is the process of transforming data into useful information by analyzing the data (JCAHO, 1997). For example, UAPs can collect data about patients by taking blood pressures, temperatures, and respiratory and pulse rates (AWHONN, 1997). Professional registered nurses analyze that data using critical thinking skills to make an assessment about patient status. Assessment requires nursing judgment, an intellectual process that the registered nurse uses to analyze data and determine the next course of nursing actions (ANA, 1996).

Nursing diagnosis, establishment of nursing care goals, and development of the nursing care plan are central to nursing practice and cannot be delegated (ANA, 1996). Selected tasks that fall within the implementation component of the nursing process may be appropriate for delegation if the nursing intervention does not require professional nursing knowledge, judgment, and skill (ANA, 1996). Evaluation of the patient's progress in relation to the plan of care cannot be delegated (ANA, 1996), but the UAP can contribute data to assist the registered nurse in making that evaluation.

To determine whether these tasks are appropriate for delegation in selected clinical situations, the registered professional nurse must consider the following factors (Adapted from ANA, 1996, and Clinical Practice, AACN, 1995):

- Patient condition
- Capabilities of the UAP
- Potential for harm
- Complexity of task
- Problem solving and critical thinking required
- Unpredictability of outcome
- Amount of clinical oversight the nurse can provide
- Level of caregiver–patient interaction
- Practice setting
- Available staffing resources

"Delegated activities must be clearly defined and thoroughly described repetitive tasks that do not require nursing judgments" (AWHONN, 1997). "The knowledge base and clinical skills of the registered professional nurse provide the foundation for nursing assessments and diagnosis, critical thinking and decision-making, outcome identification, planning, implementation, and evaluations that are requisite for high-quality outcomes for women and newborns" (AWHONN, 1997). This does not imply that UAPs are incapable of critical thinking or that they lack knowledge and clinical skills (Simpson, 1997b). However, the fundamental difference between these two care providers is the type and amount of education, depth of knowledge, and level of critical thinking possessed by the registered professional nurse compared with the UAP (AWHONN, 1997).

When the professional registered nurse delegates a selected nursing task to a UAP, the nurse is responsible for the following (AWHONN, 1998b):

- Determining if the task is suitable for delegation
- Determining whether the UAP is competent to perform the task

The task must be clearly defined and thoroughly described, be repetitive and represent routine care, be performed with predictable outcome, require little or no modification from one patient care situation to another, not involve ongoing assessment or any significant interpretation, and be within the training and competence of the UAP.

Professional Liability

In many activities of daily life, such as driving a car, the law requires exercising reasonable care for the safety of others. Failure to exercise reasonable care is negligence. Harm caused to others because of negligence is the basis for liability. Negligence by a professional (ie, nurse, physician, or attorney) is malpractice. Medical negligence is medical malpractice, and nursing negligence is nursing malpractice. For a nurse to be found guilty of professional negligence, a series of facts first must be established:

- That the nurse had a responsibility to the patient *(duty)*
- That the nurse failed to carry out that responsibility *(breach of duty)* by deviating from a standard of care
- That an injury was sustained by the patient *(damages)*
- That there was a causal relationship between the patient's injury and the nurse's breach of duty *(proximate cause)*

Duty

Establishing the duty of a nurse to a patient is generally not an area of dispute in the institutional setting. The nurse is an employee of the institution that accepts the patient into its care. A relationship exists until it is terminated by the completion of care or a patient's request to voluntarily withdraw from care.

Breach of Duty

In the legal sense, the professional standard of care requires that the nurse possess and exercise the degree of knowledge, care, and skill that other nurses would ordinarily exercise under the same or similar circumstances. The nurse should act in a way that is acceptable to professional nursing peers or to reasonably prudent nurses. This broad requirement provides room for debate about what is acceptable or reasonably prudent behavior in any given clinical situation. Frequently, establishing adherence to or violation of professional standards of care may involve differences of opinion among experts. There may be equivalently reasonable interpretations or courses of action to meet a given generic standard. However, even though there may be a substantial body of evidence based on rigorously designed research studies and published standards and guidelines for a specific area of practice, there still exists the possibility for a difference of opinions about the standard of care. When litigation ensues, experts are asked to testify to their opinions about standards of care in that particular case. The plaintiffs seek experts with opinions that are consistent with the claims brought forth in the case, and the defense seeks experts with opinions favorable to their side of the matter. These opinions often represent a complete dichotomy in their points of view. Experience, knowledge, and sometimes the integrity of nursing and medical experts vary widely.

Although professional organizations publish standards, guidelines, and clinical practice bulletins or opinions on specific topics, these organizations issue general statements in the publications that acknowledge the need for flexibility and potential variations for individual patients and individual clinical situations. The *AWHONN Standards and Guidelines for Professional Nursing Practice in the Care of Women and Newborns* states the following:

> These standards and guidelines articulate general guidelines; additional considerations or procedures may be warranted for particular patients or setting. [They] are intended to serve as a guide for optimal practice. They are not designed to establish the required standard of care for legal liability, licensure, discipline, [or] ethical matters. Nurses must act in accordance with law, institutional rules and procedures, and established intraprofessional arrangements concerning the division of duties. These standards and guidelines may change in response to changes in research and practice (AWHONN, 1998b, p. vi).

Likewise, the American College of Obstetricians and Gynecologists (ACOG) provides the following disclaimer as part of their practice bulletins:

> The information is designed to aid practitioners in making decisions about appropriate obstetric and gynecologic care. These guidelines should not be construed as dictating an exclusive course of treatment or procedure. Variations in practice may be warranted based on the needs of the individual patient, resources, and limitations unique to the institution or type of practice (ACOG, 1999, p. 1).

As such, standards serve as a frame of reference for institutions to use in developing more specific policies, procedures, and protocols. As the body of evidence continues to emerge on any clinical topic, standards and guidelines are revised accordingly by professional organizations.

Injury and Legal Causation

In addition to showing that a nurse deviated from the standard of care, the claimant must also prove that an injury occurred and that the injury was caused by the professional's negligence. Referred to as *causation,* this is often the most difficult entity for the claimant to prove. This is especially true in obstetric malpractice cases, in which, for example, it may be difficult to show that earlier recognition and intervention for a nonreassuring electronic fetal heart tracing that was present on admission would have led to a better outcome or that periods of hyperstimulation with oxytocin while the fetal heart rate (FHR) was reassuring contributed to a depressed newborn at birth.

Obstetric malpractice cases frequently involve deviations from the standard of care but with no relationship to causation. A unit policy may require documentation of maternal-fetal assessments every 15 minutes. The nurse may have been at the bedside continuously but failed to document assessments according to the policy. Documentation deficiencies are many times used to claim that the nurse fell below accepted standards of care, but rarely do documentation issues contribute to patient injury. Examples of violations of accepted standards that may be easier to demonstrate contributed to adverse outcomes involving nursing care include a hypoxemic baby born after long periods of a nonreassuring FHR with no notification of the physician or nurse midwife to allow for timely intervention; failing to have appropriate resuscitation equipment available when a baby is born depressed, delaying resuscitation; using fundal pressure when a shoulder dystocia is identified, further impacting the shoulder and delaying birth; and an adverse maternal outcome after failing to note signs and symptoms of maternal deterioration when treatment was delayed.

Standards of care violations frequently cited in perinatal litigation are listed in Display 2–4. This list is not necessarily all inclusive or limited to all potential areas of litigation.

Current Issues with Risk Management

There are multiple strategies that nurses can use to decrease professional liability. Most of these strategies involve common sense and goodwill, but some specific guidelines and recommendations can decrease the likelihood of the nurse becoming involved in a successful lawsuit. A summary of current guidelines and recommendations to decrease liability are presented here. However, if the nurse is involved in a malpractice claim through the institution or named individually, it is important to consider that the patient is trying to secure financial resources to care for herself or her injured child, seek answers to questions that have not been answered by her healthcare provider or institution, or attempt to ensure what she perceives happened to her does not happen to another woman or baby (Simpson, 1999). Anyone can be sued; being named in a suit does not necessarily imply negligence. Even if the institution through its insurance carrier decides to settle the case rather than defend the nurse in court, it does not mean that the nurse contributed to the injury or incidence in any way (Simpson, 1999).

If, however, the nurse did commit an error that resulted in an adverse outcome, the best approach is an objective account in the medical record; full disclosure to the physician, patient, and risk manager; and cooperation with the legal process if litigation proceeds (Kraman & Hamm, 1999). Ideally, consultation with the risk manager occurs as quickly as possible after

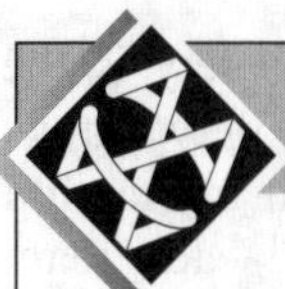

DISPLAY 2–4

Violations of Standards of Care Frequently Cited in Perinatal Litigation

Failure to

- Have in place adequate policies, procedures, and protocols for the care and treatment of women and newborns
- Provide evidence of nursing competence
- Properly triage, transfer, or discharge pregnant women
- Adequately evaluate or diagnose a condition
- Appropriately perform maternal, fetal, or newborn monitoring
- Recognize and report changes in patient condition in a timely fashion
- Troubleshoot equipment
- Interpret data
- Perform emergency interventions appropriate to the clinical situation
- Communicate data to the primary care provider and others
- Ensure the availability of the primary care provider
- Mobilize resources in a timely fashion
- Provide appropriate resuscitation
- Use the chain of command
- Provide sufficient documentation
- Ensure patient and family comprehension
- Witness informed consent
- Seek clarification or consultation (eg, medical orders, privileges, patient condition)
- Carry out medical orders

discovery of an adverse outcome. A prompt, factual explanation to the patient and family may decrease the likelihood that the adverse outcome will result in litigation. Not all adverse outcomes that are the result of medical errors are followed by litigation. Localio and colleagues (1991) estimated that there are 7.6 patient injuries caused by negligence identified for every one that results in litigation. A later study confirmed that patient injuries caused by deviations from accepted standards of care do not necessarily result in a claim (Edbril & Lagasse, 1999). Open, empathetic communication appears to be what separates an injury from a lawsuit (Hickson, Clayton, Githen, & Sloan, 1992). Effective communication between healthcare providers and patients when an error occurs may be a protective factor (Virshup, Oppenberg, & Coleman, 1999). Because early communication with effective intervention often can prevent a lawsuit or minimize the damage potential, it is important to have a system in place to identify and respond to adverse events in a timely manner (Herrington, 1997). All providers should be consistent in their communication with the patient and family. When more than one explanation is provided, the opportunity for a coordinated defense is reduced. If a claim is filed, the institution's professional liability insurance covers the actions of the nurse unless those actions are criminal. However, even when nurses have been charged with criminal offenses related to their professional nursing roles, hospitals have provided defense for the nurses involved (Kowalski, 1998).

Creating a Culture of Safety

Recent Data About Errors by Healthcare Providers

Consumer groups and the general public are aware that errors are an unfortunate common occurrence during an inpatient stay. Reports have received wide media coverage and resulted in federally sponsored initiatives to reduce the number of errors by healthcare providers and enhance patient safety. Although up to 95% of medical errors go unreported (Hallam, 2000), 42% of all Americans are aware of at least one medical error through personal involvement or through the experience of a relative or friend (National Patient Safety Foundation [NPSF], 1999). Patients rank medication errors as their top worry during inpatient stay according to a 1999 patient survey by the American Society of Health System Pharmacists (ASHP). Sixty-one percent of patients surveyed were fearful of being given the wrong medication, and 58% were afraid they would be given two or more medications that would interact in a negative way (ASHP, 1999). According to NPSF (1999), there are approximately 3 million errors per year in the inpatient setting, costing an estimated $200 billion dollars annually. An error occurs during 17% of all inpatient admissions; fortunately, only 4% result in an adverse outcome. An adverse outcome is defined as an injury caused by treatment (Buerhaus, 1999). A preventable adverse outcome can be tragic, with long-term or fatal consequences in some cases.

The most alarming data about adverse outcomes were reported by the Institute of Medicine in *To Err is Human: Building a Safer Health System* (Kohn, Corrigan, & Donaldson, 1999). Between 44,000 and 98,000 patients die every year in hospitals because of errors by healthcare providers, more than because of traffic accidents, breast cancer, and human immunodeficiency virus infection, making these types of deaths the fourth leading cause of death in the United States (Kohn et al., 1999). These deaths include mothers and babies. Along with emergency departments and perioperative services, perinatal units account for most of the claims of patient injuries and death. Many of the patient injuries related to human error are preventable. Fetal and neonatal injuries are more common than maternal injuries. Five common recurring clinical problems account for most fetal and neonatal injuries (Knox, Simpson, & Garite, 1999):

- Inability to recognize or appropriately respond to antepartum and intrapartum fetal distress
- Inability to effect a timely cesarean birth (30 minutes from decision to incision) when indicated by the fetal or maternal condition
- Inability to appropriately resuscitate a depressed baby
- Inappropriate use of oxytocin or misoprostol, leading to uterine hyperstimulation, uterine rupture, and fetal distress or death
- Inappropriate use of forceps, vacuum, or fundal pressure, leading to fetal trauma or preventable shoulder dystocia

High-Reliability Organizations: How Other Industries Promote Safe Practice

Most errors are not the result of individual recklessness or incompetence, but rather of flaws in the system (Kohn et al., 1999). An organizational culture that promotes patient safety as its first priority is needed to develop processes to identify flaws in the system and initiate strategies to minimize risk of errors. Healthcare providers are human and therefore not perfect (Lockowitz, 1997). Unfortunately, to err is human, even in the healthcare setting, where there is little tolerance for errors that result in adverse outcomes. No one goes to work planning to injure a mother or baby, but it does happen (Simpson, 2000). Rather than attempting to assign blame to an individual when an error is discovered, a more productive strategy is to determine the nature of the process or system that enabled the error to occur.

Characteristics of safe perinatal units where there is a decreased likelihood of an error occurring have been described (Knox, et al., 1999). These perinatal units function in a manner similar to what other high-risk industries have called *high-reliability organizations* (Roberts, 1990). High-reliability organizations operate highly complex and hazardous technologic systems essentially without mistakes over long periods (Roberts, 1990). Examples are nuclear power plants, airline in-flight and traffic control operations, and the technical side of the banking industry (Knox et al., 1990). In high-reliability organizations, safety is the hallmark of organizational culture. Safety ranks higher in priority than production. Team interaction is collegial rather than subordinate and each team member has an obligation to speak up if a question of safety arises (Knox et al., 1999). Communication is highly valued and rewarded. It is understood that when team members fail to engage in respectful interactions, errors can occur (Knox et al., 1999). Emergencies are rehearsed, and the unexpected is practiced. Successful operations are viewed as potentially dangerous because success leads to system simplification and shortcuts (Roberts, 1990).

Normalization of Deviance

The process by which successful operations can lead to mistakes has been characterized as the *normalization of deviance* by Vaughan (1996) in her analysis of the Challenger disaster. She concluded that all work groups continually redefine risk in the context of accidents that do not occur. Professional standards of any work group can degrade slowly and incrementally over time. Operational systems and clinical practices that are known to be risky may continue because "they get away with it" most of the time. Because accidents are rare, there is no immediate consequence for not strictly adhering to policies that are a part of the safety net to prevent their occurrence (Knox et al., 1999).

An understanding of the concept of normalization of deviance by perinatal healthcare providers is necessary to identify specific unsafe practices that have become routine over time. Examples of normalization of deviance in perinatal care include the use of fundal pressure to shorten an otherwise normal second stage of labor; increasing oxytocin dosage administration during uterine hyperstimulation; performance of amniotomy with no indication when the fetus is at high station; application of vacuum extractor using excessive pressures and timeframes; aggressive, coached, closed-glottis pushing during the second stage, with severe and variable FHR decelerations; not calling the neonatal resuscitation team when there is evidence of fetal compromise; and chronic understaffing (Knox et al., 1999; Simpson & Knox, 2000). The system becomes less safe, but the team members are not aware of this degradation until the inevitable disaster occurs.

To combat this natural tendency toward normalization of deviance, high-reliability organizations actively and continually question assumptions, promote orderly challenge of operating practices, and solicit outside views of the routine (Knox et al., 1999). Perinatal units resemble high-reliability units because they are complex, are multilayered, and include a wide variety of professionals with diverse roles and responsibilities (Knox et al., 1999). Like high-reliability organizations, they are expected by patients, family members, and society to operate without errors over long periods. Because most mothers and babies are healthy and most perinatal practices are routine and result in successful outcomes, perinatal units are especially vulnerable to normalizing deviance (Knox et al., 1999). Because most outcomes are good, near misses are not viewed as opportunities to learn how to improve the system.

Promoting Safe Perinatal Practice

To understand how to promote safe perinatal practice, characteristics of units that are at high risk for medical or nursing errors that can lead to maternal-fetal injuries are presented. Perinatal practices can be evaluated in this context, and if any of these characteristics exist, efforts can be initiated to make appropriate changes. The characteristics in Display 2–5 describe perinatal units at high risk for errors and maternal–fetal injuries. Safe perinatal units in which there are few errors that lead to maternal–fetal injuries have the characteristics described in Display 2–6 (Knox et al., 1999).

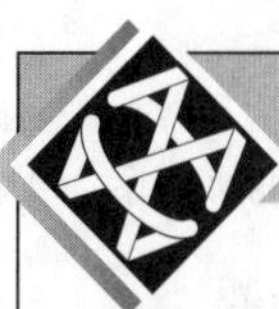

DISPLAY 2–5

Characteristics of Perinatal Units at High Risk for Errors and Maternal–Fetal Injuries

- Multiple, detailed policies and protocols exist that few follow.
- There are wide variations in practice for which clear standards and guidelines exist.
- There is ongoing nurse–physician conflict.
- Chain of command is frequently used.
- Hierarchical professional relationships exist.
- Patriarchal patient relationships exist.
- Errors are blamed on people rather than evaluating processes and unit operations.
- Abusive professional behavior is tolerated.
- Real peer review does not exist.
- Administrators are more concerned with the financial bottom line than with patient safety.
- Practices are based on what is most convenient for providers rather than what is best for mothers and babies.
- Practices are based on the "way we've always done it" instead of evidence and standards.

The characteristics of units that provide safe care are critical for minimizing maternal–fetal injuries and resultant malpractice claims (Knox et al., 1999). They are the basis for creating a culture of safety. In a culture of safety, nurses and physicians have reached consensus to practice based on evidence and standards of care. This is ideally accomplished through an interdisciplinary perinatal practice committee jointly chaired by a nurse and physician who are clinical experts with peer respect to effect change (Simpson & Knox, 1999). To prevent errors, an environment in which nurses and physicians respect each other and value input in clinical decision-making is critical. In a culture of safety, hierarchical relationships are replaced by teamwork and cohesiveness (Simpson, 2000). Different perspectives are valued and contribute to successful outcomes. Each team member has the opportunity and the obligation to add a viewpoint that others may have overlooked or not even considered, one that may prove to be the essential component of a clinical solution (Simpson & Knox, 2001). In a culture of safety, systems are designed that are geared to preventing, detecting, and minimizing the likelihood of error, rather than attaching blame to individuals (Kohn et al., 1999). Perinatal unit operations and healthcare provider relationships should be reexamined in the context of implementing a system designed for maternal–fetal safety (Simpson, 2000). Evaluation of other high-reliability industries in which safety is the number one priority can contribute to efforts to create a culture of safety in perinatal care (Knox et al., 1999).

Standards of Care and Practice Guidelines

Several governmental agencies, accreditation bodies, and professional organizations have published practice guidelines and standards of care applicable to perinatal nursing practice, including individual state nurse practice acts and JCAHO (see Chapter 1, Display 1–3). Although some standards of care are broad (eg, ANA, JCAHO), others are more inclusive and specific (eg, AWHONN, the American Association of Critical Care Nurses [AACN], the National Association of Neonatal Nurses [NANN], the Association of perioperative Registered Nurses [AORN], the American Society of Postanesthesia Nurses [ASPAN], ACOG, the American Academy of Pediatrics [AAP], the American Society of Anesthesiologists [ASA]). Institutions have written policies and procedures based on national standards and guidelines for care governing clinical practice. The goal of all standards of care and practice guidelines is the provision of safe, thera-

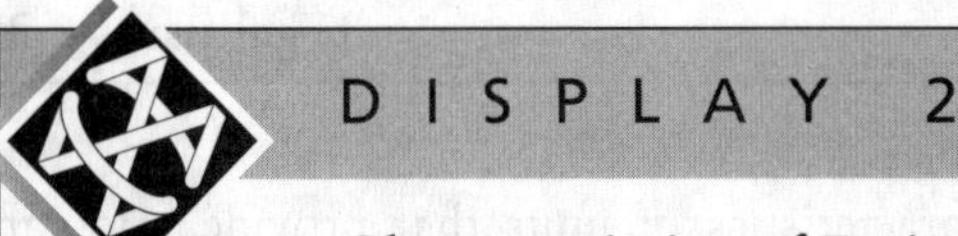

DISPLAY 2–6

Characteristics of Perinatal Units at Low Risk for Errors and Maternal–Fetal Injuries

CLEARLY STATED PURPOSE: SAFETY FIRST

- Shift reports emphasize "what if" and "what could go wrong."
- Appropriate transfer protocols for mothers and babies are in place and followed.
- Emergency preparedness (ie, practice drills for clinical situations such as emergent cesarean birth and shoulder dystocia)
- A 24-hour ability to perform an emergent cesarean birth, including in-house anesthesia coverage, a surgery team and surgeon
- Resuscitation teams are at birth if there is a question of fetal compromise.

CLEAR LANGUAGE: FETAL WELL-BEING

- Fetal well-being is defined as the presence of fetal heart rate accelerations of 15 beats per minute for 15 seconds
- Fetal well-being is required for maternal discharge, medications, oxytocin, misoprostol, ambulation, and intermittent auscultation of the fetal heart rate.
- Absence of fetal well-being requires direct physician evaluation and medical record documentation of further clinical management.

CLEAR OPERATING STYLE

- Professional standards and guidelines are the "rules of the road."
- Practices are developed by consensus in the context of a multidisciplinary perinatal practice committee.
- Minimal intervention in the context of a safety net (ie, ability to intervene in a timely manner if necessary)
- Minimal intervention acknowledges the fact that most pregnancies, labors, and births are normal and that intervention creates the potential for iatrogenic injury.

CLEAR AND CONCISE CLINICAL PROTOCOLS AND POLICIES

- A physician will come to the unit when called by a nurse.
- Electronic fetal monitoring
  - There is one mutually agreed on lanuage or nomenclature for all communication and medical record documentation.
  - Physicians and nurses participate in fetal monitoring education programs together.
  - If electronic fetal monitoring is used, it is continued until birth occurs.
  - Umbilical cord gas values are obtained if fetal status is questionable.
- Oxtocin or misoprostol
  - Recognized as potentially the most dangerous drugs in obstetrics and as preventable causes of perinatal liability
  - Protocols and practices for use of these drugs are based on ACOG/AWHONN standards and guidelines.
- Fundal pressure
  - Not used to shorten the otherwise normal second stage of labor
  - Not used when shoulder dystocia is identified
- Vaginal birth after cesarean birth (VBAC)
  - A physician is immediately available through active labor and is capable of monitoring labor and performing an emergent cesarean birth.
  - Availability of anesthesia and other necessary personnel for emergent cesarean birth
  - Close monitoring during use of oxytocin
  - No use of misoprostol
- Second–stage management
  - Aggressive, coached closed-glottis pushing is avoided.
  - Laboring down is used for women with epidurals when appropriate.
  - Management is based on fetal status.
  - Oxytocin is maintained at a rate to approximate a physiologic second stage.
  - Arbitrary time frames are not used.
- Intrapartum telephone triage
  - Advice to patients over the telephone is limited to one of two options: call your physician or certified nurse midwife, or come to the hospital to be evaluated.
- Appropriate prevention and management plans for
  - Instrumental vaginal birth
  - Meconium
  - Shoulder dystocia
  - Iatrogenic prematurity
  - Maternal and neonatal transfer

Adapted from Knox, G.E., Simpson, K.R., & Garite, T.J. (1999). High reliability perinatal units: An approach to the prevention of patient injury and medical malpractice claims. *Journal of Healthcare Risk Management, 19* (2), 27–35.

peutic, quality care by competent healthcare providers. Adherence to established standards of care and practice guidelines can decrease the likelihood of nurses being involved in situations resulting in professional liability.

Clinical Indicator and Risk Modification Programs

The most useful risk modification programs are data driven and assist with identification of significant trends in clinical practice that may expose patients to risk of injury. Well-designed, evidence-based clinical indicator sets allow identification of opportunities for improvement and document quality clinical practices and patient outcomes. Carefully collected and analyzed data are essential for meaningful risk-modification programs. Various types of risk-modification programs are used. These programs generally outline guidelines and recommendations for practices and operations known to promote safe and effective care while decreasing the risk of liability exposure. Key areas covered usually include professional standards; credentials of healthcare providers; patient rights and informed consent; prenatal care documentation; maternal–fetal monitoring; high-risk perinatal care; cesarean birth capabilities; obstetric anesthesia; neonatal resuscitation; admission, discharge, and transfer criteria; and the membership, purpose, and operations of a multidisciplinary perinatal practice committee (MMI Companies, 1998).

An adverse outcome sometimes occurs despite the best efforts of care providers. In other cases, processes were in motion that placed the patient at high risk for injury, but injury did not occur; these also are known as *near misses*. Adverse outcomes and near misses can benefit from a factual review of what happened and the possible reasons for them (Rommal, 1996). Criteria for selecting cases that include a review of the medical record and the surrounding events in a multidisciplinary team have been published by JCAHO and professional liability insurance carriers. Basic criteria include all maternal deaths, antepartum and intrapartum fetal deaths, neonatal deaths, emergent cesarean births for fetal indications not initiated within 30 minutes, and babies older than than 34 weeks' gestation transferred to the neonatal intensive care unit (MMI Companies, 1998).

A close relationship between the institution's professional liability insurance carrier and the risk manager and healthcare providers is essential to maintain an effective risk modification program. Even institutions that are self-insured usually have an excess coverage liability insurance plan. These companies can provide extensive assistance in developing programs to promote safe care and avoid the lengthy process of designing a program internally. Not only do these comprehensive programs decrease risk of errors and patient injuries, they also can result in substantial savings to the institution. In one study, institutions in full compliance with the MMI Companies Perinatal Risk Modification Guidelines had an average cost per claim that was 72 times lower than for claims paid in institutions where no guidelines were followed (mean cost per claim of $3,002 versus $218,910) (MMI Companies, 1999).

Institutional Policies and Procedures

Nationally established standards of care and practice guidelines serve as the basis for the development of institutional policies, procedures, and protocols. These documents serve many purposes within the institution, including orienting new personnel, providing a reference for nurses and physicians, serving as criteria for quality reviews, and evidencing the institution's standards of care in the legal arena.

Debate exists concerning the best way to develop unit-specific policies and procedures. The questions of which policies and procedures should be included in unit manuals and how specific they should be are frequently asked. One alternative is to identify routine unit practices and provide references to published standards, guidelines, and perinatal nursing texts for specifics, as opposed to the more traditional method of listing multiple steps in an all-inclusive policy or procedure manual (Adels & Pringle, 1992). For example, a policy concerning labor induction or augmentation may reference *AWHONN's Practice Symposium Cervical Ripening and Induction and Augmentation of Labor* (Simspon & Poole, 1998) and *ACOG's Practice Bulletin Induction of Labor* (ACOG, 1999); the procedure for cervical ripening may reference *AWHONN's Practice Symposium Cervical Ripening and Induction and Augmentation of Labor* (Simpson & Poole, 1998), *ACOG's Practice Bulletin Induction of Labor* (ACOG, 1999), *ACOG's Induction of Labor with Misoprostol*, and *ACOG's Monitoring During Induction of Labor with Dinoprostone* (ACOG, 1998). Auscultation of the FHR during labor or placement of a fetal scalp electrode or intrauterine pressure catheter may reference *AWHONN's Fetal Heart Monitoring Principles and Practices* (Feinstein & McCartney, 1997). A policy about nurse-to-patient staffing ratios can reference *AWHONN's Standards and Guidelines for Professional Nursing Practice in the Care of Women and Newborns* (1998b). Clinical protocols related to screening for and treatment of group B streptococcal disease should include the joint recommendations by the Centers for Disease Control and Prevention, AAP, and ACOG in the ACOG (1996) *Committee Opinion Prevention of Early-Onset Group B Streptococcal Disease in Newborns.* The protocol for cardiopulmonary resuscitation in pregnancy may reference *Cardiopulmonary Resuscitation in Pregnancy* (Luppi, 1999) and in *AWHONN's High Risk and Critical Care Intrapartum Nursing* (Mandeville & Troiano, 1999).

These documents should be readily available to nurses and physicians as written copies on the unit or by computer access. Advocates of this approach cite the elimination of lengthy policy and procedure manuals, cost savings related to decreased nonproductive time spent writing and revising these manuals, standardization of perinatal nursing practice, and improvement of overall quality of care as benefits. Nursing staff awareness of and adherence to standards and guidelines from professional organizations are added advantages.

Avoid lengthy policies with multiple steps that do not reflect clinical practice reality (Rommal, 1996). If very detailed policies are written, each step in the procedure or protocol should be meaningful, necessary, and consistent with evidence and standards. Healthcare providers have access to multiple sources of guidelines and protocols through various web sites on the Internet (see Chapter 1, Display 1–2). Although these sites can provide ideas or a framework for protocol development, the protocols may not be based on current evidence or be consistent with recommendations from professional organizations. Regardless of the format used to delineate institutional policies, procedures, and protocols, they should be reviewed as necessary to meet regulatory requirements or as advances in new technologies and research are identified. A mechanism should be established to facilitate notification of updates and changes in previously established institutional policies, procedures, and protocols to nurses and physicians, as well as the ability to document that the notification process has occurred.

As policies and practices are updated, copies of the previous versions should be maintained. It is important to note the date that the policy was originally initiated and when it was updated or withdrawn. If the institution is involved in litigation, it is likely that there will be a request for evidence about the policies and practices in effect at the time of the event in question.

Documentation

Medical record documentation is a vital nursing function. The nurse providing care is in control of the information included in the nursing portions of the medical record, but documentation has become one of the most time consuming of nursing activities and therefore one that is prone to omissions. Nurses often are concerned that medical record documentation forces them to focus on paperwork rather than patient care. Cumbersome documentation systems that require duplicate and triplicate entries of the same data contribute to this real problem. The ongoing challenge is to create a streamlined system for documentation that is cost effective, easy to use, efficient in terms of nursing time, and sufficiently comprehensive for current or subsequent review. There are significant ramifications for inaccuracies and omissions in medical record documentation. Documentation deficiencies may result in decreased communication among team members, denied reimbursement by insurance carriers for care rendered, lost information for statistical or outcome data for quality purposes, and in the case of litigation, increased difficulty for the defense to prove its case.

Of all strategies to decrease liability, accurate and thorough documentation may be the easiest to accomplish, but it is the most common missing piece. The medical record is often the single most important document available in the defense of a negligent action (Berry, 1999). In issues of litigation, the nurse often cannot recall the specific patient or incident and therefore must rely on written or computerized notes completed at the time of patient contact. The time from event to formal legal inquiry may involve several years, and the nurse may have limited independent recall without the documentation in the medical record. Without a complete and legible medical record, nurses may be unable to successfully defend themselves against charges of improper care (Berry, 1999; Rommal, 1996). Because lack of documentation equals a presumed lack of care, omissions are challenging to defend. According to risk-claims data from a professional liability insurance carrier, documentation ranks second only to patient monitoring and assessment in the area of nursing-related risk exposure, accounting for 20.7% of all exposures (Berry, 1999).

Litigation many times follows clinical events that result in adverse outcomes. The most complete documentation therefore is focused on the period surrounding the adverse events. During emergent situations, medical record documentation occurs retrospectively. The first priority during an emergency is to provide immediate patient care. After the mother and fetus or newborn are stable, documentation is possible. Postevent documentation should focus on reconstructing a summary of all of the assessments, actions, and communication that transpired as accurately and timely as possible. For example, after birth complicated by shoulder dystocia, it is important to note the time interval between delivery of the fetal head and the body; fetal assessment data or attempts to obtain data about fetal status during the maneuvers; the order of the maneuvers and interventions; suprapubic pressure (if used) to avoid later allegations of use of fundal pressure; times for calls for assistance and when help arrived; the condition of the newborn at birth and the immediate newborn period; any resuscitation efforts (including those who attended the newborn); and a summary of the discussion that occurred between the physician or certified nurse midwife and the woman and her family about the shoulder dystocia and subsequent condition of the newborn (Simpson, 1999). The neonatal team in attendance must be aware of the difference between suprapubic pressure and fundal pressure to avoid documenting that fundal pressure was used if this is inaccurate.

In the case of a nonreassuring FHR of acute onset resulting in an emergent cesarean birth, summary documentation should include timely recognition of the problem, nursing actions initiated for maternal or fetal resuscitation, communication with team members and their responses, time to the surgical suite and incision, and chronologies of interventions performed (including by which personnel) for newborn resuscitation, followed by a note about the details of the discussion between the physician and the woman and her family. During emergent intrapartum situations, some nurses feel that documentation directly on the FHR strip can assist them in constructing notes after patient stabilization. If this approach is used, it is important to ensure that the narrative notes written later coincide with the FHR strip annotations.

The medical record should provide a factual and objective account of care provided including direct and indirect communication with other members of the healthcare team. Only clinically relevant information should be documented. Information not related to the patient's care, such as the filing of incident reports, short staffing, or conflicts between nurses and primary care providers, should be addressed through the appropriate institutional channels rather than recorded in the medical record.

Documentation systems vary widely, and no one method has been demonstrated to be the best. Some institutions have progressed to computerized systems and paperless medical records; others use a combination of computer and paper charting. A mechanism to streamline perinatal documentation should be considered to avoid errors, improve quality, and decrease nursing time (Chez, 1997). Possible mechanisms include flow sheets, clinical pathways, checklists, summary notes, narrative notes, and computer documentation. One system that has received attention is *charting by exception.* With this method, entries are made in the medical record when there are changes or deviations from previously recorded information, and nursing time is saved by minimizing normal chart entries. Opponents of this method worry that such streamlined charting increases the institution's burden of proof in litigation to show that care was provided. No reported studies have rigorously examined the risks and benefits of charting by exception, but most experts recommend that this method be avoided during the intrapartum period and reserved for settings in which clinical situations are not as dynamic, such as postpartum and healthy newborn care.

The use of a written or computerized flow sheet as the single source of comprehensive data about maternal–fetal status, nursing interventions, and the events of labor and birth facilitates timely and accurate medical record data entry (Simpson & Poole, 1998). Well-designed flow sheets are useful tools to prompt appropriate notations and practice consistent with unit guidelines, especially in the labor and birth setting. Routine assessments and interventions can easily be documented in the flow sheet format. The practice of duplicate documentation of routine care on the FHR strip and the medical record is outdated (AWHONN, 1998b; Chez, 1997). Previously, perinatal nurses believed that there should be enough documentation on the FHR strip that the strip could "stand alone" for subsequent review. However, writing on the strip increases the amount of nursing time spent on inpatient care activities, and this practice can lead to errors in documentation and contributes to late entries on the medical record (Simpson & Poole, 1998). If the FHR strips are electronically archived, hand-written notes on the strip do not become part of the permanent medical record. As more institutions adopt computerized electronic fetal monitoring systems with typed medical record entries, this will no longer be an issue. Narrative notes should be used to document other than routine care or events that are not included on the flow sheet. Narrative notes should also be used to document any nurse–physician communication, ongoing interventions for a nonreassuring FHR that does not resolve with the usual intrauterine resuscitation techniques, significant changes in maternal status, patient concerns or requests, and complete details of emergent situations and the outcome.

Nurses should avoid using forms with preprinted times and limited space for notations. These types of forms lead to inherently inaccurate or inadequate documentation. Vital signs and other maternal–fetal assessments or emergencies do not occur at predetermined 15-minute intervals. There are times when more comprehensive documentation is required than can fit into limited, preset boxes. In cases of a reassuring FHR pattern, a few minutes may not make a difference; however, in emergencies, an accurate account is critical in recording sequential, appropriate interventions. Flow sheets also work well for mothers during the postpartum period and for newborns. Like intrapartum documentation, narrative notes should be used to document nurse–physician communication, unusual events, and significant changes in maternal or newborn status. Retrospective charting is better than no documentation, but entries after a "bad" outcome are often areas of controversy in litigation if they are written days after the event. These types of late entries often have a defensive tone. The nurse should ensure that the data entered are accurate and objective. She should not alter the medical record to include data that is not accurate, even if asked to do so by someone in a position of authority. Falsification of the medical record is dishonest and unethical, and if discovered, this action can lead to successful claims against the nurse and institution.

Incident Management

An incident can be defined as any happening that is not consistent with the routine care of a particular patient. Many adverse perinatal outcomes that result in litigation derive from perinatal incidents that are unexpected or the result of an emergency occurrence. Emergency occurrences can be categorized as actual, evolving, or perceived. Actual emergencies may include maternal hemorrhage, prolapsed cord, amniotic fluid embolism, shoulder dystocia, and neonatal asphyxia. Evolving emergencies are those that develop gradually and go unrecognized until an acute situation occurs. Examples include fetal stress progressing to severe stress, severe preeclampsia converting to overt eclampsia, and an unrecognized malpresentation going to precipitous birth without appropriate preparation. Perceived emergencies are the near misses that have the potential to result in adverse outcomes. These may include insufficient resources, inadequate communication, professional knowledge deficits, and ineffective lines of authority and responsibility.

Incident management plays an important role in reducing institutional liability and in promoting an environment of higher quality care. The goal is to objectively assess what happened (or what might have happened, such as near misses) so that problem-prone systems or operations can be identified. After identification, there are opportunities for improvement to prevent an adverse event or recurrence of the adverse event. This process requires time, extensive communication, and a systematic framework. Generally, incident management is a retrospective process that includes the examination of all of the events surrounding the incident. Key factors in the review include answers to the following questions:

- What happened?
- What were the contributing factors?
- Was it preventable or nonpreventable?
- How was it handled?
- Were sufficient resources available?
- Was there the opportunity to handle it better?
- Is there a need for remedial action?
- What is the appropriate follow-up?
- What is the required documentation?

Sentinel Events

Some incidents are of such serious nature that they are classified as sentinel events and require specific actions by JCAHO accredited institutions, including possible reporting to JCAHO. A *sentinel event* is defined by JCAHO (2000) as "an unexpected occurrence involving death or serious physical or psychological injury or the risk thereof." Serious injury includes permanent loss of limb or function (JCAHO, 2000). The "risk thereof" means that one can reasonably speculate that a recurrence of the same event carries a significant chance of a serious adverse outcome. One of two criteria must be met to apply the JCAHO sentinel event policy: the event must have resulted in a serious adverse outcome, or the event was a near miss. The subset of sentinel events that are subject to review by JCAHO includes any occurrence that meets any of the following criteria:

- The event has resulted in an unanticipated death or major loss of function not related to the natural course of the patient's illness or underlying condition.
- The event is one of the following (even if the outcome was not death or major permanent loss of function): suicide of a patient in a setting where the patient receives around-the-clock care (eg, hospital, residential treatment center, crisis stabilization center); or infant abduction or discharge to the wrong family; rape; hemolytic transfusion reaction involving administration of blood or blood products having major blood group incompatibilities; or surgery on the wrong patient or wrong body part.

Each healthcare organization is encouraged but not required to report sentinel events to JCAHO. Reporting is confidential, and limited immunity in the accreditation process is provided for reports filed within 10 days of the event. Additional examples of reportable sentinel events are intrapartum maternal death; neonatal death unrelated to a congenital condition of an infant with a birth weight greater than 2,500 g; and any patient death, paralysis, coma, or other major permanent loss of function associated with a medication error or a patient fall that results in death or major permanent loss of function (JCAHO, 2000). JCAHO may become aware of a sentinel event through communication with a patient, family member, employee of the institution, or the media. If JCAHO becomes aware (through voluntary self-reporting or otherwise) of a sentinel event, the accredited organization is expected to perform a thorough, credible root cause analysis, develop an action plan, and submit both to JCAHO within 45 calendar days of experiencing or becoming aware of a sentinel event (JCAHO, 2000). The written root cause analysis must focus primarily on systems and processes, not individual performance, and identify potential process improvements that could be made to reduce the risk of similar events occurring in the future (Kobs, 1998) (Appendix 2A).

The root cause analysis process has assisted institutions in gaining insights into their processes and risk-prone areas, but questions have been raised about the reporting of such information to an external source, especially an accrediting agency. Institutional concerns have centered on confidentiality, discoverability, and admissibility of reported information; the cumbersome format and tight timelines; the possibility that the information could be used against the reporting institution, jeopardizing accreditation; and the need for collaboration among all stakeholders (ie, legal, clinical, legislative, regulatory, and professional) to refine the process. Not all sentinel events are the result of errors. For example, a maternal death, although unexpected, may be unavoidable if the woman suddenly develops an amniotic fluid embolism or deteriorates as a result of consumptive coagulopathy. An infant weighing more than 2,500 g may not survive a complete placental abruption or prolapsed umbilical cord. The key issue is to carefully analyze the event with the goal of developing strategies to prevent future occurrences. Some adverse outcomes in perinatal care are not predictable or avoidable despite the best efforts of healthcare providers and the availability of sophisticated technology.

Staffing Resources

A policy that delineates clear staffing parameters is recommended by AWHONN (1998b). This policy should include the clinical competence of those who provide nursing care, the personnel mix, and patient census and acuity. There must be a plan to meet safe staffing needs when census and acuity are dynamic. For example, in settings in which the patient population and needs may change rapidly, as in labor and birth units, the staffing plan must be adequate to meet the changing requirements for safe care (AWHONN, 1998b). Cross-training and on-call systems are some methods to handle rapidly changing staffing requirements. In the event that there are not enough nurses to care for the patients on the unit, temporary strategies can be undertaken until there are adequate numbers of nurses to provide safe care. For example, if oxytocin is infusing and there are not enough nurses available to monitor maternal–fetal status, it should be discontinued and the physician notified that the labor induction or augmentation will be restarted when the situation resolves. An elective cesarean birth can be delayed until there are adequate staff members. An immediate priority is to maintain an environment that supports patient safety. If staffing crises are of a chronic nature, proactive steps should be taken to evaluate staffing patterns that are consistent with safe nurse to patient ratios based on scheduling of procedures and anticipated fluctuations in census and acuity (Knox, Kelley, Simpson, Carrier, & Berry, 1999).

Recommended nurse to patient ratios have been available since 1983 for perinatal nurses. These recommendations are generally considered to be the minimally accepted nurse to patient ratios for provision of safe and effective perinatal nursing care. Table 2–1 contains the recommended nurse to patient ratios according to the *Guidelines for Perinatal Care* (AAP & ACOG, 1997) and the *Standards and Guidelines for Professional Nursing Practice in the Care of Women and Newborns* (AWHONN, 1998b).

JCAHO (1998) has developed a resource for preparing for an assessment of adequate staffing during survey visits. *Addressing Staffing Needs for Patient Care* (JCAHO, 1998) covers general compliance and survey issues, staff qualifications and competence, staffing and assignment responsibilities, planning for staffing, documentation of staffing plan, design of staffing mechanisms, and staffing adequacy and nursing-specific requirements. *Principles for Nurse Staffing* (ANA, 1999) provides comprehensive guidelines and recommendations for determining adequate staffing. The ANA recommends that the following critical factors be considered in determination of appropriate staffing: number of patients, level of intensity of patients, contextual issues such as architecture and geography of the environment and available technology, and level of preparation and experience of those providing care.

An analysis of individual and aggregate patient needs should determine appropriate nurse to patient

TABLE 2–1 ■ RECOMMENDED NURSE-TO-PATIENT RATIOS ACCORDING TO THE *GUIDELINES FOR PERINATAL CARE* (AAP & ACOG, 1997) AND THE *STANDARDS AND GUIDELINES FOR PROFESSIONAL NURSING PRACTICE IN THE CARE OF WOMEN AND NEWBORNS* (AWHONN, 1998)

Nurse/Patient Ratio	Care Provided
Intrapartum	
1:2	Patients in labor
1:1	Patients in second-stage labor
1:1	Patients with medical or obstetric complications
1:2	Oxytocin induction or augmentation of labor
1:1	Coverage for initiating epidural anesthesia
1:1	Circulation for cesarean delivery
Antepartum / Postpartum	
1:6	Antepartum or postpartum patients without complications
1:2	Patients in postoperative recovery
1:3	Antepartum or postpartum patients with complications but in stable condition
1:4	Recently born infants and those requiring close observation
Newborns	
1:6–8*	Newborns requiring only routine care
1:3–4	Normal mother-newborn couplet care
1:3–4	Newborns requiring continuing care
1:2–3	Newborns requiring intermediate care
1:1–2	Newborns requiring intensive care
1:1	Newborns requiring multisystem support
1:1 or greater	Unstable newborns requiring complex critical care

*This ratio reflects traditional newborn nursery care. If couplet care or rooming-in is used, a professional nurse who is responsible for the mother should coordinate and administer neonatal care. If direct assignment of the nurse is also made to the nursery to cover the newborn's care, there may be double assigning (ie, one nurse for the mother–baby couplet and one for just the neonate, if returned to the nursery). A nurse should be available at all times, but only one nurse may be necessary, because most neonates will not be physically present in the nursery. Direct care of neonates in the nursery may be provided by ancillary personnel under the nurse's direct supervision. An adequate number of staff members are needed to respond to acute and emergency situations.

ratios. The ANA (1999) recommends considering the following specific physical and psychosocial needs of patients: age and functional ability, communication skills, cultural and linguistic diversities, severity and urgency of admitting condition, scheduled procedures, ability to meet healthcare requisites, availability of social support systems, and other specific needs identified by the patient and by the registered nurse. Adequate nurse-to-patient ratios are necessary to achieve a minimum level of quality patient care. Moving nursing away from an industrial model to a professional model would shift the industry and organizations away from the technical approach of measuring time and motion to one that examines multiple aspects of using knowledgeable nurses to provide quality care (ANA, 1999). This shift would mean the end of the "nurse is a nurse is a nurse" mentality by centering on the complexity of unit activities and levels of nurse competence needed for quality care (ANA, 1999).

Institutional Compliance with Federal Laws: Emergency Medical Treatment and Labor Act

In 1986, as part of the Consolidated Omnibus Budget Reconciliation Act (COBRA), the Emergency Medical Treatment and Labor Act (EMTALA) was passed by Congress to prevent "dumping" (ie, refusing to treat patients without insurance or financial resources who need medical care). This statute is sometimes referred to as the antidumping law. Since the statute was enacted in 1986, the Health Care Financing Administration (HCFA) issued regulations for implementation in 1992, interpretive guidelines in 1998, and special advisory bulletins on a periodic basis in an effort to clarify specific issues and obligations of institutions and healthcare providers under the law. EMTALA requirements apply to all patients, regardless of their financial status, who present for emergency services at a hospital that participates in the Medicare or Medicaid program. Three fundamental patient care obligations must be met: provide an adequate medical screening examination (MSE) for every patient; provide stabilization treatment within the capabilities of the hospital to every patient with an emergency medical condition (EMC); and transfer every patient with an EMC according to the guidelines outlined in the statute (EMTALA, 1986). These obligations also apply to pregnant women, particularly those who may be in labor.

Although the basics of the statute appear clear, this is a complex issue, made even more complex as regulations, interpretive guidelines, and special advisory bulletins are published and EMTALA cases are litigated in the court system. For example, the most recent HFCA Special Advisory Bulletin of November 1999 clarified issues with patients enrolled in managed care plans. HCFA (1999) specified that hospitals must not delay providing a MSE to managed care enrollees to get authorization to treat. There are two types of EMTALA risk exposure: private lawsuits and government administrative action. Since the 1986 statute was passed, there have been numerous lawsuits alleging improper treatment, discharge, and other EMTALA violations. The courts' opinions in these cases add to what is understood as obligations under the COBRA/EMTALA statute.

Any institution that receives Medicare or Medicaid funding must adhere to the statute. The antidumping statute is enforced jointly by HCFA and the Office of the Inspector General (OIG, 1999) of the U.S. Department of Health and Human Services (DHHS).

If institutions do not meet their obligations under the law, a complaint can be filed. One complaint can trigger a broad-reaching investigation that can result in multiple violations. Each violation has the potential for a fine of $50,000 ($25,000 for hospitals with fewer than 100 beds). For private lawsuits, there is a 2-year statute of limitations for each violation. Hospitals are directly liable for the acts of independent physicians and on-call physicians on the medical staff who are responsible for examination, treatment, or transfer of patients. However, physicians who function in these roles can also be fined individually. Hospitals are liable for the actions of their nurse employees and any other employee who may be involved in patient interactions, including admitting clerks, unit secretaries, nurses' aides, and technicians. Sanctions for violations in addition to civil monetary penalties include termination of the hospital's Medicare and Medicaid provider agreement.

Implications for the Care of Pregnant Women

The term *emergency medical condition* means "with respect to a pregnant woman who is having contractions, that there is inadequate time to effect a safe transfer to another hospital before delivery or that the transfer may pose a threat to the health or safety of the woman or unborn child" (EMTALA, 1986). According to the 1998 HCFA Interpretive Guidelines, "emergency medical conditions must be stabilized." Labor is considered an emergency medical condition. Stabilization means that it has been determined that the pregnant woman has reached the point where her continued care, including diagnostic workup and treatment, could be reasonably performed as an outpatient or as an inpatient at a later time provided the patient is given a plan for appropriate follow-up with the discharge instructions. If a woman is in labor, the hospital must deliver the baby or transfer appropriately. "Transfer appropriately" may include discharge home if a qualified professional has certified that the woman is in early labor or in false labor. Stable for discharge does not require resolution of the medical condition (pregnancy).

All pregnant women who present to the hospital for care require a medical screening examination. If, based on results of the examination, the woman is determined to be in false labor, a physician or other qualified personnel must certify that a woman is in false labor and document that certification in the medical record. If the woman presents at a hospital that does not provide obstetric services, the benefits of a transfer may outweigh the risk. If the woman with complications of pregnancy presents at a hospital that is not capable of handling high-risk pregnancies or high-risk infants, the hospital still must meet the screening, treatment, and transfer requirements. A written transfer agreement with facilities capable of caring for high-risk pregnant women and high-risk infants works best. Transfers must be effected through qualified personnel. For pregnant women, emergency medical technicians may not meet that requirement, especially if there is a risk of birth en route or the woman is medically unstable. The transferring hospital, not the receiving hospital, has the responsibility to determine the mode, equipment, and attendants for transfer.

Many hospitals have general policies that pregnant women meeting certain criteria will be seen in the labor and birth unit rather than in the emergency department. These criteria vary with institutions and may include gestational age limits and nonpregnancy-related conditions. The emergency departments of most institutions triage term labor patients with any possibility that they may be in labor directly to the labor unit. EMTALA regulations apply to women who are seen in the emergency department and in the labor and birth unit (and any other setting on hospital property). In many institutions, nurses then evaluate the woman and determine if she is in labor and assess fetal status. The EMTALA regulations allow for nurses to perform medical screening examinations under certain circumstances:

- The medical staff by-laws or rules and regulations of the institution allow medical screening examinations by nonphysicians.
- There are nursing policies defining the scope of practice and conduct of medical screening.
- There is a process in place to educate nurses who perform medical screening, including periodic validation of competence in this area.
- A discussion occurs between the nurse and physician about the results of the medical screening examination.
- Physician orders for discharge are obtained and documented in the medical record.

Discharge to home is considered a transfer under the EMTALA regulations. It is important to document certification in the medical record that the woman who is in early labor or not in labor is stable under the terms of the regulations. A log of all patients seen and their disposition ensures that accurate records are maintained to show that the statute has been followed. EMTALA regulations require that these records be kept for at least 5 years.

An EMTALA compliance program requires an understanding of the nature and intent of the law; developing numerous forms (eg, physician authorization or certification for transfer, patient acceptance of treatment, patient request for transfer, patient refusal for stabilizing treatment or transfer, transfer or discharge summary); signage requirements; record keeping (eg, transfer logs, medical records); and education of all potentially involved personnel. The U.S. DHHS web site is one source to use to keep abreast of HCFA and OIG special advisory bulletins and other updates (*http://www.dhhs.gov*). The American College of Emergency Physicians (ACEP) has another site with useful, easy to interpret information about EMTALA (*http://www.acep.org*).

Conflict Resolution

There are many challenges to achieving teamwork in the perinatal setting. It is helpful to acknowledge that no group of individuals can work together in an organization and always have the same expectations, goals, and perspectives. Conflict is an inevitable result when reality does not meet with individual expectations. Although individual expectations may differ, usually there exists among caregivers a basic commitment to quality and to the best possible outcomes for mothers and babies. Mutual trust and respect and the capacity to engage in agreeable disagreement are the hallmarks of a professional unit. When involved in a clinical or administrative situation that can potentially cause conflict, consider that both parties probably have the best interests of the patient in mind, although there may be very different approaches proposed to achieve that goal. At times, clinical practice issues arise when the "way we've always done it" conflicts with a new or an alternate approach.

Classic principles of conflict resolution can be used to successfully resolve the inevitable differences of opinion that occur in everyday clinical practice. If the conflict is not related to an emergent patient situation (ie, there is at least some time for discussion), effective communication techniques can enhance the chances of conflict resolution to the satisfaction of both parties or at least to reach a workable compromise. Taking time to listen and understand the intent of the other person is a helpful starting point. While the other person is expressing herself, give visual and verbal feedback to ensure that their concern is important and being taken seriously, such as nodding the head or saying, "I see, please go on" or summarizing what it is the other person is concerned about by saying "Let me see if I am understanding you correctly . . . ." Phrases such as "I have a different perspective" usually work better in conflict resolution than "You are wrong." Other successful strategies include a calm, collected attitude and careful consideration of the goal to be accomplished.

Communication in conflict resolution may not always be so rational and under one's control. This is especially true when dealing with difficult people, particularly those who are hostile or aggressive. These individuals manifest behavior that is abusive, abrupt, intimidating, and overwhelming. Being confronted by this behavior often catches the victim by surprise and generates feelings of helplessness. When being attacked, it is important to stand up for yourself and command respect. Calmly wait for the person to run down and then jump in and interrupt the attack. Use words that express your assertiveness. For example, saying "I am willing to discuss this with you when you are ready to speak to me with respect" may help stop the verbal attack and allow time for more respectful discussion when they are rational (Hendrickson, 1999).

Selecting the best time and place for interaction is also essential. Ideally, the setting does not allow opportunity for patients, family members, or other colleagues to overhear the discussion. The focus of the discussion should remain on the issue, preferably on the potential impact on patient care. If the conversation deteriorates beyond personal capacity to handle it or the colleague becomes verbally abusive, ending the discussion until a later time and informing a third party who has the ability to help or the responsibility to know about the interaction is helpful.

An important strategy for promoting positive long-term professional collaboration is the development of interdisciplinary specialty practice opportunities in which colleagues can come together to work toward a common goal (Simpson & Knox, 1999). This can include the development of unit guidelines, joint learning from a case review or grand rounds, examining quality or research findings, designing unit projects, or discussion of conflict resolution. When colleagues come together to identify problems, define objectives, address alternatives, integrate changes, remain patient focused, disagree agreeably, negotiate, demonstrate mutual respect, and recognize and praise positive attributes and actions, it can facilitate a professional culture for positive conflict resolution. Strategies for developing and nurturing an environment where true teamwork and collaboration among perinatal healthcare professionals can be a reality is discussed in detail in Chapter 3.

Chain of Command

Some issues of conflict in the clinical setting cannot be solved at the lowest level and do not allow the luxury of time. If, after careful deliberation, the issue is determined to be a matter of maternal–fetal well-being or there is potential for the clinical situation to deteriorate rapidly, the nurse must initiate an appropriate course of action. One example is failure of the physician to respond to a nonreassuring FHR pattern or deteriorating maternal condition. Decisive, timely nursing intervention may be necessary to avoid a potentially adverse outcome.

Knowledge and the use of the chain of command are ways to attempt to resolve differences of opinion in clinical practice settings. An example of chain of command is presented in Figure 2–1. If discussions with the physician or certified nurse midwife do not result in care appropriate for the clinical practice situation, the nurse has the responsibility to use the perinatal unit institutional chain of command to avoid harm to the mother and newborn. Frequently, this involves the staff nurse notifying the appropriately available immediate supervisory nurse (ie, charge nurse, nurse manager, or nursing supervisor) to provide assistance and then documenting in the medical record that this action has been taken. In selected instances, it may be necessary to go further up the chain of command if the situation cannot be resolved. It is important to recognize that this process may require more time than the situation can accommodate. In other words, invoking the complete use of the chain of command is generally most successful when there is an urgent situation (eg, progressively nonreassuring FHR tracing) rather than an overt emergency (eg, shoulder dystocia).

Institutions have a responsibility to support nurses who use the chain of command. Nurses may be reluctant to invoke this vehicle because of intimidation, a sense of personal or professional jeopardy, fear of retribution, or lack of confidence in the institutional lines of authority and responsibility. It is important that nurses and physicians know the institution's policy for using the chain of command and that data about its use be collected and analyzed so that the process can be optimized and personnel receive positive feedback for its appropriate use. Chain of command should not be the routine method of conflict resolution. Clinical disagreements that result in chain of command are detrimental to nurse–physician relationships. Soon after a clinical disagreement that resulted in use of the chain of command, all those involved should meet and calmly discuss what happened and why. Having an objective third party such as the risk manager present during this discussion may facilitate the interaction. Prospective plans should then be developed to avoid this situation in the future. A positive corporate culture that includes selected use of the chain of command as appropriate recognizes that when personnel are given the resources, support, and guidance that are necessary to carry out the responsibilities of their positions, everyone generally benefits: the institution, their employees, the medical staff, and the patients.

Professional Liability Insurance

Perinatal nurses continue to ask whether they should carry their own liability insurance. The question is an important one in light of increased litigation surrounding adverse perinatal outcomes. However, the prevalence of litigation has little to do with the deci-

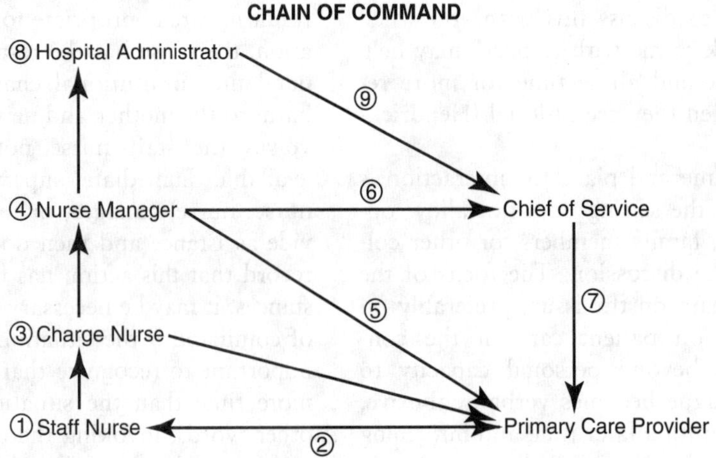

EXAMPLE

1. Conflict exists between judgment of nurse and primary care provider.
2. Direct conversation with primary care provider to verbalize/communicate conflict/concern.
3. Notification of charge nurse, who may confer with provider.
4. Notification of nurse manager.
5. Conversation with primary care provider.
6. Conversation with chief of service.
7. Chief of service confers with primary care provider.
8. Hospital administrator notified.
9. Hospital administrator confirms resolution of conflict.

WHO: Every perinatal nurse
WHAT: A mechanism (usually administrative) to resolve conflict in patient management plans
WHERE: Every patient-care setting
WHEN: Whenever there is a question regarding patient care, patient safety, or the nurse is uncertain about how to proceed in a situation of conflict
HOW: Notification of an administrative line of authority to resolve the conflict

FIGURE 2–1. Each perinatal care setting should have its own administrative chain of command to assist in conflict resolution in the management of patients. Such a chain of command is illustrated here. Adapted from Chez, B.F., Harvey, C.J., Murray, M.L. (1990). *Critical Concepts in Fetal Heart Rate Monitoring.* (p. 32). Baltimore: Williams & Wilkins.

sion-making that the individual nurse must go through. There are multiple factors for the perinatal nurse to consider.

All perinatal nurses engaged in the practice of nursing should be insured against liabilities to third parties arising out of their professional practice. The means by which a professional nurse elects to insure professional practice should be based on an informed decision. Insurance options available to nurses include reliance on the employer-provided insurance or purchase of self-insurance as an independent practitioner or as part of a group when there is no employer-provided insurance. Either option fulfills the expectation that there exists a financial responsibility for professional practice.

The issue for nurses is whether to purchase individual coverage in addition to employer-provided coverage. The nurse is an employee of the institution. An institutional liability policy covers the nurse for acts that are within the scope of employment. The nurse should assess his or her clinical practice against the established policies and procedures of the institution. The nurse is covered by the employer's policy when the nurse is acting within the employer's direction and control and within the stated scope of practice.

A fear among nurses is that the employer may attempt to recover partial damages from the nurse if the nurse is found negligent in a malpractice action. This process is referred to as *indemnification and contribution.* There are limited data on separate suits against nurses in this regard, but it has been attempted. There are valid reasons why healthcare institutions would not or should not sue nurses. Among these reasons, the nurse is an employee of the institution, and because the nurse is acting under the institution's power and control, it is responsible for all actions of the nurse. Another reason is that it makes for very poor public relations when an institution sues its own employees. If a nurse has no personal insurance policy to recover from, the suit may not be worth it from a financial standpoint.

An additional concern among nurses is the loss of personal assets if they are not separately insured. Unfortunately, there are scant data on the liability of uninsured nurses. However, many states have laws protecting money and property that are jointly held. An uninsured nurse is an unlikely financial "deep pocket" for any claimant. A final consideration for nurses is that the purchase of individual or personal coverage may make it more likely for a nurse to become involved as an individual in a malpractice action, because the nurse with significant coverage is viewed as a financial deep pocket, separate and distinct from the employer. When the employer and the nurse have policies, which policy is considered the primary coverage depends on the nature and language of the policies, and prorated contributions may result if the nurse is determined to be negligent in a malpractice action. Nurses should be knowledgeable about the conditions of their policy.

SUMMARY

As knowledge and technologic advances continue in the fields of perinatology and neonatology, responsibilities and opportunities for perinatal nurses are evolving. Keeping current with changes in practice and developing new research-based knowledge is critically important for perinatal nurses to ensure provision of quality care for mothers and babies and to avoid errors that result in patient injuries and professional liability. Developing truly collaborative relationships with physician colleagues that involve mutual respect and healthy interactions contributes to a culture of safety. Establishment of an interdisciplinary practice committee jointly led by a nurse and a physician expert where current practices and proposed practices are evaluated and discussed is essential for safe care. Practice based on evidence and standards of care from professional organizations has been shown to decrease errors by healthcare providers, maternal–fetal injuries, malpractice claims, and the dollar amount of claims that are filed (MMI Companies, 1998). Creating an environment to promote safe care requires significant professional energy to overcome the existing challenges. The investment in time and effort is worth it when the status quo is considered. Practice in a perinatal setting where patient safety is the number one priority is professionally rewarding and personally fulfilling.

REFERENCES

Adels, N., & Pringle, S. (1992). Stop re-inventing the wheel: Textbooks as procedure manuals. *Nursing Management, 23*(5), 74–75.

Afriat, C. I., Simpson, K. R., Chez, B. F., & Miller, L. (1994). Electronic fetal monitoring competency—To validate or not to validate: The opinions of experts. *Journal of Perinatal and Neonatal Nursing, 8*(3), 5–9.

American Academy of Pediatrics & American College of Obstetricians and Gynecologists. (1997). *Guidelines for perinatal care* (4th ed.). Washington, DC: Author.

American Association of Critical Care Nurses. (1995). *Delegation: A tool for success in the changing workforce*. Aliso Viejo, CA: Author.

American College of Obstetricians and Gynecologists. (1999). *Induction of labor* (practice bulletin no. 10). Washington, DC: Author.

American College of Obstetricians and Gynecologists. (1999). *Induction of labor with misoprostol* (committee opinion no. 228). Washington, DC: Author.

American College of Obstetricians and Gynecologists. (1998). *Monitoring during induction of labor with dinoprostone* (committee opinion no. 209). Washington, DC: Author.

American College of Obstetricians and Gynecologists. (1996). *Prevention of early-onset group B streptococcal disease in newborns* (committee opinion no. 173). Washington, DC: Author.

American Nurses Association. (1979). *The study of credentialing in nursing: A new approach* (vol. 1). The Report of the Committee. Kansas City, MO: Author.

American Nurses Association. (1985). *Code for nurses with interpretive guidelines*. Kansas City, MO: Author.

American Nurses Association. (1996). *Registered professional nurses and unlicensed assistive personnel*. Washington, DC: Author.

American Nurses Association. (1998). *Standards of clinical nursing practice*. Washington, DC: Author.

American Nurses Association. (1999). *Principles for nurse staffing*. Washington, DC: Author.

American Nurses Credentialing Center. (2000). *Nurses Credentialing Center certification catalog*. Washington, DC: Author.

American Society of Health System Pharmacists. (1999). *The 10 common patient concerns in hospitals and other components of health systems*. Washington, DC: Author.

Association of Women's Health, Obstetric and Neonatal Nurses. (1997). *The role of unlicensed assistive personnel in the nursing care of women and newborns*. Position statement. Washington, DC: Author.

Association of Women's Health, Obstetric and Neonatal Nurses. (1998a). *Clinical competencies and educational guidelines: Antepartum and intrapartum fetal heart rate monitoring*. Washington, DC: Author.

Association of Women's Health, Obstetric and Neonatal Nurses. (1998b). *Standards and Guidelines for Professional Practice in the Care of Women and Newborns* (5th ed.). Washington, DC: Author.

Association of Women's Health, Obstetric and Neonatal Nurses. (1999). *Interstate compact for mutual recognition of state licensure*. Position Statement. Washington, DC: Author.

Berry, M. C. (1999). Changes in the nursing environment create new liability exposures. *MMI Advisory, 15*(3), 1–4.

Booth, D., & Carruth, A. (1998). Violations of the nurse practice act: Implications for nurse managers. *Nursing Management, 29*(10), 35–40.

Buerhaus, P. I. (1999). Lucian Leape on the causes and prevention of errors and adverse outcomes in health care. *Image: Journal of Nursing Scholarship, 31*(3), 281–286.

Cary, A. H. (2000). *International survey of certified nurses in the U.S. and Canada*. Washington, DC: Nursing Credentialing Research Coalition, American Nurses' Credentialing Center.

Chally, P., & Loriz, L. (1998). Decision making in practice: A practical model for resolving the types of ethical dilemmas you face daily. *American Journal of Nursing, 98*(6), 17–20.

Chez, B. F. (1997). Electronic fetal monitoring: Then and now. *Journal of Perinatal and Neonatal Nursing, 10*(4), 1–4.

Christman, L. (1998). Who is a nurse? *Image The Journal of Nursing Scholarship, 30*(3), 211–214.

Donahue, M. P. (1996). *Nursing, the finest art: An illustrated history* (2nd ed.). St. Louis: Mosby.

Edbril, S. D., & Lagasse, R. S. (1999). Relationship between malpractice litigation and human errors. *Anesthesiology, 91*(3), 848–855.

Emergency Medical Treatment and Active Labor Act, 42 U.S.C. 1395dd (1986).

Emergency Medical Treatment and Active Labor Act, *Statutory Regulations*, 42, CFR, part 489 (1992).

Feinstein, N., & McCartney, P. (1997). *Fetal heart rate monitoring: Principles and practices*. Washington, DC: Association of Women's Health, Obstetric and Neonatal Nurses.

Freda, M. C. (1999). Now is the time. *MCN The American Journal of Maternal Child Nursing, 24*(6), 277.

Gallup Organization. (1999). *Gallup's annual honesty and ethics poll.* Princeton, NJ: Gallup Organization.

Gennaro, S., & Lewis, J. (2000). Is the BSN as the criteria for entry in professional nursing practice still worthwhile and realistic? *MCN The American Journal of Maternal Child Nursing, 25*(2), 62–63.

Geolot, D. (1999). *Nursing workforce characteristics*. Presented at the Tri-Council Meeting, May 3, Washington, DC.

Hallam, K. (2000). Hearings look at fixes for medical errors. *Modern Healthcare, 30*(5), 8–9.

Health Care Financing Administration. (1998). Interpretive guidelines: Responsibilities of Medicare participating hospitals in emergency cases. *State operations manual.* Washington, DC: Author.

Henrickson, M. (1999). Dealing with difficult people. *AWHONN Lifelines, 3*(3), 51–52.

Herrington, B. (1997). Early intervention and communication with the family when an error results in patient injury. *MMI Advisory, 13*(4), 4–5.

Hickson, G. B., Clayton, E. C., Githens, P. B., & Sloan, F. A. (1992). Factors that prompted families to file malpractice claims following perinatal injury. *Journal of the American Medical Association, 267*(10), 1359–1363.

Joint Commission on Accreditation of Healthcare Organizations. (2000). *Comprehensive accreditation manual for hospitals* Chicago: Author.

Jones, J. W., Barge, B. N., Steffy, B. D., Fay, L. M., Kunz, L. K., & Wuebker, L. J. (1988). Stress and medical malpractice: organizational risk assessment and intervention. *Journal of Applied Psychology, 73*(4), 727–735.

Knox, G. E., Kelley, M., Simpson, K. R., Carrier, L., & Berry, D. (1999). Downsizing, re-engineering and patient safety: Numbers, newness and resultant risk. *Journal of Healthcare Risk Management* 19(4), 18–25.

Knox, G. E., Simpson, K. R., & Garite, T. J. (1999). High reliability perinatal units: An approach to the prevention of patient injury and medical malpractice claims. *Journal of Healthcare Risk Management, 19*(2), 27–35.

Kobs, A. (1998). Sentinel event: A moment in time, a lifetime to forget. *Nursing Management, 29*(2), 10–13.

Kowalski, K., & Horner, M. D. (1998). A legal nightmare: Denver nurses indicted. *MCN The American Journal of Maternal Child Nursing, 23*(3), 125–129.

Kraman, S. S., & Hamm, G. (1999). Risk management: Extreme honesty may be the best policy. *Annual of Internal Medicine, 131*(12), 963–967.

Localio, A. R., Lawthers, A. G., Brennan, T. A., Laird, N. M., Hebert, L. E., Peterson, L. M., Newhouse, J. P., Weiler, P. C., & Hiatt, H. H. (1991). Relation between malpractice claims and adverse events due to negligence: Results of the Harvard Medical Practice Study III. *New England Journal of Medicine, 325*(4), 245–251.

Lockowitz, P. (1997). Examining healthcare errors: Creating a patient safety culture. *MMI Advisory, 13*(4), 1–2.

MMI Companies Inc. (1998). *Perinatal services risk modification program*. Deerfield, IL: MMI Companies.

MMI Companies Inc. (1999). *Transforming insights into clinical practice improvements: Improving patient outcomes and reducing costs: A 12 year data summary resource*. Deerfield, IL: MMI Companies.

National Certification Corporation for the Obstetric, Gynecologic, and Neonatal Nursing Specialties (NCC). (2000). *Certification program*. Chicago: National Council of State Boards of Nursing.

National Council of State Boards of Nursing. (1993). *National Council position paper on the regulation of advanced nursing practice*. Chicago, IL: Author.

National Council of State Boards of Nursing. (1995). *Delegation: Concepts and decision making process.* Chicago, IL: Author.

National Patient Safety Foundation. (1999). *Finding cures for medical error*. Chicago, IL: National Patient Safety Foundation.

Nichols, F. H. (1993). Issues in perinatal education. *AWHONN's Clinical Issues in Perinatal and Women's Health Nursing* 4(1), 55–59.

Office of the Inspector General & Health Care Financing Administration. (1999). Special advisory bulletin on the patient antidumping statute. *Federal Register, 64*(217), 61353–61359.

Phillips, M. E., & Szymanowksi, M. (1999). Should practice on a medical-surgical unit be a prerequisite for new graduates who want to be labor and delivery nurses? *MCN The American Journal of Maternal Child Nursing, 24*(6), 278–279.

Poole, J. H. (1992). Legal and professional issues in critical care obstetrics. *Critical Care Nursing Clinics of North America 4*, (4), 687–690.

Rhodes, A. M. (1997). Liability for unlicensed personnel. *MCN, the American Journal of Maternal Child Nursing, 22*(6), 327–328.

Roberts, K. H. (1990). Some characteristics of high reliability organizations. *Organizational Science, 1*(2), 160–177.

Rommal, C. (1996). Risk management issues in the perinatal setting. *Journal of Perinatal and Neonatal Nursing, 10*(3), 1–31.

Rostant, D. M. (1999). Sources and classification of law. In D. M. Rostant & R. F. Cady (Eds.), *AWHONN's Liability issues in perinatal nursing* (pp. 3–12). Philadelphia: Lippincott, Williams & Wilkins.

Simpson, K. R. (1990). A specialty certification incentive program: Costs versus benefits. *Journal of Nursing Staff Development,* 6(4), 181–185.

Simpson, K. R. (1997a). A collaborative approach to fetal assessment in the adult ICU. *American Association of Critical Care Nurses: AACN Clinical Issues. 8*(4), 558–563.

Simpson, K. R. (1997b). Unlicensed assistive personnel: What nurses need to know. *AWHONN Lifelines, 1*(3), 26–31.

Simpson, K. R. (1998a). Registered professional nurses and unlicensed assistive personnel: Delegation, supervision and staffing resources. In K. R. Simpson & P. A. Creehan (Eds.), *Competence validation for perinatal care providers: Orientation, continuing education and evaluation*. Philadelphia: AWHONN and Lippincott Williams & Wilkins.

Simpson, K. R. (1998b). Using guidelines and standards from professional organizations as a framework for competence validation. In K. R. Simpson & P. A. Creehan (Eds.), *Competence validation for perinatal care providers: Orientation, continuing education and evaluation* (pp. 2–11). Philadelphia: AWHONN and Lippincott Williams & Wilkins.

Simpson, K. R. (1999). Shoulder dystocia: Nursing interventions and risk management strategies. *MCN The American Journal of Maternal Child Nursing, 24*(6), 305–311.

Simpson, K. R. (2000). Creating a culture of safety: A shared responsibility. *MCN, The American Journal of Maternal Child Nursing, 25*(2), 61.

Simpson, K. R. (2001). EFM Competence validation: The pros and cons of traditional approaches. In C. A. Menihan & E. Zitolli (Eds.), *Evidence-based electronic fetal monitoring interpretation.* Philadelphia: Lippincott, Williams & Wilkins.

Simpson, K. R., & Creehan, P.A. (Eds.). (1998). *AWHONN's competence validation for perinatal care providers: Orientation, continuing education and evaluation.* Philadelphia: Lippincott.

Simpson, K. R., & Knox, G. E. (1999). Strategies for developing an evidence-based approach to perinatal care. *MCN The American Journal of Maternal Child Nursing, 24*(3), 122–132.

Simpson, K. R., & Knox, G. E. (2000). Fundal pressure during the second stage of labor: Clinical perspectives and risk management issues. *MCN The American Journal of Maternal Child Nursing,* (In press).

Simpson, K. R., & Knox, G. E. (2001). Perinatal teamwork: Turning rhetoric into reality. In K. R. Simpson & P. A. Creehan (Eds.), *AWHONN's Perinatal nursing* (2nd ed., pp. 57–71). Philadelphia: Lippincott Williams & Wilkins.

Simpson, K. R., & Poole, J. H. (1998). *Cervical ripening, induction and augmentation of labor: AWHONN symposium.* Washington, DC: Association of Women's Health, Obstetric and Neonatal Nurses.

Vaughn, D. (1996). *The Challenger launch decision: Risky technology, culture and deviance at NASA.* Chicago, IL: University of Chicago Press.

Ventura, S. J., Martin, J. A., Curtin, S. C., Mathews, T. J., & Park, M. M. (2000). Births: Final data for 1998. *National Vital Statistics Reports, 48*(3), 1–100.

Virshup, B. B., Oppenberg, A. A., & Coleman, M. M. (1999). Strategic risk management: Reducing malpractice claims through more effective patient-doctor communication. *American Journal of Medical Quality, 14*(4), 153–159.

APPENDIX **2 A**

Framework for Root Cause Analysis in Response to a Sentinel Event

This two-page grid is provided as an aid in organizing the steps in a root cause analysis. Not all possibilities and questions will apply in every case, and there may be others that will emerge in the course of the analysis. However, all possibilities and questions should be fully considered in your quest for the root cause.

Level of analysis	Possibilities	Questions	Findings	Risk Reduction Strategies	Measurement Strategies
What happened?	Sentinel event	What are the details of the event?			
		What area/service was impacted?			
Why did it happen? **What was the proximate cause(s)?** (Typically a "special cause" variation)	Human error	What was the error?			
	Process deficiency	What was the missing or weak step?			
	Equipment breakdown	What broke?			
	Controllable environmental factors	What factors directly affected the outcome?			
	Uncontrollable external factors	Are they truly beyond the organization's control?			
	Other	Are there any other factors that have directly influenced this outcome?			
Why did that happen? What processes were involved? (May involve "special cause" variation, "common cause" variation, or both)	Patient care process(es) (Specify)	What are the steps in the process?	Flow chart		
		What steps were involved in (contributed to) the event?	Cause-effect; change analysis; failure mode analysis		
		What is currently done to prevent failure at this step?		(eg, simplification, redundancy)	
		What is currently done to protect against a bad outcome if there is a failure at this step?	Barrier analysis	(eg, "fail-safe" design, redundancy)	
		What other areas or service are impacted?		(Generalize improvements to all applicable areas)	

Why did that happen? What systems underlie those processes? (Common cause variation here may lead to special cause variation in dependent processes.)	Human resource issues	Are staff properly qualified and currently competent for their responsibilities?			
		Is staffing adequate?			
		Does planning account for contingencies that would tend to reduce effective staffing levels?			
		Is staff performance in the operant process(es) addressed?			
		Can orientation and in-service training be improved?			
	Information management issues	Is all necessary information available when needed? accurate? complete? unambiguous?			
		Is communication among participants adequate?			
	Environmental management issues	Was the physical environment appropriate for the processes being carried out?			
		Are systems in place to identify environmental risks?			
		Are emergency and failure-mode responses adequately planned and tested?			
	Leadership issues: Corporate culture	Is the culture conducive to risk identification and reduction?			
	Encouragement of communication	Are there barriers to communication of potential risk factors?			
	Clear communication of priorities	Is the prevention of adverse outcomes adequately communicated as a high priority?			
	Uncontrollable factors	How can we protect against these?	Barrier analysis		

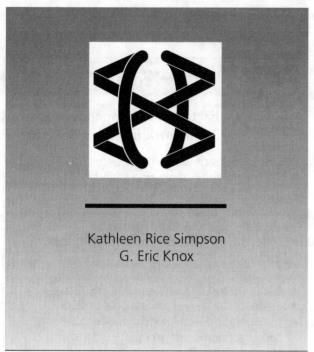

Kathleen Rice Simpson
G. Eric Knox

CHAPTER 3

Perinatal Teamwork: Turning Rhetoric Into Reality

In today's perinatal practice, "teams, teamwork, and team building" are words often said, seldom heard, and only rarely considered operational reality. Despite relentless cost, quality, and regulatory pressures, most perinatal units function as discrete and separate collections of nurses and physicians rather than as one team with mutually agreed on goals, tactics, and incentives. In extreme examples, nurse–physician relationships have been described as "strained or barely tolerable" (Palvovich-Davis, Forman, & Simek, 1998).

Because downsizing, re-engineering, and the perpetual managerial challenge of "doing more with less" will not go away, understanding how professionals can work most efficiently and effectively on clinical units remains a clear organizational imperative (Knox, Kelley, Simpson, Carrier, & Berry, 1999). Nurses and physicians, absolutely professionally dependent on each other, can no longer afford to simply coexist or, worse, sabotage each other's contribution to patient care.

Successful organizations in a wide variety of other professional and service industries, facing similar or more difficult challenges, have come to recognize multidisciplinary teams as the unifying principle that creates operational excellence and success (Katzenbach & Smith, 1993). Valuable lessons can be learned from examining how teams function in other service industries (Simpson, 2000a). Principles that are key components of their success could be applied to perinatal practice. This chapter explores several important questions. What accounts for the fact that nurses and physicians have not been able to learn what other service groups assume to be self evident? What, if anything, can be done to change the way we currently do business? How can perinatal units move from a service model of coexisting individual professions (professionals) to a team-based model of delivering perinatal services?

WHY TEAMS?

In virtually every performance domain studied, teams perform better than collections of individuals operating within confined job roles and responsibilities (Katzenbach & Smith, 1993). Whether it is customer service, innovation, product development, healthcare quality, safety in high-risk technically complex domains, healthcare resource use, or decision-making competence, the conclusion is invariably the same (Briscoe & Authur, 1998; Klein, 1998; Mannarelli, Roberts, & Bea, 1996; Roberts, 1990; Smith & Reinhart, 1991). In any situation requiring a real time combination of multiple skills, experiences, and judgment, teams—as opposed to individuals—create superior performance. Katzenbach and Smith (1993) have summarized the factors that explain the superior performance inherent in teams.

- No single individual can possess the complimentary skills and experience required to respond efficiently to operational challenges such as innovation, quality, customer service, or patient care emergencies.
- Communication established between professionals during team formation creates the basis for efficient real-time problem solving.

- Teams build trust and confidence in each member's information, intellectual challenges and differing adaptability to change.
- Importantly, working in teams that achieve significant performance goals is fun. Given the inherent external stress existing in healthcare today, maintaining a pleasant nonhostile work environment is a key component in every organization's attempt to survive.

WHY NOT TEAMS?

Given what appears to be a universal and irrefutable organizational truism, why have teams not become the predominant unit of performance in the delivery of perinatal care? The answer to this question is complex and involves many interrelated factors (Display 3–1). Some of these factors can be changed or overcome, but others represent challenges embedded in the structure of our current healthcare system.

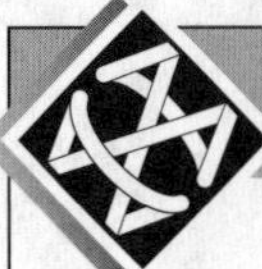

DISPLAY 3–1

Factors That Impede Teamwork in Perinatal Care

- Historic roles of women in society
- Traditional roles of physicians and nurses
- Institutional territory and politics
- Licensure and professional accountability
- Type and quantity of education
- Different styles of learning and information exchange
- Socialization of each group
- Methods and amounts of compensation
- Power of social and professional position
- Collaboration—an impediment because it assumes separation of groups
- Unresolved conflict, setting the stage for the expectation of future discord
- Inability to get common incentives

Historic Roles of Men and Women: The Gender Issue

Although women have made significant political, social, and economic progress in the past century, the historic role of women in society remains a factor in how nurses and physicians communicate, interact, and ultimately work together in the clinical setting. Ninety-five percent of nurses in the United States are women, and very few of the male nurses work in perinatal care (Geolot, 1999). This ratio of male to female professionals in the perinatal setting perpetuates the traditional male physician (dominant) and female nurse (submissive) model of interaction, rather than the equality needed for true team behavior (Bickel, 1997).

Although increasing numbers of female obstetricians—currently 60% of those entering the specialty are women (Seltzer, 1999)—could be expected to alter the historic way nurses and doctors relate to each other, observations suggest that the socialization of female physicians during medical education perpetuates the traditional male–female roles rather than creating behavior based more on female–female interaction (Pasko & Seidman, 1999). The resulting interactional dichotomy between what might be expected based on gender and the reality created by professional training is confusing and disappointing to many nurses. For example, informal conversations between female physicians and nurses about common challenges faced by working women (ie, child care difficulties and long hours away from families) that could invite camaraderie and collaboration can be quickly followed by unilateral and authoritarian "physician orders" with no input invited or desired from the nurses providing direct care. What could have been the basis for establishing the trust required for effective team performance quickly disappears under the differential socialization of the involved professionals.

Understanding the powerful effect of socialization and how resulting roles influence behavior may be helpful in explaining how gender differences have an impact on nurse–physician relationships. Kearny and White (1994) examined behaviors associated with work and categorized them as "warrior" or "villager" based on the way the people involved interact with each other and approach the tasks to be completed. Warriors are aggressive, competitive, and distrustful of others, viewing life as a struggle or contest to be won on the battlefield of living (Kearny & White, 1994). Warriors are not inclined to ask other warriors for help, fearing that would imply weakness or incompetence. However, warriors make excellent leaders because they have a firm resolve to meet their objectives, and their confident attitude inspires others to follow their directions (Kearny & White, 1994). Warriors make decisions on data they see as black or white, rarely letting emotion influence the decisions they make.

In contrast, villagers are cooperative and eager to please, even if that means giving in to the needs of others (Kearny & White, 1994). The goals of the village outweigh individual objectives or desires. Villagers reach decisions by consensus and are generous in giving praise to other team members, regardless of whether those praised are pulling their own weight on the team (Kearny & White, 1994). Villagers excel at working together, recognizing the value of cooperation, and fostering relationships. They are generally sensitive and caring, and they use these feelings to guide decision-making over more objective data (Kearny & White, 1994).

These behaviors are not determined by genetics, but rather are learned as an integral byproduct of the socialization that defines the unique culture of each society. Historically and stereotypically in U.S. society, men have been taught the characteristics and behaviors of warriors, and women have been assigned the villager role. Traditional training of nurses and physicians has reinforced these generalized societal expectations. Although the place and status of women in society and in healthcare has been altered toward more equality in recent years, the male–female and physician–nurse hierarchy and the personality types attracted to these roles remains a strong barrier to the establishment of effective service teams.

Traditional Roles of Physicians and Nurses: Who is in Charge, and How Do We Talk to Each Other?

Interaction and communication between physicians and nurses occurs in a hierarchical model (based on tradition and training) in which physicians give orders and nurses are expected to follow those orders without question (Keenan, Cooke, & Hillis, 1998). Communication of this type does not always create optimal patient care and is potentially dangerous. Examples include rapidly changing patient status for which the nurse at the bedside has more information than the physician at home or in the office; training situations in which the nurse has more experience than the physician in training; situations in which the nurse has more up-to-date knowledge than the attending physician; or situations in which the nurse has learned important information from the patient or family that the family has chosen not to communicate with the physician. In circumstances such as these, experienced nurses have developed strategies designed to overcome the fact that many physicians are not comfortable with nurses making overt diagnoses or clinical suggestions concerning how their patients should be cared for (ie, violating the expected hierarchic model of communication).

Instead of mutual direct communication leading to a plan of care developed through the wisdom and experience of two knowledgeable professionals, nurses are forced to revert to the "doctor–nurse" game to achieve what they believe is in the patient's best interest. Although this technique was first described in the literature more than 30 years ago (Stein, 1967), it was used for many years before Dr. Stein's classic article was published and is still alive and well today. Tips on how to play this game are given by experienced nurses to new graduates as part of socialization to the role of the professional registered nurse (Willis & Parish, 1997). For example, one of the most common techniques taught is how to get physicians to think it was their idea to order an intervention, medication, or laboratory test rather than that of the nurse. The doctor–nurse game avoids open disagreement or conflict and allows the nurse to give recommendations and the physician to request recommendations without appearing to do so (Peter, 2000). Nurses are expected to learn how to phrase suggestions (different for each physician) in such a way that the physician will reach the same clinical decision or course of management that the nurse thinks correct. This can be dangerous for patients and lead to adverse outcomes in multiple ways: when nurses are unable to find the right "story" or words that convey the emergent nature of an evolving clinical situation (Knaus, Draper, & Wagner, 1986); when the nurse is wrong in her assessment because of a clinical fact known to the physician but not the nurse; or when the assessment is correct but the description misunderstood by the physician. In these and other easily imagined clinical scenarios, patient care suffers because of delays and clinical miscues inherent in the dysfunctional communication adapted as part of the doctor–nurse game.

One study described common strategies used by intrapartum nurses in dealing with obstetricians. These strategies included letting them feel in control, avoiding making them feel threatened, not lying for them but not contradicting them, being tactful and subservient, and doing whatever would keep them happy (Sleutel, 2000). Using these strategies routinely serves as a powerful barrier to real communication and collaboration. The doctor–nurse game is a real problem because it does not foster the open dialogue needed to provide quality care (Peter, 2000).

In contrast, one hallmark of team behavior is clear language agreed to and understood by all members. How much better patient care would be if telephone communication with the physician were direct and to the point. "Based on my initial assessment, she probably has severe preeclampsia; would you please order preeclampsia blood work and intravenous magnesium sulfate and come in to see this patient as soon as possible?" or "Fetal status is deteriorating quickly and I need you here now." Instead, many nurses find themselves searching for the "right words or story" designed primarily to not offend the referring physician while at the same time attempting to obtain the required clinical action. The result is indirect, inefficient, and often inaccurate communication.

Physicians may not understand the real sense of clinical urgency when nurses are reluctant to communicate directly. In cases resulting in maternal–fetal injury, physicians are often quoted as saying, "If she had only told me this was a real emergency, I would have come right in, but I didn't know things were that bad." This can be a valid concern and legitimate statement if the nurse did not communicate effectively. Urgent time is lost playing the doctor–nurse game, and miscommunications are common with this approach to physician–nurse interactions.

An important by-product of this dysfunctional communication is an underlying attempt to shift blame away from yourself and onto other professionals. Mutual accountability, the hallmark of successful teams, does not develop or is easily destroyed in the resulting "culture of blame" (Leape, 1994). Ultimately, an escalating cycle of mistrust between healthcare providers is created, accentuated, and perpetuated, with resulting deterioration in patient care.

This is more than a theoretical possibility. In a classic study of how the quality of nurse–physician interactions in an intensive care setting affects patient outcomes, Knaus and colleagues demonstrated that the most powerful determinant of severity-adjusted patient death rates was how well nurses and physicians worked together in the planning and subsequent delivery of patient care (Knaus et al., 1986). They concluded that a high degree of involvement and interaction between nurses and physicians directly influences patient outcomes. A later study found that for each severity level of medical condition studied, patients were at greater risk of dying or being readmitted when nurses and resident physicians failed to communicate and effectively work together (Baggs, Ryan, & Phelps, 1992). The Institute of Medicine's report (Corrigan, Kohn, & Donaldson, 1999) of how human errors contribute to patient deaths should provide enough evidence that this is a serious problem for which we all share responsibility. It is estimated that between 44,000 and 98,000 inpatients die each year in the United States as a result of human error, more than those who die from traffic accidents, breast cancer, or human immunodeficiency virus infection, making these types of deaths the fourth leading cause of death in the United States. Corrigan et al. (1999) concluded that most errors are not the result of individual recklessness or incompetence, but rather resulted from flaws in the system. The current system of nurse–physician interaction could benefit from significant re-evaluation and fundamental change to minimize the likelihood of adverse maternal–fetal outcomes.

Institutional Politics and Organizational Structure

In addition to the factors previously discussed, institutional politics and organization structure contribute to difficulties in physician–nurse interaction. Physicians traditionally have been viewed as customers who bring patients and revenue to the healthcare system or institution. As a result, physicians are treated with a level of organizational deference and respect not afforded the registered nurse (who is a cost on the balance sheet). An institution can more easily replace a nurse than a revenue-generating physician. Historically and in the extreme, a physician could demand that a particular nurse be terminated (for good reasons or bad) and expect that the institution would cause it to happen. Conversely, physician behavior that is inappropriate and disruptive often is tolerated by those same institutions (Knox, 1999). Nurses behaving similarly would be terminated. In addition to these behavioral and operational observations, the differential status of nurses and physicians may be seen in hospital organizational charts where nursing services are placed on a lower level than that of the medical departments.

Methods and Amount of Compensation

Differences in methods and amount of compensation for nurses and physicians further divide the professions. Nurses are compensated for hours worked, and unless they are in a managerial role, responsibility and accountability for patient care end when a nursing shift is completed. Physician compensation is commensurate with years of education and 24-hour ultimate responsibility for patients under their care. This results in physicians earning 5 to 10 times more than staff nurses who provide most of the direct hands-on care. The disparity in compensation creates a professional barrier and a social barrier. There are distinct differences in lifestyles between those who are middle class and those who are upper class, and these discrepancies carry over into professional attitudes and interactions.

Wide Disparity in Level of Educational Preparation

The disparity in educational preparation between physicians and nurses affects professional working relationships in multiple ways. Differential levels of education influence clinical interactions, contribute to inequity in compensation and professional respect, and result in real or perceived differences in social status. One of the most serious challenges facing nurses today is the issue of educational criteria and entry level into professional practice. Unfortunately, according to the latest data (Geolot, 1999), 59% of registered professional nurses in the United States do not hold a 4-year college degree. This inequity in education, when compared with other healthcare disciplines, is a significant barrier to advancing the professional practice of nursing and serves as a significant barrier to teamwork. Consider that laboratory and radiation technicians are required to hold a baccalaureate degree; social workers and speech, occupational, and physical therapists require a master's degree; and pharmacists must have a doctorate in pharmacology. There is no other profession that nurses must collaborate with professionally that does not require at least a 4-year college degree.

For reasons not entirely clear, nurses do not insist that they cease to be the poorest prepared of all healthcare professions (Christman, 1998). Because nurses are the least educated, they are also the lowest earning and least respected of the healthcare professions (Gennaro & Lewis, 2000). Given the wide disparity in education between nurses and physicians, clinical discussions that involve research, outcomes, and clinical judgment can be challenging at best. Without at least a baccalaureate education, nurses have a hard time evaluating evidence and deciding how to provide care that is based on science rather than tradition (Gennaro & Lewis, 2000). Nurses need a solid background in science and the scientific method to effectively collaborate with the medical profession. Nurses also need to know how to access the latest scientific information and how to use the most appropriate technology to gather information and provide care (Gennaro & Lewis, 2000). This knowledge is critical for nurses when planning with physicians the pros and cons, risks and benefits, and expected outcomes based on what is known about interventions for specific clinical conditions (Simpson & Knox, 1999). An equal voice in clinical discussions must be the voice of one who has been educated in an institution of higher learning in a manner similar to the other members of the healthcare team. The discrepancy in educational preparation between physicians and nurses plays an important role in less than optimal professional communication and clinical interactions, and ultimately adversely affect patient outcomes.

Physicians have a paradoxical view regarding nurses increasing their level of education. When asked to list weaknesses of nurses in a survey, some physicians thought that nurses had too many credentials and spent too much time in the classroom, but others believed that nurses had low initiative and suffered from a failure to seek advanced education (Pavlovich-Davis, Forman, & Simek, 1998). In a July 1999 Harris poll, 76% of Americans indicated they expected nurses to have 4 or more years of education to be successful clinicians.

The time has come to stop arguing about the entry level into practice issue and set a date requiring nurses to hold a baccalaureate degree in nursing. Those who are currently registered nurses should be "grandfathered" to increase the likelihood of support for this initiative. Traditional arguments for moving forward simply are not compelling. Many nurses complain that they did not have the time or money to complete a 4-year degree in nursing but still want to be recognized as professional nurses. Others insist that there will not be enough nurses if a baccalaureate degree is required. The latter argument may have cause and effect reversed. Other healthcare professions with more educational requirements, such as physical therapy and pharmacology, have seen a dramatic rise in the number of highly motivated, qualified applicants seeking admission to their programs and have the opportunity to choose from an applicant pool that is diverse in terms of ethnicity and gender (Gennaro & Lewis, 2000). Nursing programs have not experienced the same increase in quality of their applicant pool. Movement toward higher and more uniform educational requirements could significantly increase the potential for the nursing profession as well as teamwork in the clinical arena.

Licensure and Professional Accountability

Licensure and professional accountability are generally not thought of when factors that inhibit collaboration between physicians and nurses are considered. However, their effect may be as powerful as any of the previously mentioned factors. Physician licensure gives authority and demands accountability for admission, discharge, treatment (including all procedures and medications), and general oversight of all patient care. In short, physicians have ultimate responsibility for patient care. Nurses provide most direct patient care ordered by physicians, but nurses do have independent responsibility for ensuring that orders received and followed are reasonable and appropriate. This differential responsibility is highlighted when litigation ensues as a result of patient injury. Nurses are responsible for their clinical judgments and interventions. It is unacceptable to "delegate up" (ie, a process whereby nurses avoid responsibility for their decisions for implementing care by invoking the authority of physicians as the basis for their decision-making) when there is a question about appropriateness of orders (Rubin, 1996). However, it is not uncommon for some nurses to claim in retrospect "the doctor made me do it," even when they were aware that the ordered course of treatment was not in the best interests of the patient. If maternal–fetal well-being is at risk, the nurse has the moral responsibility to refuse to carry out that order and should be given institutional protection from potential physician-initiated repercussions (Peter, 2000).

From the regulatory and legal perspective, a nurse is expected to know which orders given by a physician (who has many more years of education, training, and experience) are unreasonable or inappropriate (ie, should be questioned either directly with the physician) or result in a request for additional assistance (ie, chain of command) in the event of physician nonresponsiveness to a question asked by a nurse. This nursing accountability specified by licensure is in conflict with the hierarchical role of physicians giving orders and nurses following those orders without question, and it reinforces the factors previously cited that lead to the historic role definition in the first place. Licensing requirements place a nurse in the difficult theoretical position of needing to "know more" than the physician giving the order. Nurses are compelled to take steps to directly "go against" physician orders with serious institutional and professional ramifications if they are found to be wrong in retrospect. Clinical conflicts not able to be resolved by direct communication that result in chain of command initiatives, inhibit physician–nurse trust and collaboration, and use of chain of command is a strong indicator that teamwork is nonexistent in the first place.

Conclusion About Barriers to Teamwork

From the forgoing analysis, it should not be a surprise that Robert's classic (1983) study found that nurses exhibited symptoms of oppressed group behavior, with physicians as their oppressors. Nurses were found to be frustrated with their situation and powerless to effect change (Roberts, 1983). Physicians have historically viewed nurses as their "handmaidens," ready to serve but without ability to think critically or independently. Because of this social reality, it should be apparent that transforming these disparate professional groups into a team-based model of perinatal care will not be accomplished easily, nor will the transformation occur quickly or without a significant commitment of organizational resources. Nonetheless, it is our belief that if the commitment is understood, planned and budgeted appropriately, the result will be well worth the dollars and effort expended. Despite many historic, professional, and cultural differences, nurses and physicians share a powerful common goal around which effective teamwork can be developed: the best possible outcomes for mothers and babies under our care.

TEAM MEMBERS CHANGING PERCEPTIONS OF EACH OTHER: GOOD NEWS AND A FURTHER FOUNDATION FOR BUILDING EFFECTIVE PERINATAL TEAMS

Fortunately, nurse and physician perceptions of each other have improved significantly over the past decade. A study of physician–nurse relationships revealed that nurses and physicians generally have positive perceptions about each other (Pavlovich-Davis et al., 1998). Nurses and physicians were asked to describe the role of the other's profession and to list respective strengths and weaknesses. In this study, nurses described physicians as leaders and the most important members of the healthcare team, collaborative, involved, and caring (Pavlovich-Davis et al., 1998). Physicians described nurses as patient and physician advocates, emotionally supportive, and comforting to patients, the ones who provide minute-to-minute care and as partners with physicians (Pavlovich-Davis et al., 1998). Mutual respect and admiration between professionals appears to be increasing and needs to be nurtured so that teamwork becomes the model for delivering perinatal care.

WHAT IS A TEAM?

One of the most difficult tasks in creating an effective team is understanding what it is and, most important, what it is not (Katzenbach & Smith, 1993). Although chemistry of personality, getting along, and team building are important components in the creation of teams, they do not, individually or collectively, define or describe team in a functional or operational sense. Rather, *team is a discrete unit of performance*, not a positive set of values. True teams have the following identifiable characteristics:

- *Consensus (agreeing to agree):* The primary purpose of any perinatal unit can be defined very differently from different professional vantage points. Physicians and nurses simply see the world differently. For example, consider the wide range of professional viewpoints and professional activity currently existing between maternal–fetal medicine specialists and nurse midwives. Whether birth center or tertiary teaching institution, each perinatal management team needs to articulate consensus on mission, vision, goals, and objectives (Knox, Simpson, & Garite, 1999). Despite differences among professionals, it is necessary to acknowledge and respect the unique contributions that each can contribute to reaching team goals and objectives. Ultimately, if optimal outcomes for mothers and babies is the stated and desired goal, it will be necessary to develop a common methodology for creating that reality. It may not be possible to gain complete consensus. The concept of consensus is sometimes used by those who refuse to agree to anything as a barrier to stop the group from moving forward. They claim consensus means that each and every team member must agree to all points of any initiative. Consensus in that model actually means minority rule and can effectively halt any progress toward common goals. We use consensus to indicate that most of the team agrees to agree, and we acknowledge that complete consensus may be elusive in any work group despite the best efforts of the team.

- *Mutual accountability:* Each member of a team-based operational unit must be willing to hold the team rather than himself, herself, or other individual accountable for success or failure.
- *Organizational discipline*: Teams can succeed only in an organization that recognizes team rather than the individual as the operating unit, has strong overall performance standards, pushes for ever larger achievement goals, and has sufficient discipline to adhere to these principles.
- *Task:* The more demanding the performance challenge, the better is the resulting team. Creating "the best perinatal center" works much better as a catalyst for teamwork than "doing pathways" in an effort to "enhance collaboration."
- *Time:* A specific time limit is set within which ultimate goals must be achieved keeps teams on task and focused.

HEALTHCARE UNDER PRESSURE: RESULTING STRESS MAKES TEAMWORK DIFFICULT

In addition to the fundamental concepts of teams cited, Parker (1996) summarized operational characteristics of effective teams (Display 3–2). These characteristics, although logical and intuitive, are seldom seen in healthcare, in large part because of the anti-team forces cited earlier as well as the extreme challenge produced by the rapid constant change facing all of healthcare today. Under stress, the natural reaction of any professional is to revert to previous history, socialization, and teaching—all of which conflict with the fundamental operational descriptors of teamwork.

Effective teams operate in an informal, comfortable, and relaxed atmosphere (Parker, 1996), the very antithesis of the professional climate found in healthcare today. Cost pressure, staff reductions, legal and regulatory concerns, and marketplace competition all combine to create time pressure, nonaligned incentives, and potential mistrust among the professionals who must cooperate for a team to succeed. These same environmental forces serve to confuse teams in selecting and maintaining effective, necessary partnerships. Cooperating and competing simultaneously with stake holders who, at the same time, may likewise be competing and cooperating with each other, can occupy inordinate amounts of energy that could otherwise be devoted to productive team activity. The characteristics of participation, listening, civilized disagreement, consensus decisions, open communication, and shared leadership are often difficult to achieve because of the socialization and psychology of physician participants (Kassebaum & Culter, 1998). Highly individualistic, trained to be self-reliant and competitively aggressive under stress, and imbedded with a historic mistrust of hospital administration, physicians do not easily adopt to team dynamics and participation. The key ingredient necessary for effective perinatal team development is physician leadership that understands the importance and operating principle of team as the functional unit of production. Without physician leadership, nurses are forced to develop secondary, much less effective, often dysfunctional coping mechanisms for the delivery of perinatal care.

TEAM-BASED PERINATAL CARE: SELF-ASSESSMENT

Given all the factors that tend to work against effective team function in healthcare today, it is not surprising that most perinatal organizations currently resemble ineffective or nonfunctioning teams (Parker, 1996). Does your current work group exhibit any of the following characteristics?

- The mission, vision or goals of the perinatal team are not uniformly agreed on or not able to be described by all participants. Goals and vision

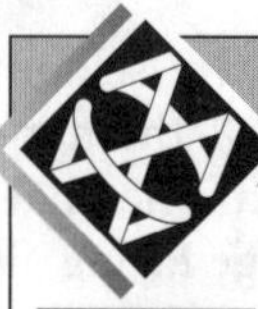

DISPLAY 3–2

Characteristics of Effective Teams

1. *Clear purpose:* The vision, mission, goal, or task of the team has been defined and is now accepted by everyone. There is an action plan.
2. *Informality:* The climate tends to be informal, comfortable, and relaxed. There are no obvious tensions or signs of boredom.
3. *Participation:* There is much discussion, and everyone is encouraged to participate.
4. *Listening:* The members use effective listening techniques such as questioning, paraphrasing, and summarizing to get out ideas.
5. *Civilized disagreements:* There is disagreement, but the team is comfortable with this and shows no signs of avoiding, smoothing over, or suppressing conflict.
6. *Consensus decisions:* For important decisions, the goal is substantial, but not necessarily unanimous, agreement through open discussion of everyone's ideas, avoidance of voting, or easy compromises.
7. *Open communication:* Team members feel free to express their feelings on the tasks and on the group's operation. There are few hidden agendas. Communication takes place outside of meetings.
8. *Clear roles and work assignments:* There are clear expectations about the roles played by each team member. When action is taken, clear assignments are made, accepted, and carried out. Work is fairly distributed among team members.
9. *Shared leadership:* Although the team has a formal leader, leadership functions shift from time to time, depending on the circumstances, the needs of the group, and skills of the members. The formal leader models the appropriate behavior and helps establish norms.
10. *External relations:* The team spends time developing key outside relationships, mobilizing resources, and building credibility with important players in other parts of the organization.
11. *Style diversity:* The team has a broad spectrum of team-player types, including members who emphasize attention to task, goal-setting, focus on process, and questions about how the team is functioning.
12. *Self-assessment:* Periodically, the team stops to examine how well it is functioning and what may be interfering with its effectiveness.

From Parker, G.A. (1996). *Team players and teamwork: The new competitive business strategy.* San Francisco: Jossey-Bass Publishers.

left unsaid produce several agendas often in conflict with each other.

- Meetings are formal, tense, and uncomfortable when multidisciplinary professionals are present.
- The ratio of output to discussion is low. Similar agenda items appear again and again.
- Conflict is downplayed or avoided rather than used as an opportunity for learning.
- Disagreements and discussion continue outside of team meetings.
- Decisions are made unilaterally after "input" was sought rather than by consensus.
- Trust among members is low or nonexistent.
- Work assignments and accountability are not specified.
- Consistent external or internal assessment of teams as a discrete unit of production is not done.

These characteristics describe most perinatal units. However, despite the inherent difficulties in building and sustaining a successful perinatal management team, it is ultimately worth the time and effort involved. Examples of excellent perinatal teamwork are found throughout the country. What follows are some features of successful perinatal services encountered by the authors in which teamwork is a reality.

A Powerful Vision Driven by Patient and Marketplace Need

"Perinatal excellence," "mothers and babies first," quality and safety first," and "faith-based perinatal care" are examples that every team member can ascribe to. The level of care (I, II, or III) delivered is not as important as the excellence in patient service provided. This passion for customer satisfaction or service is used as a means to align incentives, goals, and operations of all involved caregivers. Doing what's best for mothers and babies and doing it better than the competition can be a powerful uniting mission. Teamwork thrives on competitive challenges and a vision embracing patient or market needs is used to provide this type of challenge.

Leadership Embracing the Vision of Physicians and Nurses

Leadership must come from physicians and nurses. It could be argued that, without a significant commitment from the physician community, the team concept cannot exist. When this situation occurs, it is better to recognize that decent relationships among professional individual work groups is the best that can be hoped for. Alternative strategies should be employed and time not wasted attempting to create an illusion of a team that does not exist.

Sustainable leadership spends significant professional time learning each other's work and communication style; understands the requirements for success; and creates plausible time lines for the series of projects needed to move forward. Aside from a clear commitment to each other and the vision, the other requirement for successful leadership is the respect of most members of the obstetric department. This usually entails respect in the clinical domain as an initial requirement, with implications for the potential nurse and physician selected. From the perspective of physician leadership, the position need not be full time or salaried, but because of the time commitment involved, monetary compensation for the physician leadership is often considered.

Congruence of Parent Organizational and Perinatal Goals and Objectives

Potentially strong teams can be weakened by a parent organization not being specific in what the commitment of resources and corresponding vision for the perinatal center is. Without this understanding, team leadership can easily be caught between the nursing and private physician staff in a no win situation. Taking the time to be sure that "everyone is on the same page" is a fundamental step that must be taken before a team gets started. This can be particularly challenging when institutions with different philosophies, goals, and objectives are merged into the same healthcare system, such as merging Catholic and non-Catholic hospitals under a corporate structure in which church doctrine may or may not be the dominant framework for care and service.

Professional Competence and Capabilities

Competence and capabilities of all professionals within the perinatal center are specified and expected. In saying this, it is important to emphasize team as well as individual competence. As much side-by-side or simultaneous orientation, education, and performance metrics for physicians and nurses is specified and operationalized. The team—not individuals or single professions—is the unit of performance and should be recognized and promoted as such.

Effective Communication

Effective communication is an absolute requirement. The first and essential step toward establishing a clinical world where teamwork is reality is the development of effective team communication. Although this may sound simple, communication consists of more than just talking (eg, effective listening). Other characteristics of effective communication include mutual respect, sharing, negotiating, compromise, resolution, and moving forward based on agreements reached. Acknowledgment that different perspectives are valued and contribute to successful solutions is critical. Each healthcare team member has the potential and obligation to add a viewpoint that others may have overlooked or not even considered; one that may prove to be the essential component of a clinical solution.

One of the significant differences between nursing and medical education is the emphasis placed on teaching effective communication. Some nursing curricula devote extensive sections of course work to developing communication styles that work best with patients, family members of patients, peers, physicians, and other allied health professionals. Nurses are taught how to be collaborative and advice-seeking, whereas physicians learn to be decisive, independent, problem-solvers—qualities that do not necessarily contribute to good communication (Blickensderfer, 1996).

Nurses need to be more assertive in clinical discussions by communicating openly, honestly, and directly with physicians. Avoid the subtle, tactful recommendations about patient care made in ways designed to allow the physician to think he or she actually came to the conclusion independently. Refuse to play the doctor–nurse game. This approach is outdated and can be demoralizing and degrading when it is the primary method of communication. Although not all physicians will appreciate the changing rules, many will appreciate the more direct approach (Stein, Watts, & Howell, 1990). In today's fast-paced clinical environment, physicians have little time or patience to attempt to interpret a mixed message; major conflicts can arise when communication with nurses is inadequate or unassertive (Katzman & Roberts, 1988). Provide direct clinical observations and patient assessments to the physician and clearly ask for the order, intervention, or therapy that you believe indicated. Specifically, avoid communication techniques that imply uncertainty or a lack of confidence such as "I'm confused but I thought this was contraindicated . . ."; "I may be wrong but . . ."; or "I'm really not an expert on this, but . . ." (Blickensderfer, 1996). Never say "I'm only a nurse, but . . . ." This style of communication sets the stage for lack of respect from physician colleagues. Instead, use variations of the following types of opening phrases: "I have a different perspective . . ."; "What you are proposing is not consistent with what the patient has requested . . ."; "The patient's condition has changed since you last saw her . . ."; "I am not aware of any sound evidence to support that . . ."; or "The department has a new policy for . . . ." Open, honest, and direct communication promotes self-respect and respect from others and improves patient outcomes (Baggs et al., 1992; Knaus et al., 1986).

Multidisciplinary Perinatal Practice Committee: Instrument of Consensus

The best approach to unit policy development, clinical practice guideline establishment and unit operational issue resolution is formation of a multidisciplinary perinatal practice committee (Simpson, 1999a). The function of this committee is to allow nurses and physicians the opportunity to discuss all important topics and operational issues that affect patient outcomes (Simpson & Knox, 1999). As nurses and physicians gain mutual confidence and familiarity within this formal structure, enhanced informal communication during routine clinical interactions will follow. The practice committee has two purposes: to establish the basis for and to define current institutional practice and as knowledge, professional guidelines, or regulatory requirements change, to redefine practice accordingly (Simpson & Knox, 1999). Established regular and frequent meetings are necessary for the committee to succeed. The committee should be empowered to develop unit policies and protocols and make decisions about practice changes based on review of current literature, evidence, and standards.

Joint nurse–physician leadership of the perinatal practice committee is essential for success. Selection of these leaders should be based on peer respect, clinical expertise, and ability to influence and manage change. Because skilled clinicians are not necessarily skilled at effective group process, they may need formal development or training for effective group leadership. The key requirements for co-chairmanship of the practice committee are recognized clinical expertise, peer respect, support, and enough influence (simple positional power cannot succeed) to implement committee decisions. Committee membership should include physician representatives from pediatrics, neonatology, and anesthesiology; advanced practice nurses; and staff nurses from all clinical areas such as the labor and delivery, mother–baby, and neonatal intensive care units. Staff nurses should be selected based on their ability to be articulate and assertive and their willingness to share their perspectives with physician colleagues (Simpson & Knox, 1999). Providers from other disciplines and departments such as pharmacy, social services, grief support, lactation services, and risk management can be added as ad hoc committee members, encouraged to attend and required to participate if issues involving their departments are under consideration (Simpson & Knox, 1999).

After a committee has been formed, there are several additional considerations. A firm commitment to consistent attendance and meaningful participation by all members is necessary for committee operations. Finding a regular meeting time that is convenient for all may be difficult. Acknowledge (and plan accordingly) that the best meeting times for nurses may not always be the best times for physicians, but that for the process to truly be the result of a collaborative effort, both groups need to be actively involved. Committee consensus is required to designate the best time to meet. Flexibility is the key to success so that as many members as possible can attend regularly.

One of the important first goals of the committee is the development of a philosophy of care for childbearing women if one does not already exist (Simpson & Knox, 1999). Developing a philosophy may seem like an overwhelming task, but it need not be. A few simple statements will do (Display 3–3). This philosophy provides the framework for evaluating current clinical practice and proposing new practices and protocols. It is also very helpful in keeping committee members focused on their commitment to women and newborns in the organizational context of "what we do" and "how we do business."

Based on our collaborative consulting experience working with a variety of perinatal units and healthcare organizations, two ground rules are suggested. First, there should be an agreement that no unit oper-

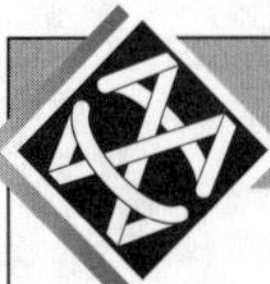

DISPLAY 3-3

Philosophy of Perinatal Care

- Birth is part of the miracle of life and thus a profound experience that belongs to the woman and her family.
- Pregnancy, labor, and birth are natural physiologic processes. Most women do well with support and selected minimal intervention.
- It is our privilege to facilitate, rather than control, the childbirth process to enhance the best possible outcomes for women and their newborns.
- Collaboration and open communication between perinatal care providers and the woman and her family during childbirth lead to informed decision making. Our goal is to meet the woman's needs and expectations within the framework of safe and effective perinatal care.
- Learning to understand, appreciate, and work with each other are critical components of establishing teamwork and collaboration in clinical practice.
- Recognizing the inherent differences in personalities and styles can enhance professional communication.

ational or practice change will be approved that is inconsistent with available research or established standards and guidelines from professional organizations. Second, when a change in practice is being considered, the person who is requesting this change is responsible for developing a proposal that includes a review of available and appropriate standards and guidelines; available literature and evidence; potential impact on unit resources (capital and staff) and clinical operations; cost-benefit analysis; and potential benefits to patients. The completed proposal should be distributed well in advance of the committee meeting where it will be discussed so members have the opportunity to gather additional data if desired. Obvious benefits of this approach include assurance that practice is evidence based, consistent with risk management principles and focused on the best possible maternal–fetal outcomes (Knox, Simpson, & Garite, 1999). An additional benefit of this formalized approach is the development of interpersonal relationships and effective methods of professional communication that carry over to discussions during everyday clinical interactions. Respectful communication between partnering professionals can only enhance the likelihood that all perspectives will be considered when deciding the best options for interventions and therapies for individual patients. The ultimate goal of the best possible outcomes is served.

Joint Educational Opportunities for Physicians and Nurses

Joint education on clinical topics is an excellent way to foster effective communication between nurses and physicians. There is potential for collegial relationship enhancement as well. Several clinical topics with opportunity for joint education include fetal assessment during labor, neonatal resuscitation, and emergency preparedness drills for cesarean birth and shoulder dystocia. Nurses and physicians interacting in the context of clinical education in these areas of practice learn to speak the same language and be in sync, with mutual role expectations during routine as well as when a perinatal crisis or emergency exists (Knox et al., 1999).

Electronic Fetal Monitoring

Joint educational programs about electronic fetal heart rate (FHR) monitoring are an ideal arena of mutual education because of the frequency of clinical disagreement between physicians and nurses in the description and interpretation of FHR patterns (Simpson, 2000b). Mutual electronic fetal monitoring (EFM) strip reviews work well because the presentation and discussion are associated with specific clinical cases and graphic display of FHR patterns. Case studies with EFM strips are more interesting and closer to daily reality in the clinical setting than a series of single topic examination lectures (Afriat et al., 1994). Responses to case study questions are more likely to result in critical thinking and interpretation than single topic exam items. A committee of attending physicians and staff nurse volunteers can be recruited to develop case studies from interesting strips of actual patients. A group process can be used to review expected responses, appropriate interpretations, and related interventions. Team discussions can lead to an increased knowledge of EFM principles for everyone involved. Not all participants need be experts with many years of clinical experience. "A new view created through differentially experienced eyes" can create excellent group learning. A willingness to volunteer should be the only criteria for participation. Joint education is an excellent opportunity to mentor those with less experience and develop collegial relationships between nurses and physicians. Any opportunity for collaboration between nurses and physicians who jointly are responsible for FHR pattern interpretation and clinical interventions should be seen as a positive step toward collaboration in everyday clinical interactions.

Developing case studies containing clinical ambiguity is an ideal avenue for clarifying ongoing clinical issues where interpretation and expectations of both provider groups are not in sync (Simpson, 2000b). Physicians may expect a series of nursing interventions for a specific FHR pattern that are not the routine of nurses on the unit. For example, there may be clinical disagreement about what to do when uterine hyperstimulation is the result of oxytocin administration but the FHR remains reassuring. Nurses may routinely decrease the oxytocin dosage or discontinue the infusion completely while physician colleagues believe the nurses are overreacting. An open discussion of the rationale based on physiologic principles and standards of care may lead to less conflict in the clinical setting (Simpson & Knox, 1999).

Development of case studies and accurate responses can lead to a common understanding of FHR pattern nomenclature that is mutually agreed on and routinely used by all providers. If not already in place, this is an opportunity to suggest adoption of a common language for FHR pattern interpretation and medical record documentation (Simpson, 2000b). There are several FHR pattern nomenclatures published in the literature, including those described in the *AWHONN Fetal Heart Monitoring Principles and Practices* text (Feinstein & McCartney, 1997), the technical bulletin from the American College of Obstetricians and Gynecologists (ACOG), *Fetal Heart Rate Patterns: Monitoring, Interpretation and Management* (ACOG, 1995), and the National Institute of Child Health and Human Development (NICHD) Research Planning Workshop (NICHD, 1997). No one EFM nomenclature has shown to be better than others, but it is important to adopt one set of unit specific definitions so that all providers are speaking the same language in oral communication and written documentation in the medical record (Menihan, 2001; Simpson, 2000b).

A clear definition of fetal well-being should guide most unit clinical decision-making and can be used to simplify communication between nurses and physicians (Knox et al., 1999). The presence of fetal well-being is sufficient criteria for maternal discharge, maternal medications, and use of oxytocin and epidural anesthesia in most clinical situations. Absence of fetal well-being necessitates direct physician evaluation with written documentation of further clinical management (Knox et al., 1999). Coming to this agreement can be a significant outcome of joint development of EFM case studies. This nurse–physician collaboration has a positive spillover effect on other daily clinical operations (Simpson & Knox, 1999).

Neonatal Resuscitation

The educational program developed by the American Academy of Pediatrics and the American Heart Association for neonatal resuscitation is valuable for all members of the perinatal healthcare team. When a baby is born depressed unexpectedly or even when potential unstable neonatal condition can be predicted, all team members need to know what to do and how to work together. This program provides structure for planning interventions based on an evidence-based algorithm and outlines roles and responsibilities of the resuscitation team in attendance. Because working together effectively as a perinatal team is critical to the best possible outcome for babies, this is an ideal opportunity to introduce joint nurse–physician education. Few could argue with the benefits of learning the appropriate management techniques in a multidisciplinary format.

Preparedness for Shoulder Dystocia and Emergent Cesarean Birth

The most critical time to be working in sync as a team is during an obstetric emergency such as shoulder dystocia or clinical conditions requiring emergent cesarean birth such as uterine rupture, placenta abruption, or prolapsed umbilical cord (Simpson, 1999b). Patient safety is enhanced on units that routinely practice for clinical emergencies (Knox et al., 1999). The American College of Obstetricians (ACOG, 1995) has developed videotape regarding shoulder dystocia that can be viewed simultaneously by nurses and physicians and used as a framework for planning preparation for this emergency. This provides an excellent chance to discuss iatrogenic interventions that can lead to shoulder dystocia such as fundal pressure (Simpson & Knox, 2000) or inappropriate use of forceps and vacuums. What to do when clinical disagreements occur related to these iatrogenic interventions can be prospectively resolved using simulation techniques. Prospective discussions about the best approach during educational programs attended by all members of the perinatal team can avoid clinical disagreements at the bedside (Simpson, 1999b).

When clinical conditions indicate the need for an emergent cesarean birth, minutes lost to ineffective communication or teamwork can have a direct impact on neonatal outcome. Practicing roles and responsibilities for emergent cesarean birth is a natural situation for joint nurse–physician education. Each member of the team needs to know what to do and how to accomplish this quickly in the context of the obstetric resources available. Cesarean birth drills are effective methods for improving teamwork and building collegial relationships. When these drills lead to successful patient outcomes during subsequent emergencies, the pleasure of working together can be celebrated. There are few situations more rewarding than emerging from a potentially deadly clinical crisis with a healthy mother and baby.

CHALLENGES AND OPPORTUNITIES WITH PERINATAL TEAMWORK

A commitment to perinatal teamwork is not a one-time pledge. Rather, it is an ongoing process that may require substantial personal change and more professional energy than other suggested methods of implementing and evaluating presumed positive changes in patient care. Unit culture may not initially support open communication and true collaboration between physicians and nurses. If the culture is one in which nurses and physicians simply coexist instead of collaborate, an opportunity for meaningful change is present. Discussions about clinical practice that are based on evidence and standards of care rather than hierarchical relationships, personal preferences and old routines can be helpful in setting the stage for collaboration, leading ultimately to real teamwork. However, taking advantage of this opportunity is not easy. Much of what is done in perinatal care is based on myths, rituals, and "the way we've always done it" (Simpson & Knox, 1999). Those who are invested in this approach will resist attempts at change. The old way is comfortable and does not require the stress of change. The concept of real teamwork in perinatal care may be foreign and therefore a threat. The process of agreeing to establish a multidisciplinary practice committee and select committee members may require months of negotiation. In some unit cultures it may be difficult initially for nurses to develop an equal voice in clinical practice development and to be viewed as a credible member of a multidisciplinary clinical practice committee. The "way we've always done it" may include physicians telling nurses about the latest research and standards of care and nurses "complying" without discussion or reviewing these data themselves.

Significant change in unit culture will not occur overnight. Professional relationships between nurses and physicians that include trust and mutual respect evolve progressively and are based on multiple interactions (Simpson & Knox, 1999). The inevitable mistakes and failures should not be allowed to derail overall positive progress. Developing and nurturing an environment that supports collaboration and teamwork may take years (increasingly made difficult by downsizing and staff turnover). It may be helpful for committee members to participate in team building exercises to enhance the likelihood of success. Initial success must be measured in small steps and implementation of simple practice changes that do not involve controversy or conflict. After members are more comfortable with the process and working together, more complex clinical practice issues can be addressed.

Based on our experience, it is not unusual for periods to exist during which it appears that nothing can be accomplished, group consensus is impossible, or even more frustrating, members revert back to the old ways of interacting and decision-making. A firm resolve to move forward and keep in focus the mutual goal of providing best possible patient care can help get through these periods. Periodic review and affirmation of the philosophy of care originally developed may be useful in getting the group back on target. Selective addition of new members or rotation of membership may help energize the committee. One key to success is to acknowledge chaos and frustration as a sign that the process is ongoing and dynamic and therefore moving in the desired direction. Eventually, if committee members are continually committed to changing to a collaborative approach of clinical decision-making, successful implementation of a team-based delivery of perinatal care will emerge (Simpson & Knox, 1999).

POTENTIAL BENEFITS OF PERINATAL TEAMWORK

Although a collaborative approach to clinical decision-making may not evolve as quickly as desired and may involve significant professional energy, ongoing investment will ultimately prove worth the effort. The ultimate advantage of perinatal teamwork is the resulting evidence-based approach to perinatal care that leads to maternal–fetal safety and a decreased likelihood of adverse outcomes. After this goal is accomplished, care practices will be defended as internal budgets become more restricted (almost guaranteed to happen), resulting clinical operations will enhance patient safety, and the number of obstetric malpractice suits and the dollar cost for each claim filed will be reduced (MMI Companies, 1998). The resulting dollar savings accruing to an organization are potentially available to be used for better patient care. Ultimately, a team-based model of delivery can ensure the public and purchasers that practices are clinically and fiscally sound and are consistent with scientific data and existing professional standards. Each of the resultant advantages of team-based care should create a better chance of organizational survival in a healthcare environment becoming increasingly complex and difficult.

SUMMARY

Perinatal teamwork can be a reality if there is commitment to this goal and cooperation in moving forward by nurses and physicians. We can no longer afford to coexist. Our collective survival is contingent on success. Mothers and babies are counting on us. If you think, "This sounds great, but it could never happen on our unit," read the chapter again and reconsider. Attempt to see things as they could be, rather than as they are. Give a copy to your physician colleagues. Nurses and physicians in leadership positions have the opportunity to act as role models so that effective communication and teamwork to establish evidence-based practice can be appreciated and used by staff nurses, attending physicians, and resident physicians during all clinical interactions. It no longer is a matter of "should" we work together effectively as a perinatal team; it is a matter of "when and how." We must leave the old ways of communicating behind and move forward together. Resolve to stop playing the doctor–nurse game. It may have been the way to interact in the 1960s but this new century requires true collaboration built on mutual respect and recognition. Together, we have the opportunity to make important positive differences in the care we deliver to mothers and babies.

REFERENCES

Afriat, C. I., Simpson, K. R., Chez, B. F., & Miller, L. (1994). Electronic fetal monitoring competency—to validate or not to validate: The opinions of experts. *Journal of Perinatal and Neonatal Nursing, 8*(3), 5–9.

American College of Obstetricians and Gynecologists. (1995). *Fetal heart rate patterns: Monitoring, interpretation and management.* (technical bulletin no. 207), Washington, DC: Author.

American College of Obstetricians and Gynecologists. (1995). *Shoulder dystocia* [videotape]. Washington, DC: Author.

Baggs, J. G., Ryan, S. A., & Phelps, C. E., Richeson, J. F., & Johnson, J. E. (1992). The association between interdisciplinary collaboration and patient outcomes in a medical intensive care unit. *Heart and Lung, 21*(1), 18–24.

Bickel, J. (1997). Gender stereotypes and misconceptions: Unresolved issues in physician's professional development. *Journal of the American Medical Association, 277*(17), 1405–1407.

Blickensderfer, L. (1996). Nurses and physicians: Creating a collaborative environment. *Journal of Intravenous Nursing, 19*(3), 127–131.

Briscoe, G., & Authur, G. (1998). CQI teamwork: Reevaluate, restructure, renew. *Nursing Management, 29*(10), 73–80.

Christman, L. (1998). Who is a nurse? *Image The Journal of Nursing Scholarship. 30*(3), 211–214.

Corrigan, J., Kohn, L., & Donaldson, M. (Eds.). (1999). *To err is human: Building a safe health system.* Washington, DC: National Academy of Sciences Press

Feinstein, N., & McCartney, P. (1997). *Fetal heart rate monitoring: Principles and practices.* Washington, DC: Association of Women's Health, Obstetric, and Neonatal Nurses.

Gennaro, S., & Lewis, J. (2000). Is the goal of a BSN as the criteria for entry into professional nursing practice still worthwhile and realistic? *MCN, The American Journal of Maternal Child Nursing, 25*(2), 62–63.

Geolot, D. (1999). *Nursing workforce characteristics.* Presented at the Tri-Council Meeting, May 3, Washington, DC.

Kassebaum, D., & Culter, E. (1998). On the culture of student abuse in medical school. *Academic Medicine, 73*(11), 1149–1158.

Katzenbach, J. R., & Smith, D. K. (1993). *The wisdom of teams.* Boston, MA: Harvard Business School Press.

Katzman, E. M., & Roberts, J. I. (1988). Nurse-physician conflicts as barriers to enactment of nursing roles. *Western Journal of Nursing Research, 10*(5), 576–590.

Kearny, K. G., & White, T. I. (Eds.). (1994). *Men and women at work: Warriors and villagers on the job.* Hawthorne, NJ: Cancer Press.

Keenan, G. M., Cooke, R., Hillis, S. L. (1998). Norms and nurse management of conflicts: Keys to understanding nurse-physician collaboration. *Research in Nursing and Health, 21*(1), 59–72.

King, T. L., & Simpson, K. R. (2001). Intrapartum fetal monitoring. In K. R. Simpson and P. A. Creehan (Eds.), *AWHONN's Perinatal Nursing* (2nd ed.). Philadelphia: Lippincott Williams & Wilkins.

Klein, G. (1998). *Sources of power: How people make decisions.* Cambridge, MA: MIT Press.

Knaus, W. A., Draper, E. A., & Wagner, D. P. (1986). An evaluation of outcome from intensive care units in major medical centers. *Annals of Internal Medicine, 104*(3), 410–418.

Knox, G. E. (1999). Doctors behaving badly and the people who let them. *Trustees, 52*(4), 18–19.

Knox, G. E., Kelley, M., Simpson, K. R., Carrier, L., & Berry, D. (1999). Downsizing, reengineering and patient safety: Numbers, newness and resultant risk. *Journal of Healthcare Risk Management, 19*(4), 18–25.

Knox, G. E., Simpson, K. R., & Garite, T. J. (1999). High reliability perinatal units: An approach to the prevention of patient injury and medical malpractice claims. *Journal of Healthcare Risk Management, 19*(2), 27–35.

Leape, L. L. (1994). Error in medicine. *Journal of the American Medical Association, 272*(23), 1851–1857.

Mannarelli, T., Roberts, K. H., & Bea, R. G. (1996). Learning how organizations mitigate risk. *Journal of Contingencies and Crisis Management, 4*, 83–92.

MMI Companies. (1998). *Transforming insights into clinical practice improvements: A 12 year data summary resource.* Deerfield, IL: MMI Companies.

National Institute of Child Health and Human Development Research Planning Workshop. (1997). Electronic fetal heart rate monitoring: Research guidelines for Interpretation. *Journal of Obstetric, Gynecologic, and Neonatal Nursing, 26*(6), 635–639.

Parker, G. A. (1996). *Team players and teamwork: The new competitive business strategy.* San Francisco: Jossey-Bass Publishers.

Pasko, T., & Seidman, B. (1999). *Physician characteristics and distribution in the workplace*. Chicago, IL: American Medical Association.

Pavlovich-Davis, S., Forman, H., & Simek, P. F. (1998). The nurse-physician relationship: Can it be saved? *Journal of Nursing Administration, 28*(7), 17–20.

Peter, E. (2000). Ethical conflicts or political problems in intrapartum nursing care. *Birth: Issues in Perinatal Care, 27*(1), 46–48.

Roberts, K. H. (1990). Some characteristics of high reliability organizations. *Organization Science, 1*(2), 160–177.

Roberts, S. J. (1983). Oppressed group behavior: Implications for nurses. *Advances in Nursing Science, 5*(4), 21–30.

Rubin, J. (1996). Impediments to the development of clinical knowledge and ethical judgment in critical care nursing. In P. Benner, C. A. Tanner & C. Chelsa (Eds.), *Expertise in nursing practice: Caring clinical judgment and ethics* (pp. 170–192). New York: Springer Publishing.

Seltzer, V. L. (1999). Changes and challenges for women in academics in obstetrics and gynecology. *American Journal of Obstetrics and Gynecology, 180*(4), 837–884.

Simpson, K. R. (1999a). Routine care during labor and birth: Is this really how we want to practice perinatal nursing or are we ready to advocate for childbearing women and insist on evidence-based care? *Mother Baby Journal, 4*(4), 5–7.

Simpson, K. R. (1999b). Shoulder dystocia: Nursing interventions and risk management strategies. *MCN, The American Journal of Maternal Child Nursing, 24*(6), 305–311.

Simpson, K. R. (2000a). Creating a culture of safety: A shared responsibility. *MCN, The American Journal of Maternal Child Nursing, 25*(2), 61.

Simpson, K. R. (2000b). EFM competence validation: The pros and cons of traditional approaches. In C. A. Menihan, E. Zitolli, & M. Lapidus (Eds.), *Evidence-based electronic fetal monitoring interpretation*. Philadelphia: Lippincott Williams & Wilkins.

Simpson, K. R., & Knox, G. E. (1999). Strategies for developing an evidence-based approach to perinatal care. *MCN American Journal of Maternal Child Nursing, 24*(3), 122–132.

Simpson, K. R., & Knox, G. E. (2000), Fundal pressure during the second stage of labor: Clinical perspectives and risk management issues. *MCN, The American Journal of Maternal Child Nursing*, (in press).

Smith, P. G., & Reinhart, D. G. (1991). *Developing products in half the time*. New York: Van Nostrand Reinhold.

Sleutel, M. R. (2000). Intrapartum nursing care: A case study of supportive interventions and ethical conflicts. *Birth, 27*(1), 38–45.

Stein, L. I. (1967). The doctor-nurse game. *Archives in General Psychiatry, 16*(6), 699–703.

Stein, L. I., Watts, D. T., & Howell, T. (1990). The doctor-nurse game revisited. *New England Journal of Medicine, 322*(8), 546–549.

Willis, E., & Parish, K. (1997). Managing the doctor-nurse game: A nursing and social science analysis. *Contemporary Nurse, 6*(3), 136–144.

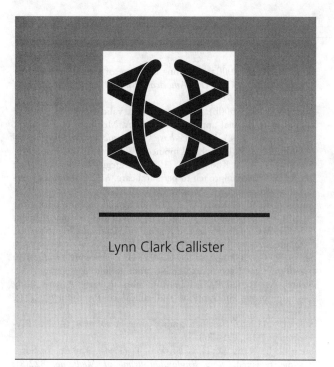

Lynn Clark Callister

CHAPTER 4

Integrating Cultural Beliefs and Practices Into the Care of Childbearing Women

Maria, a Mexican-American woman having her first baby, attended a childbirth education class where the expectant fathers learned labor support techniques. She declined to lie on the floor surrounded by other men while her husband massaged her abdomen.

Inaam, a Muslim Arabic woman experiencing her first labor, was attended by her mother and mother-in-law. As the labor slowly progressed and Inaam began to complain, the two mothers rotated between offering her loving support, chastising her for acting like a child, and praying loudly that mother and baby will be safe from harm.

Nguyet, a Vietnamese woman having her first baby, had been in the United States only a short time when she went into labor. She arrived on the birthing unit dilated 4 to 5 cm and in active labor. Nguyet and her husband Duc spoke very limited English. Her labor was difficult but she did not utter a sound. Her husband entered the birthing room only when the nurses asked him to translate for his wife. After 20 hours of labor, a cesarean birth was performed. On the mother–baby unit, Nugyet cooperated with the instructions from the nurse to cough and deep breath, but she became agitated when the nurse set up for a bed bath and began bathing her. When she was encouraged to walk, she shook her head and refused. She also refused the chilled apple juice the nurse brought to her. Because of abdominal distention and dehydration, a nasogastric tube was inserted, and intravenous fluids were restarted. No one could understand why she was so uncooperative.

Because of a nonreassuring fetal heart rate, Koua Khang needed an emergent cesarean birth. The nurse told her she would need to remove a nondescript white string bracelet from her wrist before surgery. The woman became hysterical, gesturing and trying to convey the message that the bracelet would protect her during the birth from evil spirits and should not be removed.

Cynthia, a certified nurse midwife, cared for a Mexican-American mother who finally confided in her that during her postpartum hospitalization she would go into the shower and turn on the water but was very careful not to get wet. She was following instructions from her nurse while trying to maintain her own cultural beliefs.

Mei Lin, a Chinese woman in graduate school in the United States, promised her mother she would follow traditional Asian practices after her son was born, including "doing the month" and subscribing to the "hot/cold" theory. Even though this woman was intellectually aware these practices had little scientific basis, she demonstrated her respect for her mother and her culture by honoring her mother's request.

Childbirth is a time of transition and social celebration in all cultures (Callister, 1998; Shilling, 2000). A Wintu child living in Africa, in deference to his mother, refers to her as, "She whom I made into mother." Culture also influences the experience of perinatal loss, particularly the meaning a death has in that cultural group. Healthcare beliefs and health seeking behaviors surrounding pregnancy, childbirth, and parenting are deeply rooted in cultural context. Culture is a set of behaviors, beliefs, and practices, a value system that is transmitted from one woman in the group to another. Culture is more than skin color, language, or country of origin, it provides a framework within which women think, make decisions, and act. Culture is the essence of who women are. The extent to which a woman adheres to cultural practices, beliefs, and rituals is complex and depends on acculturation and assimilation into the dominant culture within the society, social support, length of time in the United States or Canada, generational ties, and linguistic preference (DePacheco & Hutti, 1998). Even within individual cultural groups, there is tremendous heterogeneity. Although women may share a common birthplace or language, they do not always share the same cultural traditions.

Diversity is a reality in the United States and Canada. Nurses provide care to immigrants, refugees, and women from almost everywhere in the world, many of whom are of childbearing age. More than one fourth of the population of the United States now consists of individuals from culturally diverse groups, whereas only 9% of registered nurses come from racial or ethnic minority backgrounds. It is projected that, by the year 2050, minorities will account for more than 50% of the population of the United States. Each year, nearly 1 million immigrants come to the United States, and 1 of every 13 U.S. residents is foreign born. Twenty-seven percent of women living in the United States are women of color. One of the challenges for healthcare in this century is that members of racial and ethnic minorities make up a disproportionately high percentage of persons living in poverty. This poverty brings many challenges in healthcare delivery (Krostoski & Silliman, 1997; United States Bureau of Census [USBC], 1998; United States Department of Health and Human Services [USDHHS], 1997, 1998).

Clinical examples in this chapter represent only some of the possible cultural beliefs, practices, and behaviors the perinatal nurse may see in practice. It is beyond the scope of this chapter to thoroughly discuss each cultural group. Although generalizations are made about cultural groups, a stereotypical approach to the provision of perinatal nursing care is not appropriate. Cultural beliefs and practices are dynamic and evolving, and they require ongoing exploration. In any given culture, each generation of childbearing families perceives pregnancy, childbirth, and parenting differently.

CULTURAL FRAMEWORKS

A variety of cultural frameworks and cultural assessment tools have been developed to guide perinatal nursing practice. Leininger Sunrise Model (1991) is based on culture care theory. Variables include economic, educational, and technologic; religious or philosophic, kinship or social, and political or legal factors; and cultural value lifeways (Fig. 4–1). Giger and Davidhizar's The Transcultural Assessment Model (1995) includes cultural phenomena that appear in all cultural groups: communication, space, social organization, time, environmental control, and biologic variations (Fig. 4–2). Andrew and Boyle's (1995) Transcultural Nursing Model is illustrated in Figure 4–3. Purnell and Paulanka (1998) identified

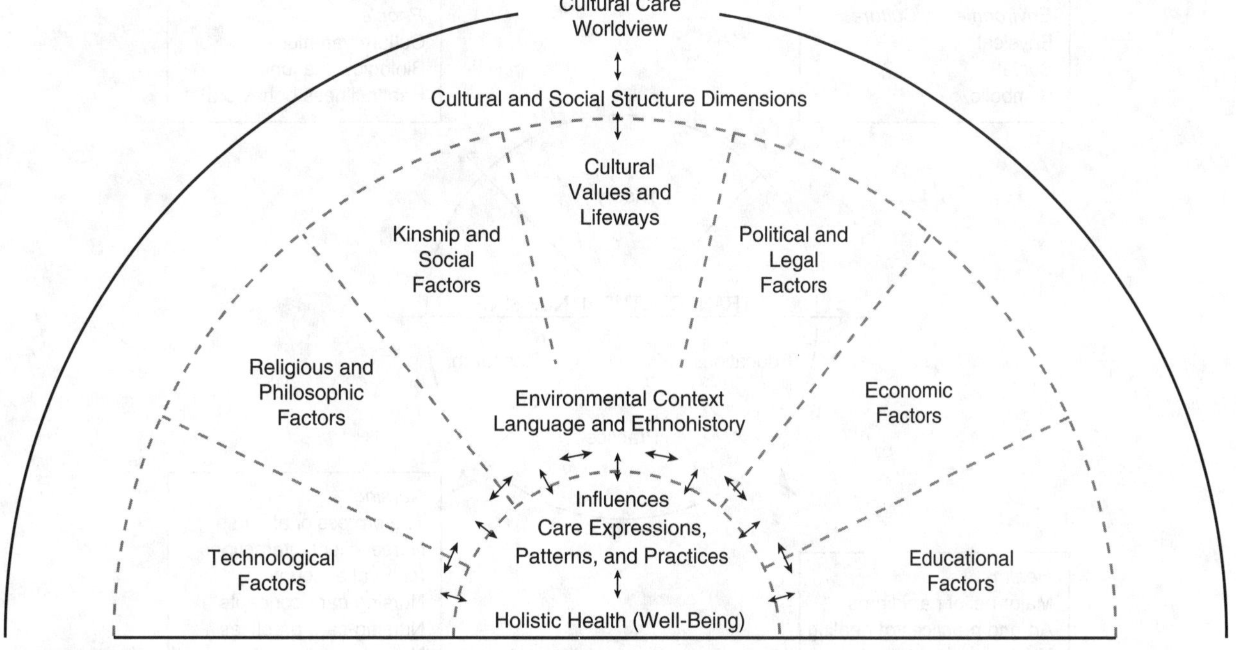

FIGURE 4–1. The sunrise model. (From Leininger, M. [1991]. *Cultural care diversity and universality.* New York: National League for Nursing.)

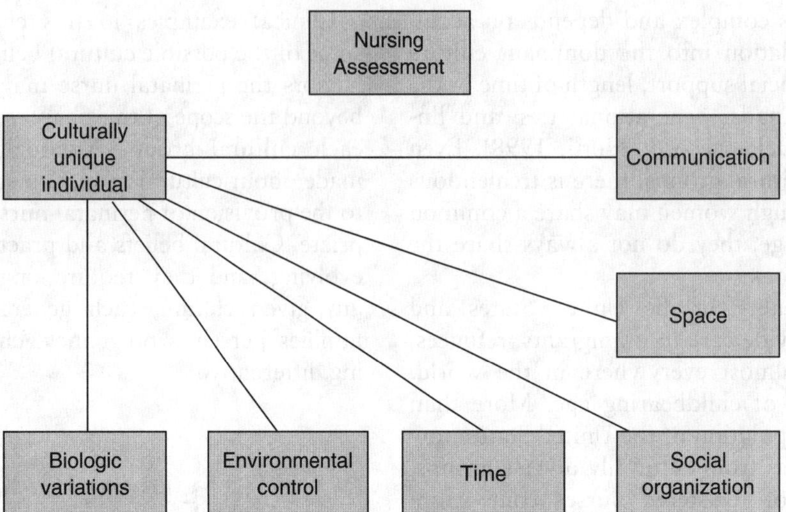

FIGURE 4–2. Giger and Davidhizar's transcultural model. (From Giger, J.N., & Davidhizar, R.E. [1995]. *Transcultural nursing: Assessment and intervention* [pp. 127–161]. St. Louis: Mosby–Year Book.)

the domains of culture as: communication, family roles and organization, workforce issues, biocultural ecology, high-risk health behaviors, nutrition, pregnancy and childbearing practices, death rituals, spirituality, healthcare practices, and healthcare practitioners. Mattson (1993) has conceptualized specific ethnocultural considerations in caring for childbearing women (Fig. 4–4). Campinha-Bacote (1994) defined the process of cultural competence in the delivery of healthcare services, including cultural awareness, skills, encounters, and knowledge (Fig. 4–5).

Balcazar, Peterson, and Krull (1997) developed the General Acculturation Index (GAI) scale. Item content areas include written and spoken language, country where childhood was spent, current circle of friends,

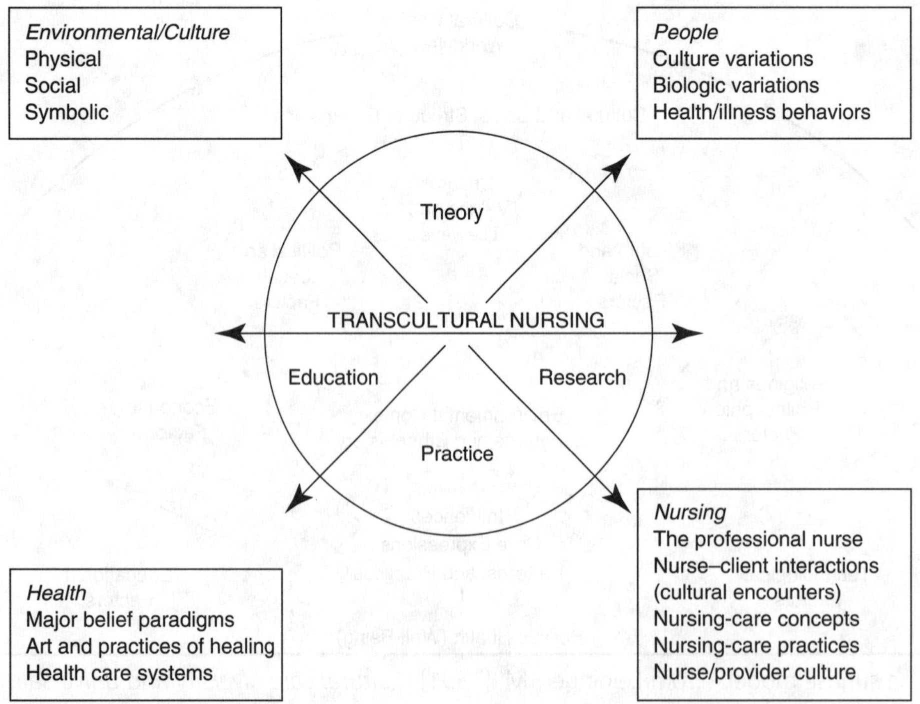

FIGURE 4–3. Transcultural nursing.

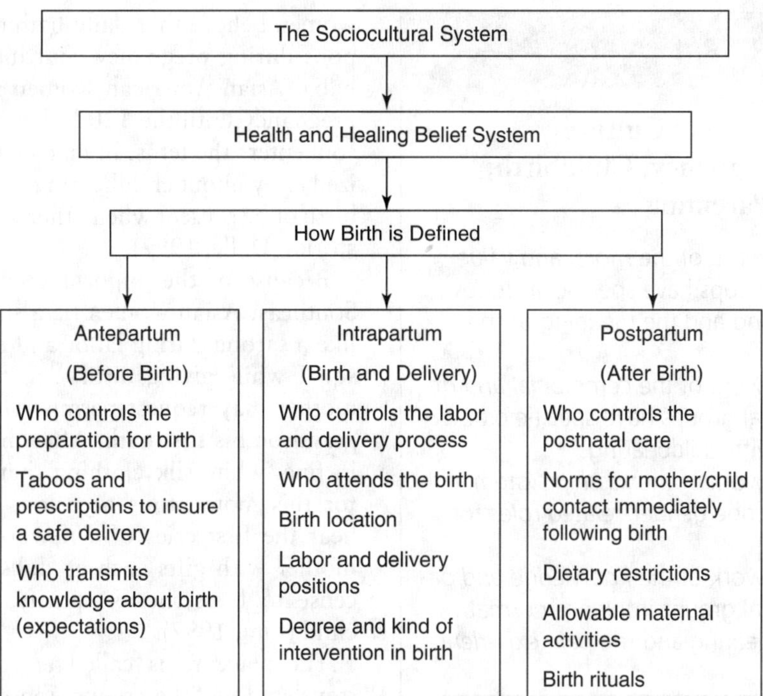

FIGURE 4–4. The sociocultural system, health and healing belief system, and how birth is defined. (From Mattson, S. [1995]. Cultural sensitive perinatal care for Southeast Asians. *Journal of Obstetric, Gynecologic, and Neonatal Nursing, 24*[5], 335–341.)

and pride in cultural background. Four assumptions define the influence culture has on pregnancy, childbirth, and parenting (Display 4–1).

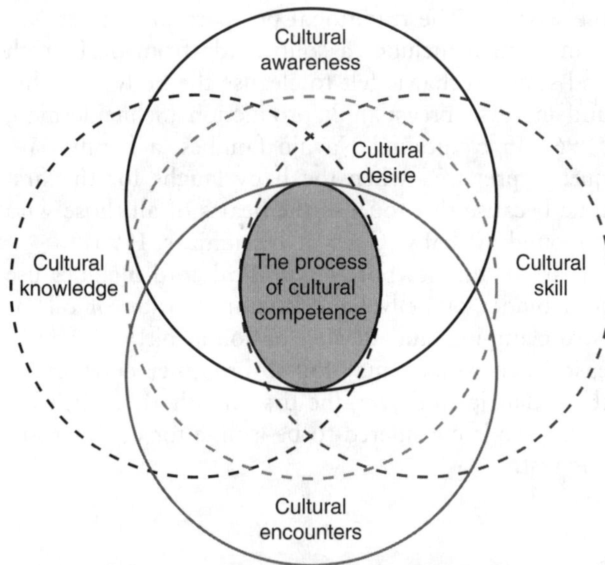

FIGURE 4–5. The process of cultural competence in the delivery of health care services. (From Campinha-Bacote, J. [1994]. *The process of cultural competence in healthcare: A culturally competent model of care.* Wyoming, OH: Transcultural CARE Associates.)

CHILDBEARING AND THE MEANING OF BIRTH

What constitutes a positive and satisfying birth experience varies from one culture to another (Chalmers & Meyer, 1994). For example, within the Japanese culture there is the belief in a process called "education of the unborn." A happy mother is thought to ensure joy and good fortune. Japanese mothers are vigilant during their pregnancy to ensure the health of the fetus because the unborn child learns, communicates, and responds in utero. The individual personality is formed before birth. Such a belief about the fetus is reflected in many cultures, with concern during pregnancy about envious spirits, birthmarks, fertility rites, and beliefs about what determines the sex of the child.

Rich meaning is created by women espousing traditional religious beliefs (Callister, Semenic & Foster, 1999; Khalaf & Callister, 1997; Semenic, Callister, & Foster, 2001). An Orthodox Jewish mother gives silent thanks in the ancient words of the Psalms following the birth of her first-born son. She believes by birthing a son she has fulfilled the reason for her creation in obedience to rabbinical law. The creation of life and giving birth represent obedience to religious law and the spiritual dimensions of the human experience.

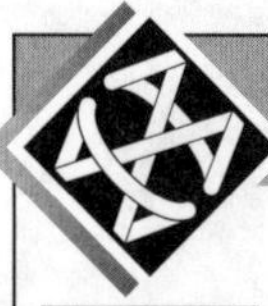

DISPLAY 4–1

Influence of Culture on Pregnancy, Childbirth, and Parenting

- Within the framework of the *moral and value system,* cultural groups have specific *attitudes* toward childbearing and the meaning of the birth experience.
- Within the framework of the *ceremonial and ritual system,* cultural groups have specific *practices* associated with childbearing.
- Within the framework of the *kinship system,* cultural groups prescribe *gender-related roles* for childbearing.
- Within the framework of the *knowledge and belief system,* cultural groups influence *normative behavior* in childbearing and the *pain experience* of childbirth.

Giving birth is an incredibly significant life event, a reflection of a woman's personal values about childbearing and child rearing, the expression and symbolic actualization of the union of the parents (Nichols, 1996). For Muslim women, giving birth fulfills the scriptural injunctions recorded in the Quran. Muslim women may be asked soon after getting married whether they "save anything inside their abdomen yet," meaning "are you pregnant?" Pregnancy in a traditional Asian family is referred to as a woman having "happiness in her body." In Latin America, if you were to ask an expectant mother when her baby is due, the direct translation from Spanish to English is, "When are you going to give to light?"

PRACTICES ASSOCIATED WITH CHILDBEARING

There are many diverse cultural rituals, customs, and beliefs associated with childbearing. American Indian mothers believe tying knots or weaving will cause birth complications associated with cord accidents. Navajo expectant mothers do not choose a name or make a cradleboard because doing so may be detrimental to the well-being of the newborn. Arabic Muslim women do not prepare for the baby in advance (ie, no baby showers, layette accumulation, or naming the unborn child), because such planning has the potential for defying the will of Allah regarding pregnancy outcomes. Filipino women believe that daily bathing and frequent shampoos during pregnancy contributes to having a clean baby. Asian American women may not disclose their pregnancy until the 120th day, when it is believed the soul enters the fetus. In many cultures, girls are socialized early about childbearing. They may witness childbirth or be present when other women repeat their birth stories (Dalle, 1997).

Because of the importance of preserving modesty, Southeast Asian women tie a sheet around themselves like a sarong during labor and express a preference to squat while giving birth. An Italian maternal grandmother may request permission to give her newborn grandson his first bath. After the bath she dresses him in fine, white silk clothing that she stitched by hand for this momentous occasion. When women in Bali hear the first cries of a newborn, they visit the new mother with gifts such as dolls, fruit, flowers, or incense to bless, honor, purify, and protect the new child (Lim, 1997).

The placenta is called *el companero* in Spanish, translated as "the companion of the child" (Vincent, 1995). There are a variety of cultural rituals associated with the disposal of the placenta. These include having it dried, burned, or buried in a specific way (Schneiderman, 1998). Although disposing of the placenta must meet with standard infection control precautions, individual family preferences should be honored as much as possible.

A variety of cultural practices influence postpartum and newborn care. Laotian women stay home the first postpartum month, near a fire or heater to "dry up the womb." The traditional postpartum diet for Korean women includes a soup made from beef broth and seaweed that is felt to cleanse the body of lochia and increase breast milk production (Schneiderman, 1996). In traditional Navajo families, a family banquet is prepared when the baby laughs for the first time because this touches the hearts of all those who surround the baby (Giger & Davidhizar, 1995).

Care of the newborn's umbilical cord includes use of a binder or belly band, the application of oil, or cord clamping, and sterile excision at birth. A Southeast Asian woman may fail to bring her newborn to the pediatrician during the first month after birth because this is considered to be a time for confinement and rest.

GENDER ROLES

Many cultural groups show strong gender preference for a son. For example, according to Confucian tradition, only a son can perform the crucial rites of ancestor worship. A woman's status is often closely tied to her ability to produce a son (Jambunathan & Stewart, 1995; Khalaf & Callister, 1997).

A Mexican-American woman may prefer that her mother or sister be present during her childbirth, rather than the father of her child. In some cultures, fathers may prefer to remain in the waiting room until after the birth. Vietnamese fathers rarely participate in the birth of their children. Only after the newborn is bathed and dressed may the father see him. In cultures in which the husband's presence during birth is not thought to be appropriate, nurses should not assume this denotes lack of paternal involvement and support.

Modesty laws and the law of family purity found in the Torah prohibit the Orthodox Jewish husband from observing his wife when she is immodestly exposed, and from touching her when there is vaginal bleeding. Depending on the specific religious sect, observance of the law varies from the onset of labor or bloody show to complete cervical dilation. Jewish husbands present at birth stand at the head of the birthing bed or behind a curtain in the room and do not observe the birth or touch their wives. In one study, only 37% of Orthodox Jewish husbands attended the birth. Although cultural factors may limit a husband's ability to physically support or coach his wife during labor and birth, Jewish women still feel supported. Husbands praying, reading Psalms, and consulting with the rabbi represent significant and active support to these women (Callister, Semenic, & Foster, 1999; Semenic, Callister, & Foster, 2001).

EXPERIENCES OF PAIN

A major pain experience unique to women is the pain associated with giving birth. Many cultural differences related to the perception of childbirth pain have been identified (Weber, 1996; York, Bhuttarowas, & Brown, 1999). Some women feel that pain is a natural part of childbirth and that the pain experience provides opportunity for important and powerful growth. Others see childbirth pain as no different from the pain of an illness or injury; it is inhumane and unnecessary to suffer.

Words used to describe the pain associated with childbirth vary. Labor pain has been described as horrible to excruciating, episiotomy pain described as discomforting and distressing, and postpartum pain described as mild to very uncomfortable (Lee & Essoka, 1998). Korean women described pain with words such as "felt like dying" or the "sky was turning yellow," or the sense of "tearing apart." Mexican American women view pain as a physical experience, composed of personal, social, and spiritual dimensions (Villarruel, 1995). Scandinavian women demonstrate a high level of resilience and hardiness when giving birth. One Finnish woman spoke of her solitary struggle to meet the increasing pain of her contractions, "We were alone, me and my pain. I focused only on the pain and how I could work with the pain" (Callister, Lauri, & Vehvilainen-Julkenen, 2000, p. 8). Women's perceptions of personal control have been found to positively influence women's satisfaction with pain management during childbirth (McCrea & Wright, 1999).

Pain behaviors also are culturally bound. Mexican-American laboring women may moan in a rhythmic way and rub their thighs and abdomen to manage the pain. In labor, Haitian women are reluctant to accept pain medication and use massage, movement, and position changes to increase comfort. Filipino women believe that noise and activity around them during labor increases labor pain. African American or black women are more vocally expressive of pain. American Indian women are often stoic, using meditation, self control, and traditional herbs to manage pain. Puerto Rican women are often emotive in labor, expressing their pain vocally.

MAJOR CULTURAL GROUPS IN THE UNITED STATES

The major cultural groups in the United States include African American/Blacks (AA/B), American Indian/ Alaska Native (AI/AN), Asian American/Pacific Islanders (AA/PI), Hispanic/Latino (H/L), and white/ Caucasian (W/C). Designation in one of these five categories is not equated with within-group homogeneity. Comparative statistical data are summarized in Table 4–1. The U.S. population by race and ethnic origin is shown in Figure 4–6 (USBC, 1998). The names used to identify these major U.S. cultural groups are those used by the U.S. Census Bureau. The following two modifications were made in the year 2000 census data. The AA/PI category was separated into two categories, Asian American or Native Hawaiian/Pacific Islander, and Latino has been added to the Hispanic category (H/L).

African American or Black

Constituting 12.6% of the population in the United States, this heterogenous group has origins in black racial groups of Africa and the Caribbean Islands, including the West Indies, Dominican Republic, Haiti,

TABLE 4–1 ■ COMPARATIVE STATISTICAL DATA

Group	Infant Mortality (per 100 live births)	Neonatal Mortality (per 100 live births)	Low-Birth-Weight Infants (%)	Preterm Births (%)		First trimester prenatal care (%)	Adequate prenatal care (%)	Maternal Mortality (per 100,000 pregnant women)	Initiating Breast-feeding (%)	Breast-feeding at 6 Months (%)
				<32 Weeks	*32–36 Weeks*					
African American/black	14.6	9.6	13	4	13	70	64	22.1	37	11
American Indian/Alaska native	9.0	3.9	6	2	10	67	57	Numbers too small to calculate	52	24
Asian-American/Pacific Islander	5.3	3.4	7	1	8	78	71	Numbers too small to calculate	Not available	Not available
Hispanic/Latino	6.3	4.1	6	2	9	71	62	6.3	61	20
White/Caucasian	6.3	4.1	6	2	8	84	75	4.2	64	24
Baseline	7.6	4.9	7	9	9	81	73	7.1	60	22

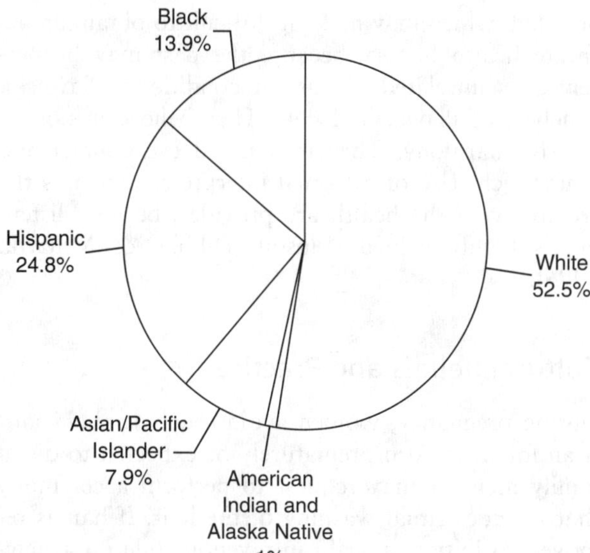

FIGURE 4–6. United States predicted population by race and ethnic origin, 2050.

and Jamaica. AA/B persons may speak French, Spanish, African dialects, and various forms of English. By 2050, the AA/B population is expected to nearly double its present size to 61 million (Jones, 1999). A disproportionate percentage of AA/Bs are disadvantaged because of poverty and low educational levels, and they are more likely to have only public insurance (Agency for Healthcare Policy and Research [AHCPR], 1998). Comparative lifetime pregnancy rates for U.S. women between the ages of 15 and 44 are 2.7 for W/Cs and 4.6 for AA/B and H/L women (Ventura, Mosher, Curtin, Abama, & Henshaw, 1999). Infant mortality rates for AA/Bs have consistently been twice those of the overall population (USDHHS, 1997). As a group, AA/Bs are at increased risk for sickle cell anemia, hypertension, and cancer of the esophagus and the stomach (Spector, 2000).

Core Values

African American/Black families display resilience and adaptive coping strategies in their struggles with racism and poverty (Johnson, 1997). They have a strong religious commitment as observed in Southern Baptist, fundamentalist, and black Muslim church communities. Fifty-one percent of AA/B families are female headed, and more than 55% of all AA/B children younger than 3 years of age are born into single-parent families (Swanson & Nies, 1997). AA/B families have extensive networks of extended families, friends, and neighbors who participate in child rearing with a high level of respect for elders (Friedman, 1998a). Children are highly valued, and as a result of extended family networks, the "mothering" a child receives comes from many sources. An example of this is the active role assumed by the maternal grandmother when an adolescent pregnancy occurs. Becoming a mother at a young age is acceptable. AA/Bs are demonstrative; comfortable with touch, physical contact, and emotional sharing; and have an orientation toward the present.

Providing healthcare to this group may be complicated by folk practices, including the belief that all animate and inanimate objects have good or evil spirits. Healers may include family, a "Granny," or a spiritualist. Folk practices may also include pica (ie, ingestion of nonfood items such as starch, clay, ashes, or plaster) and wearing of garlic, amulets, and copper or silver bracelets (Spector, 2000).

Cultural Beliefs and Practices

African American/Blacks living in poverty may demonstrate a lack of respect or fear of public clinics and hospitals (Bayne-Smith, 1997). They tend to seek prenatal care later then other women, usually after the first trimester (Locks & Boateng, 1996). The incidence of breast-feeding is related to level of maternal education and social support (Locks & Boateng, 1996). AA/B women are more expressive of pain and are usually accompanied during labor and birth by female relatives. Most have their male newborns circumcised.

Haitian women are less likely than other groups to seek prenatal care. During pregnancy, they believe they should not swallow their saliva and instead carry a "spit" cup with them. Fathers are unlikely to be present during birth, believing it is an event for women. Haitian women are encouraged by their community to breastfeed. However, some inaccurate beliefs persist such as "thick" milk causing skin rashes and "thin" milk resulting in diarrhea. During the postpartum period, women may believe that a series of three baths aids in their recovery. The first 3 days, women bathe in a special water prepared by boiling with special herbs. For the next 3 days, women bathe in water in which leaves have been soaked and warmed by the sun. After 1 month, a cold bath is taken that is believed to tighten muscles and bones loosened during the birth process. Women also believe that wearing a piece of linen or a belt tightly around the waist prevents the entry of gas into their body. Eating white foods such as milk, white Lima beans, and lobster are avoided during the postpartum period because they are believed to increase vaginal discharge and hemorrhaging. Traditionally, Haitian women do not have their newborns circumcised because they believe it decreases sexual satisfaction (Colin & Paperwalla, 1996).

West Indian countries of origin are Trinidad, Jamaica, and Barbados. Traditionally, the father of the baby is not present during labor and birth. It is common to breast-feed exclusively. Historically, male circumcision was not practiced, but as acculturation occurs, this procedure is becoming more common (Hill, 1996).

Ethiopian woman are considered to be in a delicate state after birth. To be protected from disease and harm, they remain secluded for at least 40 days. A special diet including milk and warm foods such as a gruel made of oats and honey is thought to increase breast milk production (Beyene, 1996).

American Indian and Alaskan Native

Descendants of the original peoples of North America (ie, American Indian, Eskimo, and Aleut), this group constitutes 0.9% of the population (USDHHS, 1997). There are 500 federally recognized AI nations (Hodge & Frederick, 1999) accessing healthcare from Indian Health Services and/or traditional healers (Seideman, Jacobson, Primeaux, Burns, & Weatherby, 1996). AI/AN have a higher unemployment and poverty rate than the general population. They average 9.6 years of formal education, the lowest rate of any major group in the United States (Swanson & Nies, 1997).

Urban AI/AN have a much higher rate of low-birth-weight infants compared with urban WCs and rural AI/AN and a higher rate of infant mortality than urban W/Cs. Urban AI/AN have a high incidence of risk factors associated with poor birth outcomes including delayed prenatal care, single marital status, adolescent motherhood, and use of tobacco and alcohol. These risk factors resemble the prevalence among AA/Bs except for the higher incidence of alcohol use among AI/AN. Rural AI/AN have lower rates of low-birth-weight infants and higher rates of timely prenatal care than their urban counterparts (Grossman, Krieger, Sugarman, & Forquera, 1994). As a group, AI/AN are at increased risk for alcoholism, heart disease, cirrhosis of the liver, and diabetes mellitus (Spector, 2000).

Core Values

American Indian/Alaskan Natives have a strong spiritual foundation in their lives with a holistic focus on the circular wheel of life. It is important to live in complete harmony with nature. Values include oral traditions passed from generation to generation. Elders play a dominant role in decision-making and AI/AN societies are matrilineal. AI/ANs are present oriented, which may make it difficult to obtain an accurate health history because the past may be perceived as unrelated to current conditions (Plawecki, Sanchez, & Plawecki, 1994). They believe in nonaggressive harmony. They may avoid eye contact and limit touch. Use of a formal interpreter increases the credibility of the healthcare provider, because listening is highly valued (Lipson, Dibble, & Minarik, 1996).

Cultural Beliefs and Practices

During pregnancy, women avoid touching their hair. If an infant is born prematurely or expected to die, a family member may request to perform a ceremony that includes ritual washing of the hair. If hair is removed to initiate a scalp intravenous line on a newborn, some families want the hair returned to them. The mother and newborn remain indoors resting for 20 days or until the umbilical cord falls off. The umbilical cord may be saved, because some AI/ANs believe that it has spiritual significance.

Asian American and Pacific Islander

AA/PIs are people with origins in the Far East, Southeast Asia, the Indian subcontinent, or the Pacific Islands. AA/PIs constitute 3.6% of the population in the United States, projected to be at 8.7% by 2050 (Jones, 1999). There is great diversity in the 28 AA/PI groups designated in the census (Yee, 1997). Asians comprise 95% of this population and are divided into 17 groups, speaking 32 different primary languages, plus multiple dialects. Major groups of AAs include Chinese, Japanese, Koreans, Filipinos, Vietnamese, Cambodians, and Laotians. The major groups, Chinese and Japanese, are the most long-standing groups of Asian immigrants.

Pacific Islanders comprise 5% of AA/PIs, with specific groups including Hawaiian, Samoan, Guamanian, Tongan, Tahitian, North Marianas, and Fijian (Jones, 1999). There are more than 50 subgroups speaking at least 32 different languages (Affonso, 1998). Approximately two thirds of Asians living in the United States are foreign-born (USDHHS, 1998). This group is culturally and linguistically heterogeneous. AA/PI are highly concentrated in the western states and in metropolitan areas.

There is a paucity of data regarding the health status of AA/PIs. Because they are a small minority, AA/PIs are often overlooked in healthcare services planning and research (Hong & Friedman, 1998). In relation to healthcare, AA/PI comprise the most misunderstood, underrepresented, underreported, and understudied ethnic population (Chen, 1997). They are often mistakenly referred to as the healthy minority (USDHHS, 1998). Their educational attainment has a bipolar distribution, with 39% having college degrees and 5% assessed as functionally illiterate (USDHHS, 1998). Posttraumatic stress syndrome is of concern in AA/PI refugee women, especially Hmong women who may have suffered atrocities while living in their country of origin (Chen & Hawks, 1995). Infant mortality rates are highest in Native Hawaiians (11.4/1,000 live births) (Chen, 1997). As a group, AA/PIs are at increased risk of hypertension, liver cancer, stomach cancer, and lactose intolerance (Spector, 2000).

Core Values

Values embody the philosophical traditions of Buddhism, Hinduism, and Christianity. They believe events are predestined and strive for a degree of spirituality in their lives. Core values include cohesive families, filial piety, and respect for the elderly, respect for authority, interdependence and reciprocity, interpersonal harmony and avoidance of disagreement and conflict. Saving face, fatalism, education/achievement orientation, and a strong work ethic are also core values (Hong & Freidman, 1998; Sharts-Hopko, 1995; Yee, 1997).

Asians seldom express strong reactions to emotionally arousing events, and are taught to suppress feelings to maintain harmonious relationships with others. They avoid public displays of affection except among family and close friends and have clearly defined gender roles (Engebretsen, 1997; Holroyd, Yin-king, Poi-yuk, Kwok-hong & Shuk-lin, 1997; Matocha, 1998).

Traditional therapies are often employed concurrently with Western medicine, including acupuncture, herbs, nutrition, and meditation. Asian women may believe Western medicines are too strong and may halve the prescribed dosages (Yee, 1997). Chinese women avoid oral contraceptives because of a perception that hormones may be harmful.

Cultural Beliefs and Practices

Traditional Asian healthcare beliefs and practices are Chinese in origin, with the exception of Filipino beliefs and practices being based primarily on Malaysian culture (Yee, 1997). The yin/yang polarity is a major life force and focuses on the importance of balance for the maintenance of health. Yin represents cold, darkness, and wetness; yang represents heat, brightness, and dryness. For those who subscribe to the hot/cold theory (including Asians and Hispanics), health requires harmony between heat and cold. Balance should be maintained for women to be in harmony with the environment. During pregnancy women eat "cold" foods such as poultry, fish, fruits, and vegetables. Eating "hot" foods at this time such as red peppers, spicy soups, red meat, garlic, ginger, onion, coffee, and sweets is believed to cause abortion or premature labor. A designation of "hot" or "cold" does not necessarily refer to physical temperature but the specific effects the food is believed to have on the body.

Because pregnancy is a "hot" condition, some expectant mothers espousing this theory may be reluctant to take prenatal vitamins that are considered a "hot" medication. Encouraging the woman to take her prenatal vitamins with fruit juice may resolve the problem. Some pregnant Asian women believe that iron hardens bones and makes birth more difficult, and these women resist taking vitamin preparations containing iron (Cantos & Rivera, 1996; Kulig, 1990). Many Southeast Asian women believe that exposure of the genital area is inappropriate because this is considered a sacred part of the body. They may be reluctant to have pap smears, seek prenatal care later, and communicate poorly about physical changes of pregnancy. Sexual intercourse is avoided during the third trimester because it is thought to thicken amniotic fluid, causing respiratory distress in the newborn.

Vaginal exams and an open hospital gown may be deeply humiliating and unnerving to Southeast Asian women who value humility and modesty (Affonso, 1998; Chen, 1997). Giving birth is believed to deplete a woman's body of the "hot" element (blood) and inner energy. This places her in a "cold" state for about 40 days after birth, which is assumed to be the period for the womb to heal (Fok, 1996). Rice, eggs, beef, tea, and chicken soup are foods high in "hotness" and are eaten by postpartum women.

During postpartum, pericare and hygiene are considered important, but women are discouraged from showering for several days to 2 to 4 weeks (Cantos & Rivera, 1996; Farrales, 1996; Kulig, 1990). Most women breast-feed for several years. Women in the Hmong community (originally from Laos) may choose to formula feed, inaccurately believing American women do not breast-feed because they do not see this practice in public like they did in their homelands (Johnson, 1996).

Child rearing occurs within the extended family (Choi, 1995; Howard & Berbiglia, 1997). A newborn's head is considered sacred, the essence of his being. Touching the newborn's head is distressing to parents and should be avoided. Traditionally, newborns have not been circumcised but as acculturation occurs some AA/PIs have adopted this practice.

Cambodian women avoid certain activities during pregnancy such as standing in doorways, because they believe this will cause the baby to become stuck in the birth canal. Sexual intercourse is not permitted during the third trimester. It is thought that avoidance of sexual intercourse during pregnancy will produce a more attractive baby. Vernix caseosa is believed to be sperm. Cambodian woman will not be seen cuddling their newborns; instead, the newborn is held down and away from their body. Herbal medications are prepared during the third trimester to be eaten three to four times per day during the postpartum period to restore body heat. Along with eating special foods that are thought to restore lost heat, mothers wear heavy clothing during the postpartum period. Breast-feeding is delayed for several days because colostrum is thought to be harmful for the newborn (Kulig, 1990).

Filipino women are discouraged from remaining in a dependent position late in pregnancy, because sitting or standing may cause retention of fluid. Sexual intercourse is discouraged for the last 2 months. Women eat eggs, believing that slippery foods help the baby move through the birth canal. Filipino women are accompanied in labor by a woman who has herself given birth (Cantos & Rivera, 1996).

Korean women avoid certain animal foods during pregnancy because they believe these foods can harm the newborn's character or appearance. It is believed that eating duck can cause the newborn to be born with webs between his fingers and that eating eggs causes the child to be born without a spine (Howard & Berbiglia, 1997). Dairy products are not traditionally part of the Korean diet, so care should be taken to ensure women are receiving adequate amounts of calcium during pregnancy. In the Korean culture, the new mother is perceived as being sick and in need of care. Postpartum women do not easily participate in self-care activities or care for their newborn. The husband's mother is responsible for caring for the newborn and the recovery of her daughter-in-law. The need to return the hot element to the body after childbirth is accomplished by eating a special seaweed soup made with beef broth and avoiding anything cold such as ice. The soup is thought to increase breast milk production and rid the body of lochia (Schneiderman, 1996). Korean women may refuse an ice pack or chemical cold pack for control of perineal edema because of the belief that coldness in any form may cause chronic illness such as arthritis. Women who breast-feed are reluctant to offer infants formula supplementation (Howard & Berbiglia, 1997).

Samoan women do not eat octopus or raw fish during pregnancy. In labor, women supporting the laboring woman often gently massage the abdomen of the laboring woman to relieve discomfort and determine the position of the baby (Ishida, Toomata-Mayer, & Mayer, 1996). During the postpartum the abdomen may be bound and abdominal massage performed by the midwife. Women do not carry the newborn after dark or stand in front of windows with the newborn at night. Most women choose to breast-feed, and it is customary to abstain from sexual intercourse while breast-feeding. Generally, males are circumcised.

Vietnamese women must avoid sexual intercourse and be kept warm during their pregnancy. Special hygiene practices include using salt water to wash their teeth and gums (Farrales, 1996).

Hispanic and Latino

H/L women have ethnic origins from countries where Spanish is the primary language, including Mexico, Puerto Rico, Cuba, Spain, and South or Central America. They constitute at least 10.2% of the population in the United States and are the fastest growing ethnic group (Jones, 1999). Spanish is the most common second language spoken in the United States. H/Ls are becoming the largest minority group in the United States; immigration is estimated at one million people per year. Fifty percent of undocumented immigrants are of H/L origin (Jones, 1999). Sixty-two percent are of Mexican origin (Colucciello & Woelfel, 1998). Assimilation is minimal, with strongly held cultural beliefs and behaviors (Balacazar et al., 1997; Jimenez, 1995). Traditional beliefs, values, and customs govern decision-making behaviors.

Significant increases in the H/L population are related to a natural increase (births over deaths) of 1.8%, and a fertility rate 50% higher than W/Cs. Women comprise the largest group among the H/L population in the United States, accounting for an estimated 11 million (dePacheco & Hutti, 1998). Latino women are younger than non-H/L women at the age of first pregnancy (Juarbe, 1995). The fertility rate of H/L women is 84% higher than white women and 31% higher than black women (USDHHS, 1997). Although H/L women are the most likely group of women to have children, they are the least likely to initiate early prenatal care (Conrad, Hollenbach, Fullerton, & Feigelson, 1998; Reichman & Kenney, 1998).

Forty-three percent of H/L births were to unmarried mothers, with adolescents accounting for a large percentage of those births. Two thirds of H/L births are to Mexican-American mothers (Horton, 1995). Unintended pregnancies are more common among H/Ls compared with other ethnic groups, especially among women of low socioeconomic status (Henshaw, 1998). First generation or less acculturated Mexican-American women seem to have a perinatal advantage despite low levels of maternal education, low socioeconomic status, and less than adequate prenatal care. Aspects of their culture that seem to protect them include nutritional intake, lower prevalence of smoking and alcohol consumption, extended family support, and spirituality or a religious lifestyle (Fuentes-Afflick, Hessol, & Perez-Stable, 1998; Heilemann, Lee, Stinson, Korhar, & Goss, 2000; Pollock, 1999; Miska, 1999).

There is a strong association between social support and use of contraception in H/L women (Unger & Molina, 1998). Immigrants usually favor Depo-Provera for family planning. Because there may be much distress and embarrassment about touching and inserting fingers into the vagina, diaphragms are not a good choice for family planning.

Compared with women born in the United States, foreign-born H/L women are more likely to be economically disadvantaged and uninsured, factors usually associated with poor birth outcomes when adjustments were made for maternal and healthcare factors. Although H/Ls represent only 11.6% of the population under age 65, they make up more than 21% of the uninsured population (Agency for Healthcare Policy and Research [AHCPR], 1998). With larger families and inadequate sources of income, more than 30% of H/L families have incomes below the poverty level (Fulwood, 1996). As a group, H/Ls are at higher risk for diabetes mellitus, parasitic disease, and lactose intolerance (Spector, 2000).

Core Values

In the H/L community, there are strong family ties, large and cohesive kin groups, and a family decision-making process. It is believed that the family has a meditating effect on stress (Gaffney, Choi, Jones, & Tavangar, 1997; Miska, 1999). Family values include pride and self-reliance, dignity, trust, intimacy, and respect for older family members and authority figures. H/L women usually consult their husbands, significant others, or other important family members such as godparents about major health decisions (dePacheo & Hutti, 1998). *Curanderismo* or folk medicine is frequently used. Mexican Americans may seek the services of folk healers such as herbalists, bone and muscle therapists, and midwives. These practitioners are more prevalent in border towns and may be used there as an adjunct to the established healthcare systems (Colucciello & Woelfel, 1998).

Cultural Beliefs and Practices

Pregnancy is an important family event engendering extensive physical and emotional support from family members. Motherhood is seen as the most important role a woman can achieve (de Paula, Lagana, & Gonzalez-Ramirez, 1996). Most H/L babies are wanted, cherished, and pampered. They are thought to be untouched by sin and evil (Friedman, 1998b).

H/Ls have a present orientation. This orientation effects how prenatal care is accessed. Women are frequently late for or miss prenatal appointments and may not understand how high-risk behaviors affect their long-term well-being and the well-being of the fetus. H/Ls have a sense of fatalism, believing that their destiny is controlled by fate or by the will of God. Hispanic women may see early prenatal care as unnecessary because pregnancy outcomes are beyond personal control. This sense of fatalism can also promote a sense of vulnerability and lack of control (Giachello, 1997).

During pregnancy, women maintain healthy diets and exercise, and they may take herbs and teas recommended by the herbalist. Certain folk traditions are thought to prevent birth defects. A safety pin attached to an undergarment helps protect the fetus from a cleft lip or palate. If a pregnant woman sees an eclipse (ie, a "bite" taken out of the moon), her unborn child may have a bite taken out of its mouth, resulting in a cleft lip or palate (Callister & Vega, 1998).

Some H/L women believe that unsatisfied cravings cause defects or injury to the fetus. For example, a strawberry nevus is believed to occur because the pregnant woman had an unsatisfied craving for strawberries during her pregnancy. Vitamins and iron are avoided by some women during pregnancy because they are thought to be harmful (de Paula et al., 1996). During labor, women believe that walking makes birth occur more quickly and that inactivity decreases the amount of amniotic fluid and causes the fetus to stick to the uterus, delaying the birth. Cesarean birth is feared and viewed as life threatening for the mother (de Paula et al., 1996).

Postpartum women are discouraged from taking a shower for several days (de Paula et al., 1996). Belief in the "evil eye" means that a fixed stare from a person believed to be envious may result in illness. *La manita de azabache*, a black onyx hand, may be placed on or near the newborn to ward off the envious evil eye (Rodriguez-Trias, 1997). An H/L mother may assume that a nurse who overly praises her newborn or is perceived as staring at the child can cause the child to cry excessively and be very restless. H/L women view colostrum as "bad" or "old" milk and may delay breast-feeding until several days after the birth (Riordan, 1999). Avoiding foods such as chilies and beans is thought to protect the newborn from illness (de Paula et al., 1996). Traditionally, circumcision has not been practiced, but as acculturation occurs, this practice is becoming more acceptable.

White or Caucasian

W/Cs have origins in Europe, North Africa, or the Middle East and constitute 83% of the population of the United States. There are 53 ethnic groups classified as W/C living in the United States (Jones, 1999). In many ways, W/Cs are perceived as being privileged. For example, there are substantial differences in sources of prenatal care, with 78% of W/C women receiving private care compared with 51% of Mexican-American women, 44% of AA/B women, and 47% of Puerto Rican women (Gardner, Cliver, McNeal, & Goldenberg, 1996).

W/Cs are generally acknowledged to be the dominant culture rather than a designation of "non-culture." This cultural group seems intent on accomplishments achieved in a short period contributing to a high-energy, high-stress lifestyle compared with other cultural groups that have more peaceful ways of life. Predominant belief systems accept the Western biotechnologic model of healthcare, but paradoxically, childbearing women want nurturing, supportive, and meaningful care (Callister, Vehvilainen-Julkunen, & Lauri, 1996; Callister, Lauri, & Vehvilainen-Julkinen 2000).

Core Values

Core values include individualism, self-reliance, personal achievement and independence, democratic ideals and egalitarianism, work, productivity, and materialism, punctuality, and future time orientation, as well as openness, assertiveness, and directness in communication.

NONTRADITIONAL CULTURAL GROUPS

Cultures are not limited to the obvious traditional ethnic or racial groups. Examples of other "cultures" include refugees and immigrants, the culture of poverty, women who have experienced ritual circumcision, and deeply religious women.

Immigrant and Refugee Women

Immigrant women are coping with tremendous cultural differences, personal and family development, and issues related to making transitions that may be extremely stressful (Catolico, 1997; Fraktman, 1998; Mattson, 1995; Stewart & Jambunathan, 1996). As first generation new Americans, these women have stronger ties to cultural traditions and customs than second- or third-generation Americans. For instance, they may have given birth previously in their home attended by a traditional midwife and their mother or mother-in-law. The biotechnologic environment of birthing units in the United States may be foreign and frightening (Davis-Floyd & Sargent, 1997; Downs, Bernstein, & Marchese, 1997). There may be a deep sadness for these mothers as they give birth without the assistance of their own mothers (Fraktman, 1998). Many immigrants and refugees are migrant farm workers, living in unsanitary, unsafe, and crowded conditions. Language, limitations in literacy, and cultural barriers have a negative impact on access to healthcare.

As conservators of family health, the role of immigrant women in health promotion is critical. Refugees are eligible for special refugee medical assistance during their first 18 months in the United States. After this initial coverage, those who cannot afford private health insurance and are ineligible for Medicaid benefits may become medically indigent. Limitations in literacy and language make it difficult to enter the healthcare system. Feelings of fear and paranoia creates circumstances where these women are unwilling to access care (Ferran, Tracy, Gany, & Kramer, 1999; Taylor, Ko, & Pan, 1999).

Ritually Circumcised Women

It is estimated that at least 130 million women throughout the world have been ritually circumcised. Immigrants and refugee women from developing countries in Asia (ie, Malaysia, India, Yemen, and Oman) and 28 African countries may have experienced female genital mutilation. Genital mutilation may occur at any point between the newborn period and the time a woman gives birth to her first child (Wright, 1996). These women experience extreme pain and complications during childbirth because the inadequate vaginal opening and scarring may prevent cervical dilatation and fetal passage. After giving birth in their native counties, some women experience reinfibulation (ie, suturing together of the labia) (World Health Organization, 1997). Because female circumcision is a culturally bound rite of choice, women may resent Western attitudes about this practice. Perinatal nurses need to create an environment of trust, establish rapport with male family members, ensure privacy, and be sensitive to the stoicism demonstrated toward childbirth pain (Reichert, 1998).

Deeply Religious Women

A variety of religious and spiritual beliefs and practices influence childbearing (Schott & Henley, 1996). Orthodox Jews have a rich body of traditions associated with childbearing and great reverence for childbearing and child rearing. Some Jewish women feel a moral responsibility to bring just "one more child into the world" because of the destruction of their ancestors during the Holocaust (Semenic et al., 2001). Circumcision is a Jewish ritual based on a Hebrew covenant in the Old Testament (Genesis 17:10–14). It is performed on all male children by a mohel (ie, skilled circumcisionist) on the eighth day of life (de Sevo, 1997).

For Islamic women, creating an environment that honors traditional practices according to the precepts of Islam is important. Islamic women practice a cleansing process at the end of each menstrual period (Rajaram & Rashidi, 1999). Palestinian refugee women feel a strong obligation to bear a significant number of children, especially sons, to continue the generations of the Arabic bloodline (Khalaf & Callister, 1997). A woman espousing the beliefs of the Church of Jesus Christ of Latter-day Saints (Mormon) may request her husband to lay his hands on her head and give her a blessing for strength, comfort, and well-being as she labors and gives birth (Callister, 2000). Mexican-American women often speak in terms of a person's soul or spirit (*alma* or *espiritu*) when referring to one's inner qualities (Rojas, 1996).

The sacred day of worship varies. Sunday is the Sabbath for most Christians. The Muslim's holy day is sunset Thursday to sunset Friday. Jews and Seventh Day Adventists celebrate the Sabbath from sunset on Friday to sunset on Saturday. For an Orthodox Jewish woman, honoring the Sabbath may mean not raising the head of the bed to breast-feed and not turning on the call light to request assistance. In the Orthodox culture, these acts would constitute "work." Table 4–2 provides common religious dietary prohibitions.

There is a strong relationship between health status and spiritual well-being (Rojas, 1996). Religiosity and a spiritual lifestyle have been found to be the source of powerful strength during childbearing, especially when complications occur such as fetal or neonatal demise (Miller, 1995). Spiritual beliefs and religious affiliations are effective coping mechanisms and sources of support (Callister & Khalaf, 2001; Callister et al., 1999; Rehm, 1999).

TABLE 4–2 ■ RELIGIOUS DIETARY PROHIBITIONS

Religion	Dietary Prohibitions
Hinduism	All meats are prohibited.
Islam	Pork and alcoholic beverages are prohibited.
Judaism	Pork, predatory fowl, shellfish, and blood by ingestion (eg, blood sausage, raw meat) are prohibited. Foods should be kosher (meaning "properly preserved"). All animals should be ritually slaughtered to be kosher. Mixing dairy and meat dishes at the same meal is prohibited.
Mormonism (Church of Jesus Christ of Latter-day Saints)	Alcohol, tobacco, coffee, and tea are prohibited.
Seventh-Day Adventism	Pork, certain seafood (including shellfish), and fermented beverages are prohibited. A vegetarian diet is encouraged.

BIOLOGIC AND PHYSIOLOGIC VARIATIONS BETWEEN GROUPS

There is a paucity of research identifying health differences among minority groups and the prevalence of illness among specific populations of childbearing women. As far as body structure is concerned, AA/PIs typically have small for gestational age neonates. Birth weight is lower in AA/B newborns, but size for size, they are more mature for gestational age. AA/B newborns have a mean 9 days' shorter gestation period than other ethnic groups, and there is a slowing of intrauterine growth in black infants after 35 weeks' gestation. Neonatal body proportions differ in racial groups, genetically conforming to the mother's pelvic shape (Overfield, 1985).

Mongolian spots are commonly found in AA/B, AA/PI, AI/NA, and H/L infants. Dermal practices among Southeast Asian refugees may be noticed during a physical assessment and assumed to be a sign of physical abuse. An example of a cultural practice that may be misinterpreted is "cupping." In this practice, a cup is heated and placed on the skin, leaving a circular ecchymotic area. Pinching and rubbing may produce bruises or welts. Rubbing the skin with a spoon or coin produces dermal changes. Touching a burning cigarette to the skin may also represent cultural self-care (Spector, 2000).

Chemical substances are metabolized differently from one group to another. There is an increasing incidence of alcoholism among H/Ls and AA/Bs, but Asians have the lowest alcoholism rate (Grossman et al., 1994). Most Asians and AI/NAs experience a rapid onset but slow decrease in blood acetaldehyde levels, leaving long periods of exposure to substances causing alcohol intoxication. Fetal alcohol syndrome or its effect is highest among AI/NAs. Caffeine is metabolized and excreted faster by W/Cs than Asians. The incidence of lactose intolerance is 94% in AA/PI, 90% in AA/Bs, 79% in AI/NA, 50% in H/Ls, and 17% in W/Cs. This can have a negative effect on breast-feeding, because infants may be lactose intolerant as well.

The Rh negative factor, common in Caucasians, is rare in other groups (especially Asians) and essentially absent in Eskimos. There is a high incidence of diabetes in AI tribes, whereas the disease is rare in Alaskan Eskimos (Overfield, 1985). The prevalence of insulin-dependent diabetes mellitus (IDDM) is highest among AA/Bs. Gestational diabetes mellitus (GDM) occurs in 20% of pregnant women and is not affected by race or culture.

Communicable diseases that threaten foreign-born and new immigrants, particularly those from China, Korea, the Philippines, Southeast Asia, and the Pacific, are tuberculosis and hepatitis B. Among these women, hepatitis B has a prevalence of 8% to 22%, compared with 2% for women living in the United States. Fifty percent of women who give birth to hepatitis B carrier infants in the United States are Asian foreign-born women (Chen, 1997). There is a significantly higher incidence of tuberculosis in AI/ANs and foreign born AA/PIs. The incidence of tuberculosis is four times higher among Asians than the overall population (Krotoski & Silliman, 1997). AA/PI and AI/AN women diagnosed with tuberculosis tend to be of childbearing age (Chen, 1997).

There is a higher incidence of hypertension in AA/Bs and H/Ls. The incidence of lupus is four times higher in AA/B women and twice as prevalent in H/L than in nonHispanic W/C women (Horton, 1995). Native Hawaiian and Samoan women are reported to be the most obese in the world (Chen, 1997). Sickle cell anemia occurs predominately in AA/Bs. Tay-Sachs disease is predominately found in Hasidic Jews of Eastern European descent, particularly Ashenazi and Sephardi women. Thalassemia is a genetic blood disorder found in women from the Mediterranean region, the Middle East, and Southeast Asia (Chen, 1997).

BARRIERS TO INTEGRATING CULTURE INTO NURSING CARE

Barriers to culturally competent care include values, beliefs, and customs; communication challenges; and the biomedical healthcare environment.

Differences in Values, Beliefs, and Customs

Ethnocentrism is the belief that one's own ways are the best, superior, the only way. *Cultural imposition* is the tendency to impose one's beliefs, values, and patterns of behaviors on another culture. Characteristics of caregivers that influence their ability to be culturally competent include educational level, multicultural exposure, personal attitudes and values, and professional experiences. Identifying and understanding the childbearing woman's attitudes, behaviors, values, and needs assists the perinatal nurse in identifying interventions that are culturally appropriate; acceptable to healthcare providers, the women, and their families; have the potential to increase adherence to therapeutic regimens; and will over time result in constructive changes in perinatal healthcare delivery (Jackson, 1997).

Nurses demonstrate various levels of commitment when caring for culturally diverse women on a continuum from resistant care to generalist care, to impassioned care (Kirkham, 1998). Nurses who are resistant judge behaviors, ignore client needs, and complain. Resistant nurses may ignore or resent culturally diverse women and their families. Culture is seen as an inconvenience or problem. Nurses who provide generalist care are respectful and competent but do not differentiate cultural diversities. Culture is a nonissue. They may empathize with client experiences but don't feel empowered to bring about substantial change. Racist attitudes of colleagues are tolerated. Nurses who provide impassioned care have a high degree of personal commitment to provide culturally sensitive care. These nurses go beyond accommodation to an appreciation of cultural diversity.

They are aware of the complexities of cultural competence and the variability of expressions within cultural groups. Creativity and flexibility are the hallmarks of the care they provide to culturally diverse clients. They feel empowered to make a difference through their clinical practice. Display 4–2 provides the characteristics of the culturally competent nurse.

It is essential that the nurse examines his or her own cultural beliefs, biases, attitudes, stereotypes, and prejudice and asks, "Whose birth is it anyway?" The following story is told by Khazoyan and Anderson (1994, p. 226).

> Señor Rojas sat at the bedside of his laboring wife, held her hand, and spoke soft, encouraging words to her. This was the kind of support that she desired during her labor: his presence, his attention, and his affection. Following the birth of their child, Senora Rojas expressed contentment and proudly described the support that her husband had provided. He had met her expectations. The nurses, however, expected more. They had wanted Señor Rojas to participate more actively in his wife's labor by massaging her back and assisting her with breathing techniques.

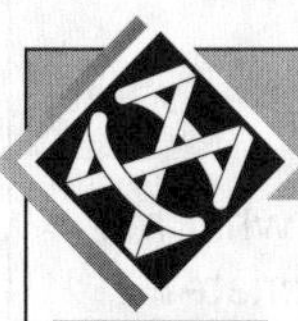

DISPLAY 4–2

Characteristics of the Culturally Competent Practitioner

- Moves from cultural unawareness to an awareness and sensitivity to her or his own cultural heritage
- Recognizes her or his own values and biases and is aware of how they may affect clients from other cultures
- Demonstrates comfort with cultural differences that exist between herself/himself and clients
- Knows specifics about the particular cultural groups she or he is working with
- Understands the historic events that may have caused harm to particular cultural groups
- Respects and is aware of the unique needs of patients from diverse communities
- Understands the importance of diversity within and between cultures
- Endeavors to learn more about cultural communities through patient interactions, participation in cultural diversity workshops and community events, readings on cultural dynamics, and consultations with community experts
- Makes a continuous effort to understand the other's point of view
- Demonstrates flexibility and tolerance of ambiguity and is nonjudgmental
- Maintains a sense of humor and an open mind
- Demonstrates a willingness to relinquish control in clinical encounters, to risk failure, and to look within for the source of frustration, anger, and resistance
- Acknowledges that the process is as important as the product

Adapted from Rorie, J.L., Paine, L.L. & Barger, M.K. (1996). Cultural competence in primary care services. *Journal of Nurse Midwifery, 41*(2), 92–100.

Communication Challenges

Communication between cultures (or lack of communication) occurs whenever a message produced in one culture must be processed into another culture. A significant barrier to culturally competent care is language and the lack of bilingual personnel and staff with culturally diverse backgrounds (Villarruel, 1999). Hospitals frequently enlist nonprofessional employees of the client's ethnic background to act as interpreters. These individuals are often unfamiliar with English medical terminology and may not be able to translate accurately. Interpreters who are members of the client's cultural group may be of a different social class than the client or may be more acculturated and anxious to appear part of the dominant culture. In some cases, interpreters may be disdainful or dismissive of the client's belief system. Using children or other family members to interpret may also lead to problems.

Healthcare Environment

This barrier includes bureaucracy (eg, difficulties with the dietary department to provide culturally appropriate diets), nonsupportive administration, lack of educational opportunities on cultural diversity, lack of translators, and rigid policies and protocols that do not support cultural diversity. Consider how difficult it is for the woman who may be living in the United States without the support of extended family (especially female family members), speaking little or no English, having limited understanding of the dominant culture, having little education, and working in a low-skills level job without benefits (Denman-Vitale & Murillo, 1999). When this woman arrives at the birthing unit, an unfamiliar environment and procedures serve only to increase her stress (Fouche, Fourie, Schoon, & Barn, 1998).

TECHNIQUES TO INTEGRATE CULTURE INTO NURSING CARE

Standards for the Joint Commission for Accreditation of Healthcare Organizations (JCAHO, 2000) suggest that understanding the cultural context in which a patient lives is important to fully appreciate their response to illness and is necessary for planning appropriate nursing and medical interventions. It is essential that culturally competent care be integrated into all standards of practice. Becoming culturally competent is a developmental process. As nurses become more sensitive to the issues surrounding healthcare and the traditional health beliefs of the women they care for, more culturally competent healthcare will be provided (Clark, 1999; Cooper, 1996).

When the cultural expectations of nurse and patient collide, both are left feeling frustrated and misunderstood. The woman's adherence to traditional practices may be seen as strange and backward to the nurse, who responds by trying to "fit" the woman into the biotechnologic Western system. For example, an AI/NA mother may avoid eye contact and fail to ask questions or breast-feed in the presence of the mother–baby nurse. For many women, including Southeast Asian women, there is "loss of face" because she feels she is responsible for confusion and cultural conflict between herself and the nurse who is perceived as a social superior. This experience may discourage her from future contact with healthcare professionals (Davis-Floyd & Sargent, 1997). Display 4–3 provides the components of a cultural assessment.

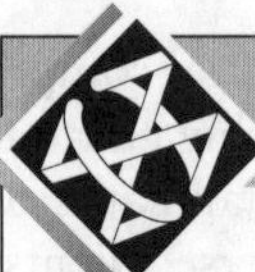

DISPLAY 4–3

Cultural Assessment of the Childbearing Woman

- How is childbearing valued?
- Is childbearing viewed as a normal physiologic process, a wellness experience, a time of vulnerability and risk, or a state of illness?
- Are there dietary, nutritional, pharmacologic, and activity prescribed practices?
- Is birth a private intimate experience or a societal event?
- How is childbirth pain managed, and what maternal and paternal behavior is appropriate?
- What support is given during pregnancy, childbirth and beyond, and who appropiately gives that support?
- How is the newborn viewed, and what are the patterns regarding care of the infant and relationships within the nuclear and extended families?
- What maternal precautions or restrictions are necessary during childbearing?
- What does the childbearing experience mean to the woman?

From Callister, L.C. (1995). Cultural meanings of childbirth. *Journal of Obstetric, Gynecologic, and Neonatal Nursing, 24* (3), 327–331.

Enhancing Communication Skills

Display 4–4 contains suggestions for communicating effectively with childbearing women and their families. It is important to remember that effective communication requires a sincere desire to understand the other person's way of seeing the world and acting (Nance, 1995). Cultural reciprocity occurs when a woman feels that she has permission to share her cultural needs, concerns, and feelings. Respect and sensitivity characterize this kind of relationship. A perinatal nurse described the following experience:

> I cared for a Mexican-American woman in perinatal testing. I was able to help her out by being her translator. Modesty was a big issue with her, and she was extremely uncomfortable with undoing her pants and showing her abdomen for the procedure. I felt that there was a unique bond and friendship that was created because of my understanding and sensitivity of her cultural values. It makes all the difference to the woman if she is able to communicate with you and you can convey that you really care.

Be considerate, polite, and speak softly. Caring behaviors and personal attention from healthcare providers are important to individuals of all cultures. Spend a few minutes talking to the woman and her family as she is admitted to the unit to build rapport. Just a greeting and knowing a few of the social words in the woman's language and use of culturally specific etiquette helps to establish rapport. It is essential to understand cultural communication patterns. For example, Native Americans may maintain silence and do not interrupt others. Hispanics appreciate interactions beginning with personal conversation or "small talk," which serves to promote trust (dePacheo & Hutti, 1998).

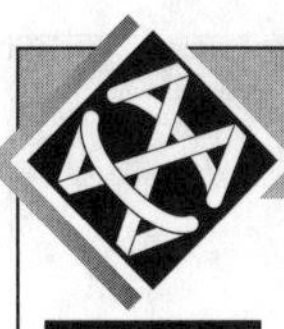

DISPLAY 4–4

Culturally Competent Communication

- Enhance communication skills.
- Develop linguistic skills.
- Determine who the family decision makers are.
- Understand that agreement does not indicate comprehension.
- Use nonverbal communication.
- Use appropriate names and titles.
- Use culturally appropriate teaching techniques.

Developing Linguistic Skills

Learning a second language is an excellent way to lower cultural barriers. A nurse described her experience caring for a Mexican-American laboring woman:

> When I stepped into the room and began to speak in my high-school-level Spanish, her face brightened and she quickly responded in a rapid flow of unintelligible (to me) foreign syllables. Soon, we were able to communicate quite well, and I became comfortable with her. I translated the physician's words and vice versa. I rubbed her leg and stroked her hair when she cried out or moaned. I'd then ask her about the pain and reassured her as much as I could.

Pay attention to changing trends in language and incorporate them into your spoken and written language. Avoid using complex words, medical terms, and jargon that are difficult to understand in any language. Keep instructions simple and repeat as necessary.

Saying "I understand" may be patronizing. Speak slowly, distinctly, and try to appear unhurried. Speak simply, and state your message sentence by sentence. Find creative ways to convey information. One mother–baby nurse described caring for a woman who spoke no English:

> I was left with hand gestures and body language for communication. It was very difficult for her to understand my actions. Her assessment was especially hard because I was unable to assess her pain, bleeding, and nipple tenderness adequately. I finally found a Spanish to English health dictionary, but this was of limited help to me because I was so bad at pronouncing the words that she still had a very difficult time understanding me. Finally, I just let her read the words from the dictionary. This was the most effective way of communicating that I could come up with. I know that she felt somewhat isolated because she had a difficult time communicating her needs to me also.

Determining Who Makes Family Decisions

Ask women whom they wish to include in their birth experience and make sure those persons are present for all discussions and participate in decision-making. Families fulfill several roles for women that include providing security and support, caregivers, advocates, and liaisons (Kennedy, DeVoe, Ramer-Henry, & West-Kowalski, 1999). Families should be treated respectfully with the goal of establishing trust. For some cultural groups, conversation should be directed toward a specific family member. It is important to identify a spokesperson in the family, often the family member most proficient in English. Ask about family roles and respect the preferences of the woman and her family. When a Mexican-American woman was asked if she wanted an epidural, the husband answered, saying it was better to have the baby unmedicated. The wife complied with this suggestion, and the nurse modeled support for the laboring woman and demonstrated respect for their decision.

For example, understanding the role of different family members in the Korean family system is important, because a woman's mother-in-law traditionally cares for her and the newborn during the postpartum period. The nurse needs to recognize that any teaching she does must include the mother-in-law.

Agreement May Not Indicate Comprehension

The woman may pretend to understand to please the nurse and gain acceptance. The woman's smile may mask confusion, and her nod of assent or "a-huh" may mean only that she hears, not that she understands or agrees. For example, a new mother who did not speak English was admitted to the mother–baby unit on the night shift. When asked if she were voiding sufficient amounts, she responded "yes." In the early morning hours, the mother began to complain of intense abdominal pain. She was catheterized and drained of more than 1200 mL of urine. The nurse made an incorrect assumption.

Nonverbal Communication

Use eye contact, friendly facial expressions, and face-to-face positions. Do not assume the woman dislikes you, does not trust you, or is not listening to you because she avoids eye contact. Koreans, Filipinos, and many other Asian groups, as well as NI/AIs, consider direct eye contact rude and confrontational. Islamic women are taught to lower their gaze with members of the opposite sex. Use touch to express caring and comfort. Nonverbal communication makes an important difference. A labor and delivery nurse said,

> I cared for a Korean first time mother who came to the hospital fully dilated and gave birth to her son unmedicated. She did not speak any English, and her young husband was obviously uncomfortable and had little understanding about what was going on. As she gave birth, I could see the pain on her face, but she was stoic. I felt powerless because of her language and cultural barriers, but I stayed with her and held her hand and encouraged her. Even though she could not understand words, I hope she understood that I really cared.

Use universally understood language, such as charades (acting out), drawings, gestures, repeating the message several times in different words, and common words. Use of simple words that are easily translated serves to improve communication (McCaffery, 1999).

Use of Names and Titles

Determine how the childbearing woman and her family wish to be addressed. Names and appropriate titles are often complex and confusing. Mexican-American clients appreciate being addressed by their last name. In the Korean culture, family members are addressed in terms of their relationship to the youngest child in the family (eg, "Sung's grandmother").

Teaching Techniques

Use visual aids and demonstrations, and assist with return demonstrations. Do not assume that the woman can read or write. Ensure that teaching or educational materials can be understood by the client and are appropriate for the woman's cultural group and educational level. Display 4–5 contains suggestions for beginning the process of developing culturally appropriate patient education material (Freda, 1997; Salt 1997). Appendix 4A contains a sampling of culturally specific educational resources.

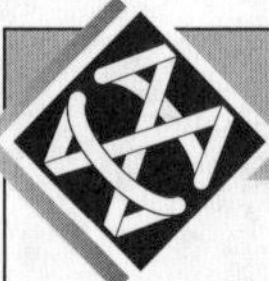

DISPLAY 4–5

Developing Culturally Appropriate Educational Material

- Be aware of your own assumptions and biases.
- Develop an understanding of the target culture, including core values.
- Work with a multicultural team.
- Develop materials in the native language rather than having materials translated.
- Have materials reviewed by members of the target cultural group.

Accommodating Cultural Practices

Stereotypical generalization involves two different dynamics; stereotyping and generalizing. Stereotypes, or believing that something is the same for everyone in a group, should be avoided. Generalizations, however, must be made to understand potential cultural beliefs and practices. The goal of individualizing care is to achieve a balance between what is indigenous to the culture and what may be specific to an individual woman. An experience that made one nurse sensitive to differences among women within the same culture was when she assumed that birth in H/L culture was exclusively a woman's experience, with little involvement by the father of the baby. She said,

> When I helped a Hispanic couple having their first baby, much to my surprise the father was right in there coaching his wife. So I supported his efforts and tried to make the birth experience what they wanted it to be.

If in doubt, ask. A culturally competent labor and delivery nurse described the following experience with a Muslim family:

> I asked the father if there was anything I should know about their customs, and he told me that, before anyone could handle the baby, [besides the physician], the father had to hold the baby and whisper a prayer into the ear of the baby to protect the baby from evil. I told him that as long

as there were no problems with the baby immediately after birth, I would hand him the baby, and if there were problems, he could "do his thing" while the baby was under the warmer and stabilized. He agreed to that. There were no problems, and the father got his wishes and I had the opportunity to attend a wonderfully rich cultural birth.

One Muslim husband stayed with his wife 24 hours each day during her hospitalization. The husband observed the tradition of prayers five times each day, which is a religious duty specified in the Holy Quran. It was challenging for the nurse as she walked into the room when he was praying on the floor on his prayer mat, but she did all she could to support these religious rituals.

In many cultures, there is a gender preference for male children. For example, a Korean mother gave birth to a healthy baby girl. Her husband was an active, supportive coach during the labor and vaginal birth. When he saw the baby girl, however, his demeanor changed, and he shouted at his wife and started to cry. The mother also cried and refused to hold or look at her newborn daughter. The father left the room, and the mother became subdued but still refused to hold the baby. Later, the nurse commented about the beautiful infant, referring to her not as a "baby girl" but as "the baby." The mother asked to hold her child. The father came back into the room, and the nurse told him his baby was perfect and beautiful. This reinforcement seemed to appease the father, who then held his infant.

It is essential to respect the wisdom of other cultures. Healthcare beliefs and practices can be divided into three categories; potentially beneficial, harmless or neutral behaviors, and those that may be potentially harmful. Examples in each category are listed in Table 4–3. Preservation of potentially helpful beliefs or practices and harmless or neutral behaviors that respect the natural wisdom of the culture should be encouraged, valued, and celebrated. Beneficial as well as harmless or neutral practices and those of unknown efficacy may increase a woman's connection to her own historical and cultural roots. For example, an East Indian pregnant woman may softly sing songs passed from generation to generation, massaging her abdomen several times a day and continuing that practice with her infant through the first year of life. Energy should be focused on changing harmful practices. For example, the motivator for a pregnant woman to discontinue a harmful practice, such as the use of certain herbs or smoking, is to appeal to her protective instincts toward her unborn child.

TABLE 4–3 ■ PERINATAL CULTURAL PRACTICES

Potentially Helpful	Harmless or Neutral	Potentially Harmful
Postpartum diet, hygiene practices	Avoidance of sexual activity during menstruation	Avoiding bathing during menstruation
Carrying the infant close in a sling	Prohibition of sexual intercourse during lactation	Avoiding iron supplements during pregnancy because of the belief that iron causes hardening of the bones and a hard labor
Breast-feeding on demand	Yarn tied around the middle finger to give hope and signify spiritual wholeness	Belief that colostrum is "dirty" or "old" and unfit for the newborn
Spacing of children by long-term breast-feeding	Keeping the mother's head covered at all times with a scarf or a wig	Prolonged bed rest after birth
Remaining active throughout labor		Placing a raisin on the umbilical cord to prevent air from entering the newborn's body
Giving birth in nonrecumbent positions	Not allowing the newborn to see his image in a mirror	Use of abdominal binders to prevent umbilical hernia
Swaddling a newborn to maintain warmth	Garlic charm around the baby's neck to offer protection from the "evil eye"	
	Eating of garlic to prevent illness	

It is essential to show genuine interest and appreciation. The culturally competent nurse seeks to understand the woman's unique way of experiencing birth and expressing what birth means. Failure of the nurse to demonstrate interest and caring toward cultural practices she does not understand causes women to lose confidence in the nurse and the larger healthcare system and may decrease adherence with suggested health promotion strategies (Zoucha, 1998).

LONG-TERM STRATEGIES

Changes are needed in nursing education, healthcare delivery, and in nursing research to increase cultural competence in perinatal nursing practice.

Nursing Education

Most nursing students have little knowledge about any culture other than their own. Changes in basic nursing education programs would begin to increase cultural competence. National nursing education standards require that educational programs prepare nurses to understand the effect cultural, racial, socioeconomic, religious, and lifestyle differences have on health status and responses to health and illness (American Association of Colleges of Nursing [AACN], 1998). Graduates should have the knowledge and skills to provide holistic care to a variety of diverse cultures. Nursing education should expose students to culturally diverse clients in a variety of settings; include theoretical and factual information about cultural groups; identify strategies and skills useful in providing nursing care to culturally diverse clients; allow students the opportunity to examine their own personal values and attitudes; and encourage linguistic skills in a second language (Lenburg et al., 1995).

Healthcare Delivery

Most healthcare systems in the United States exhibit "cultural blindness," ignoring differences as if they do not exist. Healthcare in the United States is a culture unto itself based on the dominant Western biomedical model of health beliefs and practices. In most hospitals, only "American" food is served, and there is a universal assumption that everyone seeking healthcare understands English. Nurses are in a position to challenge institutional forces that may inhibit culturally sensitive care. Suggestions include those generated by participants at the 1998 AWHONN Intrapartum Practice Summit (Display 4–6). Strategies for changing perinatal nursing unit milieu to increase cultural competence were proposed at the AWHONN 1998 Intrapartum Practice Summit (Display 4–7). Helpful communication strategies for use within a multicultural healthcare team are summarized in Display 4–8 (Giger & Mood, 1997).

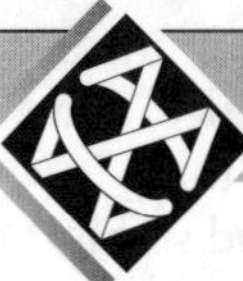

DISPLAY 4-6

Changing Institutional Forces to Facilitate Culturally Competent Care

- Changing birthing room policies and unit protocols to promote individualized and family-centered care
- Lobbying for increased resources such as translation services and cultural mediators
- Designing continuing education opportunities to increase cultural competence
- Hiring a nursing staff reflecting the culture of the community
- Generating a pool of volunteer translators who meet women prenatally and follow them through their births and the postpartum period
- Increasing the availability of language line services
- Developing innovative programs addressing the unique needs of culturally diverse populations and integrating community and acute care services for childbearing women and their families

Nursing Research

Culturally sensitive scholarship is essential (Meleis, 1996). Many cultures are silent or invisible minorities because of the lack of research on their health needs, status, beliefs, behavior, and family roles (Castillo, 1996). Cross-cultural comparative studies of childbirth demonstrate that much of the information available is medically oriented or narrowly anthropologic in focus (Jordan, 1993).

There is a need for qualitative approaches to research, with women as participants or coinvestigators rather than study subjects. Qualitative approaches include focus groups with a bilingual discussion leader, or participative research in which results are returned rapidly to participants to improve service. Such approaches are empowering and give legitimacy to health-

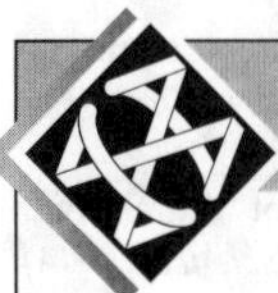

DISPLAY 4-7

Strategies Fostering Culturally Competent Care on Perinatal Nursing Units

- Educational offerings on ethnic, religious, cultural, and family diversity
- Educational offerings about available community resources
- Literature searches focused on the predominant cultural groups cared for, followed by development of a resource binder available on the unit
- Generating a culture database
- Establishing a task force to create culturally sensitive birth plans for the predominant cultural groups cared for
- Establishing cultural competencies that are part of the yearly staff evaluation
- Making cultural competence part of the interview process
- Supporting each other in frustrating situations
- Nursing grand rounds focusing on cultural issues
- Celebrating successes by peers in providing culturally competent care
- Sharing resources such as books and professional journal articles
- Discouraging negativism and discrimination on the unit
- Creating connections between community and acute care settings

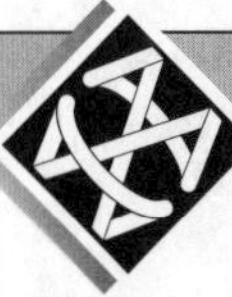

DISPLAY 4-8

Communication Within a Multicultural Health Care Team

- Assess the personal beliefs of members
- Assess communication variables from a cultural perspective
- Modify communication patterns to enhance communication
- Identify mannerisms that may be threatening and avoid using them
- Understand that respect for others and the needs they communicate is central to positive working relationships
- Use validating techniques when communicating
- Be considerate of a reluctance to talk when the subject might involve culturally taboo topics, such as sexual matters
- Use team members from a different culture as resources, but do not support a dependency by the team on those members
- Support team efforts to plan and adapt care based on communicated needs and cultural backgrounds of individual patients
- Identify potential interpreters for patients whenever necessary in order to improve communication

Adapted from Giger, J.N., & Mood, L.H. (1997). Cultural competent teamwork. In *Cultural diversity in nursing: Issues, strategies, and outcomes* (pp. 13–19). Washington DC: American Academy of Nursing.

care issues of culturally diverse women (Sword, 1999). The ideal research team includes members (ie, insiders) of the culture under study as well as nonmembers (ie, outsiders). Multidisciplinary research teams that include transcultural nurses, nurse anthropologists, sociologists, and others are effective.

There are cultural issues of specific interest to women that have the potential to improve the quality of nursing care provided to women and their quality of life. One understudied area is the measurement of biologic and physiologic differences in cultural, ethnic, and racial groups of women. Studies also are needed on the sexual and emotional complications of genital mutilation (American Medical Association Council on Scientific Affairs, 1995). Another important research priority is intervention studies designed to measure the effectiveness of strategies for providing healthcare to vulnerable populations of culturally diverse women.

SUMMARY

Nurses caring for childbearing women should be respectful of women's cultural diversity and the societal context of their lives (American Academy of Nursing [AAN], 1997). Perinatal nurses should seek to create a healthcare encounter with the childbearing woman that respects the sociocultural and spiritual context of her life and moves beyond the superficial to understand the deeper meaning of the human condition (Callister, 1995). Perinatal nurses must never lose sight of the fact that a woman's childbirth experience is not only about making a baby but also about creating a mother—a mother who is strong and competent and who trusts her own capacities because she has been cared for by a culturally competent nurse (Rothman, 1996). Giving birth has the potential to be a rich cultural and spiritual experience facilitated by such a nurse.

REFERENCES

Affonso, D. D. (1998). Asian and Pacific Islander American women. In L. A. Wallis (Ed.), *Textbook of women's health* (pp. 85–86). Philadelphia: Lippincott-Raven.

Agency for Healthcare Policy and Research (AHCPR). (1998). *Racial and ethnic differences in health, 1996*. Rockville, MD: Government Printing Office.

American Academy of Nursing (AAN) Expert Panel on Women's Health. (1997). Women's health and women's healthcare: Recommendations of the 1996 AAN Expert Panel of Women's Health. *Nursing Outlook, 45*(1), 7–15.

American Association of Colleges of Nursing (AACN). (1998). *The essentials of baccalaureate education for professional nursing practice*. Washington, DC: Author.

American Medical Association Council on Scientific Affairs. (1995). Female genital mutilation. *Journal of the American Medical Association, 274*(21), 1714–1716.

Andrew, M. M., & Boyle, J. S. (1995). *Transcultural concepts in nursing care*. Philadelphia: J.B. Lippincott.

Balacazar, H., Peterson, G. W., & Krull, J. F. (1997). Acculturation and family cohesiveness in Mexican American pregnant women: Social and health implications. *Family and Community Health, 20*(3), 16–31.

Bayne-Smith, M. (1997). Impact on traditional and cultural health practices on African American women's health. In National Institutes of Health Office for Research on Women's Health (NIH ORWH), *Agenda for research on women's health for the 21st century* (pp. 121–124). Rockville, MD: Government Printing Office.

Beyene, Y. (1996). Ethiopians & Eritreans. In J. G. Lipson, S. L. Dibble, & P. A. Minarik (Eds), *Culture & nursing care: A pocket guide* (pp. 101–114). San Francisco: UCSF Nursing Press.

Callister, L. C. (1995). Cultural meanings of childbirth. *Journal of Obstetric, Gynecologic, and Neonatal Nursing, 24*(3), 327–331.

Callister, L. C. (2000). Perinatal nursing care of Mormon women and their infants. In M. L. Moore (Ed.), *Perinatal nursing in a multi-cultural* society. White Plains, NY: March of Dimes.

Callister, L. C., & Khalaf, I. (2001). Cultural competency in the care of women and newborns. *Journal of Obstetric, Gynecologic, and Neonatal Nursing, 30*(2), in press.

Callister, L. C., Lauri, S., & Vehvilainen-Julkunen, K. (2000). A description of birth in Finland. *MCN The American Journal of Maternal Child Nursing, 25*(3), 146–150.

Callister, L. C., Semenic, S., & Foster, J. C. (1999). Cultural/spiritual meanings of childbirth: Orthodox Jewish and Mormon women. *Journal of Holistic Nursing, 17*(3), 280–295.

Callister, L. C., & Vega, R. (1998). Giving birth: Guatemalan women's voices. *Journal of Obstetric, Gynecologic, and Neonatal Nursing, 27*(3), 289–295.

Callister, L. C., Vehvilainen-Julkunen, K., & Lauri, S. (1996). Cultural perceptions of childbirth: A cross-cultural comparison of childbearing women. *Journal of Holistic Nursing, 1*(1), 66–78.

Campinha-Bacote, J. (1994). *The process of cultural competence in healthcare: A culturally competent model of care*. Wyoming, OH: Transcultural CARE Associates.

Cantos, A., & Rivera, E. (1996). Filipinos. In J. G. Lipson, S. L. Dibble, & P. A. Minarik (Eds.), *Culture & nursing care: A pocket guide* (pp. 115–125). San Francisco: University of California at San Francisco (UCSF) Nursing Press.

Castillo, H. M. (1996). Cultural diversity: Implications for nursing. In S. Torres (Ed.), *Hispanic voices* (pp. 1–12). New York: National League for Nursing Press.

Catolico, O. (1997). Psychological well-being of Cambodian women in resettlement. *Advances in Nursing Science, 19*(4), 75–84.

Chalmers, B., & Meyer, D. (1994). What women say about their birth experiences: A cross-cultural study. *Journal of Psychosomatic Obstetrics and Gynecology, 15*(4), 211–218.

Chen, M. S., & Hawks, B. L. (1995). A debunking of the myth of healthy Asian Americans and Pacific Islanders. *American Journal of Health Promotion, 9*(4), 261–268.

Chen, V. T. (1997). Asian and Pacific Island women. In K. M. Allen & J. M. Phillips (1997). *Women's health across the life span* (pp. 363–381). Philadelphia: Lippincott-Raven.

Choi, E. C. (1995). A contrast of mothering behaviors in women from Korea and the United States. *Journal of Obstetric, Gynecologic, and Neonatal Nursing, 24*(4), 363–369.

Clark, M. J. (1999). Cultural influences on community health. *Nursing in the community* (pp. 317–362). Stamford, CT: Appleton & Lange.

Colin, J. M., & Paperwalla, G. (1996). Haitians. In J. G. Lipson, S. L. Dibble, & P. A. Minarik (Eds.), *Culture & nursing care: A pocket guide* (pp. 139–154). San Francisco: USCF Nursing Press.

Colucciello, M. L., & Woelfel, V. (1998). Child care beliefs and practices of Hispanic mothers. *Nursing Connections, 11*(3), 33–40.

Conrad, J. K., Hollenbach, K. A., Fullerton, J. T., & Feigelson, H. S. (1998). Use of prenatal services by Hispanic women in San Diego county. *Journal of Nurse Midwifery, 43*(2), 90–96.

Cooper, T. P. (1996). Culturally appropriate care: Optional or imperative. *Advanced Practice Nursing Quarterly, 2*(2), 1–6.

Dalle, S. (1997). Birth in Honduras: A source of women's self esteem. *Midwifery Today,* 43AA(3), 47–48.

Davis-Floyd, R. B., & Sargent, C. F. (1997). *Childbirth and authoritative knowledge*. Berkeley: University of California Press.

Denman-Vitale, S., & Murillo, E. K. (1999). Effective promotion of breastfeeding among Latin American women newly immigrated to the United States. *Holistic Nursing Practice, 13*(4), 51–60.

de Pacheco, M. R., & Hutti, M. H. (1998). Cultural beliefs and healthcare practices of childbearing Puerto Rican American women and Mexican American women. *Mother Baby Journal 3*(1), 14–22.

de Paula, T. Laganu, K., & Gonzalez-Ramirez, L. (1996). Mexican Americans. In J. G. Lipson, S. L. Dibble, & P. A. Minarik (Eds.), *Culture & nursing care: A pocket guide* (pp. 203–221). San Francisco: UCSF Nursing Press.

de Sevo, M. R. (1997). Keeping the faith: Jewish traditions in pregnancy and childbirth. *Association of Women's Health, Obstetric, and Neonatal Nursing Lifelines, 1*(4), 46–49.

Downs, K., Bernstein, J., & Marchese, T. (1997). Providing culturally competent primary care for immigrant and refugee women: A Cambodian study. *Journal of Nurse Midwifery, 42*(6), 499–508.

Engebretsen, J. (1997). Cultural diversity and care. In B. M. Dossey (Ed.), *Core curriculum for holistic nursing* (pp. 108–118). Gaithersburg, MD: Aspen.

Farrales, S. (1996). Vietnamese. In J. G. Lipson, S. L. Dibble, & P. A. Minarik (Eds.). *Culture & nursing care: A pocket guide* (pp. 280–290). San Francisco: UCSF Nursing Press.

Ferran, E., Tracy, L. C., Gany, F. M., & Kramer, E. J. (1999). Culture and multi-cultural competence. In E. J. Kramer, S. L. Ivey, & Y. W. Ying (Eds.). *Immigrant women's health* (pp. 20–34). San Francisco: Jossey-Bass.

Fok, D. (1996). Cross cultural practice and its influence on breastfeeding—the Chinese culture. *Breastfeeding Review, 4*(1), 13–18.

Fouche, J. P., Fourie, M. C., Schoon, M. G., & Barn, R. H. (1998). The psychological needs of African women in labor in Western-oriented obstetrical care. *South African Journal of Psychology, 26*(2), 71–73.

Fraktman, M. G. (1998). Immigrant mothers: What makes them high risk? In C. G. Coll, J. L. Surrey, & K. Weingarten (Eds.), *Mothering against odds* (pp. 85–107). New York: Guilford Press.

Freda, M. (1997). Cultural competence in patient education. *Maternal Child Nursing, 22*(4), 219–220.

Friedman, M. M. (1998a). The African-American family. In *Family nursing: Research, theory, and practice* (pp. 527–545). Stanford, CT: Appleton & Lange.

Friedman, M. M. (1998b). The Hispanic-American family. In *Family nursing: Research, theory, and practice* (pp. 505–526). Stanford, CT: Appleton & Lange.

Fuentes-Afflick, E., Hessol, N. A., & Perez-Stable, E. J. (1998). Maternal birthplace, ethnicity, and low birth-weight in California. *Archives of Pediatric and Adolescent Medicine, 152*(11), 1105–1112.

Fulwood, S. (1996). Income shows first rise since 1989 as poverty falls. *Los Angeles Times*, September 27, pp. A1, A16.

Gaffney, K. F., Choi, E., Jones, G. B., & Tavangar, N. N. (1997). Stressful events and pregnant Salvadoran women: A cross cultural comparison. *Journal of Obstetric, Gynecologic, and Neonatal Nursing, 26*(3), 303–310.

Gardner, M. O., Cliver, S. P., McNeal, S. F., & Goldenberg, R. L. (1996). Ethnicity and sources of prenatal care: Findings from a national survey. *Birth, 23*(2), 84–87.

Giachello, A. L. (1997). Latino/Hispanic women. In K. M. Allen & J. M. Phillips (Eds.), *Women's health across the life span.* Philadelphia: Lippincott.

Giger, J. N., & Mood, L. H. (1997). Cultural competent teamwork. In *Cultural diversity in nursing: Issues, strategies, and outcomes* (pp. 13–19). Washington, DC: American Academy of Nursing.

Giger, J. N., & Davidhizar, R. E. (1995). *Transcultural nursing: Assessment and intervention* (pp. 127–161). St. Louis: Mosby–Year Book.

Grossman, D. G., Krieger, J. W., Sugarman, J. R., & Forquera, R. A. (1994). Health status of urban American Indians and Alaska Natives. *Journal of the American Medical Association, 271*(11), 845–850.

Heilemann, M. S. V., Lee, K. A., Stinson, J., Koshar, J. H., & Goss, G. (2000). Acculturation and perinatal health outcomes among women of Mexican descent. *Research in Nursing and Health, 232*, 118–125.

Henshaw, S. K. (1998). Unintended pregnancy in the United States. *Family Planning Perspectives, 30*, 24–29, 46.

Hill, P. (1996). West Indians. In J. G. Lipson, S. L. Dibble, & P. A. Minarik. *Culture & nursing care: A pocket guide* (pp. 291–303). San Francisco: UCSF Nursing Press.

Hodge, F., & Frederick, L. (1999). American Indian and Alaska Native populations in the United States. In R. Huff & M. Kline (Eds.), *Promoting health in multi-cultural populations* (pp. 269–289). Thousand Oaks, CA: Sage.

Holroyd, E., Yin-king, L., Pui-yuk, L. W., Kwok-hong, F. Y., & Shuk-lin, B. L. (1997). Hong Kong Chinese women's perception of support from midwives during labor. *Midwifery, 13*(2), 16–72.

Hong, G. K., & Friedman, M. M. (1998). The Asian-American family. In M. M. Friedman (Ed.). *Family nursing: Research, theory, and practice* (pp. 547–566). Stanford, CT: Appleton & Lange.

Horton, J. A. (Ed.). (1995). *The women's health data book: A profile of women's health in the United States* (2nd ed.). Washington, DC: Jacob's Institute of Women's Health.

Howard, J. Y., & Berbiglia, V. A. (1997) Caring for childbearing Korean women. *Journal of Obstetric, Gynecologic, and Neonatal Nursing, 26*(6), 665–672.

Ishida, D. N., Toomata-Mayer, T. F., & Mayer, J. F. (1996). Samoans. In J. G. Lipson, S., L, Dibble, & P. A. Minarik (Eds.), *Culture & nursing care: A pocket guide* (pp. 150–263). San Francisco: UCSF Nursing Press.

Jackson, L. E. (1997). Understanding, eliciting, and negotiating clients' multi-cultural health beliefs. In B. W. Spradley & J. A. Allender (Eds.), *Readings in community health nursing* (pp. 530–542). Philadelphia: Lippincott-Raven.

Jambunathan, J. & Stewart, S. (1995). Hmong women in Wisconsin: What are their concerns in pregnancy and childbirth. *Birth, 22*(4), 204–210.

Jimenez, S. L. M. (1995). The Hispanic culture, folklore, and perinatal health. *Journal of Perinatal Education, 4*(1), 9–16.

Johnson, L. B. (1997). Three decades of black family empirical research: Challenges for the 21st century. In H. P. McAdoo (Ed.), *Black families* (3rd ed., pp. 94–113). Thousand Oaks, CA: Sage.

Johnson, S. (1996). Hmong. In J. G. Lipson, S. L. Dibble, & P. A. Minarik (Eds.), *Culture & nursing care: A pocket guide* (pp. 155–168). San Francisco: UCSF Nursing Press.

Joint Commission for Accreditation of Healthcare Organizations. (2000). *Comprehensive accreditation manual for hospitals: the official handbook.* Chicago: JCAHCO.

Jones, F. C. (1999). Cultural influences. In M. E. Broome & J. A. Rollins (Eds.), *Core curriculum for the nursing care of children and their families* (pp. 393–409). Pitman, NJ: Janetti Publications.

Jordan, B. (1993). *Birth in four cultures.* Prospect Heights, IL: Waveland Press.

Juarbe, T. (1995). Access to healthcare for Hispanic women: A primary healthcare perspective. *Nursing Outlook, 43*(1) 23–28.

Kennedy, C. A., DeVoe, D., Ramer-Henry, K., & West-Kowalski, J. (1999). Influence of self-care education on illness behaviors and health locus of control of Mexican American women. *Women and Health, 28*(3), 1–13.

Khalaf, I., & Callister, L. C. (1997). Cultural meanings of childbirth: Muslim women living in Jordan. *Journal of Holistic Nursing, 15*(4), 373–388.

Khazoyan, C. M., & Anderson, N. L. R. (1994). Latinas' expectations of their partners during childbirth. *Maternal Child Nursing, 19*(4), 226–229.

Kirkham, S. R. (1998). Nurses' descriptions of caring for culturally diverse clients. *Clinical Nursing Research, 7*(2), 125–146.

Krostoski, D., & Silliman, J. (1997). Reproductive and middle years. In National Institutes of Health Office for Research on Women's Health (NIH ORWH), *Agenda for research on women's health for the 21st century* (pp. 61–62). Rockville, MD: Government Printing Office.

Kulig, J. C. (1990). Childbearing beliefs among Cambodian refugee women. *Western Journal of Nursing Research, 12*(1), 108–118.

Lee, M. C., & Essoka, G. (1998). Patient's perception of pain: Comparison between Korean-American and Euro-American obstetric patients. *Journal of Cultural Diversity, 5*(1), 29–40.

Leininger, M. (1991). *Cultural care diversity and universality.* New York: National League for Nursing.

Lenburg, C. B., Lipson, J. G., Demi, A. S., Blaney, D. R., Stern, P. N., Schultz, P. R., & Gage, L. (1995). *Promoting cultural competence in and through nursing education: A critical review and comprehensive plan of action.* Washington, DC: American Academy of Nursing.

Lim, R. (1997). Growing up in the sea of milk . . . Bali's ritual for babies. *The Journal of Perinatal Education, 6*(1), 49–57.

Lipson, J. G., Dibble, S. L., & Minarik, P. A. (1996). *Culture & nursing care: A pocket guide.* San Francisco: UCSF Nursing Press.

Locks, S., & Boateng, L. (1996). Black/African Americans. In J. G. Lipson, S. L. Dibble, & P. A. Minarik (Eds.), *Culture & nursing care: A pocket guide* (pp. 37–43). San Francisco: UCSF Nursing Press.

McCaffery, M. (1999). Pain control. *American Journal of Nursing, 99*(8), 18.

McCrea, H., & Wright, M. E. (1999). Satisfaction in childbirth and perceptions of personal control in pain relief during labor. *Journal of Advances in Nursing, 29*(4), 877–884.

Matocha, L. K. (1998). Chinese Americans. In L. D. Purnell & B. J. Paulanka (Eds.). *Transcultural healthcare* (pp. 163–188). Philadelphia: F.A. Davis.

Mattson, S. (1995). Cultural sensitive perinatal care for Southeast Asians. *Journal of Obstetric, Gynecologic, and Neonatal Nursing, 24*(5), 335–341.

Mattson, S. (1993). Ethnocultural considerations in the childbearing period. In S. Mattson & J. E. Smith (Eds.). *Core curriculum for maternal newborn nursing* (pp. 81–97). Philadelphia: W.B. Saunders.

Meleis, A. I. (1996). Culturally competent scholarship: Substance and rigor. *Advances in Nursing Science, 19*(2), 1–16.

Miller, M. A. (1995). Culture, spirituality, and women's health. *Journal of Obstetric, Gynecologic, and Neonatal Nursing, 24*(3), 257–263.

Miska, K. J. (1999). Mexican American family processes: Nurturing, support, and socialization. *Nursing Science Quarterly, 12*(2), 138–142.

Nance, T. A. (1995). Intercultural communication: Finding common ground. *Journal of Obstetric, Gynecologic, and Neonatal Nursing, 24*(3), 249–255.

Nichols, F. H. (1996). The meaning of the childbirth experience: A review of the literature. *Journal of Perinatal Education, 5*(4), 71–77.

Overfield, T. (1985). *Biologic variation in health and illness.* Menlo Park, CA: Addison Wesley.

Plawecki, H. M., Sanchez, T. R., & Plawecki, J. A. (1994). Cultural aspects of caring for Navajo Indian clients. *Journal of Holistic Nursing, 12*(3), 291–306.

Pollock, S. E. (1999). Health related hardiness in different ethnic populations. *Holistic Nursing Practice, 13*(3), 1–10.

Purnell, L. D., & Paulanka, B. J. (1998). Purnell's model for cultural competence. In *Transcultural healthcare* (pp. 7–51). Philadelphia: F.A. Davis.

Rajaram, S. S., & Rashidi, A. (1999). Asian-Islamic women and breast cancer screening. *Women and Health, 28*(3), 45–58.

Reichert, G. A. (1998). Female circumcision. *Association of Women's Health, Obstetric, and Neonatal Nursing (AWHONN) Lifelines, 2*(3), 29–34.

Rehm, R. S. (1999). Religious faith in Mexican-American families. *Image: Journal of Nursing Scholarship, 31*(1), 33–38.

Reichman, N. E., & Kenney, G. M. (1998). Prenatal care, birth outcomes, and newborn hospitalization costs: Patterns among Hispanics in New Jersey. *Family Planning Perspectives, 30*(4), 182–187, 200.

Riordan, J. (1999). The cultural context of breastfeeding. In J. Riordan and K. G. Auerbach (Eds.), *Breastfeeding and human lactation* (pp. 29–51). Boston: Jones & Bartlett.

Rodriguez-Trias, H. (1997). Latinas/Hispanic women and research issues: Impact of traditional and cultural health practices. In National Institutes of Health Office for Research on Women's Health (NIH ORWH), *Agenda for research on women's health for the 21st century* (pp. 130–140). Rockville, MD: Government Printing Office.

Rojas, D. Z. (1996). Spiritual well-being and its influence on the holistic health of Hispanic women. In S. Torres (Ed.), *Hispanic voices* (pp. 213–229). New York: National League for Nursing Press.

Rothman, B. K. (1996). Women, providers, and control. *Journal of Obstetric, Gynecologic, and Neonatal Nursing, 25*(2), 253–256.

Salt, K. (1997). Melting pot: Respecting multi-cultural diversity in your classroom. *Childbirth Instructor Magazine* 2nd quarter, 31–33.

Schneiderman, J. U. (1996). Postpartum nursing for Korean mothers. *Maternal Child Nursing, 21*(3), 155–158.

Schneiderman, J. U. (1998). Rituals of placental disposal. *Maternal Child Nursing, 23*(3), 142–143.

Schott, J., & Henley, A. (1996). *Culture, religion, and childbearing in a multi-racial society.* Oxford, UK: Butterworth Heinemann.

Seideman, R., Jacobson, S., Primeaux, M., Burns, P., & Weatherby, F. (1996). Assessing American Indian families. *MCN The American Journal of Maternal Child Nursing, 21*(6), 272–279.

Semenic, S., Callister, L. C., & Foster, J. C. (2001). Giving birth: Voices of Orthodox Jewish women. *Journal of Obstetric, Gynecologic, and Neonatal Nursing, 30*(2), in press.

Sharts-Hopko, N. C. (1995). Birth in the Japanese context. *Journal of Obstetric, Gynecologic, and Neonatal Nursing, 24*(4), 343–351.

Shilling, T. (2000). Cultural perspectives on childbearing. In F. H. Nichols & S. S. Humenick. *Childbirth education: Practice, research, and theory* (pp. 138–154). Philadelphia: W.B. Saunders.

Spector, R. E. (2000). *Cultural diversity in health and illness* (5th ed.). Upper Saddle River, NJ: Prentice Hall Health.

Stewart, S., & Jambunathan, J. (1996). Hmong women and postpartum depression. *Healthcare for Women International, 17*(4), 319–330.

Swanson, J. M., & Nies, M. A. (1997). Cultural influences in the community. *Community health nursing: Promoting the health of aggregates* (pp. 524–572). Philadelphia: W.B. Saunders.

Sword, W. (1999). A socio-ecological approach to understand barriers to prenatal care for women of low income. *Journal of Advanced Nursing, 29*(5), 1170–1177.

Taylor, F. M. A., Ko, R., & Pan, M. (1999). Prenatal and reproductive healthcare. In E. J. Kramer, S. L. Ivey, & Y. W. Ying (Eds.), *Immigrant women's health* (pp. 121–135). San Francisco: Jossey-Bass.

Unger, J. B., & Molina, G. B. (1998). Contraceptive use among Latina women: Social, cultural, and demographic correlates. *Women's Health Issues, 8*(6), 357–369.

United States Bureau of Census, Population Division (USBC). (1998). *United States population estimates, 1990 to 1997.* Rockville, MD: Government Printing Office.

United States Department of Health and Human Services (USDHHS). (1997). Advance Report of Final Mortality Statistics, 1995. *Monthly Vital Statistics Report, 45*(11).

United States Department of Health and Human Services. (1998). *Healthy people 2010 objectives.* Rockville, MD: Government Printing Office.

Ventura, S. J., Mosher, W. D., Curtin, S. C., Abama, J. C., & Henshaw, S. (1999). Highlights of trends in pregnancies and pregnancy rates by outcome: Estimates for the United States, 1976–1996. *National Vital Statistics Report, 47*(29), 1–9.

Villarruel, A. M. (1999). A perspective on Latino healthcare. In V. D. Ferguson (Ed.). *Case studies in cultural diversity* (pp. 47–58). Boston: Jones & Bartlett.

Villarruel, A. M. (1995). Mexican-American cultural meanings, expressions, self care and dependent-care activities associated with experiences of pain. *Research in Nursing and Health, 18*(5), 427–436.

Vincent, P. (1995). Traditional and modern thought about the placenta. *Midwives, 108*(1293), 325–327.

Weber, S. F. (1996). Cultural aspects of pain in childbearing women. *Journal of Obstetric, Gynecologic, and Neonatal Nursing, 25*(1), 67–72.

Office of Health Communications and Public Relations, World Health Organization. (1997). *Fact Sheet N-153, Female genital mutilation*. Geneva: World Health Organization.

Wright, J. (1996). Female genital mutilation: An overview. *Journal of Advanced Nursing, 24*(2), 251–259.

Yee, B. W. K. (1997). Influence of traditional and cultural health practices among Asian women. In National Institutes of Health Office for Research on Women's Health (NIH ORWH). *Agenda for research on women's health for the 21st* century (pp. 150–165). Rockville, MD: Government Printing Office.

York, R., Bhuttarowas, P., & Brown, L. P. (1999). Nursing in Thailand and its relationship to childbearing practices. *MCN The American Journal of Maternal Child Nursing, 2*(3), 145–150.

Zoucha, R. D. (1998). The experiences of Mexican Americans receiving professional nursing care. *Journal of Transcultural Nursing, 9*(2), 34–44.

APPENDIX **4 A**

Culture Care Resources

CLINICAL HANDBOOKS

Bolane, J.E. (1999). *Labor and birth: Terms, techniques, problem solving.* Waco TX: Childbirth Graphics. (Pocket glossary of labor and birth terms and interactions. Translated into Spanish, French, Tagalog, Vietnamese, Chinese, and Korean.)

Lipson, J.G., Dibble, S.L., & Minarik, P.A. (1996). *Culture and nursing care: A pocket guide.* San Francisco: University of California at San Francisco. (Not specific to perinatal nursing.)

Schrefer, S. (1994). *Quick reference to cultural assessment.* St. Louis: Mosby–Year Book. (Not specific to perinatal nursing.)

GENITAL MUTILATION/RITUAL CIRCUMCISION

RAINBO—Research, Action, and Information Network for Bodily Integrity of Women Task Force on Caring for Circumcised Women http://www.rainbo.org

PERINATAL SPANISH TEACHING MATERIALS

Beginnings: Una Guia Practica Durante Su Embararazo by Lisa Nixon

http://www.prenataled.com/newsletters/v3n10/frames.htm

El Embarazo, El Parto Y Tu by Linda B. Jenkins, RN, BSN, PHN, ACCE

http://www.birthpre.com Spanish videos also available from this source

Childbirth Graphics, (800) 299-3366, ext. 295, Fax (888) 977- 7653

LANGUAGE LINE SERVICES

AT&T (800) 752-0093 www.languageline.com
Available seven days a week, 24 hours a day
Translation from English into more than 140 languages

1. Subscribed interpretation (organizations, frequent use)
2. Membership interpretation (organizations, predictable need)
3. Personal interpreter (individuals, occasional use)

MATERNAL AND INFANT CARE ISSUES

http://www.lib.iun.indiana.edu/trannurs.htm

http://www.hslib.washington.edu/clinical/ethnomed/peri.html

Global Institute for Nursing and Health. To subscribe, access list-subscribe@ginh.org

PROFESSIONAL JOURNALS

Cross Cultural Issues

Journal of Cultural Diversity

Journal of Multi-cultural Nursing

Journal of Transcultural Nursing

Western Journal of Medicine

SPANISH TRANSLATOR

Master/Maestro Ingles translator, available at Radio Shack

PART 2

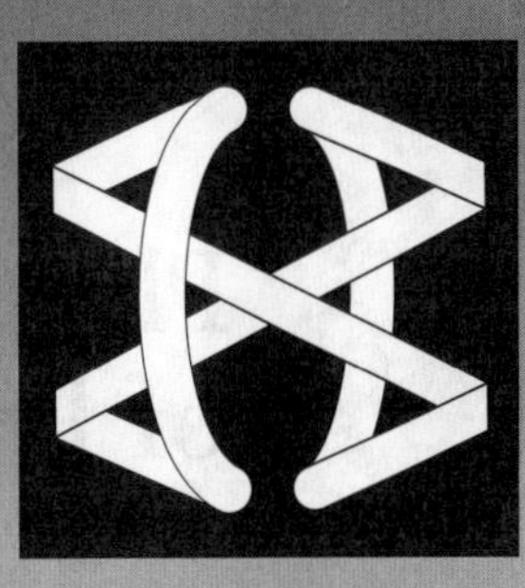

ANTEPARTUM

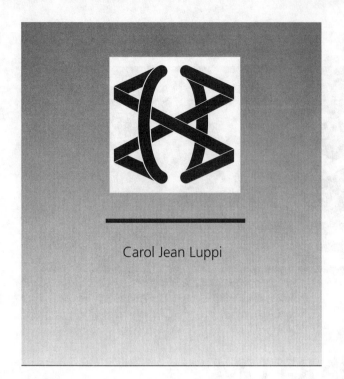

Carol Jean Luppi

CHAPTER 5

Physiologic Changes of Pregnancy

Pregnancy is a dynamic state. The woman experiences dramatic physiologic changes to meet the demands of the developing fetus and to prepare for birth and lactation. Maternal adaptations during pregnancy are attributed to significant hormonal influences and secondary mechanical pressures exerted by the growing fetus and enlarging uterus. These changes maintain the woman's normal physiologic function and facilitate fetal development. Physiologic changes in pregnancy affect physical examination findings and laboratory values. An understanding of normal physiologic changes of pregnancy is essential for discriminating between normal and abnormal states. Laboratory values and physical findings considered normal in the nonpregnant woman may not be normal for women during pregnancy. The following review of physiologic changes during pregnancy provides baseline information to guide the perinatal nurse in conducting an accurate and thorough assessment of the pregnant woman.

REPRODUCTIVE HORMONAL CHANGES DURING PREGNANCY

Hormones play major roles in the endocrine system of the human body. They are responsible for maintaining homeostasis, for regulation of growth and development, and for cellular communication. Reproductive hormones are produced by endocrine glands, are transported by the blood to their target cells throughout the pregnant woman's body, and mediate many of the significant physiologic adaptations to pregnancy.

Human Chorionic Gonadotropin

Human chorionic gonadotropin (hCG) is secreted by the blastocyst and the placenta. It stimulates progesterone and estrogen production by the corpus luteum until the developed placenta assumes this role. There is a pattern of hCG secretion. It is initially high and can be used to detect early pregnancy. The level diminishes and plateaus as the pregnancy progresses. Eventually, the placenta becomes the major source of estrogen and progesterone, and the corpus luteum is no longer required. In multiple pregnancies, hCG levels are more than twice as high as in singleton pregnancies (Liu & Rebar, 1999).

Human Placental Lactogen

Human placental lactogen (hPL), formally known as human chorionic somatomammotropin, is produced by the syncytiotrophoblast of the placenta. Unlike hCG levels, serum hPL levels rise concomitantly with placental growth. The hormone is an antagonist of insulin (Lui & Rebar, 1999). It increases the amount of free fatty acids available for metabolic needs and decreases maternal metabolism of glucose. When maternal glucose is limited, hPL reserves glucose for fetal use, and free fatty acids are used preferentially by the mother. This preferred breakdown of free fatty acids results in increased levels of ketones and therefore causes pregnant women to be more prone to develop ketosis with decreased food intake.

Estrogen

Estrogens are steroid hormones secreted by the ovaries during early pregnancy. By 7 weeks' gestation, more than one half of the estrogen is secreted by the placenta. Estrogen stimulates the growth of the uterine muscle mass. Luteinizing hormone (LH) and follicle-stimulating hormone (FSH) are inhibited by high concentrations of progesterone in the presence of estrogen. The presence of estrogen prevents further follicular development during pregnancy. Estrogens affect the renin-angiotensin-aldosterone system and stimulate production of hormone-binding globulins in the liver during pregnancy. They prepare the breasts for lactation, increase blood flow to the uterus, and may be involved in the timing of the onset of labor (Casey, Winkel, Porter, & MacDonald, 1983). Estrogens also play an important role in fetal development.

Estriol is the primary estrogen produced by the placenta during pregnancy. Maternal serum estriol levels increase to between 12 and 20 mg/mL by the end of pregnancy because of a decreased affinity for sex hormone–binding globulin. Maternal estriol levels were historically used as an index of adequate fetal and placental function; however, numerous problems with interpretation have limited their usefulness.

Progesterone

Initially produced by the corpus luteum and then by the placenta, progesterone plays a crucial role in supporting the pregnancy. It maintains the secretory endometrium required for implantation and discourages uterine contractions by acting on uterine smooth muscle to inhibit prostaglandin production (Bagchi & Kumar, 1999). Progesterone may also aid in maintaining the pregnancy by inhibiting T-lymphocyte–mediated processes that are associated with tissue rejection and by creating a barrier to penetration of pathogens into the uterus. Progesterone also relaxes venous walls to accommodate the increase in blood volume and aids in the development of acini and lobules of the breasts for lactation.

Relaxin

Relaxin is secreted primarily by the corpus luteum and in small amounts by the placenta and decidua. It is detectable by the first missed menstrual period. Relaxin is believed to contribute to the inhibition of uterine activity, diminishing the strength of uterine contractions, softening of the cervix, and producing the long-term effect of remodeling collagen. The role of relaxin is not completely understood.

Prostaglandins

Prostaglandins are lipid substances found in high concentrations in the female reproductive tract and in the decidua during pregnancy. Prostaglandins are part of a family of substances (ie, eicosanoids) synthesized from arachidonic acid, which is present in plasma membrane phospholipids. This family includes prostaglandins, thromboxanes, and leukotrienes. These substances are produced in response to a stimulus to the plasma membrane. The eicosanoid is released immediately and acts locally. Prostaglandins affect smooth muscle contractility. The interplay between thromboxane and prostacyclin is believed to contribute to hypertensive disorders in pregnancy (Walsh, 1985).

Prostaglandins play an important role in the onset of labor. Prostaglandin (phospholipase A_2) activity in the amnion is decreased in women in labor compared with women not in labor (Skannal, Eis, Brockman, Siddiqi, & Myatt, 1997). Production of arachidonic acid metabolites may be elevated at term and in preterm labor, suggesting that they can stimulate contractility of smooth muscle. Animal studies have shown that prostaglandin receptors may also be involved in the onset of labor because the receptor for prostaglandin $F_{2\alpha}$ ($PGF_{2\alpha}$) is not found when parturition is delayed (Sugimoto et al., 1997). These physiologic data support the use of various prostaglandins for cervical ripening and induction of labor when indicated. Prostaglandin E_2 (PGE_2) dissolves collagen bundles and increases submucosal edema (Gibb, 1998). PGE_2 gel (Prepidil) is widely used for cervical ripening and is instilled into the cervix or the posterior fornix of the vagina (Simpson & Poole, 1998). The intracervical product contains 0.5 mg of the prostaglandin dinoprostone that is dispensed in a syringe containing 2.5 mL of gel. There is extensive experience with administering PGE_2 gel intravaginally in a dose of 2 to 5 mg. A vaginal pessary that provides sustained release of PGE_2 (Cervidil) has been available since 1995 and has the added benefit of convenient removal using the attached string in the event of hyperstimulation of uterine activity or a nonreassuring fetal response.

For the past few years, PGE_1 (misoprostol) has been used for cervical ripening. Current recommendations are for intravaginal administration of misoprostol (American College of Obstetricians and Gynecologists [ACOG], 1999). Oral administration remains under investigation.

Further evidence of the role of prostaglandins in parturition is supported by the use of prostaglandin synthase-1 inhibitors to attempt to prevent preterm labor. Indomethacin is one prostaglandin synthase inhibitor that has been used with various degrees of success to decrease myometrial contractility and prolong pregnancy.

Prolactin

Prolactin is released from the anterior pituitary. The hormone is responsible for the increase and maturation of ducts and alveoli and for initiation of lactation. During pregnancy, there is a marked increase of prolactin because of the effects of angiotensin II, gonadotropin-releasing hormone, and vasopressin on the pituitary. However, the higher amounts of estrogen found during pregnancy inhibit lactation by direct action on the mammary glands. After the major source of estrogen and progesterone is eliminated by delivery of the placenta, the anterior pituitary produces large amounts of prolactin, which stimulates the breast to begin lactation. The serum prolactin concentration begins to rise in the first trimester and by term may reach 10 times the nonpregnant concentration (Lui & Rebar, 1999). After birth, prolactin levels reach 200 to 250 ng/mL and then return to prepregnancy levels of less than 25 ng/mL in non–breast-feeding mothers (Liu & Park, 1988).

CARDIOVASCULAR SYSTEM

The cardiovascular system undergoes numerous and profound adaptations during pregnancy (Table 5–1), some of which are mediated by reproductive hormones. Cardiovascular anatomy, blood volume, cardiac output, and vascular resistance are altered to accommodate the additional maternal and fetal circulatory requirements. Increased ventricular wall muscle mass, an increased heart rate, cardiac murmurs, and dependent peripheral edema are evidence of these anatomic and functional changes. Physical symptoms may occur during pregnancy in response to normal cardiovascular changes. Some women report palpitations, lightheadedness, or decreased tolerance for activity (Milne, Howie, & Pack, 1978; Wolfe et al., 1989). Cardiovascular adaptations have a significant impact on all organ systems.

Heart

The position, appearance, and function of the heart change during pregnancy. When the growing uterus exerts pressure on the diaphragm, the heart is displaced upward, forward, and to the left. The first-trimester increase in ventricular muscle mass and the second- and early third-trimester increase in blood volume cause the heart to enlarge (Crapo, 1996; Thompson et al., 1986). The point of maximal impulse is deviated to the left at the fourth intercostal space. During the first few days postpartum, the left atrium also appears to be enlarged because of the increased blood volume that occurs after birth.

The maternal heart rate begins to increase at 4 to 5 weeks' gestation and peaks in the third trimester with an increase of 15 to 20 beats/min above baseline (Robson, Hunter, Boys, & Dunlop, 1989). In twin pregnancies, the maternal heart rate at term increases as much as 40% above nonpregnant rates (Crapo, 1996). Heart rate and atrial size return to normal prepregnancy values in the first 10 days postpartum, whereas left ventricular size normalizes after 4 to 6 months (Robson, Hunter, Moore, & Dunlop, 1987).

TABLE 5–1 ■ CARDIOVASCULAR CHANGES DURING PREGNANCY

Parameter	Change
Heart rate	Increases 15% (10–20 bpm)
Blood volume	Increases 45% (1,450–1,750 mL)
Plasma volume	Increases 45% (1,200–1,300 mL)
Red cell mass	Increases 20%–30% (250–450 mL)
Cardiac output	Increases 30%–50% (6.2 ± 1.0 L/min)
Stroke volume	Increases 50%
Systemic vascular resistance	Decreases 21%
Colloid oncotic pressure	Decreases 20% (23 mmHg)

During the second trimester of pregnancy, a change in heart sounds and a systolic murmur may be heard in approximately 90% to 95% of pregnant women because of the increased cardiovascular load. Phonocardiographic studies as early as the 1960s documented alterations in maternal heart sounds (Cutforth & MacDonald, 1966). Ninety percent of pregnant women have a wider split in the first heart sound and an audible third heart sound. The first heart sound generally becomes louder in all pregnant women. Around 30 weeks' gestation, the second heart sound also demonstrates an audible splitting. About 5% of pregnant women also have an audible fourth heart sound. Systolic murmurs are auscultated in more than 95% of pregnant women. However, systolic murmurs greater than grade 2/4 and any type of diastolic murmur are considered abnormal. Systolic murmurs can be best auscultated along the left sternal border and result from aortic and pulmonary artery blood flow (Limacher, Ware, O'Meara, Fernandez, & Young, 1985).

Blood Volume

To support maternal and fetal circulation, blood volume increases approximately 25% to 52% (1,450 to 1,750 mL) by 32 weeks' gestation (Crapo, 1996). The volume increases beginning in the first trimester, reaches a peak in the third trimester, and returns to a prepregnant volume 2 to 3 weeks postpartum. Blood volume is greater in multiple gestations (2,000 to 2,500 mL) and increases proportionally according to the number of fetuses (Duvekot, Cheries, Pieters, Menheere, & Peters, 1995). The increased blood volume is necessary to provide adequate blood flow to the uterus, fetus, and maternal tissues; to maintain blood pressure; to assist with temperature regulation by increasing cutaneous blood flow; and to accommodate blood loss at birth. This elevated blood volume results from increases in plasma volume and red cell mass.

Plasma volume increases approximately 45% to 50% (1,200 to 1,600 mL) by term, and red cell mass increases 20% to 30% (250 to 450 mL). The rapid increase in plasma volume and later rise in red blood cell (RBC) volume results in relative hypervolemia hemodilution, often referred to as *physiologic anemia of pregnancy* (Brown & Gallery, 1994). This is not true pathologic anemia. Hemodilution is believed to reduce the risk of thrombus formation by decreasing blood viscosity and enhancing uteroplacental circulation (Koller, 1982). Even with increased RBC production, hemoglobin values decrease during pregnancy (12 to 16 g/dL of blood), and the hematocrit values also decrease (37% to 47%). This decrease is more obvious during the second trimester, when the rapid increase in blood volume occurs.

One proposed mechanism for expansion of blood volume is hormonal stimulation of plasma renin activity and aldosterone levels (Barron & Lindheimer, 1984), which stimulates tubular reabsorption of sodium and a subsequent increase in total body water (Davison, 1985). Total body water increases by 6 to 8 L, of which 4 to 6 L are extracellular (Fuschino, 1992).

To prevent hemorrhage immediately after childbirth, the uterus contracts, shunting blood from uterine vessels into the systemic circulation, and causing an autotransfusion of approximately 1,000 mL. The rise in cardiac output is accompanied by a reflex decrease in heart rate, and stroke volume is therefore greatly increased and remains elevated for 1 to 2 weeks after birth (Crapo, 1996). The average blood loss is 500 to 600 mL for a vaginal birth and 800 to 1,200 mL for a cesarean birth or vaginal birth of multiples (Fuschino, 1992). Blood loss during birth accompanied by the postpartum diuresis reduces the plasma volume during the first several days postpartum (Metcalfe, McAnulty, & Ueland, 1981), and the plasma volume returns to prepregnant levels 2 to 3 weeks postpartum.

Cardiac Output

Cardiac output is the product of heart rate, blood volume, cardiac contractility, vascular resistance, and maternal position. Cardiac output increases 30% to 50% during pregnancy and reaches a volume of 5 to 7 L/min (Clark et al., 1989). Cardiac output increases beginning as early as 8 weeks' gestation, peaks in the second trimester, and then plateaus until term. In early pregnancy, the increase in cardiac output primarily results from an increase in stroke volume. As pregnancy progresses, the increase in cardiac output results from the increase in heart rate and stroke volume (Robson et al., 1989). Changes in cardiac output during the intrapartum period depend on maternal position, type of anesthesia, and method of birth.

Maternal position can greatly influence cardiac output, most dramatically during the third trimester. In the supine position, pressure exerted on the inferior vena cava from the gravid uterus decreases venous return and results in decreased cardiac output. This position may lead to supine hypotension with diaphoresis and possible syncope. Early studies showed that changing from the supine position to the lateral position could increase cardiac output 25% to 30% (Ueland & Hansen, 1969), with a resultant increase in uterine and renal blood flow. Studies demonstrate that right and left lateral positions optimize cardiac output (not just the left lateral position as was previously believed) (Clark et al., 1991). In summary, cardiac output is optimized in the lateral position, somewhat decreased in the sitting position, and markedly decreased in the supine position (Clark et al., 1991).

Cardiac output rises progressively during labor (Robson, Dunlop, Boys, & Hunter, 1987). During the first stage of labor, approximately 300 to 500 mL of blood are shunted from the uterus into the systemic circulation with each contraction. This is responsible for a 12% to 31% rise in cardiac output in the first stage of labor and a 49% rise in the second stage (Robson, Dunlop et al., 1987). The autotransfusion that occurs at this time maintains cardiac output even with a decrease in heart rate. Cardiac output progressively decreases and returns to nonpregnant levels by 6 weeks postpartum (Fuschino, 1992). Cardiac output normalizes to prelabor values 1 hour after birth (Robson, Hunter et al., 1987).

Epidural anesthesia causes a sympathectomy and a marked decrease in peripheral vascular resistance that may cause a decrease in venous return, resulting in decreased cardiac output. An intravenous fluid bolus before epidural placement may mitigate these effects. A well-managed epidural block decreases pain, anxiety, and bearing-down efforts and prevents a rapid rise in cardiac output (Ueland & Metcalfe, 1975). General anesthesia decreases cardiac output, whereas local or paracervical anesthesia is associated with a rise in cardiac output (Ueland & Hansen, 1969). Table 5–2 summarizes the increases in cardiac output during labor and birth.

TABLE 5–2 ■ INCREASES IN CARDIAC OUTPUT DURING LABOR AND BIRTH

Labor Phase or Stage	Increase Above Prelabor Values
Latent phase	15%
Active phase	30%
Second stage	45%
Immediately after birth	65%

Distribution of Blood Flow

Most of the increase in blood volume during pregnancy is distributed to the uterus, kidneys, breasts, and skin. The uterus accommodates one third of the additional blood volume at term (approximately 500 mL/min). The kidneys receive approximately 400 mL/min, a 30% increase. Glandular growth, distended veins, and tissue engorgement reflect increased blood flow to the breasts. Hyperemia of the cervix and vagina is also evident. Blood flow to the maternal skin increases to accommodate the additional heat loss requirements created by the active metabolism of the fetus (Beinder, Huch, & Huch, 1990). This increased blood flow can result in alterations in nail and hair growth, increased nasal congestion, increased risk of epistaxis, sensations of warm hands and feet, and other associated symptoms.

Blood Pressure

Maternal position during blood pressure (BP) measurement significantly affects BP values. Sitting or standing BP measurement shows minimal change in systolic blood pressure (SBP) throughout pregnancy. Diastolic blood pressure (DBP), measured in the sitting or standing positions, gradually decreases by approximately 5 to 10 mm Hg over the first-trimester values. In the left lateral recumbent position, SBP decreases 5 to 10 mm Hg, and DBP decreases 10 to 15 mm Hg. BP reaches its lowest point in the second trimester and returns to prepregnant levels by the third trimester (Crapo, 1996).

Different methods of DBP measurement produce significantly different readings. DBP measurements can vary as much as 15 mm Hg with the use of different methods: a mercury cuff with Korotkoff sounds assessed with a stethoscope, intraarterial catheters, or automated BP devices (Kirshon, Lee, Cotton, & Giebel, 1987). Accurate comparison of BP values depends on consistent techniques of measurement and consistent maternal positioning.

The renin-angiotensin-aldosterone system plays an important role in regulation of BP and blood volume in pregnancy and is discussed later in the renal section of this chapter.

Systemic Vascular Resistance

Systemic vascular resistance (SVR) and pulmonary vascular resistance decrease during pregnancy by approximately 21% and 34%, respectively. The uteroplacental vascular system is a low-resistance network that accommodates a large percentage of maternal cardiac output. Progesterone and prostaglandins relax smooth muscle and produce vasodilation. Uterine vascular resistance also decreases during pregnancy and enhances uterine blood flow. SVR decreases in early pregnancy (ie, 5 weeks' gestation), is lowest at 14 to 24 weeks' gestation, and gradually increases by term. The mean SVR may approximate nonpregnant values at term (Clark et al., 1989).

Hematologic Changes

To meet additional oxygen requirements of pregnancy, RBC volume increases approximately 17% to 32%. Normal hematocrit values for pregnancy are between 36% and 41% (Pritchard, 1965). Plasma volume increases to a greater degree than the erythrocyte volume; therefore, the hematocrit decreases approximately 4% to 7%. This decrease is most obvious during the second trimester, when the rapid increase in blood volume occurs.

Hemoglobin levels during pregnancy are between 12 and 16 g/dL (Pritchard, 1965). With the increase in the number of RBCs, the need for iron for the production of hemoglobin also increases. Approximately 500 mg of iron is needed for the increases in maternal RBCs, and 300 mg of iron is needed for fetal RBC production. Gastrointestinal absorption of iron is increased during pregnancy, but additional iron supplementation is nonetheless necessary to maintain maternal iron stores. If iron stores are initially low and supplemental iron is not added to enhance the diet, iron deficiency anemia may result (Mashburn, Graves, & Gillmor-Kahn, 1992). There is controversy surrounding the efficacy and benefit of oral iron supplementation during pregnancy (Beard, 2000). One study recommended that normal hemoglobin values should be derived from women who have consumed iron supplementation during pregnancy, and the investigators cite the lowest normal hemoglobin value as 11.0 g/dL in the first trimester and 10.5 g/dL in the later trimesters (Milman, Byg, & Agger, 2000).

Leukocyte production also increases in pregnancy. An average white blood cell (WBC) count in the third trimester is 6,000 to 16,000/mm^3. Labor and early postpartum levels may reach 20,000 to 30,000/mm^3 without an infection (Priddy, 1997). The increase in WBC count begins with an increase in the neutrophilia count during the second month, and the level returns to the normal range for nonpregnant women by 6 days postpartum. Slight increases in eosinophil levels and slight decreases in basophil levels have also been reported (Kilpatrick & Laros, 1999).

Coagulation and fibrinolytic systems undergo significant changes during pregnancy. Pregnancy is considered a hypercoagulable state because of increased levels of several essential coagulation factors and placental factors that inhibit fibrinolysis. Increases occur in factors I (fibrinogen), V, VII, VIII, IX, X, and XII. Placental inhibiting factors decrease plasma fibrinolytic activity (Bonnar, McNichol, & Douglas, 1969). Bleeding time, prothrombin time (PT), partial thromboplastin time (PTT), and clotting time remain unchanged despite an increase in clotting factors. Table 5–3 summarizes the changes in clotting factors during pregnancy.

Platelet counts range between 150,000/mm^3 and 400,000/mm^3, with a gradual decrease throughout pregnancy and then an increase in the early postpartum period (Crapo, 1996). The net effect of these alterations places pregnant women at increased risk for thrombus formation and consumptive coagulopathies (Gerbasi, Bottoms, Farag, & Mammen, 1990). After birth, coagulation is initiated to prevent hemorrhage. Fibrinogen and platelet counts decrease as platelet plugs and fibrin clots form to provide hemostasis.

In summary, women with normal cardiovascular function should be able to accommodate the dramatic cardiovascular changes associated with pregnancy. Women with cardiovascular disease are at increased risk for various complications during pregnancy, labor, or the postpartum period, in part because of alterations in volume and cardiac output and the potential for coagulopathies.

RESPIRATORY SYSTEM

Changes in the respiratory system are essential to accommodate increased maternal–fetal ventilatory requirements and to ensure adequate gas exchange to meet maternal and fetal metabolic needs. The respiratory system must provide an increased amount of oxygen and efficiently remove carbon dioxide.

Structural Changes

Pressure from the uterus shifts the diaphragm upward approximately 4 cm, decreasing the length of the lungs. To adjust to this decreased length, the anteroposterior diameter of the chest enlarges by 2 cm. Increased pressure from the uterus widens the substernal angle 50%, from 68 to 103 degrees, and causes the ribs to flare out slightly. The circumference of the thoracic cage may increase 5 to 7 cm, compensating for the decreased lung length (Harvey, 1999). Many of these changes are probably caused by hormonal influence, because they occur before pressure is exerted from the growing uterus.

Despite the mechanical elevation of the diaphragm in pregnancy, breathing remains diaphragmatic. Certain components of lung volume are altered. Table 5–4 summarizes the changes in respiratory function during pregnancy.

Lung Volume

The volume of the lungs is decreased because of the elevated diaphragm, which reduces total lung volume (ie, amount of air in lungs at maximal inspiration) by 5% and residual volume (ie, amount of air in lungs

TABLE 5–3 ■ CLOTTING FACTORS DURING PREGNANCY

Parameter	Change
Fibrin	Increases 40% at term
Plasma fibrinogen	Increases 50%, 300–600 mg/dL
Clotting time	Unchanged
Coagulation factors V,VII, VIII, IX, X, XII	Increases
Coagulation factors XI, XIII	Decreases slightly
Prothrombin time	Increases slightly or unchanged
Platelets	Unchanged, 140,000–440,000/mm^3

TABLE 5-4 ■ RESPIRATORY CHANGES DURING PREGNANCY

Parameter	Change
Tidal volume	Increases 30–40%, from 500–700 mL
Vital capacity	Unchanged
Inspiratory reserve volume	Unchanged
Expiratory reserve volume	Decreases 20%
Respiratory rate	Unchanged or slight increase
Functional residual capacity	Decreases 20%
Total lung volume	Decreases 5%
Residual volume	Decreases 20%
Minute ventilation	Increases 40%
pH	Slight increase to 7.40–7.45
Oxygen consumption	Increases 15–20%
PaO_2	104–108 mmHg
$PaCo_2$	27–32 mmHg

after maximum expiration) by 20%. Functional residual capacity (ie, amount of air remaining in the lungs at resting expiratory level, permitting air for gas exchange between breaths) is reduced by 20% (Puranik et al., 1994). Tidal volume (ie, amount of air inspired and expired with normal breath) increases 30% to 40% (450 to 600 mL/min) during pregnancy and compensates for decreases in expiratory reserve volume and residual volume. Vital capacity (ie, maximum amount of air that can be forcibly expired after maximum inspiration) and inspiratory reserve volume (ie, maximum amount of air that can be inspired at end of normal inspiration) remain unchanged. Expiratory reserve volume (ie, maximal amount of air that can be expired from the resting expiratory level) falls 20% during pregnancy (Puranik et al., 1994).

Ventilation

The net effect of these lung volume changes is that there is no change in maximum breathing capacity during pregnancy. Spirometric measurements used for the diagnosis of respiratory problems do not change and remain useful for evaluation when needed. Minute ventilation (ie, amount of air inspired in 1 minute) increases 48% during late pregnancy and reaches 6.5 to 10 L/min at term. Progesterone stimulates ventilation by lowering the carbon dioxide threshold of the respiratory center and may also act as a primary stimulant to the respiratory center independent of carbon dioxide sensitivity and threshold. Minute ventilation is the product of the respiratory rate and the tidal volume. In pregnancy, the increase in minute ventilation is caused by an increase in tidal volume, because the respiratory rate remains unchanged or increases only slightly (Puranik, 1994). During labor, tidal volume can reach 40 L/min.

Oxygen and Carbon Dioxide Exchange

Oxygen consumption increases 15% to 20% (ie, approximate increases of 50 mL/min at term) during pregnancy to meet increasing oxygen demand in maternal and fetal tissues. This oxygen demand is met by the increase in minute ventilation described previously and by increased cardiac output. Increased minute ventilation increases arterial partial pressures of oxygen (PaO_2) and decreases alveolar carbon dioxide tension. The PaO_2 during pregnancy is mildly elevated to between 104 and 108 mmHg, and carbon dioxide levels in arterial vessels ($PaCO_2$) are decreased to between 26 and 32 mmHg (Thornberg, Jacobson, Giraud, & Morton, 2000). The decrease in $PaCO_2$ is accompanied by an equivalent fall in plasma bicarbonate concentration. Decreased carbon dioxide levels in the blood leads to higher pH values that are compensated for by renal excretion of bicarbonate (Lucius, Gahlenbeck, Kleine, Fabel, & Bartels, 1970), and the woman is maintained in a normal pH range of 7.4 to 7.45. The result of these changes is mildly elevated PaO_2 and decreased $PaCO_2$ and serum bicarbonate levels compared with normal values for nonpregnant women. The acid-base status during pregnancy reflects a mild renal-compensated respiratory alkalosis.

Oxygen consumption increases as pregnancy advances and is greater for multiple gestations. The fetus and reproductive tissues use 50% of the oxygen consumed. Oxygen consumption and respiratory rate further increase during labor. Respiratory rate during pregnancy is essentially unchanged (Harvey, 1999).

Pregnant women can report symptoms that are secondary to changes within the respiratory system. Fifty percent of women report feeling shortness of breath at some time during their pregnancies (Milne et al., 1978). The exact cause of this dyspnea is unclear, but theories regarding hyperventilation, the effects of progesterone, increased oxygen consumption, and decreased $PaCO_2$ levels have been proposed. Symptoms of nasal stuffiness and epistaxis are also common for pregnant women and are related to vascular congestion resulting from increased levels of estrogen.

RENAL SYSTEM

The renal system undergoes structural and functional changes during pregnancy. Changes in renal function accommodate the increased metabolic and circulatory requirements of pregnancy. The renal system excretes maternal and fetal waste products. Pressure placed on the renal system and the relaxation effect progesterone has on vascular tissue enhance the ability of the renal system to accommodate the cardiovascular changes of pregnancy.

Structural Changes

Increased renal vascular and interstitial volumes and hormonal influences during pregnancy lengthen the kidneys by 1 to 1.5 cm (Beydoun, 1985). The relaxing effects of progesterone on smooth muscle have been historically considered to be responsible for the dilation of the renal calyces, pelves, and ureters (ie, hydroureter of pregnancy) (Hytten & Leitch, 1971). This muscular relaxation coupled with increased urine volume and stasis is associated with an increased risk of urinary tract infection.

Later in the gestation, the growing uterus and the ovarian vein plexus place pressure on the ureters and bladder. The ureters become dilated, elongated, and more tortuous, with increased changes in the portions above the pelvic rim. The urethra also lengthens. Dilation of the right side is more pronounced than that on the left because of the cushioning that occurs on the left side and the dextrarotation of the uterus because of the sigmoid colon (Beydoun, 1985). This uterine obstructive effect is considered to be the cause of the physiologic hydronephrosis and hydroureter of pregnancy (MacNeily, Goldenberg, Allen, Ajzen, & Cooperberg, 1991).

During the second trimester, hyperemia of pelvic organs, hyperplasia of all muscles and connective tissues, and the gravid uterus elevate the bladder trigone and cause thickening of the interuretic margin (Hytten & Leitch, 1971). The bladder is displaced forward and upward in late pregnancy. Mechanical pressure placed on the bladder by the gravid uterus changes it from a convex to a concave organ. Reports of urinary retention capacity and bladder pressures are inconsistent; studies have reported decreased capacity and increased urinary bladder pressures (Iosif, Ingemarsson, & Ulmsten, 1980), as well as decreased pressures associated with a hypotonic bladder (Beydoun, 1985).

Pressure on the renal system can impair drainage of blood and lymph and can impede urine flow, which increases risk of infection and trauma during pregnancy. Renal volumes normalize with the first week after birth. However, hydronephrosis and hydroureter may take 3 to 4 months to return to normal (Fried, Woodring, & Thompson, 1983).

Renal Blood Flow and Glomerular Filtration Rate

Renal plasma flow (RPF) increases 35% to 60% by the end of the first trimester because of increased blood volume and cardiac output and the lowered peripheral vascular resistance caused by progesterone. RPF then progressively decreases by term to a level 50% greater than nonpregnant values (Hytten & Leitch, 1971). Women lying in the supine position can have decreased RPF in late pregnancy (Sturgiss, Dunlop, & Davison, 1994) compared with values obtained while in lateral positions. The glomerular filtration rate (GFR) begins to rise after 6 weeks of gestation and peaks by the end of the first trimester at 40% to 50% greater than nonpregnant levels (Duvekot et al., 1993). Animal studies suggest that the rise in GFR results from vasodilation of preglomerular and postglomerular resistance vessels without any alteration in glomerular capillary pressure (Baylis, 1987).

The renal clearance of many substances is elevated during pregnancy with a related decrease in serum levels (Table 5–5). Amino acids, glucose, electrolytes, and water-soluble vitamins are excreted in amounts higher than in nonpregnant women. Serum urea and creatinine levels decline because of increased GFR. Blood urea nitrogen levels fall 25%. Serum uric acid levels decrease in early pregnancy and rise after 24 weeks (Lind, Godfrey, Otun, & Phillips, 1984).

Fluid and Electrolyte Balance

Kidneys play a significant role in the regulation of sodium and potassium content in the body. Serum potassium values are influenced by elevated plasma aldosterone levels, which increase potassium excretion, and by increased progesterone levels, which prevent potassium excretion (Lindheimer, Richardson, Ehrlich, & Katz, 1987). Loss of sodium is compensated for by changes in tubular reabsorption, keeping sodium levels carefully balanced.

Renal sodium is the primary determinant of volume homeostasis. The filtered load of sodium increases from nonpregnant levels of 20,000 mEq/day to approximately 30,000 mEq/day during pregnancy (Davison, 1985). Increases in GFR, increases in antidiuretic hormone and atrial natriuretic factor, decreases in plasma albumin, elevated progesterone and

TABLE 5–5 ■ LABORATORY MEAN VALUES DURING PREGNANCY: RENAL FUNCTION

	Nonpregnant	Pregnant	
Blood			
Serum creatinine	0.6–1.2 mg/dL	Decreases to	
		First trimester	0.73 mg/dL
		Second trimester	0.58 mg/dL
		Third trimester	0.53 mg/dL
Blood urea nitrogen	8–20 mg/dL	Decreases to	
		First trimester	11 mg/dL
		Second trimester	9 mg/dL
		Third trimester	10 mg/dL
Uric acid	4.5–5.8 mg/dL	Decreases to	
		First trimester	3.1 mg/dL
		Second trimester	2.0–3.0 mg/dL
		Increases to	
		Term	4.5–5.8 mg/dL
Urine			
Creatinine clearance	90–130 mL/min/1.73 m^2	Increases to 150–200 mL/min/1.73 m^2	
Urea		Increases	
Uric acid	250–750 mg/24 hr	Increases	
Glucose	60–115 mg/dL	Increases	

prostaglandin levels, and decreased vascular resistance all contribute to sodium excretion during pregnancy.

An additional 2 to 6 mEq of sodium are reabsorbed each day for fetal and maternal stores. A gradual increase to 950 mEq of sodium is normally retained during pregnancy to meet fetal needs (Harvey, 1999). The physiologic changes that cause excretion of sodium are accompanied by increases in tubular reabsorption of sodium to avoid sodium depletion. Increases in aldosterone, estrogen, and cortisol all contribute to sodium reabsorption (Davison, 1985). These hormones, which are regulated by the renin-angiotensin-aldosterone system, promote sodium absorption and are evident in the first trimester of pregnancy.

Fluid volume and blood pressure regulation is mediated by the renin-angiotensin-aldosterone system, which is dramatically changed in pregnancy. Aldosterone acts on the renal cortical collecting ducts to cause sodium reabsorption. Aldosterone is controlled by a specialized region of the kidney, which secretes the peptide hormone renin in response to decreases in blood pressure, sodium contents of the renal tubules, and stimulation of the sympathetic nervous system. Renin release converts angiotensinogen to angiotensin I. Angiotensin I is cleaved in the lungs by angiotensin-converting enzyme (ACE) to form angiotensin II. Angiotensin II is a potent stimulator of aldosterone secretion and a potent vasodilator. Angiotensinogen, plasma renin activity, plasma renin concentration, angiotensin II concentration, and aldosterone levels are increased in pregnancy. It also has been reported that the myometrium and the chorion synthesize renin (Roberts, 1999). Increased plasma levels of aldosterone promote water and sodium retention, which results in the natural volume-overload state of pregnancy. Despite the elevated levels of angiotensin II in pregnancy, blood pressure is not elevated in normal pregnancy because of altered vascular resistance. Various studies show that women with preeclampsia lose this decreased sensitivity to angiotensin, and blood pressure rises (Whalley, Everett, Gant, Cox, & MacDonald, 1983). However, there is no clear relationship between the components of the renin-angiotensin-aldosterone system and preeclampsia.

Glycosuria and Amino Acid Excretion

Renal absorption of glucose and amino acids is not enhanced during pregnancy. Renal tubules are unable to resorb the dramatic increase (10 to 100 times prepregnancy values) in glucose load; therefore, glycosuria during pregnancy is common. Excess glucose is excreted in the urine and may not be considered pathogenic during pregnancy (Davison, 1985). Clinical management of the woman with diabetes requires

TABLE 5–6 ■ AMINO ACID EXCRETION PATTERNS

Unchanged	Increase	Double, Then Decrease or Remain Stable
Arginine	Alanine	Cystine
Asparagine	Glycine	Leucine
Glutamic acid	Histidine	Lysine
Isoleucine	Serine	Phenylalanine
Methionine	Threonine	Taurine
Ornithine		Tyrosine

serum glucose evaluation rather than urine glucose evaluation during pregnancy. A unique pattern of selective amino acid excretion and reabsorption is seen in pregnancy (Monga, 1999). Specific amino acid excretion may be increased, decreased, or unaffected (Table 5–6).

Proteinuria

There may be an increase in excreted protein during pregnancy because of the increased GFR when the protein-filtered load exceeds the tubular resorptive capacity. Urinary protein measurements should not be considered abnormal until 24-hour urine values greater than 250 mg are reached. Levels higher than 250 mg/24 hours may indicate renal disease, preeclampsia, or urinary tract infection (Misiani et al., 1991).

GASTROINTESTINAL SYSTEM

Nutritional requirements during pregnancy increase, and changes in the gastrointestinal system occur to meet these demands. The alimentary tract is altered physiologically and anatomically during pregnancy. Many of the common discomforts of pregnancy can be attributed to the gastrointestinal system. Sensitivity to taste and smell can also lead to gastrointestinal discomfort. Ptyalism may increase or become excessive. Hyperemia and softening of the gums may cause them to bleed easily.

Esophagus

After the uterus is large enough to alter the positioning of the stomach and intestines, the lower esophageal sphincter function is hindered by displacement into the thorax. However, the major explanation for altered lower esophageal sphincter function is the hormonally induced changes in sphincter smooth muscle tone. Gastrointestinal tone, lower esophageal sphincter tone, and motility of the stomach are decreased during pregnancy because of the relaxing effect of progesterone on smooth muscle.

Nausea and Vomiting

Nausea and vomiting during early pregnancy affect 50% to 80% of pregnant women (Soules et al., 1980). Several theories about the cause of nausea and vomiting have been proposed, including relaxation of the smooth muscle of the stomach, elevated levels of steroid hormones and hCG (Jordan et al., 1999), and emotional tension (Peebles-Kleiger, 2000). Soules and colleagues (1980) found no relationship between the levels of hCG and the incidence of severity of nausea and vomiting in healthy pregnant women or in women with molar pregnancies. Lazuras (1994) found that in pregnancies in which hCG levels were unusually elevated, nausea and vomiting were likely to be more frequent and severe. Treatment is supportive and involves instructing the woman to avoid foods that trigger nausea and to eat smaller meals more frequently.

Hyperemesis gravidarum is a more pronounced form of nausea and vomiting and is associated with weight loss, electrolyte imbalance, ketonemia, and dehydration. Any underlying illness should be excluded, and hospitalization for fluid and electrolyte replacement may be necessary.

Stomach

The gravid uterus displaces the stomach. Progesterone decreases stomach muscle tone and motility and causes delayed gastric emptying. Relaxation of the esophageal sphincter permits reflux of gastric contents into the esophagus, causing pyrosis (ie, heartburn). Gastric reflux is more common later in pregnancy. Because increased estrogen production causes decreased secretion of hydrochloric acid, peptic ulcer formation during pregnancy is uncommon. Early research found that gastric acid secretion is decreased in the beginning of pregnancy, and significant increases were documented in the third trimester and during lactation (Hunt & Murray, 1958).

Small and Large Intestines

The intestines are pushed upward and laterally. The appendix is displaced superiorly. Increased progesterone levels during pregnancy relax gastrointestinal tract tone and decrease intestinal motility, allowing increased absorption from the colon. Absorption of nutrients from the small intestine has not been studied in human pregnancy. Animal studies have shown increased absorption of vitamin B_{12} (Brown, Robertson, & Gallagher, 1977), increased transport of certain amino acids, and increased small intestinal weight (Burdett & Reek, 1979) in addition to the increased absorption of iron previously mentioned.

Reduced motility, mechanical obstruction by the uterus, and increased water absorption from the colon cause feces to become hard and dry, making constipation a common problem. Hemorrhoids may develop when there is straining during bowel movements related to constipation, and from the increased pressure exerted on the vessels below the level of the uterus.

Liver

Liver size and morphology apparently do not change during pregnancy, but liver function is altered (Bynum, 1977). Hepatic blood flow increases in pregnancy, but the percentage of circulating blood volume reaching the liver remains unchanged. Tests of liver function during pregnancy produce values that would suggest hepatic disease in nonpregnant women.

Serum concentration of many proteins produced by the liver increases during pregnancy in response to estrogen and hemodilution. Fibrinogen levels increase by 50% by the end of the second trimester. Serum levels of bilirubin, aspartate aminotransferase (AST), and alanine aminotransferase (ALT) are unchanged in normal pregnancy (Bynum, 1977) (Table 5–7). Plasma albumin concentration decreases to 3.0 g/dL compared with 4.3 g/dL in the nonpregnant woman. Such a decrease in nonpregnant patients could indicate liver disease. Serum alkaline phosphatase activity and serum cholesterol concentration can be twice the normal range or even higher in multiple gestations (Carter, 1990; Sadovsky & Zuckerman, 1965). This elevation results from the increased levels of placental alkaline phosphatase isoenzymes.

Gallbladder

Gallbladder size and function are altered during pregnancy. Elevated progesterone levels cause the gallbladder to be hypotonic and distended. Gallbladder smooth muscle contraction is impaired and may lead to stasis. Emptying time is slow after 12 weeks' gestation. In the second and third trimesters, fasting and residual volumes are twice as great as in the nonpregnant woman, and the rate at which the gallbladder empties is much slower (Radberg et al., 1989). Hypercholesterolemia may follow and predispose the pregnant woman to gallstone formation (Harvey, 1999).

TABLE 5–7 ■ LIVER FUNCTION DURING PREGNANCY

Parameter	Normal Range	Change
Increase		
Alkaline phosphatase		Progressive to 2–4 times greater by term
Fibrinogen		50% by second trimester Progressive to term
Globulins, alpha and beta		Progressive to term
Lipids		Progressive to term
Decrease		
Albumin		20% during first trimester
Globulins, gamma		Minor or unchanged
Unchanged		
Bilirubin	0.1–1.2 mg/dL	
Aspartate aminotransferase (AST [SGOT])	0–35 U/L	No change; may be lower than nonpregnant reference levels
Alanine aminotransferase (ALT [SGPT])	0–35 U/L	No change; may be lower than nonpregnant reference levels
5-Nucleotidase		
Prothrombin time	11–15 seconds	Unchanged or slight increase

METABOLIC CHANGES

In normal pregnancies, profound metabolic changes occur to provide for the development and growth of the fetus. Adequate maternal weight gain and normal pancreas, glucose, and fat metabolism are important factors in normal fetal growth and development.

Weight Gain

In the past two decades, there has been increased awareness about the relationship between maternal weight gain and infant birth weight. Prenatal care, socioeconomic factors, and adequate nutrition influence pregnancy outcome. Women who are underweight before conception and women who have inadequate weight gain during pregnancy are at greater risk for having a low-birth-weight infant. The risk is greatest for women with both factors (Abrams & Pickett, 1999). Maternal obesity and excessive weight gain during pregnancy has been associated with fetal macrosomia (Abrams & Pickett, 1999). A nutritional assessment should be made at the initial prenatal visit, with referral to a registered dietitian as needed. If the woman is financially unable to meet her nutritional needs, a referral to the Women, Infants, and Children (WIC) program is indicated. Table 5–8 summarizes the approximate weight gain distribution that occurs during pregnancy. The woman's prepregnancy height and weight determine her actual caloric intake needs. On average, the increased demands of pregnancy require an additional 300 kcal each day. Women who are pregnant with twins or higher-order multiples need an additional 300 kcal per fetus each day. There are differences in suggested weight gain based on prepregnancy weight and body mass index. Women who are underweight before pregnancy are encouraged to gain more weight than women who are overweight before conception. Recommended weight gain is 28 to 40 pounds for underweight women, 25 to 35 pounds for normal-weight women, and 15 to 25 pounds for overweight women (Institute of Medicine, 1990).

TABLE 5–8 ■ WEIGHT INCREASE DISTRIBUTION DURING PREGNANCY

Source	Pounds
Fetus, placenta, amniotic fluid	11
Uterus, breasts	2
Blood volume	4
Maternal stores	5
Tissue, fluid	3

Pancreas and Glucose Metabolism

Early in pregnancy, the effects of estrogen and progesterone most likely induce a state of relative hyperinsulinemia. In the absorptive state, estrogen stimulates beta cell hyperplasia and hypertrophy, resulting in an increased response to glucose and hyperinsulinemia. In the initial anabolic phase, the increased level of insulin promotes tissue storage of glycogen, increased fat synthesis, fat cell hypertrophy, and inhibition of lipolysis (Boden, 1996). As pregnancy advances, increased insulin resistance is observed along with continued hyperinsulinemia. Insulin antagonism is caused by hPL and other placental hormones (ie, progesterone, estrogen, cortisol, and prolactin) that oppose the action of insulin and promote maternal lipolysis (Buchanan & Kitzmiller, 1994). Decreased sensitivity to insulin in the liver and peripheral tissues leads to persistent hyperglycemia after meals. This hyperinsulinemia and hyperglycemia of pregnancy has been referred to as a *diabetogenic state*. During late pregnancy, the earlier anabolic metabolism is replaced by a phase of catabolic metabolism. Maternal lipid stores are used as the source of glucose and nutrients for fetal growth.

The National Diabetes Data Group defines gestational diabetes mellitus (GDM) as carbohydrate intolerance with onset or diagnosis during pregnancy. Up to 40% to 50% of women with GDM will develop diabetes within 10 years of the pregnancy (O'Sullivan, 1982). Selective screening for diabetes is recommended after a risk assessment during the first prenatal visit (American Diabetes Association [ADA], 2000). Women with a history of GDM, marked obesity, glycosuria, or a strong family history of diabetes should have a 1-hour 50-g glucose screen as soon as possible. If this value is less than or equal to 140 mg/dL (ie, negative screen), the woman is retested at 24 to 28 weeks' gestation, when the diabetogenic effect of pregnancy is detectable. Women who are younger than 25 years of age and have a normal weight before pregnancy, no history of abnormal glucose testing, poor obstetric outcome, family history of diabetes in a first-degree relative, and are not members of an ethnic group with a high prevalence of diabetes (eg, Hispanic American, Native American, African American of Pacific Islander) do not require diabetes screening (ADA, 2000). All other women should have screening performed at 24 to 28 weeks' gestation (ADA, 2000). A blood glucose level greater than or equal to 140 mg/dL (7.8 mmol/L) 1 hour after a 50-g glucose load demonstrates the need for a 100-g 3-hour oral glucose tolerance test. GDM is diagnosed if two or more values are elevated.

In early pregnancy, type 1 (immune-mediated) diabetics may require less insulin as the circulating glucose levels are reduced because of fetal uptake of glucose. In later pregnancy, women with Type 2 diabetes may require exogenous insulin to maintain optimal glucose levels because of the increase in insulin-antagonist placental hormones and insulin resistance. GDM usually does not manifest in the first trimester because the insulin antagonism is not significant until approximately 26 weeks' gestation (Hollingsworth, 1985).

Maternal morbidity is not increased in patients with GDM, but maternal morbidity is increased for type 1 and type 2 diabetics (Reece, Homko, & Hagay, 1995). Hypertensive disease is increased among advanced diabetic classifications (Kendrick, 1999). The incidence of diabetic ketoacidosis (DKA) is increased during pregnancy because accelerated fat breakdown enhances the formation of ketones (Kendrick, 1999). Treatment goals during pregnancy focus on achieving and maintaining euglycemia and avoiding hypoglycemia. Antenatal testing provides insight into fetal well-being.

Fat Metabolism

Fats are stored in the early months of pregnancy, whereas later in pregnancy, fat mobilization correlates with the increased use of glucose and amino acids by the fetus (Herrera, 2000). Fats are more completely absorbed during pregnancy, and the demand for carbohydrates increases. In the second half of pregnancy, plasma lipids increase, but triglycerides, cholesterol, and lipoproteins decrease soon after the birth. The ratio of low-density proteins (LDL) to high-density proteins (HDL) increases during pregnancy.

ENDOCRINE SYSTEM

Thyroid Gland

Increased vascularity and hyperplasia of glandular tissue during pregnancy result in increased gland size and activity. The production, circulation, and disposal of thyroid hormone are altered in pregnancy (Lazarus, 1994). Estrogen levels of pregnancy cause an increase in serum thyroxine (T_4) binding globulin. Chorionic gonadotropin stimulates production of T_4 and triiodothyronine (T_3). A study reported free T_4 levels falling as pregnancy progresses and early pregnancy T_4 levels below the lower end of the nonpregnant normal range (McElduff, 1999). The placenta mediates the accelerated degradation of thyroid hormone (Brent, 1997). Serum protein-bound iodine increases from a nonpregnant level of 5 to 12 μg/dL to a level of 9 to 16 μg/dL during pregnancy (Burrow, Fisher, & Larsen, 1994).

A diagnosis of hyperthyroidism occurs in 2 of 1,000 pregnancies and is challenging because normal signs of symptoms of pregnancy include heat intolerance, tachycardia, wide pulse pressure, and vomiting, mimicking hyperthyroidism. Poor metabolic control during pregnancy can result in preterm labor, fetal loss, or thyroid crisis, necessitating early recognition and treatment. Diagnosis of abnormal thyroid function requires a complete pattern of thyroid studies (Brent, 1997). Hypothyroidism has been associated with spontaneous abortion, preeclampsia, and mental retardation in children. Iodine supplementation has been found to decrease the incidence of cretinism in populations with high endemic levels of the condition (Mahomed & Gulmezoglu, 2000).

Parathyroid Glands

Traditional radioimmunoassays reported an increase in concentration of parathyroid hormone (PTH) during pregnancy, with levels peaking between 15 and 35 weeks and returning to normal after birth. Immunoradiometric assays for PTH reveal a decrease during pregnancy that is apparently balanced by increased parathyroid-related protein (PTHrp) from the fetus and placenta (Seki, Wada, Nagata, & Hagata, 1994).

Regulation of calcium is closely related to magnesium, phosphate, PTH, vitamin D, and calcitonin levels. Any alteration in one is likely to alter the others. Increases in serum ionized calcium or magnesium suppress PTH levels, whereas decreases in serum ionized calcium or magnesium stimulate the release of PTH (Hosking, 1996).

Pituitary Glands

The anterior pituitary enlarges somewhat and returns to its usual size after delivery. FSH stimulates ovum growth, and LH affects ovulation. Both FSH and LH are inhibited during pregnancy. Thyrotropin and adrenotropin alter metabolism to support the pregnancy. Prolactin is responsible for initial milk production during lactation.

The posterior pituitary is an outgrowth of the hypothalamus, and posterior pituitary hormones (ie, oxytocin and vasopressin) are stored in axon terminals. Oxytocin influences contractility of the uterus, and after birth, it stimulates milk ejection from the breasts. Vasopressin (ie, antidiuretic hormone) causes vasoconstriction when released in large amounts, which increases blood pressure. The major role of vasopressin is its antidiuretic action in the regulation of water balance. Secretion of vasopressin is controlled by changes in plasma osmolarity and blood volume. Plasma levels of vasopressin do not change during pregnancy despite the changes in blood volume, indicating that vasopressin is secreted at a lower plasma osmolality in pregnancy. In addition to this change in secretion, metabolic clearance of vasopressin increases at the end of the first trimester and continues until mid-pregnancy. An increased level of circulating vasopressinase is also found at this time (Lindheimer, Barron, & Davison, 1991).

Adrenal Glands

Few structural changes occur in the adrenal glands during pregnancy, but steroidogenesis is altered. The plasma level of corticotropin-releasing hormone progressively increases in the second and third trimesters of pregnancy. Circulating cortisol levels regulate carbohydrate and protein metabolism. Renin activity increases early, peaks by the end of the first trimester, and declines in the third trimester to accommodate increased sodium excretion. Total testosterone levels also increase in pregnancy because of an increase in sex hormone–binding globulin. Free testosterone levels are low normal before 28 weeks' gestation, however.

NEUROLOGIC SYSTEM

In general, there are no nervous system changes during pregnancy, although several discomforts reported by pregnant women are associated with the nervous system. Mild frontal headaches may occur in the first and second trimesters and may be caused by tension or may be related to hormonal changes because no other cause can be found. Severe headache, especially after 20 weeks' gestation, may be associated with preeclampsia. This type of headache is a result of cerebral edema from vasoconstriction. Dizziness may result from vasomotor instability, postural hypotension, or hypoglycemia, especially after prolonged periods of sitting or standing. Paresthesia of the lower extremities can occur because of pressure from the gravid uterus, interfering with circulation. Excessive hyperventilation, resulting in lower $PaCO_2$ levels, creates a tingling sensation in the hands (Harvey, 1999).

INTEGUMENTARY SYSTEM

Skin changes induced by pregnancy include vascular alterations, variations in nail and hair growth, connective tissue changes, and altered pigmentation. Blood flow to the skin increases three to four times above prepregnant levels. Vascular spider nevi appear on the face, neck, chest, arms, and legs. These are small, bright red elevations of the skin radiating from a central body. Spider nevi are related to increased subcutaneous blood flow and potentially to increased estrogen levels in the tissues (Foucar, Bentley, Laube, & Rosai, 1985). Palmar erythema is a normal vascular change in pregnancy, but it has also been associated with liver and collagen vascular diseases.

During early pregnancy, the number of hairs in the growth phase remain stable. In the later stages of pregnancy, hormonal levels apparently increase the number of hairs in the growing phase and decrease the number of hairs in the resting phase. After birth, the proportion of hairs that enters the resting phase doubles, and women experience an increase in hair loss 2 to 4 months postpartum. Occasionally, nail growth may be affected, and nail changes include transverse grooving, softening, and increased brittleness (Wong & Ellis, 1989).

Striae gravidarum (ie, stretch marks) may occur on the skin of the breasts, hips, and upper thighs and are usually most pronounced on the abdomen. Striae, which result from the normal stretching of the skin and softening and relaxing of the dermal collagenous and elastic tissues during the last months of pregnancy, occur in about 50% of pregnant women (Madlon-Kay, 1993).

Increases in estrogen and progesterone may cause an increase in melanocyte-stimulating hormone, causing hyperpigmentation in the integumentary system. Darkening of the nipples, areolae, and the perianal and genital areas occurs. The linea alba becomes the linea nigra and divides the abdomen longitudinally from the sternum to the symphysis. Melasma (ie, "mask of pregnancy," previously referred to as chloasma) appears as irregularly shaped brown blotches on the face, with a masklike distribution on the cheekbones and forehead and around the eyes. Chloasma is thought to result from elevated serum levels of estrogen and progesterone, which also stimulate melanin deposits. Chloasma disappears after pregnancy but may reappear with excessive sun exposure or with oral contraceptive use (Grimes, 1995).

MUSCULOSKELETAL SYSTEM

Early in pregnancy, the ligaments of the pregnant woman soften from the effects of progesterone and relaxin (Musumeci & Villa, 1994). This softening, especially evident in the sacroiliac, sacrococcygeal, and pubic joints of the pelvis, facilitates birth. The center of gravity changes with advancing pregnancy because of the increase in weight gain, fluid retention, lordosis, and mobilization of ligaments. To accommodate the increased weight of the uterus, the lumbodorsal spinal curve is accentuated, and the woman's posture changes. The rectus abdominis muscle may separate because of the pressure exerted by the growing uterus, producing diastasis recti.

Increased PTH levels enhance gastrointestinal absorption and decrease renal excretion of calcium. In normal pregnancy, there is no loss of bone density (Musmeci & Villa, 1994). Calcium intake recommendations during pregnancy are similar to those for nonpregnancy. Calcium intake should be 1.3 g/day in the last trimester and during lactation for women younger than 18 years old or 1 g/day for women older than 19 years of age (Institute of Medicine, 1998).

REPRODUCTIVE SYSTEM

Uterus

Before pregnancy, the uterus is a small, semisolid, pear-shaped organ that weighs 50 to 70 g. During pregnancy, the uterus becomes globular and increases in length. At term, the uterus weighs approximately 1,000 to 1,200 g because of hypertrophy of the myometrial cells. One sixth of the total maternal blood volume flows through the vascular system of the uterus. During the first few months of pregnancy, the wall of the uterus thickens by means of hyperplasia and hypertrophy in response to elevated estrogen and progesterone levels. The myometrial hypertrophy ends by the fifth month, and the muscle wall thins, allowing palpation of the fetus. The size and number of blood vessels and lymphatics increase.

The causes of activation and stimulation of the uterus are the subject of a large volume of research, but the exact causes remain unknown. There is an increase in excitability, responsiveness, and coordination of the uterine muscle in labor. After the uterus is activated, the muscle fibers respond to oxytocin and prostaglandins. Activation is thought to be affected by the fetal production of ion channels, oxytocin and prostaglandin receptors, and gap junctions (Challis, Lye, & Gibb, 1997). The activation stage is thought to be mediated by increased estrogen output and progesterone withdrawal. Chapter 9 provides a comprehensive discussion of the initiation of labor.

Placental blood flow is essential for adequate fetal growth and survival. By term, the blood flow from the uterine and ovarian arteries to the uterus is approximately 500 to 700 mL/min, 80% of which is directed to the placental bed. Maternal position, maternal arterial pressure, and uterine contractility influence uterine blood flow. The decidual portion of the spiral arteries is altered by the trophoblast, and they greatly increase in diameter to increase perfusion to the placental implantation site.

Cervix

The cervix undergoes changes characterized by increased vascularity and water content, softening, and dilation (Norman, Ekman, & Malmstrom, 1993). Estrogen stimulates glandular tissue of the cervix, which increases the number of cells. Early in pregnancy, increased vascularity causes a softening and a bluish discoloration of the cervix known as Chadwick's sign. Endocervical glands, which occupy one half of the mass of the cervix at term, secrete a thick, tenacious mucus that forms the mucous plug and prevents bacteria and other substances from entering the uterus. This mucous plug is expelled before the onset of labor and may be associated with a bloody show. Hyperactive glandular tissue also causes an increase in the normal mucus production during pregnancy.

Ovaries

Ovulation ceases during pregnancy. Cells that line the follicles, known as thecal cells, become active in hormone production and serve as the interstitial glands of pregnancy. The corpus luteum persists and secretes progesterone until the 10th to 12th week, which maintains the endometrium until adequate progesterone is secreted by the placenta.

Vagina

Vaginal epithelium and muscle layers undergo hypertrophy, increased vascularization, and hyperplasia during pregnancy in response to estrogen levels. Loosening of the connective tissue and thickening of the mucosa increase vaginal secretions. These secretions are thick, white, and acidic and play a role in preventing infection. By the end of pregnancy, the vaginal wall and perineal body become relaxed enough to permit stretching of the tissues to accommodate the birth of the infant.

Breasts

Breasts increase in size and nodularity to prepare for lactation. Nipples become more easily erectile, and veins are more prominent. Areolar pigmentation increases. Montgomery's follicles, the sebaceous glands located in the areola, hypertrophy. Striae may develop as the breasts enlarge. Colostrum, a yellow secretion rich in antibodies, may leak from the nipples during the last trimester of pregnancy. Feelings of fullness, tingling, and increased sensitivity begin in the first few weeks of gestation.

HOST DEFENSE AND IMMUNITY

One mystery in pregnancy is the process by which the mother's immune system remains tolerant of the foreign paternal antigens in the fetus and yet maintains adequate immune competence against microorganisms. Overall, the maternal immune system has a somewhat reduced resistance to infection because of the decrease in cellular immune response and the decreased efficiency and activity of T lymphocytes. Case reports have indicated that pregnant women may be more susceptible to a large number of infections, including hepatitis, influenza, varicella, variola, cytomegalovirus infection, polio, listeriosis, streptococcal infections, gonorrhea, salmonellosis, leprosy, malaria, and coccidioidomycosis (Silver & Branch, 1999). However, changes in the maternal immune system promote fetal growth and development, and data indicate that pregnant women do not have substantial impairment of systemic immunity.

Immunity refers to all mechanisms used by the body as protection against agents that are foreign to the body, including microorganisms, chemicals, drugs, and environmental substances such as pollen, animal hair, and dander. The first line of defense involves body systems that come in contact with the environment. The skin, digestive system, and respiratory system provide nonspecific defenses. Unique cells and chemical mediators are also involved in defense. Leukocytes are important for immune responses in the body. They are the most numerous of immune system cells and are grouped into three categories: polymorphonuclear granulocytes, mononuclear phagocytes, and lymphocytes. Polymorphonuclear granulocytes include neutrophils, eosinophils, and basophils. Mononuclear phagocytes function primarily as phagocytes and secrete toxic chemicals for extracellular killing. They also process and present antigens to helper T cells, as well as produce cytokines (eg, interleukin-1) involved in the inflammatory response and in T-cell activation. Lymphocytes include T lymphocytes (ie, helper T cells [CD4] and cytotoxic T cells [CD8]) and B lymphocytes. Helper T cells secrete cytokines (eg, interleukin-2), whereas cytotoxic T cells bind antigen on infected or altered cells and destroy the cell. B lymphocytes bind antigen to their plasma membrane receptors, called immunoglobulins, to initiate an antibody-mediated immune response. B lymphocytes differentiate into plasma cells, which secrete plasma membrane receptors in the form of soluble antibody. Table 5–9 summarizes the changes in these immune system components.

The placenta separates the maternal–fetal blood and lymph systems, and this barrier limits the flow of

TABLE 5–9 ■ MATERNAL CELLULAR AND HUMORAL IMMUNITY IN PREGNANCY

Immune System Component	Function	Alteration in Pregnancy
B-cell numbers	Bind antigen to immunoglobulins to initiate cell-mediated immune response	No change
T-cell numbers and subsets	Helper T cells (CD4) secrete cytokines. Cytotoxic T cells (CD8) bind antigen on infected or altered cells and destroy the cell.	No change
T-cell function		No change or decreased
Natural killer cell function	Produce interleukin-2 and interferon-γ	Decreased
IgG	Mediates agglutination, opsonization, and complement activation; can cross placenta	No change or decreased
IgM	Primary immune response; mediates agglutination and complement activation; secreted into mucous membranes and skin and provides first line of defense against ingested and inhaled pathogens; can cross into breast milk	No change
IgA		No change

cytotoxic cells and cytotoxic antibodies to the fetus. The fetal trophoblast plays an important role in evading recognition by the maternal immune system by inhibiting proliferation of cytotoxic T cells and natural killer (NK) cells. The trophoblast cells use three major mechanisms to achieve this effect: expression of FAS ligand, expression of complement regulator proteins, and failure to express major histocompatibility complex (MHC) molecules (Sargent, 1993).

The trophoblast expresses FAS ligand that protects the fetus. Any maternal immune cells that express FAS undergo apoptosis at the interface of the placenta and decidua. The trophoblast also expresses complement regulator proteins CD46, CD55, and CD59 (Weetman, 1999).

Trophoblast cells fail to express MHC class I or II molecules, and this may be the major reason the fetus is not targeted by the maternal immune system. The absence of MHC class I and II molecules prevents maternal T-cell activation and cytotoxic T-cell destruction (Daya, Rosenthal, & Clark, 1987). Extravillous cytotrophoblast cells produce a large amount of an immunosuppressive factor (from a nonclassic MHC gene encoding HLA-G) that inhibits the proliferation of cytotoxic T cells and NK cells (Menu, Kaplan, Andreu, Denver, & Chaouat, 1989). Cytokines, prostaglandin E_2, steroid hormones, estrogen, hCG, and various pregnancy-specific proteins also exert immunosuppressive effects. Adaptations to the maternal immune system are necessary for fetal survival and allow the pregnant woman to adequately respond to a large number of infectious diseases.

SUMMARY

Significant physical, metabolic, and structural changes occur from conception until weeks into the postpartum period. A thorough understanding of these changes facilitates assessment of normal pregnancy progression. Recognition of variations from normal may result in early identification of risk factors and potential complications. Prompt management can be initiated to help ensure optimal outcomes for both mother and fetus.

REFERENCES

Abrams, B., & Pickett, K. E. (1999). Maternal nutrition. In R. K. Creasy & R. Resnik (Eds.), *Maternal-fetal medicine* (4th ed., pp. 122–131). Philadelphia: W.B. Saunders.

American College of Obstetricians and Gynecologists. (1999). *Induction of labor* (Practice Bulletin No. 10). Washington, DC: Author.

American Diabetes Association. (2000). Gestational diabetes mellitus (Clinical practice recommendations 2000). *Diabetes Care, 23*(Suppl. 1), S1–116.

Bagchi, I. C., & Kumar, S. (1999). Steroid-regulated molecular markers of implantation. *Seminars in Reproductive Endocrinology, 17*(3), 235–240.

Barron, W. M., & Lindheimer, M. D. (1984). Renal sodium and water handling in pregnancy. *Obstetric & Gynecologic Annals, 13*, 35–69.

Baylis, C. (1987). The determinants of renal hemodynamics in pregnancy. *American Journal of Kidney Disease, 9*(4), 260–264.

Beard, J. L. (2000). Effectiveness and strategies of iron supplementation during pregnancy. *American Journal of Clinical Nutrition, 71*(5, Suppl.), 1288S–1294S.

Beinder, E., Huch, A., & Huch, R. (1990). Peripheral skin temperature and microcirculatory reactivity during pregnancy. *Journal of Perinatal Medicine, 18*(5), 383–390.

Beydoun, S. N. (1985). Morphologic changes in the renal tract in pregnancy. *Clinical Obstetrics and Gynecology, 28*(2), 249–256.

Boden, G. (1996). Fuel metabolism in pregnancy and in gestational diabetes mellitus. *Obstetrics and Gynecology Clinics of North America, 23*(1), 1–10.

Bonnar, J., McNichol, G. P., & Douglas, A. S. (1969). Fibrinolytic enzyme system and pregnancy. *British Medical Journal, 3*(677), 387–389.

Brent, G. A. (1997). Maternal thyroid function: Interpretation of thyroid function tests in pregnancy. *Clinical Obstetrics and Gynecology, 40*(1), 3–15.

Brown, J., Robertson, J., & Gallagher, N. (1977). Humoral regulation of vitamin B_{12} absorption by pregnant mouse small intestine. *Gastroenterology, 72* (5, Pt. 1), 881–888.

Brown, M. A., & Gallery, E. D. (1994). Volume homeostasis in normal pregnancy and pre-eclampsia: Physiology and clinical implications. *Baillieres Clinical Obstetrics and Gynaecology, 8*(2), 287–310.

Buchanan, T. A., & Kitzmiller, J. L. (1994). Metabolic interaction of diabetes and pregnancy. *Annual Review of Medicine, 45*, 245–260.

Burdett, K., & Reek, C. (1979). Adaptation of the small intestine during pregnancy and lactation in the rat. *Biochemical Journal, 184*(2), 245–251.

Burrow, G. N., Fisher, D. A., & Larsen, P. R. (1994). Maternal and fetal thyroid function. *New England Journal of Medicine, 331*(16), 1072–1078.

Bynum, T. E. (1977). Hepatic and gastrointestinal disorders in pregnancy. *Medical Clinics of North America, 61*(1), 129–138.

Carter, J. (1990). Liver function in normal pregnancy. *Australian and New Zealand Journal of Obstetrics and Gynaecology, 30*(4), 296–302.

Casey, M. L., Winkel, C. A., Porter, J. C., & MacDonald, P. C. (1983). Endocrine regulation of the initiation and maintenance of parturition. *Clinics in Perinatology, 10*(3), 709–721.

Challis, J. R., Lye, S. J., & Gibb, W. (1997). Prostaglandin and parturition. *Annals of the New York Academy of Sciences, 26*(828), 254–267.

Clark, S. L., Cotton, D. B., Lee, W., Bishop, C., Hill, T., Southwick, J., Pivarnik, J., Spillman, T., DeVore, G. R., Phelan, J., Hankins, G. D., Benedetti, T. J., & Trolley, D. (1989). Central hemodynamic assessment of normal term pregnancy. *American Journal of Obstetrics and Gynecology, 161*(6, Pt. 1), 1439–1442.

Clark, S. L., Cotton, D. B., Pivarnik, J. M., Lee, W., Hankins, G. D., Benedetti, T. J., & Phelan, J. P. (1991). Position change and central hemodynamic profile during normal third-trimester pregnancy and postpartum. *American Journal of Obstetrics and Gynecology, 164*(3), 883–887.

Crapo, R. O. (1996). Normal cardiopulmonary physiology during pregnancy. *Clinical Obstetrics and Gynecology, 39*(1), 3–16.

Cutforth, R., & MacDonald, C. B. (1966). Heart sounds and murmurs in pregnancy. *American Heart Journal, 71*(6), 741–747.

Davison, J. M. (1985). The physiology of the renal tract in pregnancy. *Clinical Obstetrics and Gynecology, 28*(2), 257–265.

Daya, S., Rosenthal, K. L., & Clark, D. A. (1987). Immunosuppressor factor(s) produced by decidua-associated suppressor cells: A proposed mechanism for fetal allograft survival. *American Journal of Obstetrics and Gynecology, 156*(2), 344–350.

Duvekot, J. J., Cheriex, E. C., Pieters, F. A., Menheere, P. P., & Peeters, L. H. (1993). Early pregnancy changes in hemodynamics and volume homeostasis are consecutive adjustments triggered by a primary fall in systemic vascular tone. *American Journal of Obstetrics and Gynecology, 169*(6), 1382–1392.

Foucar, E., Bentley, T. J., Laube, D. W., & Rosai, J. (1985). A histopathologic evaluation of nevocellular nevi in pregnancy. *Archives of Dermatology, 121*(3), 350–354.

Fried, A. M., Woodring, J. H., & Thompson, D. J. (1983). Hydronephrosis of pregnancy: A prospective sequential study of the course of dilatation. *Journal of Ultrasound in Medicine, 2*(6), 255–259.

Fuschino, W. (1992). Physiologic changes of pregnancy: Impact on critical care. *Critical Care Nursing Clinics of North America, 4*(4), 691–701.

Gerbasi, F. R., Bottoms, S., Farag, A., & Mammen, E. F. (1990). Changes in hemostasis activity during delivery and the immediate postpartum period. *American Journal of Obstetrics and Gynecology, 162*(5), 1158–1163.

Gibb, W. (1998). The role of prostaglandins in human parturition. *Annals of Medicine, 30*(3), 235–241.

Grimes, P. E. (1995). Melasma: Etiologic and therapeutic considerations. *Archives of Dermatology, 31*(12), 1453–1457.

Harvey, M. (1999). Physiologic changes during pregnancy. In L. K. Mandeville & N. H. Troiano (Eds.), *AWHONN's high risk and critical care intrapartum nursing*. Philadelphia: Lippincott, Williams & Wilkins.

Herrera, E. (2000). Metabolic adaptations in pregnancy and their implications for availability of substrates to the fetus. *European Journal of Clinical Nutrition, 54*(Suppl. 1), S47–S51.

Hollingsworth, D. R. (1985). Maternal metabolism in normal pregnancy and pregnancy complicated by diabetes mellitus. *Clinical Obstetrics and Gynecology, 28*(3), 457–472.

Hosking, D. J. (1996). Calcium homeostasis in pregnancy. *Clinical Endocrinology, 45*(1), 1–6.

Hunt, J. N., & Murray, F. A. (1958). Gastric function in pregnancy. *Journal of Obstetrics and Gynaecology of the British Empire, 65*(1), 78–83.

Hytten F. E., & Leitch I. (1971). *The physiology of human pregnancy* (2nd ed.). Oxford: Blackwell Scientific.

Iosif, S., Ingemarsson, I., & Ulmsten, U. (1980). Urodynamic studies in normal pregnancy and in puerperium. *American Journal of Obstetrics and Gynecology, 137*(6), 696–700.

Institute of Medicine. (1998). *Dietary reference intakes: Calcium, phosphorous, magnesium, vitamin D, and flouride*. Washington, DC: National Academy Press.

Institute of Medicine. (1990). *Nutrition during pregnancy: Weight gain and nutrient supplements*. Washington, DC: National Academy Press.

Jordan, V., Grebe, S. K., Cooke, R. R., Ford, H. C., Larsen, P. D., Stone, P. R., & Salmond, C. E. (1999). Acidic isoforms of chorionic gonadotrophin in European & Somoan woman with hyperemesis gravidarum and who may be thyrotropic. *Clinical Endocrinology, 50*(5), 619–627.

Kendrick, J. M. (1999). Diabetes mellitus during in pregnancy. In L. K. Mandeville & N. H. Trioano (Eds.), *AWHONN's high risk and critical care intrapartum nursing*. Philadelphia: Lippincott, Williams & Wilkins.

Kilpatrick, S. J., & Laros, R. K. (1999). Maternal hematologic disorders. In R. K. Creasy & R. Resnik (Eds.), *Maternal-fetal medicine*. (4th ed., pp. 935–963). Philadelphia: W.B. Saunders.

Kirshon B., Lee W., Cotton, D. B., & Giebel, R. (1987). Indirect blood pressure monitoring in the postpartum patient. *Obstetrics and Gynecology, 70*(5), 799–801.

Koller, O. (1982). The clinical significance of hemodilution during pregnancy. *Obstetrical and Gynecological Survey, 37*(11), 649–652.

Lazarus, J. H. (1994). Thyroxine excess and pregnancy. *Acta Medica Austriaca, 21*(2), 53–56.

Limacher, M. C., Ware, J. A., O'Meara, M. E., Fernandez, G. C., & Young, J. B. (1985). Tricuspid regurgitation during pregnancy: Two-dimensional and pulsed Doppler echocardiographic observations. *American Journal of Cardiology, 55*(8), 1059–1062.

Lind, T., Godfrey, K. A., Otun, H., & Phillips, P. R. (1984). Changes in serum uric acid concentrations during normal pregnancy. *British Journal of Obstetrics and Gynaecology, 91*(2), 128–132.

Lindheimer, M. D., Richardson, D. A., Ehrlich, E. N., & Katz, A. I. (1987). Potassium homeostasis in pregnancy. *Journal of Reproductive Medicine, 32*(7), 517–522.

Lindheimer, M. D., Barron, W. M., & Davison, J. M. (1991). Osmotic volume control of vasopressin release in pregnancy. *American Journal of Kidney Diseases, 17*(2), 105–111.

Lucius, H., Gahlenbeck, H., Kleine, H. O., Fabel, H., & Bartels, H. (1970). Respiratory functions, buffer system and electrolyte concentrations of blood during human pregnancy. *Respiration Physiology, 9*(3), 311–317.

Liu, J. H., & Park, K. H. (1988). Gonadotropin and prolactin secretion increases during sleep during the puerperium in nonlactating woman. *Journal of Clinical Endocrinology and Metabolism, 66(4)*, 839–845.

Liu, J. H., & Rebar, R. W. (1999). Endocrinology of pregnancy. In R. K. Creasy & R. Resnik (Eds.), *Maternal-fetal medicine* (4th ed., pp. 379–391). Philadelphia: W.B. Saunders.

MacNeily, A. E., Goldenberg, S. L., Allen, G. J., Ajzen S. A., & Cooperberg, P. L. (1991). Sonographic visualization of the ureter in pregnancy. *Journal of Urology, 146*(2), 298–301.

Madlon-Kay, D. J. (1993). Striae gravidarum: Folklore and fact. *Archives of Family Medicine, 2*(5), 507–511.

Mahomed, K., & Gulmezoglu, A. M. (2000). *Maternal iodine supplements in areas of deficiency* (Cochrane Review). In: Cochrane Library, Issue 2.

Mashburn, J., Graves, B. W., & Gillmor-Kahn, M. (1992). Hematocrit values during pregnancy in a nurse-midwifery caseload. *Journal of Nurse-Midwifery, 37*(6), 404–410.

McElduff, A. (1999). Measurement of free thyroxine (T_4) levels in pregnancy. *Australian and New Zealand Journal of Obstetrics and Gynaecology, 39*(2), 158–161.

Menu, E., Kaplan, L., Andreu, G., Denver, L., & Chaouat, G. (1989). Immunoactive products of human placenta: I. An immunoregulatory factor obtained from explant cultures of human placenta inhibits CTL generation and cytotoxic effector activity. *Cellular Immunology, 119*(2), 341–352.

Metcalfe, J., McAnulty, J. H., & Ueland, K. (1981). Cardiovascular physiology. *Clinical Obstetrics and Gynecology, 24*(3), 693–710.

Milman, N., Byg, K. E., & Agger, A. O. (2000). Hemoglobin and erythrocyte indices during normal pregnancy and postpartum in 206 women with and without iron supplementation. *Acta Obstetricia et Gynecologica Scandinavica, 79*(2), 89–98.

Milne, J. A., Howie, A. D., & Pack, A. I. (1978). Dyspnoea during normal pregnancy. *British Journal of Obstetrics and Gynaecology, 85*(4), 260–263.

Misiani, R., Marchesi, D., Tiraboschi G., Gualandris, L., Pagni, R., Goglio, A., Amuso, G., Muratore, D., Bertuletti, P., & Massazza, M. (1991). Urinary albumin excretion in normal pregnancy and pregnancy-induced hypertension. *Nephron, 59*(3), 416–422.

Monga, M. (1999). Maternal cardiovascular and renal adaptation to pregnancy. In R. K. Creasy, & R. Resnik (Eds.), *Maternal-fetal medicine* (4th ed., pp. 783–792). Philadelphia: W.B. Saunders.

Musumeci, R., & Villa, E. (1994). Symphysis pubis separation during vaginal delivery with epidural anesthesia: Case report. *Regional Anesthesia, 19*(4), 289–291.

Norman, M., Ekman, G., & Malmstrom, A. (1993). Prostaglandin E_2-induced ripening of the human cervix involves changes in proteoglycan metabolism. *Obstetrics and Gynecology, 82*(6), 1013–1020.

O'Sullivan, J. B. (1982). Body weight and subsequent diabetes mellitus. *Journal of the American Medical Association, 248*(8), 949–952.

Peebles-Kleiger, M. J. (2000). The use of hypnosis in emergency medicine. *Emergency Medicine Clinics of North America, 18*(2), 327–338.

Priddy, K. D. (1997). Immunologic adaptations during pregnancy. *Journal of Obstetric, Gynecologic and Neonatal Nursing, 26*(4), 388–394.

Pritchard, J. A. (1965). Changes in the blood volume during pregnancy and delivery. *Anesthesiology, 26*(4), 393–399.

Puranik, B. M., Kaore, S. B., Kurhade, G. A., Agrawal, S. D., Patwardhan, S. A., & Kher, J. R. (1994). A longitudinal study of pulmonary function tests during pregnancy. *Indian Journal of Physiology and Pharmacology, 38*(2), 129–132.

Radberg, G., Asztely, M., Cantor, P., Rehfeld, J. F., Jarnfeldt-Samsioe, A., & Svanvik, J. (1989). Gastric and gallbladder emptying in relation to the secretion of cholecystokinin after a meal in late pregnancy. *Digestion, 42*(3), 174–180.

Reece, E. A., Homko, C. J., & Hagay, Z. (1995). When the pregnancy is complicated by diabetes. *Contemporary Obstetrics and Gynecology, 43*, 43–61.

Roberts, J. M. (1999). Pregnancy-related hypertension. In R. K. Creasy & R. Resnik (Eds.). *Maternal–fetal medicine* (4th ed., pp. 833–872). Philadelphia, PA: W. B. Saunders.

Robson, S. C., Dunlop, W., Boys, R. J., & Hunter, S. (1987). Cardiac output during labour. *British Medical Journal, 295*(6607), 1169–1172.

Robson, S. C., Hunter, S., Moore, M., & Dunlop, W. (1987). Haemodynamic changes during the puerperium: A Doppler and M-mode echocardiographic study. *British Journal of Obstetrics and Gynaecology 94*(11), 1028–1039.

Robson, S. C., Hunter, S., Boys, R. J., & Dunlop, W. (1989). Serial study of factors influencing changes in cardiac output during human pregnancy. *American Journal of Physiology, 256*(4, Pt. 2), H1060–H1065.

Sadovsky, E., & Zuckerman, H. (1965). An alkaline phosphatase specific to normal pregnancy. *Obstetrics and Gynecology, 26*(2), 211–214.

Sargent, I. L. (1993). Maternal and fetal immune responses during pregnancy. *Experimental and Clinical Immunogenetics, 10*(2), 85–102.

Seki, K., Wada, S., Nagata, N., & Nagata, I. (1994). Parathyroid hormone-related protein during pregnancy and the perinatal period. *Gynecologic and Obstetric Investigation, 37*(2), 83–86.

Silver, R. M., & Branch, D. W. (1999). The immunology of pregnancy. In R. K. Creasy & R. Resnik (Eds.), *Maternal-fetal medicine* (4th ed., pp. 72–89). Philadelphia: W.B. Saunders.

Simpson, K. R., & Poole, J. H. (1998). *Cervical Ripening and Induction and Augmentation of Labor* (Symposium). Washington, DC: Association of Women's Health, Obstetric and Neonatal Nurses.

Skannal, D. G., Eis, A. L., Brockman, D., Siddiqi, T. A., & Myatt, L. (1997). Immunohistochemical localization of phospholipase A_2 isoforms in human myometrium during pregnancy and parturition. *American Journal of Obstetrics and Gynecology, 176*(4), 878–882.

Soules, M. R., Hughes, C. L., Jr., Garcia, J. A., Livengood, C. H., Prystowsky, M. R., & Alexander, E., 3rd. (1980). Nausea and vomiting of pregnancy: Role of human chorionic gonadotropin and 17-hydroxyprogesterone. *Obstetrics and Gynecology, 55*(6), 696–700.

Sturgiss, S. N., Dunlop, W., & Davison, J. M. (1994). Renal haemodynamics and tubular function in human pregnancy. *Baillieres Clinical Obstetrics and Gynaecology, 8*(2), 209–234.

Sugimoto, Y., Yamasaki, A., Segi, E., Tsuboi, K., Aze, Y., Nishimura, T., Oida, H., Yoshida, N., Tanaka, T., Katsuyama, M., Hasumoto, K., Murata, T., Hirata, M., Ushikubi, F., Negishi, M., Ichikawa, A., & Narumiya, S. (1997). Failure of parturition in mice lacking the prostaglandin F receptor. *Science, 277*(5326), 681–683.

Thompson, J. A., Hayes, P. M., Sagar, K. B., & Cruikshank, D. P. (1986). Echocardiographic left ventricular mass to differentiate chronic hypertension from preeclampsia during pregnancy. *American Journal of Obstetrics and Gynecology, 155*(5), 994–999.

Thornberg, K. L., Jacobson, S. L., Giraud, G. D., and Morton, M. J. (2000). Hemodynamic changes in pregnancy. *Seminars in Perinatology, 24*(1), 11–14.

Ueland, K., & Hansen, J. M. (1969). Maternal cardiovascular hemodynamics: III. Labor and delivery under local and caudal anesthesia. *American Journal of Obstetrics and Gynecology, 103*(1), 8–18.

Ueland, K., & Metcalfe, J. (1975). Circulatory changes in pregnancy. *Clinical Obstetrics and Gynecology, 18*(3), 41–50.

Walsh, S. W. (1985). Preeclampsia: An imbalance in placental prostacyclin and thromboxane production. *American Journal of Obstetrics and Gynecology, 152*(3), 335–340.

Weetman, A. P. (1999). The immunology of pregnancy. *Thyroid, 9*(7), 643–646.

Whalley, P. J., Everett, R. B., Gant, N. F., Cox, K., & MacDonald, P. C. (1983). Pressor responsiveness to angiotensin II in hospitalized primigravid women with pregnancy induced hypertension. *American Journal of Obstetrics and Gynecology, 145*(4), 481–483.

Wolfe, L. A., Hall, P., Webb, K. A., Goodman, L., Monga, M., & McGrath, M. J. (1989). Prescription of aerobic exercise during pregnancy. *Sports Medicine, 8*(5), 273–301.

Wong, R. C., & Ellis, C. N. (1989). Physiologic skin changes in pregnancy. *Seminars in Dermatology, 8*(1), 7–11.

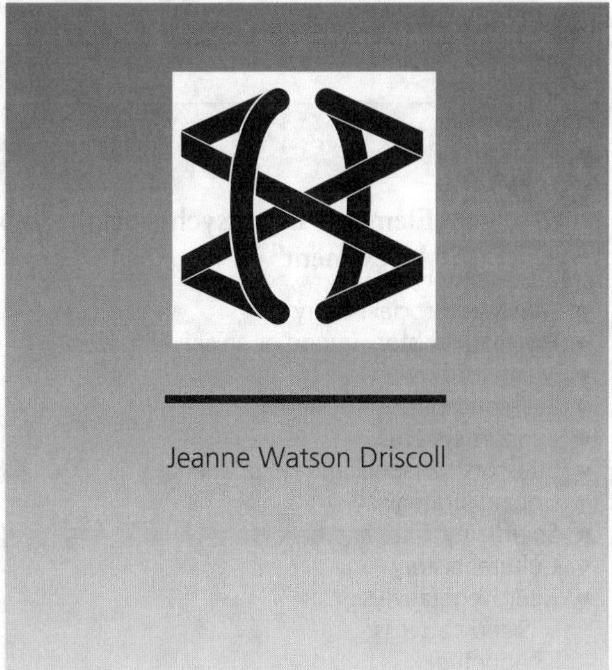

Jeanne Watson Driscoll

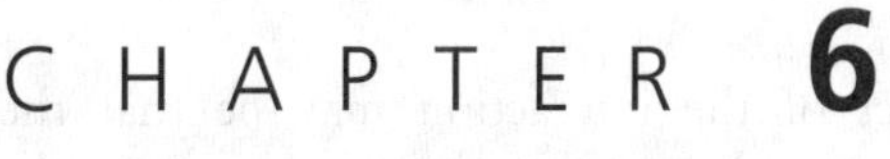

CHAPTER 6

Psychosocial Adaptation to Pregnancy and Postpartum

The goal of psychosocial care is the integration and normalization of the pregnancy and postpartum experience. It is hoped that, with caring concern, the emotional development of the new family will be encouraged, supported, and valued. Many changes occur during pregnancy and postpartum. The woman experiences changes in physiology, body size, body shape, relationships, roles, and responsibilities. The partner also undergoes changes in roles, relationships, responsibilities, and coping strategies. Pregnancy, childbirth, and the postpartum experience are life events. The way in which they are experienced is influenced by past events in women's lives. The experiences of childbirth and the postpartum period influence future life experiences (Clement, 1998).

Although family development is an ongoing process that occurs during pregnancy and postpartum, it is not the focus of this chapter; this chapter focuses on the psychosocial aspects of the woman as she progresses through the normal process of pregnancy and postpartum. The purpose here is to provide the perinatal nurse with an overview of these normal psychosocial experiences so that she or he can provide comprehensive care to the woman and her family. It is by knowledge of normal experiences that the nurse is able to recognize deviations that may require referrals to multidisciplinary colleagues for collaborative, quality, holistic care.

As the woman moves through her pregnancy, the perinatal nurse provides anticipatory education and guidance regarding the physiologic, psychological, and spiritual journey. One cannot stress enough the significance of the role the nurse plays as confidant, information provider, and supporter.

ASPECTS OF PSYCHOSOCIAL NURSING CARE

Each woman is unique. To her pregnancy she brings experiences, relationships, and realities as she perceives them. It is this unique experiential history that makes her who she is. It is this identity of self that forms the foundation for her development of the maternal self and adaptation to the maternal role.

Psychosocial Assessment

The perinatal nurse plays an important role in the woman's psychosocial adaptation. A psychosocial relationship develops based on trust, mutuality, security, validation, and support. The nurse's knowledge of normal developmental and psychosocial processes allows for rapid identification of problems or alterations in the experience. Critical to the adaptation process are the concepts of care and communication. It is important for the woman to feel she is "heard" and validated. The perinatal nurse needs to be actively involved in the interaction, clarifying communications frequently and avoiding assumptive thinking. For instance, some people commonly say "You know what I mean." If the nurse does not understand what the woman is saying, her response should be, "No, I don't know what you mean. Help me understand what you are saying or feeling." This communication strategy places the responsibility onto the woman to describe her experience in her words and her reality.

The nurse needs to establish an atmosphere in which the woman can freely ask questions and engage in discussions about things that concern her. The most difficult aspect of the interaction may be that the nurse will, at times, have to sit with the woman as she "bares her soul" while the nurse knows there is no magic to make the woman feel better. It is important to validate the woman's uncertainties without paternalism, indifference, or judgment. Nursing actions should be directed at supporting, facilitating, and encouraging the woman's personal exploration and understanding of the experience so that she can integrate this significant life event in to her reality.

Because there are transference issues in any relationship, the nurse's self-awareness is a necessity. If the nurse is unaware of his or her own issues, they may be projected onto the woman. The result may be that the woman does not feel safe. Such projections can lead to misinformation, lack of concern, validity, and disconnected relationships. If the nurse finds that she or he is reacting to something that has been said, it is imperative that the reactions be processed through self-inquiry or with consultation. For example, the fact that a nurse has been pregnant does not mean that she knows how every pregnant woman feels. It merely means that the nurse knows what she personally felt. A situation when projection may occur is during the admission of a 16-year-old primipara when the admitting nurse has a daughter of the same age. Self-awareness is especially important because many healthcare providers are the same age as their patients and at similar stages in development. Healthy, clear boundaries are necessary for the development of a therapeutic relationship.

Emphasis of the psychosocial assessment is on normalcy, health, universality, strengths, and developmental concepts, rather than on the formulation of a psychiatric diagnosis. The physiologic aspects of pregnancy often get more attention than the psychosocial aspects, but pregnancy and postpartum are holistic experiences. The mind, body, and soul are affected by these major changes and transitions. The perinatal nurse can use the holistic model to provide total care for this woman.

Psychosocial assessment is dynamic and ongoing. The process includes the pregnant woman, her family, and the nurse. The focus of the assessment is to gather biopsychosocial-spiritual and cultural data. It is from these data that nursing diagnoses can be identified, care plans developed in collaboration with the woman and her family, strategies developed, implemented, and evaluated.

Because the psychosocial assessment is an ongoing process, assessment is made at every visit. Key elements to be included in a psychosocial assessment are listed in Display 6–1.

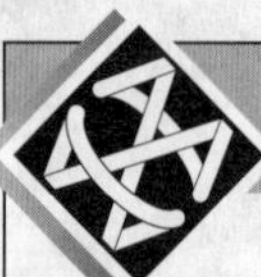

DISPLAY 6–1

Elements of a Psychosocial Assessment

- Family and social history
- Psychiatric history (mood or anxiety disorders)
- Mental status
- Self-concept or self-esteem
- Support systems
- Stressors: personal and occupational
- Coping strategies
- Spirituality: faith and beliefs
- Cultural history
- Neurovegetative signs:
    - Sleep patterns
    - Appetite
    - Energy or motivation
    - Mood or anxiety state
    - Sexual desires
- Knowledge of pregnancy experience

The style of obtaining information is derived from the interviewing skills of the clinician. It may be helpful to use permission-giving statements such as "Many woman have told me they have some periods when they cry. Has this happened to you?" This allows the woman to hear that the nurse is open to her worries and concerns and that she does not have to be "fine." The timing and location of the interview are also important. If there is limited time for interaction and more time is necessary for disclosure and discussion, make another appointment. This strategy validates the woman's issues and demonstrates the nurses' caring and concern.

Collaborative Care and Referral

A critical aspect of holistic care planning is the coordination of the multidisciplinary team to provide care for this woman and her family. Often, women present with issues, needs, or concerns that are beyond the realm of the perinatal nurse. These issues may require collaboration with the members of the psychiatric or mental health specialties, nutrition services, social services, or community agencies.

There is a strong correlation between the onset of mood and anxiety disorders before pregnancy and their exacerbation in the postpartum period (Sichel & Driscoll, 1999). All too often, when women talk about mood swings and increased anxiety during pregnancy, the reports of these uncomfortable symptoms are devalued with statements such as, "It's just because of your hormones. It will go away after you have the baby." This type of paternalistic remark denigrates the importance of the woman's feelings and may silence her. It is important for perinatal healthcare providers to be aware that a woman with previous mood and anxiety disorders is at high risk for reoccurrence of these disorders during pregnancy and postpartum (Sichel & Driscoll, 1999). A history of mood and anxiety disorders mandates coordination of the woman's care in a holistic manner, involving mind, body, and soul. If the perinatal nurse is vigilant about the adaptation and attainment processes during pregnancy, referrals to multidisciplinary colleagues can be made as appropriate to facilitate this woman's journey to motherhood.

The perinatal nurse should be aware of community mental health resources. This may require developing a resource list, talking with providers, and developing referral relationships.

ADAPTATIONS DURING PREGNANCY

In the following sections, the psychosocial aspects of pregnancy are presented. Ongoing assessment of mood and anxiety levels in addition to the need for information and support is mandatory. Offering anticipatory guidance about physiologic and psychological changes during pregnancy supports the woman as she moves through a period of transition between two lifestyles and two states of being: the woman without child and the woman with child (Lederman, 1996).

Reva Rubin, in her classic work (1984), described tasks that a woman needs to accomplish during her pregnancy. These tasks include ensuring a safe passage for herself and her child; ensuring social acceptance of child by significant others; increasing affinity ties in the construction of the image and identity of the "I" and the "you"; and exploring the meaning of the transitive act of giving and receiving. Regina Lederman (1996) described seven psychosocial variables that are relevant to a woman's transition into self during pregnancy. These include acceptance of pregnancy; identification with a motherhood role; relationship with her mother and partner or husband; preparation for labor; and prenatal fears of loss of control and self-esteem in labor. The perinatal nurse plays a significant role in the facilitation of a woman's attainment of these tasks and as well as helping her to navigate the psychosocial transitions. It is through the establishment of a strong professional relationship of care and concern that this relationship develops and grows.

First Trimester

Experience of the Mother

Myriad physiologic symptoms occur in the first trimester, and it is a time of strange feelings and secrets. The woman may know that she is pregnant as a result of a home pregnancy test, or she may deny the possibility until she requests a pregnancy test. Often, the nurse calls the woman to tell her the test result is positive. Psychosocial assessment begins at this initial nurse–patient contact. What was her response to the news that she is pregnant: shock, disbelief, joy, anticipation, denial, or fear? Major areas of assessment are listed in Display 6–2.

"The task of the first trimester is progressive movement of the woman from a state of conflict and ambivalence to one of acceptance of the pregnancy, the child, and the motherhood role" (Lederman, 1990, p. 281). The nurse promotes this transition through concern, care, and support. Many women share that they are not sure what to feel. Moods can range from high to low, calm to panic, happy to sad, and acceptance to denial. She may feel a bit detached, emotionally labile, nauseous, fatigued, anxious, and concerned.

Often, women describe the feelings of the first trimester as "like being on a roller coaster." Ambivalence is high. "This is what I thought I wanted; why do I feel so confused and sick?" Anticipatory guidance helps the woman resolve some of these feelings. If this is her first pregnancy, she needs consistent in-

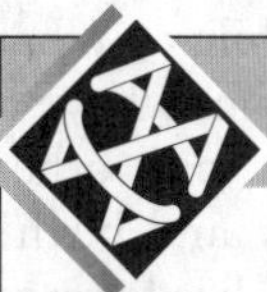

DISPLAY 6–2

Assessment Issues in the First Trimester

- Mood and anxiety changes
- Meaning of the pregnancy (personal)
- Physical concerns or issues
- Partner or significant other's response
- Sexuality: issues or concerns
- Concerns regarding pregnancy or postpartum experience
- Relationship with family
- Support system
- Coping strategies
- Neurovegetative signs:
  - Sleep patterns
  - Appetite
  - Energy or motivation
- Spirituality: beliefs and values

formation and support. If she is a multiparous woman, how did she experience her other pregnancies? Has she had any abortions? Were they spontaneous or elective? What was her response at that time? Does she have live children? Has she had a stillborn infant? The woman's history affects this pregnancy experience.

Today, with regular use of amniocentesis, the woman may delay attachment to the pregnancy until results of an amniocentesis are available, usually at about 20 weeks of pregnancy. So for almost 20 weeks, she may remain disconnected from her feelings and emotions in an effort to protect herself from potential pain and disappointment. If she has a history of miscarriage, she may be afraid to become attached to the pregnancy until she passes the "critical week" when she lost the other pregnancy. It is not uncommon for women with histories of loss to delay attachment until they see a live baby at birth.

Developing a therapeutic relationship with the woman takes work. Key aspects of this relationship include the development of trust, confidence, mutuality, active listening, and empowerment. Pregnancy is a time of emotional changes, and she needs a "safe place" to share her thoughts and concerns. Suggest that she begin a journal of her pregnancy experiences as a place to share personal thoughts. What about the father of the baby? What are his thoughts? How does she think he is doing with this new information? Meeting with the woman's partner or significant other provides additional information to help the nurse with the complete family assessment. Ascertain any misconceptions, needs for information, and feelings about the pregnancy. What is his availability? What about other support people? Does the woman have a best friend or confidant, or can she talk with other women who have experienced pregnancy and birth? What about her concepts of spirituality; is her faith or belief system helpful to her?

The woman needs validation and support. A major nursing role is to "listen" to the woman's experience. What does it feel like for her? All too often, she feels as though the people in the physician's office care only about the urine samples, her vital signs, and weight status. She is nervous and will do well with permission to feel, anticipatory information, and support as she moves through this first trimester.

Role of the Nurse

The role of the nurse during the first trimester includes the following tasks:

- Begin psychosocial assessment at initial contact; assess the woman's response to pregnancy.
- Promote the woman's accomplishment of the first task of pregnancy by showing concern and giving care and support.
- Give anticipatory guidance related to the experiences of the first trimester.
- Continue to make assessments by interviewing the partner or significant other.
- Validate the woman's concerns and support her emotional state.

Second Trimester

Experience of the Mother

As she moves into the second trimester, the pregnant woman begins to feel fetal activity. She may have seen an image of the fetus by ultrasound, but now she feels the baby move. "Fantasies during pregnancy, expressed as descriptions of the unborn child, are believed to be a key component in maternal–child relational and concomitant maternal role formation" (Sorenson & Schuelke, 1999). What are her fantasies? Who does she imagine her baby looks like? What does she think it will be like to have a baby? It is by asking these types of questions that role development may be facilitated. Building on prior assessments, Display 6–3 contains issues critical to the second trimester.

The woman is dealing with issues related to body changes. She begins to wear maternity clothes and people ask her about her pregnancy; it is no longer a secret. She may need to do some grief work and talk about the loss of her body shape and size. The perinatal nurse must exercise caution and not project per-

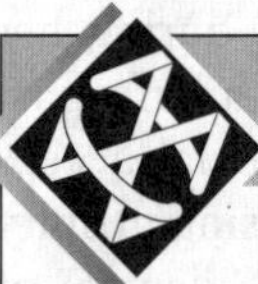

DISPLAY 6–3

Assessment Issues in the Second Trimester

- Mood and anxiety changes
- Feelings and perceptions about fetal movements
- Feelings about body changes and body image
- Attachment to fetus
- Neurovegetative signs:
  - Sleep patterns
  - Appetite
  - Energy or motivation
- Relationship with partner or significant other
- Sexuality: issues and concerns
- Relationship with work and family
- Knowledge about the pregnancy experience
- Spirituality: faith and beliefs

sonal feelings onto the woman. For example, the perinatal nurse may say, "You must be excited about feeling the baby move." However, the woman may feel as though there is an alien inside; it is more frightening than exciting. Now she knows that the nurse thinks that she should be excited, so she better not reveal how she really feels. She is afraid the nurse may think something is wrong with her if she is not excited. She is vulnerable and needs to feel safe and confident that her feelings are heard in a nonjudgmental way.

Pregnant women have increased vulnerability to emotional nuances in relationships. They perceive from the nurse's looks, innuendos, and responses whether or not they are being valued. Women have been socialized to be other-centered, so she may need help focusing on her needs, wants, and concerns (Miller, 1986). It is hard to share the feelings that may not seem "nice." If the nurse reacts negatively to the woman's feelings, it will close the door to the woman's development of trust, mutuality, and confidence in her own feelings as valid and real. Permission-giving statements should be used, such as, "In my clinical practice, women have shared with me that they are not too excited about the changes in their body. How do you feel about this?" This allows her to know that you have heard some negative things and that perhaps it is safe for her to disclose her real feelings, contrary to what she has been told she should feel.

Although the second trimester is often thought to be a time of tranquility and quiescence, the pregnant woman may be experiencing increased anxiety as the baby makes his or her presence known. She begins to feel better physiologically and her focus may shift from her self-concern to baby-concern. The woman is more aware of her changing body size and her perception of her body space. She may be more anxious about these changes. She may begin to have some fears or phobias about something happening. If the nurse feels that the woman's anxieties and concerns are getting in the way of her healthy day to day functioning, a referral to a psychiatric or mental healthcare provider may be necessary. This lets the woman know that her concerns and fears are valued and that the goal is to provide holistic care.

The pregnant woman may tell you that she is having weird, sometimes frightening, dreams about "strangers" entering her life. When one stops to think about it, there is a stranger in her life. A woman's perception of her unborn child develops through watching images during ultrasound examinations or the personal characteristics the woman imagines in response to fetal movements. For example, many women describe in detail the attributes of their baby based on ultrasound images or cycles of fetal activity. If fetal sex is known as a result of ultrasonography or genetic testing, more gender-specific traits can be imagined. It is not unusual for women to report, "He's a wild one," or "She likes to keep me up at night." Encourage her to share her perceptions and dreams with her partner or another significant person in her life. Tell the woman that it often helps to just talk about them. Let her know that some women find it worthwhile to write about their dreams and feelings in a journal during pregnancy. Benefits of keeping a journal include the woman's ability to review entries at a later date and analyze the development of her impressions as the pregnancy progresses.

Anticipatory information and education about the childbirth experience begin to be of importance now. It is time to register for prepared childbirth classes. Attending these classes appeals to the cognitive side of the process because she is becoming informed about her body and the upcoming labor and birth. Sometimes, a secondary gain of childbirth classes is development of new friendships among the participants based on shared experiences. These relationships often carry over into the postpartum period and beyond.

Role of the Nurse

The role of the nurse during the second trimester includes the following tasks:

- Continue ongoing psychosocial assessments of the woman and her partner or significant other.
- Encourage verbalization regarding grief process (eg, body image).
- Maintain a nonjudgmental attitude.
- Refer to a psychiatric care provider if anxieties seem greater than normal.
- Encourage the woman to share dreams, thoughts, and feelings with a close friend or her partner or keep a personal journal.
- Provide anticipatory guidance regarding normal changes and concerns.
- Provide information regarding childbirth classes for the woman and her partner.

Third Trimester

Experience of the Mother

During the third trimester, frequency of visits to healthcare providers increases. The woman may begin to ask more questions and verbalize increased concerns about what will happen during labor and birth.

The major issues of the third trimester are birth preparation and the baby's well-being. The mother may begin to experience an approach-avoidance conflict related to childbirth and the possible consequences that may evolve such as pain and loss of control (Rofe, Blittner, & Lewin, 1993). Display 6–4 describes assessment issues pertinent to this trimester.

During this trimester, some women experience physical discomforts because of body size and physiologic changes. They worry about what will happen when they go into labor. Role responsibilities are changing. The woman may be leaving work to begin maternity leave, a role change that may affect daily interaction with adults and potentially her identity. She may begin to talk about her fear of losing control during labor and birth. "What if I scream?" "How will I know when I am in labor?" "I won't leave the house!" "What if my water breaks in the mall?" Her anxieties begin to rise. Ongoing assessment of her anxiety level is necessary. It is important to validate her concerns and support her normalcy. If the nurse feels that the woman's mood is more intense than usual, referral may be necessary for evaluation by the psychiatric or mental health team. If she does have a history of postpartum mood and anxiety disorders, this is a good time to have her meet with the psychiatric treatment team so that her care plan could be developed for prophylaxis postpartum (Sichel & Driscoll, 1999).

Her dreams may begin to include fears of being stuck or trapped, fears of some harm happening to her or the baby, and concerns for survival. It is not uncommon at this time for the woman to experience increased anxiety secondary to hearing other women's stories of their birth experiences. She worries about her performance and about the "awful" things that might happen. She needs to have a safe place to share her concerns and worries.

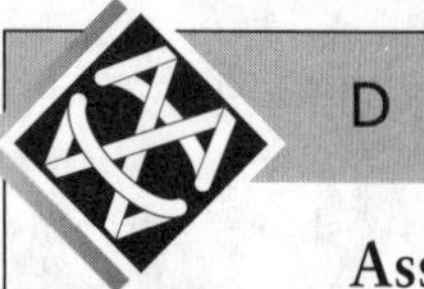

DISPLAY 6–4

Assessment Issues in the Third Trimester

- Mood and anxiety changes
- Physical changes
- Attachment to the fetus
- Body image or self-concept
- Expectations of self and partner about labor and birth
- Neurovegetative signs:
    - Sleep patterns
    - Appetite
    - Energy or motivation
- Relationship with partner or significant other
- Sexuality: issues and concerns
- Relationship with family and work
- Spirituality: faith and beliefs

It is important to discuss and plan for the postpartum experience. What about support? Who is going to help her? What are her expectations of the experience? If there are other children, who will take care of them and help her after she gets home with the new baby? Assist the woman to develop lists of things to do and people she needs to contact and enlist support from before birth. If she will be breast-feeding, encourage her to attend breast-feeding support groups before birth to promote relationship and resource development.

Role of the Nurse

The role of the perinatal nurse continues to be one of assessment, information, and support. The nurse's role in the third trimester includes the following tasks:

- Continue ongoing psychosocial assessment of the woman and her partner or significant other.
- Support and reinforce information obtained in childbirth education classes.
- Facilitate verbalization of concerns related to employment status and role changes.
- Encourage sharing of feelings and concerns with her partner or significant other.
- Provide anticipatory education regarding the postpartum experience.
- Facilitate planning for help at home after the birth.
- Encourage her to obtain information about new mothers' support groups and breast-feeding support groups.

ADAPTATIONS DURING LABOR AND BIRTH

Experience of the Mother

The labor and birth experience is a critical turning point. The mother makes the major physical and psychological transition to birth. The onset of labor can be a scary experience, especially when she realizes that there is no way back. Often, she calls with the first twinges and asks, "What should I do?" She needs a lot of support and gentle guidance. She is concerned about her well-being, that of her baby, and of her partner. She is afraid that she will "lose it," and she wants to "be a good patient." Her sense of reality is intense.

If she is having her baby in the hospital or birth center, it is important that the perinatal nurse orient the woman and her partner to the unit and talk with them about their hopes and desires for this birth experience. The establishment of an empathic, therapeutic relationship is necessary to provide the woman with the connection and concern that she needs to proceed in the labor experience. Anticipatory guidance and information sharing need to be ongoing, as she may lose sense of time because of the crisis of labor. Continual assessment of her psychosocial ability to stay focused and connected to the experience is important. Pay close attention to the interaction between the laboring woman and her support person so that you will be available as needed to support them both.

Each woman will labor and birth in a unique way, and nursing care should be individualized rather than routine. Similarly, there is no behavior or response that one would expect to see after the birth. Some women will be jubilant and excited, want to hold their baby, count fingers and toes, and breast-feed. Other women need to go into themselves to regroup on an intrapersonal level. There is no one right way. One woman, after a precipitous birth experience, when asked if she wanted to hold her new baby, said, "Not yet; give me some time to get myself together. I can't believe this is over." With all the pressure about "bonding," it is important for the nurse to support the individual new mother's request at this time. This is the beginning of the conflicts of new motherhood: do I take care of myself, or do I put the baby first? Klaus, Kennell, and Klaus (1995) found that the care the woman receives at this phase appears to affect her attitudes, feelings, and responses to her family, herself, and especially her new baby to a remarkable degree. The psychosocial assessment issues of this experience are listed in Display 6–5.

Role of the Nurse

The role of the nurse during adaptation to the labor and birth experience is intense and critical. The woman may be scared, vulnerable, or excited. She may even regress in response to the stress of the situation. The role of the nurse during labor and birth includes the following tasks:

- Establish an empathic relationship based on trust.
- Orient the laboring woman and her support person to the unit or birth center.
- Facilitate the interaction between the woman and her labor support person.

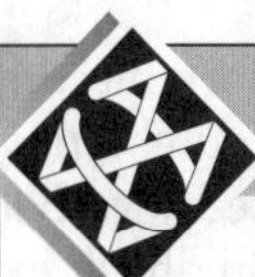

DISPLAY 6–5

Assessment Issues During Labor and Birth

- Mood and anxiety changes
- Coping strategies
- Adjustment to the environment
- Relationship with partner or significant other
- Assess ability to focus and work with the labor process
- Cultural aspects of childbirth
- Spirituality: faith and beliefs

- Provide ongoing psychosocial assessment.
- Provide anticipatory guidance regarding the labor experience.
- Encourage attachment to the baby after it is born, in relation to the new mother's needs.

ADAPTATIONS IN THE POSTPARTUM PERIOD

The birth occurs. The family has a new member. The new mother begins her physiologic recovery, relationship development with the "real" baby, and psychological adaptation to motherhood.

During this early postpartum period, it is important for the perinatal nurse to observe the maternal–newborn attachment process and identify behavior patterns that may indicate the need for further follow-up care. It is critical to differentiate behaviors related to maternal exhaustion or discomfort from real problems with attachment. For example, the woman who asks that her baby spend the night in the nursery so she can get some rest is probably physically exhausted from the labor and birth, and the woman who does not want to hold her baby after a cesarean birth may be having significant incisional pain. Each woman is unique and responds to her newborn in her own way. A series of interactions are necessary for accurate assessment of maternal–newborn attachment. Nursing assessment should also focus on maternal confidence in basic newborn care skills such as comforting strategies, formula or breast-feeding, bathing, and diapering. Encouragement and reinforcement may be necessary as the new mother tries to learn all she needs to know about newborn care in the very short time she is hospitalized.

The new mother needs time to share her labor and birth experience (Rubin, 1984). This is often done by calling all of her friends on the phone or by meeting other new mothers in the perinatal unit and chatting. She is putting meaning into the experience by verbalizing her reality. This integration of the childbirth experience into her self-system is a major issue of the early postpartum experience (Rubin). There is the need to talk about and process reality versus fantasy. There is an element of loss as she begins to mourn the imagined childbirth experience (Driscoll, 1990; Nicolson, 1999). The perinatal nurse plays a significant role in the validation and clarification of the experience for this woman by listening and supporting her evolving maternicity.

Today, with the reality of shortened postpartum lengths of stay, the new mother has to move quickly from self-concern to other-concern: her newborn. It is important that her physical and psychological needs be met so that she will be better able to focus on her newborn's care. She may become intensely focused on the cognitive learning needs related to newborn feeding and physical care. The new mother may verbalize anxiety and concern. If so, she needs to be heard and her concerns must be validated. The newly evolving relationship with the newborn is based on connection and care. If she has difficulty with these beginning skills, it may alter her self-esteem and maternal development (Driscoll, 1993). The woman brings with her many performance expectations that need to be discussed and clarified. Mercer (1986) described maternal role attainment as a process that takes a period of about 10 months to develop. During this postpartum phase, the new mother attaches to her newborn, gains competence as a mother, and expresses gratification in the mother–infant interaction. This adaptation can be delayed or altered if the woman's health and mental status is less than optimal. The reality of the current healthcare delivery system is that much of the work of the postpartum maternal adjustment and role attainment is done after discharge. Referral to community resources and discharge planning are imperative in the total care plan.

Emotionally, these early days can be disconcerting. It is supposed to be such an exciting time, but she may be experiencing alternating periods of crying and joy, irritability, anxiety, headaches, confusion, forgetfulness, depersonalization, and fatigue. She may have the "baby blues." Between 70% and 80% of new mothers may experience this transitory mood disorder. Unfortunately, this phenomenon occurs so frequently that it is often considered normal and therefore does not get the attention that it deserves. It is felt that this disorder is related to the normal physiologic and psychosocial changes that occur in the process of becoming a new mother. There is a rapid drop in pregnancy hormones after delivery of the placenta, which may alter biochemical neurotransmitters in the brain (Sichel & Driscoll, 1999). This transitory mood disorder can greatly affect the new mother and her family, especially if they are unaware of the possibility or what to do about it. Assessment issues relevant to the postpartum experience are listed in Display 6–6.

Women and their families need information about normal mood changes after childbirth. They should be aware that with much support, reassurance, rest, and good nutrition, these labile moods usually balance out, and the woman will begin to feel better and feel more organized and confident. However, if the moods do not stabilize by about 21 days, referral should be made to the psychiatric or mental health team specialists in postpartum mood and anxiety disorders (Suri & Burt, 1997).

A study of first-time mothers surveyed during the postpartum period revealed a 63% incidence of depressive disorders of early onset and lengthy duration (McIntosh, 1993). Most affected women reported that they did not seek help because they felt their depression was caused by the stress of becoming a mother; they thought it was a normal reaction. An additional reason women cited for not talking to a professional healthcare provider about their feelings was the fear that they would be labeled as mentally ill and considered an unfit mother (McIntosh). Perinatal nurses must be proactive in identifying women with mood or anxiety disorders during the postpartum period to facilitate early intervention and referral to psychiatric or mental health specialists.

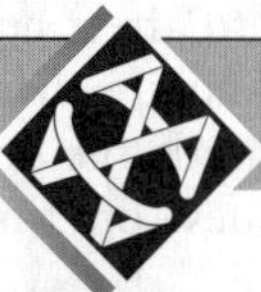

DISPLAY 6–6

Assessment Issues During the Postpartum Period

- Mood and anxiety states
- Perceptions of the birth experience
- Maternal-newborn attachment
- Relationship with partner or significant other
- Neurovegetative signs:
    - Sleep patterns
    - Energy or motivation
    - Pain levels
- Coping strategies
- Support systems
- Cultural aspects of childbearing
- Knowledge about postpartum process after discharge
- Spirituality: faith and beliefs

Postpartum Depression

Postpartum depression (PPD) is a mood disorder that is estimated to affect 3% to 30% of women (Sichel & Driscoll, 1999). Symptoms of postpartum depression may include anxiety, irritability, fatigue, a demoralizing sense of failure, feelings of guilt, sleep disorders, appetite changes, suicide ideation, and excessive concerns about the baby. Treatment for postpartum depression and related mood and anxiety disorders may include antidepressant agents, antianxiety agents, psychotherapy, counseling, and support groups. With appropriate intervention, prospects for recovery are excellent.

Postpartum Psychosis

The most serious psychiatric disorder that can occur after the birth of a baby is postpartum psychosis. This is an organic psychosis that affects 1 or 2 women per 1,000 births. This disorder is a psychiatric emergency. The woman can demonstrate symptoms of psychosis within 1 to 2 days after the birth of her baby. The signs and symptoms of psychosis are sleep disturbances, confusion, agitation, irritability, hallucinations, delusions, and potential for suicide or infanticide. Hospitalization is mandatory. With aggressive treatment most women recover from this disorder (Sichel & Driscoll, 1999).

Postpartum Anxiety Disorders

Anxiety disorders may present as a panic disorder or obsessive compulsive disorder (OCD). Often, women with a history of panic disorder experience exacerbations postpartum. The symptoms include palpitations, pounding heart, rapid heart rate, sweating, trembling, sensations of smothering, shortness of breath, feeling of choking, chest pain or tightness, nausea, dizziness, lightheadedness, feeling detached, fear of dying or of going crazy, numbness in fingers, and chills or hot flashes. These episodes begin to occur regularly, out of the blue, and interfere with the woman's every day living. Treatment includes antianxiety medications, antidepressant medications, and cognitive-behavioral strategies (Sichel & Driscoll, 1999).

OCD is a disorder that is typified by repetitive thoughts and behaviors that have no particular meaning and over which sufferers have little or no control. Postpartum onset of OCD often presents in the postpartum period. The woman describes the onset of ego-alien thoughts that something harmful might happen to the baby. She cannot get the thought out of her mind, and she begins to imagine that she could be capable of doing the harm, which increases her anxiety. In response to these thoughts, women develop avoidance behaviors so they "will not act on my thoughts." Anxiety symptoms surge and depression can occur. This is not a psychotic disorder, the woman knows that these thoughts are bizarre. We are not sure of the cause of this disorder, but there may be some correlation between the rapid drops of estrogen and the oxytocin levels in the brain (Sichel & Driscoll, 1999). Treatment includes antidepressants, antianxiety agents, and cognitive-behavioral strategies.

It cannot be stressed enough that women and their families need anticipatory information about postpartum mood disorders so that prompt identification and early treatment can be initiated. A heightened awareness among perinatal healthcare providers regarding the incidence of postpartum mood and anxiety disorders, knowledge of common signs and symptoms, and the prospects for recovery can contribute to successful outcomes for affected women and their families.

Discharge planning has become a critical issue in this time of shortened length of stay. Before discharge from the hospital, the woman should be given a list of telephone numbers of her care providers as well as any emergency services that she may need. It is important to go over the key support people with the new mother and her partner during discharge teaching.

Role of the Nurse

The role of the perinatal nurse during the postpartum experience is changing continually in response to current lengths of stay. Hospitals are developing home-discharge programs, private home health agencies are being established, and most postpartum care occurs in the community. The nurse has several tasks during the postpartum period:

- Continue ongoing psychosocial assessment of woman and her partner or significant other.
- Assess and facilitate maternal attachment.
- Encourage verbalization of birth experience to promote integration.
- Assess and facilitate family development.
- Assess support systems and networks in the family and community.
- Provide education about normal postpartum emotional adjustments and provide anticipatory guidance regarding postpartum mood and anxiety disorders.
- Make referrals to psychiatric or mental healthcare providers who specialize in perinatal psychiatric care if needed.

SUMMARY

Psychosocial adaptation to pregnancy and postpartum is a dynamic process. The nurse plays a significant role in the promotion and facilitation of this experience in a healthy way. It is a time when the woman is open to great psychological growth and relies on the healthcare team for information and support. The nurse needs to be aware of the normal process to identify those that are abnormal. It is helpful in the assessment of mood, anxiety, and emotional states to remember three words: frequency, duration, and intensity. If the woman says she is having difficulty functioning in her activities of daily living and having a tough time coping because of emotional, mood, or anxiety changes, referral is necessary. The referral process needs to be managed in an empowering, supportive way. Letting her know that she is valued and that her concerns and feelings are important is a way for the perinatal nurse to give the woman the message that she deserves good care. Appropriate healthcare provider attitudes support the referral process.

Because of the rapid changes in the healthcare delivery system and decreasing lengths of stay, it is imperative for the perinatal nurse to actively pursue, nurture, and promote collaborative relationships with colleagues in the community. This active communication and relational approach to the care of this new mother and her family promotes, facilitates, and encourages healthy maternal and paternal psychosocial adaptation and adjustment.

REFERENCES

Clement, S. (1998). *Psychological perspectives on pregnancy and childbirth.* New York: Churchill Livingstone.

Driscoll, J. W. (1990). Maternal parenthood and the grief process. *Journal of Perinatal and Neonatal Nursing, 4*(2), 1–10.

Driscoll, J. W. (1993). The transition to parenthood. In C. S. Fawcett (Ed.), *Family psychiatric nursing* (pp. 97–108). St. Louis: C.V. Mosby.

Lederman, R. P. (1990). Anxiety and stress in pregnancy: Significance and nursing assessment. *NAACOG's Clinical Issues in Perinatal and Women's Health Nursing, 1*(3), 279–288.

Lederman, R. P. (1996). *Psychosocial adaptation in pregnancy.* (2nd ed.). New York: Springer Publishing.

Klaus, M. H., Kennell, J. H., & Klaus, P. H. (1995). *Bonding: building foundations of secure attachment and independence.* Reading, MA: Addison-Wesley Publishing.

McIntosh, J. (1993). Postpartum depression: Women's help seeking behavior and perceptions of cause. *Journal of Advanced Nursing, 18*(2), 178–184.

Mercer, R. T. (1986). *First-time motherhood: Experiences from teens to forties.* New York: Springer-Verlag.

Miller, J. B. (1986). *Toward a new psychology of women* (2nd ed.). Boston: Beacon.

Nicolson, P. (1999). *Post-natal depression: psychology, science, and the transition to motherhood.* New York: Routledge.

Rofe, Y., Blittner, M., & Lewin, I. (1993). Emotional experiences during the three trimesters of pregnancy. *Journal of Clinical Psychology, 49*(1), 3–12.

Rubin, R. (1984). *Maternal identity and the maternal experience.* New York: Springer-Verlag.

Sichel, D., & Driscoll, J. W. (1999). *Women's Moods.* New York: William Morrow.

Sorenson, D. S., & Schuelke, P. (1999). Fantasies of the unborn among pregnant women. *Maternal Child Nursing, 24*(2), 92–97.

Suri, R., & Burt, V. K. (1997). The assessment and treatment of postpartum psychiatric disorders. *Journal of Practical Psychiatry and Behavioral Health, 3*(2), 67–77.

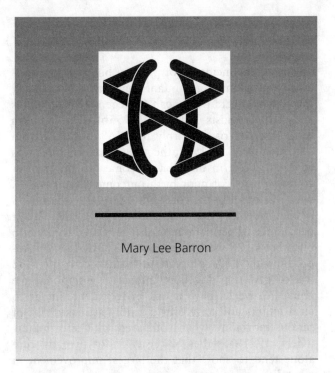

Mary Lee Barron

CHAPTER 7

Antenatal Care

Quality prenatal care includes education and support for the pregnant woman, ongoing maternal–fetal assessment, preparation for parenting, and promotion of a positive physical and emotional family experience. Prenatal care has several goals:

- Maintenance of maternal–fetal health
- Accurate determination of gestational age
- Ongoing risk assessment and risk-appropriate intervention
- Woman and family education about pregnancy, birth, and parenting
- Rapport with the childbearing family
- Referral to appropriate resources.

BIRTH IN THE UNITED STATES

With the arrival of the 21st century, an examination of natality trends in the United States over the past several decades provides a basis for understanding current challenges and goal setting in prenatal care. Important trends to examine are the effect of the postwar baby boom on age distribution of women of childbearing age and patterns of childbearing among women of various ages. Studies have shown that prenatal care has the greatest impact on those women who are at highest risk of poor pregnancy outcome such as adolescents and unmarried and minority women (Horton, 1995).

Birth Rate Trends

Since the baby boom of the late 1940s, 1950s, and early 1960s, the birth rate in the United States has steadily declined. A reversal of that trend occurred between 1986 and 1990, when the annual number of births in the United States increased overall by 11% (Ventura, Martin, Taffel, Matthews, & Clarke, 1995). In 1990, there were 4,158,212 births in the United States, the highest number since the baby boom years. However, since the peak in 1990, crude birth rates declined about 7% between 1990 and 1997 (Ventura, Martin, Curtain, Matthews, & Park, 2000). In 1998, the last year for which data are available, there were 3,941,553 births, representing a birth rate of 14.6 per 1,000 (Ventura et al., 2000).

Although the overall birth rate has declined, the number of births to women between ages 30 and 44 has continued to increase because as the population ages, there are more women in that age group (Ventura et al., 2000). Birth rates for women in their thirties increased to 87.4 per 1,000 women between the ages of 30 and 34 years, up 2%, and to 37.4 per 1,000 women between the ages of 35 and 39 years, up 4% (Ventura et al., 2000). The rates for these age groups are at their highest in at least three decades. The birth rate for women between the ages of 40 and 44 years increased in 1998 to 7.3 per 1,000 (Ventura et al., 2000).

Birth rates for adolescents between the ages of 15 and 19 has declined by 18% between 1991 and 1998 (Ventura et al., 2000). The birth rate for young teenagers (15 to 17 years) is at 30.4 per 1,000, a record low. Birth rates for women in their twenties, the principal childbearing years, has remained relatively stable over the past 25 years. The birth rate for unmarried women (15 to 44 years) in 1998 was 44.3 births per 1,000 unmarried women, representing 1,293,567 births, the highest number ever reported (Ventura et al., 2000). Births to unmarried women (15 to 44 years) comprised one third of the total births in the United States for 1998.

Social Trends

Social trends to consider related to U.S. natality statistics include decreased family size and an increased number of women in the work force. Family size, roles, and living environments have been affected by recent economic and technologic changes. Factors influencing family dynamics include high divorce rates, increased age at first marriage, increased number of female-headed households, and an increased number of women of childbearing age who live alone. Consideration must be given to data on chemical dependency, homelessness, and poverty. Growth in illicit drug use among women of childbearing age and their partners has contributed to epidemics of acquired immunodeficiency syndrome (AIDS) and other sexually transmitted diseases. Socioeconomic factors, such as an increase in the poverty rate and a decline in health-care insurance coverage, have created barriers to prenatal care and affected pregnancy outcomes (Maloni, Cheng, Liebl, & Maier, 1996; March of Dimes, 1993). Nearly one third of births in the United States is subsidized by Medicaid (Carpenter, 1995), but because of differences in state eligibility requirements and systems barriers to access, many poor women still do not receive prenatal care.

Infant Mortality

The infant mortality rate refers to the number of deaths in children younger than 1 year of age per 1,000 live births. Although incidence of infant deaths during the first year of life has decreased dramatically since the turn of the century, the rate of decline has been slower in recent years. In 1995, the United States ranked 25th among developed countries in infant mortality, a further decrease from the 22nd ranking of 1991 (NCHS, 1999). The United States did not reach its 1990 goal of 9 deaths per 1,000 live births, but by 1995, the infant mortality rate declined to 7.1 deaths per 1,000 live births. In 1997, the rate was 7.2 deaths per 1,000 live births (MacDorman & Atkinson, 1999). Reductions in infant mortality were seen in all race and education groups examined, although the decline occurred more steadily in some groups than others. The U.S. African American infant mortality rate (14.2) remains at 2.3 times the rate for Caucasian infants (6.0) (MacDorman & Atkinson, 1999).

Preterm birth, before 37 completed weeks' gestation, continues to be a significant cause of perinatal mortality and morbidity. During the past 25 years, advances in neonatal intensive care have improved outcomes for small neonates. Advances in perinatal care have allowed for increased lengths of gestation in women at risk for preterm birth. Despite technologic advances, the incidence of preterm birth of appropriate for gestational age infants has not declined over the past 40 years (American College of Obstetricians and Gynecologists [ACOG], 1995b). The preterm birth rate has risen sharply to 11.6% in 1998 from 11.0% in 1996. In 1981, the rate of preterm birth was at 9.4%. Preterm birth has become the single most common cause of poor birth outcome (Display 7–1), with 7% of all births contributing to more than 60% of infant death (Moore & Freda, 1998). The highest percentage of perinatal mortality is related to preterm birth before 28 weeks' gestation (ACOG, 1995b). Approximately 80% of preterm births occur after 32 weeks' gestation. Liveborn infants of gestational age above 32 weeks have a risk in mortality similar to term infants and have only a mildly increased risk of serious morbidity when compared with term infants (Kiely, 1991). Studies of the effect of prenatal care alone tend to show that the largest improvement in mortality occurs in term newborns, not those that are born preterm (Tyson, Guzick, & Rosenfeld, 1990).

Maternal Mortality

Numerous definitions of maternal death by professional organizations, individual states, government agencies, and the World Health Organization (WHO) have contributed to inconsistencies and inaccuracies in reporting maternal mortality statistics. The Centers for Disease Control and Prevention (CDC) estimate

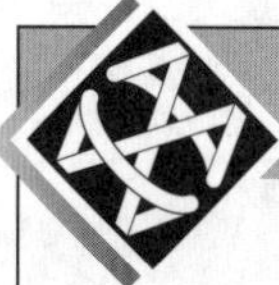

DISPLAY 7–1

Preterm Delivery and Neonatal Mortality

- Seventy-six percent of neonatal deaths are infants born preterm (< 37 weeks' gestation).
- Preterm infants (< 37 weeks) are 30 times as likely to die in the neonatal period as term infants (37–41 weeks).
- Low-birth-weight infants (< 2,500g) are 23 times as likely to die during the first year of life as infants born weighing 2,500g or more.
- Very-low birth-weight infants (< 1,500g) are 95 times as likely to die during the first year of life as infants born weighing 2,500g or more.

From National Center for Health Statistics. (2000). 1997 Final natality and linked birth/infant death rate. White Plains, NY: March of Dimes Perinatal Data Center.

there is approximately 37% underreporting of maternal deaths in the United States (Atrash, Rowley, & Hogue, 1992). The CDC's definitions of maternal deaths are as follows:

- *Pregnancy-associated maternal death:* the death of any woman from any cause, while she is pregnant or within 1 calendar year of termination of pregnancy, regardless of duration and site of pregnancy;
- *Pregnancy-related maternal death:* the death of any woman resulting from complications of the pregnancy itself, the chain of events initiated by the pregnancy that led to the death, or aggravation of an unrelated condition by the physiologic or pharmacologic effects of the pregnancy that subsequently caused death (Ellerbrock, Atrash, Hogue, & Smith, 1988)

Although maternal mortality has decreased dramatically in the past 50 years, deaths of pregnant women and recently pregnant women remain an important public health concern. Women continue to experience preventable pregnancy-related deaths. Older women and African American women, at greater risk 50 years ago, remain at greater risk today (Berg, Atrash, Koonin, & Tucker, 1996).

In 1998 (the last year for which data are available), a total of 281 were reported to have died of maternal causes. This does not include all deaths occurring to pregnant women, but only to those deaths reported on the death certificate and assigned to the cause of death as complications of pregnancy, childbirth, and the puerperium (ICD-9 nos. 630–676). It excludes deaths occurring more than 42 days after the termination of a pregnancy and deaths of pregnant women because of nonrelated causes (eg, accidents). The maternal mortality rate was 7.1 deaths per 100,000 live births (Murphy, 1999). African American women continue to have a substantially higher risk of maternal death than white women. In 1998, the maternal mortality rate was 17.1, more than three times the rate of 5.1 for white women, a ratio essentially unchanged since 1975 (Atrash et al., 1992; Murphy, 1999).

Maternal mortality rates have traditionally been reported as deaths rate per 100,000 live births, but this statistical methodology does not result in a true rate. Although all maternal deaths, regardless of outcomes, are included in the numerator, only live births are included in the denominator. These data actually reflect a maternal mortality ratio. In 1988, the CDC proposed the following statistical measures of pregnancy-related mortality to facilitate comparisons and identify groups at special risk: pregnancy mortality ratio—the number of pregnancy-related deaths per 100,000 live births; pregnancy mortality rate—the number of pregnancy-related deaths per 100,000 reported pregnancies; and outcome-specific pregnancy mortality rate—the number of deaths related to a specific outcome per 100,000 pregnancies that resulted in the same outcome (Ellerbrock, Atrash, Hogue, & Smith, 1988). Outcome-specific pregnancy mortality rates can be used to determine risk associated with specific pregnancy outcomes (live birth, stillbirth, ectopic pregnancy, molar pregnancy, abortion, and undelivered). Although these data can improve accuracy, data on the actual number of pregnancies are difficult to obtain. Legal abortions are reported in the United States, but spontaneous abortions may not be reported, especially if they occur early in gestation. When comparing across countries, it is important to clarify the denominator (ie, live births or all reported pregnancies).

ACCESS TO PRENATAL CARE

Although use of prenatal care has increased in the 1990s, many women in the United States receive little or no prenatal care even though there has been social support for the importance of prenatal care since the early 1900s (Kogan et al., 1999). In 1998, 4% of all pregnant women in the United States received late or no prenatal care (Ventura et al., 2000). In *Guidelines for Perinatal Care* by the American Academy of Pediatrics [AAP] and ACOG (1997), late prenatal care is defined as beginning care after the fifth month of pregnancy or beginning earlier but receiving fewer than half of the visits recommended. For 2000, the target for first-trimester care was to be raised from a 1987 baseline of 76% to 90% of all live births. Although there has been a steady increase over the past 9 years, only 82.8% of pregnant women began care in the first trimester in 1998 (Ventura et al., 2000). Racial disparity remains a concern: 73% of black women and 74% of Hispanic women, compared with 88% of white women, received early prenatal care. Women beginning care in the third trimester and women receiving no prenatal care are at increased risk of poor pregnancy outcomes. Regular prenatal care is associated with reduced infant mortality and favorable outcomes on measures of child health such as birth weight.

Many programs have been developed in an effort to improve birth outcomes in the United States. Most have focused on the antepartum period, with emphasis on increasing use of prenatal care. Opportunities for intervention before pregnancy have received less attention.

Because many women become pregnant unintentionally, education about preconception health should be a component of care for all women of childbearing age (ACOG, 1995a). Information can be provided during routine healthcare visits, following discussion of family planning methods. It is estimated that almost 60% of pregnancies in the United States are unplanned at the time of conception (Institute of Medicine, 1995). Identification of medical complications that increase risks to the woman and fetus allow opportunity for early intervention. Women with preexisting conditions such as diabetes, phenylketonuria, seizure disorders, or infectious diseases can especially benefit from preconception health counseling (ACOG, 1995a). All women need information about the use of folic acid to prevent neural tube defects, the importance of avoiding certain prescription medications, and strategies to promote dietary and lifestyle changes before they become pregnant (ACOG, 1995a; March of Dimes, 1999). Family planning services and school-based nurses are in strategic positions to promote the importance of a planned pregnancy and early comprehensive prenatal care (Jamieson & Buescher, 1992). In a study of factors in the use of prenatal services by low-income African American women, an unanticipated finding was that many women delayed care because they were not aware of the pregnancy (Burks, 1992). Seeking early and frequent care was determined by the presence of known risk factors or symptoms (Burks, 1992).

Factors Influencing the Decision to Seek Prenatal Care

Relatively little is known about factors that influence a pregnant woman's decisions about initiating and continuing prenatal care. Key demographic factors associated with insufficient prenatal care include poverty, being unmarried, age younger than 20 years, higher parity, and having less than a high school education. In one study, ethnicity was not a significant predictor of the woman's decision to initiate prenatal care when other demographic variables were controlled (Goldenburg, Patterson, & Freese, 1992); however, in the United States, African American and Hispanic women generally receive prenatal care later than Caucasian women. The percentage of African American women (39.4%) who did not receive prenatal care in the first trimester during 1990 was nearly twice that of Caucasian women (20.8%) (CDC, 1995a). Fortunately, this disparity is changing and in 1996 the gap was only a 3% difference in these two groups, with 19.6 % of African American women and 16.7% of Caucasian women not receiving first-trimester prenatal care. The CDC suggests that differences in pregnancy-related morbidity, access to and use of healthcare services, and content and quality of prenatal care may be possible explanations for this disparity. It is often difficult or impossible to separate the effects of poverty, marital status, or other socioeconomic factors from the decision to seek prenatal care (Goldenberg, Patterson, & Freese, 1992; March of Dimes, 1993). Variables that influence use of prenatal care and are associated with the previously mentioned demographic variables have been identified in a number of studies and include the following: an unintended pregnancy, little perceived value attached to prenatal care, a tenuous connection to the healthcare system, negative experiences with healthcare providers, financial difficulties, and ambivalence or fear regarding the pregnancy (Goldenberg et al, 1992; Harvey & Faber, 1992; March of Dimes, 1999). In a study examining why some low-income women (enrolled in Medicaid managed care) take advantage of prenatal care and others do not, "personal factors" were more likely to determine whether she gets adequate prenatal care than sociodemographic factors such as her race or income level. Women were 3.5 times more likely to get inadequate prenatal care if they experienced physical violence, were "too tired" (2.2 times), had an unsupportive partner (1.9 times), or if they did not enroll in a plan until after the pregnancy began (2.0 times) (Gazmararian, Arrington, Bailey, Schwarz, & Koplan, 1999). Sociodemographic factors (age, race, marital status, income) and system factors (adequate transportation, appointment times) were not associated significantly with when and how often women sought prenatal care. In an earlier study of prenatal care the prevalence of delayed entry associated with physical violence was 18.1% and was seen in older women (older than 25 years) and women of *higher socioeconomic status* (Dietz, Gazmararian, Goodwin, Bruce, Johnson, & Rochat, 1997).

Trends in Provider Selection

In the recent past, the focus of prenatal care concerned collection and evaluation of laboratory values and physical measurements (ie, preeclampsia model). This approach did not address what a diverse population of women may need in terms of health education, counseling, and social support (Maloni, Cheng, Liebl, & Maier, 1996; McClanahan, 1992). Minimal progress in the decline of the infant mortality rate in the United States in recent years has stimulated a shift in focus from "high-tech" care to primary prevention. High-quality prenatal care (ie, a multidisciplinary effort), including financial access to such care for poor women, is recognized as a key strategy for improving birth outcome (Handler & Rosenberg, 1992).

Advanced practice nurses (APNs) such as women's healthcare nurse practitioners (WHCNPs), family nurse practitioners (FNPs), and certified nurse midwives (CNMs), are actively involved in providing primary care. Healthcare reform has spotlighted all advanced practice roles as being capable of providing safe and cost-effective care (Fenton, 1998). Not only are APNs competent to perform physical assessments, but they also focus on psychosocial support, counseling, and education; this focus has had a positive effect on pregnancy outcome (McClanahan, 1992).

Perinatal clinical nurse specialists (CNSs) practice in an advanced role, primarily in the inpatient setting. Major functions of the CNS are consultation, patient and staff education, research, and coordination and delivery of nursing care to families requiring intensive nursing support. The perinatal nurse practitioner (PNNP) is a newer role for advanced practice nurses in the perinatal specialty. PNNPs practice collaboratively with perinatalogists and obstetricians in the care of high-risk pregnant women in acute care and ambulatory care settings.

Rural areas, underserved by physicians, are the testing grounds for new models that allow nurses to function independently. Rural hospitals are relying more heavily on outpatient services for revenue, and APNs are viewed as the most economic providers of such care. Direct reimbursement for services and legal authority to write prescriptions are necessary for independent practice. Every state has some type of prescriptive authority (Pearson, 2000). Reimbursement issues are more complex even though the U.S. Congress approved direct reimbursement for nurse practitioners in rural areas and Medicaid reimbursement for certified nurse midwives and pediatric and family nurse practitioners. Reimbursement administration varies from state to state.

Because there is an overlap between nursing and medical practice, conflict may arise. However, there are many collaborative practices that offer a multidisciplinary approach to prenatal care. Consumers benefit when they know more about nursing care and choices of healthcare providers. In recent years, consumers have become more aware of the existence of advanced practice nurses, and the terms nurse practitioner and nurse midwife have almost become household words (Fenton, 1998). Some subgroups (ie, adolescents and women with medical complications) especially benefit from comprehensive care. At a minimum, comprehensive care should use multidisciplinary caregivers such as nurses and physicians with obstetric and pediatric education in providing prenatal care, with other professionals (eg, social workers, health educators, nutritionists, lay community members) to meet the diverse needs of the pregnant woman (Maloni, Cheng, Liebl, & Maier, 1996). Collaboration complements the expertise of nurses and physicians. The woman benefits by receiving higher quality and more individualized care.

EFFECTS OF PRENATAL CARE ON BIRTH OUTCOME

Early, adequate prenatal care has long been associated with improved pregnancy outcomes. Continued contact with the pregnant woman through comprehensive prenatal care provides an ideal opportunity for the healthcare provider to assess for and identify potential problems that may place the woman and fetus at risk. Risk-appropriate prenatal care further enhances the possibility of a positive pregnancy outcome among women who are at increased medical or social risk (ACOG, 1995b). However, 50% of all preterm births occur in women with *no identifiable risk factors* (Creasy, 1999). The nurse should view those women with risk factors to be higher risk than those without but should avoid concentrating her or his efforts on only those in a high-risk category.

More data are needed about which components of prenatal care are protective against adverse maternal–infant outcomes. A study examining the relationship of prenatal care and the risk of having a second preterm or low-birth-weight infant suggests the lack of scientific knowledge of causal factors for preterm birth and low-birth-weight infants contributes to the inability to design prenatal care programs that are more effective in preventing poor outcomes (Raine, Powell, & Krohn, 1994). Until the underlying pathophysiology of preterm birth and the risks related to socioeconomic and lifestyle factors are fully understood, prenatal care should be directed toward early identification, education, and intervention, with frequent contact between the pregnant woman and her primary healthcare provider.

Definition of Adequate Prenatal Care

General guidelines for prenatal care have been established (AAP & ACOG, 1997); however, these recommendations are not consistently followed by all healthcare providers (Baldwin et al., 1994). Traditionally, prenatal care has been evaluated using the number of prenatal visits, gestational age at entry into prenatal care, or a combination of these factors. If the number of prenatal visits is used as the sole evaluation criteria, women who deliver premature infants and therefore have fewer prenatal visits are misclassified. Lack of differentiation between women who seek prenatal care late in pregnancy and those women who have one or two early visits and then lose contact with the healthcare system further complicates the evaluation of adequate prenatal care and reporting of vital statistics. Attempts have been made to develop new indices for evaluating the effectiveness of prenatal care in light of the increasing preterm birth rate and paradoxically, the increased use of prenatal care (Alexander & Kotelchuck, 1996; Kogan et al., 1998; Kotelchuck, 1994). However, these new indices look at intensive use (ie, more prenatal visits than standard recommendation). There has not yet been an index to examine characteristics of pregnancies (ie, presence of bacterial infection of the genitourinary tract or poor health before pregnancy) and the content of the care (ie, education regarding risk of preterm birth or more frequent laboratory analysis of urine) used to address those characteristics and related to perinatal outcome.

Another important aspect to consider in evaluating the effectiveness of prenatal care is the discrete nature of prenatal care. Intensive use of prenatal care does not impact a woman's preconceptional health. The stressful and impoverished environment in which many minority and low-income woman live may be a fundamental factor that influences pregnancy outcome (Misra & Guyer, 1998).

Adequate prenatal care is a comprehensive process in which problems associated with pregnancy are identified and treated. Education and support are provided. Three basic components of adequate prenatal care have been identified: early and continuing risk assessments, health promotion, and medical and psychosocial interventions with follow-up (Expert Panel on the Content of Prenatal Care, 1989). Comprehensive services include health education; nutrition education; the Women, Infants, and Children's (WIC) program; social services assessment; medical risk assessment; and referral as appropriate. To provide optimal, individualized care, nurses must recognize the effect of pregnancy on a woman's life span. Pregnancy has been viewed as a discrete event, with little or no relationship to a woman as she ages (Walker & Tinkle, 1996). Although a woman's preconceptional health has an impact on pregnancy, it is also true that childbearing is an event that may affect her long-term health. It is important to consider pregnancy within the larger context of women's health (Walker & Tinkle, 1996).

PRENATAL RISK ASSESSMENT

The goal of risk assessment is to identify women and fetuses at risk for developing antepartum, intrapartum, postpartum, or neonatal complications to promote risk-appropriate care, enhancing perinatal outcome. The underlying causes of preterm labor and intrauterine growth restriction are not fully understood. Because of these limitations, a perfect risk-assessment system has not been identified (Edenfield, Thomas, Thompson, & Marcotte, 1995; Enkins, 1994). However, a large body of knowledge regarding risk factors associated with prematurity and low birth weight has developed. These factors include demographic, medical, obstetric, sociocultural, lifestyle, and environmental risks. It is important to note that many risk factors have been identified in studies of women who develop complications of pregnancy or deliver preterm; however, no firm cause and effect relationship between some of the commonly associated risk factors and poor outcome has been established (Enkins, 1994). For example, marital status or low income does not cause poor pregnancy outcomes; however, many women who are unmarried or live in poverty do experience complications of pregnancy. Risk-assessment tools may be helpful in distinguishing between women at high and low risk (Display 7–2). Unfortunately, the predictive value of these tools is limited. Enthusiasm for risk assessment must be tempered with reality. A significant number of problems occur in women not identified as high risk, and conversely, some women undergo unnecessary hospitalizations, cesarean sections, false diagnoses of disease, and unmeasured psychological impact that result from inaccurate screening (Murphy, 1994). Approximately one third of the potential complications of pregnancy occur during the intrapartum period and are not predictable by current risk-assessment systems (AAP & ACOG, 1997; Auman & Baird, 1993). Risk assessment orients the provider toward areas in which intervention can have a positive impact on perinatal outcomes. The nurse's knowledge of prenatal risk assessment allows for anticipatory planning, individualized education, and appropriate referral. Outcomes of risk assessment provide guidelines by which the effectiveness of the care can be evaluated (Maloni, Cheng, Liebl, & Maier, 1996). The nurse's role in prenatal care is discussed within these parameters.

Initial Prenatal Visit

Antepartum assessment begins with the first prenatal visit. Generally, a woman with an uncomplicated pregnancy is examined approximately every 4 weeks for the first 28 weeks of pregnancy, every 2 to 3 weeks until 36 weeks' gestation, and weekly thereafter. Women with medical or obstetric problems may require closer surveillance. Intervals between visits are determined by the nature and severity of the problem (AAP & ACOG, 1997).

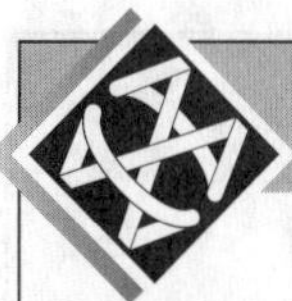

DISPLAY 7–2

Risk Assessment

OBSTETRIC HISTORY

- History of infertility
- Grand multiparity
- Incompetent cervix
- Uterine or cervical anomaly
- Previous preterm labor or preterm birth
- Previous cesarean birth
- Previous macrosomic infant
- Two or more spontaneous or elective abortions
- Last pregnancy <1 year before present conception
- Previous hydatidiform mole or choriocarcinoma
- Previous infant with neurologic deficit, birth injury, or congenital anomaly
- Previous ectopic or spontaneous abortion
- Previous stillborn/neonatal death
- Previous multiple gestation
- Previous prolonged labor
- Previous low birth weight infant
- Previous midforceps delivery
- DES exposure in utero

MEDICAL HISTORY

- Cardiac disease
- Metabolic disease
- Gastrointestinal disorders
- Chronic hypertension
- Seizure disorders
- Malignancy
- Reproductive tract anomalies
- Emotional disorders, mental retardation
- Family history of severe inherited disorders
- Previous surgeries, particularly involving the reproductive organs
- History of abnormal Pap smear
- Pulmonary disease
- Renal disease, repeat urinary tract infections, bacteriuria
- Endocrine disorders
- Hemoglobinopathies
- Sexually transmitted diseases
- Surgery during pregnancy

CURRENT OBSTETRIC STATUS

- Inadequate prenatal care
- Intrauterine growth-restricted fetus
- Large for gestational age fetus
- Pregnancy-induced hypertension, preeclampsia
- Polyhydramnios
- Placenta previa
- Abnormal presentation
- Maternal anemia
- Weight gain <10 lb
- Weight loss ≥5 lb
- Overweight or underweight
- Immunization status
- Fetal or placental malformations
- Abnormal fetal surveillance tests
- Rh sensitization
- Preterm labor
- Multiple gestation
- Premature rupture of membranes
- Abruptio placentae
- Postdatism
- Fibroids
- Fetal manipulation
- Cervical cerclage
- Sexually transmitted diseases
- Maternal infection

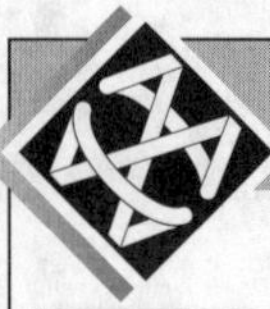

DISPLAY 7–2 (cont.)

Risk Assessment

PSYCHOSOCIAL FACTORS

Inadequate finances	Poor housing
Social problems	Unwed, father of baby uninvolved or unsupportive
Adolescent	Minority status
Poor nutrition	Parental occupation
More than 2 children at home, no help	Inadequate support systems
Unacceptance of pregnancy	Dysfunctional grieving
Attempt or ideation of suicide	Psychiatric history
Domestic violence	

DEMOGRAPHIC FACTORS

Maternal age <16 or >35 years	Education <11 years

LIFESTYLE

Smokes >10 cigarettes/day	Alcohol intake
Substance abuse	Heavy lifting, long periods of standing
Long commute	Unusual stress
Nonuse of seat belts	No in-home smoke detectors

The initial prenatal visit is of vital importance and requires careful attention to detail. The nurse is obligated to practice within the framework of professional standards, such as the Association of Women's Health, Obstetric and Neonatal Nurses (AWHONN) *Standards and Guidelines (1998)* and *Guidelines for Perinatal Care* (AAP & ACOG, 1997), which provide guidelines for practice in the ambulatory care setting. During the first prenatal visit, baseline health data are obtained and assessed, a patient-centered relationship is established, and the plan of care is initiated. Risk assessment during the initial prenatal visit should include the following:

- A careful family medical history, individual medical history, and reproductive health history
- A comprehensive physical examination designed to evaluate potential risk factors
- Appropriate prenatal laboratory screening
- Individualized, risk-appropriate laboratory evaluation
- Fetal assessment as developmentally appropriate (eg, fetal heart rate [FHR], fetal activity, kick counts) and individualized fetal surveillance as indicated (eg, nonstress test [NST], ultrasonography, biophysical profile [BPP])

Medical and Obstetric History

Assessment of health factors that may influence pregnancy outcome includes careful evaluation of the woman's individual medical, gynecologic, obstetric, psychosocial, and environmental history. Pertinent family history of the woman and her partner is necessary for complete evaluation. Maternal–family reproductive health history (eg, preeclampsia, hypertension, preterm birth) may be particularly significant. Chronic conditions (ie, diabetes, hypertension, or cardiac disease) are known to be affected by the additional physiologic stress of pregnancy. Likewise, factors such as a recent history of frequent sexually transmitted diseases (STDs) or chemical dependency may be indicative of lifestyle behaviors that threaten maternal–fetal well-being.

Obstetric history, such as length of previous labors, birth weight, gestational age, history of preterm labor or preterm birth, operative birth, grand multiparity, elective or spontaneous abortion, previous stillbirth, or uterine or cervical anomaly may indicate potential risks for the current pregnancy (Fogel & Lewallen, 1995). These risk factors should be applied within the context of the gestational age. For example, a history of preterm birth would not be a pertinent risk to a woman who is presently at 37 weeks' gestation but is relevant when the woman is at 20 weeks' gestation. Familial history, including cardiac disease, diabetes, bleeding disorders, etc., should be noted. The woman may also be affected by her mother's obstetric history. There is a familial predisposition to develop preeclampsia. Daughters born to mothers who maintained their pregnancy through use of diethylstilbestrol (DES) may have uterine anomalies that increase their risk for preterm labor. However, these women are now aging beyond childbearing years. The pregnant woman's and the father's family medical and genetic history serve to guide counseling and testing for predisposed genetic complications.

Socioeconomic Factors

Demographic factors, such as maternal age and education, have been linked to pregnancy outcomes. Optimal childbearing age is considered to be between 20 and 30 years of age, with an increased risk of perinatal morbidity after age 35. Children born to mothers younger than 19 or older than 35 years of age have an increased risk of prematurity, congenital anomalies, and risks from other complications of pregnancy (Fogel & Lewallen, 1995). The incidence of genetic anomalies such as Down syndrome increases with advanced maternal age (Hook, 1981). Number of years of completed maternal education has been correlated with birth weight, perinatal mortality and morbidity, and neonatal neurologic sequelae (Auman & Baird, 1993). In general, as years of maternal education increase, incidence of perinatal mortality and morbidity decrease. Not surprisingly, adolescents are more likely to begin prenatal care later than adults (Kogan et al., 1998). Pregnant women who have more education are more likely to start prenatal care early and have more visits (United States Department of Health and Human Services [USDHHS], 1998). This association may be a reflection of education as an indicator of socioeconomic status. A disproportionate number of women of childbearing age are uninsured or underinsured. Women in lower socioeconomic groups tend to initiate prenatal care later than their middle socioeconomic group counterparts (Maloni et al., 1996; York & Brooten, 1992).

Financial barriers have been identified as the most important factor contributing to maternal inability to receive adequate prenatal care (Maloni et al., 1996). Although many women qualify for Medicaid insurance, the process may be so burdensome that women often do not register. Access to prenatal care is complicated by numerous negative institutional practices such as extended wait times for the first visit, daytime hours only appointments, and transportation difficulties (Maloni et al., 1996).

Maternal and paternal occupation and employment status has been linked to perinatal outcome. Overall, the highest incidence of perinatal loss occurs in families where the father is not present. In families where the father is present, the incidence of perinatal loss is higher when the father is a semiskilled or manual laborer, and lower in families where the father is a professional or a farmer (Auman & Baird, 1993). Multiple studies suggest marital status is associated with incidence of low birth weight. In a study evaluating perinatal outcomes of nearly 15,000 singleton pregnancies, women who were separated, divorced, or widowed had 43% more low-birth-weight infants than women who were married (McIntosh, Roumayah, & Bottoms, 1995).

Women in low-income positions or employed as unskilled laborers are at increased risk for preterm labor. The woman's occupation may require long commutes, heavy work, or long periods of standing or sitting, all of which contribute to the risk of preterm labor. However, decreasing or eliminating work during pregnancy may place the woman at greater socioeconomic risk by threatening her livelihood. Socioeconomic factors influence gestational age at entry to prenatal care, nutritional status, and availability of support systems.

Lifestyle Factors

Lifestyle or behavior factors significantly affect women's health in general and perinatal health specifically. Approximately 8% to 10% of birth defects occur because of environmental factors such as maternal infection, disease, or exposure to chemicals, drugs, or alcohol (Beckman & Brent, 1986; Robins & Mills, 1993). An exact cause for the defect can be determined in less than 50% of the cases (ACOG, 1997). All of these factors can be linked to lifestyle issues and can be affected by positive healthcare decisions (Pletsch, 1990). Careful assessment of the woman's daily routine provides valuable information about potential lifestyle risk factors.

Use of prescription or over-the-counter medications and use of nonmedical doctors and nontraditional therapies such as homeopathy, acupuncture, acupressure, massage, exercise, folk remedies, relaxation techniques, biofeedback, spiritual healing, and prayer should be assessed. This provides the nurse with a more complete picture of the woman's approach to heath care and allows her to identify potentially harmful practices (Wheeler, 1997). If there is a potential substance or practice about which there is a question of teratogenicity the nurse can contact the Organization of Teratology Information Services at its toll-free number (1-888-285-3410) for more information. This organization is a national service that can refer the pregnant woman or nurse to local resources or, if none is available, can answer the question itself. Counseling regarding possible teratogenic influences should be performed in a factual yet sympathetic and supportive way so the woman is not unduly alarmed or burdened with guilt (ACOG, 1997).

The impact of nutrition on maternal and fetal well-being cannot be underscored. The special physiology of a female creates variable nutrient requirements during different stages of the life cycle. A healthy well-nourished female has a surplus of all nutrients. This surplus can be crucial in the first trimester of pregnancy, when the ability to eat is impaired by hormonal shifts and the tissues and organs of the embryo are being differentiated. This is a time when adequate nutrition is believed to help against some birth defects (Gutierrez, 1994). Many women in the United States do not consume the recommended daily allowance (RDA) in their daily diet (Lemone, 1999). For example, folic acid requirements are increased to 5 to 10 times normal during pregnancy, and dietary intake may not meet these requirements. Deficiencies in folic acid may have devastating effects in the formation of neural tube defects in the baby (March of Dimes, 1999). Nutritional practices influence every pregnancy as well as influence the woman's lifetime risk for diabetes mellitus, cardiovascular disease, osteoporosis, and several types of cancer (ACOG, 1993a, 1994a, 1996c). Specific complications of pregnancy such as preeclampsia, preterm birth, intrauterine growth restriction, and low-birth-weight infants can be correlated to nutritional status.

Many women today are influenced by cultural pressures that promote dieting and therefore limit their intake of essential nutrients, which may compromise nutritional status (Gutierrez, 1994). Underweight women or women who fail to gain the recommended 25 to 40 pounds during pregnancy are at greater risk for delivering low-birth-weight babies (ACOG, 1993a). Overweight women and women who exceed the recommended prenatal weight gain are at risk for developing preeclampsia, gestational diabetes, or for delivering a large-for-gestational age infant, increasing the risk for perinatal morbidity and mortality (Cnattinghaus, Berstrom, Lipworth, & Kramer, 1998; Wolfe, 1998).

Nutritional care during the antepartum period should include assessment of nutritional risk factors (Display 7–3), nutritional assessment, nutritional counseling, and nutrient supplements as appropriate. The nutrition assessment includes diet information (13-day recall), monitoring weight gain, and hematologic assessment. Assessment of usual dietary patterns provides a basis for understanding nutritional health. Variations from the normal dietary routine, such as eating disorders, food shortages, and metabolic disorders such as diabetes, warrant additional interventions. Women who have eating disorders may be reticent to reveal this information. This assessment may require a number of prenatal visits and a building of a trusting relationship between the nurse and the woman. After an eating disorder is revealed, the nurse should ask the woman how she manages eating food and meals, as well as what is her attitude toward eating (eg, preoccupation with food, feeling guilty after eating, engaging in dieting, enjoyment of food).

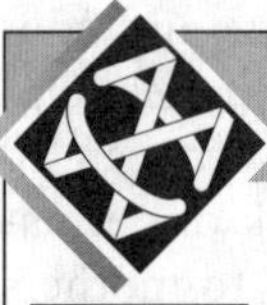

DISPLAY 7–3

Risk Factors for Nutritional Problems

- Low income
- Adolescence
- Cigarette smoking
- Substance abuse
- Frequent dieting, fasting, or meal skipping
- Vegan (completely vegetarian) diet
- Pica
- High parity
- Menorrhagia
- Physical or mental illness
- Use of certain medications, such as phenytoin
- Mental retardation
- Problems with chewing, swallowing, or mobility
- Decreased sense of smell or taste
- Elderliness
- Disability
- Cancer and treatment
- Chronic diseases

From American College of Obstetricians and Gynecologists. (1996). *Nutrition and women* (educational bulletin no. 229). Washington, DC: Author.

Many pregnant women experience pica or olfactory cravings during pregnancy. Some women are embarrassed to tell the nurse about these cravings, yet they may significantly interfere with dietary intake of proper nutrients during pregnancy. Pica and olfactory cravings are not limited to any one group, educational level, race, ethnic group, income level, or religious belief (Cooksey, 1995); however, the type of substance ingested does seem to culturally influenced (Harvey & Moretti, 1993; Herbert, Dodds, & Cefalo, 1993).

Another aspect of the nutritional assessment is the use of vitamins and herbs. Because herbs and vitamins are considered dietary supplements these products are not regulated in the same manner that prescription and over-the-counter medications are. Often the products are labeled as "natural," and the woman may conclude that the product is therefore not harmful. Excesses of one nutrient can alter the need for, absorption of, or use of other nutrients. Supernutrient regimens and or megadoses of vitamins cannot ensure a healthy pregnancy and may be harmful.

The Institute of Medicine (1990) and ACOG (1993a) recommend a weight gain for women, based on their prepregnant weights and single births (Table 7–1). A weight gain of 35 to 45 pounds is recommended for women with twins (ACOG, 1993a; Institute of Medicine, 1990). Weight gain should be carefully monitored during each prenatal visit. Weight gain or loss may be indicative of maternal nutritional status or development of complications. Excessive weight gain, weight loss, or inadequate weight gain indicates a need for consultation with a nutritionist. The *pattern* of weight gain is as important as the *total amount*. Second-trimester weight gain is more predictive of infant birth weight than total maternal weight gain (Abrams & Selvin, 1995). Weight gain of 5 or more pounds in 1 week after 20 weeks' gestation requires evaluation for preeclampsia (ACOG, 1996a).

Cigarette smoking has been linked to an increased incidence of low birth weight and prematurity. In the United States, 12.9% of pregnant women are smokers, with the highest concentration occurring in the 18- to 24-year-old age group. Maternal smoking among teenagers rose again for the fourth consecutive year to 19.2%. A higher percentage of white teens (29.8) are smokers than black teens (7.0) (Ventura et al., 2000). Among black and white women, rates for low-birth-weight infants are double those for nonsmokers (Guyer, Strobino, Ventina, MacDorman, & Martin, 1996). However, in one study, less than 20% of pregnant women who smoked quit when pregnancy was confirmed (Hebel, Fox, & Sexton, 1988). From a preventative perspective, it is not enough to discourage smoking in pregnant women. The focus must be on discouraging smoking in any woman of childbearing age who may potentially become pregnant (Moore & Freda, 1998). During pregnancy, many women are more highly motivated to stop or decrease their smoking; however, simply providing information may not be enough for the pregnant woman with a long history of smoking. For pregnant smokers a smoking cessation program may be a good adjunct to support the woman in her efforts. A nurse actively working (eg, frequent telephone follow-up) with the woman to cease smoking using a variety of strategies (eg, distracting activities) has also shown promise (Moore, Elmore, Ketener, Wagoner, & Walsh, 1995).

TABLE 7–1 ■ RECOMMENDATIONS FOR WEIGHT GAIN DURING PREGNANCY

Prepregnant Status	Weight Gain	
Underweight	28–40 lb	(12.7–18.2 kg)
Average weight	25–35 lb	(11.4–15.9 kg)
Overweight	15–25 lb	(6.8–11.4 kg)
Obese	15 lb	(6.8 kg)

From Institute of Medicine. (1990). *Nutrition during pregnancy.* Washington, DC: National Academy Press and from American College of Obstetricians and Gynecologists. (1993). *Nutrition during pregnancy* (technical bulletin no. 179). Washington, DC: Author.

Substance abuse (ie, alcohol and illicit drugs) can have disastrous effects in pregnancy. Alcohol use has been identified as the leading preventable cause of birth defects (DHHS, 1991). The most recent data from the National Institute on Drug Abuse suggest that more than 1 million children per year are exposed to alcohol and illicit drugs during gestation (USDHHS, 1999). One population-based study estimated the prevalence of perinatal drug use at 5.2%, alcohol use at 6.7%, and self-reported smoking at 8.8% (Vega, Bohdan, Hwang, & Noble, 1993). Across multiple studies, most researchers agree that infants prenatally exposed to illicit substances or alcohol exhibit intrauterine growth retardation, prematurity, and impaired neurobehavioral functioning (Chasnoff, 1998).

Substance abuse or chemical dependency affects all body systems and can cause cardiac, pulmonary, gastrointestinal, and psychiatric complications. Use of unsterile drug paraphernalia contributes to infection and disease transmission. When substance abuse occurs during pregnancy, maternal risk of abruptio placenta, preterm labor, sudden cardiac death, and stroke is increased (Chasnoff, 1989). Substance abusers rarely abuse a single substance (ACOG, 1994c). The woman's lifestyle when using drugs, which may include alcohol abuse, cigarette smoking, inadequate prenatal care, poor nutrition, and sexual promiscuity, further complicates the pregnancy (Brown & Zuckerman, 1991). Robins and Mills' (1993) comprehensive review of research on the effects of substance exposure in utero found that overall there is enough data to suggest substance exposure adversely affects some pregnancies. However, individual research studies have found the effects of substance exposure in utero to be transitory. It is difficult to determine to what extent complications of pregnancy may be attributed to actual drug use or to lifestyle factors associated with drug use (Robins & Mills). Because substance abuse or chemical dependency can adversely affect the health of the woman and the fetus, it is essential to include drug use assessment and education strategies in prenatal and women's healthcare encounters (Appendix 7A).

A moderate level of physical activity, in the absence of medical or obstetric complications, maintains cardiorespiratory and muscular fitness throughout pregnancy (ACOG, 1994b). Many women are committed to exercising regularly and wish to continue throughout the pregnancy. Overall exercise benefits the woman psychologically and physically. Activities that cause excessive fatigue such as heavy work, job-related stress, or daily automobile, train, or bus commutes may stimulate uterine contractions and increase the risk of perinatal complication (Papiernik, 1993).

Areas to ask about in the nature of the woman's job include sitting or standing continuously, lifting heavy objects, perceived problems with ventilation, and exposure to toxic chemicals or radiation. Hobbies and the home environment should be assessed. Information that influences counseling includes exposure to potential teratogens and sources of stress. One study found that unemployed women had higher preterm labor rates than their employed counterparts (Mamelle, Laumon, Munoz, & Collin, 1989). Household tasks may be a source of fatigue equal to or greater than job-related fatigue. Household stress is further influenced by home ownership (ie, private or government housing); quality of comfort (eg, heat, water); housekeeping burden; and number and age of children (Mamelle et al., 1989). Unusual stressful events, such as death of a significant family member or friend, job loss, or a problematic relationship with the baby's father may increase risk of poor pregnancy outcome. The nurse should be aware that many women continue to work under hazardous or stressful conditions out of economic necessity but that they will attempt to minimize any known risk factors or job environment as much as possible.

Psychosocial screening of every woman presenting for prenatal care is an important step toward improving the woman's health and the birth outcome. In this way, the nurse can identify areas of concern, validate major issues, and make suggestions for possible changes. Depending on the nature of the identified problem, a referral may be made to an appropriate member of the healthcare team. A woman may be reluctant to share information until a trusting relationship has been formed. Questions asked at the first prenatal visit bear repeating with ongoing prenatal care. She may need reassurance as to the confidentiality of the information. For example, if she reveals she uses cocaine, would she be turned over to the judicial system and possibly jailed? The nurse is obligated to know how to answer the woman when these issues arise.

Pregnancy affects the entire family, and therefore assessment and intervention must be considered in a family-centered perspective. Stress has been suggested as a potential contributor to physical complications during pregnancy and birth, including prolonged labor, increased use of intrapartum analgesics and barbiturates, and other complications. Maternal anxiety has also been associated with interference in fetal and newborn development (Lederman, 1990). Other symptoms of dysfunctional family relationships, such as violence toward the pregnant woman, child abuse, or psychosomatic illnesses, are also indicative of risk and warrant investigation. In a study of pregnant adolescents, those who were abused gave birth to infants with significantly lower birth weights than those who were not abused. Abused adolescents had significantly more previous miscarriages, substance use, and triage visits during pregnancy. Identification of the abused adolescent and their social resources during pregnancy may enhance prediction of infants at high risk as well as provide opportunities for intervention (Renker, 1999). Appendix 7B provides an abuse assessment tool.

Addressing psychosocial issues during pregnancy has the potential to reduce costs to the individual and to society but there have been no screening tools that are widely available that have been shown to have high degrees of sensitivity and specificity (ACOG, 1999b). One particularly well-regarded screening system was developed by the Healthy Start Program of the Florida Department of Health and has been refined and in use since 1992. This tool is a concise (9 questions) way to open the questioning about perinatal psychosocial risk factors (Display 7–4). If the patient answers in a way indicative of risk to any of the questions, the nurse can further explore the topic with the woman. It is possible to identify women prenatally that are at risk for experiencing parenting difficulties. Asking the woman how she thinks her pregnancy is progressing and questions about her preparations for the care of the baby opens up areas to discuss that

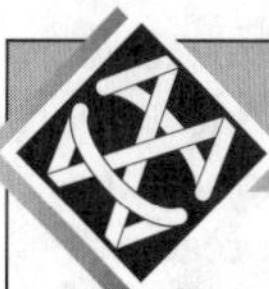

DISPLAY 7–4

Psychosocial Screening Tool

1. Do you have any problems that prevent you from keeping your health care appointments?
2. How many times have you moved in the past 12 months? 0, 1, 2, 3, more than 3
3. Do you feel unsafe where you live?
4. Do you or any members of your household go to bed hungry?
5. In the past 2 months, have you used any form of tobacco?
6. In the past 2 months, have you used drugs or alcohol (including beer, wine, or mixed drinks)?
7. In the past year, has anyone hit you or tried to hurt you?
8. How do you rate your current stress level—low or high?
9. If you could change the timing of this pregnancy, would you want it earlier, later, not at all, or no change?

From American College of Obstetricians and Gynecologists. (1999). *Psychosocial risk factors: Perinatal screening and intervention.* (ACOG educational bulletin no. 255). Washington, DC: Author.

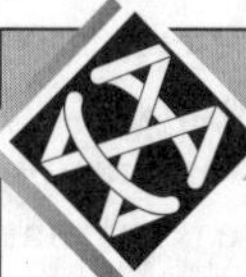

DISPLAY 7–5

Predisposing Factors for Postpartum Depression

Stressful life event during pregnancy and/or puerperium

- Loss of loved one (fetus, newborn, partner, or other child)
- Illness of partner, parent, or child
- Financial difficulties
- Job loss
- Move of household

Problematic interpersonal relationships (particularly with partner)
Inadequate social support from partner, family, friends
History of sexual abuse and/or domestic violence
Personal history of poor psychological adjustment before or after pregnancy
High levels of anxiety, neurotic behavior, and depression or emotional distress
Personal and/or family history of psychopathology, particularly depression

Adapted from Scarr, E., & Sammons, L. (1999). Postpartum depression. In W.L. Star, M.T. Shannon, L.N. Sammons, L. Lommel, & Y. Gutierrez (Eds.), *Ambulatory obstetrics: Protocols for nurse practitioners/nurse midwives* (3rd ed.). San Francisco: School of Nursing, University of California.

may provide insight into positive or negative reactions to the experience of pregnancy and preparation for parenthood The woman is given the opportunity to verbalize thoughts about the changes she is experiencing, fantasies about the baby, and acceptance of pregnancy and the child by the family. Predisposing risk factors for the development of postpartum depression have been identified (Display 7–5).

Culture

Cultural assessment is an important part of prenatal care. Cultural beliefs and practices can affect the health status of the woman by influencing her use of healthcare services, confidence and acceptance of recommended prevention and treatment strategies, and global beliefs regarding her body, illness, religion, and so forth (Allen & Mitchell, 1997). Principal beliefs, values, and behaviors that relate to pregnancy and childbirth should be identified, taking care to avoid sweeping generalizations about cultural characteristics or cultural values. Not every individual in a culture may display certain characteristics as there are variations among cultures and within cultures. Planning culturally specific care includes information about ethnicity, degree of affiliation with the ethnic group, religion, patterns of decision-making, language, style of communication, norms of etiquette, and expectations about the healthcare system (Andrews, 1996; Ramer, 1992).

Nutritional practices and beliefs about medication are particularly significant in pregnancy. Certain behavioral differences can be expected if a culture views pregnancy as an illness, as opposed to a natural occurrence; for example, seeking prenatal care may or may not be important if pregnancy is viewed as a natural occurrence. Healthcare practices during pregnancy are influenced by numerous factors, such as the prevalence of folk remedies, indigenous healers, and the influence of professional healthcare workers. Socioeconomic status and living in an urban or rural setting affects patterns of use of home remedies and use of the healthcare system.

Without cultural awareness, nurses and other healthcare providers tend to project their own cultural responses onto women and families from different socioeconomic, religious, or educational groups. This leads caregivers to assume patients are demonstrating a certain type of behavior for the same reason that they themselves would. Moreover, healthcare providers frequently fail to recognize that medicine has its own culture, which has been dominated historically by traditional middle-class values and beliefs (ACOG, 1998). In an ethnocentric approach, caregivers sometimes believe that if members of other cultures do not share Western values, they should adopt them. An example of this is a nurse who values equality of the sexes dealing with an Asian woman who defers to the husband to make the decisions. Pressuring the woman to defy cultural values and beliefs can prove stressful for the woman and significantly interfere with a therapeutic relationship.

When a language barrier exists, the woman may be reluctant to provide information if the interpreter is male, a relative, or a child of the pregnant woman. Reviewing the goals and purposes of the interview with the interpreter in advance generally enhances the interaction with the woman (Wheeler, 1997). Gender is an important factor in health beliefs. In many cultures, a male physician would not be allowed to examine a woman, much less deliver her baby.

Nurses cannot expect to be culturally competent for every woman they care for. However, culturally sensitive behaviors can enhance prenatal care. If a particular ethnic group dominates the population it is a professional responsibility to learn as much about that culture so as to provide optimal care. A cultural assessment should include the following points (adapted from Seidel, Ball, Dains, & Benedict, 1998):

- *Health beliefs and practices:* assessment of methods used to maintain health (ie, hygiene and self-care practices), treatment of illness, attitude toward necessity of prenatal care, family member responsible for healthcare decisions, and healthcare topics that are taboo for discussion
- *Religious influences and special rituals:* assessment of religious preference, significant persons she looks to for guidance, any special practices with regard to birth (eg, baptism for a dying baby), religious view of pregnancy when not married
- *Language and communication:* assessment of oral and written language spoken in the home and elsewhere, appropriate nonverbal communication such as touch and eye contact and its meaning, and culturally appropriate ways to enter and leave situations
- *Parenting styles and role of the family:* assessment of who is making the decisions in the family, composition of the family, attitude toward marriage and divorce, role and attitude toward children, special beliefs toward conception, pregnancy, childbirth, lactation, and child rearing
- *Dietary practices:* assessment of food preferences, person responsible for food preparation, forbidden foods by culture or religion, required foods for special rite or custom, method used to prepare food, specific beliefs concerning food's role in causing or curing illness

Current Pregnancy Status

Assessment of current pregnancy status includes analysis of current pregnancy history, psychosocial factors, nutritional status, and laboratory data; a review of symptoms that may reflect medical or pregnancy complications; and a complete physical examination. Symptom review includes questions about nausea and vomiting, headache, abdominal or epigastric pain, visual changes, fever, viral illness, vaginal bleeding, dysuria, cramping, and other concerns. This screening process incorporates assessment of historical and social factors with current health status. Evaluation of current pregnancy status provides baseline data that guides planning for future evaluation and health promotion activities.

The physical examination is comprehensive and covers a review of the cardiovascular, respiratory, neurologic, endocrine, gastrointestinal, reproductive, and genitourinary systems. Particular attention should be directed to the anthropometric assessment including the woman's height, weight, and pelvimetry data because these physical characteristics can influence the pregnancy course and birth (Witter, Caulfield, & Stoltzfus, 1995). Pelvic examination includes measurement of cervical length, a Pap smear, and assessment for sexually transmitted diseases. The abdominal examination compares data from the woman's report of her last menstrual period with physical findings. Depending on weeks of gestation, the FHR may be auscultated.

Selected laboratory data are valuable to the assessment process. Biochemical information provides information about current prenatal health, as well as general wellness status. Evaluation of specific laboratory data is discussed later in this chapter.

Ongoing Prenatal Care

Subsequent prenatal visits should be structured to promote continuous, rather than episodic, risk assessment. Each prenatal visit should include a maternal–fetal physical assessment, including vital signs, weight, fundal height, FHR, and fetal movement (Display 7–6), as well as a review of pertinent laboratory data,

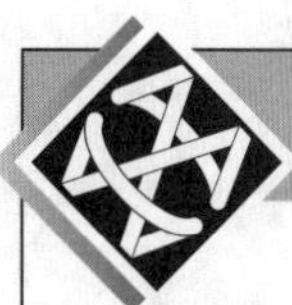

DISPLAY 7–6

Schedule of Prenatal Care

INITIAL PRENATAL VISIT

Intake Assessment

- Comprehensive medical and reproductive health history
- Comprehensive family history
- History of current pregnancy
- Psychosocial assessment (by social worker if possible)
- Nutrition assessment (by nutritionist if possible)
- Comprehensive physical examination

Biochemical Evaluation

- Complete blood count (CBC)
- Blood type and Rh; antibody screen
- PAP smear
- Gonorrhea culture
- *Chlamydia* test
- Serology (RPR, VDRL)
- Rubella (unless previously noted to be immune)
- Hepatitis B surface antigen (HBsAg)
- Urinalysis
- Urine culture and sensitivity
- Sickle cell screen (for women of African, Asian, or Middle Eastern descent)
- Tay-Sachs screening (for women of Jewish or French-Canadian ancestry)
- Glucose challenge test (GCT) if woman is at risk, as indicated by
  - History of fetal demise
  - Recurrent spontaneous abortion
  - History of prior macrosomic infant (birth weight >4,000g)
  - History of gestational diabetes
  - Maternal family history of diabetes (1st degree relatives)
  - Obesity
- Offer HIV testing (provide pretest counseling)
- PPD (tuberculin screen)
- Obtain if indicated
  - TORCH titers
  - Group B *Streptococcus* culture
  - Ultrasound examination

SUBSEQUENT VISITS

Assessment (each visit)

- Vital signs
- Urine dipstick for glucose, albumin, and ketones
- Weight
- Fundal height
- Fetal heart rate (FHR)
- Fetal movement
- Leopold's maneuvers to evaluate fetal lie/presentation
- Assess presence or absence of edema

15–20 weeks

- Maternal serum α-fetoprotein (MSAFP)
- Begin preterm birth prevention education
- One-hour glucose challenge test (GCT) as indicated by risk

20–24 weeks

- Preterm birth prevention education

24–28 weeks

- Cervical examination at 28 weeks as indicated by risk status
- One-hour 50g GCT
- Ongoing education about preterm birth prevention and warning signs of pregnancy complications
- Initiate education regarding contraceptive options

28–36 weeks

- CBC at 28 weeks for selected at-risk women
- Blood group antibody screen at 28 weeks if Rh negative; RhoGAM if indirect Coombs negative

dating data, the problem list, and the woman's response to recommended interventions (eg, smoking cessation). At return prenatal visits, risk factors must be analyzed to evaluate their relevance to the gestational age. For example, if a woman has a history of preterm labor and is at 37 weeks' gestation in the current pregnancy, this risk factor would no longer be relevant. Conversely, new risk factors may develop during the pregnancy, such as preeclampsia or placenta previa. Ongoing antenatal care is a dynamic

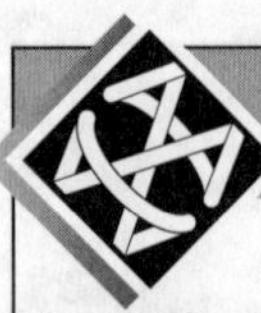

DISPLAY 7–6 (cont.)

Schedule of Prenatal Care

28–36 weeks
- Cervical examination at 32 weeks as indicated by risk status
- Follow-up visit with dietition/nutritionist
- Breast assessment/educational preparation for breast-feeding
- Ongoing education about preterm birth prevention and warning signs of pregnancy complications
- Initiate parenting education

36–40 weeks
- CBC if Hbg <11g/dL or Hct <33% at 28 weeks
- Repeat GC, *Chlamydia,* RPR, HIV, HBsAg if indicated
- Initiate education about signs of labor, preparation for birth (after 37 weeks' gestation)

Adapted from American Academy of Pediatrics & American College of Obstetricians and Gynecologists. (1997). *Guidelines for perinatal care* (4th. ed.). Elk Grove Village, IL: Author and from Shannon, M.T. (1999). Initial prenatal visit. In W.L. Star, M.T. Shannon, L.N. Sammons, L. Lommel, & Y. Gutierrez (Eds.). *Ambulatory Obstetrics: Protocols for nurse practitioners/nurse midwives* (3rd. ed.). San Francisco: School of Nursing, University of California.

process in which risk factors may change from month to month. Achieving healthy pregnancy outcomes is a multifaceted and sometimes complex process. Nurses are credible sources of information who are nonthreatening confidants as the woman and her partner sort through information and decision-making during pregnancy (Raines, 1996). Nurses need to recognize the benefits, limitations, and social implications of the variety of maternal and fetal surveillance techniques offered.

Particular attention should be given to evaluation of blood pressure trends. During pregnancy, blood pressure values decrease slightly during the second trimester but return to early pregnancy values by the third trimester. Ideally, during preconception care or early prenatal care, a baseline blood pressure is noted. It is important to evaluate and document blood pressure measurements in the same arm with the woman in the same position (ie, sitting or semi-Fowler's) with the blood pressure cuff at the level of the heart. Use of the same device for assessing blood pressure is also critical to accuracy. Consistency in blood pressure monitoring allows for more accurate assessment and comparison across prenatal visits. Traditionally, an elevation of systolic blood pressure of 30 mmHg or an elevation of 15 mmHg for diastolic blood pressure over prepregnancy or first-trimester measurements was thought to be predictive of the development of preeclampsia, but data suggest this criteria may be of questionable value for diagnosis (Villar & Sibai, 1989). The predictive validity of elevated mean arterial pressure (MAP) during the second trimester is also low. There is a high incidence of false-positive results (MAP value >90 mmHg) for women who remain normotensive during pregnancy (Roberts, 1994; Villar & Sibai, 1989). When there is a change in blood pressure, the woman should be assessed for the concurrent development of proteinuria, headaches, dizziness, visual disturbances, epigastric pain, or edema.

Basic fetal surveillance includes assessment of fundal height, FHR, and fetal activity. Fundal height is the measurement of the uterus from the symphysis pubis to the top of the fundus. The measurement of the fundal height in centimeters (±2 cm) should correlate with gestational age between 22 and 34 weeks. Fundal height less than gestational age may be indicative of intrauterine growth restriction (IUGR). Fundal height greater than for gestational age may indicate multiple gestation, polyhydramnios, fibroids, or other conditions that cause uterine distension. Fetal activity is an indirect measure of central nervous system function and is predictive of fetal well-being.

Selected biochemical screens may be repeated at specific intervals during pregnancy (Table 7–2). Subsequent prenatal visits usually include urinalysis by dipstick for evidence of proteinuria, glucosuria, and ketonuria. Although it is common practice, there are few data to suggest routine urinalysis by means of dipstick provides useful clinical information or is predictive of women who will develop complications of pregnancy (Hooper, 1996; Gribble, Fee, & Berg, 1995). After a baseline complete blood cell count (CBC) is obtained, periodic assessment of hematocrit and hemoglobin values may be indicated for certain at-risk populations.

Based on medical and obstetric history, clinical symptoms, and assessment information, more extensive laboratory data may be indicated, including screen-

TABLE 7–2 ■ COMMON PRENATAL LABORATORY TESTS

Test	Timing	Significant Values
Complete blood count		
Hematocrit	Initial visit, 28, 36 weeks	<32%
Hemoglobin	Initial visit, 28, 36 weeks	<11g/dL
White blood cell count	Initial visit, 28, 36 weeks	>15,000/mm^3
Type and Rh	Initial visit	Mother Rh–, Father Rh+
Antibody screen	Initial visit, 36 weeks	Positive
Serology	Initial visit, 36 weeks	Positive
Rubella	Initial visit	≤1:8; significant rise 50 g
50 g 1hr glucose challenge test	24–28 weeks	>140 g/dL
HBsAg	Initial visit, as indicated	Positive
Urinalysis	Initial visit	Positive
Urine culture and sensitivity	Initial visit	Positive
Urine		
Glucose/protein	Each visit	>2+
Pap smear	Initial visit	Abnormal cervical cytology
Group B Strep culture	36 weeks	Positive
GC/*Chlamydia* probe	Initial visit, 36 weeks	Positive
Rh antibody	Initial visit, 28 weeks	Negative
HIV	Initial visit (offer), 36 weeks	Positive
Maternal serum α-fetoprotein	15–20 weeks	≥2.0 (multiples of the median)
Sickle cell screen, Hgb electrophoresis	Initial visit	Positive for trait/anemia
Tay-Sachs screen	Initial visit	Carrier
PPD (tuberculin screen)	Initial visit	Positive

Adapted from Barron, M. L. (1998). *Nursing assessment of the pregnant woman: Antepartal screening and laboratory evaluation.* (Nursing Module). White Plains, NY: March of Dimes Birth Defects Foundation.

ing for sexually transmitted diseases (AAP & ACOG, 1997). Data indicate risk of maternal–fetal transmission of the human immunodeficiency virus (HIV) can be reduced by prophylactic administration of zidovudine during the antepartum and intrapartum periods to pregnant women who are HIV seropositive and to their infants (Carpenter et al., 1996). All pregnant women should be offered screening for HIV to initiate timely treatment (AAP & ACOG, 1997; CDC, 1995b). Appropriate counseling and referral services should be available for women with positive test results.

Serum glucose evaluation before 28 weeks' gestation may be indicated based on family history or maternal factors such as previous macrosomic infant, previous unexplained fetal loss, advanced maternal age, maternal obesity, or previous gestational diabetes mellitus (GDM) (Herbert, Dodds, & Cefalo, 1993). Pregnant women who have not been identified as glucose intolerant should have a Glucose Screening Test (GST) between 24 and 28 weeks' gestation (ACOG, 1994b). A level of about 140 mg/dL 1 hour after consuming a 50-g glucose load warrants further evaluation with an oral glucose tolerance test (OGTT) (Reece & Coustan, 1995). An alternative to the 50-g glucose beverage that may be offered to the woman is 28 jelly beans (ie, 50 g of simple carbohydrate). Women report fewer side effects after a jelly bean challenge than after a 50-g glucose beverage challenge (Lamar et al., 1999). Diagnosis of GDM is based on two or more abnormally elevated venous plasma glucose values (Reece & Coustan, 1995). Women diagnosed with GDM require education about appropriate nutrition, self-management, and self-glucose monitoring and referral for appropriate medical care and counseling.

Risk status in pregnancy is a dynamic process that affects clinical and nonclinical parameters (Muerer & Taren, 1993). Psychosocial factors, socioeconomic factors, and lifestyle patterns also require ongoing evaluation. Employment status, family economic status, and relationship status could change from visit to visit. These changes affect the woman's psychosocial stress level, potentiating existing risk factors. In general, factors with potential to affect the pregnancy are in a constant state of fluctuation and require continued surveillance.

Laboratory Assessment

Laboratory data such as CBC, urinalysis, blood type & Rh, antibody screen, rubella titer, rapid plasma reagin test (RPR), hepatitis B surface antigen (HBsAg), gonorrhea and *Chlamydia* testing, and cervical cytology should be obtained from all pregnant women. Additional laboratory tests (eg, STD screens, group B streptococci, TORCH titers, tuberculin testing, toxicology screens, and genetic screens) should be performed as indicated, based on historical indicators or clinical findings (AAP & ACOG, 1997; ACOG, 1992a).

Maternal serum alpha-fetoprotein (MSAFP) screening should be offered to all pregnant women between 15 and 20 weeks' gestation (Baumann & McFarlin, 1994). Screening should be voluntary, and the patient should be counseled about its limitations and benefits. The American College of Obstetricians and Gynecologists recommends screening for AFP but only within a coordinated system that includes quality control, counseling, follow-up, and high-resolution sonographic facilities (ACOG, 1996b).

AFP is a protein that is produced in the fetal yolk sac during the first trimester and in the fetal liver during later gestation. Abnormally elevated MSAFP levels have been associated with birth defects and chromosomal anomalies, such as open neural tube defects, open abdominal defects, and congenital nephrosis (ACOG, 1996b). High MSAFP levels also may result from multiple gestations. Low MSAFP levels have been associated with Down syndrome and other chromosomal anomalies (ACOG, 1996b). Double-marker screening (ie, AFP and human chorionic gonadotropin [hCG]) and triple-marker screening (ie, AFP, hCG, and estriol) are also available to screen for trisomy 21 and neural tube defects, although these are more costly and not offered as frequently as the MSAFP. Average hCG levels are higher and unconjugated estriol levels are lower in Down syndrome pregnancies. The hCG and estriol levels are lower in trisomy 18 pregnancies. Benefits of double and triple screening include increased accuracy in diagnosis because more parameters are evaluated; triple screening detects approximately 60% of pregnancies with trisomy 21, with a false-positive rate of approximately 5% (Hendricks, Von Eschen, & Grady, 1995). However, this method still fails to detect Down syndrome in women younger than 35 years of age (ACOG, 1996b). The woman should be made aware of the tests available, including benefits and risks of each procedure.

Hemoglobin electrophoresis is used to detect genetic hemoglobin disorders, including sickle cell anemia, sickle cell disease, and thalassemia. These recessive inherited conditions occur in the United States primarily in families of African descent but can also be found in families of Asian, Middle Eastern, or Mediterranean area descent (Larrabee & Cowan, 1995). Women of African descent are routinely screened for these disorders. Although prevalence of sickle cell trait is common among African Americans (8 to 12%), information related to inheritance patterns is not well known to those at risk. Display 7–7 and Figure 7–1 provide teaching tools that may be helpful in explaining the genetic transfer of sickle cell trait and sickle cell disease to women and their partners (Larrabee & Cowan, 1995).

Tay-Sachs disease is another recessive disorder seen in families of Jewish ancestry. This disease causes poorly metabolized lipid substances to accumulate with resultant fatty deposits causing neural tissue degeneration within 6 months of birth and death by 5 years of age (Paritsky, 1985). Approximately 1 in 30 Ashkenazi Jews is a carrier, and this group should be screened prenatally (Baumann & McFarlin, 1994).

Prenatal Diagnosis

Prenatal diagnostic evaluation should be considered for families with any of the following: maternal age of 35 years or more; a family history of chromosomal anomalies; parental balanced translocation carrier; the mother a known or at-risk carrier for X-linked disorder; parents who are carriers of an autosomal recessive disorder detectable in utero; a parent affected with an autosomal dominant disorder detectable in utero; a family history of neural tube defects (Bauman & McFarlin, 1994; Matthews & Smith, 1993; Pletsch, 1994) (Display 7–8 and Table 7–3).

Amniocentesis

Amniocentesis is the collection of a sample of amniotic fluid from the amniotic sac for identification of genetic diseases, selected birth defects, and fetal lung maturity; therapy for polyhydramnios; and progressive evaluation of isoimmunized pregnancies. Amniocentesis for genetic evaluation may be performed between 15 and 20 weeks' gestation. Genetic amniocentesis allows for detection of chromosomal anomalies, biochemical disorders, neural tube defects, some ventral wall defects, and DNA analysis for a number of single gene disorders. Early amniocentesis between 11 and 14 weeks' gestation is offered at some centers with outcomes similar to mid-trimester amniocentesis (Cunningham, MacDonald, Gant, Leveno, & Gilstrap, 1997). Before testing, families should be given information about indications for amniocentesis, how the procedure is done, risks involved, and ramifications of findings.

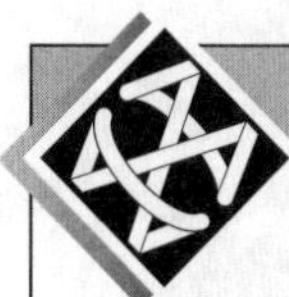

DISPLAY 7–7

Patient Teaching Tool for Genetic Transfer of Sickle Cell Disease/Trait

1. Two parents affected with sickle cell trait:

   SA+SA = 25% of children will have sickle cell disease
   50% of children will have sickle cell trait
   25% of children will not be affected by the trait or disease

2. One parent affected with sickle cell trait, one parent affected with sickle cell disease:

   SA+SS = 50% of children will have sickle cell disease
   50% of children will have sickle cell trait
   0% of children will not be affected by the trait or disease

3. Two parents affected by sickle cell disease:

   SS+SS = 100% of children will have sickle cell disease
   0% of children will have sickle cell trait
   0% of children will not be affected by the disease

4. One parent affected by sickle cell disease, one parent unaffected:

   SS+AA = 100% of children will have sickle cell trait
   0% of children will have sickle cell disease
   0% of children will not be affected by trait

5. One parent affected by sickle cell trait, one parent unaffected:

   SA+AA = 50% of children will have sickle cell trait
   50% of children will not be affected by the trait
   0% of children will not be affected by sickle cell disease

SA, sickle cell trait; SS, sickle cell disease; AA, unaffected.
From Larrabee, K. & Cowan, M. (1995). Clinical nursing management of sickle cell disease and trait during pregnancy. *Journal of Perinatal and Neonatal Nursing, 9* (2) 29–41.

Chorionic Villus Sampling

Chorionic villus sampling (CVS) involves the removal of a small sample of chorionic (placental) tissue through a catheter inserted through the cervix. The villi are harvested and cultured for chromosomal analysis and processed for DNA and enzymatic analysis as indicated. Results are available in 4 days. CVS is ideally performed between 10 and 12 weeks' gestation. Severe limb deformities have been associated with CVS performed between 56 and 66 days' gestation (Cunningham et al., 1997). As with amniocentesis, information about benefits and risks must be provided before the procedure.

Ultrasonography

Ultrasonography (ie, fetal imaging by intermittent high-frequency sound waves) is the most commonly used prenatal diagnostic procedure. Approximately 70% of pregnant women in the United States have at least one ultrasound examination during pregnancy (ACOG, 1993b). Indications vary widely and depend on gestational age and on type of diagnostic information sought. During early pregnancy, ultrasound is frequently used to determine presence of an intrauterine gestational sac, fetal number, and cardiac activity and to measure crown-rump length. Ultrasound during the second and third trimesters can be useful when there is a discrepancy between the woman's last menstrual period and uterine size, to detect fetal anatomic defects, and for placental localization and amniotic fluid volume estimates (ACOG, 1993b). When maternal or fetal complications are suspected or identified, ultrasonography serves as a valuable tool to confirm the diagnosis and follow-up on fetal status. Ultrasonography is also used to guide the obstetrician during other diagnostic procedures such as CVS, amniocentesis, and fetal blood sampling.

Controversy exists about the benefits of routine ultrasound examination for all pregnant women. Advocates suggest routine screening can decrease incidence of labor induction for suspected postdate pregnancies

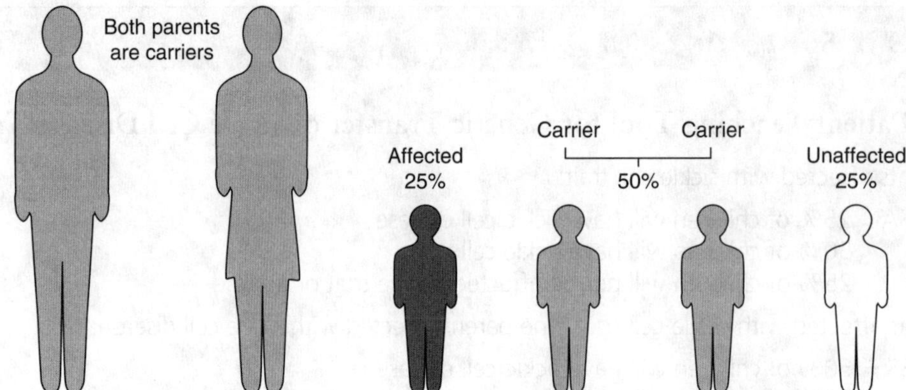

FIGURE 7–1. The inheritance pattern of offspring when both parents are carriers of an autosomal recessive gene.

and avoid undiagnosed fetal anomalies and twin gestations. Based on a cost-benefit analysis, ACOG (1993b) does not support routine ultrasonography for women with no identified maternal or fetal risk factors.

Fetal Blood Sampling

Fetal blood sampling, also known as percutaneous umbilical blood sampling (PUBS) or cordocentesis, allows direct evaluation of fetal blood obtained from the umbilical cord. Using ultrasonography to guide placement, a needle is inserted into one of the umbilical vessels (usually the vein), and a small amount of blood is withdrawn. Valuable information can be gained from analysis of fetal blood, including prenatal diagnosis of fetal blood disorders, isoimmunization, metabolic disorders, infections, and karyotyping (Cunningham, et al., 1997). Cordocentesis can also be used for fetal therapies such as red blood cell and platelet transfusions.

Biochemical Markers

Fetal fibronectin (fFN), a protein secreted by the trophoblast, can be detected by use of a monoclonal antibody: FDC-6. The exact function is unknown, but this protein is thought to play a role in mediating placental–uterine attachment. Fetal fibronectin is normally present in the cervical or vaginal fluid before 20 weeks' gestation. However, after 20 weeks, the presence of fFN may indicate a disruption of the attachment of the fetal membranes, and therefore it has been investigated as an early marker for preterm birth.

Revah, Hannah, and Sue-A-Quan (1998), in their summary review of the research on the utility of fFN, made several conclusions. The sensitivity of fFN as a predictor for delivery within 7 to 10 days was 98% in symptomatic women. However, the positive predictive value was only 15%, probably because some women with symptoms of premature labor do not experience preterm birth. For asymptomatic women, the sensitivity was only 58%. If asymptomatic women are screened for fFN, 42% who deliver within the next 7 to 28 days will have a negative test result.

The specificity for symptomatic women was more than 80%. For symptomatic women, a negative test result for fFN should be useful in ruling out the likelihood of delivery within the next 7 to 10 days. For asymptomatic women, testing for fFN is unlikely to be useful as many women at risk will be misclassified as normal (Moore, 1999; Revah, Hannah, and Sue-A-Quan, 1998).

Testing for fetal fibronectin is simple but requires a pelvic examination. The specimen for analysis is collected from the cervix and posterior fornix of the vagina using a sterile polyester swab. If the woman has had intercourse in the prior 24 hours, the specimen should not be collected at that time. To avoid the effect of a cervical examination, the specimen should be collected before any cervical evaluation other than the gentle manipulation that is required to obtain the specimen. Results are usually available in 24 hours. A level of fFN greater than 50 ng/mL, measured by use of an enzyme-linked immunosorbent assay, is the most commonly used indicator of a positive test (Cunningham et al., 1997; Moore, 1999; Revah, Hannah, & Sue-A-Quan, 1998).

In pregnancy, estriol (a form of estrogen) is present in plasma at 9 weeks' gestation. Estriol rises throughout pregnancy but is accelerated before preterm and term birth. Researchers have postulated that an early increase in serum estriol, reflected in levels of estriol in saliva, may indicate preterm labor. Salivary estriol levels of more than 2.1 ng/mL of saliva are considered positive (Moore, 1999). Salivary estriol is collected by the woman between 9:00 AM and 8:00 PM. Before the collection (at least 1 hour after eating, drinking,

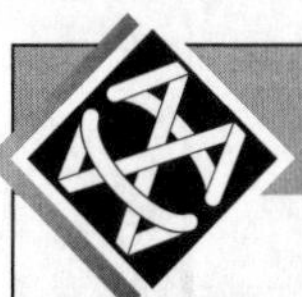

DISPLAY 7–8

Conditions With Incidences and Carrier Frequencies Calling for Prenatal Diagnosis and Counseling

Conditions	*Carrier Frequencies*	*Prenatal Diagnostic Methods*
Couples at an increased risk		
Maternal age >35 years		
Balanced chromosome rearrangement		
Previous child with chromosome abnormality		
Low maternal serum α-fetoprotein		
Family history of birth defects and/or mental retardation		
Congenital heart disease	8/1,000	Echocardiography
Neural tube defect	1.5/1,000	US, AC
Cleft lip and/or palate	1/700	US
Multiple congenital anomalies		US
Mental retardation		
Family history of known or suspected mendelian genetic disorder		
Cystic fibrosis	1/2,500 (whites) to 1/17,000 (blacks)	CVS
Hemophilia A	1/10,000 males	
Hemophilia B	1/1,500–1/2,000 males	FBS
Duchenne muscular dystrophy	1/4,000 males	CVS, AC
Becker muscular dystrophy		CVS, AC
Ethnicity		
African population		
Sickle cell disease	1/600 U.S. blacks	
Trait carriers	1/12	CVS, AC
Mediterranean/Indian: β-thalassemia		CVS, AC
Jewish: Tay-Sachs disease		
Ashkenazic Jews	1/3,600	
Trait carriers	1/30	
General population	1/360,000	
Trait carriers	1/300	CVS
Exposure to possible teratogens		
Alcohol		US
Radiation		US
Occupational chemical exposures		US
Toxoplasmosis		US, FBS
Rubella		US, FBS
Cytomegalovirus		US
Syphilis		US
Insulin-dependent diabetes mellitus		US
Epileptic disorder: drugs		US, AC
Patients with low or high levels of maternal serum α-fetoprotein		US, AC
Fetal abnormalities diagnosed by ultrasonogram		CVS, AC, FBS
Consanguinity		US
Multiple pregnancy losses, stillbirth, infertility		US
Anxiety		US

US, ultrasound; AC, amniocentesis; FBS, fetal blood sampling; CVS, chorionic villus sampling.

From Baumann, P., & McFarlin, B. (1994). Prenatal diagnosis, *Journal of Nurse-Midwifery, 39* (2) (Suppl).

TABLE 7–3 ■ PRENATAL SCREENING TESTS

Preconception	0–12 Weeks	12–24 Weeks	24–40+ Weeks
Carrier screening for cystic fibrosis (CF) Fragile X, Tay-Sachs, hemoglobinopathies	Early amniocentesis Chorionic villus sampling Ultrasound	Ultrasound Amniocentesis Serum biochemical indices: Alpha fetoprotein (AFP), human chorionic gonadotropin (HCG), estriol	Ultrasound Percutaneous umbilical cord blood sampling (PUBS) Fetal fibronectin, salivary estriol Group β-*Streptococcus* culture

Test	Indication	Risk	Accuracy	Limitations
Invasive Procedures				
CVS	Fetal karyotype, diagnosis of X-linked disease or enzymatic disorders	1% risk of fetal loss, maternal Rh isoimmunization, infection, possible limb reduction defects	99.5%; mosaicism may cause doubtful results in 2% or less	No detection of NTD defects
Amniocentesis (amnio)	History of recurrent spontaneous abortion with presence of parental balance rearrangement, fetal karyotype, amniotic AFP to diagnose amnionitis	1.0–1.5% risk of spontaneous abortion, maternal Rh isoimmunization, infection, fetal trauma, fetomaternal hemorrhage, preterm labor; 1/200–300 loss rate	99.4% accurate	Results take 2 weeks; no detection of defects caused by teratogens
PUBS	Fetal karyotype, diagnosis of blood disorders, isoimmunization, metabolic disorders, fetal infection, evaluation of hypoxia, fetal therapy	Fetal loss rate 1–2% due to infection, membrane rupture, transient fetal bradycardia; 0.8% abortion rate; bleeding at puncture site.		Anomalous or growth-retarded fetuses not as tolerant of procedure as "normal" fetuses
Serum Testing				
Carrier screening	To test for CF, Tay-Sachs, fragile X, hemoglobinopathies	Negligible for parents. Fetal risk is method dependent		
AFP	To screen for neural tube defects (NTDs), midline ventral fusion defects, risk of fetal Down syndrome	Negligible	Detects 70–80% of open NTDs, 40% of Down syndrome	Correct dating essential; does not detect closed NTDs; inevitable false positive and false negative results
Double (HCG, AFP) Triple (HCG, AFP, estriol)	To screen for Down syndrome and trisomy 18	Negligible	Detects 2/3 of Down syndrome cases, 90% of open NTDs	

From Creasy, R. & Resnick, R. (1999). *Maternal-fetal medicine: Principles and practice.* Philadelphia: W.B. Saunders and from Cunningham, F.G., MacDonald, P.C., Grant, N.F., Leveno, K.J., & Gilstrap, L.C. (1997). *Williams obstetrics,* (20th ed.) Norwalk, CT: Appleton & Lange.

smoking, chewing gum, and dental care), she rinses her mouth with water. Ten minutes later, the specimen is collected by placing a small test tube with a funnel at the top and allowing her saliva to flow into the tube. The tube is then capped and mailed to a central laboratory in envelopes provided by the company. A level of estriol greater than 2.1 ng/mL of saliva is the most commonly used indicator of a positive test (Moore, 1999; Revah, Hannah, and Sue-A-Quan, 1998).

Gingivitis or bleeding gums, not uncommon in pregnancy, affect the accuracy of the test. SalEst (ie, salivary estriol) is much easier to acquire than fFN but improper collection may invalidate the test. The directions for acquiring salivary estriol are very specific and may pose a challenge to women with low literacy skills. Determinations of fFN and salivary estriol may need to be repeated at 1- or 2-week intervals. This provides the nurse with the opportunity to review signs and symptoms of preterm labor and address any fears or anxieties the woman or family may have regarding preterm birth.

FETAL DEVELOPMENT

It is helpful to relate education about positive pregnancy outcome to fetal development. Throughout a normal pregnancy, the fetus is nourished and protected by placental functioning. This dependence on the placenta leaves the fetus vulnerable to insult from lifestyle factors such as substance abuse, smoking, and poor nutrition. However, education focusing first on the woman's own health needs is essential in establishing an environment of respect for her as an individual separate from a maternal–fetal unit.

A number of factors contribute to risks for the women and fetus throughout the pregnancy. Environmental agents may cross the placenta and affect the development of the embryo or fetus. Three critical periods of development exist: fertilization and implantation; the embryonic period, from day 18 through day 55; and the fetal stage, from day 56 through birth. Factors influencing development in the first period include the quality of the sperm and ovum, the adequacy of the intrauterine environment, and maternal stores and nutrition. A critical window exists in which cells undergoing the most rapid growth are most vulnerable to teratogenic agents. Long-term exposure to noxious agents may impair development. Approximately 10% of all human malformations are caused by environmental factors, 10% by genetic factors, and the remaining 80% are presumably the result of combination of environmental and genetic factors (Sadler, 1995).

Teratogens are agents that cause congenital anomalies in the fetus. Major teratogenic influences include medications, illicit drugs, alcohol, environmental and occupational toxins, radiation, endocrinopathies, injuries, infectious agents, hyperthermia, and nutritional deficiencies (Baumann & McFarlin, 1994). Exposure to teratogenic influences during the embryonic period can cause structural and functional defects. During the fetal period, when there is organ differentiation, structural defects and fetal growth retardation can occur (Table 7–4). Appendix 7C covers immunization during pregnancy.

Nurses interacting with the childbearing family in the prenatal period assess the well-being of the woman and the growth and well-being of the fetus. Nursing intervention is directed by the data obtained from ongoing comprehensive maternal–fetal assessments. Knowledge of beneficial and detrimental behaviors to pregnancy outcome is necessary if the nurse is to provide guidance to the childbearing family. Evaluation of the growth and development of the fetus can be shared with the parents to promote prenatal parent–infant attachment. Display 7–9 identifies normal fetal developmental events.

FETAL SURVEILLANCE

Fetal assessment is an integral component of prenatal care. Careful assessment of fetal well-being enhances perinatal outcome through early identification and intervention for fetal compromise. The goal of antepartum fetal surveillance is to prevent fetal death. Display 7–10 provides the indications for antepartum fetal surveillance. Techniques based on FHR patterns have been in use for almost 3 decades (ACOG, 1999a). Ultrasonography may be used as indicated throughout the pregnancy to assess fetal growth and development. Doppler ultrasound may be used during the second half of pregnancy to assess blood flow changes in the fetal heart, aorta, cerebrum, and the uterine and umbilical arteries and is useful in assessing intrauterine growth restriction associated with postterm gestation, diabetes mellitus, systemic lupus erythematosus, or antiphospholipid syndrome (ACOG, 1999a). Data indicate cervical ultrasonography is useful in identifying women at risk for preterm birth (Iams, et al., 1994). In one study, a cervical length of at least 30 mm, when evaluated between 24 and 35 weeks' gestation, predicted a low likelihood of preterm birth (Iams, Paraskos, Landon, Teteris, & Johnson, 1994).

(text continues on page 160)

TABLE 7–4 ■ TERATOGENIC AGENTS

Agent	Effects	Comments
Drugs and chemicals		
Alcohol	Growth restriction before and after birth, mental retardation, microcephaly, midfacial hypoplasia producing atypical facial appearance, renal and cardiac defects, various other major and minor malformations	Nutritional deficiency, smoking, and multiple drug use confound data. Risk from ingestion of one to two drinks per day is not well defined but may cause a small reduction in average birth weight. Fetuses of women who ingest six drinks per day have a 40% risk of developing some features of the fetal alcohol syndrome.
Androgens and testosterone derivatives (eg, danazol)	Virilization of female, advanced genital development in males	Effects are dose dependent and related to the stage of embryonic development at the time of exposure. Given before 9 weeks of gestation, labioscrotal fusion can be produced; clitoromegaly can occur with exposure at any gestational age. Risk related to incidental brief androgenic exposure is minimal.
Angiotensin-converting enzyme (ACE) inhibitors (eg, enalapril, captopril)	Fetal renal tubular dysplasia, oligohydramnios, neonatal renal failure, lack of cranial ossification, intrauterine growth restriction	Incidence of fetal morbidity is 30%. The risk increases with second- and third-trimester use, leading to in utero fetal hypotension, decreased renal blood flow, and renal failure.
Coumarin derivatives (eg, warfarin)	Nasal hypoplasia and stippled bone epiphyses are most common; other effects include broad, short hands with shortened phalanges, ophthalmologic abnormalities, intrauterine growth restriction, developmental delay, anomalies of neck and central nervous system	Risk for a seriously affected child is considered to be 15–25% when anticoagulants that inhibit vitamin K are used in the first trimester, especially during 6–9 weeks of gestation. Later drug exposure may be associated with spontaneous abortion, stillbirths, central nervous system abnormalities, abruptio placentae, and fetal or neonatal hemorrhage.
Carbamazepine	Neutral tube defects, minor craniofacial defects, fingernail hypoplasia, microcephaly, developmental delay, intrauterine growth restriction	Risk of neural tube defect, mostly lumbosacral, is 1–2% when used alone during first trimester and increased when used with other antiepileptic agents.
Folic acid antagonists (methotrexate and aminopterin)	Increased risk for spontaneous abortions, various anomalies	These drugs are contraindicated for the treatment of psoriasis in pregnancy and must be used with extreme caution in the treatment of malignancy. Cytotoxic drugs are potentially teratogenic. Effects of aminopterin are well documented. Folic acid antagonists used during the first trimester produce a malformation rate of up to 30% in fetuses that survive.

Drugs and chemicals (continued)		
Cocaine	Bowel atresias; congenital malformations of the heart, limbs, face, and genitourinary tract; microcephaly; intrauterine growth restriction; cerebral infarctions	Risks may be affected by other factors and concurrent abuse of multiple substances. Maternal and pregnancy complications include sudden death and placental abruption.
Diethylstilbestrol	Clear cell adenocarcinoma of the vagina or cervix, vaginal adenosis, abnormalities of cervix and uterus, abnormalities of the testes, possible infertility in males and females	Vaginal adenosis is detected in more than 50% of women whose mothers took these drugs before 9 weeks of gestation. Risk for vaginal adenocarcinoma is low. Males exposed in utero may have a 25% incidence of epididymal cysts, hypotrophic testes, abnormal spermatozoa, and induration of the testes.
Lead	Increased abortion rate, stillbirths	Fetal central nervous system development may be adversely affected. Determining preconceptional lead levels for those at risk may be useful.
Lithium	Congenital heart disease, particularly Ebstein anomaly	Risk of heart malformations due to first-trimester exposure is low. The effect is not as significant as reported in earlier studies. Exposure in the last month of gestation may produce toxic effects on the thyroid, kidneys, and neuromuscular systems.
Organic mercury	Cerebral atrophy, microcephaly, mental retardation, spasticity, seizures, blindness	Cerebral palsy can occur even when exposure is in the third trimester. Exposed individuals include consumers of fish and grain contaminated with methyl mercury.
Phenytoin	Intrauterine growth restriction, mental retardation, microcephaly, dysmorphic craniofacial features, cardiac defects, hypoplastic nails and distal phalanges	The full syndrome is seen in less than 10% of children exposed in utero, but up to 30% have some manifestations. Mild to moderate mental retardation is found in some children who have severe physical stigmata. The effect may depend on whether the fetus inherits a mutant gene that decreases production of epoxide hydrolase, an enzyme necessary to decrease the teratogen phenytoin epoxide.
Streptomycin and kanamycin	Hearing loss, eighth-nerve damage	No ototoxicity in the fetus has been reported from use of gentamicin or vancomycin.
Tetracycline	Hypoplasia of tooth enamel, incorporation of tetracycline into bones and teeth, permanent yellow-brown discoloration of deciduous teeth	Drug has no known effect unless exposure occurs in second or third trimester.
Thalidomide	Bilateral limb deficiencies, anotia and microtia, cardiac and gastrointestinal anomalies	Of children whose mothers used thalidomide between 35 and 50 days of gestation, 20% show the effect.

(continued)

TABLE 7–4 ■ TERATOGENIC AGENTS (continued)

Agent	Effects	Comments
Drugs and chemicals (continued)		
Trimethadione and paramethadione	Cleft lip or cleft palate; cardiac defects; growth deficiency; microcephaly; mental retardation; characteristic facial appearance; ophthalmologic, limb, and genitourinary tract abnormalities	Risk for defects or spontaneous abortion is 60–80% with first-trimester exposure. A syndrome, including V-shaped eyebrows, low-set ears, high arched palate, and irregular dentition, has been identified. These drugs are no longer used during pregnancy due to the availability of more effective, less toxic agents.
Valproic acid	Neural tube defects, especially spina bifida; minor facial defects	Exposure must occur before normal closure of neural tube during first trimester to produce open defect (incidence of approximately 1%).
Vitamin A and its derivatives (eg, isotretinoin, etretinate, and retinoids)	Increased abortion rate, microtia, central nervous system defects, thymic agenesis, cardiovascular effects, craniofacial dysmorphism, microphthalmia, cleft lip and palate, mental retardation	Isotretinoin exposure before pregnancy is not a risk because the drug is not stored in tissue. Etretinate has a long half-life, and effects occur long after drug is discontinued. Topical application does not have a known risk.
Infections		
Cytomegalovirus	Hydrocephaly, microcephaly, chorioretinitis, cerebral calcifications, symmetric intrauterine growth restriction, microphthalmos, brain damage, mental retardation, hearing loss	Most common congenital infection. Congenital infection rate is 40% after primary infection and 14% after recurrent infection. Of infected infants, physical effects as listed are present in 20% after primary infection and 8% after secondary infection. No effective therapy exists.
Rubella	Microcephaly, mental retardation, cataracts, deafness, congenital heart disease; all organs may be affected	Malformation rate is 50% if the mother is infected during first trimester. Rate of severe permanent organ damage decreases to 6% by midpregnancy. Immunization of children and nonpregnant adults is necessary for prevention. Immunization is not recommended during pregnancy, but the live attenuated vaccine virus has not been shown to cause the malformations of congenital rubella syndrome.
Syphilis	If severe infection, fetal demise with hydrops; if mild, detectable abnormalities of skin, teeth, and bones	Penicillin treatment is effective for *Treponema pallidum* eradication to prevent progression of damage. Severity of fetal damage depends on duration of fetal infection; damage is worse if infection is greater than 20 weeks. Prevalence is increasing; need to rule out other sexually transmitted diseases.

Toxoplasmosis	Possible effects on all systems but particularly central nervous system: microcephaly, hydrocephaly, cerebral calcifications. Chorioretinitis is most common. Severity of manifestations depends on duration of disease.	Low prevalence during pregnancy (0.1–0.5%); initial maternal infection must occur during pregnancy to place fetus at risk. *Toxoplasma gondii* is transmitted to humans by raw meat or exposure to infected cat feces. In the first trimester, the incidence of fetal infection is as low as 9% and increases to approximately 59% in the third trimester. The severity of congenital infection is greater in the first trimester than at the end of gestation. Treat with pyrimethamine, sulfadiazine, or spiramycin.
Varicella	Possible effects on all organs, inluding skin scarring, chorioretinitis, cataracts, microcephaly, hypoplasia of the hands and feet, and muscle atrophy	Risk of congenital varicella is low, approximately 2–3%, and occurs between 7 and 21 weeks of gestation. Varicella-zoster immune globulin is available regionally for newborns exposed in utero during last 4–7 days of gestation. No effect from herpes zoster.
Radiation	Microcephaly, mental retardation	Medical diagnostic radiation delivering less than 0.05 Gy* to the fetus has no teratogenic risk. Estimated fetal exposure of common radiologic procedures is 0.01 Gy or less (eg, intravenous pyelography, 0.0041 Gy).

*1 gray (Gy) = 100 rad.

From American College of Obstetricians and Gynecologists. (1997). *Teratology* (Educational bulletin no. 236). Washington, DC: Author.

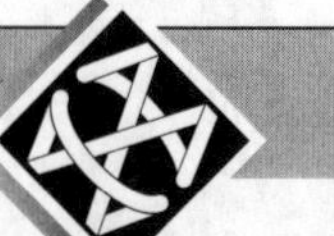

DISPLAY 7–9

Major Normal Events of the Fetal Period (9th to 40th week)

WEEKS 9 TO 12

Crown-rump length doubles between 9 and 12 weeks.
Upper limbs develop to normal proportions, while lower limbs remain less developed.
Male and female genitalia are recognizable by 12 weeks.
Production of red blood cells transfers from the liver to the spleen at 12 weeks.

WEEKS 13 TO 16

Rapid fetal growth occurs.
Fetus doubles in size.
Lanugo begins to grow.
Fingernails are formed.
Kidneys begin to secrete urine.
Fetus begins to swallow amniotic fluid.
Fetus appears human.
Placenta is fully formed.

WEEKS 17 TO 23

Fetal growth slows.
Lower limbs are fully formed.
Fetal body is covered with lanugo.
Vernix caseosa covers the body to protect the skin from amniotic fluid.
Brown fat forms.

WEEKS 24 TO 27

Skin growth is rapid, and skin appears red and wrinkled.
The eyes open, and eyelashes and eyebrows are formed.
The fetus becomes viable at 26 to 27 weeks.

WEEKS 28 TO 31

Subcutaneous fat is deposited.
If the fetus is born at this time with immature lungs, respiratory distress syndrome may occur.

WEEKS 32 TO 36

Lanugo has disappeared from the body but remains on the head.
Weight gain is steady.
Fingernails are growing.
The fetus has a good chance of surviving if born.

WEEKS 37 TO 40

Subcutaneous fat builds, and fetal contours appear round.
Both testes have descended in the male.
The skull is fully developed.

Assessment of Fetal Activity

Fetal movement counting (ie, "kick counts") has been proposed as a primary method of fetal surveillance for all pregnancies. Cessation of fetal movement is correlated with fetal death. The mother's observation of fetal movement has been validated through an 80% to 90% correlation of maternal perception of movement with movement detected on real-time ultrasonography (Moore & Piacquadio, 1989).

Several methods of fetal movement counting have been proposed; however, neither the ideal number of kicks nor the ideal duration for movement counting has been defined (ACOG, 1999). Perception of 10 distinct movements in a period of up to 2 hours is considered reassuring. After 10 movements have been perceived, the count may be discontinued. Another approach is to instruct women to count fetal movements for 1 hour three times per week. The count is considered reassuring if it equals or exceeds the woman's established baseline count (ACOG, 1999a). Freda and coworkers (1993) found no evidence that women prefer or are more compliant with either method. Regardless of technique, monitoring of fetal movement is recommended for pregnant women at high risk for antepartum fetal death beginning as early as 26 to 28 weeks' gestation. For most at-risk patients, however, initiating testing at 32 to 34 weeks is appropriate (ACOG, 1999a). Because fetal movement counting is inexpensive, reassuring, and a relatively easily taught skill, all women could benefit from instruction on fetal activity assessment.

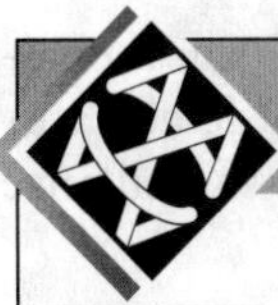

DISPLAY 7–10

Indications for Antepartum Fetal Surveillance

MATERNAL CONDITIONS

- Antiphospholipid syndrome
- Hyperthyroidism (poorly controlled)
- Hemoglobinopathies (hemoglobin SS, SC, or S-thalassemia)
- Cyanotic heart disease
- Systemic lupus erythematosus
- Chronic renal disease
- Type 1 diabetes mellitus
- Hypertensive disorders

PREGNANCY-RELATED CONDITIONS

- Pregnancy-related hypertension
- Decreased fetal movement
- Oligohydramnios
- Polyhydramnios
- Intrauterine growth restriction
- Postterm pregnancy
- Isoimmunization
- Previous fetal demise (unexplained or recurrent risk)
- Multiple gestation (with significant growth discrepancy)

From American College of Obstetricians and Gynecologists. (1999). *Antepartum fetal surveillance* (ACOG practice bulletin no. 9). Washington, DC: American College of Obstetricians and Gynecologists.

Although fetal activity is a reassuring sign, decreased fetal movement is not necessarily ominous. A healthy fetus usually has perceivable movements within 10 to 60 minutes (Lommel, 1990). However, perception of fetal movement can be influenced by many factors, including time of day, gestational age, placental location, glucose loading, maternal smoking, maternal medications, and decreased uterine space as gestation increases. Decreased fetal movement may also reflect the fetal sleep state. Early identification of conditions that can affect pregnancy outcome can minimize perinatal morbidity by allowing for the establishment of an appropriate treatment plan and referrals (AAP & ACOG, 1997). Report of decreased fetal movement is an indication for further assessment. The woman should be instructed to have something to eat and drink, rest, and focus on fetal movement for 1 hour. Four movements in 1 hour are considered reassuring. If fewer than four movements are perceived in 2 hours, the woman should call her primary healthcare provider immediately.

Nonstress Test

The NST is one of the most common methods of antenatal screening and involves electronic FHR monitoring for approximately 20 minutes. The NST is based on the premise that the normal fetus moves at various intervals and that the central nervous system and myocardium responds to movement with acceleration of the FHR. Acceleration of the FHR during fetal activity is a sign of fetal well-being (ACOG, 1999a). Various definitions of reactivity have been used. Using the most common definition, the NST is considered to be reactive when two or more FHR accelerations of 15 beats per minute above baseline and lasting at least 15 seconds occur within a 20-minute timeframe with or without perception of fetal movement by the woman (ACOG, 1999a). NSTs that do not meet this criteria are nonreactive. A reactive NST is reassuring, indicating less than a 1% chance of fetal death within 1 week of a reactive NST (Field, 1989). Most deaths within 1 week of a reactive NST fall into nonpreventable categories such as abruptio placentae, sepsis, and cord accidents. However, a nonreactive NST is not necessarily an ominous sign. Rather, the nonreactive NST indicates a need for further testing and should be followed by a contraction stress test (CST) or BPP (Gegor & Paine, 1992). The NST of the noncompromised preterm fetus (24 to 28 weeks' gestation) is frequently nonreactive, and up to 50% of NSTs may not be reactive from 28 to 32 weeks' gestation (ACOG, 1999a).

Contraction Stress Test

The CST, formerly known as the oxytocin challenge test (OCT), evaluates FHR response to uterine contractions. FHR and uterine activity are assessed by an electronic fetal monitor. A baseline monitor tracing is obtained for 20 minutes. If spontaneous uterine contractions do not occur, uterine stimulation is produced through IV oxytocin infusion or nipple stimulation, until three contractions of at least 40 seconds duration occur within a 10-minute time frame. CSTs are evaluated as follows according to the presence or absence of late decelerations (ACOG, 1999a):

- Negative CST (normal): no late or significant variable decelerations

- Positive CST (abnormal): late decelerations after 50% of contractions (even if the contraction frequency is less than three in 10 minutes)
- Equivocal or suspicious CST: intermittent late or significant variable decelerations
- Equivocal-hyperstimulatory CST: FHR decelerations that occur in the presence of contractions more frequent than every 2 minutes or lasting longer than 90 seconds
- Unsatisfactory CST: fewer than three contractions per 10 minutes or quality of tracing inadequate for interpretation

The negative CST result is reassuring and is associated with a low fetal death rate within 1 week of the negative test result. A positive CST result requires further evaluation or birth. The CST false-positive rate of 30% to 50% warrants evaluation of the CST within the context of the total clinical picture (Lommel, 1990).

Biophysical Profile

The BPP combines electronic FHR monitoring with ultrasonography to evaluate fetal well-being based on multiple biophysical variables. Five parameters are assessed: fetal muscle tone, fetal movement, fetal breathing movements, amniotic fluid volume, and FHR reactivity as demonstrated by NST. Each item has a maximum score of 2, with a summed score of 8 to 10 indicating fetal well-being (ie, reassuring). A score of 6 is considered "equivocal," and the test should be repeated the next day in a preterm fetus. A term fetus should be delivered. A score of 4 usually indicates that delivery is warranted, although for extremely premature pregnancies, management is individualized. Scores of 0 to 3 are "abnormal," with expeditious delivery considered (ACOG, 1999a). Indications for BPP are those listed for antepartum fetal surveillance with weekly testing usually recommended. A BPP may also be indicated to follow-up on a nonreactive NST.

Modified Biophysical Profile

The modified BPP combines the use of a NST as a short-term indicator of fetal well-being with the assessment of amniotic fluid index as an indicator of long-term placental function. The amniotic fluid index (AFI) is the sum of the measurements of the deepest cord-free amniotic fluid pocket in each of the four abdominal quadrants. An AFI value greater than 5 cm generally is considered to represent an adequate volume of fluid. A modified BPP is considered reassuring if the NST is reactive and the AFI is greater than 5 but abnormal if the NST is nonreactive or the AFI is 5 or less (ACOG, 1999a). The modified BPP is less cumbersome and appears to be as predictive of fetal status as other approaches of biophysical fetal surveillance (AAP & ACOG, 1997; ACOG, 1999a).

PLAN FOR NURSING CARE AND INTERVENTION

Nursing interventions are based on nursing diagnoses and a collaborative approach to the identification of strengths and problems. Together, the nurse and woman set goals and strategize ways to implement a plan of care to meet these goals. During the antepartum period, nursing care typically includes comfort promotion (eg, measures to relieve discomforts caused by the physiologic changes of pregnancy), family adaptation in planning the addition of a new member, and encouraging behaviors to enhance maternal and fetal well-being. Providing information, especially for the woman pregnant for the first time, is an important aspect of antepartum care. The nurse has the opportunity and the responsibility to teach the woman and her family about beneficial and detrimental lifestyle practices, potential risks, and care required to promote maternal and fetal well-being. The nurse in ambulatory care provides anticipatory planning, assesses all available data, and structures education and nursing interventions accordingly. Inherent in competent perinatal nursing practice is the ability to differentiate between normal pregnancy variations and high-risk complications, and the initiation of appropriate nursing interventions.

COLLABORATIVE MANAGEMENT AND FOLLOW-UP

Total care management of the childbearing family requires cooperation, collaboration, and communication across disciplines. Risk factors must be evaluated in terms of individual risk versus benefit to be effective. Healthcare providers are charged with the task of finding the goodness of fit between the recommended healthcare regimen and the individual's reality to optimize outcome. Case management allows for a single healthcare professional to coordinate healthcare management in collaboration with the pregnant woman.

Case Management

The childbearing woman and her family are the core of the perinatal healthcare team. Family-centered perinatal care is a model of care based on the philosophy that the physical, social, spiritual, and economic needs of the total family unit should be integrated and considered collectively (AWHONN, 1998). The nurse's role as case manager, advocate, and educator is of primary importance in facilitating a family-friendly system that validates the woman's own knowledge and promotes empowered healthcare decision-making.

Nutrition

The nutritionist is a valuable asset to the prenatal healthcare team. Nutrition assessment and counseling is a vital component of prenatal care. The woman may benefit from regularly scheduled appointments with the nutritionist during an early prenatal visit and again at 28 weeks' gestation. Additional visits with the nutritionist should be scheduled as indicated (eg, for inadequate or excessive weight gain, anemia, metabolic disorders such as GDM). Weight-gain charts, 24-hour diet recall, or simple, self-report dietary assessment tools are valuable education resources.

Nutritional status may change because of availability of appropriate foods and financial resources for groceries. The most significant food shortages for low-income women occur at the end of the month, when federal and local resources are depleted or when food is shared among a disproportionate number of household members. Likewise, religious practices may dictate fasting during specific times of the year (ie, Lent or Ramadan), limiting the woman's food intake. Awareness and ongoing assessment of these factors allows for timely interventions and appropriate referral to nutrition counseling, social work, and community support services. Referrals to food and nutrition supplement programs may be warranted. Women in the United States should be referred to the Special Supplemental Feeding Program for WIC. Other supplemental food and nutrition programs are available to childbearing families on a regional or local basis. The prenatal healthcare team must be knowledgeable about such resources in their area.

Social Services

The emphasis on individualized, holistic prenatal care, encompassing physiologic and psychosocial needs, promotes a prevention-oriented model of care (Young, 1990). Today's families may face unemployment, homelessness, chemical dependency, increased family and neighborhood violence, and lack of support systems that may precipitate crises and affect perinatal outcome. Early recognition of potential risk allows for prompt intervention and referral. The role of the perinatal social worker is critical in providing interventions that relieve stress, provide for woman's basic needs, follow crisis situations, and facilitate healthcare decision-making. Social work referrals are appropriate for pregnant women experiencing medical, psychological, or socioeconomic crises. Psychosocial and socioeconomic factors are evaluated on a continuing basis, with referral to social services as needed. Chapter 6 provides a more extensive discussion of psychological factors related to pregnancy.

From a practical point of view, pregnant women have much to benefit from a team approach. The woman has access to health professionals offering expertise in a specific area, and the perinatal team may be more likely to thoroughly assess and plan for a woman's individual needs. A pregnant woman may communicate about some concern to a nutritionist or social worker regarding a problem area that she did not reveal to the physician or nurse. With professional collaboration and communication among team members problems can be better identified and addressed.

Education and Counseling

Educational and health promotional activities that include the father must be integrated into prenatal care. Prenatal education should focus not only on a positive labor and birth experience but, more importantly, on laying the groundwork for a successful pregnancy outcome and family experience (AWHONN, 1998). Education regarding nutrition, sexuality, stress reduction, lifestyle behaviors, and hazards in the work place is appropriate to include in prenatal education (Display 7–11). Chapter 18 provides a more comprehensive review of prenatal education.

Early identification of conditions that can affect pregnancy outcome can minimize perinatal morbidity by allowing for the establishment of an appropriate treatment plan and referrals (AAP & ACOG, 1997). Women must receive information regarding risk factors, warning signs, and criteria for provider notification. One study of the effect of prenatal education on birth outcome in a high-risk population found that lack of advice to call the healthcare provider if preterm labor was suspected emerged as a more important predictor of preterm labor or low-birth-weight risk than lack of education in recognition of preterm labor (Libbus & Sable, 1991). In this population of high-risk, potentially disenfranchised women, the permission to act on their own instinct and self-knowledge was found to be of equal or greater value than specific educational content (Libbus & Sable). Routine prenatal care should include education to enhance recognition of warning signs of preterm labor

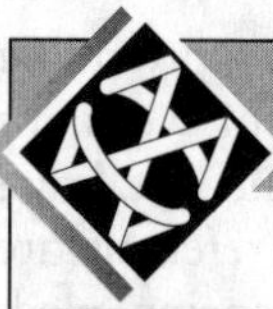

DISPLAY 7–11

Prenatal Education Topics

FIRST TRIMESTER

Smoking cessation	Teratogen avoidance
Alcohol avoidance	Nutrition
Illicit drug avoidance	Seat belt use
Work and rest patterns	Safer sex
Physiologic changes of pregnancy	Sexuality
Emotional changes of pregnancy	Discomforts of pregnancy
Healthy lifestyle	Importance of early prenatal care
Screening, diagnostic tests	What to expect during prenatal care
Nipple assessment, breast-feeding promotion	

Warning signs of pregnancy complications
Criteria and mechanism for notification of health care provider
(Information may be given at individual prenatal care visit or early pregnancy class)

SECOND TRIMESTER

Smoking cessation	Teratogen avoidance
Alcohol avoidance	Nutrition
Illicit drug avoidance	Prenatal laboratory tests
Physiologic changes of pregnancy	Sexuality
Emotional changes of pregnancy	Healthy lifestyle
Discomforts of pregnancy	Family roles
Fetal growth and development	Infant car seat use
Breast-feeding promotion	Childbirth education
Perineal exercises	Clothing choices/shoes
	Body mechanics

Preterm birth prevention
Preeclampsia precautions

THIRD TRIMESTER

Smoking cessation	Teratogen avoidance
Alcohol avoidance	Nutrition
Illicit drug avoidance	Prenatal laboratory tests
Physiologic changes of pregnancy	Sexuality
Emotional changes of pregnancy	Reproductive health
Discomforts of pregnancy	Healthy lifestyle
Fetal growth and development	Newborn care
Breast-feeding promotion	Childbirth education
Postpartum self-care choices	
Postpartum emotional changes	

Preparation for childbirth
Where to go—Who to call

Adapted from Expert Panel on the Content of Prenatal Care. (1989). *Caring for our future: The content of prenatal care.* Washington DC: Public Health Service and from Meurer, J., & Taren, D.L. (1993). Prevention and public health in Obstetrics. In R.A. Knuppel & J.E. Drukker. *High risk pregnancy: A team approach.* Philadelphia: W.B. Saunders.

and preeclampsia (see Chapter 8), fever, rupture of membranes or leaking of fluid, decreased fetal movement, vaginal bleeding, persistent nausea and vomiting, and signs and symptoms of viral or bacterial infection.

With current postpartum lengths of stay, it is increasingly difficult to teach the woman and family all they need to know about maternal–newborn care during hospitalization. The last trimester of pregnancy may be a potentially effective time to introduce maternal–newborn care content, including parenting issues and family planning information. Because there is no accurate way to predict which women will develop postpartum emotional disorders, all childbearing women and family members should be provided information about postpartum depression and where to seek help.

Confidence-building strategies that promote breast-feeding are an important component of prenatal nutrition education. Providing information about breast-feeding convenience, infant benefits, and potential formula cost savings can enhance maternal motivation. Acknowledging that some women may feel embarrassed or uncomfortable about breast-feeding and providing tips for discreet breast-feeding techniques are also helpful approaches. Anticipated length of breast-feeding is an important prenatal factor associated with breast-feeding duration (O'Campo, Faden, Geilen, & Wang, 1992). There is a positive correlation between increased breast-feeding duration and increased maternal confidence (O'Campo et al., 1992). A session with the nutritionist, focusing on nutrition during lactation, may be helpful in encouraging initiation of breast-feeding and a successful breast-feeding experience. Chapter 16 provides more discussion about breast-feeding.

The childbearing continuum is a transition involving each family member. Childbirth education provides the opportunity for enhancement of family systems and facilitation of empowered behaviors that will last a lifetime (Starn, 1993). Thirty years ago, the first childbirth education classes began as a means to provide information for women wishing to be awake, active participants in the birth of their child. Since then, childbirth education focusing on coping strategies for labor has been shown to decrease use of anesthesia in labor and enhance maternal confidence and satisfaction. Today, childbirth education goes well beyond basics to include information about birth as a natural process; environments that enhance the woman's ability to give birth; care options; and most importantly, the tools necessary to make informed healthcare decisions that are appropriate for individual families. Childbirth education has expanded in some centers to meet consumers' need for information concerning preconception wellness, care provider and birthing options, and maternal–newborn care during the postpartum period. Current, accurate information, effective coping skills, and intact support systems fostered by childbirth education provide families with the skills to explore alternatives and make informed decisions that are congruent with their personal goals (Lothian, 1993). It is important that childbirth education is available to all women. Perinatal nurses are challenged to move childbirth education from traditional services to time frames and locations that meet consumer needs.

Health Promotion

Preconception health promotion is increasingly recognized as an important factor influencing perinatal outcome. Anticipatory guidance and health promotion information are most useful when provided before conception. Health promotion and health education, beginning with children in school, is essential to improving pregnancy outcome for the next generation (March of Dimes, 1993). Programs should emphasize healthy lifestyle behaviors, self-esteem, and decision-making skills. If women have not been exposed to this information before pregnancy, healthcare professionals should seize the opportunity to provide information and experiences that promote these activities during prenatal care. Awareness of reproductive risk, healthy lifestyle behaviors, and reproductive options is essential in improving pregnancy outcome. Reproductive awareness dialogue should be incorporated into general medical care for men and women (March of Dimes, 1993).

Prenatal care provides numerous opportunities for increasing reproductive awareness from a woman's health perspective. Aside from providing valuable information regarding the current pregnancy, laboratory evaluation also provides indicators of general health status and opportunities for health promotion. Screening tests that allow for health promotion are also offered during pregnancy. For example, the woman with a negative HBsAg result may be offered the hepatitis B immunization series during her pregnancy, and the woman with a negative rubella titer result may plan to receive rubella vaccine after birth at discharge from the postpartum unit (ACOG, 1992b). HIV testing and counseling is available and should be offered to all women (AAP & ACOG, 1997; CDC, 1995b). HIV pretest counseling should include assessment of individual risk, benefits of testing, test procedure and meaning of results, and confidentiality of procedure. Posttest counseling should include discussion of results, limitations of results, review of potential modes of transmission, and discussion regarding risk-reduction behaviors and safe-sex practice.

SUMMARY

Nursing care during the prenatal period is multifaceted, requiring knowledge of the psychosocial tasks and issues surrounding the childbearing continuum, as well as knowledge of normal physiologic processes and potential risks. Anticipatory guidance during the prenatal period can have a significant impact on perinatal outcome. Education based on individual assessment empowers women and underscores their partnership in healthcare decision-making. The goal of prenatal care must go a step farther than targeting a positive physical outcome. Rather, we must work toward providing care and education that facilitates holistic family wellness.

REFERENCES

Abrams, B., & Selvin, S. (1995). Maternal weight gain pattern and birth weight. *Obstetrics and Gynecology, 86*(2), 163–169.

Allen, K., & Mitchell, J. (1997) *Women's health across the lifespan: A comprehensive perspective.* Philadelphia: Lippincott-Raven.

Alexander, G., & Kotelchuck, M. (1996). Quantifying the adequacy of prenatal care: A comparison of indices. *Public Health Reports, 111*(5), 408–418.

American Academy of Pediatrics & American College of Obstetricians and Gynecologists. (1997). *Guidelines for perinatal care* (4th ed.). Elk Grove Village, IL: Author.

American College of Obstetricians and Gynecologists. (1992b). *Guidelines for hepatitis B virus screening and vaccination during pregnancy* (committee opinion no. 1110). Washington, DC: Author.

American College of Obstetricians and Gynecologists. (1993a). *Nutrition during pregnancy* (technical bulletin no. 179). Washington, DC: Author.

American College of Obstetricians and Gynecologists. (1993b). *Ultrasonography in pregnancy* (technical bulletin no. 200). Washington, DC: Author.

American College of Obstetricians and Gynecologists. (1994a). *Diabetes and pregnancy* (technical bulletin no. 200). Washington, DC: Author .

American College of Obstetricians and Gynecologists. (1994b). *Exercise during pregnancy and the postpartum period* (technical bulletin no. 189). Washington, DC: Author.

American College of Obstetricians and Gynecologists. (1994c). *Substance abuse in pregnancy* (technical bulletin no. 195). Washington, DC: Author.

American College of Obstetricians and Gynecologists (1995a). *Preconceptional care* (technical bulletin no. 205). Washington, DC: Author .

American College of Obstetricians and Gynecologists. (1995b). *Preterm labor* (technical bulletin no. 206). Washington, DC: Author.

American College of Obstetricians and Gynecologists (1996a). *Hypertension in pregnancy* (technical bulletin no. 219). Washington, DC: Author.

American College of Obstetricians and Gynecologists. (1996b). *Maternal serum screening* (technical bulletin no. 228). Washington, DC: Author.

American College of Obstetricians and Gynecologists. (1996c). *Nutrition and women* (educational bulletin no. 229). Washington, DC: Author.

American College of Obstetricians and Gynecologists. (1997). *Teratology* (educational bulletin no. 236). Washington, DC: Author.

American College of Obstetricians and Gynecologists. (1998). *Cultural competency in health care* (committee opinion no. 201). Washington, DC: Author.

American College of Obstetricians and Gynecologists. (1999a). *Antepartum fetal surveillance* (ACOG practice bulletin no. 9). Washington, DC: Author.

American College of Obstetricians and Gynecologists. (1999b). *Psychosocial risk factors: Perinatal screening and intervention* (ACOG educational bulletin no. 255). Washington, DC: Author.

Andrews, M. (1996). Transcultural nursing: Theoretical perspectives. In M. Andrews & J. Boyle (Eds.), *Transcultural concepts in nursing care* (pp. 54–59). Philadelphia: J.B. Lippincott.

Atrash, H. K., Rowley, D., & Hogue, C. J. (1992). Maternal and perinatal mortality. *Current Opinion in Obstetrics and Gynecology, 4*(1), 61–71.

Auman, G. E., & Baird, M. M. (1993). Risk assessment for pregnant women. In R. A. Knuppel & J. E. Drukker (Eds.), *High-risk pregnancy: A team approach* (pp. 8–35). Philadelphia: W.B. Saunders.

Association of Women's Health, Obstetric and Neonatal Nurses. (1998). *Standards and guidelines for professional nursing practice in the care of women and newborns* (5th ed.). Washington, DC: AWHONN.

Baldwin, L. M., Raine, T., Jenkins, L. D., Hart, G., & Rosenblatt, R. (1994). Do providers adhere to ACOG standards? The case of prenatal care. *Obstetrics and Gynecology, 84*(4, Pt. 1), 549–556.

Barron, M. L. (1998). *Nursing assessment of the pregnant woman: Antepartal screening and laboratory evaluation.* (Nursing Module). White Plains, NY: March of Dimes Birth Defects Foundation.

Baumann, P., & McFarlin, B. (1994). Prenatal diagnosis. *Journal of Nurse-Midwifery, 39*(Suppl. 2), 35–51.

Beckman, D. A., & Brent, R. L. (1986). Mechanisms of known environmental teratogens: Drugs and chemicals. *Clinics in Perinatology, 13*(3), 649–687.

Brown, E. R., & Zuckerman, B. (1991). The infant of the drug abusing mother. *Pediatric Annals, 20*(10), 555–563.

Carpenter, C., Fischl, M., Hammer, S., Hirsch, M., Jacobsen, D., Katzenstein, D., Montaner, J., Richman, D., Saag, M., Schooley, R., Thompson, M., Vella, S., Yeni, P., & Volberding, P. (1996). Antiretroviral therapy for HIV infection. *Journal of the American Medical Association, 276*(2), 146.

Carpenter, M. B. (1995). The impact of legislation designed to reduce infant mortality. *Journal of Perinatal and Neonatal Nursing, 9*(1), 19–30.

Centers for Disease Control and Prevention. (1995a). Differences in maternal mortality among black and white women—United States, 1990. *Morbidity and Mortality Weekly Report, 44*(1), 6–7, 13–14.

Centers for Disease Control and Prevention. (1995b). USPHS recommendations for HIV counseling and voluntary testing for pregnant women. *Morbidity and Mortality Weekly Report, 44*(RR-7) 1–15.

Chasnoff, I. (1998). Silent violence: Is prevention a moral obligation? *Pediatrics, 102*(1), 145–148.

Chasnoff, I. J. (1989). Drug use and women: Establishing a standard of care. *Annals of the New York Academy of Sciences, 562*, 208–210.

Cnattinghaus, S., Bergstrom, R., Lipworth, L., & Kramer, M. (1998). Prepregnancy weight and the risk of adverse pregnancy outcomes. *New England Journal of Medicine, 338*(3), 147–152.

Cooksey, N. (1995). Pica and olfactory cravings of pregnancy: How deep are the secrets? *Birth: Issues in Perinatal Care, 22*(3), 129–137.

Creasy, R., & Resnick, R. (1999). *Maternal-fetal medicine: Principles and practice.* Philadelphia: W.B. Saunders.

Cunningham, F. G., MacDonald, P. C., Gant, N. F., Leveno, K. J., & Gilstrap, L. C. (1997). *Williams obstetrics* (20th ed.). Norwalk, CT: Appleton & Lange.

Dietz, P. M., Gazmararian, J. A., Goodwin, M. M., Bruce, F. C., Johnson, C. H., Rochat, R. W. (1997). Delayed entry into prenatal care: Effect of physical violence. *Obstetrics and Gynecology, 90*(2), 221–224.

Edenfield, S. M., Thomas, S. D., Thompson, W. O., & Marcotte, J. J. (1995). Validity of the Creasy risk appraisal instrument for prediction of preterm labor. *Nursing Research, 44*(2), 76–81.

Ellerbrock, T., Atrash, H. K., Hogue, C. J., & Smith, J. (1988). Pregnancy mortality surveillance: A new initiative. *Contemporary Obstetrics and Gynecology, 31*(6), 23–34.

Enkins, M. W. (1994). Risk in pregnancy: The reality, the perception, and the concept. *Birth, 21*(3), 131–134.

Expert Panel on the Content of Prenatal Care. (1989). *Caring for our future: The content of prenatal care.* Washington, DC: Public Health Service.

Fenton, M. (1998). In C. Sheehy & M. McCarthy (Eds.), *Advanced practice nursing: Emphasizing common roles* (foreword). Philadelphia: F.A. Davis.

Fogel, C. I., & Lewallen, L. P. (1995). High-risk childbearing. In C. I. Fogel & N. F. Woods (Eds.), *Women's health care: A comprehensive handbook* (pp. 427–453). Thousand Oaks, CA: Sage.

Freda, M. C., Mikhail, M., Mazloom, E., Polizzotto, R., Damus, K., & Merkatz, I. (1993). Fetal movement counting: Which method? *MCN, The American Journal of Maternal Child Nursing, 18*(6), 314–321.

Gazmararian, J. A., Arrington, T. L., Bailey, C. M., Schwarz, K. S., Koplan, J. P. (1999). Prenatal care for low-income women enrolled in a managed-care organization. *Obstetrics and Gynecology, 94*(2), 177–185.

Gegor, C. L., & Paine, L. L. (1992). Antepartal fetal assessment techniques: An update for today's perinatal nurse. *Journal of Perinatal & Neonatal Nursing, 5*(4), 1–15.

Goldenberg, R. L., Patterson, E. T., & Freese, M. P. (1992). Maternal demographics, situational, and psychosocial factors and their relationship to enrollment in prenatal care: A review of the literature. *Women & Health, 19*(2–3), 133–151.

Gribble, R. K., Fee, S. C., & Berg, R. L. (1995). The value of routine urine dipstick screening for protein at each prenatal visit. *American Journal of Obstetrics and Gynecology, 173*(1), 214–217.

Gutierrez, Y. (1994). Nutrition in health maintenance and health promotion for primary care providers. San Francisco, CA: University of California, San Francisco School of Nursing.

Guyer, B., Strobino, D., Ventina, S., MacDorman, M., & Martin, J. (1996). Annual summary of statistics. *Pediatrics, 98*(6, Pt. 1), 1007–1019.

Handler, A., & Rosenberg, D. (1992). Improving pregnancy outcomes: Public versus private care for urban, low-income women. *Birth*, 123–130.

Harvey, M. & Moretti, M. L. (1993). Maternal adaptatins to pregnancy, in R. Knuppel & J. Drukker (Eds.). *High-risk pregnancy: A team approach* (pp. 224–243). Philadelphia, PA: W. B. Saunders.

Harvey, S. M., & Faber, K. S. (1992). Obstacles to prenatal care following implementation of a community-based program to reduce financial barriers. *Family Planning Perspectives, 25*(1), 32–36.

Hebel, J. R., Fox, N. L., & Sexton, M. (1988). Dose response of birth weight to various measures of maternal smoking during pregnancy. *Journal of Clinical Epidemiology, 41*(5), 483–489.

Hendricks, S. K., Von Eschen, M., & Grady, M. C. (1995). Preconception counseling and care of common medical disorders. In D. P. Lemcke, J. Pattison, L. A. Marshall, & D. S. Crowley (Eds.), *Primary care of women* (pp. 518–530). Norwalk, CT: Appleton & Lange.

Herbert, W., Dodds, J., & Cefalo, R. (1993). Nutrition in pregnancy. In R. A. Knuppel & J. E. Drukker (Eds.), *High risk pregnancy: A team approach* (pp. 8–35). Philadelphia: W.B. Saunders.

Hook, E. B. (1981). Rates of chromosome abnormalities at different maternal ages. *Obstetrics and Gynecology, 58*(3), 282–285.

Hooper, D. (1996). Detecting GDM and pre-eclampsia: Effectiveness of routine urine screening for glucose and protein. *Journal of Reproductive Medicine, 41*(12), 885–888.

Horton, J. (Ed.). (1995). *The women's health data book: A profile of women's health in the United States* (2nd ed.). Washington, DC: Elsevier.

Iams, J. D., Paraskos, J., Landon, M. B., Teteris, J. M., & Johnson, F. F. (1994). Cervical sonography in preterm labor. *Obstetrics and Gynecology, 84*(1), 40–45.

Institute of Medicine. (1990). *Nutrition during pregnancy.* Washington, DC: National Academy Press.

Institute of Medicine. (1995). *The best intention: Unintended pregnancy and the well-being of children and families.* Washington, DC: National Academy Press.

Jamieson, D. J., & Buescher, P. A. (1992). The effect of family planning participation on prenatal care use and low birth weight. *Family Planning Perspectives, 24*(5), 214–218.

Kiely, M. (Ed.). (1991). *Reproductive and perinatal epidemiology.* Boca Raton, FL: CRC Press.

Kogan, M., Martin, J., Alexander, G., Kotelchuck, M., Ventura, S., Frigoletto, F. (1998). The changing pattern of prenatal care utilization in the United States, 1981–1995, using different prenatal care indices. *Journal of the American Medical Association, 279*(20), 1623–1628.

Kotelchuck, M. (1994). An evaluation of the Kessner adequacy of prenatal care index and a proposed adequacy of prenatal care utilization index. *American Journal of Public Health, 84*(9), 1314–1320.

Lamar, M., Kuehl, T., Cooney, A., Justin, G., Hollerman, S., & Allen, S. (1999). Jelly beans as an alternative to a fifty-gram glucose beverage for gestational diabetes screening. *American Journal of Obstetrics and Gynecology, 181*(5, Part 1), 1154–1157.

Larrabee, K., & Cowan, M. (1995). Clinical nursing management of sickle cell disease and trait during pregnancy. *Journal of Perinatal and Neonatal Nursing, 9*(2), 29–41.

Lederman, R. P. (1990). Anxiety and stress in pregnancy: Significance and nursing assessment. *NAACOG's Clinical Issues in Perinatal and Women's Health Nursing, 1*(3), 279–288.

Libbus, M. K., & Sable, M. R. (1991). Prenatal education in a high-risk population: The effect on birth outcomes. *Birth, 18*(2), 78–82.

Lommel, L. (1990). Antepartal fetal surveillance. In W. L. Star, M. T. Shannon, L. N. Sammons, L. Lommel, & Y. Gutierrez (Eds.), *Ambulatory obstetrics: Protocols for nurse practitioners/nurse midwives* (2nd ed.). San Francisco: School of Nursing, University of California.

Lothian, J. A. (1994). Is childbirth education obsolete? *The Journal of Perinatal Education, 3*(2), 5–6.

MacDorman, M. F., & Atkinson, J. O. (1999). Deaths: Final data for 1997. *National Vital Statistics Reports, 47*(19), 1–105.

Maloni, J. A., Cheng, C. Y., Liebl, C. P., & Maier, J. S. (1996). Transforming prenatal care: Reflections on the past and present with implications for the future. *Journal of Obstetric, Gynecologic, and Neonatal Nursing, 25*(1), 17–23.

Mamelle, N., Laumon, B., Munoz, F., & Collin, D. (1989). Life style. In E. Papiernik, L. G. Keith, J. Bouyer, J. Dreyfus, & P. Lazar (Eds.), *Effective prevention of preterm birth: The French experience at Hagenau* (pp. 73–86). White Plains, NY: March of Dimes Birth Defects Foundation.

March of Dimes Birth Defects Foundation. (1993). *Toward improving the outcome of pregnancy: The 90's and beyond.* White Plains, NY: March of Dimes Birth Defects Foundation.

March of Dimes. (1999). *Folic acid fact sheet.* White Plains, NY: March of Dimes Birth Defects Foundation.

Matthews, A. L., & Smith, A. C. M. (1993). Genetic counseling. In R. A. Knuppel & J. E. Drukker (Eds.), *High-risk pregnancy: A team approach* (pp. 664–703). Philadelphia: W.B. Saunders.

McClanahan, P. (1992). Improving access to and use of prenatal care. *Journal of Obstetric, Gynecologic, and Neonatal Nursing, 21*(4), 280–284.

McIntosh, L. J., Roumayah, N. E., & Bottoms, S. F. (1995). Perinatal outcome of broken marriages in the inner city. *Obstetrics and Gynecology, 85*(2), 233–236.

Meuerer, J., & Taren, D. L. (1993). Prevention and public health in obstetrics. In R. A. Knuppel & J. E. Drukker (Eds.), *High-risk pregnancy: A team approach.* Philadelphia: W.B. Saunders.

Misra, D., & Guyer, B. (1998). Benefits and limitations of prenatal care: From counting visits to measuring content. *Journal of the American Medical Association, 279*(20), 1623–1628.

Moore, M. L., Elmore, T., Ketener, M., Wagoner, S., & Walsh, K. (1995). Reduction and cessation of smoking in pregnant women. The effect of a telephone intervention. *Journal of Perinatal Education* 4(1), 35–39.

Moore, M., & Freda, M. (1998). Reducing preterm and low birth weight birth: Still a nursing challenge. *MCN, The American Journal of Maternal-Child Nursing, 23*(4), 200–208.

Moore, T. R., & Piacquadio, K. (1989). A prospective evaluation of fetal movement screening to reduce the incidence of antepartum fetal death. *American Journal of Obstetrics and Gynecology, 160*(5, Pt. 1), 1075–1080.

Murphy, P. (1994). Risk, risk assessment and risk labels. *Journal of Nurse-Midwifery, 39*(2), 67–69.

Murphy, S. (1999). Deaths: Final data for 1998. *National Vital Statistics Reports 48*(11), 1–95.

O'Campo, P., Faden, R. R., Geilen, A. C., & Wang, M. C. (1992). Prenatal factors associated with breastfeeding duration: Recommendations for prenatal interventions. *Birth, 19*(4), 195–201.

Papiernik, E. (1993). Prevention of preterm labor and delivery. *Balliere's Clinical Obstetrics and Gynecology, 7*(3), 499–521.

Paritsky, J. F. (1985). Tay-Sachs: The dreaded inheritance. *American Journal of Nursing, 8*(3), 260–264.

Pearson, L. (2000). Annual update of how each state stands on legislative issues affecting advanced nursing practice. *Nurse Practitioner, 25*(1), 16–28.

Pletsch, P. (1990). Birth defect prevention: Nursing interventions. *Journal of Obstetric, Gynecologic, and Neonatal Nursing, 19*(6), 482–488.

Pletsch, P. (1994). The genetic code and fetal development. In K. A. May & L. R. Mahlmeister (Eds.), *Maternal and neonatal nursing: Family centered care* (pp. 251–274). Philadelphia: J.B. Lippincott.

Raine, T., Powell, S., & Krohn, M. A. (1994). The risk of repeating low birth weight and the role of prenatal care. *Obstetrics and Gynecology, 84*(4, Pt. 1), 485–489.

Raines, D. (1996). Fetal surveillance: Issues and implications. *Journal of Obstetric, Gynecologic, and Neonatal Nursing, 25*(7), 559–563.

Ramer, L. (1992). *Culturally sensitive caregiving and childbearing families.* White Plains, NY: March of Dimes Birth Defects Foundation.

Reece, E., & Coustan, D. (1995). *Diabetes in pregnancy* (2nd ed.). New York: Churchill Livingstone.

Renker, P. R. (1999). Physical abuse, social support, self-care, and pregnancy outcomes of older adolescents. *Journal of Obstetric, Gynecologic, and Neonatal Nursing, 28*(4), 377–387.

Revah, A., Hannah, M., & Sue-A-Quan, A. (1998). Fetal fibronectin as a predictor of preterm birth: An overview. *American Journal of Perinatology, 15*(11), 613–621.

Roberts, J. (1994). Current perspectives on preeclampsia. *Journal of Nurse-Midwifery, 39*(2), 70–90.

Robins, L. N., & Mills, J. L. (Eds.). (1993). Effects of in utero exposure to street drugs. *American Journal of Public Health, 83*(Suppl.), 9–32.

Sadler, T. W. (1995). *Medical embryology.* Baltimore: Williams & Wilkins.

Scarr, E., & Sammons, L. (1999). Post-partum depression. In W. L. Star, M. T. Shannon, L. N. Sammons, L. Lommel, & Y. Gutierrez (Eds.), *Ambulatory obstetrics: Protocols for nurse practitioners/nurse midwives* (3rd ed.). San Francisco: School of Nursing, University of California.

Seidel, Ball, Dains, & Benedict (1998) *Mosby's Guide to Physical Examination* (4th ed.). CV Mosby: Philadelphia

Tyson, J., Guzick, D., & Rosenfeld, C. R. (1990). Prenatal care evaluation and cohort analyses. *Pediatrics, 85*(2), 195–204.

United States Department of Health and Human Services (USDHHS). (1998). *Health, United States, 1998 with socioeconomic status and health chartbook* (Department of Health and Human Services publication no. [PHS] 98–1232). Hyattsville, MD: National Center for Health Statistics.

United States Department of Health and Human Services (USDHHS). (1999). Annual National Drug Survey Press release. *HHS News* Aug. 18.

Villar, M. A., & Sibai, B. M. (1989). Clinical significance of elevated mean arterial blood pressure in second trimester and threshold increase in systolic or diastolic blood pressure during third trimester. *American Journal of Obstetrics and Gynecology, 160*(2), 419–423.

Ventura, S., Martin, J., Curtain, S., Matthews, M., & Park, M. (2000). Births: Final data for 1998. National Vital Statistics Reports. *National Center for Health Care Statistics, 48*(3), 1–19.

Ventura, S., Martin, J., Taffel, S., Matthews, M., & Clarke, S., (1995). Advance report of final natality statistics, 1993. *Monthly Vital Statistics Report, 44*(Suppl. 3), 1–2.

Walker, L., & Tinkle, M. (1996). Toward an integrative science of women's health. *Journal of Obstetric, Gynecologic, and Neonatal Nursing, 25*(5), 379–382.

Wheeler, L. (1997). *A practical guide to prenatal and postpartum care.* Philadelphia: J.B. Lippincott.

Witter, F. R., Caulfield, L. E., & Stoltzfus, R. J. (1995). Influence of maternal anthropometric status and birth weight on the risk of cesarean delivery. *Obstetrics and Gynecology, 86*(6), 947–951.

Wolfe, H. (1998). High prepregnancy body mass index—A maternal-fetal risk factor. *New England Journal of Medicine, 338*(3), 191–192.

York, R. & Brooten, D. (1992). Prevention of low birthweight. *NAACOG's Clinical Issues in Perinatal and Woman's Health, 3*(1), 13–24.

APPENDIX 7A

Perinatal Substance Abuse Assessment Guide

Drug and alcohol use among women of childbearing age presents many challenges to healthcare professionals. Maternal chemical dependence has been associated with numerous medical, obstetric, and neonatal complications. Comprehensive assessment strategies are necessary to identify women at risk for or currently using drugs and alcohol in pregnancy. Thorough assessment includes observation of the woman's physical appearance and behavioral characteristics, as well as a complete medical, obstetric, psychosocial, and substance abuse history. The following information provides recommendations and suggested approaches to assessment that may lead to early identification of substance abuse.

MEDICAL HISTORY

Factors associated with chemical dependence may include a history of

Cellulitis	Septicemia	Undocumented seizure disorder or blackouts
Cirrhosis	Pneumonia	Victim of physical or sexual abuse
Depression	Acute hypertension	Recent sexually transmitted disease
Endocarditis	Suicide attempt	Multiple drug allergies
Hepatitis	HIV infection	Use of mood-altering prescription drugs
Pancreatitis	AIDS	

OBSTETRIC HISTORY

Factors associated with chemical dependence may include a history of

Abruptio placentae	Low birth weight	Meconium staining
Unexplained fetal death	Spontaneous abortion	Premature rupture of membranes
Preeclampsia or eclampsia	Placental insufficiency	Unexplained preterm labor or preterm delivery
Gestational diabetes	Amnionitis	Sudden infant death syndrome

PRESENT PREGNANCY

Factors associated with chemical dependence may include

Preterm labor	Inactive or hyperactive fetus	Late, no, or sporadic prenatal care
Poor weight gain	Spotting or bleeding	Sexually transmitted diseases

PSYCHOSOCIAL HISTORY

Family personal factors associated with chemical dependence may include

Dysfunctional family	Psychiatric history	History of marked emotional deprivation
Drunk driving record	Lack of religiosity	Minimal coping and communication skills
Arrest record	Self-destructive behaviors	Self-induced social isolation
Low self-esteem	Previous child in foster care	Family history of substance abuse

Unstable lifestyle	Major depressive episodes	Poor relationship with family members

Partner has history of or current substance abuse problem

PHYSICAL APPEARANCE AND DEMEANOR

Aspects of the physical appearance associated with chemical dependency include

Untidy appearance	Pupil changes	Looks physically exhausted
Track marks	Abscesses	Inflamed or indurated nasal mucosa
Rhinitis	Cardiac arrhythmias	Thrombophlebitis or sclerosed veins
Alcohol on breath	Weight loss	Liver or abdominal tenderness
Edema of extremities	Fundal size less than dates	Lung congestion or diminished breath sounds

BEHAVIORAL CHARACTERISTICS

Behavioral characteristics associated with chemical dependency include

Behavioral Cues

Slurred speech	Inappropriate behavior	Agitation or restlessness
Emotional lability	Ataxia	Nystagmus
Mistrust of authority figures or other professionals		

Coping Mechanisms

Denial	Rationalization	Minimizing
Blaming		

Withdrawal or Crash Symptoms

Increased respiratory rate	Lacrimation	Diaphoresis
Yawning	Diarrhea	Rhinorrhea
Tremors/muscle spasms	Piloerection	Irritability
Anxiety	Dilated pupils	Insomnia
Nausea or vomiting	Tachycardia	Abdominal cramps
Anorexia	Chills or flushing	Hypertension
Weakness		

SUBSTANCE ABUSE HISTORY

The substance abuse history is an effective means for assessment of risk status of all pregnant women. It is important that the substance abuse history is conducted in a nonthreatening, nonjudgmental manner. The following questions provide an outline for substance abuse assessment, which may be helpful in guiding the assessment process.

Tobacco

- Have you ever smoked cigarettes?
- Before you found out you were pregnant, how many cigarettes did you smoke per day?
- How many cigarettes do you smoke in one day?
- Are there times when you seem to smoke more?

Alcohol

- Have you ever drunk alcohol (ie, beer, wine, wine coolers, mixed drinks, or hard liquor)?
- Before you found out you were pregnant, how many drinks did you have per day? Per week?
- How many beers, glasses of wine, or glasses of hard liquor do you drink per week now?
- How many beers, glasses of wine, or glasses of hard liquor do you drink per day?
- What other types of beverages containing alcohol, such as wine coolers, champagne, champalle, mixed drinks (eg, margaritas, wine spritzers) do you like to drink?
- Are there times when you seem to drink more often?

Over-the-Counter Medications

- How often do you use over-the-counter medications (eg, aspirin, Tylenol)?
- How often have you taken over-the-counter medications during this pregnancy?
- What have you taken these medications for?
- How often do you take sleeping pills, diet pills, laxatives, water pills, cough medicine, antihistamines, or other medications?
- When was the last time you used any of these medications? Reason?

Prescription Medications

- How often have you taken prescription medications during this pregnancy?
- Are you currently taking medications requiring a prescription? What are they?
- Why are you taking them? How often?
- Were the medications prescribed for you?
- Who prescribed them?
- Does your obstetrician know that you are taking them?
- Does the prescribing physician know that you are pregnant?
- Are there times when you tend to use more of this medication?

Illicit Drugs

It is important to be familiar with drugs available in your area and interview regarding list of specific drugs (eg, crack, cocaine, marijuana, speed, primos).

- Have you ever used marijuana, cocaine, or other illegal drugs?
- How often did you use the drug (name specifics) before you found out you were pregnant?
- How often have you used this drug during this pregnancy?
- Are there times when you use more?
- How do you take the drug (eg, intravenously, smoke, snort)?
- When was the last time you used this drug?

Other Helpful Questions

Significant other or family members' past or current substance abuse history is also a recognition cue. The following questions may be helpful:

- Does your significant other or family member use drugs or alcohol?
- What are you doing while they are using or partying?
- Where are you when they are using?

If answers to the previous questions indicate the need for further exploration of drinking and drugging patterns, asking the following questions may be helpful.

- Have you ever tried to cut down your use of ___________? What was that like for you?
- Do you feel annoyed by criticism of your drinking or drug use?
- Do you feel guilty about your drinking or drug use?
- Do you ever experience memory lapses (blackouts)?
- Do you get sick from drinking or drug use afterward?
- Do you ever regret what you have done while drinking or using drugs?
- Do you ever use ___________ first thing in the morning to steady your nerves or get rid of a hangover?
- Do you ever get shaky or edgy if you don't use ___________?

REFERENCES

Chappel, J.N. (1987). Alcohol and drug dependencies: How to spot; what steps to take. *Consultant,* 27 (4), 60–75.

Chasnoff, I.J. (1987). Perinatal effects of cocaine. *Contemporary OB/GYN, 26*(5), 163–179.

Chisum, G.M. (1990). Nursing interventions with the antepartum substance abuser. *Journal of Perinatal and Neonatal Nursing, 3* (4), 26–33.

Finkellstein, N., Duncan, S.A., Derman, L., & Smeltze, J. (1990). *Getting sober, getting well.* Cambridge, MA: The Women's Alcoholism Program of C.A.S.P.A.R.

Glans, J.C., & Woods, J.R. (1991). Obstetrical issues in substance abuse. *Pediatric Annals, 20*(10), 531–539.

Hoegerman, G., & Schnoll, S. (1991). Narcotic use in pregnancy. *Clinics in Perinatology, 18*(1), 51–73.

Ryall, J. (1989). Eliciting a history of pathological drinking from women. *A&D News,* 1–4.

Starr, K.L., & Chisum, G.M. (1992). The chemically dependent pregnant woman. In L.K. Mandeville, & N.H. Troiano (Eds.), *High risk intrapartum nursing* (pp. 115–145). New York: J.B. Lippincott.

APPENDIX **7 B**

Abuse Assessment

These questions may help you when assessing female clients for abuse. For some women, answering "sometimes" to abuse questions is easier than yes or no.

1.	Do you know where you could go or who could help you if you were abused or worried about abuse	Yes	No	
2.	Are you in a relationship with a man who physically hurts you?	Yes	No	
3.	Does he threaten you with abuse?	Yes	No	Sometimes
4.	Has the man you are with hit, slapped, kicked or otherwise physically hurt you?	Yes	No	Sometimes
5.	If yes, has he hit you since you've been pregnant?	Yes	No	Not applicable
6.	If yes, did the abuse increase since you've been pregnant?	Yes	No	Not applicable
7.	Have you ever received medical treatment for abuse injuries?	Yes	No	Not applicable
8.	Were you pregnant at the time?	Yes	No	Not applicable

Actions Suggestive of Abuse

When assessing for abuse, some women may be uncomfortable with the topic and may exhibit some of the behaviors below. For some women these behaviors may be suggestive of abuse and disclosure of battering may follow at a later date.

1.	Laughing/"tittering"	Yes	No
2.	No eye contact *(not applicable in some cultures)*	Yes	No
3.	Crying	Yes	No
4.	Sighing	Yes	No
5.	Minimizing statements	Yes	No
6.	Searching/engaging eye contact *(fear)*	Yes	No
7.	Anxious body language *(standing to leave, dropped shoulders, depressed)*	Yes	No
8.	Anger, defensiveness	Yes	No
9.	Comments about emotional abuse	Yes	No
10.	Comments about "friend" who is abused	Yes	No

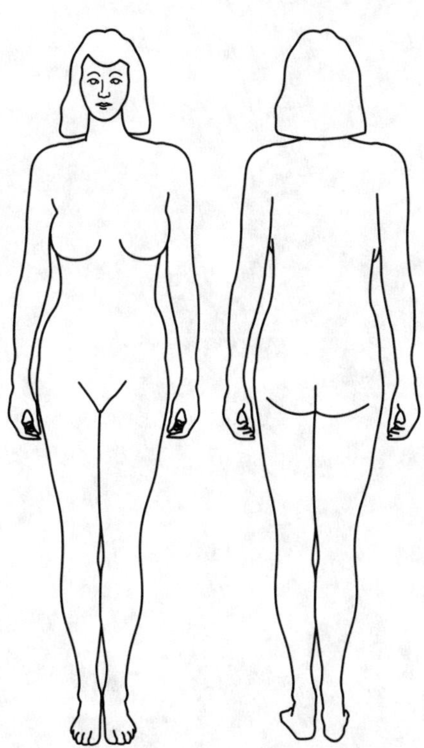

If you've been abused, remembering the last time he hurt you, mark the place where he hit you on the body map above.

From A. S. Helton. (1987). *Protocol of Care for the Battered Woman*, (pp. 8–9). White Plains, N.Y.: March of Dimes Birth Defects Foundation.

APPENDIX **7 C**

Immunization During Pregnancy

Immunobiologic Agent	Risk from Disease to Pregnant Woman	Risk from Disease to Fetus or Neonate	Type of Immunizing Agent	Risk from Immunizing Agent to Fetus	Indications for Immunization During Pregnancy	Dose Schedule	Comments
Measles	Significant morbidity; low mortality; not altered by pregnancy	Significant increase in abortion rate; may cause malformations	Live attenuated virus vaccine	None confirmed	Contraindicated (see immune globulins)	Single dose SC, preferably as measles-mumps-rubella*	Vaccination of susceptible women should be part of postpartum care
Mumps	Low morbidity and mortality; not altered by pregnancy	Probable increased rate of abortion in first trimester	Live attenuated virus vaccine	None confirmed	Contraindicated	Single does SC, preferably as measles-mumps-rubella	Vaccination of susceptible women should be part of post-partum care
Poliomyelitis	No increased incidence in pregnancy, but it may be more severe if it does occur.	Anoxic fetal damage reported; 50% mortality in neonatal disease	Live attenuated virus (oral polio vaccine [OPV] and enhanced-potency inactivated virus [e-IPV] vaccine)†	None confirmed	Not routinely recommended for women in United States except persons at increased risk for exposure	*Primary:* Two doses of e-IPV SC at 4–8 week intervals and a third dose 6–12 months after the second dose. *Immediate protection:* One dose OPV orally (in outbreak setting)	Vaccine indicated for susceptible pregnant women traveling in endemic areas or in other high-risk situations
Rubella	Low morbidity and mortality; not altered by pregnancy	High rate of abortion and congenital rubella syndrome	Live attenuated virus vaccine	None confirmed	Contraindicated	Single dose SC, preferably as measles-mumps-rubella	Teratogenicity of vaccine is theoretic, not confirmed; vaccination of susceptible women should be part of post-partum care.

Immunobiologic Agent	Risk from Disease to Pregnant Woman	Risk from Disease to Fetus or Neonate	Type of Immunizing Agent	Risk from Immunizing Agent to Fetus	Indications for Immunization During Pregnancy	Dose Schedule	Comments
Yellow fever	Significant morbidity and mortality; not altered by pregnancy	Unknown	Live attenuated virus vaccine	Unknown	Contraindicated	Single dose SC	Postponement of travel preferable to vaccination, if possible
Influenza	Possible increase in morbidity and mortality during epidemic of new antigenic strain	Possible increased abortion rate; no malformations confirmed	Inactivated virus vaccine	None confirmed	Women with serious underlying diseases; public health authorities to be consulted for current recommendation	One dose IM every year	
Rabies	Near 100% fatality; not altered by pregnancy	Determined by maternal disease.	Killed virus vaccine	Unknown	Indications for prophylaxis not altered bypregnancy; each case considered individually	Public health authorities to be consulted for indications, dosage, and routeof administration	
Hepatitis B	Possible increased severity during third trimester	Possible increase in abortion rate and prematurity; neonatal hepatitis can occur; high risk of newborn carrier state	Recombinant vaccine	None reported	Before and after exposure for women at risk for infection	Three- or four-dose series IM	Used with hepatitis B immune globulin for some exposures; exposed newborn needs vaccination as soon as possible

Cholera	Significant morbidity and mortality; more severe during third trimester	Increased risk of fetal death during third-trimester maternal illness	Killed bacterial vaccine	None confirmed	Indications not altered by pregnancy; vaccination recommended only in unusual outbreak situations	Single dose SC or IM, depending on manufacturer's recommendations, when indicated	
Plague	Significant morbidity and mortality; not altered by pregnancy	Determined by maternal disease	Killed bacterial vaccine	None reported	Selective vaccination of exposed persons	Public health authorities to be consulted for indications, dosage, and route of administration	
Pneumococcus	No increased risk; during pregnancy, no increase in severity of disease	Unknown	Polyvalent polysaccharide vaccine	No data available on use during pregnancy	Indications not altered by pregnancy; vaccine used only for high-risk individuals	In adults one SC or IM dose only; consider repeat dose in 6 years for high-risk individuals	
Typhoid	Significant morbidity and mortality; not altered by pregnancy	Unknown	Killed or live attenuated oral bacterial	None confirmed	Not recommended routinely except for close, continued exposure or travel to endemic areas	Killed: *Primary:* Two injections SC at least 4 weeks apart. *Booster:* Single dose SC or ID (depending on type of product used) every 3 years Oral: *Primary:* Four doses on alternate days *Booster:* Schedule not yet determined	

(continued)

Immunobiologic Agent	Risk from Disease to Pregnant Woman	Risk from Disease to Fetus or Neonate	Type of Immunizing Agent	Risk from Immunizing Agent to Fetus	Indications for Immunization During Pregnancy	Dose Schedule	Comments
			Toxoids				
Tetanus-diphtheria	Severe morbidity; tetanus mortality 30%, diphtheria mortality 10%; unaltered by pregnancy	Neonatal tetanus mortality 60%	Combined tetanus-diphtheria toxoids pre ferred; adult tetanus-diphtheria formulation	None confirmed	Lack of primary series, or no booster within past 10 years	*Primary:* Two doses IM at 1–2 month interval with a third dose 6–12 months after the second *Booster:* Single dose IM every 10 years, after completion of primary series	Updating of immune status should be part of antepartum care.
			Specific Immune Globulins				
Hepatitis B	Possible increased severity during third trimester	Possible increase in abortion rate and prematurity; neonatal hepatitis can occur; high risk of carriage in newborn	Hepatitis B immune globulin	None reported	Postexposure prophylaxis	Depends on exposure; consult Immunization Practices Advisory Committee recommendations (IM)	Usually given with HBV vaccine; exposed newborn needs immediate postexposure prophylaxis.
Rabies	Near 100% fatality; not altered by pregnancy	Determined by maternal disease	Rabies immune globulin	None reported	Postexposure prophylaxis	Half dose at injury site, half dose in deltoid	Used in conjunction with rabies killed virus vaccine
Tetanus	Severe morbidity; mortality 21%	Neonatal tetanus mortality 60%	Tetanus immune globulin	None reported	Postexposure prophylaxis	One dose IM	Used in conjunction with tetanus toxoid

Varicella	Possible increase in severe varicella pneumonia	Can cause congenital varicella with increased mortality in neonatal period; rarely causes congenital defects	Varicella-zoster immune globulin (obtained from the American Red Cross)	None reported	Can be considered for healthy pregnant women exposed to varicella to protect against maternal, not congenital, infection	One dose IM within 96 hours of exposure	Indicated also for newborns of mothers who developed varicella within 4 days before delivery or 2 days after delivery; approx. 90–95% of adults are immune to varicella; not indicated for prevention of congenital varicella
			Specific Immune Globulins				
Hepatitis A	Possible increased severity during third trimester	Probable increase in abortion rate and prematurity; possible transmission to neonate at delivery if mother is incubating the virus or is acutely ill at that time	Standard immune globulin	None reported	Postexposure prophylaxis	0.02 mL/kg IM in one dose ofimmune globulin	Immune globulin should be given as soon as possible and within 2 weeks of exposure; infants born to mothers who are incubating the virus or are actually ill at delivery should receive one dose of 0.5 mL as soon as possible after birth.

(continued)

Immunobiologic Agent	Risk from Disease to Pregnant Woman	Risk from Disease to Fetus or Neonate	Type of Immunizing Agent	Risk from Immunizing Agent to Fetus	Indications for Immunization During Pregnancy	Dose Schedule	Comments
Measles	Significant morbidity, low mortality; not altered by pregnancy	Significant increase in abortion rate; may cause malformations	Standard immune globulin	None reported	Postexposure prophylaxis	0.02 mL/kg IM in one dose of immune globulin up to 15 mL	Unclear if it prevents abortion; must be given within 6 days of exposure

SC, subcutaneously; PO, orally; IM, intramuscularly; ID, intradermally.

*Two doses necessary for adequate vaccination of students entering institutions of high education, newly hired medical personnel, and international travelers.

†Inactivated polio vaccine recommended for nonimmunized adults at increased risk

From American College of Obstetricians and Gynecologists. (1991). *Immunization during pregnancy* (technical bulletin no. 160). Washington, DC: Author.

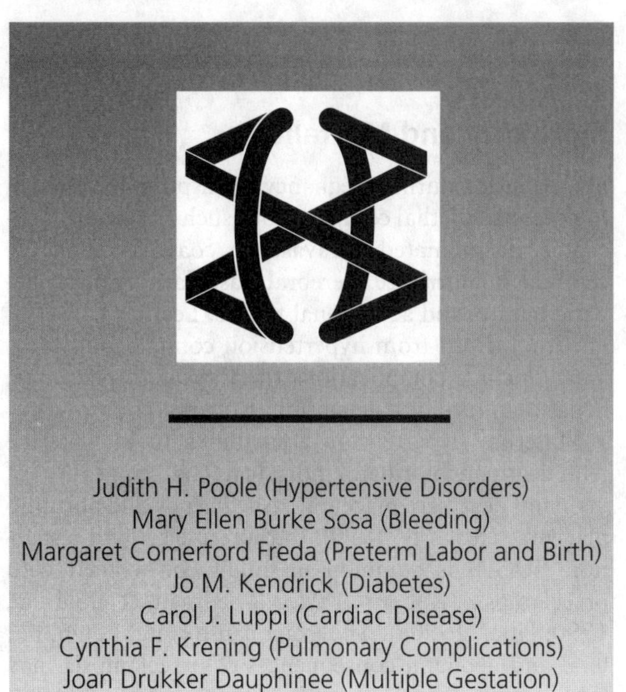

Judith H. Poole (Hypertensive Disorders)
Mary Ellen Burke Sosa (Bleeding)
Margaret Comerford Freda (Preterm Labor and Birth)
Jo M. Kendrick (Diabetes)
Carol J. Luppi (Cardiac Disease)
Cynthia F. Krening (Pulmonary Complications)
Joan Drukker Dauphinee (Multiple Gestation)
Mary Ellen Burke Sosa (Maternal Transfer)

CHAPTER 8

High-Risk Pregnancy

Pregnancy, labor, and birth are natural processes. Most women do well with periodic assessment, supportive measures, and encouragement. Healthy pregnant women require minimal intervention. However, complications during pregnancy do occur, frequently with little or no warning. Life-threatening events such as hemorrhage from a placenta previa or abruption, diabetic ketoacidosis, peripartum cardiomyopathy, preterm labor at 26 weeks' gestation, or an eclamptic seizure place the woman and fetus at risk for significant morbidity and mortality.

Providing safe and effective care for the woman during pregnancy requires a joint effort from all members of the healthcare team, with each member contributing unique skills and talents to promote optimal outcomes for mothers and babies. The nurse in the perinatal setting must quickly assess and identify changes in maternal–fetal condition and adjust care accordingly. Comprehensive nursing assessments and interventions are essential in recognizing alterations from the normal process during the antepartum, intrapartum, and postpartum periods. Anticipatory nursing care is invaluable in preventing a complication from becoming a crisis. Notifying the primary healthcare provider immediately of signs or symptoms of alterations from expected clinical progression during pregnancy can facilitate early intervention and determine the proper course and place of treatment.

This chapter covers the care of women with selected high-risk conditions during pregnancy: hypertension, bleeding, preterm labor and birth, diabetes, cardiovascular disease, pulmonary complications, and multiple gestation. Suggestions are made for home care management of women in stable condition and guidelines for maternal transfer to a tertiary center.

HYPERTENSIVE DISORDERS

Significance and Incidence

Hypertensive disorders of pregnancy are the most common medical complications during pregnancy, labor, birth, and the postpartum period. Preeclampsia is a significant contributor to maternal and perinatal morbidity and mortality, complicating approximately 5% to 8% of all pregnancies not terminating in first-trimester abortions (Egerman & Sibai, 1999; Myatt & Miodovnik, 1999). For women with a history of chronic hypertension or renal disease predating pregnancy, the occurrence of preeclampsia is 25% (Jones & Hayslett, 1996). The rate of pregnancy-related hypertension rose for the sixth consecutive year in the United States during 1997, from a rate of 35.9 per 1,000 births in 1996 to 36.8 in 1997 (Ventura, Martin, Curtin, Mathews, & Park 2000). The rate for pregnancy-related hypertension has increased for all ages, races, and ethnic groups during the 1990s; rates for chronic hypertension and eclampsia have remained unchanged (Ventura et al., 2000). Maternal race influences the rate of hypertension complicating pregnancy, with the highest rates seen for Native Americans (48.1/1,000) and African-American (39.7/1,000) women. Asian or Pacific Islander women have the lowest rate for hypertension complicating pregnancy (20.1/1,000) (Ventura et al., 2000) (Table 8–1). Age distribution graphs as a U-shaped curve, with women younger than 20 years and older than 40 years of age having the highest rates of hypertension (Table 8–2).

In the United States, pregnancy-associated hypertension is a leading cause of maternal death. Final mortality data for 1997 reported a total of 327 maternal deaths, producing a rate of 8.4 deaths per 100,000 live births (Hoyert, Kochanek, & Murphy, 1999). The overall rate of maternal death from preeclampsia or eclampsia is 1.6 per 100,000, which is one of the leading specific causes of death identified; the rate of obstetric pulmonary embolism–specific maternal death is also 1.6. There is a large disparity between rates of maternal death by race. African-American women are more likely to die of preeclampsia. The overall maternal death rate for African-American women was 20.8 per 100,000 in 1997, compared with 5.8 for white women and 18.3 for all other races. Of those maternal deaths from preeclampsia or eclampsia, the maternal mortality rate was 1.1 for whites, 4.5 for African Americans, and 3.8 for all other races (Hoyert et al., 1999).

TABLE 8–1 ■ RATES OF PREGNANCY-INDUCED HYPERTENSION BY MATERNAL RACE

Maternal Race	Rate per 1,000 Live Births*
All races	36.8
Caucasian	37.1
African American	39.7
American Indian	48.1
Asian or Pacific Islander	
Total	20.1
Chinese	14.4
Japanese	18.4
Hawaiian	28.8
Filipino	28.8
Other	18.7
Hispanic	
Total	26.8
Mexican	25.7
Puerto Rican	28.1
Cuban	30.0
Central and South American	27.1
Other or unknown Hispanic	36.9
Non-Hispanic	
Total	39.1
White	40.1
Black	39.8

*Rates reported as number of live births with specified medical risk factor per 1,000 live births by specified group. From Ventura et al., 2000

Morbidity and Mortality

Hypertension during pregnancy predisposes the woman to potentially lethal complications such as abruptio placentae, disseminated intravascular coagulation (DIC), cerebral hemorrhage, cerebral vascular accident, hepatic failure, and acute renal failure. Leading causes of maternal death from hypertension complicating pregnancy include complications from abruptio placentae, hepatic rupture, and eclampsia (Roberts, 1999).

Maternal hypertension contributes to intrauterine fetal death and perinatal mortality. The main causes of neonatal death are placental insufficiency and abruptio placentae (Roberts, 1999). Intrauterine growth restriction (IUGR) is common in infants of women with preeclampsia (Roberts, Taylor, Friedman, & Goldfien, 1990; Sibai, 1990a). The exact cause is unknown, but fetal and neonatal consequences of preeclampsia may be related to the changes in the uteroplacental unit. Histologic findings of placentas from pregnancies complicated by preeclampsia are consistent with poor uteroplacental perfusion, which can lead to chronic hypoxemia in the fetus (Roberts, 1999).

Risk Factors

Preeclampsia is a subtle and insidious disease process unique to human pregnancy. The signs and symptoms of preeclampsia become apparent relatively late in the course of the disease, usually during the third trimester of pregnancy. However, the underlying pathophysiology may be present as early as 8 weeks of gestation (Friedman, Taylor, & Roberts, 1991).

Historically, several well-defined risk factors have been identified for the development of preeclampsia (Display 8–1). Although risk factors are identified, the individual predictive values of the risk factors for screening and risk identification purposes have not been verified. Women should not be arbitrarily labeled as low- or high-risk patients based solely on historical risk factors.

Age

The incidence of preeclampsia is reported to increase in the teenage population and for the older pregnant woman. The risk of developing preeclampsia for the nulliparous adolescent younger than 19 years is significantly higher than in women older than 19 years of age (Butler & Alberman, 1958; Goldberg & Craig, 1983; Guzick et al., 1987; Montagu, 1979; Taylor, 1988; Ventura et al., 2000). However, this association has not been identified independent of other risk factors, especially parity. Because a higher proportion of pregnancies, especially first pregnancies, are in women of younger age, more cases of preeclampsia occur in this age group. Age may be significant only in that older women are more likely to enter pregnancy with preexisting medical complications, such as undiagnosed hypertension, and the teenage population may be at risk because of coexisting lifestyle risk factors (Mittendorf, Lain, Williams, & Walker, 1996).

Race

Maternal race is often identified in conjunction with socioeconomic status; therefore, it is difficult to identify its independent significance in relation to preeclampsia. African-American women have been identified to be at a higher risk for developing preeclampsia (Cunningham & Leveno, 1988; Guzick et al., 1987; Ventura et al., 2000). However, the prevalence of hypertension is generally more common among African Americans. The association between race and preeclampsia may not be race related but more closely associated with the prevalence of unrecognized preexisting chronic hypertension (Roberts, 1999). The presence of preexisting chronic hypertension may help explain why women 35 years or older have a significantly (70%) greater risk of preeclampsia than their counterparts between the ages of 30 and 34 years (Saftlass, Olson, Franks, Atrash, & Pokras, 1990).

Socioeconomic Status

Socioeconomic status, contrary to past belief, is not a predisposing factor to the development of preeclampsia (Baird, 1977; Chesley, 1978; Davies, 1971; Nel-

TABLE 8–2 ■ RATES OF PREGNANCY-ASSOCIATED HYPERTENSION BY MATERNAL AGE*

Maternal Age (years)	Chronic Hypertension	Pregnancy-Induced Hypertension	Eclampsia
All races			
All ages	6.9	36.8	3.3
<20	2.5	42.8	4.9
20-24	4.1	37.0	3.5
25–29	6.1	35.7	3.0
30–34	8.6	33.6	2.7
35–39	13.9	37.2	3.1
40–54	23.0	46.2	4.2
White			
All ages	6.0	37.1	3.1
<20	2.1	42.7	4.4
20–24	3.5	38.0	3.3
25–29	5.4	36.6	2.9
30–34	7.3	33.6	2.7
35–39	11.4	36.7	3.0
40–54	18.7	44.8	4.1
African American			
All ages	12.2	39.7	4.6
<20	3.4	44.1	6.0
20–24	6.5	35.2	4.5
25–29	11.8	36.8	4.0
30–34	20.8	41.0	3.7
35–39	35.2	46.5	4.2
40–54	55.8	58.4	5.4

*Rates reported as number of live births with specified medical risk factor per 1,000 live births by specified group. From Ventura, et al., 2000

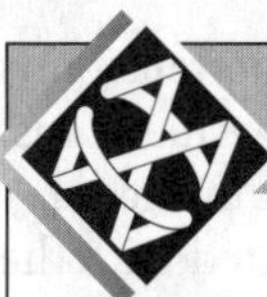

DISPLAY 8–1

Risk Factors for the Development of Preeclampsia

- First pregnancy or a pregnancy of a new genetic make-up (Chesley & Cooper, 1986; Cunningham & Leveno, 1988)
- Multiple gestation (Thompson, Lyons, & Makowski, 1987)
- Preexisting diabetes, collagen vascular disease, hypertension, or renal disease (Mabie, Pernoll, & Biswas, 1986; Cunningham, Cox, Harstad, Mason, & Pritchard, 1990; Siddiqi, Rosenn, Mimouni, Khoury, & Miodovnik, 1991)
- Hydatiform mole (Page, 1939)
- Fetal hydrops (Barron, 1991)
- Maternal age (Spellacy, Miller, & Winegar, 1988)
- African-American race (Cunningham & Leveno, 1988)
- Family history of pregnancy-induced hypertension (Chesley & Cooper, 1986)
- Antiphospholipid syndrome (Branch, Silver, Blackwell, Reading, & Scott, 1992)
- Angiotension gene T235 (Ward et al., 1993)
- Socioeconomic status (Guzick et al., 1987)
- Failure to demonstrate hemodilution (Hays, Cruikshank, & Dunn, 1985)
- Failure to demonstrate a decrease in systemic vascular resistance and second-trimester mean arterial pressures (Ales, Norton, & Druzin, 1989; Gavette & Roberts, 1987)
- Use of contraceptives that prevent exposure to sperm (Klonoff-Cohen, Savitz, Cefalo, & McCann, 1989; Robillard et al., 1994)
- Not having oral sex (Dekker, Robillard, & Hulsey, 1998; Dekker & Sibai 1998; Dekker, 1999)
- Pregnancy achieved through artificial donor insemination (Dekker, Robillard, & Hulsey, 1998)
- Partner who fathered a preeclamptic pregnancy in another woman (Lie et al., 1998)
- Obesity or insulin resistance (Schaffir, Lockwood, Lapinski, Yoon, & Alvarez, 1995; Khan and Daya, 1996; Ness and Roberts, 1996; Dekker, Robillard, & Hulsey, 1998)
- Thrombophilic disorders, including hyperhomocysteinemia (Branch, Andres, Digre, Rote, & Scott, 1989; Pattinson, Kriegler, Odendaal, Muller, & Kirsten, 1989; Branch, 1990; Branch, Dudley, & Mitchell, 1991; Branch, Dudley, LaMarche, & Mitchell, 1992; Branch, Silver, Silver, Blackwell, Reading, & Scott, 1992; Out et al., 1992; Dizon-Townson, Nelson, Easton, & Ward, 1996; Yamamoto, Takahashi, Geshi, Sasamori, & Mori, 1996; Grisaru, Zwang, Peyser, Lessing, & Eldor, 1997; Lindoff, Ingemarsson, Martinsson, Segelmark, Thysell, & Astedt, 1997; Dizon-Townson, Major, & Ward, 1998)

son, 1955). Eclampsia, however, is clearly a disease of lower socioeconomic status (Davies et al., 1970; Nelson, 1955).

Lower socioeconomic status is associated with poorer diets and an increase in smoking (Redman, 1995). The association between maternal nutritional status and risk for preeclampsia is inconclusive (Belizán & Villar, 1980; Brewer, 1974, 1976; Chaudhuri, 1971; Fitzgibbon, 1922; Lu et al., 1981; Ross et al., 1954). Belizán and Villar (1980) and Chaudhuri (1971) reported that dietary deficiencies, especially calcium and certain vitamins, are important in the pathogenesis of preeclampsia based on observations in animal models. The roles of calcium and vitamins in the pathogenesis of preeclampsia are being examined in prospective clinical trials (Levine & CPEP Study Group, 1997). Brewer (1974, 1976) reported that protein deprivation played an etiologic role in preeclampsia. However, the results reported by Brewer have been questioned because the incidence of preeclampsia was no different from the incidence in the general population during the study time frame. The role of a specific link between a nutritional deficit and the development of preeclampsia remains controversial.

Socioeconomic status and cigarette smoking are associated because the prevalence of smoking increases in the lower socioeconomic classes. Smoking has been reported to reduce the incidence of preeclampsia in several studies (Duffus & MacGillivray, 1968; Mittendorf et al., 1996; Sibai et al., 1995). Although smoking increases perinatal mortality, smoking appears to diminish the maternal responses to the placental problems of preeclampsia (Redman, 1995). Like maternal age and race, the independent contribution of socioeconomic status to the risk for developing preeclampsia is unclear.

Gravidity and Parity

A woman pregnant for the first time is six to eight times more likely to develop preeclampsia (Chesley, 1978; Taylor, 1988). The incidence of preeclampsia ranges from 10% to 14% in the primigravid woman, compared with 5.7% to 7.3% in the multigravid woman (Long, Abell, & Beischer, 1979; Villar & Sibai, 1989). A previous pregnancy may afford a protective effect on the incidence of preeclampsia in subsequent pregnancies. Second-trimester abortion, compared with first-trimester abortion, also appears to afford some protection in subsequent pregnancies (Campbell, MacGillivray, & Carr-Hill, 1985). However, if the woman has a new partner for a subsequent pregnancy, this protective effect is not seen (Beer, 1978; Dekker, 1999; Feeney & Scott, 1980). The reported incidence for preeclampsia among nulliparous women (3.2%) and multiparous women with a change in paternity (3%) are similar but increased when compared with multiparous women with no change in paternity (1.9%) (Dekker, 1999). A Norwegian study reported that men who fathered a pregnancy complicated by preeclampsia were nearly twice as likely to father a pregnancy complicated by preeclampsia in a different woman (Lie et al., 1998).

Among parous women, the risk for developing preeclampsia is increased if preeclampsia complicated a previous pregnancy (Dekker, 1999). The risk of preeclampsia in a second pregnancy is 10 to 15 times greater for women when the disease is recurrent compared with women for whom the first pregnancy was normal (Campbell, 1985; Davies et al., 1970; Dekker, 1999). One of the few factors that may help identify the woman at risk for early-onset preeclampsia is a history of previous preeclampsia (Moore & Redmon, 1983).

Gestational Age at First Prenatal Visit

Mittendorf and colleagues (1996) suggest women entering prenatal care after the first trimester are at increased risk for developing preeclampsia. The unadjusted odds ratio for beginning prenatal care after the first trimester was 1.9 (95% CI: 1.4–3.0). However, Eskenazi, Fenster, and Sidney (1991) found no association between initiation of prenatal care after the first trimester and preeclampsia.

Family History of Pregnancy-Induced Hypertension

A frequently overlooked characteristic of preeclampsia is the tendency of the condition to occur in daughters and sisters of women with a history of preeclampsia. Adams and Finlayson (1961) found a fourfold increase in the occurrence of proteinuric preeclampsia in sisters of women who had preeclampsia in their first pregnancy compared with sisters of women without the disease. Chesley and colleagues found the occurrence of preeclampsia in sisters, daughters, and granddaughters of women who had preeclampsia to be higher than the daughters-in-law (Chesley, 1984; Chesley & Cooper, 1986). The risk of eclampsia among daughters of women who were eclamptic is eight times higher than the risk among daughters of women who did not suffer from eclampsia (Chesley, Annitto, & Cosgrove, 1968). These findings may indicate a genetic predisposition for preeclampsia.

The pattern of inheritance is unclear, but researchers have suggested that a single recessive gene for which the woman is homozygous may be responsible for the susceptibility for preeclampsia (Chesley & Cooper, 1986). The single-gene theory has been challenged because identical twins do not have concordant histories (Thornton & Onwude, 1991). Several studies have also reported an association between preeclampsia and the presence of the histocompatibility leukocyte antigen DR4 (Kilpatrick, Liston, Gibson, & Livingstone, 1989; Redman, Bodmer, Bodmer, Beilin, & Bonnar, 1978; Simon et al., 1988). The genotype of the fetus may also be significant, suggesting the possibility that the father of the child could contribute genetically to preeclampsia (Liston & Kilpatrick, 1991).

Chronic Disease

There is disagreement about the incidence of superimposed preeclampsia among women with chronic hypertension, but most investigators agree that preeclampsia is more common in this situation (Chesley, 1978; Chesley & Cooper, 1986). Women with chronic hypertension that predates the pregnancy are three to seven times more likely to develop superimposed preeclampsia than women who are normotensive (Chesley & Annitto, 1947; Guzick et al., 1987). Women with a history of pregestational diabetes mellitus (Garner, D'Alton, Dudley, Huard, & Hardie, 1990; Siddiqi, Rosenn, Mimouni, Khoury, & Miodovnik, 1991; White, 1935) and hypertension associated with chronic renal disease are at increased risk for preeclampsia (Felding, 1969). Later research identified an association between the presence of antiphospholipid antibodies (Branch et al., 1989; Branch et al., 1992) and an angiotensinogen gene (Ward et al., 1993) with an increased incidence of preeclampsia. A history of migraine headaches may also predisposes the woman to preeclampsia (Marcoux, Berube,

Brisson, & Fabia, 1992; Moore & Redmon, 1983) and eclampsia (Rotten, Sachtleben, & Friedman, 1959).

Pregnancy Complications

A pregnancy complicated by a multifetal gestation, fetal hydrops, or hydatidiform mole is at increased risk for the development of preeclampsia. The incidence of preeclampsia is increased five times in a pregnancy with a twin gestation (Barron, 1991; Thompson, Lyons, & Makowski, 1987). Nonimmune fetal hydrops may increase the risk for preeclampsia by as much as 50% (Barron, 1991). For the woman diagnosed with a hydatidiform mole, a well-known association exists between the molar pregnancy and the onset of preeclampsia (Page, 1939; Slattery, Khong, Dawkins, Pridmore, & Hague, 1993). One report suggests that the primiparous woman who has a urinary tract infection (UTI) complicating pregnancy is five times more likely to have preeclampsia than the primiparous woman who does not have a UTI during pregnancy (Mittendorf et al., 1996).

Definitions

Terminology used to describe the hypertensive disorders of pregnancy is associated with imprecise usage, causing confusion for healthcare providers caring for women with hypertensive complications during pregnancy and childbirth. The American College of Obstetricians and Gynecologists' technical bulletin, *Management of Preeclampsia,* outlines current accepted terminology for the hypertensive disorders of pregnancy (American College of Obstetricians and Gynecologists [ACOG], 1996). Clinically, there are two basic types of hypertension during pregnancy—chronic hypertension and pregnancy-induced hypertension (PIH)—with the distinction based on the onset of hypertension in relation to the pregnancy.

Chronic Hypertension

Chronic hypertension is hypertension present before the pregnancy, diagnosed before 20 weeks' gestation, or hypertension continuing beyond 42 days postpartum (ACOG, 1996).

Pregnancy-Induced Hypertension

PIH is the onset of hypertension, generally after the 20th week of pregnancy, appearing as a marker of a pregnancy-specific vasospastic condition (Roberts, 1999). These two types of hypertension (chronic hypertension and PIH) may occur independently or simultaneously.

Once PIH is present, hypertension is further classified according to the maternal organ systems affected. The practitioner must keep in mind that hypertension during pregnancy represents a continuum of disease processes. Hypertension may be the first sign, but the underlying pathophysiology can involve all major organ systems.

Preeclampsia

Preeclampsia is characterized by renal involvement, as evidenced by the onset of proteinuria. The disease process is said to be mild or severe on the basis of maternal or fetal findings. If signs and symptoms of preeclampsia or eclampsia occur in women with chronic hypertension, the diagnosis of superimposed preeclampsia or eclampsia is made.

HELLP Syndrome

HELLP syndrome is characterized by hepatic involvement as evidenced by hemolysis, elevated liver enzymes, and low platelet counts.

Eclampsia

Eclampsia is characterized by the onset of seizure activity or coma in the woman diagnosed with PIH, with no history of preexisting neurologic pathology.

Transient Hypertension

Transient hypertension is the development of hypertension during pregnancy, labor, or the first 24 hours postpartum without other signs of preeclampsia or chronic hypertension.

Pathophysiology of Preeclampsia

Preeclampsia has been called the "disease of theories." There is not one established cause. Research is ongoing to identify the pathophysiology of this process. Although the exact mechanism is unknown, preeclampsia is thought to occur because of changes within the maternal cardiovascular, hematologic, and renal systems.

Normal physiologic adaptations to pregnancy include an increase in plasma volume, vasodilation of the vascular bed, decreased systemic vascular resistance, elevation of cardiac output, and increased prostacyclin production. Physical assessment findings consistent with these changes are dilutional anemia, lower systemic blood pressures and mean arterial pressure, a slight increase in heart rate, and peripheral edema. In preeclampsia, these normal adaptations are altered. Instead of plasma volume expansion and hemodilution, there is a decrease in circulating plasma volume resulting in hemoconcentration. Women with preeclampsia have inadequate plasma volume expansion, with an average plasma volume 9% below expected values for mild disease and up to 40% below normal with severe disease (Duvekot, Cheriex, Pieters, Menheere, & Peeters, 1993; Hays, Cruikshank, & Dunn, 1985; Sibai, Anderson, Spinnato, & Shaver, 1983). Further intravascular volume depletion may occur from endothelial injury and leaking capillaries. This may result in increased blood viscosity, leading to a decrease in maternal organ perfusion, including the uteroplacental unit. The reduction in plasma volume may be more closely related to IUGR than hypertension (Sibai et al., 1983). The vascular bed demonstrates increased sensitivity to vasoactive substances, resulting in vasoconstriction and increased vascular tone. Vasoconstriction results in increased systemic vascular resistance and hypertension. This hypertension is further aggravated by arterial vasospasms; the underlying mechanism for observed signs and symptoms of the disease process. The cumulative effect of decreased intravascular volume and vasoconstriction leads to a decreased organ perfusion. As the process worsens, hemolysis may also compromise tissue oxygen delivery.

Vasoconstriction and a further increase in cardiac output above the normal pregnancy elevation (Easterling, Benedetti, Schmucker, & Millard, 1990) results in arterial vasospasms, endothelial damage, and an imbalance in endothelial prostacyclin and thromboxane ratios (Sibai, 1991; Zeeman, Dekker, van Geijn, & Kraayenbrink, 1992). Tables 8–3 and 8–4 provide highlights of the pathophysiology of disease progression and multiple organ system involvement. Figure 8–1 demonstrates the pathophysiologic changes related to preeclampsia.

Clinical Manifestations of Pregnancy-Induced Hypertension

Historically, the classic triad for preeclampsia has included hypertension, proteinuria, and edema. However, not all of these parameters must be present for the diagnosis of PIH. Hypertension and proteinuria are the most significant indicators. Edema is significant only if hypertension, proteinuria, or signs of multisystem organ involvement are present.

The clinical manifestations of PIH are directly related to the presence of vascular vasospasms. These vasospasms result in endothelial injury, red blood cell destruction, platelet aggregation, increased capillary permeability, increased systemic vascular resistance, and renal and hepatic dysfunction.

Hypertension

Although controversy exists about the most appropriate definition of hypertension, ACOG (1996) defines hypertension as a sustained blood pressure elevation of 140/90 mm Hg after the 20th week of gestation that is recorded on two or more measurements. The use of elevations above baseline values to define hypertension is of questionable value for the diagnosis of preeclampsia. MacGillivary, Rose, and Rowe (1969) reported that 73% of nulliparous women with normal pregnancies had an increase in diastolic blood pressure of more than 15 mm Hg during pregnancy, and 57% of these women had an increase in diastolic pressure of more than 20 mm Hg. Later studies have confirmed these findings (Moutquin et al., 1985; Villar & Sibai, 1989), suggesting that further study is required to determine the degree of elevation that is significant for the prediction of preeclampsia.

Earlier research suggests that an increase in mean arterial pressure in the second trimester (MAP-2) of more than 85 mm Hg is useful in identifying the women at risk for developing hypertension during pregnancy (Page & Christianson, 1976). Several investigators have correlated an elevation of MAP-2 with an increased risk for maternal hypertension and for fetal and neonatal risks (Ales, Norton, & Druzin, 1989; Chesley & Sibai, 1987; Gavette & Roberts, 1987; O'Brien, 1990, 1992). However, more definitive research is needed.

Proteinuria

Proteinuria is defined as the excretion of 0.1 g of protein per liter (100 mg/L) in a random urine specimen, 0.3 g/L (300 mg/L) in a 24-hour specimen, or 1 to 2+ on a dipstick determination (ACOG, 1996). Proteinuria indicates a worsening of the disease process, increasing the risk of adverse outcome for the woman and fetus. There is a positive correlation between the degree of proteinuria and perinatal mortality and fetal growth restriction (Tervila, Vartianen, Timonen, & Kauppinen, 1975). The concentration of urine protein is extremely variable. Urinary protein concentration is influenced by factors such as contamination of the specimen with vaginal secretions, blood, or bacteria; urine specific gravity and pH; exercise; and posture. Urine dipstick

TABLE 8–3 ■ PHYSIOLOGIC AND PATHOPHYSIOLOGIC CHANGES ASSOCIATED WITH PREECLAMPSIA

Feature	Normal Pregnancy	Preeclampsia Alterations
Blood volume	50%↑	Smaller ↑
Plasma volume	50%↑	Little or no change
Red cell mass	20%↑	Hemoconcentration
Cardiac output	40%–50%↑ Widening pulse pressure	Variable ↓ Vascular compliance
Blood pressure	↓ Initially with return to prepregnant values by third trimester	Hypertension
Peripheral vascular resistance	↓ Total peripheral resistance ↑ Venous capacitance	↑ Resistance ↑ Vascular reactivity Vasospasms
Renal function	↑	↓
RPF	75%↑	↓
GFR	50%↑	↓
BUN	↓	↑
Creatinine clearance	↑	↓
Serum creatinine	↓	↑
Uric acid	↓	↑
Renin-angiotensin-aldosterone system	Markedly activated and responds appropriately to posture and salt intake	Plasma renin concentration and activity suppressed Loss of antagonists (vasodilators) to AII Increased sensitivity to vasoactive substances
Coagulation system		Normal with mild disease
Fibrinogen	↑	Normal initially, then ↓
Factors VII, VIII, IX, X	All ↑	Increase in ratio of von Willebrand factor to factor VII, coagulant activity increased leading to consumption of factor VI
Fibrinolytic activity	↓	↑
Platelet count	Normal	↓
Bleeding time	Normal	Prolonged

RPF=renal plasma blood flow; GFR=glomerular filtration rate; BUN=blood urea nitrogen
AII=angiotensin II; ↑=increased; ↓=decreased.
Adapted from Roberts, J. (1994). Current perspectives on preeclampsia. *Journal of Nurse-Midwifery, 39*(2), 76.

evaluation is a poor quantifier of protein excretion. Studies comparing traditional urine dipstick analysis to 24-hour urine protein quantitation to determine proteinuria found that in routine clinical practice a finding of "negative" or "trace" proteinuria misses significant proteinuria in up to 40% of hypertensive women. Evaluation of total protein excretion should be done by 24-hour urine protein quantitation rather than urinalysis or dipstick analysis (Brown & Buddle, 1995; Kuo, Loumantakis, & Gallery, 1992; Meyer, Mercer, Friedman, & Sibai, 1994).

Edema

Edema is a common finding of pregnancy and is not necessary for the diagnosis of PIH. Dependent edema in the absence of hypertension or proteinuria is generally related to changes in interstitial and intravascular hydrostatic and osmotic pressures that facilitate movement of intravascular fluid into the tissues. Intracellular and extracellular edema represents a generalized and excessive accumulation of fluid in tissue. As vasospasms worsen, capillary en-

TABLE 8–4 ■ PREECLAMPSIA PATHOPHYSIOLOGY AS A MULTIORGAN SYSTEM DISEASE

System	Effect of Preeclampsia	Clinical Implications
Vascular Bed		
Endothelial dysfunction Altered coagulation Altered response to vasoactive substances	Increased release of cellular fibronectin, growth factors, VCAM-1, factor VIII antigen, and peptides Endothelial cell injury initiates coagulation by intrinsic pathway (contact adhesion) or extrinsic pathway (tissue factor) Decreased production of prostacyclin and alteration in prostacyclin/thromboxane ratio	Endothelial dysfunction present before clinical signs of disease Increased thrombus formation, including pulmonary and cerebral emboli Vasoconstriction and vasospasm Increased sensitivity to vasoactive substance Capillary permeability, which contributes to edema formation
Cardiovascular and Pulmonary		
↑ Vascular resistance ↑ Cardiac output and stroke volume ↓ Colloid osmotic pressure	Arteriolar narrowing ↑ Sympathetic activity ↑ Levels of endothelin-1, a vasoconstrictor ↑ Sensitivity to endogenous pressors, including vasopressin, epinephrine, and norepinephrine ↑ Capillary permeability Further depletion of intravascular colloids through capillary permeabililty and renal excretion of proteins	Increased blood pressure Hyperdynamic cardiac activity Epidurals can be used safely but must be cautious if using ephedrine to correct hypotension Subendocardial hemorrhages occur in >50% of women who die of eclampsia At risk for pulmonary edema, myocardial ischemia, left ventricular dysfunction
Renal		
Proteinuria Altered function	Slight decrease in glomerular size Diameter of glomerular capillary lumen decreased Glomerular endothelial cells are greatly enlarged and may occlude the capillary lumen Glomular capillary endotheliosis; thickening of renal arterioles	Proteinuria plus hypertension is the most reliable indicator of fetal jeopardy, indicative of glomerular dysfunction ↑ Serum uric acid secondary to a ↓ urate clearance (uric acid better predictor of outcome than blood pressure) ↓ Creatinine clearance with an elevation of serum creatinine levels ↑ BUN mirrors changes in creatine clearance and is a function of protein intake and liver function Urine sediment analysis may not be beneficial At risk for oliguria, ATN, renal failure
Hepatic		
Hepatic dysfunction Hepatic rupture	Changes consistent with hemorrhage into hepatic tissue	Elevations of liver function tests; association of microangiopathic anemia and elevations of AST/ALT

(continued)

TABLE 8–4 ■ PREECLAMPSIA PATHOPHYSIOLOGY (continued)

System	Effect of Preeclampsia	Clinical Implications
	Later changes consistent with hepatic infarction ↑ Hepatic artery resistance Fibrin deposition Hepatocellular necrosis	carries ominous prognosis for mother and fetus HELLP syndrome Possible elevations in bilirubin Signs of liver failure: malaise, nausea, epigastric pain, hypoglycemia, hemolysis, anemia
Hematologic		
Thrombocytopenia Altered platelet function Hemolysis	↑ Platelet destruction ↑ Platelet aggreability ↓ Platelet life span Hemolytic anemia Destruction of RBCs in microvasculature	Platelets <100,000 increase risk of coagulopathy Platelets <50,000 increase risk of hemorrhage Platelets <20,000 increase risk for spontaneous bleeding Decreased oxygen carrying capacity and organ oxygenation
Central Nervous System		
Hyperreflexia	May indicate increasing CNS involvement but not diagnostic of disease Alteration of cerebral autoregulation with seizures ↑ Intracranial pressures	Cerebral edema with severe disease Signs of CNS alterations: headache, dizziness, changes in vital signs, diplopia, scotomata, blurred vision, amaurosis, tachycardia, alteration in level of consciousness
Fetal or Neonatal		
Fetal intolerance to labor Preterm birth Oligohydramnios IUGR IUFD Abruptio placentae	Alteration in placental function At risk for indicated preterm birth secondary to maternal disease process	Must monitor for signs of fetal compromise Monitoring for IUGR and IUFD At risk for abruptio placentae, oligohydramnios, nonreassuring FHR patterns
Uteroplacental		
Spiral arteries Changes consistent with hypoxia	Abnormal invasion Retain nonpregnant characteristics Limited vasodilatation Vessel necrosis	Decreases in uteroplacental perfusion Increased risk for fetal compromise and IUGR

ALT = alanine aminotransferase; AST = aspartate aminotransferase; ATN = acute tubular necrosis; BUN = blood urea nitrogen; CNS = central nervous system; FHR = fetal heart rate; IUFD = intrauterine fetal death; IUGR = intrauterine growth restriction; RBC = red blood cells; VCAM-1 = vascular cell adhesion molecule-1; ↑ = increased; ↓ = decreased.

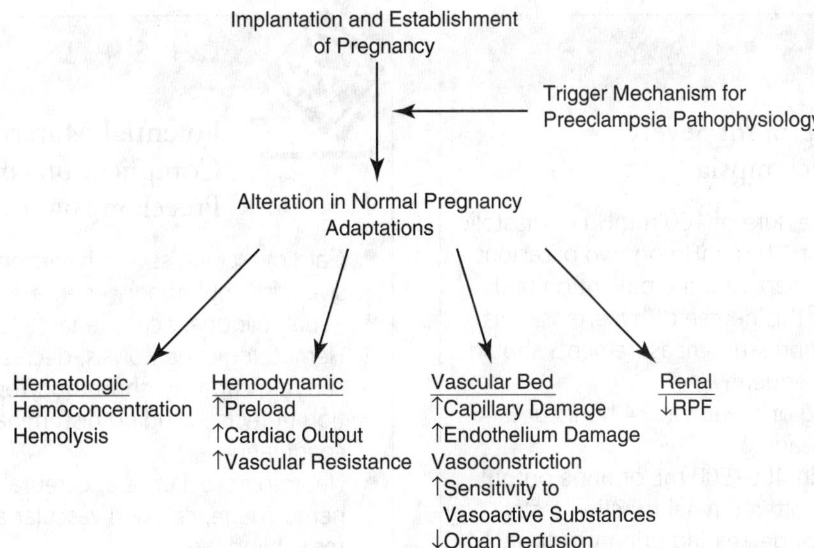

FIGURE 8–1. Pathophysiology of preeclampsia.

dothelial damage results in increased systemic capillary permeability (ie, leakage), which facilitates hemoconcentration and increases the risk of pulmonary edema.

Mild Versus Severe Preeclampsia

To identify the progression of PIH from mild to severe disease, nursing management requires accurate and thorough observation and assessments. Display 8–2 lists criteria for severe preeclampsia and Display 8–3 gives the potential maternal and fetal complications of severe preeclampsia.

While caring for women with hypertensive disorders of pregnancy, nursing assessments focus on identification of the disease progression. PIH is a systemic disease in which one or more organ systems are involved. The wide range of symptoms and multiple organ system involvement can sometimes result in misdiagnosis and delay in treatment. Cocaine intoxication, lupus nephritis, chronic renal failure, and acute fatty liver of pregnancy are examples of conditions that may mimic preeclampsia and eclampsia (O'Brien, Mercer, Friedman, & Sibai, 1993; Simpson, Luppi, & O'Brien-Abel, 1998). Women with chronic hypertension or any preexisting medical condition that predisposes to the development of hypertension are at increased risk for superimposed preeclampsia and eclampsia. Care of the woman with severe preeclampsia or HELLP syndrome is best referred to a tertiary perinatal center.

Nursing Assessment and Interventions for Preeclampsia

The only definitive therapy for preeclampsia is birth. The decision to initiate birth versus expectant management must be individualized. Decisions for management are determined by maternal and fetal status and gestational age.

Home Care Management

Mild preeclampsia may be managed at home with frequent follow-up care, including telephone contact between the woman and a high-risk perinatal nurse and periodic nurse home visits. Criteria for home management vary with the primary perinatal healthcare provider and home care agency. The woman must be in a stable condition with no evidence of worsening maternal or fetal status. Diagnostic criteria and considerations suggested for home care referral for management of women with mild PIH can be found in Appendix 8A.

Inpatient Management

Women with mild preeclampsia may be evaluated in the inpatient setting and remain hospitalized. Women with severe preeclampsia or eclampsia are managed in the hospital. A woman with a fetus at an early gestational age, usually less than 34 weeks, is generally managed in a tertiary center because of the ability to provide advanced neonatal care if delivery is indicated.

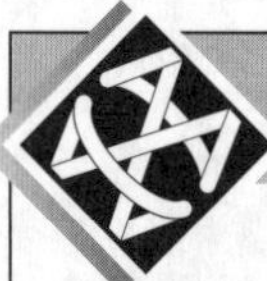

DISPLAY 8–2

Criteria for Severe Preeclampsia

- Systolic blood pressure of 160 mmHg or diastolic blood pressure of 110 mmHg on two occasions at least 6 hours apart with the patient on bed rest. However, if this degree of hypertension is sustained, blood pressure measurements should be taken more frequently.
- Proteinuria of 5 g or greater in 24 hours or 3–4+ on the dipstick reading.
- Oliguria: less than 400–500 mL of urine output over 24 hours or altered renal function tests. Look for trends of decreasing urinary output. A kidney that is adequately perfused and oxygenated should produce a minimum of 30 mL/h or 100 mL/4 h of urine.
- Elevated serum creatinine >1.2
- Intrauterine growth restriction
- Cerebral or visual disturbances, including (but not limited to) altered level of consciousness, headache, scotomata, or blurred vision (magnesium sulfate may cause headache or blurred vision if serum concentration is in the high therapeutic range)
- Impaired liver function demonstrated by right upper quadrant or epigastric pain and/or altered liver function tests (increased aspartate transaminase [AST or SGOT] or alanine transaminase [ALT or SGPT] liver enzymes). With significant hepatic involvement, there is increased risk for coagulation defects and hypoglycemia.
- Thrombocytopenia: platelet count <150,000/mm^3; coagulopathies generally not present until platelet counts drop below 100,000/mm^3
- Pulmonary or cardiac involvement: may manifest as pulmonary edema, cyanosis, chest pain, cardiac dysrhythmias
- Development of eclampsia
- Development of HELLP syndrome

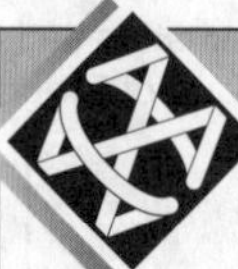

DISPLAY 8–3

Potential Maternal and Fetal Complications of Severe Preeclampsia

- Cardiovascular: severe hypertension, hypertensive crisis, pulmonary edema
- Renal: oliguria, acute renal failure
- Hematologic: hemolysis, decreased oxygen-carrying capacity, thrombocytopenia, coagulation defects including disseminated intravascular coagulation
- Neurologic: eclampsia, cerebral edema, cerebral hemorrhage, cerebral vascular accidents, amaurosis (blindness)
- Hepatic: hepatocellular dysfunction, hepatic rupture, hypoglycemia
- Uteroplacental: abruptio placentae, fetal growth restriction, fetal death, fetal intolerance to labor

Nursing care involves accurate and astute observations and assessments. Comprehensive knowledge regarding pharmacologic therapies, management regimens, and possible complications is also required.

The most important aspect of care for women with hypertension in pregnancy is recognition of the abilities of the facility and the obstetric and neonatal staff to handle potential emergencies. The decision to transfer a patient to a perinatal center should be based on the level of care required for the woman or should be made because the fetus is preterm and neonatal support will be required. It is best not to attempt expectant management of patients with severe preeclampsia (antepartum or postpartum) unless in a tertiary care center. However, providers of obstetric care, regardless of level of care provided, must be able to stabilize the woman before transport.

Controversial Management Protocols: Use of Colloids and Diuretics

Some management protocols are considered to be inappropriate in the care of women with preeclampsia. Diuretics and administration of high concentrations of colloid solutions (eg, albumin, Hespan) should not be used to decrease peripheral edema because of further depletion of intravascular volume and an increased risk of pulmonary edema and uteroplacental insufficiency (Clark, Cotton, Hankins, & Phelan, 1997; Dildy, Phelan, & Cotton, 1992; Repke, 1993). Intravenous fluid therapy is not without risk in the management of a woman with preeclampsia. Administration of intravenous fluids decreases intravascular colloid osmotic pressure (Gonik & Cotton, 1984), but the administration of colloid solutions, such as Hespan or albumin, is not indicated. The administration of colloid solutions theoretically increases intravascular colloid osmotic pressure, but the proteins in these solutions leak into the tissues as a result of capillary injury and increased capillary permeability. There is a resulting alteration in the hydrostatic and osmotic forces that potentiate the development of pulmonary edema and further depletion of intravascular volume (Kirshon et al., 1988). The administration of colloids in any clinical situation in which endothelial injury and capillary permeability complicate the disease process is contraindicated.

Valium is no longer the first-line agent to stop seizure activity because of the depressant effect on the fetus and depression of the maternal gag reflex. Seizure precautions should be followed according to institution protocol. It is important to avoid insertion of a padded tongue blade to the back of the throat; a nasopharyngeal airway may be appropriate, if available. Heparin should not be administered as prophylaxis against coagulopathies, because it increases the risk for intracranial bleeding.

Antepartum Management

Antepartum management of the woman diagnosed with mild preeclampsia remains controversial. Key to the debate is whether the woman should be hospitalized or ambulatory management is appropriate. In the face of severe disease, the woman should be hospitalized with the timing of birth dictated by maternal and fetal status.

Historically, women diagnosed with mild preeclampsia were admitted to the hospital for two reasons: to prevent eclampsia and to improve perinatal outcome (Gilstrap, Cunningham, & Whalley, 1978). However, researchers have questioned the practice of routine hospitalization of women diagnosed with mild preeclampsia. Mathews, Agarwal, and Shuttleworth (1980) and Crowther, Bouwmeester, and Ashurst (1992) reported no differences in maternal or perinatal outcomes for women with mild preeclampsia managed in hospitals compared with those managed expectantly on an outpatient basis. ACOG (1996) recognizes that outpatient management for women with mild preeclampsia is a viable option for those who agree to follow established protocols, can have frequent office or home visits, and can perform blood pressure monitoring.

The role of antihypertensive medication in the expectant management of women with mild preeclampsia is controversial. Antihypertensive regimens reported in prospective and retrospective studies include hydralazine, methyldopa, nifedipine, prazosin, diuretics, and β blockers (Cruickshank, Robertson, Campbell, & MacGillivray, 1992; Gruppo di Studio Iperensione in Gravidanza, 1998; Plouin et al., 1988, 1990; Rubin et al., 1983; Sibai, 1996; Sibai, Barton, Akl, Sarinoglu, & Mercer, 1992; Sibai, Gonzalez, Mabie, & Moretti, 1987). Although each of these studies examined the effect of different antihypertensive agents, none reported a better perinatal outcome compared with management without antihypertensives. There are insufficient data to support prophylactic use of antihypertensive therapy in the management of mild preeclampsia.

Traditionally, women diagnosed with severe preeclampsia remote from term are delivered expeditiously. Although this approach may allow recovery from the disease process for the woman, it may not improve fetal and neonatal outcomes. The use of conservative management for severe preeclampsia remote from term has suggested that pregnancy may be prolonged to gain fetal maturity without increased risk to the woman (Fenakel et al., 1991; Friedman, Schiff, Lubarsky, & Sibai, 1999; Odendaal, Pattinson, Bam, Grove, & Kotze, 1990; Schiff, Friedman, & Sibai, 1994; Sibai, Mercer, Schiff, & Friedman, 1994). With strict criteria for patient selection and intensive maternal and fetal surveillance, pregnancy may be prolonged. Table 8–5 provides the selection criteria for expectant management of severe preeclampsia remote from term.

Activity Restriction

Activity restriction, varying from frequent rest periods with legs elevated to complete bed rest in the full lateral position, is frequently prescribed for women with PIH. While on bed rest, blood pressure decreases, and interstitial fluid is mobilized into the intravascular space, enhancing flow to the uterus and kidneys.

Controversy exists about whether the reduction of systolic blood pressure associated with bed rest improves maternal or fetal outcomes. For pregnancies complicated with nonproteinuric hypertension, bed rest does not appear to significantly improve outcome; however, for women with proteinuric preeclampsia, bed rest does seem to have some benefit. It is unclear whether bed rest in a hospital setting improves outcomes because of concurrent intensive inpatient maternal–fetal assessments and appropriate medical intervention or is beneficial when considered as an independent factor (Goldenberg et al., 1994).

Ongoing Assessment

Preeclampsia can appear to occur without warning or be recognized with the gradual development of symptoms. A key goal is early identification of women at risk for development of preeclampsia.

TABLE 8–5 ■ EXPECTANT MANAGEMENT SELECTION CRITERIA FOR PATIENTS WITH SEVERE PREECLAMPSIA REMOTE FROM TERM

Management Approach (if one or more of the clinical findings present)	Clinical Findings
Expedite birth (within 72 hours)	*Maternal* • Uncontrolled hypertension • Eclampsia • Platelet count <100,000/μL • AST or ALT >2 times upper limit of normal with epigastric pain or RUQ tenderness • Pulmonary edema • Compromised renal function • Abruptio placentae • Persistent severe headache or visual changes *Fetal* • Repetitive late or severe variable decelerations • BPP ≤4 on two occasions 4 hours apart • AFI ≤2 cm • Ultrasound estimated fetal weight ≤5th percentile • Reverse umbilical artery diastolic flow
Consider expectant management	*Maternal* • Controlled hypertension • Urinary protein of any amount • Oliguria (<0.5 mL/kg/h) that resolves with routine fluid/food intake • AST or ALT >2 times upper limit of normal without epigastric pain or RUQ tenderness *Fetal (all findings required)* • BPP ≥6 • AFI >2 cm • Ultrasound fetal weight >5th percentile

AFI = amniotic fluid index; ALT = alanine aminotransferase; AST = aspartate aminotransferase; BPP = biophysical profile; RUQ = right upper quadrant.
Data from Friedman et al., 1999; Schiff et al., 1994; and Sibai et al., 1994.

A review of the major organ systems adds to the database for detecting changes from baseline in blood pressure, weight gain, pattern of weight gain, increasing edema, and presence of proteinuria. The nurse should note whether the woman complains of unusual, frequent, or severe headaches; visual disturbances; or epigastric pain. Lack of specific reliable diagnostic tests hinders early detection and treatment of preeclampsia.

Accurate and consistent blood pressure assessment is important for establishing a baseline and monitoring subtle changes throughout the pregnancy. Blood pressure readings are affected by maternal position and measurement techniques. Consistency must be ensured with the use of proper equipment and cuff size, correct maternal positioning, a rest period before recording the pressure, and recording of Korotkoff phases IV (ie, muffling sound) and V (ie, disappearance of sound) (Barton, Witlin, & Sibai, 1999). Korotkoff phase IV is typically 5 to 10 mm Hg higher than phase V. Ideally, blood pressure measurements should be recorded with the woman in a semi-Fowler's position with the arm at heart level. If the initial measurement indicates an elevation, the woman should be allowed to relax and have a repeat measurement performed, again in a semi-Fowler's position (ACOG, 1996). Use of electronic blood pressure devices produces different values than those obtained with a manual cuff and stethoscope. Electronic blood pressure devices systematically underestimate diastolic pressure values by approximately 10 mm Hg and overestimate systolic pressure values by approximately 4 to 6 mm Hg. These differences are related to the normal hemodynamic changes that occur during pregnancy and the subsequent changes in Korotkoff phases sounds able to be heard with the human ear compared with the electronic device. There is a widening of pulse pressure when using electronic blood pressure devices compared with manual readings; however, mean arterial pressure is unchanged (Marx, Schwalbe, Cho, & Whitty, 1993). The main points to remember are that blood pressure measurements should be taken in a consistent manner and that assessment focuses on trends, rather than a single reading.

Presence of edema, in addition to hypertension, warrants additional investigation. Edema, assessed by distribution and degree, is described as dependent or pitting. If periorbital or facial edema is not obvious, the pregnant woman is asked if it was present when she awoke.

Deep tendon reflexes (DTRs) are evaluated if preeclampsia is suspected. The biceps and patellar reflexes and ankle clonus are assessed and the findings recorded. The evaluation of DTR is especially important if the woman is being treated with magnesium sulfate; absence of DTR is an early indication of impending magnesium toxicity.

Proteinuria is determined from dipstick testing of a clean-catch or catheter urine specimen. A reading greater than +1 on two or more occasions at least 4 hours apart should be followed by a 24-hour urine collection (Brown & Buddle, 1995). A 24-hour collection for protein and creatinine clearance is more reflective of true renal status, because proteinuria is a later sign in the course of preeclampsia. Urine output is assessed for volume of at least 25 to 30 mL/hour or 100 mL/4 hours. Placement of an indwelling Foley catheter with a urometer facilitates accurate assessment of fluid balance and early signs of renal compromise.

An important ongoing assessment is determination of fetal status. Uteroplacental perfusion decreases in women with preeclampsia, thereby placing the fetus in jeopardy. The spiral arteries of the placental bed are subject to vasospasm. When this occurs, perfusion between maternal circulation and the intervillous space is compromised, decreasing blood flow and oxygenation to the fetus. Oligohydramnios, IUGR, fetal compromise, and intrauterine fetal death all are associated with preeclampsia. The fetal heart rate (FHR) should be assessed for baseline rate, variability, and reassuring versus nonreassuring patterns. The presence of abnormal baseline rate, decreased or absent variability, or late decelerations indicates fetal intolerance to the intrauterine environment. The presence of variable decelerations, antepartum or intrapartum, suggests decreased amniotic fluid volumes (ie, oligohydramnios), increasing the risk of umbilical cord compression, and fetal compromise. Biophysical or biochemical monitoring for fetal well-being may be ordered. These tests include fetal movement counting, nonstress testing (NST), contraction stress test, biophysical profile (BPP), and serial ultrasonography (Phelan, 1991). As long as the fetus continues to grow in an appropriate manner, it can be inferred that the placenta and uterine blood flow are appropriate.

Uterine tonicity is evaluated for signs of labor and abruptio placentae. If labor is suspected, a vaginal examination for cervical changes is indicated. Preterm contractions or a tense, tender uterus may be early indications of an abruptio placentae.

Assessments target signs of deterioration from mild preeclampsia to severe preeclampsia or eclampsia. Signs of liver involvement (eg, epigastric pain, elevated liver function test, thrombocytopenia), renal failure, worsening hypertension, cerebral involvement, and developing coagulopathies must be assessed and documented. Respirations are assessed for rales (ie, crackles) or diminished breath sounds, which may indicate pulmonary edema. Noninvasive assessment parameters include level of consciousness, blood pressure, hemoglobin oxygen saturation (ie, pulse oximetry), electrocardiogram (ECG) findings, and urine output. Invasive hemodynamic monitoring with a flow-directed pulmonary artery catheter (Swan-Ganz) may be indicated in selected patients (Clark et al., 1997).

Laboratory Tests

The nurse assists in obtaining a number of blood and urine specimens to aid in the diagnosis of preeclampsia, HELLP syndrome, or chronic hypertension. No known laboratory tests predict the development of preeclampsia (Gavette & Roberts, 1987). Laboratory abnormalities are nonspecific in preeclampsia, but changes can reflect underlying multiorgan system dysfunctions (Barton et al., 1999). Thrombocytopenia is the most common hematologic abnormality, but routine assessment of the other coagulation factors is not recommended until the platelet concentration is less than 100,000/mm^3. Unless a preexisting coagulopathy is present, the woman is not at an increased risk for developing a coagulopathy until the platelet level falls below 100,000/mm^3 (Leduc, Wheeler, Kirshon, Mitchell, & Cotton, 1992). Baseline laboratory test information is useful in the early diagnosis of preeclampsia and for comparison with results obtained to evaluate progression and severity of disease. Display 8–4 provides the common laboratory assessments for a woman with hypertension during pregnancy.

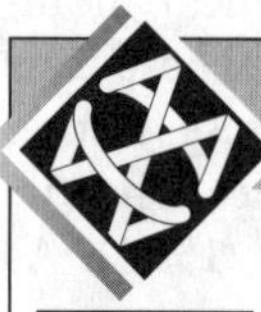

DISPLAY 8–4

Laboratory Values Assessed for Women With Hypertension During Pregnancy

- Complete blood count
  - Hemoglobin
  - Hematocrit
  - Platelet count
- Chemistry
  - Electrolytes
  - Blood urea nitrogen (BUN)
  - Serum creatinine
  - Serum albumin
  - Uric acid
  - Serum calcium
  - Serum sodium
  - Serum magnesium
  - Liver function tests: lactate dehydrogenase, aspartate aminotransferase, alanine aminotransferase
- Urine
  - Urinalysis for protein
  - 24-hour creatinine clearance may be measured in patients with chronic hypertension or renal disease
  - 24-hour urine for sodium excretion
  - Specific gravity
- Coagulation profile
  - Platelet count
  - Prothrombin and partial thromboplastin times
  - Fibrinogen
  - Fibrin split or fibrin degradation products
  - Bleeding time
  - D-dimer

Pharmacologic Therapies

Pharmacologic therapies are instituted for two purposes: seizure prophylaxis and antihypertensive management.

Magnesium Sulfate

Magnesium sulfate ($MgSO_4$) is the drug of choice in the management of preeclampsia to prevent seizure activity. $MgSO_4$ is administered as a secondary infusion by an infusion-controlled device to achieve serum levels of approximately 5 to 8 mg/dL (4 to 7 mEq/dL). The loading dose is a 4- to 6-g intravenous bolus over 15 to 30 minutes, followed by a maintenance infusion of 2 to 3 g/hour.

The action of $MgSO_4$ as an anticonvulsant is controversial, but it is thought to decrease neuromuscular irritability and block the release of acetylcholine at neuromuscular junctions, depressing the vasomotor center and thereby depressing central nervous system (CNS) irritability.

Side effects of $MgSO_4$ are dose dependent and include flushing, nausea, vomiting, headache, lower maternal temperature, blurred vision, respiratory depression, and cardiac arrest. The effect of $MgSO_4$ on fetal heart baseline variability is controversial.

Nursing responsibilities and assessments for women receiving $MgSO_4$ include

- Assessing maternal baseline vital signs, DTR, and urinary output before initiation of therapy and reassessing per institution protocol
- Preparing $MgSO_4$ according to protocol
- Establishing the primary intravenous line and intravenously administering $MgSO_4$ piggyback by means of a controlled-infusion device
- Documenting $MgSO_4$ infusion in grams per hour
- Continuous fetal assessment
- Keeping calcium gluconate (1 g of a 10% solution) at bedside
- Being cautious with concurrent administration of narcotics, CNS depressants, calcium channel blockers, and β blockers; discontinuing $MgSO_4$; and notifying the physician if signs of toxicity occur (including loss of DTRs, respiratory depression, oliguria, respiratory arrest, and cardiac arrest) or if the woman complains of shortness of breath or chest pain

Phenytoin

Phenytoin (Dilantin) has also been proposed for eclampsia prophylaxis; however, it is not a first-line therapy in the United States. Clinical studies have not demonstrated better results with phenytoin compared with $MgSO_4$ (The Eclampsia Collaborative Group,

1995). Because of a lack of experience with phenytoin and the significant maternal side effects, $MgSO_4$ remains the first-line drug in the United States.

Antihypertensive Therapy

Pharmacologic therapies directed at the control of significant hypertension include a variety of agents. Several general precautions should be considered when antihypertensive agents are ordered: antihypertensive therapy is initiated when blood pressure is sustained at greater than 110 mm Hg diastolic to prevent maternal cerebral vascular accident; the effect of the agent may depend on intravascular volume status, and hypovolemia resulting from increased capillary permeability and hemoconcentration may need correction before the initiation of therapy; and diastolic blood pressure should be maintained between 90 and 100 mm Hg to maintain uteroplacental perfusion.

Hydralazine Hydrochloride

Hydralazine hydrochloride (Apresoline) is considered by many to be the first-line agent to decrease hypertension. Dosage regimens vary, but intermittent intravenous boluses generally work equally as well as continuous infusions; there is also less chance of rebound hypotension with intermittent boluses. Side effects of hydralazine include flushing, headache, maternal and fetal tachycardia, palpitations, and uteroplacental insufficiency with subsequent fetal tachycardia and late decelerations. Because hydralazine increases maternal cardiac output and heart rate, hypertension may worsen.

Labetalol

Labetalol has been used in place of hydralazine for the management of hypertension. Dosage regimens vary, based on physician experience and preference. Labetalol is contraindicated in women with asthma and those with greater than first-degree heart block (Chez & Sibai, 1994). Because of labetalol's α- and β-adrenergic blockage, transient fetal and neonatal hypotension, bradycardia, and hypoglycemia are possible.

Postpartum Management

Immediate postpartum curettage has been associated with a more rapid recovery for women with severe preeclampsia, although more research is needed in this area (Magann et al., 1993). Most women are clinically stable within 48 hours after birth. However, because of the risk of eclampsia during the first 24 to 48 hours postpartum, careful monitoring is essential and should include frequent assessments of vital signs, level of consciousness, DTRs, urinary output, and laboratory data. Intravenous $MgSO_4$ is usually continued for 24 hours postpartum. It is important to be alert for early signs and symptoms of complications of preeclampsia such as postpartum hemorrhage, DIC, pulmonary edema, HELLP syndrome, increased intracranial pressure, and intracranial hemorrhage. Intensity of monitoring and progression of activity are based on the patient's condition. After vital signs and mental status are stable, laboratory data indicate condition is improving, urinary output is reassuring, and intravenous $MgSO_4$ is discontinued, the frequency of maternal assessments can be decreased from 1 to 2 hours to 4 to 8 hours, the Foley catheter is removed, and the patient is encouraged to ambulate. It is important to provide assistance and assess stability during initial ambulation, after bed rest, and after intravenous administration of $MgSO_4$ during the intrapartum and postpartum period. Efforts should be made to initiate maternal–newborn attachment by bringing the newborn, if stable, to visit the mother. Photographs of the newborn can be taken and provided to the woman if the maternal or newborn condition prevents visitation.

HELLP Syndrome

HELLP syndrome, a multisystem disease, is a form of severe preeclampsia in which the woman presents with a variety of complaints and exhibits common laboratory markers for a syndrome of hemolysis (H), elevated liver enzymes (EL), and low platelets (LP). This subset of women progresses from preeclampsia to the development of multiple organ involvement and damage. The complaints range from malaise, epigastric pain, nausea, and vomiting to nonspecific viral syndrome–like symptoms. On presentation, these patients are generally in the second or early third trimester and initially may show few signs of preeclampsia. Because of the presenting symptoms, these patients often receive a nonobstetric diagnosis, delaying treatment and increasing maternal and perinatal morbidity and mortality (Sibai, 1990b; Weinstein, 1982, 1985). Assessments and management of the woman diagnosed with HELLP syndrome are the same as for the woman with severe preeclampsia.

Eclampsia

Eclampsia is the development of seizures or coma or both in a woman with signs and symptoms of preeclampsia. Other causes of seizures must be excluded. Eclampsia can occur antepartum, intrapartum, or postpartum; approximately 50% of cases occur antepartum (Fairlie & Sibai, 1993). The immediate care during a seizure is to ensure a patent airway. Once this has been attained, adequate oxygenation must be maintained by use of supplemental oxygen. $MgSO_4$ (and amobarbital sodium for recurrent convulsions) is given according to the institutional protocol (Sibai, 1990c). Aspiration is a leading cause of maternal morbidity after an eclamptic seizure. After initial stabilization and airway management, the nurse should anticipate orders for a chest radiograph and possibly arterial blood gas (ABG) determinations to exclude the possibility of aspiration. Rapid assessments of uterine activity, cervical status, and fetal status are performed. During the seizure, membranes may rupture, and the cervix may dilate because the uterus becomes hypercontractile and hypertonic. If birth is not imminent, the timing and route of delivery and the induction of labor versus cesarean birth depend on maternal and fetal status. All medications and therapy are merely temporary measures.

BLEEDING

Significance and Incidence

Hemorrhagic complications during pregnancy are a significant causative factor in adverse maternal–fetal outcomes. Although bleeding can cause considerable problems for the mother, the fetus is especially at risk. Major maternal blood loss can result in negative alterations in maternal hemodynamic status and maternal–fetal exchange. Maternal blood loss decreases oxygen-carrying capacity and adversely affects oxygen delivery to the fetus. When bleeding affects blood flow to the placenta, the fetus is at risk for progressive physiologic deterioration (ie, hypoxemia, hypoxia, asphyxia, and death). This risk is directly related to the amount and duration of blood loss. Other fetal risks related to maternal hemorrhage include blood loss, anemia, and preterm birth. Bleeding that is fetal in origin is always significant because of the small volume of fetal blood. Total blood volume in the fetus is approximately 80 to 100 mL/kg, and rapid exsanguination can result in severe neurologic injury or fetal death.

Significant bleeding is an obstetric emergency. Although the physiologic changes of pregnancy prepare the woman for blood loss at birth, complications unique to pregnancy can lead to blood loss that exceeds the ability of those compensatory adaptations to protect the mother and fetus. Major blood loss predisposes the woman to an increased risk of hypovolemia, anemia, infection, and preterm labor and birth. The nurse must be alert to the symptoms of hemorrhage and shock and be prepared to act quickly to minimize blood loss and hasten maternal and fetal stabilization. Approximately up to 15% of maternal cardiac output (1 L/min) flows through the placental bed at term; unresolved bleeding can result in maternal exsanguination in 8 to 10 minutes (O'Brien, 1993; Thorp, 1993). In addition to the physiologic implications of bleeding during pregnancy, the mother experiences emotional distress as she worries about the outcome for herself and her baby. Although maternal mortality decreased significantly during the 20th century, hemorrhage remains a major cause of maternal death in all parts of the world. Maternal mortality rates in the United States during the past 15 years have remained consistent at approximately 7.5 to 8.4 per 100,000 live births (Centers for Disease Control and Prevention [CDC], 1999), but hemorrhage still accounts for almost 30% of maternal deaths (Berg, Atrash, Koonin, & Tucker, 1996). The risk for maternal mortality is consistently higher among African-American women, which may reflect social, economic, and cultural barriers to healthcare.

Approximately one in five pregnancies is complicated by bleeding; the incidence and cause of bleeding varies by trimester (Thorp, 1993). Most bleeding occurring in the first trimester of pregnancy is related to spontaneous abortion and is generally not life threatening. Ectopic pregnancy is the leading cause of life-threatening hemorrhage during the first trimester. Antepartum hemorrhage of unknown origin after 24 weeks' gestation is associated with a higher incidence of preterm labor and birth and congenital anomalies (Chan & To, 1999). Hemorrhage during the antepartum period usually results from disruption of the placental implantation site (involving a normally implanted placenta or placenta previa) or uterine rupture (spontaneous or trauma related) (Clark, 1997). Most serious obstetric hemorrhage occurs in the postpartum period as a result of uterine atony after placental separation. Other causes of postpartum hemorrhage include retained placenta, uterine rupture, uterine inversion, genital tract trauma, and coagulopathy (Clark, 1997).

The reported incidence of placenta previa at birth varies widely. This variation results from differences in the time of diagnosis. Symptomatic placenta previa is identified in approximately 0.05% of pregnancies at birth (Clark, 1999). Low implantation of the placenta is much more common during early pregnancy, but most of these cases resolve or are not found to be clinically significant as pregnancy progresses (Frederiksen, Glassenberg, & Stika, 1999; Taipale, Hiilesmaa, & Ylostalo, 1997). Up to 45% of placentas can be classified as low lying during the second trimester by routine ultrasonography, because it is difficult to determine which placentas cross the cervical os during ultrasonographic examination in early pregnancy. By the third trimester, visualization by ultrasonography is more accurate, and those placentas mistakenly thought to be implanted on both sides of the cervical os are drawn upward by the growth of the underlying myometrium (Clark, 1999).

Placenta accreta is an uncommon abnormality of placental implantation and is one of the most serious complications of placenta previa. In addition to placenta previa, prior uterine surgery significantly increases the risk of placenta accreta. With placenta previa, the risk of developing placenta accreta is 10% to 25% for women with a history of one prior cesarean birth and rises to more than 50% for women with two or more cesarean births or second-trimester pregnancy terminations (Clark, 1999).

The incidence of abruptio placentae varies in the literature according to the population studied and diagnostic criteria. In the United States, reported ranges are between 0.2% to 2.7% of all pregnancies after the second trimester (Ananth, Savitz, & Williams, 1996). The average rate is one case of abruptio placentae per 120 births (0.83%) based on all available data. A placental abruption significant enough to cause fetal death is less common (1 in 420 births), but as use of cocaine has increased, fetal death associated with abruptio placentae has risen in selected populations (Clark, 1999). Risk of recurrence in subsequent pregnancies has been reported to be as high as 5.5% to 16.6%. This rate is approximately 30 times higher than for pregnant women without a history of a prior abruptio placentae. The risk of recurrence for women with a history of two placental abruptions increases to approximately 25% (Clark, 1999).

Vasa previa, in which umbilical arteries and veins abnormally implanted throughout the amnion traverse the cervical os in front of the presenting part of the fetus at the time of rupture, is a rare but life-threatening complication for the fetus (Oyelese, Turner, Lees, & Campbell, 1999). The reported incidence is approximately 1 in 3,000 births (Clark, 1999). Rupture of the vessels during spontaneous or artificial rupture of membranes usually leads to fetal exsanguination or severe neurologic fetal injury before recognition of the cause of bleeding and before an emergent cesarean birth can be accomplished. Up to 75% of cases of ruptured vasa previa result in fetal death (Clark, 1999).

Uterine rupture is another significant cause of maternal hemorrhage. The risk of uterine rupture with a prior low transverse incision is 0.2% to 1.5% (American College of Obstetricians and Gynecologists [ACOG], 1999c). The occurrence of uterine rupture depends on the number, type, and location of the previous incisions (ACOG, 1999c; Wing & Paul, 1999). Miller, Diaz, and Paul (1994) found the risk of uterine rupture nearly tripled for women with a history of more than two prior low transverse cesarean births compared with women with one prior cesarean birth (0.06% versus 1.7%). The incidence of rupture of a vertical scar from a prior cesarean birth varies but has been reported to be as high as 7% (ACOG, 1999c; Shipp et al., 1999). The risk of uterine rupture for women with a T-shaped incision from a prior cesarean birth is between 4% and 9% (ACOG, 1999c).

Waiting for spontaneous labor (avoiding cervical ripening agents and oxytocin) appears to significantly decrease the risk of uterine rupture for women attempting vaginal birth after cesarean birth (VBAC) (Holt & Mueller, 1997; Leung, Farmer, Leung, Medearis, & Paul, 1993; Rageth, Juzi, & Grossenbacher, 1999; Zelop, Shipp, Cohen, Repke, & Leiberman, 2000). There are enough data to suggest that prostaglandins E_1 and E_2 and high rates of oxytocin infusion increase the risk for rupture (Blanco, Collins, Willis, & Prien, 1992; Grubb, Kjos, & Paul, 1996; Johnson, Oriol, & Flood, 1991; Norman, & Ekman, 1992; Rosen, Dickinson, & Westhoff, 1991). Because of the significant risk of uterine rupture with the use of misoprostol for cervical ripening or induction (Bennett, 1997; Cunha, Bughalho, Bisque, & Bergstrom, 1999; Plaut, Schwartz, & Lubarsky, 1999; Sciscione, Nguyen, Manley, Shlossman, & Colmorgen, 1998; Wing, Lovett, & Paul, 1998), ACOG (1999a, 1999b) does not recommend misoprostol for women attempting VBAC.

The incidence of uterine inversion is approximately 1 case in 3,600 births (Abouleish, Joumaa, Lopez, & Gupta, 1995). Improper management of the third stage of labor increases the likelihood of iatrogenic uterine inversion.

Postpartum hemorrhage remains one of the leading causes of maternal death worldwide. Early postpartum hemorrhage (≤24 hours after birth) is most frequently caused by uterine atony, retained placental fragments, lower genital tract lacerations, uterine rupture, uterine inversion, placenta accreta, and coagulopathies. Late postpartum hemorrhage (>24 hours to 6 weeks after birth) is more likely to be caused by infection, placental site subinvolution, retained placental fragments and coagulopathy (ACOG, 1998b). The incidence of postpartum hemorrhage after cesarean birth is approximately 6.4% compared with 3.9% after vaginal birth (ACOG, 1998b).

Definitions and Clinical Manifestations

The definitions, cause, pathophysiology, and clinical manifestations of the most frequently occurring causes of bleeding in pregnancy are described in the following sections. A diagnosis-specific summary of expected management is included. A more detailed summary of nursing interventions for bleeding during pregnancy concludes this section.

Placenta Previa

Placenta previa is the abnormal implantation of the placenta in the lower uterine segment. Asymptomatic placenta previa is often diagnosed during routine ultrasound performed in the second trimester. Most cases no longer demonstrate placenta previa by the third trimester (Taipale et al., 1997), although these women are at increased risk for other obstetric complications such placental abruption, IUGR, and hemorrhage (Clark, 1999). The term *placental migration* (a misnomer) has been used to describe the apparent "movement," but as the uterus grows, the placenta moves upward with the growth of the placenta and away from the os. The placenta does not actually move. It has been theorized that the placental tissue that surrounds the cervical os does not develop as well as the placental tissue that is in the myometrium (Clark, 1999; Taipale et al., 1997). By the end of 40 weeks of pregnancy, the incidence of placenta previa is approximately 0.05% (Clark, 1999; Taipale et al., 1997). The most significant risk factors include prior uterine surgery resulting in uterine scarring and history of a prior placenta previa (Ananth, Smulian, & Vintzileos, 1997; Chelmow, Andrew, & Baker, 1996; Macones, Sehdev, Parry, Morgan, & Berlin, 1997; Miller, Chollet, & Goodwin, 1997). Late development and implantation of the ovum, more frequently occurring in older women, may also play a role in placenta previa. Display 8–5 lists the risk factors associated with placenta previa.

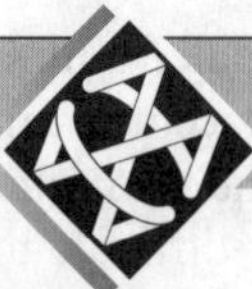

DISPLAY 8–5

Factors Associated with Placenta Previa

- Previous placenta previa
- Previous cesarean birth
- Induced or spontaneous abortions involving suction curettage
- Multiparity
- Advanced maternal age (>35 years)
- Cigarette smoking
- Multiple gestation
- Fetal hydrops fetalis
- Large placenta
- Uterine anomalies
- Fibroid tumors
- Endometritis
- African-American or Asian ethnicity

Placental implantation has traditionally been classified as normal, low-lying, partial placenta previa and total placenta previa (Fig. 8–2). Clark (1999) proposed a new classification system: placenta previa: the placenta covers the internal os in the third trimester; marginal placenta previa: the placenta is within 2 to 3 cm of the internal os but does not cover the os). The rationale for this classification system is the ambiguity and lack of clinical utility of the term *low-lying placenta*. Until recently there had been no accepted definition of how close the placenta must be to mandate cesarean birth or double setup examination. It is now known that there is no increased risk of intrapartum hemorrhage if the distance from the lower margin of the placenta to the internal os is at least 2 to 3 cm. With this classification system, the term low-lying placenta would be reserved for cases in which the exact relationship of the placenta to the cervical os has not been determined or for cases of apparent placenta previa before the third trimester. As the ability to more accurately visualize placental location increases because of advancements in ultrasound technologies, this classification system may be adopted in clinical practice.

Clinical Manifestations

Painless uterine bleeding during the second or third trimester characterizes placenta previa. The first significant bleeding episode may occur before 30 weeks' gestation; some women never exhibit bleeding as a symptom until labor develops (Clark, 1999). Rarely is the first episode life threatening or a cause of hypovolemic shock. The bright red bleeding may be intermittent or continuous. After the bleeding episode, women may demonstrate "spotting" of bright red or dark brown blood on the peripad.

Diagnosis

The standard for the diagnosis of placenta previa is an ultrasound examination. It may be a transabdominal, transvaginal, or translabial ultrasound. Transvaginal ultrasound provides precise information regarding the placement of the placenta in relation to the cervical

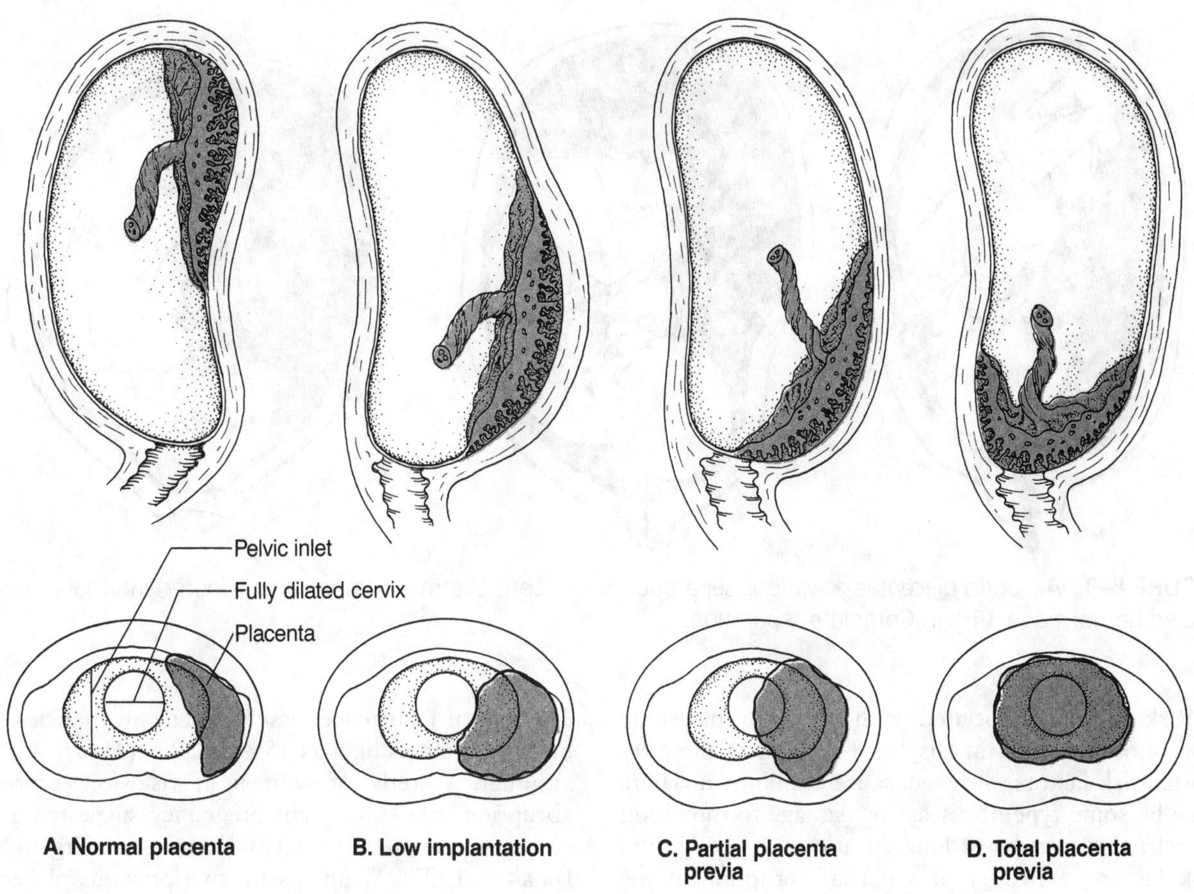

FIGURE 8–2. Placenta previa.

os (Taipale et al., 1997). If ultrasound reveals a normally implanted placenta, a speculum examination is performed to exclude local causes of bleeding (eg, cervicitis, polyps, carcinoma of the cervix), and a coagulation profile is obtained to exclude other causes of bleeding. Diagnosis of placenta previa has increased dramatically with the advent of ultrasound, especially with the vaginal transducer. It is most often diagnosed before the onset of bleeding when an ultrasound examination is performed for other indications.

Management

Conservative management is usually possible when the fetus is not mature and maternal status is stable. When survival is likely and fetal lung maturity is achieved, birth can be accomplished. Most births are by cesarean section, although vaginal birth may be achieved if the placental edge does not completely cover the cervical os. This type of vaginal birth occurs in the operating room with personnel and equipment available for a cesarean birth if needed (ie, a double setup).

Patients are frequently hospitalized with the initial bleeding episode. Those with recurrent bleeding episodes, recurrent uterine activity associated with bleeding, or evidence of fetal or maternal compromise usually remain hospitalized until birth. Women who experience an initial bleeding episode that resolves, are hemodynamically stable, demonstrate fetal well-being, and have emergency services readily available to them are candidates for expectant management as outpatients (Love & Wallace, 1996; Wing, Paul, & Millar, 1996).

Abruptio Placentae

Abruptio placentae, or premature separation of the placenta, is the detachment of part or all of the placenta from its implantation site, typically occurring after the 20th week of pregnancy (Fig. 8–3). Premature separation of the placenta is a serious event and accounts for about 15% of all neonatal deaths (Ananth et al., 1996; Witlin, Saade, Mattar, & Sibai, 1999). More than 50% of these deaths are the result of preterm birth. Other causes of fetal death include intrauterine hypoxia and asphyxia.

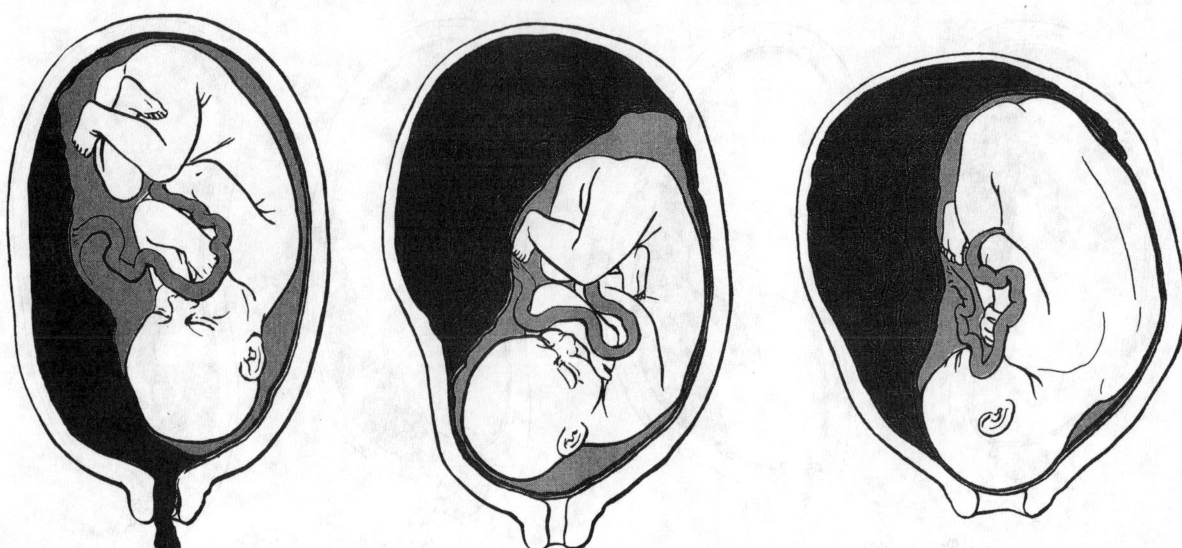

FIGURE 8–3. Abruptio placentae at various separation sites. (*Left*) External hemorrhage. (*Center*) Internal or concealed hemorrhage. (*Right*) Complete separation.

Risk factors associated with abruptio placentae abruption are listed in Display 8–6. Despite these reported risk factors, the exact cause is unknown. There may be some type of disease or damage to the blood vessels; this may be of long duration. Of the known risk factors, a history of a partial abruption in the current pregnancy is a significant risk for the woman.

DISPLAY 8–6

Factors Associated with Abruptio Placentae

- Partial abruption of current pregnancy
- Prior abruptio placentae
- Rapid decompression of the uterus, such as birth of the first of multiple fetuses and amniotic reduction therapy in polyhydramnios
- Hypertension
- Preterm premature rupture of membranes <34 weeks' gestation
- Prior cesarean birth
- Blunt abdominal trauma
- Multiparity
- Cocaine use
- Cigarette smoking
- Extremely short length of the umbilical cord
- Uterine anomalies
- Uterine fibroids at the placental implantation site
- Use of intrauterine pressure catheters during labor

The risk of recurrence in subsequent pregnancies has been reported as high as 15% to 30% (Thorp, 1993), although a study of women at risk for recurrent abruption in a subsequent pregnancy suggested a recurrence rate of only 4.4% (Rasmussen, Irgens, & Dalaker, 1997). Women with two previous placental abruptions have a risk of recurrence ranging between 19% and 40% (Rasmussen et al., 1997). Women with severe preeclampsia and eclampsia are at high risk for abruptio placentae. This high-risk status includes women with mild pregnancy-induced or chronic hypertension. Approximately 50% of placental abruptions severe enough to cause fetal death are associated with hypertension (Clark, 1999). Quantitative proteinuria and the degree of blood pressure elevation are not predictive of an abruption (Witlin et al., 1999). Investigators concluded that the greatest morbidity occurred in preeclamptic women with preterm gestations not receiving prenatal care (Witlin et al., 1999).

Clinical Manifestations

Abruptio placentae is suspected in the woman presenting with sudden-onset, intense, often localized, uterine pain or tenderness with or without vaginal bleeding. Another common presentation is preterm contractions with or without vaginal bleeding in the absence of abdominal pain. The woman may also present with painless vaginal bleeding, although this is uncommon. In mild cases, the pain from abruption may be difficult to distinguish from the pain of labor contractions. In many cases, pain is localized to the area of the abruption. When placental implantation is posterior, lower back pain may be more prominent than uterine tenderness. Occasionally, nausea and vomiting may occur. Visible blood loss from an abruptio placentae may not be proportional to the area of placental detachment because blood may become trapped behind the placenta. If the abruption is located centrally, no bleeding is visualized initially. Approximately 10% of women present with concealed hemorrhage (Clark, 1999). Marginal separations and large abruptions are associated with bright red bleeding and are almost always accompanied by contractions that are usually of low amplitude and high frequency (Clark, 1999). Contractions may be difficult to record if there is an increase in uterine resting tone or early in gestation. Palpation for uterine contractions or hypertonus is necessary. The woman may present with preterm contractions with an occult abruption. Fetal assessment by electronic fetal monitoring is accomplished before obtaining a full uterine ultrasound because most abruptions cannot be accurately identified with ultrasonography. In a retrospective study of 167 patients presenting with bleeding between 13 and 26 weeks' gestation, only 31% demonstrated an identifiable intrauterine clot (Signore, Sood, & Richards, 1998).

The fetal response to abruptio placentae depends on the volume of blood loss and the extent of uteroplacental insufficiency. Anticipatory nursing care includes being alert to the possibility of an abruption in the presence of any or all of the following: fetal tachycardia; bradycardia; loss of variability; presence of late decelerations; decreasing baseline (especially from tachycardia to a normal or near normal baseline with minimal or absent variability); a sinusoidal FHR pattern; low-amplitude, high-frequency contractions; uterine hypertonus; and abdominal pain.

The mother's serum or vaginal blood may be tested for the presence of fetal cells. Fetal-to-maternal transfer of blood is documented by the presence of fetal cells in maternal serum. Depending on fetal age and size, the number of fetal cells present in maternal blood can be calculated to estimate the fetal blood loss. Formulas for this calculation can be found in the maternal–fetal medicine literature and in laboratory manuals.

Women with an abruption may demonstrate very rapid labor progress (Mahon, Chazotte, & Cohen, 1994). However, for women who are not at term or not in labor, the pregnancy may be continued if the abruption is small and the fetus is stable. Chronic abruptio placentae may develop, with the woman experiencing episodic bleeding, subjecting the fetus to prolonged stress. Risk of developing DIC exists during abruption because of release of thromboplastin from the site into the maternal bloodstream.

Diagnosis

The diagnosis of abruptio placentae is based on the woman's history, physical examination, and laboratory studies. Examination of the placenta at delivery confirms the diagnosis. Ultrasonography is used to exclude placenta previa; however, it is not diagnostic for abruption (Clark, 1999; Lowe & Cunningham, 1990). Abruptions are classified as partial, marginal (ie, only the margin of the placenta is involved), or total (ie, complete).

Management

Treatment depends on maternal and fetal status. In the presence of fetal compromise, severe hemorrhage, coagulopathy, poor labor progress, or increasing uterine resting tone, an emergent cesarean birth is performed. In an older but reliable study, 22% of all perinatal deaths from abruption occurred after the patient was hospitalized, with 30% occurring in the first 2 hours (Knab, 1978). If the mother is hemodynamically stable, the fetus is alive with a reassuring FHR tracing, or if the fetus is dead, a vaginal birth may be attempted. If the mother is hemodynamically unstable, attempts are first directed at maternal stabilization.

Fluid resuscitation may be aggressive in the presence of hemorrhage. Blood replacement products and lactated Ringer's solution are infused in quantities necessary to maintain a urine output of 30 to 60 mL/hour and a hematocrit of approximately 30%. Some experts suggest 1 unit of blood replacement for every 4 L of intravenous fluid. With rapid volume intravenous infusions, the nurse anticipates the possibility of pulmonary edema due lower colloid osmotic pressure in pregnancy.

Abnormal Placental Implantation

Abnormal adherence of the placenta occurs for unknown reasons but is thought to be the result of zygote implantation in a zone of defective endometrium. Abnormal adherence of the placenta is diagnosed in only about 1 of every 12,000 births. At least 15% of cases of abnormally adherent placenta (all types) are associated with placenta previa (Zahn & Yeomans, 1990). The risk is increased with the number of previous cesarean births, increasing to 67% in a patient with four or more cesarean births presenting with placenta previa (Clark, Koonings, & Phelan, 1985). Patients with one cesarean birth presenting with placenta previa in a second pregnancy have a 24% risk of placenta accreta (Clark et al., 1985). Other risk factors include elevated maternal serum α-fetoprotein (MSAFP) and free β-human chorionic gonadotropin (hCG) levels in the second trimester and advanced maternal age.

Placenta accreta occurs when there is a lack of decidua basalis, so that the placenta is implanted directly into the myometrium. Complete accreta occurs when the entire placenta is adherent; partial accreta occurs with one or more cotyledons adherent; and focal accreta occurs with one piece of a cotyledon adherent. *Placenta increta* is the abnormal invasion of the trophoblastic cells into the uterine myometrium. *Placenta percreta* occurs when the trophoblast cells penetrate the uterine musculature, and the placenta develops on organs in the vicinity of the percreta. The placenta percreta can adhere to the bladder and other pelvic organs and vessels. Figure 8–4 demonstrates abnormal adherence of the placenta.

Placenta accreta, increta, and percreta tend to occur if there is lack of decidua basalis in the area of uterus where the placenta would normally implant. Elevated MSAFP in the second trimester has been associated with abnormal adherence of the placenta (Hung et al., 1999; Wheeler, Anderson, Kelly, & Boehm, 1996). It is theorized that MSAFP can diffuse more easily over the increased surface area. Because ultrasound is routinely performed for a woman with an elevated MSAFP level, placenta accreta, increta, or percreta may be diagnosed prenatally (Hung et al., 1999). Placenta increta has been diagnosed by ultrasound as early as 18 weeks (Wheeler et al., 1996), and placenta percreta has been diagnosed in the first trimester with magnetic resonance imaging (Thorp, Wells, Wiest, Jeffries, & Lyles, 1998).

The diagnosis of an abnormally adherent placenta was made historically when manual separation of a retained placenta was attempted. If the placenta does not separate readily (even a portion), rapid surgical intervention may be indicated. The mother with an abnormally attached placenta is at increased risk for hemorrhage; 90% of women lose more than 3,000 mL of blood intraoperatively (Hudon, Belfort, & Broome, 1998).

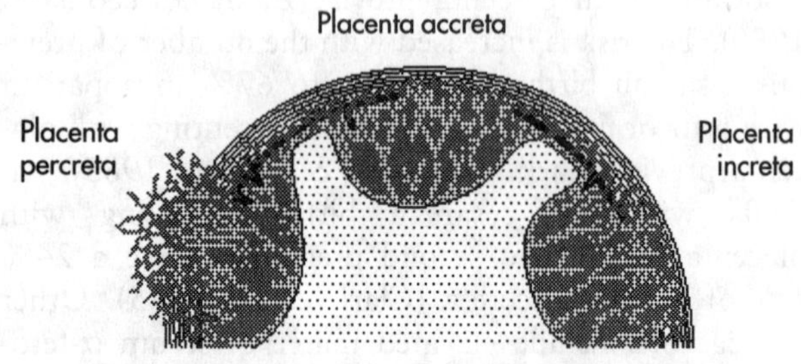

FIGURE 8–4. Abnormal adherence of the placenta.

Patients who are diagnosed before birth are treated by a multidisciplinary team to minimize complications. The goal is to prevent shock, thrombosis, infection, and adult respiratory distress syndrome (ARDS). Patients may receive erythropoietin before the surgery, and thrombosis prevention, antibiotics, and fluid resuscitation during the surgery. Hemodynamic monitoring is continuous. It is recommended that 8 to 10 units of packed red blood cells be available in the operating room, with the blood bank maintaining the same amount (Hudon et al., 1998). Anesthesia, surgery, and urology services are involved in the cesarean hysterectomy. Radiology may be needed if selective embolization of the hypogastric arteries with an absorbable gel is performed to reduce blood loss (Dubois, Garel, Grignon, Lemay, & Leduc, 1997; Hudon et al., 1998).

Patients diagnosed at the time of birth are at higher risk for developing the previously described complications, as well as for an increased risk of maternal death. Mobilization of nursing and medical staff, blood bank, surgery, and radiology is necessary immediately to perform the cesarean hysterectomy.

Vasa Previa

Vasa previa is the result of a velamentous insertion of the umbilical cord. With vasa previa, the umbilical cord is implanted into the membranes rather than the placenta. The vessels then traverse within the membrane, crossing the cervical os before reaching the placenta. The umbilical vein and arteries are not surrounded by Wharton jelly, so they have no supportive tissue. The umbilical blood vessels are at risk for laceration; this occurs most frequently during rupture of the membranes (Oyelese et al., 1999). The sudden appearance of bright red blood at the time of spontaneous or artificial rupture of the membranes, coupled with the sudden onset of a nonreassuring FHR pattern, should immediately alert the nurse to the possibility of vasa previa. Immediate cesarean section is indicated in the presence of vasa previa. Vasa previa rupture may also occur before or after rupture of the membranes; the diagnosis is considered for women with limited antenatal bleeding and nonreassuring FHR patterns. Risk factors associated with vasa previa are listed in Display 8–7.

Although it rarely occurs (generally 1 in 3000 births or 1 in 50 cases in which there is a velamentous insertion of the cord), vasa previa is associated with high incidence of fetal morbidity and mortality because fetal bleeding rapidly leads to shock and exsanguination (Oyelese et al., 1999; Sherer & Anyaegbunam,

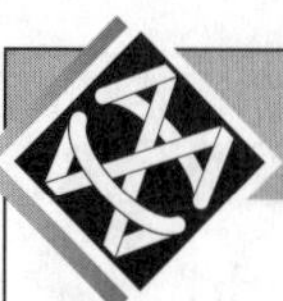

DISPLAY 8–7

Factors Associated with Vasa Previa

- Succenturiate-lobed placenta
- Bilobed placenta
- Placenta previa
- In vitro fertilization
- Multiple gestation
- Fetal anomaly

1997). Vasa previa is occasionally diagnosed before rupture of the membranes by examiners palpating a pulsing vessel, directly visualizing a vessel, or identifying fetal blood cells in vaginal blood. Diagnosis before birth may be made with transvaginal color Doppler ultrasound in patients with known risk factors. If noted, planned cesarean birth is accomplished. In the case of an antenatal bleed, a number of laboratory tests are available to determine if the blood is maternal or fetal. Because the fastest test (Ogita) still takes 5 minutes (Odunsi, Bullough, Henzel, & Polanska, 1996; Oyelese et al., 1999), these tests have limited clinical utility during labor because of the short time required from rupture to birth to save the fetus.

Uterine Rupture

Uterine rupture may be a catastrophic event for the woman and fetus, whether related to rupture of a uterine scar from prior uterine surgery, hyperstimulation, trauma, or rarely, spontaneous rupture of the uterus. The terms *uterine rupture* and *uterine dehiscence* are sometimes used interchangeably in the literature. Uterine rupture refers to the actual separation of the uterine myometrium or previous uterine scar, with rupture of the membranes and extrusion of the fetus or fetal parts into the peritoneal cavity. Dehiscence refers to a partial separation of the old scar, but the fetus usually remains inside the uterus. Excessive bleeding usually occurs with uterine rupture, whereas bleeding is generally minimal with dehiscence.

Uterine rupture occurs most frequently in women with a previous uterine incision through the myometrium. Hyperstimulation or hypertonus of the uterus by oxytocin or prostaglandin administration can cause uterine rupture. Invasive or blunt trauma, seen in women after a motor vehicle accident, battery, fall or with knife, or gunshot wound, are additional causes of uterine rupture. Uterine rupture may also occur spontaneously with no history of uterine surgery or terminations of pregnancy. The pathophysiology related to spontaneous rupture is not fully understood. Display 8–8 describes the risk factors associated with uterine rupture.

Clinical Manifestations

The clinical presentation of the woman experiencing a uterine rupture depends on the specific type of rupture. The clinical picture may develop over several hours, with the woman complaining of abdominal pain and tenderness, vomiting, syncope, vaginal bleeding, tachycardia, pallor, or changes in the FHR pattern. Uterine contractions usually continue without a decrease in tone (Menihan, 1998). The most common sign of rupture is a nonreassuring FHR tracing (ACOG, 1999c). Fetal bradycardia may be the first indication of uterine rupture (Menihan, 1999). If unrecognized, bleeding can quickly cause maternal hypotension and shock.

A violent or traumatic rupture may be apparent almost immediately in the woman who complains of sharp, tearing pain, "like something has given way." There may be an inability on the part of the practitioner to reach the presenting part on vaginal examination. Uterine contractions may be absent, and the fetus palpated through the abdominal wall. Bleeding may be vaginal, into the abdominal cavity or both. Intraabdominal bleeding is suspected if the woman has a tense, acute abdomen with shoulder pain. Signs of shock appear soon after a catastrophic rupture, and complete cardiovascular collapse rapidly follows without prompt intervention.

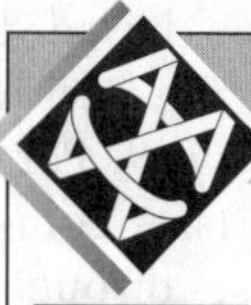

DISPLAY 8–8

Factors Associated with Uterine Rupture

- Previous uterine surgery
- High dosages of oxytocin
- Prostaglandin preparations (eg, misoprostol, dinoprostone)
- Hyperstimulation
- Hypertonus
- Grand multiparity
- Blunt or penetrating abdominal trauma
- Midforceps rotation
- Maneuvers within the uterus
- Obstructed labor
- Abnormal fetal lie
- Previous termination(s) of pregnancy

Dehiscence of a prior lower segment cesarean scar is usually asymptomatic initially. The woman may continue to have contractions without further dilation of the cervix; if an intrauterine pressure catheter is in place for labor assessments, there may be little or no change in intrauterine pressure or resting tone pressures. If the dehiscence extends past the scar tissue, the woman may begin to complain of pain in the lower abdomen that is unrelieved with analgesia or epidural anesthesia. Prolapse of the umbilical cord can occur through the dehiscence resulting in fetal bradycardia or repetitive variable decelerations after each contraction.

Diagnosis

The key to diagnosis is suspicion that uterine rupture has occurred. The nurse immediately should inform the primary healthcare provider at the first suspicion of a uterine rupture. Diagnosis is confirmed at birth.

Management

Treatment includes maternal hemodynamic stabilization and immediate cesarean birth. If possible, the uterine defect is repaired, or hysterectomy is performed. Uterine rupture is discussed further in Chapters 9 and 10.

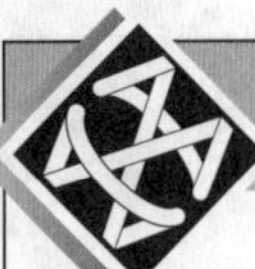

DISPLAY 8–9

Factors Associated With Uterine Inversion

- Uterine atony
- Abnormally adherent placental tissue
- Fetal macrosomia
- Fundal placentation
- Uterine anomalies
- Use of oxytocin
- Use of fundal pressure
- Traction on the umbilical cord
- Abnormally short umbilical cord

Inversion of the Uterus

Inversion of the uterus (ie, turning inside out) after birth is a potentially life-threatening complication. The incidence of uterine inversion is approximately 1 case in 2,500 to 3,600 births (Abouleish et al., 1995; ACOG, 1998b).

Fundal pressure and traction applied to the cord may result in inversion. Other factors associated with inversion of the uterus are listed in Display 8–9. Partial inversion occurs when the fundus inverts. A complete inversion occurs when the fundus passes through the opening of the cervix, and the uterus is totally inverted if the vagina also inverts (Brar, Greenspoon, Platt, & Paul, 1989). Although proper management of the third stage of labor prevents most uterine inversions, some are spontaneous and others unavoidable. Regardless of the precipitating factor, once an inversion occurs, prompt recognition and correction is necessary to reduce maternal morbidity and mortality.

Clinical Manifestations

In addition to possible visualization of the inversion, the primary presenting symptoms of uterine inversion are hemorrhage and hypotension. The woman may experience sudden, acute pelvic pain. Attempts to massage the fundus are unsuccessful because the fundus has inverted into the uterus or vaginal vault, or it is visible at or through the introitus.

Management

Uterine inversion is an emergent situation requiring immediate attempts to replace the uterus. If attempts to replace the uterus are not quickly successful, administration of tocolytics (eg, terbutaline, nitroglycerin) or general anesthesia may be necessary (ACOG, 1998b). Monitoring of maternal vital signs is extremely important because these agents may exacerbate maternal hypotension. Uterine inversion may occasionally recur during a subsequent birth.

Management of this condition involves initiating fluid resuscitation to prevent shock that invariably is out of proportion to the blood loss; there may be a vagal component from peritoneal traction (Dayan & Schwalbe, 1996). The uterus is replaced after the woman has received tocolysis or is under deep anesthesia. Oxytocin is withheld until the uterus has been repositioned. Abdominal or vaginal surgery may be necessary to reposition the uterus if successful manual replacement fails. Blood replacement therapy is administered as indicated. Broad-spectrum antibiotic therapy and placement of a nasogastric tube may be initiated.

Postpartum Hemorrhage

Postpartum hemorrhage is defined as a 10% change in hematocrit from admission assessment to postpartum data or the need to administer a transfusion of red blood cells (ACOG, 1998b). Estimated blood loss is traditionally underestimated by 30% to 50% (ACOG, 1998b). Treatment is based on clinical signs and symptoms (Veronikis & O'Grady, 1994). Postpartum hemorrhage is a leading cause of maternal morbidity and mortality. Complications of postpartum hemorrhage depend on the severity of the hemorrhage and range from anemia to death.

Postpartum hemorrhage can result from uterine atony; abnormal implantation of the placenta; lacerations of the cervix, vagina, or perineum; uterine inversion; and DIC. The most common cause is uterine atony. Early postpartum hemorrhage occurs after the delivery of the placenta, up to 24 hours after birth; late postpartum hemorrhage occurs 24 hours to 6 weeks after birth. Late postpartum hemorrhage is associated with subinvolution of the uterus and with retained placental tissue that may be the result of abnormal placental implantation. Display 8–10 lists the risk factors for postpartum hemorrhage. A thorough discussion of postpartum hemorrhage is found in Chapter 12.

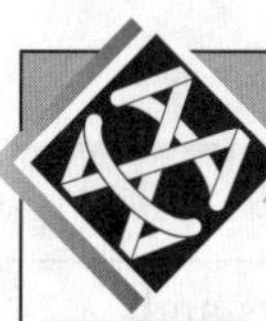

DISPLAY 8–10

Factors Associated With Postpartum Hemorrhage

Uterine atony
Precipitous labor
Intraamniotic infection
Macrosomia
Multifetal gestation
History of uterine atony
Retained products of conception
Clotted blood in uterus
Polyhydramnios
Prolonged labor
High parity
Oxytocin induction or augmentation
Anesthesia effects
Trauma to genital tract: large episiotomy, including extensions; lacerations of the perineum, vagina, or cervix; ruptured uterus
Genital tract lacerations
Genital tract hematoma
Compound presentation
Precipitous birth
Forceps birth
Vacuum extraction
Episiotomy extension
Coagulation defects
Prostaglandin ripening or induction
Sepsis
Poorly perfused myometrium because of hypotension, hemorrhage, conduction anesthesia

Uterine Atony

Uterine atony is marked hypotonia of the uterus. Because of the increased blood flow to the placenta in late pregnancy (approximately 500 to 750 mL/min), failure of the uterus to contract after placental separation can result in significant blood loss very rapidly. Traditional methods to prevent uterine atony by uterine massage or administration of oxytocin are common. Carbetocin, a synthetic analogue of oxytocin with a long half-life, may be administered as an intravenous or intramuscular one-time dose, although it is an experimental drug (Dansereau et al., 1999).Various dosages of misoprostol (100 mcg to 400 mcg) per rectum have been reported in the literature as a successful alternative to the traditional drugs used for postpartum hemorrhage related to uterine atony. Research about misoprostol for postpartum hemorrhage is ongoing.

Uterine atony is more likely to occur when the uterus is overdistended (eg, multiple gestation, macrosomia, polyhydramnios). In such conditions, the uterus is "overstretched" and contracts poorly. Other causes of atony include induction or augmentation of labor, traumatic birth, halogenated anesthesia, tocolytics, rapid or prolonged labor, intraamniotic infection, and multiparity.

Lacerations of the Birth Canal

Lacerations of the birth canal are the second major cause of postpartum hemorrhage (ACOG, 1998b). Birth canal lacerations may include injuries to the labia, perineum, vagina, and cervix. Lacerations secondary to birth trauma occur more commonly with operative vaginal birth (ie, forceps or vacuum assisted). Other risk factors include fetal macrosomia, precipitous labor and birth, and episiotomy (ACOG, 1998b). Prevention, recognition, and prompt, effective treatment of birth canal lacerations are vital. Lacerations may be anticipated if the uterus is well contracted but bleeding remains brisk. Hematoma formation may conceal the blood loss; the woman may develop shock in the absence of other signs of hemorrhage. Pelvic pain may be the woman's only complaint.

Continued bleeding despite efficient postpartum uterine contractions call for reinspection of the birth canal. Continuous bleeding from so-called minor sources may be just as dangerous as a sudden loss of a large amount of blood, because it may be ignored until shock develops.

Management

The first step in the treatment of uterine bleeding is to evaluate the uterus to determine if it is firmly contracted. Intravenous access must be obtained if not already established. Generally, 20 to 40 units of oxytocin in 1 L of crystalloid solution are given intravenously at 10 to

15 mL/min. This infusion is usually continued at least 3 or 4 hours. If the uterus initially fails to respond to oxytocin, 0.2 mg of methylergonovine given intramuscularly produces tetanic uterine contractions and is effective in treating hemorrhage from uterine atony. However, its use is contraindicated in the presence of hypertension. If methylergonovine fails or is contraindicated, 15-methyl-prostaglandin $F_{2\alpha}$ may be administered in the absence of maternal asthma or systemic lupus. Most hemorrhage can be controlled after one or two injections of 0.25 mg of 15-methyl-prostaglandin $F_{2\alpha}$ by intramuscular or intramyometrial routes, depending on the type of birth. Table 8–6 lists the uterotonic agents used for postpartum hemorrhage. Intrauterine irrigation with the same agent by means of a Foley catheter has also been reported to be successful (Kupferminc et al., 1998).

Blood transfusion for blood replacement and treatment of shock may be urgently needed. The use of cell-saver technology, in which the patient's blood is collected during surgery, washed, and transfused back to the patient, has been used since the early 1970s but has only recently been studied for use in obstetrics. A multicenter trial documented that there are no increased risks of complications in patients who underwent autologous blood collection and autotransfusion during cesarean birth (Rebarber, Lonser, Jackson, Copel, & Sipes, 1998; Rebarber, Odunsi, Baumgarten, Copel, & Sipes, 1998).

The interior of the uterus is explored so that retained products of conception can be removed and possible rupture of the uterus diagnosed. If the blood being lost fails to clot, DIC may be developing, and prompt, appropriate treatment may be life saving. The treatment for DIC is to cure the underlying problem. Figure 8–5 provides a management plan for postpartum hemorrhage.

Nursing Assessment

A medical history is usually available in the prenatal record and can be assessed for previous bleeding or bleeding disorders. Assessment of the woman who is bleeding begins with careful evaluation of amount and color of blood loss, character of uterine activity,

TABLE 8–6 ■ UTEROTONIC AGENTS USED FOR POSTPARTUM HEMORRHAGE

Medication	Dose	Primary Route (Alternate)	Frequency of Dose	Side Effects	Comments and Contraindications
Oxytocin	10–40 U in 1,000 mL of normal saline or lactated Ringer's solution	IV (IM, IMM)	Continuous infusion	Usually none, but nausea, vomiting, and water intoxication have been reported	No contraindications
Methylergonovine	0.2 mg	IM (IMM)	Every 2–4 h	Hypertension, hypotension, nausea, vomiting	Contraindications include hypertension and toxemia
15-m-PGF_{2a}	0.25 mg	IM (IMM)	Every 15–90 min, not to exceed 8 doses	Vomiting, diarrhea, nausea, flushing or hot flashes, chills or shivering	Contraindications include active cardiac, pulmonary, renal, or hepatic disease
Dinoprostone (PGE_2)	20 mg	PR	Every 2 h	Vomiting, diarrhea, nausea, fever, headache, chills or shivering	Should be avoided in hypotensive patient because of vasodilatation; if available, 15-m-$PGF_{2\alpha}$ is preferable

15-m-$PGF_{2\alpha}$ = 15-methyl-prostaglandin $F_{2\alpha}$; IM = intramuscular; IMM = intramyometrial; IV = intravenous; PR = per rectum.
Adapted from American College of Obstetricians and Gynecologists. (1998). Postpartum hemorrhage (Education Bulletin No. 243). Washington, DC: Author.

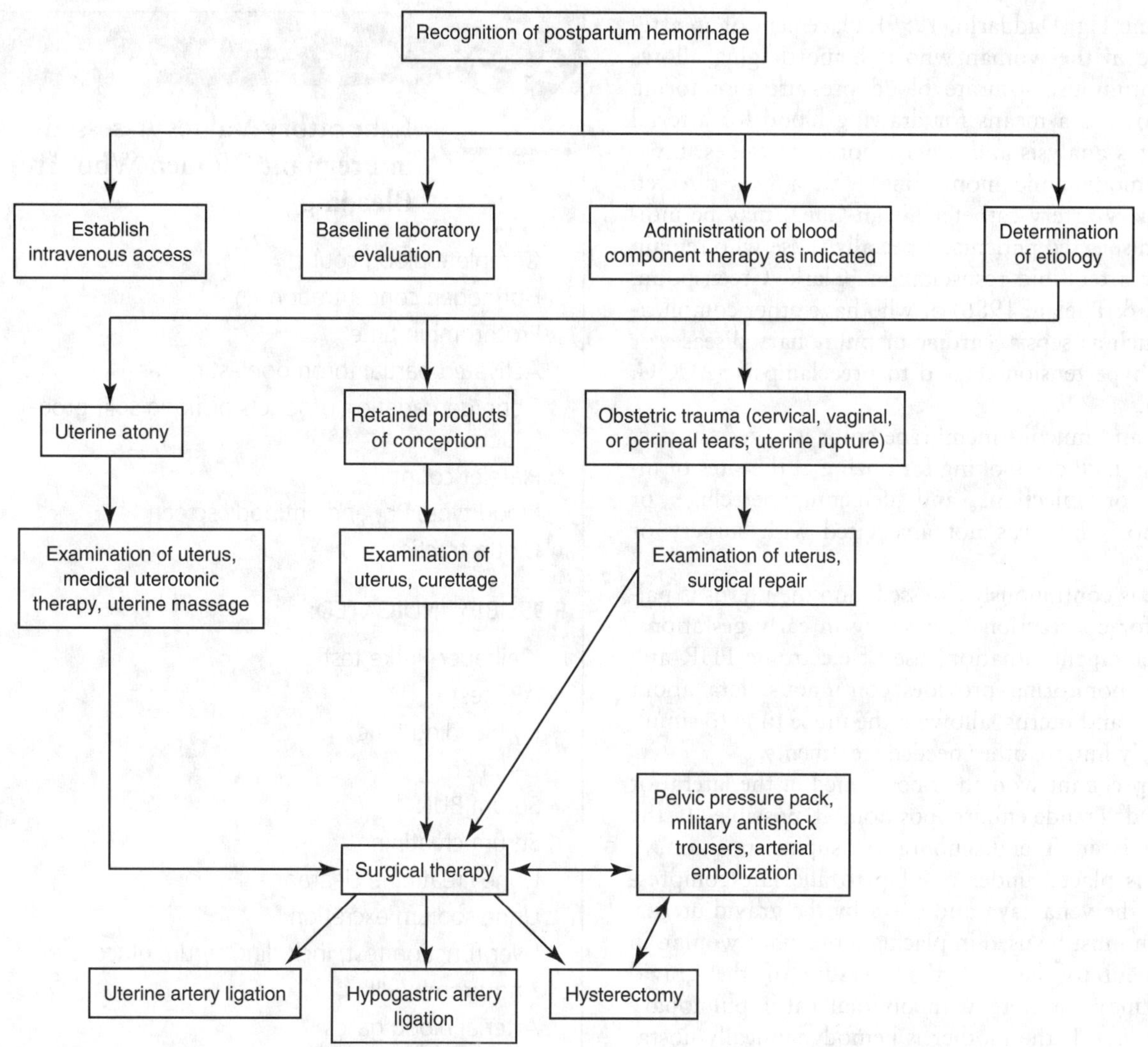

FIGURE 8–5. Management plan for postpartum hemorrhage. (American College of Obstetricians and Gynecologists. 1998. Postpartum hemorrhage. Educational Bulletin No. 243. Washington DC: Author.)

presence of abdominal pain, stability of maternal vital signs, and fetal status. Bright red vaginal bleeding suggests active bleeding, and dark or brown blood may indicate past blood loss.

Vital signs are important in assessing amount of blood loss. Maternal or fetal tachycardia and maternal hypotension suggest hypovolemia; however, hypotension is a late sign. Historically, the frequency of vital signs depends on patient stability. Vital signs are usually repeated every 15 minutes until the bleeding is controlled and the vital signs remain or return to normal. Vital signs are performed more frequently (every 1 to 5 minutes) when there is evidence of instability, including systolic blood pressure less than 90 mm Hg, maternal tachycardia, and decreasing level of consciousness.

When using an automatic blood pressure cuff, ensure that the Doppler is directly over the brachial artery for an accurate recording. However, in severe hypotensive states, the automatic blood pressure device is less accurate. Many automatic blood pressure monitors calculate mean arterial pressure (MAP = systolic blood pressure + 2 × diastolic blood pressure ÷ 3), which provides a quick number for reference and is a more stable parameter of hemodynamic function. The normal value for mean arterial pressure in the second trimester of pregnancy is approximately 80 mm Hg (Page & Christianson, 1976) and is 90 mm Hg at term (Cunningham et al., 1997).

When the blood pressure cannot be assessed with a blood pressure cuff, systolic blood pressure may be estimated by the presence of a radial, femoral, or brachial pulse. The presence of a radial pulse is associated with a systolic blood pressure of approximately 80 mm Hg, a femoral pulse with a blood pressure of 70 mm Hg, and a carotid pulse with a blood pressure of 60 mm Hg (Daddario, 1999). Placement of an arterial line in the woman who is hemorrhaging allows for continuous, accurate blood pressure monitoring and provides a means for drawing blood for arterial blood gas analysis and other laboratory values. Invasive hemodynamic monitoring with a flow-directed pulmonary artery catheter (Swan-Ganz) may be indicated in selected patients, especially those who remain oliguric after fluid resuscitation (Clark, Greenspoon, Aldahl, & Phelan, 1986) or who have other complications such as sepsis, cardiac or pulmonary disease, or severe hypertension related to preeclampsia (ACOG, 1998b).

Skin and mucous membrane color is noted. Inspection also includes looking for oozing at the sites of incisions or injections and detecting petechiae or ecchymosis in areas not associated with surgery or trauma.

FHR is continuously assessed, and the uterus is palpated for contractions, especially in early gestations. In an emergent situation, use of electronic FHR and uterine monitoring provides continuous data about the fetus and uterus, allowing the nurse time to simultaneously initiate other needed treatments.

The pregnant woman is positioned in the lateral or modified Trendelenburg position, if possible. If the patient is in Trendelenburg or supine position, a wedge is placed under one hip to alleviate compression of the vena cava and aorta by the gravid uterus. Caution must be used in placing a pregnant woman in Trendelenburg because the pressure of the gravid uterus may interfere with optimal cardiopulmonary functioning. If the mother is hemodynamically unstable, oxygen is administered, preferably by nonrebreathing face mask at 10 to 12 L/min to maintain maternal–fetal oxygen saturation. Mentation is assessed frequently and provides additional indication of maternal blood volume and oxygen saturation.

Blood is drawn to assess maternal hemoglobin, hematocrit, platelet count, and coagulation profile. Display 8–11 lists the blood tests commonly ordered for the woman who is bleeding. In an emergent situation, blood may be drawn into a plain red-top (clot) tube and then visually evaluated for clot formation. Treatment for a significant coagulopathy should be initiated if no signs of clotting are evident within 4 to 8 minutes (Clark, 1999). Fresh-frozen plasma, whole blood, and cryoprecipitate may be administered; platelets are not usually given unless the platelet count decreases to less than 30,000 cells/mm^3. Table 8–7 lists blood replacement products, factors present, and the expected effect per unit administered.

Circulating volume is usually restored with intravenous crystalloid solution administration. Two large-bore intravenous lines are needed for fluid replacement and administration of drug therapies. Blood and blood products are administered as needed or as soon as they are available. Breath sounds are auscultated before fluid volume replacement if possible to provide a baseline for future assessment. Massive fluid replacement during pregnancy or the immediate postpartum period for the woman who is hemorrhaging increases the potential for development of pulmonary edema. However, fluid replacement is necessary to restore circulatory volume, and the nurse anticipates and assesses for the development of peripheral or pulmonary edema and treatment with furosemide as needed. Initial crystalloid fluid replacement is 3 mL for each 1 mL of blood loss (ACOG, 1998b).

Oxygen saturation can be monitored with a pulse oximeter. Pulse oximeters are an adjunct to assessment; they are not always accurate, especially in a patient in

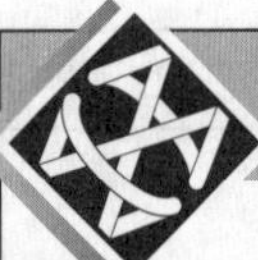

DISPLAY 8–11

Laboratory Values Assessed in Pregnant Women Who Are Bleeding

- Complete blood count
- Fibrinogen concentration
- Prothrombin time
- Activated partial thromboplastin time
- Fibrin degradation products or fibrin split products
- Platelet count
- Blood type, Rh, and antibody screen
- Clot retraction

POSSIBLY INDICATED:

- Kleihauer-Betke test
- APT test
- Ivy bleeding time
- D-dimer
- Serum BUN
- Serum creatinine
- Urine creatinine clearance
- Urine sodium excretion
- Liver function test, including serum glucose
- Antithrombin III
- Arterial blood gases
- Urine or serum drug screen

TABLE 8–7 ■ BLOOD REPLACEMENT PRODUCTS

Component	Volume/Unit*	Factors Present	Effect/Unit
Fresh whole blood	500	Red blood cells, all procoagulants	Increase hematocrit 3%
Packed red blood cells	200	Red blood cells only	Increase hematocrit 3%
Fresh-frozen plasma	200–400	All procoagulants, no platelets	Increase fibrinogen 25 mg/dL
Cryoprecipitate	20–50	Fibrinogen, factors VIII and XIII	Increase fibrinogen 15–25%
Platelet concentrate	35–60	Platelets, small amounts of fibrinogen, factors V and VIII	Increase platelet count by about 8,000/mm^3

*Volume depends on individual blood bank.

From Clark, S. L. (1999). Placenta previa and abruptio placenta. In R. Creasy & R. Resnick (Eds.) *Maternal-fetal medicine* (4th ed., pp. 616–631). Philadelphia: WB Saunders.

hypovolemic shock. In the hemorrhagic patient, blood flow to the extremities is decreased, and the oxygen saturation displayed may not accurately reflect tissue oxygenation status. Blood gas analysis may therefore be necessary to determine oxygen status. Pulmonary artery monitoring is achieved with a Swan-Ganz catheter, which is also used for blood gas retrieval. A maternal oxygen saturation level of at least 95% and a PaO_2 of at least 65 mm Hg as determined by blood gas analysis are necessary for the fetus to maintain adequate oxygenation (Barth, 1997).

Continuous ECG monitoring is indicated for the woman who is hypotensive or tachycardiac, continuing to bleed profusely, or in shock. Maternal hypovolemia leading to hypoxia and acidosis may result in maternal heart rate dysrhythmias, including premature ventricular contractions, tachycardia, and atrial or ventricular fibrillation.

A Foley catheter with a urometer is inserted to allow for hourly assessment of urine output. The most objective and least invasive assessment of adequate organ perfusion and oxygenation is urinary output of at least 30 mL/hour (Clark, 1999). Attempts should be made to maintain urine output above 0.5 mL/kg per hour (ACOG, 1998b). In addition to volume, urine is assessed for the presence of blood, protein, and for specific gravity.

Nursing Interventions

Evaluation and management of acute episodes of bleeding during pregnancy usually occur in the inpatient setting. An exception is spotting during early gestation. After stabilization and a period of hospitalization, selected women may be managed at home.

Home Care Management

Controversy exists concerning home care management of women with placenta previa and marginal separation of the placenta; however, women in stable condition increasingly are being cared for in the home, with visits by perinatal nurses or daily provider-initiated phone contact. Criteria for home care management vary with the primary perinatal provider and home care agency. The woman must be in stable condition with no evidence of active bleeding and have resources to be able to return to the hospital immediately if active bleeding resumes. Bed rest at home remains a controversial topic; there are few data to determine how much time a women should be in bed or if bed rest affects outcome in a positive manner. Complete or partial bed rest has long-term deleterious effects on the woman physically and psychologically (Gupton, Heaman, & Ashcroft, 1997; Maloni, 1998).

Appendix 8A lists the diagnostic criteria and considerations for home care referral for management of women with antepartum bleeding.

Inpatient Management

When the woman is admitted to the hospital, the nurse begins assessment of the bleeding. The woman with acute bleeding requires continuous, ongoing nursing assessments and interventions. Maternal vital signs are assessed frequently according to individual clinical situations. Careful assessments are mandatory. Vital signs and noninvasive assessments of cardiac output (eg, skin color, skin temperature, pulse oximetry, mentation, urinary output) are obtained frequently to observe for signs of declining hemodynamic status.

Because a nonreassuring FHR pattern may be the first sign of maternal or fetal hemodynamic compromise electronic, FHR and uterine activity monitoring should be continuous. It is important to appreciate how rapidly maternal–fetal status can deteriorate as a result of maternal hemorrhage. Blood is shunted away from the uterus when the mother experiences hypotension or hypovolemic shock. Because of the potential for maternal–fetal mortality, it is essential to be prepared for an emergent birth at all times when caring for a pregnant woman who is bleeding. Supportive staff necessary for an emergency cesarean birth (ie, anesthesia personnel, operating room team, and neonatal resuscitation team) should be notified and on standby (if possible, in the hospital). Hemorrhage from placenta previa, abruptio placentae, or uterine rupture requires expeditious birth. Two large-bore intravenous catheters (at least 18 gauge) are placed if the woman is experiencing heavy bleeding. If consistent with institution policy, a 14- or 16-gauge intracatheter should be considered. The need to replace fluids and blood is determined by a number of parameters, including vital signs, amount of blood loss, mental status, laboratory values, and fetal condition.

Fluid replacement consists of administering lactated Ringer's or normal saline solution, packed red blood cells, fresh-frozen plasma, and possibly platelets. Blood product replacement therapy is anticipated, and communication with the blood bank is essential. Significant hemorrhage resulting in syncope or hypovolemic shock generally necessitates transfusion.

Blood type, Rh, and antibody screen should be obtained on admission; crossmatching is ordered as necessary. The use of blood components, rather than whole blood, is usually a better treatment option because it provides only the specific components needed (ACOG, 1998b). By using only the specific products required for the emergency, blood resources are conserved, and there is a decreased risk of blood replacement complications. Transfusion reactions may be demonstrated by chills, fever, tachycardia, hypotension, shortness of breath, muscle cramps, itching, convulsions, and ultimately cardiac arrest. The woman is assessed throughout the procedure. In the event of a reaction, the transfusion is immediately discontinued, and the intravenous line flushed with normal saline. Treatment is then based on clinical symptoms. The development of anaphylaxis should be considered and appropriate treatment available.

Careful fetal surveillance is critical to ensure fetal well-being during transfusion of multiple blood products. The increased incidence of uteroplacental insufficiency is related to complications of coagulation factor replacement therapy (Simpson, Luppi, & O'Brien-Abel, 1998). Administration of multiple replacement blood products leads to increased intravascular fibrin formation. Deposition of fibrin in the decidual vasculature of the chorionic villi may cause fetal compromise.

Because of the normal hemodynamic changes that occur, pregnant women may lose up to one fourth of their fluid volume before displaying signs of shock (Clark, 1999). Women who are bleeding should be monitored carefully for the actual amount of blood loss, although this is sometimes difficult to assess in an emergent situation. Sheets or pads can be inspected and weighed. Accurate intake and output measurement and documentation is critical. Ideally, one nurse is assigned to monitor intake and output during a period of massive fluid and blood replacement. In an emergent situation in which the obstetrician and anesthesiologist may be ordering or adding replacement fluid to multiple intravenous lines, it becomes essential that one nurse records and maintains a running total of intake and output in addition to signing for blood products and overseeing administration.

The woman may develop a coagulopathy. Display 8–12 lists the risk factors for DIC. Pulmonary edema and renal failure, as evidenced by oliguria proceeding to anuria, must be anticipated. Systolic blood pressures of less than 60 mm Hg are associated with acute renal failure. The woman is at risk for development of acute tubular necrosis from lack of perfusion to the kidneys (ie, prerenal failure). Prolonged periods of severe hypotension may result in renal cortical necrosis. Urine output of less than 30 mL/hour should be reported to the primary care provider immediately.

In the case of severe hemorrhage, control of abdominal bleeding may be achieved by the placement of

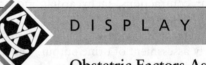

DISPLAY 8–12

Obstetric Factors Associated With Disseminated Intravascular Coagulation

- Abruptio placentae
- Hemorrhage
- Preeclampsia or eclampsia
- Amniotic fluid embolism
- Saline termination of pregnancy
- Sepsis
- Dead fetus syndrome
- Cardiopulmonary arrest
- Massive transfusion therapy

medical antishock trousers (MAST suit), which are used in emergency and trauma units to control bleeding. Consensus does not exist about the benefits of using MAST suits; however, they are used in many institutions. Care must be taken not to put any pressure on the lower abdomen.

Hemorrhagic and Hypovolemic Shock

Hemorrhagic and hypovolemic shock is an emergent situation in which the perfusion of body organs may become severely compromised and death may ensue. Aggressive treatment is necessary to prevent adverse sequelae (eg, cellular death, fluid overload, ARDS, oxygen toxicity). Common clinical symptoms of inadequate intravascular volume (ie, hypovolemia) that necessitates blood replacement include evidence of hemorrhage (ie, loss of a large amount of blood externally or internally in a short period of time); evidence of hypovolemic shock (ie, increasing pulse, cool clammy skin, rapid breathing, restlessness, and reduced urine output); or a decrease in hemoglobin and hematocrit below acceptable level for trimester of pregnancy or the nonpregnant state.

Aggressive fluid and blood replacement is not without risk. The 24 hours after the shock period are critical. Observe for fluid overload, ARDS, and oxygen toxicity. Transfusion reactions may follow administration of blood or blood components. Even in an emergency, each unit should be checked per hospital protocol. Rapid transfusion with cold blood can chill the woman and cause vasoconstriction, arrhythmia, or arrest. Banked blood may be calcium deficient, increasing the risk for arrhythmias and further bleeding. Potassium levels may increase to dangerous levels. Laboratory values for other parameters are usually checked at least every 4 to 6 hours or as indicated by the woman's condition. Display 8–13 suggests a management plan for hypovolemic shock (Clark, 1997). Infection is another complication of hemorrhage. Causes may include surgical procedures, multiple pelvic examinations, anemia, and loss of the white blood cell component of the blood. It is anticipated that the patient may receive prophylactic antibiotics or treatment for signs of infection.

Hemorrhagic disorders in pregnancy are nursing and medical emergencies requiring rapid and efficient

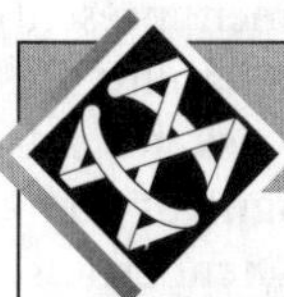

DISPLAY 8–13

Management Plan for Obstetric Hypovolemic Shock

GOALS:

- Maintain systolic blood pressure ≥90 mmHg, urine output ≥0.5 mL/kg/h, and normal mental status.
- Eliminate source of hemorrhage.
- Avoid overzealous volume replacement that may contribute to pulmonary edema.

MANAGEMENT:

- Establish two large-bore intravenous lines.
- Place woman in Trendelenburg position (wedge under hip if undelivered).
- Rapidly infuse 5% dextrose in lactated Ringer's solution while blood products are obtained.
- Infuse fresh whole blood or packed red blood cells, as available.
- Infuse platelets and fresh frozen plasma only as indicated by documented deficiencies in platelets (<30,000/mL) or clotting parameters (fibrinogen, prothrombin time [PT], partial thromboplastin time [PTT].
- Search for and eliminate the source of hemorrhage.
- Use invasive hemodynamic monitoring if the woman fails to respond to clinically adequate volume replacement.
- Critical laboratory tests include complete blood count, platelet count, fibrinogen, PT, PTT, and arterial blood gas determinations.

Adapted from Clark, S. L. (1997). Hypovolemic shock. In S. L. Clark, D. B. Cotton, G. D. V. Hankins, & J. P. Phelan (Eds.), *Critical care obstetrics* (3rd ed. pp. 412–422). Malden, MA: Blackwell Scientific.

teamwork from all members of the healthcare team. Perinatal nurses play an important role in the initial assessments, early interventions, and stabilization of the woman. Recognition that blood loss out of proportion to the patient's clinical presentation is important because initial vital signs may remain within normal range in the presence of a significant hemorrhage. Anticipating that a woman who is bleeding may rapidly proceed to hypovolemic shock can prevent complications and decrease maternal and fetal morbidity and mortality.

Maternal Trauma

The perinatal nurse may encounter pregnant women who have experienced trauma because, in some cases, they are directly admitted to the labor and delivery unit or to an obstetric triage unit. In most institutions, women with major trauma are stabilized in the emergency department with the assistance of perinatal healthcare providers who are called to the department for consultation, whereas women with minor trauma may be sent directly to the labor and delivery unit. The focus of this discussion is women who present with seemingly minor or non–life-threatening trauma. A thorough knowledge of the normal physiologic changes during pregnancy, complications of bleeding and preterm labor, and maternal–fetal assessment is necessary to provide optimum care for pregnant women after trauma.

Approximately 6% to 8% of women experience trauma during pregnancy (ACOG, 1998a; Curet, Schermer, Demarest, Bieneik, & Curet, 2000). Approximately two thirds of all trauma events during pregnancy are the result of motor vehicle accidents. Motor vehicle accidents are the most significant cause of fetal death due to trauma (ACOG, 1998a). The incidence and severity of injuries can be reduced by appropriate use of automobile safety restraints, but not all pregnant women use safety restraints while driving or riding as a passenger in a car. Other significant causes of trauma during pregnancy are falls and direct assaults to the abdomen. Domestic violence is becoming an increasing source of trauma during pregnancy. Data about incidence of domestic violence have been difficult to accumulate because of reporting issues and the frequency of inaccurate description of the causative factors for injury given by the woman. Various sources cite rates of domestic violence ranging between 1% and 20% of pregnant women (ACOG, 1998a). The Centers for Disease Control and Prevention estimate that up to 300,000 pregnant women in the United States each year are victims of domestic violence (Jones, 2000). Fetal loss resulting from blunt abdominal trauma may occur because of abruptio placentae or other placenta injury, direct fetal injury, uterine rupture, maternal shock, maternal death, or a combination of these events (ACOG, 1998a).

Nursing assessment and interventions for the pregnant woman who has experienced trauma are based on the clinical situation and maternal–fetal status. A thorough history is essential and should include the nature of the trauma event, condition and symptoms at time of injury, and current clinical symptoms. The principles of management of preterm labor and complications of bleeding are applied based on the clinical situation. Ongoing maternal–fetal assessments and accurate reporting of findings to the primary healthcare provider are important.

Fortunately, most women who experience trauma suffer only minor injures that would not require inpatient evaluation for the nonpregnant population. However, approximately 5% to 25% of women who experience minor trauma have an adverse maternal or fetal outcome (Curet et al., 2000). Minor or non–life-threatening injuries are associated with a fetal loss rate of 1% to 5% (Pearlman, 1997). Up to 50% of fetal losses related to trauma occur in women with seemingly minor or nonsignificant injuries (ACOG, 1998a). Careful evaluation of maternal–fetal status is warranted when pregnant women present with reports of any type of trauma. Reliability of methods to predict which women are at risk for adverse outcomes remains low. The usual signs of complications, including bleeding, uterine tenderness, contractions, and loss of amniotic fluid, are valuable, but they may not be present in all cases (Curet et al., 2000). Use of ultrasound to exclude abruptio placentae has the potential to miss 50% of cases (Reis, Sander, & Pearlman, 2000). Continuous electronic fetal monitoring (EFM) is useful for ongoing evaluation of fetal status and uterine activity. Recommended duration of continuous EFM after trauma ranges from 6 hours to 24 hours based on clinical signs and symptoms and the mechanism of injury (ACOG, 1998a; Curet et al., 2000). Monitoring should be continued, and further evaluation is warranted if uterine contractions, a nonreassuring FHR pattern, vaginal bleeding, significant uterine tenderness or irritability, serious maternal injury, or rupture of the membranes occurs (ACOG, 1998a). The decision to continue inpatient evaluation, discharge to her home, or transfer to another facility should be made in collaboration with the primary healthcare provider, consistent with maternal–fetal status and as outlined in the federal Emergency Medical Treatment and Labor Act (EMTALA) regulations (see Chapter 2).

PRETERM LABOR AND BIRTH

Significance and Incidence

Despite active research since the early 1980s into the cause, diagnosis, management, and prevention of preterm labor and birth, the rate of preterm birth in the United States increased from 9.4% in 1981 to 11.6% in 1998, representing an overall increase of 23% (Ventura, Martin, Curtin, Mathews, & Park, 2000). Although preterm births for singleton pregnancies have also increased slightly, the significant rise in preterm births in recent years has been influenced largely by the increase in the number of women with multiple gestations. Twins and higher-order multiples are more likely to be born preterm and are at much greater risk for having low birth weight (LBW). Approximately 55% of women pregnant with twins give birth preterm (Kogan et al., 2000). The rate of preterm birth for women with triplets is 90%, rising to 99% for higher-order multiples (Ventura et al., 2000).

Preterm birth is responsible for 75% of neonatal deaths not caused by congenital anomalies (American College of Obstetricians and Gynecologists [ACOG], 1995). As the second leading cause of infant mortality (birth defects is first) and because it is one of the most serious complications of pregnancy, preterm labor and birth are appropriate targets for intensive research and will remain so in the foreseeable future. Based on what has been learned from the research, it is doubtful that one causative factor will be discovered. All indications are that preterm labor has multiple causes, including social factors, physiologic factors, medical history factors, and illness factors (Goldenberg & Rouse, 1998). Preterm labor is one of the last symptoms in a cascade of biochemical events that lead to preterm birth. Preterm birth is an end-stage symptom of a multifactorial disease (Katz & Farmer, 1999).

The rise in rates of preterm birth exists in stark contrast to the dramatic drop in rates of infant mortality since the 1950s. In 1997, the rate of infant mortality for the United States was 7.2% (MacDorman & Atkinson, 1999); in 1950, it was 29.2% (March of Dimes, 1997). The favorable change in infant mortality rates correlates with the emergence of the science of neonatal care. More infants are now living past their first birthday despite being born at earlier gestational ages.

Preterm birth, LBW, and very low birth weight (VLBW) occur frequently and contribute to multiple morbidities and mortality in the affected infants. In 1999, more than 300,795 LBW (<2,500 g) infants and more than 57,388 VLBW (<1,500 g) infants were born in the United States (Curtin & Martin, 2000). Sixty-five percent of the LBW infants and 95% of the VLBW infants were born preterm (Curtin & Martin, 2000). An infant born weighing less than 1500 g is 200 times more likely to die before the end of the first year of life than infants weighing more than 2500 g (ACOG, 1995). Those VLBW infants who survive are 10 times more likely to be neurologically impaired (ACOG, 1995). At least 50% of infants born at or before 25 weeks' gestation suffer severe neurologic disabilities (Wood et al., 2000).

There are significant health costs related to preterm birth. Annually, preterm birth results in approximately 6.5 million inpatient days in the neonatal intensive care unit (NICU), 10.2 billion dollars in NICU inpatient costs, and 820 million dollars in maternal inpatient costs (Cole, 2000; MacDorman & Atkinson, 1999; Nicholson, Frick, & Powe, 2000; St. John, Nelson, Cliver, Bishnoi, & Goldenberg, 2000). An infant born between 24 and 29 weeks' gestation generates inpatient costs ranging from $45,000 to $250,000. The costs for infants born between 30 and 35 weeks' gestation ranges from $24,000 to $40,000. Average lifetime costs related to complications of preterm birth before 30 weeks' gestation are estimated to be more than $500,000.

Definitions

Preterm labor is defined as cervical change or effacement and uterine contractions that occur between 20 and 36 weeks of pregnancy (American Academy of Pediatrics [AAP] & ACOG, 1997). Diagnosis of preterm labor, according to the Guidelines for Perinatal Care (ACOG & AAP, 1997) involves the following factors: 20 to 36 weeks' gestation, documented uterine contractions, and documented cervical effacement of 80% *or* cervical dilation of more than 1 cm. Uterine irritability without cervical dilation or effacement therefore is not preterm labor.

The terms *preterm birth* and *low birth weight* are often used interchangeably, but they are different. Preterm birth is any birth that occurs before 37 completed weeks of pregnancy. LBW refers to birth weight alone, despite gestational age. A LBW infant is born at or below 2,500 g. Preterm infants may be, but do not have to be, LBW (eg, a 35-week gestational-age baby of a diabetic mother could be 3,000 g but is still at risk for the health problems inherent in being born prematurely). LBW babies may be born before 37 weeks but can also be born at term (eg, a 41-week gestational-age baby weighing 1,800 g because of IUGR). Risk factors, causes, and outcomes for LBW, growth restriction, and preterm birth are interrelated.

LBW and IUGR are significant predictors of perinatal morbidity and mortality. The effects of IUGR are more pronounced for infants born preterm. Preterm LBW infants are two to three times more likely to die in the first year of life compared with term LBW infants (Cogswell & Yip, 1995).

Preterm infants are twice as likely to die by their first birthday and are more likely to suffer morbidity such as respiratory distress syndrome, intraventricular hemorrhage, and necrotizing enterocolitis than infants born at term (March of Dimes, 1997). Although all infants born preterm are at risk for health problems, infants born before 32 weeks (about 2% of all infants) are at the highest risk for neonatal death (Goldenberg & Rouse, 1998).

A report based on a multicenter registry of 4,593 VLBW infants (501 to 1500 g) provides an updated picture of morbidity and mortality in that category (Stevenson et al., 1998). Based on these data, at each gestational age, a lower birth weight carried a higher mortality risk; males were at greater risk for death than female infants at all gestational ages and weights; respiratory distress syndrome was the most frequent morbidity, occurring in 52% of VLBW infants; 30% had intracranial hemorrhages, with 24% of infants between 501 and 750 g having severe hemorrhage; and 21% had necrotizing enterocolitis (Stevenson et al., 1998).

Risk Factors for Preterm Labor and Birth

In a classic work in this field, the Institute of Medicine (IOM, 1985) published the known risks at that time for preterm labor and birth. That list, modified to include some of the risks discovered more recently, is given in Display 8–14. Some factors related to preterm birth have greater risk than others. For example, a woman with a history of one prior preterm birth has a three times greater risk of a subsequent preterm birth (IOM, 1985). Two or more prior preterm births

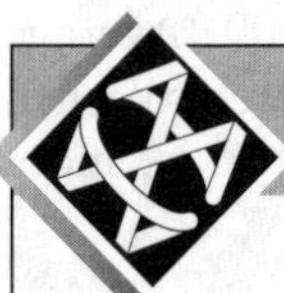

DISPLAY 8–14

Risk Factors for Preterm Labor and Birth

- Demographic risk factors
  - African-American race (doubles the risk)
  - Maternal age younger than 17 or older than 34 years
  - Low socioeconomic status
  - Unmarried
  - Low level of education
- Medical risks predating this pregnancy
  - History of a prior preterm birth (triples the risk)
  - Multiple abortions
  - Uterine anomalies
  - Low prepregnancy weight for height
  - Parity (0 or greater than 4)
  - Diabetes
  - Hypertension
- Medical risks in current pregnancy
  - Multiple gestation
  - Infections
  - Incompetent cervix
  - Short interpregnancy interval
  - Urinary tract infections
  - Bleeding in the first trimester
  - Placenta previa
  - Abruptio placentae
  - Anemia
  - Fetal anomalies
  - Premature rupture of membranes
- Behavioral and environmental risks
  - Diethylstilbestrol (DES) exposure
  - Smoking
  - Poor nutrition
  - Alcohol or other substance use
  - Late or no prenatal care
  - Domestic violence
  - Air pollution
- Other risks
  - Stress
  - Long working hours
  - Inability to rest

Adapted from the Institute of Medicine. (1985). *Preventing low birthweight.* Washington, DC: National Academy Press.

increase the risk to six times that of a woman without a prior preterm birth (ACOG, 1995). Smoking increases the risk of preterm birth by 40% (Wisborg, Henriksen, Hedegaard, & Secher, 1996). A woman who smokes more than 15 cigarettes per day probably will have an infant weighing 200 to 300 g less than if she did not smoke (Moore & Zaccaro, 2000). Alcohol use during pregnancy increases risk of preterm birth by 40%. Inadequate maternal nutrition and low weight gain during pregnancy increases the risk of having a LBW infant by 60% (Shieve et al., 2000) and the risk of preterm birth by 60% (Carmichael & Abrams, 1997).

Although the problem of increasing rates of preterm birth across the United States is alarming, more alarming still is the variation in rates of preterm birth among races. In 1998, the preterm birth rate for Caucasians was 10.2%, but for African Americans, it was 17.6% (Ventura et al., 2000). In addition to race-based differences, rates of singleton preterm birth are known to be higher for women who have already experienced preterm birth, are socially disadvantaged, have low levels of education, live with stress, have a low weight gain during pregnancy (especially during the third trimester), receive late or no prenatal care, have short interpregnancy intervals (<18 months), smoke, and are subjected to domestic violence (Basso, Olsen, Knudsen, & Christensen, 1998; Carmichael & Abrams, 1997; Cnattingius, Grnanth, Petersson, & Harlow, 1999; Copper et al., 1996; Curry, Perrin, & Wall, 1998; Lieberman, Lang, Ryan, Monson, & Schoenbaum, 1989; McFarlane & Gondolf, 1998; Moore, Elmore, Ketner, Wagoner, & Walsh, 1995; Vitoratos et al., 1997). Some of these factors, such as domestic violence, have not received much attention in the literature for interventions to prevent preterm birth, despite the fact that nursing research has shown that women in domestic violence situations are clearly at higher risk (Parker, McFarlane, & Soeken, 1994). Each year, up to 300,000 pregnant women in the United States are victims of domestic violence; violence is more common among pregnant women than many conditions for which they are routinely screened (Jones, 2000).

Risk Factors as Screening Methods to Predict Preterm Labor and Birth

The use of known risk factors to determine which women may experience preterm birth has been a common strategy in research conducted during the past two decades (Goldenberg & Rouse, 1998). One of the first major research studies about screening for pregnancy risk factors modified a risk scoring system first developed by Emil Papiernik (1989) in France, and used it to target interventions for women at highest risk for preterm labor (Herron, Katz, & Creasy, 1982). Although this scoring system was subsequently used for almost a decade in clinical settings attempting to identify women who might give birth prematurely, subsequent research has shown that risk scoring tools do not predict all preterm births. Fifty percent of all preterm births cannot be predicted by risk assessment (Collaborative Group on Preterm Birth Prevention, 1993; Main & Gabbe, 1989; U.S. Public Health Service, 1989).

The inability to prevent preterm birth for women who are identified at risk, in part, results from the fact that most risk factors that can be identified are not able to be modified or "treated." For example, most studies have suggested that African-American race, extremes of maternal age, economic and social disadvantages, unmarried status, history of multiple abortions, uterine anomalies, low maternal height for weight, and history of a prior preterm birth increase the risk of preterm birth significantly. Women with these risk factors comprise about 25% of those who give birth preterm. Approximately 50% of women who give birth preterm do not have risk factors that can be identified during pregnancy. It is essential that preterm birth prevention efforts be directed at all pregnant women. Although specialized care for women with many risk factors may be effective in helping the small subset of women with identified risk factors to give birth closer to term, routine prenatal care must contain a component of preterm birth prevention (ie, education about signs and symptoms of preterm labor and what to do should they occur) if the rate of preterm birth is ever to be decreased.

Biochemical Markers

The search for early predictive factors for preterm labor and birth has recently included the use of biochemical markers, most notably fetal fibronectin and salivary estriol. Fetal fibronectin testing for preterm labor was approved by the U.S. Food and Drug Administration (FDA) in 1995, and salivary estriol testing was approved by the FDA in 1998. Fetal fibronectin is a extracellular matrix glycoprotein produced in the decidual cells of the uterus (Moore, 1999). Fetal fibronectin is thought to be the trophoblastic "glue" in the formation of the uteroplacental junction. It is normally absent from vaginal secretions from 24 to 36 weeks of pregnancy. Fetal fibronectin found in vaginal secretions between 24 weeks and 34 weeks at a level greater than 50 ng/mL is a predictor of preterm labor (Lockwood et al.,

1991). It has been theorized that preterm labor breaks the bonds between the placenta and the amniotic membranes, causing a release of fetal fibronectin into the vaginal secretions. Several factors may affect accuracy of the results of fetal fibronectin testing. These factors include sexual activity within 24 hours of sample collection, cervical examination within 24 hours of sample collection, vaginal bleeding, intraamniotic and vaginal infections, and use of douches (Moore, 1999). It is thought that fetal fibronectin testing may be useful in determining which women with symptoms of preterm labor require treatment.

Salivary estriol is another biochemical marker being studied for its predictive value in preterm labor. Estriol is an estrogen produced by trophoblasts from the fetal adrenal and liver steroid precursors and converted into estriol in the placenta. Levels of estriol present in maternal saliva have been shown to increase just before preterm labor begins (Moore, 1999). An advantage of salivary estriol testing is the ability of the woman to collect the sample herself at home, but detailed education about sample collection is needed for accurate results. The woman places a funnel against her lower lip and allows saliva to flow into the test tube. The sample is then mailed directly to the laboratory for analysis. Women are instructed to wait at least 1 hour after eating, smoking, chewing gum, or caring for her teeth or gums. The sample is collected 10 minutes after the woman rinses her mouth with water. Samples are collected during the daytime hours (between 9 AM and 8 PM) to avoid the normal nighttime surges of estriol. A level greater than 2.1 ng/mL is considered positive. Factors that affect accuracy of testing even when the woman follows all instructions include administration of antenatal steroids, multiple gestation, active gingivitis, and bleeding gums (Moore, 1999). Results are trended based on five recommended samples collected over a 10-week period from 26 to 35 weeks' gestation. Salivary estriol is thought to be useful in predicting the onset of preterm labor and for allowing initiation of treatment before clinical signs and symptoms occur.

The discovery of these two markers was initially met by much enthusiasm by the healthcare community because it fueled speculation that preterm labor could be prevented by testing women for the presence of one of these biochemical markers (ie, if present, the woman would probably give birth prematurely). Further study has shown, however, that the negative predictive value of both of these tests is high (up to 95% for fetal fibronectin; up to 98% for salivary estriol), whereas the positive predictive value is low (25% to 40% for fetal fibronectin; 7% to 25% for salivary estriol). This means that both tests may be effective in predicting who will not experience preterm labor rather than who will experience it. Because the cost of each test is high (fetal fibronectin test costs approximately $230; each salivary estriol test costs approximately $90 and must be repeated every 2 weeks for perhaps 10 weeks at a total cost of $450), the cost of instituting these tests on a routine basis for all pregnant women to discover who will not experience preterm labor (89% of all pregnant women) is prohibitive for the healthcare system (Moore, 1999). Nevertheless, some researchers have suggested that appropriate use of fetal fibronectin testing can be clinically and financially beneficial. The use of fetal fibronectin testing reduced the number of preterm labor admissions for one institution and resulted in an associated savings of $486,000 in a 1-year period (Joffe et al., 1999). Other researchers found that rapid fetal fibronectin testing may offer more cost savings when compared with treatment of all women with threatened preterm labor and may prevent similar numbers of cases of respiratory distress syndrome and neonatal deaths (Mozurkewich, Naglie, Krahn, & Hayashi, 2000). More data are needed about screening for preterm labor using biochemical markers before widespread use can be recommended.

Cervical Length Assessment

Another risk factor for preterm labor is short cervical length. A cervical length of less than 30 mm as measured by ultrasound seems to predict some instances of preterm labor (Crane, Van den Hof, Armson, & Liston, 1997; Hartmann, Thorp, McDonald, Savita, & Granados, 1999; Yost, Bloom, Twicker, & Leveno, 1999). However, to compare measurements of cervical length, at least two or more ultrasound tests must be performed. Cervical length measurement as a screening tool for selected women at high risk for preterm labor and birth may be beneficial, but costs of the procedure are significant. More study is needed with samples large enough to provide adequate power to determine whether short cervical length can predict preterm labor and birth in women with a history of preterm birth.

Pathophysiology and Causes of Preterm Labor

Despite the fact that some of the risk factors for some preterm labor are known, the exact cause of preterm labor remains unknown. Multifactorial issues must be considered (Goldenberg & Rouse, 1998). Not all preterm births can or should be prevented. About 25% of preterm births are intentional and occur because of health problems of the mother or the fetus (eg, IUGR, preeclampsia, abruptio placentae); another 25% of preterm births follow rupture of membranes (a cause not known to be preventable). The remaining 50% of preterm births may be preventable (Goldenberg & Rouse, 1998).

Many experts believe that infection plays a part in many preterm labors (Goldenberg & Williams, 1996; Hauth, Goldenberg, Andrews, DuBard, & Copper, 1995; Hillier et al., 1995). There has been much speculation in the literature about the role of bacterial vaginosis in the cause of preterm labor and the role that metronidazole might play in the treatment or prevention of preterm labor (Carey et al., 2000). When infections are present in the cervical, vaginal, or urinary systems, the risk of preterm birth increases, but research using trials of antibiotic therapy, including metronidazole, have not reduced rates of preterm birth (Carey et al., 2000; Fiscella, 1996; Gibbs, Romero, Hillier, Eschenbach, & Sweet, 1992; Mercer & Lewis, 1997). With this in mind, nurses should encourage women to receive prenatal care on a regular basis so that infections can be treated promptly.

The pathophysiology of preterm labor is unclear. Because biomedical research has not discovered the cause of labor at term, it has also not determined the pathophysiologic causes of preterm labor. There are many hypotheses concerning the pathophysiology, including cytokine release and prostaglandin effect of myometrial contractions (Lopez-Bernal, Watson, Phaneuf, & Europe-Finner, 1993); corticotropin-releasing hormone activation because of stress (Lockwood, 1994; Wadhwa, Porto, Garite, Chicz-DeMet, & Sandman, 1998); oxytocin sensitivity (Lopez-Bernal et al., 1993); and smooth muscle reaction to estrogen and progesterone (Valenzuela, Germain, & Foster, 1993). All causes remain hypothetical.

Clinical Manifestations and Nursing Assessment for Preterm Labor

Nurses who work with women during the prenatal period should be prepared to educate women about the early symptoms of preterm labor. Intrapartum nurses must understand the sometimes imperceptible nature of preterm labor to assess women who present with subtle symptoms. When women complain about early symptoms of preterm labor, they are in danger of being told by family or those in the healthcare system that these symptoms represent "normal discomforts of pregnancy." Research has shown that some women wait hours or days before contacting a provider after preterm labor symptoms have begun, not realizing that their symptoms could be something serious (Freston et al., 1997; Iams, Stilson, Johnson, Williams, & Rice, 1990). Waiting too long to see a healthcare provider could result in inevitable preterm birth without the added benefit of the administration of antenatal glucocorticoids and ultimately result in an infant being born at higher risk for respiratory distress syndrome and intraventricular hemorrhage. Prenatal healthcare providers need to teach women that the symptoms, when felt between 20 weeks and 37 weeks of pregnancy, should be reported to a healthcare provider promptly. In addition to teaching the symptoms in a didactic fashion, it is essential that the nurse in the antepartum or intrapartum setting establish a therapeutic relationship with the pregnant woman so she will feel comfortable reporting vague, nonspecific complaints and will come in or call her primary healthcare provider if she experiences any of the following signs or symptoms of preterm labor:

- Uterine cramping (menstrual-like cramps, intermittent or constant)
- Uterine contractions every 10 to 15 minutes or more frequently
- Low abdominal pressure (pelvic pressure)
- Dull low backache (intermittent or constant)
- Increase or change in vaginal discharge
- Feeling that the baby is "pushing down"
- Abdominal cramping with or without diarrhea

When any of these symptoms is experienced, the woman should be instructed to stop what she is doing, lie down on her side, drink 2 to 3 glasses of water or juice, and wait 1 hour. If the symptoms get worse, she should call the healthcare provider. If the symptoms go away, she should tell the healthcare provider at the next visit what happened, and if the symptoms come back, she should call the healthcare provider.

Perinatal nurses must listen carefully when pregnant women between 20 and 37 weeks' gestation complain of these symptoms, assess for cervical effacement or dilation as well as uterine contractions, and encourage them to call their provider or come back to the hospital if the symptoms reappear. Women who are between 24 to 34 weeks' gestation who present with any symptoms of preterm labor are candidates for antenatal glucocorticoid therapy.

Nursing Interventions Used to Prevent Preterm Birth

Education About Signs and Symptoms of Preterm Labor

Educating women about signs and symptoms of preterm labor has been a hallmark of preterm birth prevention programs since the early 1980s (Herron et al., 1982). At its onset, the woman may think that preterm labor symptoms are a "normal discomfort of pregnancy," in part because physicians, nurse midwives, childbirth educators, and nurses continue to teach women about Braxton-Hicks contractions, expecting the women to decide whether the contractions experienced are normal or abnormal. Nursing research (Patterson, Douglas, Patterson, & Bradle, 1992) has shown that women taught in this fashion experience "diagnostic confusion" when faced with the symptoms of preterm labor and may not notify their healthcare provider because they think that the contractions they are experiencing are normal. If the goal in teaching women is to ensure prompt notification of the provider when early, subtle symptoms of preterm labor appear, use of the term *Braxton-Hicks contractions* for women before 37 weeks' gestation should be removed from prenatal teaching (Hill & Lambertz, 1990).

Because all pregnant women must be considered at risk for preterm labor, it is essential that nurses teach pregnant women how to detect the early symptoms of preterm labor (Davies et al., 1998; Freda, Damus, & Merkatz, 1991; Freston et al., 1997; Moore & Freda, 1998). Nurses providing care to pregnant women should use the literature to understand the best methods for teaching early recognition of preterm symptoms. Reassessment for symptoms at each subsequent prenatal visit is also essential. Patient education regarding any symptoms of contractions or cramping between 20 and 36 weeks' gestation should include telling the woman that these symptoms are not normal discomforts in pregnancy and that contractions or cramping that do not go away should prompt the woman to contact her healthcare provider.

Although many nurses teach their patients in a one-on-one manner, the use of a standardized videotape for teaching women about preterm symptoms has been shown by nursing research to be effective in teaching women this information (Freda, Damus, Andersen, Brustman, & Merkatz, 1990). Nurses can feel confident in using patient education materials that have been scientifically evaluated, such as the March of Dimes videotape *Helpful Hints: Some Ideas to Help Prevent Preterm Labor* and its accompanying patient education booklet (Freda, Damus, et al., 1990). No matter which method of patient education is used, it is imperative that nurses in prenatal settings make concerted efforts to teach all pregnant women about how to recognize early preterm labor.

Sometimes, patient education cannot be offered in person but can still be effective. A randomized, controlled trial demonstrated that education offered by nurses on the telephone can result in a 26% decrease in LBW births and a 27% decrease in preterm births among African-American women (Moore et al., 1998). This study demonstrates the power of nursing care, nursing support, and patient education in the care of women at highest risk for preterm birth.

Reinforcement of the signs and symptoms of preterm labor should occur at each subsequent prenatal visit along with a review of any symptoms that may have been experienced since the last visit. Some women who experience preterm labor wait for hours or days to call a healthcare provider, significantly delaying their time of entry into the healthcare system when some proactive action could be taken (Freston et al., 1997; Iams et al., 1990). Prompt notification of the healthcare provider is essential, because the use of antenatal glucocorticoids given to hasten fetal lung maturity is the most effective therapy for avoiding neonatal health problems such as respiratory distress syndrome (Leviton et al., 1999; National Institutes of Health Consensus Development Panel, 1995).

The message about the importance of educating pregnant women about preterm labor symptoms has not permeated the healthcare system. Davies et al. (1998) surveyed all prenatal care providers in Eastern Ontario and found that only one half of family physicians and obstetricians even discussed signs and symptoms of preterm labor with their prenatal patients; only 10% of family physicians and 40% of obstetricians distributed educational materials to their patients about preterm labor. In their focus groups of women who had delivered preterm, the researchers found that all of the women wished they had known more about how to recognize symptoms of preterm labor (Davies et al., 1998).

Lifestyle Modification

Evidence exists that some women experience more preterm symptoms when engaged in certain activities. When women are able to modify those lifestyle factors, they have fewer preterm births (Freda, Andersen et al., 1990; Katz, Gill, & Newman, 1986; Lynam & Miller, 1992). Activities such as stair climbing, sexual activity, riding long distances in automobiles or public transportation, carrying heavy objects, hard physical work, and inability to rest when tired have been associated with increased preterm birth (Hobel et al., 1994; Iams et al., 1990; Katz, Goodyear, & Creasy, 1990; Papiernik, 1989). Nurses who teach women about symptoms of preterm labor should assess whether symptoms increase when these or other activities are performed and work with women to find ways to help them eliminate those activities or at least decrease their frequency.

Smoking Cessation

Smoking is a lifestyle factor strongly associated with preterm birth and LBW. It is one of the few risk factors that can be altered by pregnant women. Although the effects of smoking on risk of preterm birth and LBW have been known for more than 40 years (Simpson, 1957), between 15% and 29% of women in the United States smoke during their pregnancy (ACOG, 2000). Smoking accounts for more LBW infants than any other risk factor (Goldenberg, 1994). It is estimated that there would be a 10% reduction in perinatal mortality and an 11% reduction in LBW if smoking during pregnancy were eliminated (ACOG, 2000).

The physiologic effects of smoking occur as a result of transient intrauterine hypoxemia. When the pregnant woman smokes, carbon monoxide crosses the placenta and binds with maternal and fetal hemoglobin, producing carboxyhemoglobin. Carboxyhemoglobin interferes with the normal binding process of oxygen to the hemoglobin molecule, reducing the ability of the blood to carry adequate levels of oxygen to the fetus (O'Campo, Davis, & Gielen, 1995; Secker-Walker, Vacek, Flynn, & Mead, 1997). There appears to be a dose-response relationship between smoking and the occurrence of preterm birth and LBW (Ellard, Johnstone, Prescott, Ji-Xian, & Jian-Hua, 1996; Nordentoft et al., 1996; Wisborg et al., 1996). The most pronounced effects are seen in women who smoke more than 15 cigarettes per day (Nordentoft et al., 1996; Wisborg et al., 1996). There is evidence, however, that even passive smoking can affect fetal growth (Ellard et al., 1996; Secker-Walker et al., 1997).

The effects of smoking on birth weight seem to be most prominent during the last trimester of pregnancy (Ellard et al., 1996; Groff, Mullen, Mongoven, & Burau, 1997). Infants born to women who stop smoking or reduce the number of cigarettes smoked after 28 weeks can be comparable in weight and size to infants born to women who never smoked (Goldenberg, 1994; O'Campo et al., 1995). An opportunity to reduce the risk of preterm birth and LBW exists if education for pregnant women about the effects of smoking on the fetus begins early in pregnancy. One of the most effective interventions to reduce smoking during pregnancy is to encourage the woman to institute a no-smoking policy at home (Mullen, Richardson, Quinn, & Ershoff, 1997; O'Campo et al., 1995). No-smoking policies in the workplace have also been shown to decrease the number of cigarettes smoked by pregnant women who work outside their home (O'Campo et al., 1995). Benefits of these approaches include fewer opportunities to smoke, avoidance of passive smoke of other smokers, and avoidance of the temptation to smoke when others smoke (Ellard et al., 1996; O'Campo et al., 1995). Although smoking cessation programs during pregnancy have not shown to permanently change smoking habits, there have been promising results of behavioral changes during pregnancy (Mullen et al., 1997; Nordentoft et al., 1996; O'Campo et al., 1995). At least 90% of pregnant women who smoke indicate a desire to quit during pregnancy (Lowe, Windsor, Balanda, & Woolby, 1997; O'Campo et al., 1995). An essential component of a comprehensive preterm birth prevention program is encouragement to stop smoking or reduce the number of cigarettes smoked by providing education about the effects of smoking to pregnant women and suggesting concrete strategies for behavioral changes. Even a reduction in the number of cigarettes smoked by all pregnant women who smoke may translate into a significant improvement in the LBW rate in the United States.

Several investigators have studied the effects of smoking. Mittendorf et al. (1994) found that cigarette smoking could be causative in up to 34% of preterm births. Moore et al. (1995) studied women at high risk for preterm birth and found that the preterm birth rate was 9.2% among nonsmokers, 14.4% for women who smoked less than one-half pack of cigarettes each day, and 20.4% for women who smoked one-half pack or more of cigarettes each day. They also found that cigarette smoking was associated with significantly higher rates of LBW (Moore & Zaccaro, 2000).

Nursing interventions to assist women to stop smoking have also been reported in the literature. In a study done in the early 1990s, O'Connor and colleagues (1992) evaluated two nursing interventions to promote smoking cessation: a 2-hour evening group session and a 20-minute individual session during a prenatal appointment. They found that the women who smoked and were assigned to the 20-minute individual session during prenatal care had two to three times higher rates of smoking cessation than those assigned to the evening group session. Moore et al. (1995) also instituted a nursing intervention to help women to stop smoking The intervention consisted of telephone support from nurses one to three times each week. In this study, 61.5% of the women stopped or significantly reduced their smoking with this nursing support. The success of these nursing interventions suggests that nurses can have a major impact on smoking habits of pregnant women and should provide nurses with the impetus to work more diligently toward helping women stop smoking.

There has been interest in using nicotine replacement products as smoking cessation aids for pregnant women. The use of these products has not been sufficiently evaluated for efficacy and safety during pregnancy (ACOG, 2000). Nicotine gum and patches should be considered for use during pregnancy only when nonpharmacologic treatments have failed and the risks and benefits have been clearly explained to the woman (ACOG, 2000).

Healthy Diet and Adequate Maternal Weight Gain

There is a positive linear relationship between maternal weight gain and newborn weight (ACOG, 1996b). Inadequate maternal weight gain during pregnancy is a significant factor contributing to IUGR and LBW (Seidman, Ever-Hadani & Gale, 1989; Schieve et al., 2000) and increases the risk of preterm birth by approximately 60% (Abrams, Newman, Key, & Parker, 1989; Carmichael & Abrams, 1997). Like smoking, inadequate maternal weight gain is a risk factor that can potentially be altered by the pregnant woman. Encouragement during the prenatal period to eat a well-balanced diet has been shown to be effective in enhancing maternal weight gain for pregnant women (Brown, Watkins, & Hiett, 1996). Women who lack financial resources to support an adequate diet may be eligible to participate in the Supplemental Food Program for Women, Infants, and Children (WIC) and should be referred to appropriate social services to assist in application.

All women can benefit from prenatal education focused on healthy nutritional practices (ACOG, 1996b; Brown et al., 1996). Nurses who care for women during the prenatal period should include nutritional assessment and dietary counseling as a component of care. For complex dietary issues related to food allergies, preferences such as a vegetarian diet, or specific maternal conditions such as diabetes, referral to a dietitian may be warranted.

Maternal smoking has also been associated with inadequate maternal weight gain (Ellard et al., 1996; Hellerstedt, Himes, Stroy, Alton, & Edwards, 1997; Nordentoft et al., 1996). For women who smoke during pregnancy, it is unclear whether the inadequate maternal weight gain is a result of smoking or in itself contributes further to risk of LBW infants (Nordentoft et al., 1996).

Bed Rest

It is common for bed rest therapy to be prescribed when preterm labor is suspected. Bed rest is suggested despite the fact that there is no evidence to support its effectiveness in preventing preterm birth (Maloni, Chance, Zhang, Cohen, Betts, & Grange, 1993; Goldenberg & Rouse, 1998; Goldenberg et al., 1994). Maloni et al. (1993) have shown that after only 3 days of bed rest muscle tone decreases, calcium is lost, and glucose intolerance develops. After longer periods of bed rest, women experience bone demineralization, constipation, fatigue, anxiety, and depression (Maloni et al., 1993). Bed rest may cause more harm than therapeutic benefit. Goldenberg et al. (1994) have shown that bed rest has a major financial impact for families and for society in lost wages, household help expenses, and hospital costs. Women suspected of being at risk for preterm labor are often cared for at home, sometimes being asked to endure months of bed rest. Nursing interventions for care of the woman at home are listed in Display 8–15 and in Appendix 8A.

Home Uterine Activity Monitoring

Home uterine activity monitoring (HUAM) is a system of care to detect preterm labor using a combination of recording of uterine activity with a tocodynamometer and daily telephone calls from a healthcare provider (usually a perinatal nurse) to offer the woman support and advice (ACOG, 1996a). The recording of uterine activity is transferred to the healthcare provider by telephone for rapid evaluation. The premise of HUAM is that women have an identifiable increase in uterine contractions before the onset of overt preterm labor and that pregnant women do not usually recognize these early contractions (ACOG, 1996a). Advocates of HUAM believe that early identification of uterine contractions allows for earlier treatment of preterm labor by tocolytic agents and other therapies. Some experts believe that administration of tocolytic agents before cervical changes is more likely to be successful in preventing preterm birth and allows time for administration of antenatal steroids.

HUAM has been used since the early 1980s to attempt to prevent preterm birth in women at high risk, but numerous prospective studies do not support its efficacy (ACOG, 1996a; Brown et al., 1999; Dyson et al., 1998; Grimes & Shulz, 1992). The early studies suggested that there was a 24- to 48-hour window of opportunity to prevent preterm births (Katz et al., 1986; Morrison, Martin, Martin, Gookin, & Wiser, 1987). In these studies, an increase in contraction frequency was detected 1 to 2 days before preterm birth. The researchers felt HUAM could be effective in detecting this increase in uterine activity, allowing for treatment before cervical changes occurred leading to preterm birth. Later data suggest that the period dur-

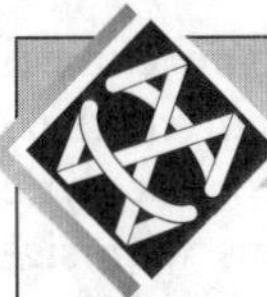

DISPLAY 8–15

Home Care Management for Women Prescribed Bed Rest as Therapy

- Assist the family in becoming involved in the nursing care plan.
- If the family is not available, suggest that the woman ask friends for help during this time.
- Hydration is essential; suggest that a cooler be kept by the bed.
- Bed rest can lead to muscle wasting; teach passive limb exercises.
- Anxiety and depression are common during bed rest; teach the family to expect this and talk about their feelings.
- The woman should be in a place where she can interact with her family rather than in a bedroom alone.
- Instruct the woman not to do any nipple preparation for breast-feeding; nipple stimulation can cause uterine contractions.
- Some women find that keeping a journal helps them deal with the isolation and boredom of bed rest.
- Household jobs that can be done in a reclining position (eg, paying bills, mending, folding laundry) help the woman feel more a part of the family.
- This is a good time to provide short educational videotapes about all aspects of pregnancy, labor, birth, and parenting.
- A home computer with Internet access can help the woman keep in touch with friends and can be educational.
- Encourage the woman to develop a support system of people with whom she can talk and vent her feelings.

ing which contractions are detected by HUAM or self-palpation is limited to 12 to 24 hours before overt preterm labor (Iams, Johnson, & Parker, 1994).

The early studies suffered from small sample sizes and errors in methodology and statistical analysis (Grimes & Shulz, 1992). When HUAM monitoring was studied using a more rigorous design, including prospective randomization and larger sample sizes, its benefits as a preterm birth prevention intervention were not supported (ACOG, 1996a). Prospective randomized clinical trials with sufficient sample size and statistical power to detect significant differences in outcomes in women at risk for preterm labor using HUAM have been been conducted (Brown et al., 1999; Dyson et al., 1998). Their findings demonstrated that the use of HUAM, even with nursing support on the telephone, did not reduce the rate of preterm births and was a very expensive intervention. Daily provider initiated telephone contact usually included with HUAM services may be effective in reducing the incidence of preterm birth in a select group of women prospectively identified as at risk for preterm birth, but confirmatory data are needed (ACOG, 1996a). Based on published research about efficacy, ACOG (1996a, 1998) does not recommend the use of HUAM for singleton or multiple pregnancies. According to ACOG (1996a), it has not been clearly demonstrated that HUAM can affect the rate of preterm birth, and the use of this expensive system and subsequent treatment has the potential for substantially increasing costs. Questions about the value of HUAM have generated much controversy within the research community (Roberts & Morrison, 1998).

Intravenous Hydration

One common strategy used in the inpatient setting to reduce preterm contractions is intravenous hydration. Significant amounts of intravenous fluids are usually administered to increase vascular volume and because, anecdotally, it is thought that uterine contractions are quieted by hydration. A literature review concluded that there is no evidence that this strategy is effective (Freda & DeVore, 1996). One possible reason that intravenous hydration therapy was not found to be effective in inhibiting uterine activity in the studies published is the small sample sizes of these studies and the inability to detect a significant difference in outcomes. Similar to bed rest therapy, however, intravenous fluid therapy is a traditional treatment that continues to be used. This therapy is not without side effects. Nurses should be cautious when administering intravenous fluids for this purpose, because if uterine activity continues, the next treatment could be intravenous administration of tocolytic agents, which carry a possible side effect of pulmonary edema. Careful attention to intake and output and auscultation of the lungs are essential to monitor for the development of pulmonary edema.

Tocolytic Therapy

The promise of pharmacologic agents to reduce the rate of preterm birth has not become reality for many reasons. The most important is that approximately 90% of pregnant women who present to the labor and birth unit with reports of uterine activity are not candidates for tocolysis because of advanced cervical dilation or spontaneous rupture of membranes (Creasy & Merkatz, 1990). Another group of pregnant women for which tocolytics are not beneficial are those with complications of pregnancy that necessitate preterm birth such as preeclampsia, cardiac disease, intraamniotic infection, or other maternal illnesses. Contraindications for the use of tocolysis for preterm labor are listed in Display 8–16.

Several classes of drugs have been used in an effort to stop preterm labor, although none has been shown to be effective for more than 24 to 48 hours (Goldenberg & Rouse, 1998; Sciscione et al., 1998; Viamontes, 1996). It is thought that the optimal use of tocolytic therapy is to gain the 24-hour window of time necessary for the full effect of antenatal glucocorticoids administered to the mother (Goldenberg & Rouse, 1998). The best way to improve neonatal outcomes is to ensure birth in a center capable of caring for a preterm infant and prescription of antenatal glucocorticoids to decrease the risk of respiratory distress syndrome and other neonatal complications (Katz & Farmer, 1999).

Controversy exists in the literature and in clinical practice about the risk–benefit data for tocolytic therapy. Three meta-analyses on the efficacy of tocolytic therapy suggest minimal benefit to the fetus with significant maternal risks (Higby, Xenakis, & Pauerstein, 1993; Macones, Berlin, & Berlin, 1995; Macones, Sehdev, Berlin, Morgan, & Berlin, 1997). A prospective, randomized study about the efficacy of terbutaline pumps in preventing preterm birth suggests tocolytic therapy by subcutaneous infusion pump works no better than a saline placebo (Wenstrom, Weiner, Merrill, & Niebyl, 1995). Oral terbutaline therapy after successful intravenous tocolytic cessation of uterine activity does not contribute to increased length of gestation (How et al., 1995; Rust, Bofill, Arriola, Andrews, & Morrison, 1996).

All tocolytic agents place the mother at some risk (Display 8–17), and this risk is increased greatly if dual tocolytic therapy is used, especially when administered intravenously. Careful, expert nursing care is essential for all women who receive tocolytic therapy (Display 8–18). The most common life-threatening complication of tocolytic therapy is pulmonary edema. Approxi-

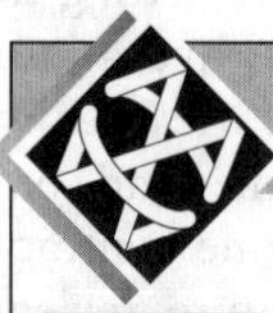

DISPLAY 8–16

Contraindications to Tocolysis for Preterm Labor

GENERAL CONTRAINDICATIONS*

- Acute fetal distress (except intrauterine resuscitation)
- Intraamniotic infection
- Eclampsia or severe preeclampsia
- Fetal demise (singleton)
- Fetal maturity
- Maternal hemodynamic instability

CONTRAINDICATIONS FOR SPECIFIC TOCOLYTIC AGENTS

Beta-mimetic agents

- Maternal cardiac rhythm disturbance or other cardiac disease
- Poorly controlled diabetes, thyrotoxicosis, or hypertension

Magnesium sulfate

- Hypocalcemia
- Myasthenia gravis
- Renal failure

Indomethacin

- Asthma
- Coronary artery disease
- Gastrointestinal bleeding (current or past)
- Oligohydramnios
- Renal failure
- Suspected fetal cardiac or renal anomaly

Nifedipine

- Maternal liver disease

*Relative and absolute contraindications to tocolysis are based on the clinical circumstances and should take into account the risks of continuing the pregnancy versus those of birth.

From American College of Obstetricians and Gynecologists. (1996). *Preterm birth* (Technical Bulletin No. 206). Washington, DC: Author.

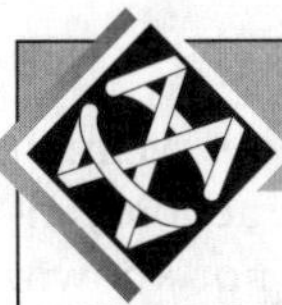

DISPLAY 8–17

Potential Complications of Tocolytic Agents

Beta-adrenergic agents
- Hyperglycemia
- Hypokalemia
- Hypotension
- Pulmonary edema
- Cardiac insufficiency
- Arrhythmias
- Myocardial ischemia
- Maternal death

Magnesium sulfate
- Pulmonary edema
- Respiratory depression*
- Cardiac arrest*
- Maternal tetany*
- Profound muscular paralysis*
- Profound hypotension*

Indomethacin
- Hepatitis†
- Renal failure†
- Gastrointestinal bleeding†

Nifedipine
- Transient hypotension

*Effect is rare and seen with toxic levels.
†Effect is rare and associated with chronic use
From American College of Obstetricians and Gynecologists. (1996). *Preterm birth* (Technical Bulletin No. 206). Washington, DC: Author.

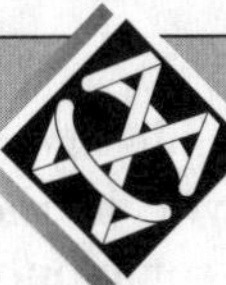

DISPLAY 8–18

Nursing Care for Women Receiving Tocolytic Therapy

- Know the contraindications and potential complications of tocolytic therapy.
- Encourage the woman to assume a sidelying position to enhance placental perfusion.
- Explain the purpose and common side effects of the drug.
- Assess maternal vital signs according to institutional protocol.
- Notify the provider if the maternal pulse exceeds 120.
- Assess for signs and symptoms of pulmonary edema.
- Assess intake and output at least every hour (unless on low-dose maintenance therapy).
- Limit intake to 2,500 mL per day (90 mL/hour).
- Provide psychosocial support.

mately 3% to 5% of all women who receive intravenous tocolytic therapy develop pulmonary edema, but the risk is greater for women with undiagnosed intraamniotic infection (21%) and for women with twin gestations (25%) (Monga & Creasy, 1995). Pulmonary edema is a significant cause of maternal mortality in the United States (National Center for Health Statistics, 1998). It is estimated that 5% of women who develop pulmonary edema from tocolytic therapy do not survive (Monga & Creasy, 1995). In 1997 and 1998, the FDA issued warnings to healthcare providers about the potential risks of using terbutaline pumps to prevent preterm birth, citing one related maternal death and lack of evidence for clinical efficacy (Nightingale, 1998). Available data do not support the role of tocolytic agents in reducing the incidence of preterm labor, increasing the interval from onset to birth, or reducing the incidence of preterm birth (ACOG, 1995; Macones et al., 1995, 1997), but they are frequently used as a secondary intervention in the United States.

If tocolytics are used, careful guidelines should be observed (Katz & Farmer, 1999):

- Maternal and fetal well-being must be established before initiating tocolytic therapy.
- The causes of preterm labor should be evaluated and treated when possible.
- The risk–benefit ratio for the mother and fetus must be reevaluated on an ongoing basis.
- When tocolytics are given before pulmonary maturity, antenatal corticosteriods should also be considered in every case.
- Long-term use of tocolytic therapy is difficult to justify.
- The safest tocolytic should be used for the shortest amount of time possible.

Because tocolytics are only effective in stopping labor for 24 to 48 hours and are associated with significant long-term effects on the mother's cardiovascular system and carbohydrate metabolism and on the fetal cardiovascular system, discontinuing tocolytic therapy should be considered after the uterus is quiet (Katz & Farmer, 1999).

Beta-Mimetics

Ritodrine hydrochloride (Yutopar) is the only agent approved by the FDA for use as a tocolytic in the United States. Terbutaline (Brethine) is commonly used for tocolysis as well, although its use is considered "off label" (ie, used for a purpose other than that approved by the FDA). Ritodrine and terbutaline are β agonists; they stimulate β-receptor cells located in smooth muscle. Theoretically, these agents work by relaxing the smooth muscle, which decreases or stops uterine contractions. The β receptors are also located in smooth muscle in the cardiovascular, pulmonary, and gastrointestinal systems. Effects of β-mimetic agents are related directly to dosage and route of administration (Higby et al., 1993). Maternal side effects are common and uncomfortable. Fetal side effects are thought to be the same as those in the mother because they rapidly cross the placenta. These β-mimetic agents are contraindicated in patients with known cardiac disease. The β-mimetic agents may be administered subcutaneously or intravenously as a secondary infusion, after baseline assessments (eg, electrolytes, blood urea nitrogen, creatinine, serum glucose, ECG status) are obtained and a meticulous intake and output record is started. The infusion is titrated according to institutional protocol until uterine activity ceases, maximum dosages are reached, or the patient experiences severe side effects. Decreases in blood pressure, a widening pulse pressure, and maternal tachycardia develop in most patients. Use of oral β-mimetic agents has not been associated with a significant increase in length of gestation (Lewis, Mercer, Salama, Walsh, & Sibai, 1996). Terbutaline pump therapy for women cared for in the home is ordered frequently in certain geographic areas of the United States. It has been studied often but has not been shown to be effective in prolonging pregnancy (Guinn, Goepfert, Owen, Wenstrom, & Hauth, 1998).

Conscientious nursing care for the woman receiving β-mimetic therapy is essential and includes ongoing assessment and monitoring of side effects. Maternal pulse rate must be monitored for any patient who is administered a β-mimetic agent. A pulse rate of 120 beats/min or greater may warrant continuous ECG monitoring and discontinuation of tocolytic therapy. A heart rate greater than 120 beats/min is associated with a decreased ventricular filling time and therefore with decreased cardiac output. Over time, if the left ventricular filling time is decreased, less blood is pumped to the myocardium, resulting in decreased myocardial perfusion. This is reflected by the patient's complaints of chest heaviness, shortness of breath, or chest pain. Myocardial infarction may result if the agent is not discontinued.

Magnesium Sulfate

Intravenous $MgSO_4$ is a commonly used intervention in intrapartum settings for preterm contractions, although the exact mechanism of action is not known. This drug, just as terbutaline, is used on an off-label basis for this purpose. Theoretically, magnesium interferes with calcium uptake in the cells of the myometrium. Because myometrial cells are thought to need calcium to contract, decreasing the amount of calcium decreases or stops contractions. $MgSO_4$ relaxes smooth muscle throughout the body, and a decrease in blood pressure may be observed with the administration of a loading dose or at high infusion rates. Many practitioners feel comfortable using this agent because they have experience in its administration for the prevention of eclamptic seizures. Institutional protocols differ widely for how this drug is used in women with preterm contractions. Maternal side effects include flushing, headache, nausea and vomiting, shortness of breath, chest pain, and pulmonary edema. Oral administration of a variety of magnesium preparations, such as magnesium gluconate, has not been shown to increase length of gestation (Ricci, Hariharan, Helfgott, Reed, & O'Sullivan, 1991).

Calcium Channel Blockers

Calcium channel blockers are another class of drugs that have been used to suppress contractions. They cause the myometrial muscle to relax by interfering with the movement of extracellular calcium into the calcium channels of the cells. This prevents the electrical system from passing the current through the cells, preventing a contraction. These agents, especially nifedipine (Procardia) and nicardipine (Nicardipine), have been compared with ritodrine, and no differences in prolongation of pregnancy were found (Garcia-Velasco & Gonzales Gonzales, 1998). The use of calcium channel blockers for inhibiting preterm labor in the United States remains limited. Common fetal side effects associated with its use include decreased uteroplacental blood flow, fetal hypoxia, and fetal bradycardia. Calcium channel blockers have also been associated with maternal hepatotoxicity when administered for preterm labor (Higby et al., 1993).

Prostaglandin Inhibitors

Prostaglandin is a naturally produced agent that is thought to cause uterine contractions and cervical ripening in term pregnancies. Because little prostaglandin has been found in women who are not in labor, the use of drugs that inhibit the production of prostaglandin has been hypothesized as a possible treatment for preterm labor (Higby et al., 1993). Several types of prostaglandins affect uterine contractions and cervical ripening. The most well-known and well-studied prostaglandin inhibitor for use as a tocolytic agent is indomethacin (Besinger, Niebyl, Keyes, & Johnson, 1991). Indomethacin competes with other factors in a long-term process whereby prostacyclin is the end product blocking the production of prostaglandin. Indomethacin is not without fetal effects, however. After 34 weeks' gestation, indomethacin may cause premature closure of the fetal ductus arteriosis, increasing the risk of fetal pulmonary hypertension (Higby et al., 1993). Indomethacin also impairs fetal renal function that may result in oligohydramnios. The use of this drug for prevention of preterm birth remains controversial. Some in the research community have found that the risk to the fetus by using indomethacin is less than the multiple morbidities associated with a birth at less than 32 weeks' gestation (Macones & Robinson, 1998).

Antenatal Glucocorticoid Administration

It has been known since the early 1970s that use of intramuscular injections of glucocorticoids given to a woman at least 24 hours before the birth of a preterm infant can accelerate fetal lung maturity. The medical community, however, did not use this information in any widespread manner to change practice, with only about 17% of practitioners stating they routinely used antenatal glucocorticoids in 1995 (Leviton et al., 1999). It was not until the National Institutes of Health Consensus Development Panel (1995) published a report and distributed it widely to healthcare providers that this evidence-based clinical practice began to be adopted. There is clear evidence that, aside from reducing rates of respiratory distress syndrome, use of antenatal glucocorticoids also decreases rates of intraventricular hemorrhage in preterm infants (Goldenberg & Rouse, 1998).

All pregnant women between 24 and 34 weeks' gestation with any possibility of preterm labor are appropriate candidates for antenatal glucocorticoid therapy. Because it takes 24 hours for the benefits of treatment to occur, the timely administration of this drug is imperative. The two glucocorticoids used are betamethasone and dexamethasone. Betamethasone is given intramuscularly in two doses of 12 mg each that are 24 hours apart. The current recommendation is to use one course of antenatal glucocorticoid treatment, but some providers believe that weekly administration of the drug is beneficial. Some studies have examined the efficacy of two or more courses of antenatal glucocorticoids, finding conflicting results (Banks et al., 1999; Elimian, Verma, Visintainer, & Tejani, 2000; French, Hagan, Evans, Godfrey, & Newnham, 1999). Because the long-term side effects of multiple courses for the pregnant woman and for the fetus remain unknown, the use of two or more courses of this drug is not recommended.

Nursing can play an important part in assuring that all eligible women receive this medication, as has been shown by a study sponsored by the Agency for Health Care Policy and Research (Leviton et al., 1999). Because many physicians continue to avoid the use of this drug despite scientific evidence of its effectiveness, nurses need to be aware of the literature regarding appropriate antenatal glucocorticoid use, discuss this with other healthcare professionals with whom they work, and encourage the use of antenatal glucocorticoids for all women who appear for triage and are between 24 and 34 weeks' gestation. The only exception to this eligibility is women with known chorioamnionitis (NIH, 1995). Because the drug needs 24 hours to have an effect on fetal lung maturity, time is of the essence in administering the drug to women who could possibly give birth preterm.

DIABETES

Significance and Incidence

Diabetes mellitus occurs in approximately 4% of all pregnancies and affects approximately 154,000 pregnant women in the United States annually (Engelgau, Herman, Smith, German, & Aubert, 1995). Gestational diabetes mellitus (GDM) affects most of these pregnancies (88%, 135,000), and the remaining cases are pregnant women with preexisting type 2 diabetes (7%, 12,000) and type 1 diabetes (4%, 7,000). Maternal diabetes rates vary by race or ethnicity and age, with a prevalence of 25.3 per 1,000 U.S. women overall (Centers for Disease Control and Prevention [CDC], 1998). Caucasian women have the lowest age-adjusted rate at 24.3 per 1,000. Native American and Alaskan Natives have the highest rate of maternal diabetes at 52.4 per 1,000, African-American women have a rate of 27.5 per 1,000, and Hispanic and Asian or Pacific Islander women slightly higher at 28.3 per 1,000 (CDC, 1998). Although the rate of diabetes in U.S. women of childbearing age is lower than that for women not born in the United States, it is increasing because of immigration of women with higher rates of type 2 diabetes (Harris et al., 1998). Diabetes in pregnancy is rare in women younger than 20 years of age (8.3 per 1,000) but steadily increases to 65.6 cases per 1,000 women between the ages of 40 and 49 years (CDC, 1998).

The rate of perinatal mortality with gestational diabetes remains similar to that for nondiabetic women, but perinatal morbidity such as neonatal asphyxia (15%), hypoglycemia (20%) and other metabolic abnormalities, and respiratory distress syndrome (15%) occur more often (Cordero & Landon, 1993). Maintenance of euglycemia throughout pregnancy in GDM reduces the risk of these hyperglycemia-related fetal and neonatal abnormalities, but there is still an increased risk for fetal macrosomia (40%) with resultant traumatic or cesarean delivery (Blank, Grave, & Metzger, 1995). First-trimester control in women with pregestational diabetes is vital in reducing the risk of macrosomia (Raychaudhuri & Maresh, 2000; Rey, Attie, & Bonin, 1999). *Macrosomia* is defined as a weight greater than the 90th percentile for gestational age and a birth weight of 4,000 g (8 pounds, 13 ounces) or more. Other factors such as morbid maternal obesity and postmaturity are also associated with fetal macrosomia and, when combined with insulin-controlled diabetes, lead to an even higher occurrence. Fetal macrosomia predisposes the newborn to a variety of traumatic injuries such as shoulder dystocia with associated risk for facial palsy, cephalohematoma, subdural hemorrhage, brachial plexus injury, and clavicle fracture (Tyrala, 1996; Uvena-Celebrezze & Catalano, 2000). Fetal macrosomia contributes to an excessively high rate of cesarean births (41%), with resultant increased surgical morbidity in the mother (Persson & Hanson, 1996).

Although comprehensive obstetric care and intensive metabolic management have reduced perinatal risk in pregnancies complicated by type 1 and 2 diabetes, morbidity and mortality still remain higher than in the general population. Congenital defects and unexplained fetal death account for the increased fetal and neonatal mortality (Reece & Homko, 2000). Preconception and early pregnancy glycemic control as evidenced by a lower glycosylated hemoglobin (Hgb A_{1C}) during the period of organogenesis greatly reduces the risk of birth defects (McElvy et al., 2000; Reece & Homko, 2000). When GDM is detected in the first trimester with an elevated Hgb A_{1c} and fasting hyperglycemia, the risk for congenital defects approaches that of women with pregestational type 1 diabetes (Schaefer et al., 1997). No specific congenital malformations are associated with diabetes, but defects in offspring of women with preexisting diabetes have been found to be more severe, usually multiple, and more often fatal (Kendrick, 1999).

In addition to the risk of fetal macrosomia for all women with diabetes, the other extreme of weight (IUGR) with an occurrence of 20% is a significant risk for infants born to women who have vascular complications of diabetes (Tyrala, 1996). Retinopathy and nephropathy associated with hypertension and poor renal function may contribute to uteroplacental insufficiency that leads to infants that are small for their gestational age. PIH, to which women with diabetes (with or without vascular disease) are predisposed, also decreases uterine blood flow, compromising intrauterine fetal growth. Congenital defects are associated with IUGR and poor glycemic control. Maintaining tight control (ie, an average blood glucose of 86 mg/dL) can help to avoid IUGR (Tyrala, 1996).

Neonatal metabolic abnormalities occur with a higher frequency in offspring of women with diabetes. Hypoglycemia, defined as a blood glucose of 35 mg/dL in term infants and 25 mg/dL in preterm infants, occurs during the first few hours of life in 25% to 40% of infants of diabetic mothers (Reece & Homko, 1994). Preterm and large for gestational age infants are at greatest risk for the development of hypoglycemia in the neonatal period. Chronic maternal hyperglycemia leads to excessive insulin production in the fetus (ie, hyperinsulinemia), which lowers plasma glucose and inhibits glycogen release from the fetal liver as a normal physiologic response to hypoglycemia. This combination contributes to the risk for hypoglycemia development in the first 24 hours of life when transplacental glucose is interrupted by cutting the umbilical cord. Early detection and prompt treatment prevent the severe neurologic sequelae associated with hypoglycemia.

Approximately 3% to 5% of infants of diabetic mothers exhibit polycythemia, which is defined as a venous hematocrit of greater than 65% (Tyrala, 1996). Polycythemia occurs as a result of chronic hyperglycemia, hyperinsulinemia, and hyperketonemia and causes increased oxygen consumption and decreased fetal arterial oxygen content (Tyrala, 1996). Erythropoietin production increases, increasing red blood cell production (Tyrala, 1996). Hyperbilirubinemia occurs in 20% of infants of mothers with diabetes without a definitive explanation. It is seen more frequently when maternal diabetes is severe and in the presence of neonatal polycythemia and prematurity (Uvena-Celebrezze & Catalano, 2000). Hypocalcemia and hypomagnesemia are other metabolic abnormalities frequently seen in infants of women with type 1 and 2 diabetes. The exact cause of hypocalcemia is unknown but occurs with a high frequency in cases of respiratory distress and in the presence of prematurity. Hypomagnesemia may be seen in conjunction with hypocalcemia and is believed to be the result of polyuria in association with hyperglycemia (Reece & Homko, 1994).

Strict maternal glycemic control has decreased the incidence of respiratory distress syndrome significantly, but other factors such as iatrogenic prematurity due to early delivery as a result of maternal or fetal compromise continue to contribute to the risk.

Fetal surfactant production is inhibited by hyperinsulinemia, which occurs more frequently in poor metabolic control and is the underlying mechanism for respiratory distress syndrome in this group (Uvena-Celebrezze & Catalano, 2000; Wiznitzer & Reece, 1999).

Risks during pregnancy for the mother include an increased incidence of hypoglycemia as a result of stricter control (Reece, Homko, & Hagay, 1995; Rosenn & Miodovnik, 2000). Hypoglycemia does not seem to cause problems for the fetus unless blood sugar levels are chronically low, but hypoglycemia does threaten the well-being of the mother. Educational efforts focusing on appropriate management of nausea and vomiting and frequent contact with the diabetes management team during periods of insulin adjustment can decrease this risk.

Diabetic ketoacidosis (DKA) is a rare complication for women with gestational diabetes and has a low incidence in women with overt diabetes. However, the occurrence of DKA carries serious morbidity and mortality for the mother and the fetus (Garner, 1995; Hagay, 1994; Kilvert, Nicholson, & Wright, 1993). Fetal loss may occur through spontaneous abortion in the first and early second trimester or as an intrauterine fetal death during an episode of DKA in late second and third trimester. Total fetal loss rate is approximately 22% (Kilvert et al., 1993). Improved perinatal management has decreased the fetal loss rate to 9% in the past decade (Cullen, Reece, Homko, & Silvan, 1996). Fetal outcomes in cases of DKA seem to be related to the stability of the diabetes mellitus during pregnancy. There are significant differences in fetal mortality in women with brittle diabetes compared with women with better controlled diabetes. In one study, spontaneous abortion rate in the brittle group was reported at 48% with DKA and 10% in the stable group (Kent, Gill, & Williams, 1994). The stillbirth rate for the brittle group was 5%, with no stillbirths associated with DKA in the stable group. Decreasing the morbidity and mortality of DKA requires prevention, early detection, and prompt and aggressive management.

Women with microvascular complications, poor glycemic control, and a longer duration of diabetes have poorer outcomes. Retinopathy affects approximately 20% to 27% of reproductive-age women, and this microvascular complication of diabetes is frequently encountered in pregnancy (Reece, Homko, & Hagay, 1996). Retinopathy progresses during pregnancy, requiring continued surveillance and treatment with photocoagulation for proliferative retinopathy (Klein, Moss, & Klein, 1990). Nephropathy is a more serious microvascular complication that has been associated with the adverse outcomes of intrauterine growth retardation, congenital malformations, preterm delivery, and intrauterine fetal death (Rosenn & Miodovnik, 2000). Hypertension almost universally develops if not present at conception and may include edema, superimposed PIH, and renal failure without meticulous care (Rosenn & Miodovnik, 2000). Macrovascular complications of diabetes such as coronary artery, peripheral vascular, and cerebral artery disease are rarely seen in reproductive-age women but are contraindications to pregnancy because of the significant maternal mortality risk (Hagay & Weissman, 1996; Wiznitzer & Reece, 1999). Gastroparesis or gastropathy is a neuropathic complication that also is a contraindication to pregnancy because of the very high risk for severe maternal and fetal malnourishment (Rosenn & Miodovnik, 2000). This condition occurs as a result of autonomic neuropathy directed at the gut, which causes delayed gastric emptying and absorption of nutrients. Mothers who continue pregnancy with gastroparesis may require total parenteral nutrition. Autonomic neuropathy directed at the cardiovascular system results in a lack of compensatory response to a decrease in blood pressure, posing a serious threat to fetal and maternal well-being, and is a relative contraindication to pregnancy (Macleod, Smith, Sonksen, & Lowy, 1990; Rosenn & Miodovnik, 2000).

Definitions and Classification

Patients with diabetes during pregnancy can be divided into two groups. The first group consists of women who have preexisting or pregestational diabetes (type 1 or 2). The terms insulin-dependent diabetes mellitus (IDDM) and non–insulin-dependent diabetes (NIDDM) are no longer used to classify type 1 and 2 diabetes, respectively (American Diabetes Association [ADA], 1997). GDM comprises the second group and is defined as carbohydrate intolerance of any degree with onset or first recognition during pregnancy (ADA, 1999c). GDM has been subdivided further to designate those women who are diet controlled (GDM A_1) or insulin controlled (GDM A_2) (Hagay & Reece, 1992).

Type 1 diabetes occurs as a result of autoimmunity directed at the β cells of the pancreas after an environmental trigger that results in a total lack of insulin production. Exogenous insulin administration and diet therapy are the mainstays of treatment. This disease usually occurs in people younger than 30 years of age. Type 2 diabetes is characterized by insulin resistance and decreased insulin production and requires diet, exercise, weight management, and oral hypoglycemic agents or insulin as treatment regimens. Type 2 diabetes is seen less frequently in pregnancy because the age of diagnosis is usually in women beyond the reproductive years (≥45 years of age). Oral hypoglycemics have not been studied extensively during pregnancy and may contribute to fetal hyperinsulinemia and are not recommended for use during pregnancy at this time. Glucose intolerance diagnosed at a gestational age of 20 weeks or less may represent undiagnosed preexisitng type 2 diabetes, but this diagnosis should not be made during pregnancy. These women should be monitored as if they have pregestational diabetes.

Priscilla White (1949) developed a classification system that was used to determine pregnancy prognosis for women based on the extent of microvascular disease and duration of type 1 or 2 diabetes. White's classification system is still used for descriptive purposes only, because the classification does not consider the level of glycemic control or comprehensive obstetric management, both of which greatly influence perinatal outcome.

Pathophysiology

Profound metabolic changes occur in normal pregnancy to allow for a continuously feeding fetus in an intermittently feeding mother. These alterations must be understood to comprehend the effects that diabetes has on a progressively changing metabolic state. In early pregnancy, β-cell hyperplasia results in increased insulin production as a result of progesterone and estrogen increases, which also contributes to increased tissue sensitivity to insulin. This hyperinsulinemic state allows increased lipogenesis and fat deposition in early pregnancy in preparation for the dramatic rise in energy needs of the growing fetus in the latter half of pregnancy. As a result of these changes and nausea and vomiting, the mother has an increased risk for episodes of hypoglycemia in the first trimester. In women with type 1 and insulin-controlled type 2 diabetes, exogenous insulin needs are decreased.

The second half of pregnancy is characterized by accelerated growth of the fetus and rapidly increasing levels of maternal and placental diabetogenic hormones, which include human placental lactogen, cortisol, estrogen, progesterone, and prolactin (Boden, 1996). Insulin resistance and increased insulin production result from increased circulating levels of insulin-antagonizing hormones. Increased insulin needs in women with type 1 and 2 diabetes and the appearance of glucose intolerance in women who have limited pancreatic reserve due to predisposing risk factors are the result of these normal metabolic changes of pregnancy (Buchanan & Kitzmiller, 1994). This constitutes the diabetogenic state of pregnancy—hyperglycemia in the presence of hyperinsulinemia—which allows a continuous supply of glucose to passively diffuse to the fetus transplacentally (Lesser & Carpenter, 1994).

The anabolic phase (ie, fat storage) of the first 20 weeks of pregnancy is followed by a catabolic phase (ie, fat breakdown or lipolysis) in the latter half of pregnancy (Lesser & Carpenter, 1994). This state is referred to as accelerated starvation because of the rapid switch from carbohydrate to lipid metabolism during fasting as a fuel source for the mother, preferentially reserving glucose and amino acids for the developing fetus (Boden, 1996). Fat breakdown increases circulating fatty acids, triglycerides, and ketones, predisposing the woman with type 1 diabetes to an increased risk for the earlier development of ketoacidosis and starvation ketosis than in women with GDM and type 2 diabetes (Buchanan & Kitzmiller, 1994). The decreased buffering capacity of pregnancy for acids leads to the earlier development of DKA. Hepatic glucose production increases by 16% to 30% during the latter half of pregnancy to meet the fetal and placental demands during maternal fasting (Butte, 2000).

In the absence of vascular disease, the pathologic manifestations of diabetes in pregnancy are usually the result of maternal hyperglycemia. Excessive hyperglycemia as a result of insulin deficiency with a corresponding increase in counterregulatory hormones (ie, glucagon, epinephrine, growth hormone, and cortisol) contributes to the development of DKA. Factors in pregnancy that trigger the release of these hormones and development of DKA are fasting, infection, stress, emesis, dehydration, steroid administration (Bouhanick, Biquard, Hadjadj, & Roques, 2000), and adrenergic agonist administration for the treatment of preterm labor (Harvey, 1992). Continuous subcutaneous insulin infusion (CSII) pump failure and poor patient compliance have also led to the development of DKA during pregnancy. Nausea and vomiting of pregnancy with decreased caloric intake has been found to be a major contributor to DKA (Cullen et al., 1996). Excessive hyperglycemia results from increased hepatic glucose production and decreased peripheral glucose use (Chauhan & Perry, 1995). Urinary excretion of potassium, sodium, and water occurs as a result of osmotic diuresis due to excessive plasma glucose. Fat metabolism leads to increased circulating levels of free fatty acids and ketone bodies, which quickly overwhelm the maternal buffering system, and metabolic acidosis results (Whiteman, Homko, & Reece, 1996).

Maternal hyperglycemia during the time of organogenesis may result in spontaneous abortion or congenital malformations (Reece & Homko, 2000). Sustained or intermittent maternal hyperglycemia later in pregnancy stimulates fetal hyperinsulinemia as a normal fetal physiologic response to elevated blood glucose with pathologic consequences. Fetal hyperinsulinemia mediates accelerated fuel use and excessive growth, leading to macrosomia (Moore, 1999). Maternal hyperglycemia also contributes to fetal hypoxia. The exact mechanism for this is unknown but may be the result of placental constriction or from accelerated fetal metabolism and increased oxygen use beyond availability (Moore, 1999). Fetal hyperinsulinemia also inhibits the release of surfactant that is necessary for pulmonary maturation resulting in respiratory distress syndrome. Maternal hyperglycemia is also associated with other neonatal metabolic abnormalities. Polyhydramnios, hypertension, UTIs, pyelonephritis, and monilial vaginitis are maternal complications of hyperglycemia.

Screening and Diagnosis of Gestational Diabetes Mellitus

Screening for gestational diabetes is recommended between 24 and 28 weeks' gestation, when the diabetogenic hormones are exerting a significant influence on insulin performance. Women without risk factors for GDM do not require screening (ADA, 1999c; American College of Obstetricians and Gynecologists [ACOG], 1994). Display 8–19 lists characteristics of women who are at low risk for developing gestational diabetes. Women younger than 25 years of age with any other risk factor for GDM should be tested. Risk factors identifying women who should be tested before 24 weeks are listed in Display 8–20. Women whose early test results are negative should be retested after 24 weeks.

Evaluation for GDM may be performed in a one- or two-step approach (Metzger & Coustan, 1998). The two-step approach consists of ingestion of a 50-g glucose solution (glucola) without consideration of time of day or last meal and obtaining a plasma or serum glucose level 1 hour after ingestion. If the test result is positive, a diagnostic 3-hour oral glucose tolerance test (OGTT) (100 g) is administered after an 8-hour fast preceded by 3 days of unrestricted diet and activity. A high carbohydrate load for 3 days before the test is no longer recommended (Entrekin, Work, & Owen, 1998). Plasma glucose determinations are made after fasting and at 1-, 2-, and 3-hour intervals. In the one-step approach, the screening 50-g test is omitted, and the diagnostic 3-hour OGTT is administered. The 75-g OGTT is another approach for diagnosis that has not been tested extensively in terms of relating outcomes to cutoff points and has not been endorsed by any diabetes groups in the United States (Metzger & Coustan, 1998).

The positive thresholds of 130 and 140 mg/dL have been used for the screening glucola. A value of 130 mg/dL identifies approximately all women with gestational diabetes, whereas a cutoff of 140 mg/dL misses 10% (ACOG, 1994; Metzger & Coustan, 1998). Using 130 mg/dL requires 15% of women to proceed with the diagnostic OGTT, and a cutoff of 140 mg/dL requires 25% of women to have the diagnostic test. The decision for which cutoff to use should be based on cost effectiveness and risk factors in the population to be tested. Regardless of the threshold to be used, women should refrain from smoking or eating and should remain seated during testing. A result of 200 mg/dL on the glucose challenge is considered diagnos-

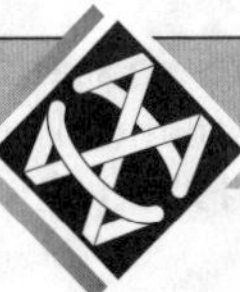

DISPLAY 8–20

Criteria for Early Screening for Gestational Diabetes Mellitus

- Diabetes symptoms: polydipsia, polyuria, polyphagia, fatigue, sudden weight loss
- Persistent glycosuria
- Obesity (>150% ideal)
- Polyhydramnios
- Oral beta-mimetic therapy
- Corticosteroid therapy
- Persistent vaginal candidiasis
- Infant with congenital anomalies
- First-degree relative with type 2 diabetes
- Previous glucose intolerance
- History of unexplained fetal death or stillborn
- Multiple spontaneous abortions
- History of fetal macrosomia (>4,000 g)

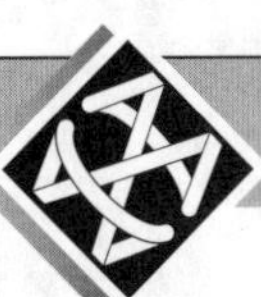

DISPLAY 8–19

Characteristics of Women at Low Risk for Gestational Diabetes Mellitus

- Younger than 25 years of age
- Normal body weight
- No family history of diabetes mellitus
- Not a member of an ethnic or racial group with higher prevalence (eg, Hispanic, African American, Native American, Asian)

tic, alleviating the need for OGTT. However, research has challenged this diagnostic threshold (Atilano, Lee-Parritz, Lieberman, Cohen, & Barbieri, 1999; Shivvers & Lucas, 1999).

Carpenter and Coustan's (1982) criteria (Table 8–8) are recommended for diagnosis of gestational diabetes by the ADA and ACOG (ACOG, 1994; Metzger & Coustan, 1998). Diagnosis is based on meeting or exceeding two thresholds. One abnormal value has been associated with adverse outcomes with 30% of these women exhibiting two abnormal values 1 month later (Langer, Brustman, Anyaegbunam, & Mazze, 1987; Neiger & Coustan, 1991). Women who fail the glucose challenge but pass the oral glucose tolerance test warrant closer surveillance with diet therapy and blood glucose monitoring or by repeat testing because of a much higher risk of macrosomia without treatment (Bevier, Fischer, & Jovanovic, 1999). Women who have a fasting plasma glucose level of 120 mg/dL can be diagnosed with this cutoff after a repeat test for confirmation and should not be administered the 100-g glucola (Metztger & Coustan, 1998). Obtaining a Hgb A_{1c} value is a prudent approach to determine whether hyperglycemia predates the measurement, which is very likely increasing the risk for the infant and the need for a more aggressive fetal surveillance.

Alternative methods for diagnosing GDM have been studied that are more economical and palatable to women. A 50-g serving of jelly beans equivalent to the 50-g glucose drink yielded similar glucose responses with fewer side effects (Lamar et al., 1999). In another jelly bean study, less than 50 g of jelly beans were given, which required lowering the threshold (Boyd, Ross, & Sherman, 1995). Each of these studies had small sample sizes, and the participants were not in a group of women with higher diabetes prevalence, both of which could affect outcomes. Rates of absorption vary among women, which could result in lower values. Further research is necessary before glucose solutions for diabetes testing are abandoned.

Fasting plasma glucose (FPG) values have also been studied for prediction of GDM. A FPG concentration of more than 105 mg/dL was found to be highly predictive of positive glucose tolerance results (Atilano et al., 1999). In another study, FPG values were obtained to determine which women required the glucose tolerance test omitting the glucose challenge (Perucchini et al., 1999). These investigators found that using a FPG resulted in fewer women requiring diagnostic testing. Further investigation is necessary to replace standard testing for GDM.

Clinical Manifestations

The clinical manifestations of diabetes occur as a result of hypoglycemia and hyperglycemia. Glycemic goals for pregnancy in women with diabetes reflect the blood glucose values found in pregnant women who do not have diabetes; 60 to 90 mg/dL fasting, 60 to 105 mg/dL before a meal, and 140 mg/dL 1 hour after a meal, and 120 mg/dL 2 hours after a meal (ACOG, 1994). Symptoms of hyperglycemia include polyuria, polydipsia, blurred vision, and polyphagia. Nonspecific symptoms include weakness, lethargy, malaise, and headache (Davidson & Schwartz, 1998). Ketosis or acidosis (DKA) accompanies severe hyperglycemia, resulting in gastrointestinal symptoms of nausea, vomiting, and abdominal pain (Davidson & Schwartz, 1998). Kussmaul respirations develop in an effort to correct the ensuing metabolic acidosis. Acetone breath develops as ketone bodies are converted to acetone and excreted by the lungs. Dehydration occurs with DKA as a result of hyperglycemia, which increases the osmotic pressure in the extracellular fluid space, causing diuresis with increased urinary excretion of potassium, sodium, and water (Whiteman et al., 1996). Orthostatic hypotension, poor tissue turgor, dry mucous membranes, sunken eyeballs, disorientation, and oliguria are all clinical manifestations of

TABLE 8–8 ■ DIAGNOSTIC CRITERIA FOR GESTATIONAL DIABETES MELLITUS

100-g Oral Glucose Tolerance Test	Threshold Glucose Levels (mg/dL)
Fasting	≥95
1 hour	≥180
2 hours	≥155
3 hours	≥140

From Carpenter, M. W., & Coustan, D. R. (1982). Criteria for screening tests for gestational diabetes. *American Journal of Obstetrics and Gynecology, 144*(7), 768–773.

severe dehydration (Chauhan & Perry, 1995). Elevated hematocrit, leukocyte, and urea nitrogen levels occur as the intravascular space becomes dry and hemoconcentrated (Kendrick, 1999). As potassium levels fall, hyporeflexia is evident, and cardiac arrhythmias may develop. Altered consciousness levels, including coma, are usually present with hyperosmolarity (Davidson & Schwartz, 1998). The diagnosis of DKA is based on the laboratory findings of a blood glucose level of more than 300 mg/dL, a bicarbonate level below 15 mEq/L, and an arterial pH of less than 7.3 (Kitabchi, Young, Sacks, & Morris, 1979).

Hypoglycemia is defined as a plasma glucose level of 70 mg/dL, but significant symptoms may occur at higher levels when the patient's average blood glucose level is higher. Autonomic nervous system stimulation by hypoglycemia results in adrenergic and cholinergic symptoms of pallor, diaphoresis, tachycardia, palpitations, hunger, paresthesias, and shakiness. Moderate hypoglycemia causes glucose deprivation in the CNS as evidenced by an inability to concentrate, confusion, slurred speech, irrational behavior, slowed reaction time, blurred vision, numbness, somnolence, or extreme fatigue (Kendrick, 1999). Disorientation, loss of consciousness, seizures, and coma may result from severe hypoglycemia.

Nursing Assessments and Interventions for Diabetes Mellitus

Evaluation and management of women with diabetes, whether pregestational or gestational, generally occurs on an outpatient basis, requiring admission only during an episode of illness, DKA, or other obstetric complication. Nurses can have a profound role in education and monitoring of women with GDM and are vital members of the multidisciplinary diabetes management team. The goal of care focuses on attaining and maintaining normal blood glucose levels to improve perinatal outcome. Combination therapy used to achieve this goal includes diet, exercise, self-monitoring of blood glucose, and insulin when euglycemia is not attained. All women with type 1 diabetes require insulin as part of the treatment regimen.

Ambulatory and Home Care Management

Nursing assessment for women with pregestational diabetes should begin immediately after conception (ideally before conception) and continue throughout the perinatal period. The assessment of women with pregestational diabetes should include a thorough history of diabetes type, duration of disease, self-care practices, acute and chronic complication assessment, and a review of current log of glucose values. Knowledge deficits should be identified and an individualized teaching plan outlined during this initial assessment. Psychosocial issues should be explored, evaluated periodically, and appropriate referrals made. Display 8–21 lists information that should be discussed with women who have pregestational diabetes. Home care management for women with diabetes is discussed in Appendix 8A.

Women who have been diagnosed with GDM need immediate counseling and education. Display 8–22 includes topics that nurses should discuss in the educational session. The diagnosis alone may bring excessive anxiety and fear. Appropriate education and support from the nurse educator should allay the woman's concerns and empower her with the resources she needs to adapt to the diabetic regimen re-

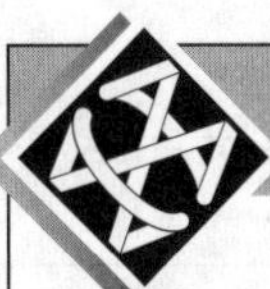

DISPLAY 8–21

Educational Guidelines for Women With Pregestational Diabetes Mellitus

- Glycemic goals for pregnancy and effect pregnancy has on diabetes
- Metabolic management (ie, exercise, nutrition, and insulin) and metabolic monitoring and logging guidelines
- Potential for maternal complications without vascular disease: hypoglycemia, ketoacidosis, polyhydramnios, cesarean birth; with vascular disease: hypertension, pregnancy-induced hypertension, edema, prolonged hospitalization, bed rest, renal failure, cesarean birth
- Potential for fetal or neonatal complications: intrauterine growth restriction, respiratory distress syndrome, macrosomia, birth trauma, prematurity, intrauterine fetal death, neonatal metabolic disturbances
- Significance of hemoglobin A_{1c} for congenital defects or spontaneous abortion
- Guidelines for ketone testing
- Use of reflectance meter with quality controls and use of autolancing device
- Sick day management and appropriate treatment of hypoglycemia
- Signs and symptoms of diabetic ketoacidosis and contributing factors
- Schedule of antenatal visits and testing

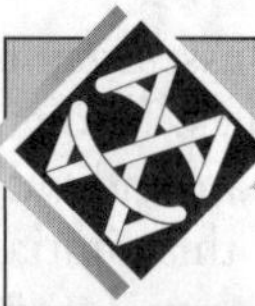

DISPLAY 8–22

Educational Guidelines for Women With Gestational Diabetes Mellitus

- Explanation of abnormal results from prenatal glucose test
- Role of glucose and insulin transport and effect pregnancy has on diabetes
- Potential poor outcomes: macrosomia, polyhydramnios, preterm birth, birth trauma, cesarean birth, neonatal metabolic derangements
- Glycemic goals for pregnancy
- Metabolic management (ie, exercise, nutrition, and possibly insulin) and metabolic monitoring with logging guidelines
- Use of reflectance meter with quality controls
- Use of autolancing device
- Guidelines for ketone testing
- Frequency of office visits and schedule of antenatal testing

ducing the risks for perinatal complications. Including family and significant others in the education and care of women with GDM provides another foundational support.

Nutrition Therapy

Nutrition therapy is an integral and vital component in the care of women with diabetes. Therapeutic goals for nutritional intervention are blunting of postprandial hyperglycemia and adequate nourishment of mother and fetus without excessive weight gain or ketosis. Current recommendations for dietary management include 24 to 30 kcal/kg for normal-weight women, 40 kcal/kg for underweight women, and 24 kcal/kg for overweight women (Jovanovic, 2000). These calories should be consumed in three meals and three snacks and should contain less than 40% carbohydrates, 20% to 25% protein, and 35% to 40% predominately monounsaturated and polyunsaturated fats (Jovanovic-Peterson & Peterson, 1996). A 25- to 35-pound weight gain is encouraged for women with normal prepregnancy weight, 15- to 25-pound weight gain for overweight women, 28 to 40 pounds for underweight women, and 15 pounds or less for morbidly obese women. Aspartame is the preferred nonnutritive sweetener in pregnancy except in women with phenylketonuria (ADA, 1993). Saccharin products cross the placenta freely, although no adverse effects have been found in humans at normal consumption rates (ADA, 1993). Women should be on a prenatal vitamin supplement with 400 μg of folic acid or 4 mg with a positive family history for neural tube defects, additional iron if anemic, and supplemental calcium for those women who do not consume enough dietary calcium.

Nutritional counseling should be individualized and culturally sensitive. Significant others and family members should be included in educational sessions to provide support. The person who prepares the meals must be a part of counseling and financial constraints determined, although a nutritional diet should not pose a financial burden. The registered dietitian should meet with the woman during each trimester to assess any dietary problems and to reevaluate nutritional needs after the initial session. More frequent visits are required for women with excessive or low weight gain or when discrepancies are encountered by the nurse when reviewing the woman's glucose log at prenatal visits.

Exercise Therapy

Exercise may be used adjunctively with dietary management of diabetes (ADA, 1999b). The glucose-lowering mechanism of exercise is unknown but may be related to increased insulin sensitivity, improved first-phase insulin release, and increased caloric expenditure (Carpenter, 2000; Langer, 2000). Specific types of exercise that are most beneficial for glucose control have not been determined, although a minimum of three episodes per week for 20 minutes seems to be necessary (Langer, 2000). Women with pregestational diabetes who are poorly controlled or who have any evidence of vascular disease should avoid exercise during pregnancy because risks outweigh any benefits. Walking and swimming are two forms of exercise with minimal risk and may be the exercise of choice for previously sedentary women. Safety considerations before implementing an exercise program should be thoroughly discussed, particularly for women with pregestational diabetes. Display 8–23 lists general guidelines for education of women who plan to exercise during their pregnancy. Women should be counseled to discontinue exercise if uterine activity occurs. The nurse should review the glucose log to evaluate the effect of exercise on blood sugar values and make appropriate food or insulin adjustment recommendations. The feet and lower extremities should be inspected for blisters, bruising, or other evidence of trauma. Exercise change may be required or a change in footwear needed.

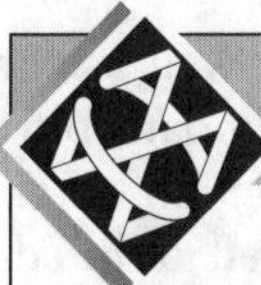

DISPLAY 8–23

Exercise Guidelines

- Proper footwear with silica gel or air midsoles
- Polyester or polyester-cotton blend socks to promote dryness and prevent blisters
- Wear a visible diabetes identification
- Carbohydrate (CHO) consumption when blood pressure <100 mg/dL and have CHO snack readily available
- Blood glucose before and after exercise
- Adequate hydration during and after exercise
- Consult healthcare provider to assist with insulin adjustments

Metabolic Monitoring

Metabolic monitoring during pregnancy is directed at detecting hyperglycemia and making pharmacologic, dietary, or activity adjustments to minimize adverse effects in the fetus. Daily self-monitoring of blood glucose in women with gestational diabetes has been found to be superior to intermittent office monitoring (ADA, 1999c). Daily self-monitoring allows the woman to know immediately the effect of food intake or activity on her blood sugar. In women with GDM, blood sugar levels should be checked at a minimum after fasting and 1 to 2 hours after each meal. One-hour postprandial glucose determinations are recommended when insulin Lispro (not FDA approved) is used because it peaks sooner than regular insulin (Jovanovic, 2000). Postprandial blood glucose determinations appear to be the most influential in the development of fetal hyperinsulinemia rather than preprandial values (ADA, 1999c). Table 8–9 lists the target glycemic values for pregnancy. These values are usually easily attainable in women with GDM and type 2 diabetes but may be unrealistic in women with type 1 diabetes who have hypoglycemia unawareness and are more difficult to control. Women with pregestational diabetes should check their blood sugar levels four to eight times daily, depending on their level of control. These determinations may be obtained fasting, preprandial, postprandial, at bedtime, and at 2 AM to 3 AM for women with a history of nocturnal hypoglycemia. Titration of insulin is smoother when based on multiple blood glucose determinations.

Women with GDM and type 2 diabetes who are on hypocaloric diets (<1,800 kcal/day) should test their urine daily from the first void for ketones to exclude starvation ketosis (ADA, 1999c). Calories should be added at the bedtime snack if ketones are detected. Women with type 1 diabetes are asked to test their urine for ketones daily from the first void and with any blood glucose level of 180 mg/dL or greater because of the increased risk for ketoacidosis. They should also be instructed to call their healthcare provider if they detect moderate levels of ketones.

All women with diabetes are asked to keep a log of their blood sugars, insulin dosages, exercise or activity level, food intake with any abnormal values (high or low), and ketone checks when necessary. These logs allow the nurse and healthcare provider to accurately evaluate and make necessary adjustments at office visits. These visits should occur weekly for women having insulin adjustments or those with identified problems. Telephone contact may be necessary to supplement visits. Visits should occur every other week for women with well-controlled diabetes, whether pregestational or gestational, until the latter half of the third trimester.

The care and use of a reflectance meter should be reviewed with the woman. Blood glucose values from a reflectance meter are 14% below laboratory plasma glucose determinations. Some meters are calibrated to provide plasma values by increasing the capillary result. Nurses need to know the limits of the reflectance meters their patients are using. For women who are newly diagnosed with GDM, a more intensive instructional session should be provided. Reflectance meters that have memory capability are important so that the nurse can correlate the values in the meter to those recorded by the woman. Studies have shown that a significant number of patients supply false blood sugar values, which can be detrimental to perinatal outcome if not detected (Langer & Mazze, 1986; Mazze et al., 1984; Moses, 1986). If false blood glucose readings have been reported, fears or contribu-

TABLE 8–9 ■ GLYCEMIC GOALS FOR PREGNANCY

Timing	Plasma Glucose Levels (mg/dL)
Fasting	60–90
Preprandial	60–105
Postprandial	1 hour: 130–140 2 hours: ≤120
2 to 6 AM	60–90

From American College of Obstetricians and Gynecologists. (1994). *Diabetes and pregnancy* (Technical Bulletin No. 200). Washington, DC: Author.

tory psychosocial issues should be explored. Sometimes, an underlying fear of insulin by women with GDM contributes to this phenomenon. These women need additional support and education and possibly referral for counseling.

Pharmacologic Therapy

Insulin is the only pharmacologic agent shown to reduce fetal morbidity in conjunction with nutrition therapy in women with pregestational or gestational diabetes (ADA, 1999c). Oral hypoglycemic agents are not recommended for use during pregnancy because they readily cross the placenta and may contribute to fetal hyperinsulinemia. Insulin requirements during pregnancy increase dramatically from the first to third trimester as the anti-insulin hormones rise and peripheral resistance increases. Requirements in the first trimester may be slightly reduced because of the nausea and vomiting of pregnancy. The first-trimester insulin requirement is 0.7 U/kg of ideal body weight, 0.8 U/kg in the second, and 0.9 U/kg in the third (Homko & Khandelwal, 1996). Twin gestations require a doubling of insulin requirements throughout pregnancy (Jovanovic, 2000). Insulin usually is administered in two divided doses per day, although intensive management in type 1 diabetes may require three to four daily injections. These dosages are merely recommended averages requiring titration to blood glucose levels and activity for individualized management. Morbidly obese women with GDM or type 2 diabetes may require more than 1 U/kg to achieve euglycemia. A decrease in insulin requirements in the third trimester may be an indication of poor placental perfusion and a reduction in anti-insulin hormones warranting immediate and comprehensive fetal evaluation (Miller, 1994).

When women who have pregestational diabetes become pregnant, an educational session should be scheduled as soon as possible with the diabetes educator and registered dietitian after or in conjunction with the initial prenatal visit. The session should include all aspects of insulin therapy, including a demonstration by the woman of the correct method for drawing up and self-injection of insulin. Oral hypoglycemic agents should be discontinued in pregnant women with type 2 diabetes. Oral hypoglycemic agents are contraindicated during pregnancy. These women require more extensive education regarding insulin and additional support with this new aspect of their diabetes management. Human insulins are associated with a shorter duration of activity, more rapid onset, less evidence of allergy, and are the only recommended insulins for use during pregnancy. Women who are on animal insulin need conversion to human insulin. Injection sites should be observed for correct regional rotation, as well as for identifying evidence of lipohypertrophy or lipoatrophy, bruising, and signs and symptoms of infection or allergy. Display 8–24 lists issues to be reviewed in the educational session about insulin.

Appropriate management of hypoglycemia should be reviewed with women with pregestational diabetes. They need an explanation that the occurrence will increase with intensive management during pregnancy. The level at which symptoms occur should be determined. If women have hypoglycemia unawareness, the risk for a potentially fatal nocturnal episode must be avoided. General guidelines for treatment of hypoglycemia during pregnancy include treatment with one carbohydrate exchange for a blood glucose of 60 mg/dL and treatment with two exchanges (liquid and solid preferably) at a level of 40 to 60 mg/dL. Blood glucose should be tested again 15 minutes after treatment of hypoglycemia. Retreatment should occur if the blood glucose level has not risen. Including protein with the carbohydrate decreases the risk for rebound hypoglycemia and provides a more consistent and stable blood glucose level after treatment. Women with evidence of gastroparesis should use liquids for initial treatment of hypoglycemia because of their slower digestion. Carbohydrates ingested for treatment of hypoglycemia should be in addition to the regularly prescribed diet so that glucagon stores may be replenished. Family members and significant others should be instructed on the use of injectable glucagon, and two kits should be readily available at all times.

Nurses should also review sick day management and provide written guidelines. Understanding ap-

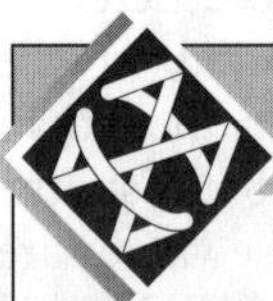

DISPLAY 8–24

Educational Guidelines for Insulin Therapy

- Glycemic goals for treatment
- Onset, peak, and duration of action of insulins to be administered
- Inspection, storage, and traveling with insulin
- Timing of injections, injection technique, site selection, and regional rotation
- Glucagon use and appropriate administration by family or significant other
- Appropriate sick day management
- Prevention strategies and appropriate management of hypoglycemia
- Syringe disposal guidelines

propriate self-care strategies during episodes of nausea and vomiting of early pregnancy is vital to prevent the development of ketoacidosis. Display 8–25 contains specific information that nurses should review with women about sick day management.

For women with GDM who fail to achieve euglycemia (see Table 8–9) with diet and exercise, insulin therapy should be initiated. Insulin is initiated when FBS values are 105 mg/dL or higher and 2-hour postprandial blood glucose values are 120 mg/dL or higher (ACOG, 1994). Insulin is required for 30% to 60% of women with GDM (Langer et al., 1994). Women with early-onset GDM have higher glycemic values and need for insulin therapy (Bartha, Martinez-Del-Fresno, & Comino-Delgado, 2000). The educational session should follow the guidelines for insulin therapy in women with pregestational diabetes (see Display 8–24). Women who are injecting insulin for the first time are very fearful and require much support and encouragement from the nurse and family members. Occasionally, a woman may not be able to correctly draw her insulin. In those situations, a home health referral can be made, another family member taught, or the nurse can draw the appropriate insulin to be refrigerated before use. Prefilled syringes may be safely refrigerated for up to 30 days. For women with needle phobias, self-injectors may be used.

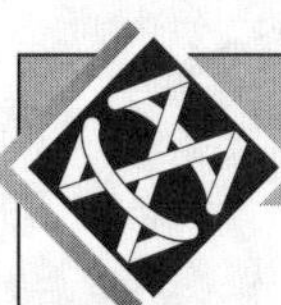

DISPLAY 8–25

Sick Day Management Educational Guidelines

- Insulin should be given even with vomiting.
- Urine ketones should be checked every 4 to 6 hours and the healthcare provider notified of moderate results.
- Blood glucose levels should be checked every 1 to 2 hours.
- Healthcare provider should be notified of blood glucose levels ≥200 mg/dL.
- Liquids or soft foods should be consumed equal to the carbohydrate value of the prescribed diet (sugar free for blood glucose levels of >120 mg/dL).
- A sipping diet of 15 to 30 g (CHO) per hour may be consumed during periods of vomiting.
- Call the healthcare provider if liquids are not tolerated.
- Review signs and symptoms of ketoacidosis to report abdominal pain, nausea and vomiting, polyuria, polydipsia, fruity breath, leg cramps, altered mental status, and rapid respirations.

Continuous Subcutaneous Insulin Infusion

Another method for intensive metabolic management in pregnancy is the use of CSII, or the insulin pump. An insulin pump involves an electronic device that is programmed to deliver a continuous low-dose amount of basal regular insulin subcutaneously through an implanted catheter. Boluses are given for meals and snacks based on carbohydrate intake in a predetermined ratio to insulin. The catheter is changed every 3 to 4 days. The use of CSII in pregnancy requires careful patient selection, and only those who are very motivated and capable of using a sophisticated electronic device should be chosen. The risk for pump use during pregnancy is pump malfunction that can lead to the rapid development of DKA. This risk can be reduced by educating the woman to self-inject regular insulin and check the pump for blood glucose levels of 200 mg/dL. Switching from conventional insulin therapy to pump therapy can be done on an inpatient or outpatient basis, individualizing the decision according to the level of family support and needs of the woman. Forty percent of the total daily insulin dose (less 25%) is given for a basal rate, with the remaining 60% given as boluses with 20% at breakfast, 15% before lunch, and 15% before dinner (Jornsay, 1998). Another method for determining the insulin dose for CSII is based on patient weight and gestational age. Dosing is based on 0.8 U/kg in the first trimester, 1.0 U/kg in the second trimester, and 1.2 U/kg in the third trimester and then reducing by 20% (Gabbe, 2000). Boluses for snacks may or may not be required. Single basal rates are not recommended on initiation because of the increased risk of nocturnal hypoglycemia; therefore, a lower basal rate should be infused during the nighttime hours (Jornsay, 1998). At a minimum, blood glucose levels should be checked while fasting, before a meal, after a meal, and at bedtime after the first 24 hours. During the first 24 hours, blood glucose values should be obtained hourly to allow for basal manipulation to more closely reflect the woman's diurnal variations. Checks are required at 2 AM to 3 AM during nighttime adjustments to avoid hypoglycemia.

Lispro is a rapid-acting insulin recommended for pump use but has not been approved for use during pregnancy (ADA, 1999a; Bloomgarden, 1999). However, a study of Lispro use in pregnancy found that the immunologic effects were similar to regular insulin, and its use was recommended by the investigators (Jovanovic et al., 1999). Buffered regular is recommended for pump use during pregnancy. Close contact with the diabetes management team becomes a vital component of successful insulin pump therapy during pregnancy.

Fetal Assessment

The best method and the appropriate time to begin antepartum fetal assessment for pregnant women with diabetes have yet to be determined. Most recommend beginning some form of fetal assessment in the third trimester for women with pregestational diabetes (ACOG, 1994; ADA, 1999a). Testing of women with GDM controlled by diet may be delayed until near term (Landon, 2000). Those controlled by insulin should begin earlier in the third trimester, or 32 weeks as has been suggested (Homko, 1998; Landon, 2000). Fetal movement counting is a simple, inexpensive, and appropriate test to begin in all pregnant women with diabetes in the beginning of the third trimester. Women with vascular disease need more intensive fetal and maternal surveillance, requiring NST, contraction stress testing, or BPP (Landon, 2000). Table 8–10 provides a sample schedule to consider for fetal testing in women with diabetes.

TABLE 8–10 ■ FETAL SURVEILLANCE FOR WOMEN WITH DIABETES

Gestational Age (weeks)	Type 1 or 2: Poorly Controlled or With Vascular Disease	Type 1 or 2: Well-Controlled, no Vascular Disease	GDM A_1 (Diet Controlled)	GDM A_2 (Insulin Controlled)
6–8	Sonographic estimation of gestational age	Same		
16–19	Maternal serum alpha-fetoprotein	Same	Same	Same
20–22	High-resolution sonography, fetal echocardiography	High-resolution sonography	High resolution sonography	High-resolution sonography
26–28	Sonographic assessment of interval growth	Same		
28	Twice-daily fetal movement counting (FMC), weekly nonstress test (NST)	FMC	FMC	FMC
32	Twice-weekly NST or weekly biophysical profile, sonographic assessment of interval growth	Weekly NST, increase to then twice weekly at 34–36 weeks		Weekly NST, then increase to twice weekly at 34–36 weeks
36–38	Sonographic estimation of fetal weight	Sonographic estimation of fetal weight	Sonographic estimation of fetal weight and weekly NST	Sonographic estimation of fetal weight
36–39	Consider amniocentesis and delivery with worsening disease			
39–40	Elective delivery without amniocentesis	Elective delivery without amniocentesis	Consider elective delivery if cervix favorable and for large for gestational age (LGA) fetus	Consider elective delivery if cervix favorable and for LGA fetus

Inpatient Management

Women with diabetes require hospitalization during periods of poor control for intensive insulin adjustment, particularly if they are in the critical time of organogenesis (6 to 8 weeks' gestation). Hospitalization may also be required during periods of illness for women with dehydration and are always required for those with DKA. Initiation of CSII therapy may or may not be an indication for hospitalization. Women with type 1 diabetes with vascular disease may require hospitalization during the third trimester for more intensive maternal and fetal surveillance.

Diabetic Ketoacidosis

The incidence, pathophysiology, predisposing factors, and signs and symptoms of ketoacidosis have been discussed in previous sections. This section focuses on the nursing interventions in the management of DKA that are vital to maternal and fetal survival. Care of women in DKA should occur in a tertiary care facility with the support services that can provide the required intensive care. Nurses in community hospitals should be capable of stabilizing the woman in preparation for, and during transport to, an appropriate facility.

Table 8–11 lists specific interventions nurses use in the care of women experiencing DKA. Initial treatment measures focus on rehydration, which improves tissue perfusion, insulin delivery, and a physiologic lowering of blood glucose by hemodilution. After intravenous access is established, insulin is administered as ordered to lower blood glucose. Caution should be exercised in lowering the blood glucose, because too rapid a fall results in the serious complication of cerebral edema. With improvement of the intravascular status, fluid shifts result in a potassium deficit that requires replacement. Nurses should continually assess the woman for signs and symptoms of hypokalemia and monitor electrolyte levels in preparation for replacement. Adequate urinary output must also be maintained with potassium replacement to avoid hyperkalemia. In addition to monitoring laboratory electrolyte status, the complete blood cell count and differential also should be monitored, as well as the clinical status for signs and symptoms of infection. Evidence of infection requires prompt and aggressive treatment for DKA treatment to be effective.

Fetal monitoring, even in previable gestations, provides an indication of hydration and perfusion status and should be instituted immediately. Nonreassuring fetal status is expected but resolves as the mother is stabilized and should not be an indication for emergent cesarean birth, which could further compromise the mother (Chauhan & Perry, 1995). Maternal oxygenation status should be monitored continually and oxygen administered based on blood gas determinations, bedside oxygen saturation levels, and fetal status. Uterine activity also is associated with severe dehydration but resolves in most cases with improved perfusion. Treatment for preterm labor should not be considered in the absence of cervical change, because the use of β-adrenergic agonists or steroids worsens the clinical picture by antagonizing insulin. Magnesium sulfate is the drug of choice for treatment because it does not interfere with the action of insulin.

After DKA has been corrected, the underlying cause—whether infection or poor self-care practices—should be discussed with the mother and family, outlining early detection and prevention strategies. For mothers whose infants did not survive, intensive grief support and follow-up should be provided.

Intrapartum Management: Pregestational and Gestational Diabetes Mellitus

Intrapartum management of women with diabetes requires skilled nursing care to prevent maternal and neonatal complications. Plasma glucose levels should be maintained at 80 to 120 mg/dL or 70 to 110 mg/dL for capillary blood determinations (Homko, 1998). Hyperglycemia in labor contributes to the development of neonatal hypoglycemia. Blood glucose should be assessed on the first laboratory blood draw and then checked at the bedside every 1 to 2 hours for all women who have previously been controlled by insulin. Women with GDM who have been controlled by diet may have their blood glucose levels checked every 2 to 4 hours. Ketones should be checked with every void or every 4 hours if euglycemia is maintained.

Intravenous access should be established early so that hydration can be maintained and insulin administered when necessary. Women with GDM and type 2 diabetes may not require insulin during labor. Those with type 1 diabetes will require glucose and insulin at some point. If, on admission, the blood glucose level of a woman with type 1 diabetes is 70 mg/dL or below, an infusion with 5% dextrose should be initiated at a rate of 100 to 125 mL/hour (Hagay & Reece, 1992). Levels above 70 mg/dL require an infusion of normal saline at the same rate. Insulin administration according to institutional protocol should be initiated when the blood glucose level reaches 120 mg/dL. Women who present in spontaneous labor who have taken their intermediate acting insulin may not require insulin during labor but will need a glucose infusion on admission to avoid hypoglycemia.

TABLE 8–11 ■ NURSING MANAGEMENT OF DIABETIC KETOACIDOSIS

Treatment	Nursing Intervention
Fluid resuscitation	1. Obtain large-bore peripheral access. 2. Anticipate need for hemodynamic monitoring. 3. Administer fluids as ordered, usually 1,000 to 2,000 mL of normal saline over 1 to 2 hours, then 200 to 250 mL/hour. 4. Assess for signs and symptoms of pulmonary edema—dyspnea, tachypnea, wheezing, cough. 5. Assess for hypovolemia; check vital signs every 15 minutes; report decrease in blood pressure, increased pulse rate, decrease in central venous and pulmonary capillary wedge pressure, and slow capillary refill. 6. Insert Foley catheter for oliguria or anuria and send specimen for urinalysis, culture, and sensitivity. 7. Hourly intake and output—report <30 mL/hour. 8. Administer 5% dextrose solution at blood glucose level of 200 to 250 mg/dL to prevent hypoglycemia.
Insulin therapy	1. Administer intravenous insulin as ordered—10 to 20 U of regular insulin as bolus, then 5 to 10 U/hour. 2. Hourly capillary blood glucose determinations (lab correlation with each draw). 3. Double dosage as ordered if 10% blood glucose decrease is not achieved in 1 hour. 4. Notify physician when blood glucose level of 200 mg/dL is reached, anticipating a decrease in insulin infusion rate to 1 to 2 U/hour. 5. Monitor for cerebral edema—headache, vomiting, deteriorating mental status, bradycardia, sluggish pupillary light reflex, widened pulse pressure.
Electrolyte replacement	1. Obtain electrocardiogram and report ST segment depression, inverted T waves, and appearance of U waves after T waves. 2. Obtain hourly laboratory electrolyte levels. 3. Anticipate potassium replacement within 2 to 4 hours.
Oxygenation	1. Establish the airway. 2. Anticipate placement of the peripheral arterial catheter. 3. Obtain initial arterial blood gases, then hourly until pH of 7.20 maintained. 4. Administer oxygen at 8 to 10 L/min by a non-rebreathing face mask to maintain oxygen saturations of 95%. 5. Anticipate the need for intubation/mechanical ventilation. 6. Use continuous pulse oximetry. 7. Administer bicarbonate as ordered for pH of 7.10.
Fetal or uterine monitoring	1. Left lateral recumbent position. 2. Apply external fetal or uterine monitoring (EFM). 3. Observe EFM for evidence of fetal compromise. 4. Observe for uterine activity. 5. Administer tocolytics as ordered ($MgSO_4$, drug of choice). 6. Avoid beta-adrenergic agonists and steroids.

Adapted from Kendrick, J. M. (1997). Diabetes in pregnancy (Nursing Module). White Plains, NY: March of Dimes Birth Defects Foundation.

An intravenous dosage of 1 unit of regular insulin per hour usually is all that is necessary with titrations based on blood glucose determinations. Polyvinyl tubing should be flushed thoroughly to allow saturation of the insulin to the tubing, allowing the prescribed dose to be infused consistently. Glucose and insulin should be maintained on pumps to avoid overdosage of either solution. Because of the higher risk for operative birth, no oral intake should be allowed intrapartally for women with diabetes.

Women with vascular disease may be fluid restricted so that total intravenous intake should be maintained at 70 mL/hour, requiring a more concentrated insulin admixture. Insulin is partially catabolized in the kidney, and in women with nephropathy, the action is unpredictable, requiring closer surveillance of blood sugar levels. Prehydration for conduction anesthesia or intravenous boluses should use non–glucose-containing solutions and be administered more slowly in the presence of vascular disease. Lactated Ringer's solution should be avoided in women with type 1 diabetes because of its gluconeogenic properties (Hirsch, McGill, Cryer, & White, 1991).

Most women with diabetes have scheduled induction or cesarean births. Early morning admissions are preferred, withholding the morning insulin dosage and with glucose and insulin initiated when indicated. Cervical ripening and induction procedures should follow institutional protocols and physician orders. Continuous EFM should be used and assessed for signs of fetal compromise. Labor abnormalities that would indicate potential cephalopelvic disproportion should be monitored closely. Nurses caring for women during labor with diabetes should prepare for assisted birth and the possibility of shoulder dystocia. The birth of a potentially high-risk neonate should also be anticipated and preparation made for full resuscitation. A neonatal team should be present at the birth or immediately available.

Hypoglycemia during labor is usually avoided with close monitoring but should be recognized and treated aggressively. Observation for signs and symptoms of hypoglycemia should be a continuous nursing assessment. Display 8–26 contains typical signs and symptoms of mild and moderate hypoglycemia. Concentrated dextrose solutions (10% and 50%) should be maintained at the bedside. Treatment should be initiated at a blood glucose level of 60 mg/dL by discontinuing insulin and administering 300 mL of 5% dextrose over 10 to 15 minutes or, if fluid restricted, 10 mL of 50% dextrose (Kendrick, 1999). The blood sugar should be rechecked after the bolus and further treatment administered if the blood glucose remains low. If the woman becomes unconscious, the physician should be notified immediately and 50% dextrose infused intravenously over 5 to 10 minutes (Kendrick, 1999). Vital signs should be assessed every 5 to 10 minutes during episodes of hypoglycemia, including blood glucose checks, until a threshold of 80 mg/dL is reached. Insulin should be resumed when the blood glucose level reaches 120 mg/dL according to a laboratory assessment or 110 mg/dL for a capillary blood glucose determination.

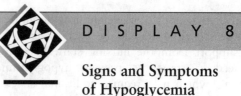

DISPLAY 8–26

Signs and Symptoms of Hypoglycemia

- Pallor
- Diaphoresis
- Tachycardia
- Palpitations
- Hunger
- Paresthesias
- Shakiness
- Cold, clammy skin
- Mental confusion and irritability
- Blurred vision
- Somnolence
- Slowed reaction time
- Extreme fatigue

Postpartum Management: Pregestational Diabetes Mellitus

Insulin requirements decrease in the immediate postpartum period when the levels of circulating anti-insulin placental hormones drop (Kjos, 2000). Insulin and glucose infusions should be discontinued immediately after a vaginal birth. After cesarean births, the insulin infusion should be decreased by 50% until eating is resumed (Miller, 1994). With oral intake, subcutaneous insulin can be resumed at the prepregnancy dosage or based on postpartum weight (Neiger & Kendrick, 1994). Strict glycemic control can be relaxed in the postpartum period, with testing of blood glucose reverting to the prepregnancy pattern. Women with type 2 diabetes who will not be breast-feeding may resume oral hypoglycemic agents. Those who choose to breast-feed require continued insulin administration; there is no transfer into breast milk.

Caloric needs mandate recalculation based on postpartum body weight and on possible lactation requirements. For obese women, a program for exercise and dietary management for weight loss should be outlined. Breast-feeding should be encouraged with adequate support from the nursing staff. Lactating mothers need assistance to prevent hypoglycemia while nursing, which may require additional snacks. Breast-feeding also increases insulin requirements because of the insulin antagonistic properties of prolactin. Contraceptive options should be explored with the woman and her partner and pregnancy planning encouraged to allow for preconception care to decrease the risks for spontaneous abortion and congenital defects in future pregnancies. Counseling and education should be provided regarding long-term consequences of diabetes and the need for glycemic control to decrease adverse sequelae.

Women with diabetes have a higher incidence of postpartum infection. Therefore, nurses should observe for signs and symptoms and notify the physician if they occur. Women who have delivered a macrosomic infant or have had prolonged or induced labors should be closely monitored for hemorrhage.

Postpartum Management: Gestational Diabetes Mellitus

Most women revert to normal glucose tolerance in the postpartum period. Reclassification of glycemic status should be obtained at the 6-week postpartum visit for nonlactating mothers. An FPG determination can be obtained at the postpartum examination. If the level is normoglycemic (<110 mg/dL), repeat testing should occur at a minimum of 3-year intervals or when pregnancy is being considered (ADA, 1999c). Women with impaired fasting glucose (IFG) or impaired glucose tolerance (IGT) should be tested at more frequent intervals (ADA, 1999c). An FPG value of 110 mg/dL or higher requires repeat testing on another day. The FPG test is the preferred method because of the lower cost, convenience, and ease of administration (ADA, 1999c). However, studies have shown a lower sensitivity using FPG alone to diagnose overt diabetes (Conway, & Langer, 1999; Kousta et al., 1999). A 75-g, 2-hour OGTT is another method for diagnostic testing. Table 8–12 lists the criteria for diagnosis of diabetes mellitus from FPG, 75-gram OGTT, and random testing. The stricter criteria for diagnosis of diabetes adopted by ADA in 1997 has resulted in a doubling of diagnoses in the postpartum period with lower degrees of impairment (Conway & Langer, 1999).

The risk for development of overt diabetes after GDM increases with time. Risk factors related to the development of overt diabetes within 5 years of the index pregnancy include gestational age at diagnosis, level of glycemia at the first postpartum visit, obesity, another pregnancy, and impairment of pancreatic β-cell function (ADA, 1999c). Counseling should be provided to women with a history of GDM in the postpartum period for risk-reducing strategies such as weight reduction by diet and exercise. Women also need to know the signs and symptoms of hyperglycemia that would warrant testing for diabetes such as polyuria, polydipsia, polyphagia, persistent vaginal candidiasis, frequent UTIs, excessive fatigue and hunger, or sudden weight loss. Women also should be informed that the risk for GDM development in subsequent pregnancies has been reported as high as 70% (Major, de Veciana, Weeks, & Morgan, 1998). Development of subsequent GDM is associated with obesity, insulin use with previous GDM, higher parity, increased weight gain between pregnancies, and shorter periods between pregnancies (<24 months) (Major et al., 1998). Testing for diabetes is encour-

TABLE 8–12 ■ CRITERIA FOR DIAGNOSIS OF DIABETES MELLITUS

Normoglycemia	IFG and IGT	Diabetes Mellitus
FPG <110 mg/dL	FPG ≥110 mg/dL and <126 mg/dL (IFG)	FPG ≥126 mg/dL
2-hour plasma glucose <140 mg/dL	2-hour plasma glucose ≥140 mg/dL and <200 mg/dL (IGT)	2-hour plasma glucose ≥200 mg/dL
		Symptoms of the disease and casual plasma glucose of ≥200 mg/dL

FPG = fasting plasma glucose; IFG = impaired fasting glucose; IGT = impaired glucose testing.
Adapted from American Diabetes Association (1999c). Gestational diabetes mellitus. *Diabetes Care,* 22 (Suppl. 1), S74–S76.

aged before conception or in the first trimester, with early prenatal care to allow intensive management of overt diabetes, which carries a higher perinatal risk than for GDM.

CARDIAC DISEASE

Significance and Incidence

Cardiac disease in pregnancy is rare and complicates 1% of all pregnancies, but the leading cause of nonobstetric maternal mortality in this country is cardiovascular disease (Rochat, Koonin, Atrash, & Jewett, 1988). The incidence and significance of diverse cardiovascular lesions and diseases varies widely. The incidence of acquired and congenital heart disease is changing (Hsieh, Chen, & Soong, 1993; deSwiet, 1993) and will likely continue to change. One case of congenital heart disease is seen in approximately every 100 live births (Hoffman, 1995). Congenital cardiac lesions include atrial septal defects, ventricular septal defects, patent ductus arteriosus, tetralogy of Fallot, coarctation of the aorta, and Eisenmenger's syndrome. Mitral stenosis and aortic stenosis are examples of acquired cardiac diseases caused by rheumatic fever. Valvular stenosis is caused by scar tissue found on the valve leaflets and chordae tendineae of the affected valve. The scar tissue is caused by the body's immune response to the group A streptococci bacteria that causes rheumatic fever. Technologic and scientific advances have limited the impact of rheumatic fever and increased the survival rate for women with congenital cardiac disease. Additional acquired cardiac diseases have an impact on pregnancy.

Coronary artery disease is rare in women of childbearing years because of hormonal protection against coronary atherosclerosis (Sullivan & Ramanathan, 1985). Risk factors include diabetes mellitus, steroid-dependent lupus erythematosus (Bruce, Urowitz, Gladman, & Hallett, 1999), cardiac transplantation (Weis & von Scheidt, 2000), and use of oral contraceptives agents (Ratnoff & Kaufman, 1982). Severe consequences of coronary artery disease and myocardial infarction are also rare in pregnancy. The incidence of myocardial infarction in pregnancy is approximately 1 in 10,000 pregnancies (Mabie & Freire, 1995). The consequence of myocardial infarction in pregnancy varies widely, depending on the timing of the infarction in relation to birth.

Marfan syndrome also has a wide variety of outcomes that are related to the degree of aortic root dilation (Mayet, Steer, & Somerville, 1998). Cardiovascular anomalies related to Marfan syndrome include aortic root dilation, coarctation of the aorta, aortic regurgitation, patent ductus arteriosus, hypertension, and cardiomegaly. The most serious maternal risk during pregnancy and birth is acute aortic dissection. Because Marfan syndrome is an autosomal dominant disorder, there is a risk of the offspring inheriting the disorder. The incidence of Marfan syndrome is 4 to 6 cases per 10,000 persons. Risk is not related to sex, race, or ethnicity (Felblinger & Akers, 1998).

The reported incidence of peripartum cardiomyopathy varies. Sources cite an incidence of 1 case per 1,300 to 5,000 pregnancies (Cunningham et al., 1986; Homans, 1985; Pierce, Price, & Joyce, 1963). The challenges of diagnosis and controversy about the cause lead to the variations in reported statistics. Peripartum cardiomyopathy is categorized as dilated cardiomyopathy within the last month of pregnancy to 6 months after birth (Pearson et al., 2000). Most cases occur within the first 3 months postpartum. Historically, the damage to the cardiac chambers that caused the rapid dilation was attributed to an autoimmune response to viral myocarditis. There is evidence to suggest that up to 20% of cases may be genetic (McMinn & Ross, 1995). Other forms of cardiomyopathy, including hypertrophic obstructive cardiomyopathy (Autore et al., 1999), are also seen during pregnancy.

Dilated cardiomyopathy and myocarditis are associated with acquired immunodeficiency syndrome (Bestetti, 1989; Rerkpattanapipat, Wongpraparut, Jacods, & Kotler, 2000). These complications rarely cause cardiac failure; nonetheless, the increased incidence of human immunodeficiency virus infection during pregnancy substantiates the importance of careful cardiac assessment.

Nursing care for the woman whose pregnancy is complicated by cardiac disease is based on sound knowledge of the cardiovascular system and the pertinent physiologic adaptations to pregnancy (Table 8–13), as well as a thorough understanding of the psychosocial aspects of pregnancy, postpartum, chronic illness, and acute illness. Pregnant woman with cardiac disease require an individualized assessment that includes careful evaluation of physical and psychosocial status. The impact of the dynamic physiologic and psychosocial adaptations to pregnancy and the potential or actual complications of pregnancy require ongoing evaluation (Luppi, 1999). This evaluation ideally includes a prepregnancy risk factor assessment and counseling, evaluation at each prenatal appointment, a comprehensive assessment during admission for labor and birth, and continued vigilance during the postpartum period. Each wo-

TABLE 8–13 ■ NORMAL PHYSIOLOGIC CHANGES OF PREGNANCY

Body System	Change
Cardiovascular System	
Total blood volume	Increased 35%
Plasma volume	Increased 45%
Red cell volume	Increased 20%
Cardiac output	Increased 40% (positional)
Heart rate	Increased 15%
Systolic blood pressure	Unchanged
Systemic vascular resistance	Decreased 15%
Central venous pressure	Unchanged
Pulmonary capillary wedge pressure	Unchanged
Ejection fraction	Unchanged
Femoral venous pressure	Increased 15%
Uterine blood flow	Increased 20–40%
Respiratory System	
Minute ventilation	Increased 50%
Alveolar ventilation	Increased 70%
Tidal volume	Increased 40%
Respiratory rate	Increased 10–15%
Functional residual capacity	Decreased 20%
Residual volume	Decreased 20%
Oxygen consumption	Increased 20%
Arterial pH	Slightly increased (Average, 7.40–7.45)
PaO_2 (mmHg)	Increased (104–108 mmHg)
$PaCO_2$ (mmHg)	Decreased (27–31 mmHg)
Renal System	
Renal blood flow	Increased 50% (by 4th month)
Glomerular filtration rate	Increased 50% (by 4th month)
Upper limit of blood urea nitrogen	Decreased 50%
Upper limit of serum creatinine	Decreased 50%
Hepatic System	
Total plasma protein concentration	Decreased 20%
Pseudocholinesterase concentration	Decreased
Coagulation factors	Mainly increased
Gastrointestinal System	
Gastric emptying	Delayed
Gastric fluid volume/acidity	Increased
Gastroesophageal sphincter tone	Variable changes

Adapted from Luppi, C. J. (1999). Cardiopulmonary resuscitation in pregnancy. In L. K. Mandeville & N. H. Trioano (Eds.), *High risk intrapartum and critical care nursing* (2nd ed., pp. 353–379).

man presents different challenges for the healthcare team. Each cardiovascular condition is unique; however, there are general guidelines for nursing care. There is also specific terminology related to the care of pregnant women with cardiovascular disease (Display 8–27).

Cardiovascular Physiology and Terminology

Function

The cardiovascular system consists of the heart and the circulatory system. This system is responsible for transport of nutrients such as oxygen and glucose and elimination of waste products such as carbon dioxide and urea. Nutrients and waste products move between the blood and the surrounding tissues by diffusion. This complex system has other important functions such as communication (by means of hormones, cytokines, and other chemicals), immunity, and coagulation. The cardiovascular system also plays an important role in body temperature regulation. Cardiovascular pathology has the potential to seriously compromise all of these functions.

Bulk Flow

The cardiovascular system moves blood through the vascular network by bulk flow. Bulk flow requires a pressure gradient that is generated by the pumping action of the heart. The pressure gradient is influenced by the amount of flow and any resistance to flow. The radius of the vessels of the cardiovascular system is the most critical variable for determination of resistance. Viscosity of the blood and the length of the vessel also affect resistance. Any interruption in the pumping action of the heart or the pressure gradient alters blood flow. Various cardiac lesions and diseases as well as obstetric complications may affect the pumping action of the heart. Any lesion or disease state that is associated with rhythm disturbances also influences the pumping action of the heart.

Cardiovascular System Anatomy

The cardiovascular system consists of the pulmonary system and the systemic system. The right side of the heart pumps blood to the lungs (ie, venous return to right atrium to right ventricle to pulmonary artery to

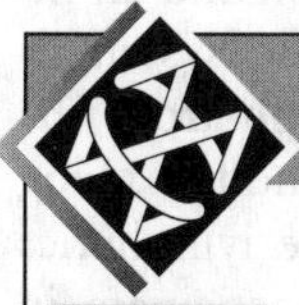

DISPLAY 8–27

Terminology

Inotrope:	Substance that affects myocardial contractility Positive inotrope = increased force of myocardial contraction Negative inotrope = decreased force of myocardial contraction
Chronotrope:	Substance that affects heart rate Positive chronotrope = increased heart rate Negative chronotrope = decreased heart rate
Dromotrope:	A substance that affects atrioventricular (AV) conduction velocity Positive dromotrope = increased AV velocity Negative dromotrope = decreased AV velocity
Preload:	Maximal ventricular volume at the end of diastole Right heart = central venous pressure (CVP) Left heart = pulmonary capillary wedge pressure (PCWP)
Afterload:	Resistance against which the heart must pump Right heart = pulmonary vascular resistance (PVR) Left heart = systemic vascular resistance (SVR)
Agonist:	Drug or substance that produces a predictable response; stimulates action
Antagonist:	Agonist that exerts an opposite action to another; blocks action
Cardiac output:	Heart rate multiplied by stroke volume
Stroke volume:	End diastolic volume minus end systolic volume

pulmonary capillaries to pulmonary vein). The volume entering the right side of the heart (ie, right preload) is reported as central venous pressure. The amount of resistance the right heart must pump against is reported as pulmonary vascular resistance. The left side of the heart pumps blood to the body (ie, pulmonary vein to left atrium to left ventricle to aorta). The volume entering the left side of the heart (ie, left preload) is reported as pulmonary capillary wedge pressure. The amount of resistance the left heart must pump against is reported as systemic vascular resistance. The left and right ventricles are separated by the interventricular septum. Figure 8–6 is a linear illustration of blood flow through the heart. Anatomic accuracy has been altered for purposes of clarity. Pathology in the right side of the heart has physiologic ramifications in the forward circulation of blood to the lungs and oxygenated blood into the systemic circulation. In some cases, right-sided pathology may have an impact on the return of blood to the heart when blood is forced backward into the system. Pathology in the left side of the heart has physiologic ramifications in the forward circulation of blood to the body and may have an impact on the circulation of blood if forward flow is impaired. The coronary vessels that branch off the aorta provide the blood supply to the heart. Cardiovascular disease and obstetric complications can seriously affect the circulation of blood throughout the body.

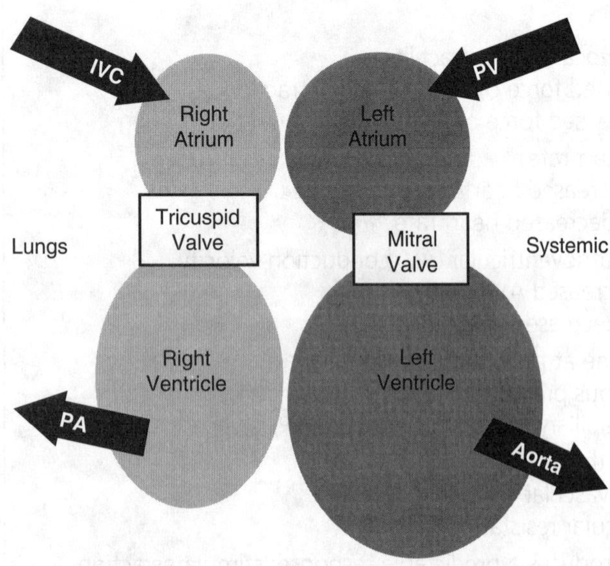

FIGURE 8–6. Linear illustration of blood flow through the heart. (Anatomic accuracy has been altered for purposes of clarity.)

Innervation

The heart is innervated by the autonomic nervous system (ie, sympathetic and parasympathetic nervous systems) and is affected by epinephrine secreted by the adrenal medulla. Epinephrine generally stimulates β-adrenergic receptors and causes the same response as norepinephrine. A review of the autonomic nervous system is summarized in Display 8–28. Many intrinsic and extrinsic factors stimulate the autonomic nervous system and affect cardiovascular function.

Vascular System

The vascular system consists of arteries, arterioles, capillaries, veins, and the lymphatic system. Arteries are low-resistance vessels that function as conduits for blood flow and as a pressure reservoir that maintains blood flow during diastole. Arteries regulate blood flow. The sympathetic nervous system innervates arterioles causing vasoconstriction. The parasympathetic nerves do not generally innervate arteriole smooth muscle (except in the external genitals, gut, and salivary glands). Capillaries are thin-walled vessels with a large cross-sectional area to deliver nutrients and eliminate wastes. The capillaries regulate the distribution of extracellular fluid. Veins are low-resistance conduits that return blood to the heart. The sympathetic nervous system innervates venous smooth muscle and causes vasoconstriction and an increase in venous pressure. The lymphatic system is a network of vessels that transport lymph from the tissues to the blood and the lymph nodes along those vessels. The major functions of the lymphatics are to regulate blood volume and to participate in defense mechanisms and absorption of fats from the gut.

Cardiac Homeostasis

The function of the cardiovascular system depends on a complex set of homeostatic mechanisms that control mean arterial pressure, cardiac output, systemic vascular resistance, and pulmonary vascular resistance. Pathology that affects any of these can alter the functioning of the cardiovascular system. The physiologic adaptations to pregnancy that modify these variables are discussed in Chapter 5. Pregnant women with cardiac disease require careful physical evaluation of the function of the cardiovascular system. The intricate function of the cardiovascular system affects every other system in the body and may have serious ramifications for the pregnant woman and her fetus.

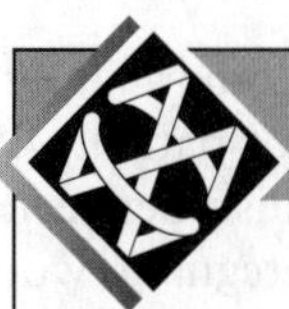

DISPLAY 8–28

Autonomic Nervous System Review

SYMPATHETIC DIVISION

- Fight or flight response
- Mobilizes the body; allows the body to function under stress
- **Neurotransmitters:** epinephrine, norepinephrine
- **Receptors**
  - Alpha-1: vascular smooth muscle, vasoconstriction
  - Alpha-2: skeletal blood vessels, inhibits release of norepinephrine
  - Beta-1: heart, increased heart rate, conduction, and contractility
  - Beta-2: lungs, smooth muscle of bronchi and skeletal blood vessels, relaxation of bronchi and vasodilation
  - Dopaminergic: coronary arteries and renal, mesenteric and visceral vessels, dilation
- **Synonymous terms:** adrenergic, sympathomimetic, catecholamine, anticholinergic, parasympatholytic, cholinergic blocker
- **Opposite terms:** sympatholytic, anti-adrenergic, sympathetic blocker, adrenergic blocker

PARASYMPATHETIC DIVISION

- "Feed and breed" response
- Restoration of body resources
- **Neurotransmitter:** acetylcholine
- **Receptors**
  - Nicotinic: skeletal muscle
  - Muscarinic: smooth muscle
    - Bronchi: constriction, increased secretion
    - Eye: pupillary constriction
    - Salivary glands: increased salivation
    - Heart: decreased heart rate
    - Gastrointestinal tract: increased secretion, increased peristalsis
- **Synonymous terms:** cholinergic, parasympathomimetic, sympathetic blocker, cholinomimetic, sympatholytic, adrenergic blocker
- **Opposite terms:** parasympatholytic, anticholinergic, cholinergic blocker, vagolytic

Obstetric Complications

Risk Factor Assessment and Counseling Before Pregnancy

Assessment of cardiovascular risk factors related to pregnancy and subsequent preconception (optimally) or antenatal counseling are traditionally based on three factors (Gianopoulos, 1989): the type of cardiovascular disorder, the degree of the woman's functional ability, and the incidence of pregnancy complications. Preconception and antenatal counseling are traditionally based on a mortality risk classification system illustrated in Display 8–29. Risk depends on the specific type of cardiac disorder and its severity. Maternal mortality data suggest that the most significant risk is seen with women with pulmonary hypertension, endocarditis, coronary artery disease, cardiomyopathy, and sudden arrhythmia (deSwiet, 1993). Preconception counseling has the benefit of allowing intervention for cardiac disorders that can be repaired or virtually repaired. Delay in pregnancy for up to a year is recommended when the woman selects this option (Shabetai, 1999).

The current trend for some women to delay childbearing adds significant risks to pregnancy in general (Hogberg, Innala, & Sandstrome, 1994) and especially for women with cardiovascular disease. Complications and progression of cardiovascular disease increase with maternal age. Conditions related to cardiovascular problems such as diabetes and hypertension are more likely to occur in women of advanced maternal age. Other factors that increase cardiovascular risk and are related to age include smoking, hyperlipidemia, and sedentary lifestyle. Maternal mortality rates for women older than 35 years are five times greater than that of women who are younger than 34 years. Parity and age also affect risk of mortality. A 35-year-old primiparous woman has a 20-fold greater risk than a multiparous woman who is younger than age 35 (Hansen, 1986). Most obstetric complications have an impact on risk status for the woman with cardiovascular disease.

The woman's functional ability is typically assessed using the New York Heart Association (Criteria Committee of the New York Heart Association [NYHA], 1979) system as shown in Table 8–14. Women are clas-

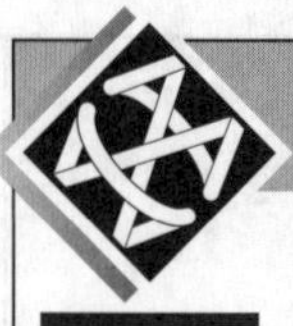

DISPLAY 8–29

Mortality Risk Associated With Pregnancy

Group I: Mortality <1%

Atrial septal defect
Ventricular septal defect (uncomplicated)
Patent ductus arteriosus
Pulmonic and tricuspid disease
Corrected tetralogy of Fallot
Biosynthetic valve prosthesis (porcine and human allograft)
Mitral stenosis, New York Heart Association (NYHA) class I and II

Group II: Mortality 5–15%

Mitral stenosis with atrial fibrillation
Mechanical valve prosthesis
Mitral stenosis, NYHA class III or IV
Aortic stenosis
Coarctation of the aorta (uncomplicated)
Uncorrected tetralogy of Fallot
Previous myocardial infarction
Marfan syndrome with normal aorta

Group III: Mortality 25–50%

Eisenmenger's syndrome
Pulmonary hypertension
Coarctation of the aorta (complicated)
Marfan syndrome with aortic involvement

sified on the basis of their symptoms of cardiac function failure. Up to 40% of women advance to a higher NYHA classification during pregnancy (Clark, 1991). This progression to a higher NYHA classification should be addressed at any risk counseling session, because the NYHA classification affects maternal mortality statistics. The incremental nature of the cardiovascular adaptations to pregnancy requires that the woman be assessed for any signs of deteriorating cardiovascular function at every healthcare provider encounter.

Nursing Assessment

The normal physiologic changes that occur during pregnancy can be similar to those of underlying cardiac disease. Fatigue, shortness of breath, orthopnea, peripheral edema, and palpitations may be observed in healthy pregnant women. These symptoms suggest congestive heart failure in the nonpregnant patient. A careful evaluation is necessary to distinguish between normal and abnormal findings. If the pregnant woman reports progressive limitation of physical activity because of worsening dyspnea, chest pain that occurs during exercise or increased activity, or syncope that is preceded by palpitations or physical exertion, underlying cardiac disease should be suspected. Display 8–30 lists the signs and symptoms of cardiac disease.

The woman's history and current physical status are analyzed in relation to cardiovascular physiology and function. Initial review includes examination of her specific medical, surgical, social, and family history. A review of her particular cardiovascular disorder, previous therapies, current medications, NYHA classification, and her knowledge base regarding all the aspects of her assessment are particularly pertinent. Past hospital admissions for medical stabilization or surgery are significant. Alcohol, drug, and tobacco use and presence of psychosocial support systems are obvious social issues. A woman's occupation can also provide useful information about functional status and environmental risk factors.

The nurses' knowledge of various methods and tools for cardiac assessment are prerequisites for a complete cardiovascular assessment. Physical assessment includes usual the methods of a head-to-toe inspection with specific attention paid to cardiovascular function. Evidence of tissue hypoxia or hypoglycemia, increased levels of carbon dioxide and urea, temperature instability, coagulopathy, or altered immunity can be signs of cardiac disease. Risk factors or physical evidence of pathologic blood flow should be assessed. This includes assessment of the pumping capabilities of the heart and vascular resistance. PIH is a notable example of impaired vascular resistance and increased viscosity of the blood that alters the bulk flow of blood.

A thorough understanding of maternal–fetal and cardiovascular anatomy, physiologic processes, and the clinical significance of the data are essential for optimum nursing care. Maternal positions that cause aortocaval compression influence accurate assessment.

Noninvasive assessment parameters include level of consciousness, blood pressure, oxygen saturation (SaO_2), ECG findings, and urine output. A cardiovascular assessment minimally includes auscultation of heart, lungs, and breath sounds; identification of pathologic edema; evaluation of respiratory rate and rhythm; evaluation of cardiac rate and rhythm; body weight assessed at the same time of day and on

TABLE 8–14 ■ NEW YORK HEART ASSOCIATION FUNCTIONAL CLASSIFICATION SYSTEM

Class	Description
I	Asymptomatic No limitation of physical activity
II	Asymptomatic at rest; symptomatic with heavy physical activity and exertion Slight limitation of physical activity
III	Asymptomatic at rest; symptomatic with minimal or normal physical activity Considerable limitation of physical activity
IV	Symptomatic at rest; symptomatic with any physical activity Severe limitation of physical activity

From Criteria Committee of the New York Heart Association. (1979). *Nomenclature and criteria for diagnosis of diseases of the heart and great vessels (8th ed.).* New York: New York Heart Association.

the same scale; assessment of skin color, temperature, and turgor; and capillary refill check. All pregnant women with preexisting cardiac disease should have a baseline 12-lead ECG and may require 5-lead cardiac monitoring during labor and birth. Certain disorders and advanced degrees of cardiovascular illness may require invasive hemodynamic monitoring using pulmonary artery catheters, peripheral arterial catheters, or central venous pressure monitors. Invasive hemodynamic monitoring is recommended for all woman designated in the NYHA class III or IV. Many women require continuous cardiac rhythm monitoring. Blood pressure readings are affected by maternal position and measurement techniques. Consistent equipment and cuff size and appropriate maternal position are significant. Electronic blood pressure may cause a widening of the pulse pressure compared with manual readings; however, the mean arterial pressure is unchanged (Marx, Schwalbe, Cho, & Whitty, 1993).

Assessment of the respiratory system reflects the function of the right heart. Auscultation of diminished breath sounds, rales, or rhonchi may reflect right cardiogenic pulmonary edema. Tachypnea, tachycardia, and anxiety are often early signs of edema and may be present before a cough or abnormal breath sounds. Abnormal skin and mucous membrane color may indicate problems with oxygenation and perfusion.

Kidney function is also assessed for adequacy of peripheral perfusion. Urinary output should be at least 25 to 30 mL/hour. Laboratory evaluation of renal function in and perfusion includes electrolytes, blood urea nitrogen, serum creatinine, protein, and uric acid levels. In acute situations, an indwelling Foley catheter with urometer can assist with assessment of fluid balance and indicate signs of inadequate renal perfusion.

Assessment of the CNS may reveal signs of inadequate blood flow. Restlessness, apprehension, anxiety, or changes in level of consciousness may indicate compromised blood flow and oxygenation of the brain.

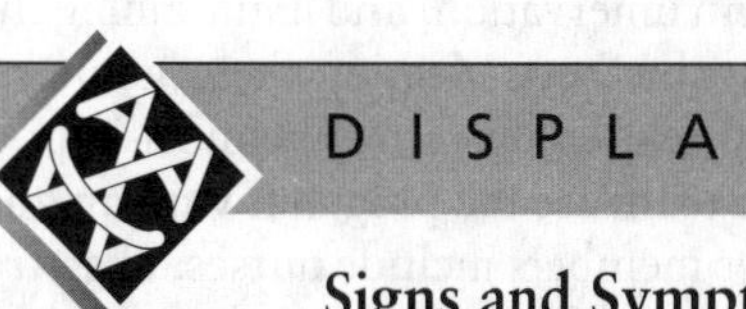

Signs and Symptoms of Cardiac Disease

History
- Progressive or severe dyspnea
- Dyspnea at rest
- Paroxysmal nocturnal dyspnea
- Angina or syncope with exertion
- Hemoptysis

Physical examination
- Loud systolic murmur or click
- Diastolic murmur
- Cardiomegaly, including parasternal heave
- Cyanosis or clubbing
- Persistent jugular venous distension
- Features of Marfan syndrome

Electrocardiogram
- Dysrhythmia

From Landon, M. B. (1996). Cardiac and pulmonary disease. In S. G. Gabbe, J. R. Niebyl, & J. L. Simpson (Eds.). *Obstetrics: Normal and problem pregnancies* (3rd ed., pp. 997–1024). New York: Churchill Livingstone.

Fetal assessment is a sensitive indicator of adequate cardiac function (Patton et al., 1990). Fetal movement counting, NST, contraction stress testing, BPP, and serial ultrasonography are all methods that evaluate uterine and placental perfusion (Simon, Sadovshy, Aboulafia, Ohel, & Zajicek, 1986). In an acute setting, continuous EFM is used to evaluate the FHR for baseline rate, variability, and specific patterns. An abnormal FHR baseline, minimal or absent FHR variability, and late deceleration patterns may indicate inadequate uteroplacental perfusion. Optimizing the hemodynamic status of the mother and avoiding aortocaval compression enhances uteroplacental perfusion and fetal oxygenation.

Clinical Management

The goals of clinical management for the woman whose pregnancy is complicated by cardiovascular disease mirror the goals for optimum uteroplacental perfusion. A stable mother is more likely to have a well-nourished baby. Optimizing cardiovascular function includes maintaining cardiac pump function, controlling vascular volume and resistance, limiting pathologic autonomic nervous system innervation, and maintaining the integrity of the vascular bed. Meeting these goals requires a coordinated team approach. The most important members of the team are the pregnant woman and her family, but other members include nurses, obstetricians, perinatologists, cardiologists, anesthesiologists, and neonatologists. Communication among team members is essential to attain a unified approach to this challenge. Decisions about timing and type of birth; anesthetic options and requirements; maternal–fetal priorities; and management strategies for potential obstetric complications need to be addressed as soon as possible. These plans may need to be reviewed during any unforeseen complications. Antepartum home care management for women with cardiac disease is discussed in Appendix 8A.

Optimum cardiac function is measured by cardiac output. Variables of cardiac output include preload, afterload, contractility, and heart rate. Manipulation of medications and intravascular volume may be necessary to optimize preload and afterload. Factors that can alter preload and afterload are summarized in Table 8–15 (Elkayam, Ostrzega, Shotan, & Mehra, 1995; DeAngelis, 1985). Ephedrine and intravenous fluid bolus are routinely used to control hypotension related to intrapartum epidural analgesia in normal pregnancy (Shnider, DeLorimier, Holl, Chapler, & Morishima, 1968). Because ephedrine may increase cardiac stress by increasing heart rate, phenylephrine has been recommended for women with many cardiac disorders (Ralston, Shnider, & DeLorimier, 1974). Tachycardia increases myocardial oxygen demands and decreased chamber filling time; therefore, phenylephrine is recommended to treat hypotension for ischemic and valvular disease.

Heart rate is affected by factors stimulating the autonomic nervous system. Certain medications may be needed when cardiac dysrhythmias are influencing heart rate and cardiac output. Commonly used antiarrhythmic medications include bretylium tosylate, digoxin, lidocaine, procainamide, propranolol, and verapamil. Cardioversion, direct pacing, and defibrillation may be required to correct serious dysrhythmias. Control of anxiety, pain, temperature, and many other variables can optimize heart rate. Cardiac output can be compromised by decreased stroke volume when there is diminished filling time due to tachycardia. A slow rate also compromises cardiac output, because cardiac output is determined by heart rate and stroke volume.

Numerous medications have been shown to modify the function of the heart by increasing or decreasing contractility. Calcium, catecholamines, dopamine,

TABLE 8–15 ■ FACTORS THAT AFFECT PRELOAD AND AFTERLOAD

Increase in Preload	Decrease in Preload	Increase in Afterload	Decrease in Afterload
Mitral insufficiency	Mitral stenosis	Aortic valve stenosis	Vasodilating substances
Left ventricular damage	Decreased intravascular volume	Peripheral arterial vasoconstriction	Hemorrhage
Increased intravascular volume	Conduction anesthesia	Hypertension	Conduction anesthesia
Vasoconstricting substances	Vasodilating substances	Polycythemia	Maternal position
Maternal position	Maternal position	Vasoconstricting agents	Decreased intravascular volume
		Maternal position	

dobutamine, epinephrine, digitalis, and norepinephrine have a positive inotropic effect. Barbiturates, propranolol, and quinidine have a negative inotropic effect.

Different levels of clinical intervention are based on the woman's ability to tolerate the cardiovascular stress of pregnancy, birth, and postpartum period. The woman's cardiovascular system is challenged by the cardiac output demands and fluid shifts surrounding birth. The nurse's assessment of cardiovascular parameters is crucial during this time. During labor, each uterine contraction increases cardiac output by 15%. Table 8–16 illustrates that the first 5 minutes after birth is the period of maximal cardiac output and hence maximum cardiovascular stress. The combination of diminished aortocaval compression by the uterus and the increased circulating blood volume that has been diverted from the placenta produce an immediate 65% increase in cardiac output. Epidural anesthesia can minimize the sudden changes in cardiovascular physiology, as well as minimizing the catecholamine production during labor. Generally, a vaginal birth is recommended and pain relief in labor is required for many cardiac disorders. Cesarean birth is reserved for the usual obstetric indications. Additional benefits of epidural anesthesia are potential avoidance of the risks of general endotracheal anesthesia should the need arise for emergent cesarean birth and avoidance of the Valsalva maneuver during second-stage pushing because of the ability to allow passive fetal descent.

During vaginal or cesarean birth, women with selected cardiac lesions are given antibiotics to prevent bacterial endocarditis. The American College of Obstetricians and Gynecologists (ACOG) recommends antibiotic prophylaxis during vaginal birth. A regimen of ampicillin and gentamycin or vancomycin should be administered before birth and for three doses after birth (ACOG, 1992). Thromboembolism prophylaxis is also an issue with selected cardiac disorders, including women with valvular heart disease, artificial heart valves, severe cardiomyopathy, and a history of thromboembolic cardiovascular disease. Heparin has been identified as the anticoagulant agent of choice. Heparin does not cross the placenta and is not associated with adverse fetal outcome (Ginsberg & Hirsh, 1995). Unfractionated heparin and low-molecular-weight heparin (LMWH) are used safely during pregnancy. Maternal complications of long-term unfractionated heparin therapy include bleeding, thrombocytopenia, and reversible osteoporosis. Use of LMWH during pregnancy has increased as the incidence of these side effects have been reduced (Weitz, 1997). Dosing does not require repeated phlebotomy for laboratory testing, and LMWH offers more consistent thromboembolism protection (Meschengieser, Fondevila, Santarelli, & Lassari, 2000). There is controversy in the literature about whether the increased body mass and glomerular filtration rate in pregnancy require increased LMWH dosages. A variety of management plans exist that address the risk of hemorrhage surrounding birth and the risk of intraspinal bleeding related to regional anesthesia for the anticoagulated woman (Chan & Ray, 1999).

TABLE 8–16 ■ PERIPARTUM CARDIAC OUTPUT

Stage of Labor	Cardiac Output Increase
Early first*	15%
Late first*	30%
Second*	45%
Postpartum—first 5 minutes	65%
Postpartum—60 minutes	40%

*An additional 15% increase accompanies each uterine contraction.

PULMONARY COMPLICATIONS

Pulmonary diseases have become more prevalent in general and during pregnancy. Pregnant women are more susceptible to injury to the respiratory tract for several reasons, including alterations in the immune system that involve cell-mediated immunity and mechanical and anatomic changes involving the chest and abdominal cavities (Goodrum, 1997). The cumulative effect is decreased tolerance to hypoxia and acute changes in pulmonary mechanics. Increased circulating levels of progesterone during pregnancy result in maternal hyperventilation and greater tidal volume without corresponding changes in vital capacity or respiratory rate. Oxygen consumption and minute ventilation increase as functional residual capacity and residual volume decrease with expanding abdominal girth. Total lung capacity is preserved, however, because of rib flaring and unimpaired diaphragmatic excursion. Pregnancy is characterized by a state of chronic compensated respiratory alkalosis. Normal maternal hyperventilation during pregnancy lowers maternal P_{CO_2} and minimally increases blood pH. The increase in blood pH increases the oxygen affinity of maternal hemoglobin and facilitates elimination of fetal carbon dioxide, but appears to impair release of maternal oxygen to the fetus. The high levels of estrogen and progesterone during pregnancy facilitate a shift in the oxygen dissociation curve back to the right, thereby stimulating oxygen release to a fetus that has an increased affinity for oxygen. These physiologic adaptations ensure that a fetus has every advantage from increased oxygen release and adequate blood gas exchange. When pulmonary complications occur during pregnancy, an understanding of the normal physiologic changes and their implications for maternal–fetal status is essential for developing appropriate interventions and treatment.

Asthma during pregnancy increases risk of preterm birth, IUGR, and maternal–fetal morbidity and mortality. Ongoing maternal–fetal assessment and aggressive treatment for exacerbations are required to avoid adverse outcomes. Treatment of asthma during pregnancy is challenging for the healthcare team, but patient education and collaboration between the pregnant woman and healthcare providers increase the likelihood of successful outcomes. Although pregnancy is complicated by pneumonia infrequently, there are serious maternal and fetal hazards with bacterial and viral lung infections. When the pregnant woman develops pneumonia, prompt assessment and diagnosis and the rapid initiation of supportive care to improve oxygenation along with appropriate antimicrobial therapy can result in the best possible outcome for mother and fetus.

Asthma

Significance and Incidence

Asthma affects approximately 7% of women of childbearing age. Between 1% and 4% of pregnant women have bronchial asthma, making it the most common respiratory disorder and potentially one of the most serious diseases complicating pregnancy (Cydulka et al., 1999; Greenberger, 1992; Mays & Leiner, 1995; Terr, 1998; Witlin, 1997). The incidence of asthma has risen by more than 30%, and the mortality rate from asthma has risen by 46% since the 1980s (ACOG, 1996). Appropriate management of asthma during pregnancy is important because of the significant risks for the mother and fetus. Goals when managing the woman with asthma during pregnancy include maintaining optimal respiratory status and function, preventing frequent episodes of wheezing requiring emergency therapy, and preventing repeated episodes of hospitalizations for status asthmaticus requiring intubation (Greenberger, 1992).

During pregnancy, approximately one third of women with asthma will improve, one third will experience worsening of their symptoms, and one third remain unchanged (Schatz, 1992, 1999). After birth, 75% of asthmatic women return to their prepregnancy asthmatic status. The disease itself has a variable natural history, creating the variability of expression during pregnancy. History of asthma severity in previous pregnancies may predict the severity of asthma in subsequent pregnancies (Brown & Halonen, 1999). There can be significant risks of asthma for the mother and her fetus. Maternal complications reported among asthmatics include hyperemesis, vaginal bleeding, hypertensive disorders, a predisposition to infections, gestational diabetes, preterm rupture of membranes, preterm labor, and having a LBW infant (Alexander, Dodds, & Armson, 1998; Coleman & Rund, 1997; Kallen, Rydhstroem, & Aberg, 2000; Minerbi-Codish, Fraser, Avnun, Glezerman, & Heimer, 1998). There is little risk to the fetus with well-controlled asthma. However, exacerbations causing hypoxia and decreased uterine blood flow increase the incidence of IUGR, preterm birth, and neonatal mortality (Coleman & Rund, 1997; Mays & Leiner, 1995). Asthma has been associated with a fetal death rate twice that of pregnant women without asthma (Juniper & Newhouse, 1993). Severe or uncontrolled asthma can be life-threatening for a woman and her fetus during pregnancy. Effective control can ensure a pregnancy outcome close to that of the general population (Greenberger, 1992; Schatz, 1999).

Definition

Asthma is a chronic pulmonary disorder in which the tracheobronchial tree is hyperresponsive to a multitude of stimuli. This results in edema of the bronchial wall, airway diameter reduction, and secretions that are thick and tenacious (Perlow, Montgomery, Morgan, Towers, & Porto, 1992). A variety of stimuli can cause response of the airways, including allergens, environmental irritants such as smoke or pollution, viral respiratory infections, cold air, exercise, food additives, and emotional stress. Common triggers of asthma exacerbations (Brown & Halonen, 1999; Mays & Leiner, 1995) are listed in Table 8–17.

Pathophysiology

The precise cause of airway inflammation and hyperresponsiveness is unknown. When triggered by external stimuli, inflammatory cells infiltrate bronchial tissue and release chemical mediators such as prostaglandins, histamine, cytokines, bradykinin, and leukotrienes (Mays & Leiner, 1995). Ultimately, airway smooth muscle responsiveness is increased because of these mediators. Narrowing of the airway

TABLE 8–17 ■ COMMON TRIGGERS OF ASTHMA EXACERBATIONS

Allergens	Pollens, molds, animal dander, house-dust mites, cockroach antigen
Irritants	Strong odors, cigarette smoke, wood smoke, occupational dusts and chemicals, air pollution
Medical conditions	Sinusitis, viral upper respiratory infections, esophageal reflux
Drugs, additives	Sulfites, nonsteroidal anti-inflammatory drugs, aspirin, beta blockers, contrast media
Other	Emotional stress, exercise, cold air, menses

lumen and airway hyperresponsiveness may be a result of the development of bronchial mucosal edema, excess fluid and mucous, inflammatory cellular infiltrates, and smooth muscle hypertrophy and constriction (Clark, 1993). During asthma exacerbations, there is decreased expiratory airflow, increased functional residual capacity, increased pulmonary vascular resistance, hypoxemia, and hypercapnia (Clark, 1993). The fetus can be negatively affected during acute episodes of asthma in which there is maternal arterial hypoxemia and the potential for uterine artery vasoconstriction (Coleman & Rund, 1997). Rapid and profound decreases in fetal oxygen saturation and resultant fetal hypoxia occur with clinically significant decreases in maternal PaO_2 below 60 mm Hg (Clark, 1993; Witlin, 1997). Despite surviving in an environment of low oxygen tension, the fetus has very little oxygen reserve.

Clinical Manifestations

The clinical manifestation of asthma is easily recognized. The woman may have only one or a combination of symptoms. Signs of respiratory distress are obvious and include shortness of breath, wheezing, nonproductive coughing, flaring nostrils, chest tightness, and use of accessory respiratory muscles. There may be scant or copious sputum, which is usually clear. Reports of nocturnal awakenings with asthma symptoms are common. Nonspecific stimuli such as an upper respiratory infection or a respiratory irritant may have provoked the exacerbation. Cyanosis, lethargy, agitation, intercostal retractions, and a respiratory rate greater than 30 per minute indicate hypoxia and impending respiratory arrest (Mays & Leiner, 1995).

Nursing Assessment

Guidelines for assessment of the severity of asthma before therapy is initiated have been developed by The National Heart, Lung, and Blood Institutes of Health (Sheffer, 1991). This classification system, like many others, was developed without specific consideration of pregnancy, but it may be helpful when assessing an adult patient with asthma. Patients are identified as mild, moderate, or severe asthmatics. Mild asthmatics experience exacerbations with coughing and wheezing no more than two times each week. There may be an intolerance of vigorous exercise. Women with moderate asthma experience more symptoms than women classified as having mild asthma. Severe exacerbations are infrequent with emergent care required less than three times each year. Severe asthmatics experience daily wheezing, and require emergency treatment more than three times per year. Women with severe asthma have poor exercise tolerance.

Identification of the woman with severe asthma is important so a plan of care and intensive treatment can be initiated early. Without comprehensive early treatment, there is significant risk to the mother and fetus. Characteristics of maternal history that should alert healthcare providers to an increased risk of a potentially fatal asthma exacerbation (Mays & Leiner, 1995) are listed in Display 8–31. Nursing evaluation

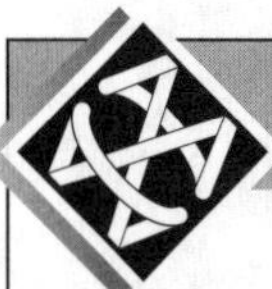

DISPLAY 8–31

Markers for Potentially Fatal Asthma

- History of systemic steroid therapy >4 weeks
- Three recent emergency room visits for asthma
- History of multiple hospitalizations for asthma
- History of hypoxic seizure, hypoxic syncope, or intubation
- History of admission to an intensive care unit for asthma

of the symptoms of asthma begins with clinical assessment of signs of respiratory distress. Significant findings include dyspnea, cough, wheezing, chest tightness, nasal flaring, presence of sputum, and tachycardia. Intercostal retractions or a respiratory rate greater than 30 per minute indicate moderate to severe asthma. Pulsus paradoxus of more than 15 mm Hg is an indication of severe asthma. If pulsus paradoxus is present, blood pressure is audible only during expiration. To make this assessment, carefully observe the woman's breathing, noting when systole first appears and the millimeter level of mercury until pulsations are heard during inspiration and expiration. Lung auscultation usually reveals bilateral expiratory wheezing. Occasionally, on inspiration or expiration, only rhonchi are heard. Rales are rarely auscultated in asthmatics. Detailed clinical findings are listed in Display 8–32.

Clinical evaluation is an invaluable assessment parameter in asthma, but laboratory findings are also useful in determining severity of an asthma attack and distinguishing it from other respiratory conditions. The most beneficial tools are pulmonary function tests such as peak expiratory flow and measurements of oxygen saturation and arterial blood gases. Predicted values of peak expiratory flow rate are unchanged during pregnancy and range from 380 to 550 L/min. An individual baseline should be established for each woman when her asthma is under control. Evaluation of exacerbations can be made by comparing baseline with current peak flow values. Peak expiratory flow values that are more than 50% below personal baseline require immediate attention (Mays & Leiner, 1995). Maternal oxygen saturation monitoring is a simple, noninvasive measure of oxygenation. Values that remain below 95% are significant for an exacerbation of asthma that requires attention. For the fetus to maintain normal levels of oxygenation, maternal oxygen saturation should be at least 95%.

During pregnancy, evaluations of arterial blood gases can help to establish severity of an asthma attack, with attention focused primarily on the pH and PCO_2 to define severity. A mild attack is characterized by an elevated pH and a PCO_2 below normal for pregnancy. The combination of normal pH, low PO_2, and normal PCO_2 for pregnancy indicates a moderate asthma attack. A low PO_2, low pH, and a high PCO_2 are most significant for severe respiratory compromise. When maternal arterial PO_2 falls below 60 mm Hg, the fetus is in severe jeopardy, and risk of fetal demise is increased (Huff, 1989).

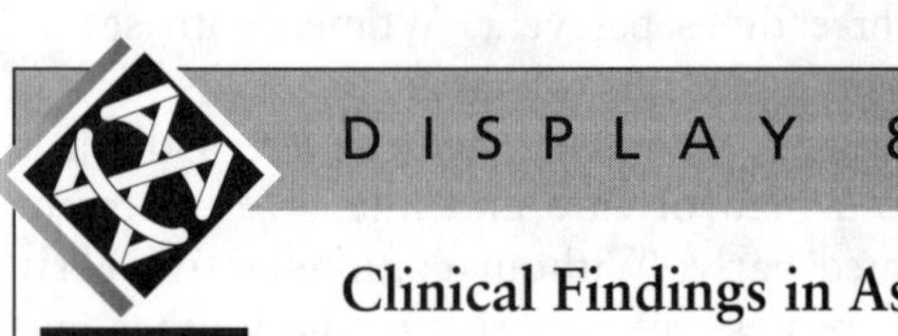

Clinical Findings in Asthma

SYMPTOMS

Shortness of breath, chest tightness, cough
Recurrent episodes of symptoms
Nocturnal awakenings from symptoms
Waxing and waning of symptoms

AUSCULTORY FINDINGS

Diffuse wheezes
Diffuse rhonchi
Longer expiratory phase than inspiratory phase

SIGNS OF RESPIRATORY DISTRESS

Rapid respiratory rate (>30 breaths/min)
Pulsus paradoxus >15 mmHg
Retractions intercostally or supraclavicularly
Lethargy
Confusion or agitation
Cyanosis

Nursing Interventions

The goals of therapeutic interventions for pregnant women with asthma are to maintain normal pulmonary function, control symptoms, prevent exacerbations, avoid adverse outcomes, avoid adverse effects of medications, and ensure the birth of a healthy baby (Witlin, 1997). Four integral components are important for effective management of asthma in pregnant women: patient education, objective assessment of maternal lung function and fetal well-being, control of environmental factors, and pharmacologic therapy (Clark, 1993).

Patient Education

Education should be designed to assist women to gain the motivation, confidence, and skill to keep their asthma under control. Much of the day-to-day management of asthma is the responsibility of the woman. A comprehensive knowledge base and patient comfort with the management are essential. Educational topics (National Heart, Lung, and Blood Institute National Asthma Education Program Working Group on Asthma and Pregnancy, 1993) include the following:

- Signs and symptoms of asthma
- Airway changes
- Avoiding asthma triggers
- Effects of pregnancy on the disease, and the disease on pregnancy
- Peak flow meters and metered dose inhalers
- Role of medications
- Adverse effects of medications
- Managing exacerbations
- Emergency care

Individualized education throughout pregnancy should be guided by assessment of the woman's understanding of her asthma assessment and management plan and her level of cooperation. It is essential to highlight the changes that pregnancy has on asthma and its treatment. When there is active participation by the healthcare provider, the patient, and her family, asthma control can be maximized.

Ongoing Maternal and Fetal Assessment

It is important to identify the pregnant woman with potentially fatal asthma so that maternal or fetal death can be avoided through greatly intensified treatment. Potentially fatal asthma includes a history of any one of the factors (Greenberger, 1992, Mays & Leiner, 1995) listed in Display 8–31. In addition to the subjective and objective measurements of the severity of a woman's asthma, ongoing fetal assessment is equally important. Serial ultrasonography beginning early in pregnancy to monitor trends in fetal growth and antepartum fetal testing such as NSTs and BPPs based on maternal–fetal status are essential to ensure fetal well-being for the moderate or severe asthmatic patient (Cousins, 1999).

Environmental Control

Identification of triggering factors for asthma in each woman is an important aspect of nonpharmacologic management that may improve clinical status, prevent acute exacerbations, and decrease the need for pharmacologic intervention. More than 75% of asthmatics report known reactions to common inhaled allergens (Dombrowski, 1997). Historic information and prior skin testing may give important information regarding common triggers such as pollens, molds, house dust mites, animal dander, and cockroach antigens. Other common asthma irritants include air pollutants, strong odors, food additives, and tobacco smoke. It is particularly important for the pregnant asthmatic woman to cease smoking during her pregnancy (Kurinczuk, Parsons, Dawes, & Burton, 1999). Education about the risks of smoking, including an increased severity of her asthma, bronchitis, or sinusitis and the need for increased medication, can be helpful in motivating the woman to stop smoking. In addition to the association between smoking and respiratory complications, smoking increases the risk of preterm birth and LBW. Although most women indicate a desire to quit smoking during pregnancy, this goal is not often met for a number of reasons. The section about Preterm Labor covers risks of smoking during pregnancy and smoking cessation programs in detail.

Viral respiratory infections, vigorous exercise, and emotional stress are common stimuli of severe asthma. Drugs such as aspirin, β blockers, nonsteroidal antiinflammatory medications, radiocontrast media, and sulfites have been implicated as asthma triggers as well. Once the woman has been assisted to identify common asthma triggers, exposure to allergens or irritants can be minimized.

Pharmacologic Therapy

The goals of asthma therapy include protection of airways from irritant stimuli, prevention of pulmonary and inflammatory response to allergen exposure, relief of bronchospasm, and resolution of airway inflammation to reduce airway hyperresponsiveness and improve pulmonary function (Dombrowski, 1997). Undertreatment is an ongoing problem in the care of pregnant asthmatic women. All medications used commonly in asthma management are generally considered safe and effective during pregnancy and lactation (Mays & Leiner, 1995, Moore-Gillon, 1994; Shatz et al., 1997). These drugs have been widely used for many years without evidence of teratogenic effect, and asthma should be treated just as aggressively in pregnant women as in nonpregnant patients. Pharmacotherapy is enhanced by appropriate environmental control measures and immunotherapy for the significant number of asthmatics with an allergic component to their disease (Terr, 1998). However, environmental control of asthma is frequently inadequate, and drug therapy is the hallmark of asthma management. Inhalation therapy is usually more effective than systemic treatment, because asthma is an airway disease. Aerosolized medications are ideal because they deliver the drug directly to the airways minimizing systemic side effects.

Bronchodilators

The use of β_2 agonists for powerful bronchodilation has been the mainstay of chronic and acute asthma therapy for decades. The onset of action is rapid, making them especially useful during early phases of asthma. Most of the β_2 agonists available are safe for use during pregnancy. Terbutaline is commonly prescribed and no association with congenital birth defects has been found (Briggs, Freeman, & Yaffe, 1998). Each of these drugs functions similarly and cause common side effects such as maternal tachycardia, maternal tremor, widened pulse pressure, restlessness, anxiety, and increased water retention. Continuous parenteral infusions may result in more serious side effects. Adverse reactions include tachyphylaxis, cardiac arrhythmias, and paradoxical bronchoconstriction (Mabie, 1996). Other than transient hypoglycemia and tachycardia, few direct adverse effects have been seen in the fetuses or neonates of women treated with β_2 agonists (Briggs et al., 1998). Inhaled β_2 agonists taken only as needed are usually sufficient to control women with mild, intermittent asthma. If symptoms disappear and pulmonary function normalizes, these medications can be used indefinitely. Prolonged use may result in rapid tolerance and limited usefulness. Women are candidates for antiinflammatory therapy if they require the use of a β_2 agonist more than three times each week (Clark, 1993). Because of the success of inhalation therapy, systemic aminophylline and theophylline are rarely used today. Sustained-release theophylline may be helpful for the pregnant woman whose symptoms are primarily nocturnal, because of its long-acting properties.

Antiinflammatory Therapy

One of the greatest advances in asthma treatment in the past decade has been the availability of inhaled corticosteroids (Kerstjens et al., 1992). For those who have required frequent β-agonist therapy, these medications are now considered first-line therapy. To minimize systemic effects and improve respiratory tract penetration, inhaled corticosteroids are administered with a spacer. At recommended doses, these medications act without systemic side effects to effectively reduce mucus secretion and airway edema. They may increase bronchodilator responsiveness while inhibiting many of the mediators of inflammation (Mays & Leiner, 1995).

Unlike the immediate acting bronchodilators, the effects of inhaled corticosteroids are gradual. After 2 to 4 weeks of use, full effects of symptom suppression and peak expiratory flow rate improvement are seen. Patient education is vital to ensure that the woman will continue her antiinflammatory therapy until the medication achieves maximum effectiveness. The most common side effect of inhaled steroids is hoarseness; it disappears when therapy is stopped. Other uncommon side effects include throat irritation, cough, and oral thrush (Mays & Leiner, 1995). Infrequent effects such as easy bruising, skin thinning, and low serum cortisol levels have been reported. Cromolyn and nedocromil are nonsteroidal antiinflammatory agents that work by preventing the release of inflammatory mediators through stabilization of mast cells. Neither produces any side effects. Although nedocromil has not been used during human pregnancy, cromolyn is an FDA category B drug (Mabie, 1996). Neither is as strong as inhaled corticosteroids in preventing asthma symptoms.

Corticosteroids

A course of oral corticosteroids may be effective when maximum doses of bronchodilators and antiinflammatory agents fail to control asthma. If a prednisone "burst" or tapering dose fails to relieve symptoms or prevent frequent recurrence, severe asthmatics require additional therapy. Oral corticosteroids may be needed chronically or used in short tapering courses. There are many side effects for the 5% of asthmatics who require stabilization with chronic therapy. Some of the unfavorable side effects include osteoporosis, hypertension, weight gain, delayed healing, immune suppression, diabetes mellitus, cushingoid appearance, cataracts, and adrenal atrophy (Mabie, 1996). Some of these side effects can be minimized with alternate-day therapy. The developing fetus has not experienced teratogenic effects from long-term steroid use in several studies (National Heart, Lung, and Blood Institute National Asthma Education Program Working Group on Asthma and Pregnancy, 1993). When compared with chronic treatment, short-term steroid use carries virtually no risk of serious side effects. A 7- to 10-day course of steroids assists with rapid control of an exacerbation of asthma, while giving time for inhaled antiinflammatory agents to reach full effectiveness.

Immunotherapy

Pregnant women with asthma who have allergens responsive to desensitization may benefit from allergen immunotherapy. Pollens, dust mites, and some fungi are aeroallergens that have been effectively suppressed with the use of allergy injections (Dykewicz, 1992). Maintenance dose injections may continue for a pregnant woman who is not reacting regularly and continues to benefit from the immunotherapy (Greenberger, 1992; Mays & Leiner, 1995). Because there is a 6- to 7-month interval before clinical benefits are seen and significant risk of a systemic reaction, pregnancy is not a time for initiation of immunotherapy.

Other Therapies

Antihistamines may be useful in the woman with a clear allergic stimulus to her asthma. Less is known about teratogenic effects on the fetus with newer medications, so caution must be used during pregnancy.

The safest decongestant for use during pregnancy appears to be pseudoephedrine. Pseudoephedrine is routinely used in the treatment of rhinitis. Pregnant women with asthma should be cautioned about use of over-the-counter medications, because many of the medications contain vasoconstrictors that may cause fetal abnormalities and decreased uterine blood flow (National Heart, Lung, and Blood Institute National Asthma Education Program Working Group on Asthma and Pregnancy, 1993). The influenza vaccine is indicated for women with chronic asthma after the first trimester. Because it is an inactivated virus, the vaccine poses no risk to the fetus.

Antepartum Care

When women have had exacerbations of asthma during pregnancy, vigilant fetal surveillance is important, especially after 20 weeks' gestation (Cousins, 1999). At each prenatal visit, confirmation that fundal height and fetal size are consistent with expected normal values based on current gestation age is crucial. Serial ultrasounds, BPPs, and electronic fetal heart monitoring are used to monitor fetal status on an ongoing basis (Cousins, 1999). Fetal movement counting may be initiated.

Inpatient Management

Acute Exacerbations

Rapid reversal of exacerbations of asthma is critical in the pregnant woman. The following are important when caring for women with exacerbations:

- Oxygen administration initiated to maintain PaO_2 as close to normal as possible (>60 mm Hg or SpO_2 >95%)
- Ongoing maternal pulse oximetry
- Baseline arterial blood gases
- Continuous EFM
- Baseline pulmonary function tests performed to gather baseline information
- β-agonist inhalation therapy every 20 minutes should be initiated (Clark, 1993). If initial bronchodilator treatments fail to result in adequate response, high-dose intravenous corticosteroids are the mainstay of therapy.

Uterine contractions are not uncommon during an exacerbation of asthma. $MgSO^4$ is the tocolytic of choice if cervical change is noted. Use of $MgSO_4$ therapy may enhance bronchodilation as well. β-Agonist therapy with terbutaline may be used to control preterm labor unless the woman already uses a β-agonist inhaler. For these women, terbutaline should be avoided to minimize the potential serious additive side effects of combined β-agonist therapy. Nonsteroidal antiinflammatory medications such as indomethacin may exacerbate asthma and are contraindicated. Antibiotics may be used to cover atypical pneumonia or secondary bacterial infection. Strict intake and output is necessary to minimize risk of fluid overload from β-mimetic therapy and intravenous steroids and avoid pulmonary edema. Ongoing care of the woman with an acute exacerbation is based on her response to the initial treatment plan.

Labor and Birth

Ten percent of women with asthma experience an exacerbation during the intrapartum period (Mabie, Barton, Wasserstrum, & Sibai, 1992). The risk of dyspnea or wheezing can be minimized through ongoing asthma medication during labor and the postpartum period. An exacerbation during labor is treated no differently than at other times. Control of the asthma is a priority for safety of the mother and her fetus. Continuous assessment of maternal oxygen saturation by pulse oximeter is important to attempt to maintain values above 95%. Oxygen should be administered by mask if saturation falls below this level. Additional information can be obtained from arterial blood gases. Air exchange is enhanced through patient positioning in a semi-Fowler's or high-Fowler's position. Potential for fluid overload can be avoided through strict intake and output measurements. Oxytocin is the drug of choice for the induction of labor, because prostaglandin $F_{2\alpha}$ is a known bronchoconstrictor (Mabie, 1996). The use of prostaglandin E_2 for cervical ripening intracervically or intravaginally has not been reported to result in bronchospasm. The pain relief method of choice for women in labor with asthma is epidural analgesia. Epidural analgesia can reduce oxygen consumption and may enhance the effects of bronchodilators (National Heart, Lung, and Blood Institute National Asthma Education Program Working Group on Asthma and Pregnancy, 1993). Meperidine and morphine sulfate are contraindicated because they may result in bronchospasm. A vaginal birth is safest for all women, but particularly for women with asthma. If operative birth is necessary, regional anesthesia is preferred. Use of methylergonovine for postpartum hemorrhage can cause bronchoconstriction and should be avoided.

Pneumonia in Pregnancy

Significance and Incidence

The incidence of pneumonia during pregnancy is similar to that of the nonpregnant population, but the disease course is often more virulent and the mortality rates from some pathogens is high. The spectrum of causative pathogens is similar to that of the nonpregnant population, and the management does not differ in general from the nonpregnant state. Pneumonia is an uncommon infection in pregnant women, but the complications for mother and fetus can be serious. It is difficult to estimate the true incidence of pneumonia during pregnancy because of variability of the rates in published studies. In some studies, the incidence of viral and bacterial pneumonia during pregnancy is estimated as 0.04% to 1% and may be on the rise (Maccato, 1991). This increase reflects the poor health of childbearing women in some communities, postponed childbearing, and the epidemic of human immunodeficiency virus, amplifying the number of pregnant women at risk for opportunistic lung infections. Pneumonia has also been strongly associated with asthma, prior lung disease, anemia, and illicit drug use (Berkowitz & Lasale, 1990; Munn, Groome, Atterbury, Baker, & Hoff, 1999).

Pneumonia is the leading cause of maternal mortality from nonobstetric infection in the peripartum period (Rodrigues & Niederman, 1992). Although the introduction of antimicrobial therapy has significantly decreased maternal mortality (Maccato, 1989; Riley, 1997), risk of maternal and fetal morbidity continues. Some viral pneumonias may be more virulent during pregnancy than in the nonpregnant patient. Maternal complications of pneumonia during pregnancy include preterm labor, empyema, bacteremia, pneumothorax, atrial fibrillation, and respiratory failure requiring intubation (Madinger, Greenspoon, & Ellrodt, 1989; Munn et al., 1999). Pneumonia has not been related to any congenital syndrome in neonates, but antepartum respiratory infection has been associated with increased incidence of complicated preterm birth. The loss of maternal ventilatory reserve normally seen in pregnancy coupled with maternal fever, tachycardia, respiratory alkalosis, and hypoxemia seen with respiratory infections can be adverse for fetuses. Reports of preterm birth, small for gestational age infants, and fetal death have been attributed to pneumonia during pregnancy (Nolan & Hankins, 1995; Riley, 1997; Rodrigues & Niederman, 1992).

Varicella pneumonia may occur in up to 20% of adults with varicella (chickenpox) infection. The mortality rate for varicella pneumonia during pregnancy may exceed 35% (ACOG, 1996) because women with varicella pneumonia are at risk for multiple complications such as bacterial superinfection, ARDS, endotoxin shock, and bronchiolitis obliterans organizing pneumonia (Chandra, Patel, Schiavello, & Briggs, 1998). The neonatal death rate for varicella pneumonia is between 9% and 20% (Grant, 1996). Pregnant women with varicella pneumonia should be hospitalized, especially if they develop complications (Baren, Henneman, & Lewis, 1996).

Definition

Pneumonia is an inflammation of the alveoli and bronchioles of the lower respiratory tract resulting in consolidation and exudation. It may be primary or secondary and may involve one or both lungs. The microorganisms that give rise to pneumonia are always present in the upper respiratory tract, and unless resistance is lowered, they cause no harm. Bacterial and viral pneumonias and aspiration pneumonitis are the most commonly seen pneumonias during gestation (Rodrigues & Niederman, 1992) (Display 8–33). Alteration in maternal immune status to prevent rejection of the developing fetus is the major factor predisposing women to severe pneumonic infections during pregnancy.

Pathophysiology

Pneumonia develops when host defenses are overwhelmed by an organism invading the lung parenchyma. Although a number of defense mechanisms protect lower airways from pathogens, infection leads to increased permeability of the capillaries. This

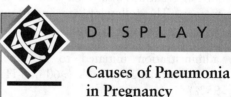

Causes of Pneumonia in Pregnancy

Pneumococcus
Haemophilus influenzae
No pathogen identified
Legionella species
Mycoplasma pneumoniae
Chlamydia pneumoniae
Viral pathogens
  Influenza A
  Varicella
Aspiration
Fungi

Adapted from Rodrigues, J., & Niederman, M. S. (1992). Pneumonia complicating pregnancy. *Clinics in Chest Medicine, 13*(4), 679–691.

causes alveolar and interstitial fluid accumulation, resulting in abnormal chest radiograph findings. Air space pneumonia, interstitial pneumonia, and bronchopneumonia are commonly seen on the chest radiograph of patients with pneumonia. Radiographic patterns differ based on the infective agent and can be helpful in diagnosing the cause of pneumonia.

Clinical Manifestations

Bacterial Pneumonia

The most common causative bacterial pathogen for pneumonia in pregnancy is *Streptococcus pneumoniae.* It is responsible for approximately 50% of cases of bacterial pneumonia during pregnancy and approximately two thirds of all pneumonias during pregnancy (Rigby & Pastorek, 1996). Women with bacterial pneumonia during pregnancy most often present with a history of upper respiratory infection. They frequently have abrupt onset of fever above 101°F and chills. Pleuritic chest pain, productive cough, and rusty sputum are other common symptoms. Blood cultures are positive in approximately 25% of cases (Neu & Sabath, 1993). *Haemophilus influenzae* is the second most common bacterium identified in patients with bacterial pneumonia, and symptoms are similar to those caused by to *S. pneumoniae.* Women with chronic obstructive pulmonary diseases and chronic bronchitis are at greatest risk. There are numerous other uncommon pneumonia pathogens that may be seen in childbearing women, including *Mycoplasma pneumoniae, Chlamydia pneumoniae, Moraxella catarrhalis, Klebsiella pneumoniae,* and *Escherichia coli.* These organisms produce atypical pneumonia syndrome, which is characterized by gradual onset, less toxicity, lower fever, nonproductive cough, malaise, and a patchy or interstitial infiltrate (Maccato, 1991). *Legionella pneumophila* may cause a pneumonia with the typical acute course or the atypical symptoms described with the less common pathogens. Underlying chronic illness, advancing age, and cigarette smoking appear to be significant predisposing factors. When a superimposed pulmonary infection follows a viral pneumonia, *Staphylococcus aureus* is frequently responsible. This organism may also spread by the hematogenous route related to intravenous catheters, intravenous drug abuse, or infective endocarditis. The onset of this pneumonia is usually abrupt, and the course is rapid. Pleuritic chest pain and purulent sputum production are evident.

Pneumonia from anaerobic organisms is usually caused by aspiration during induction or emergence from general anesthesia for an operative birth. The aspiration of particulate matter and gastric acid causes an immediate chemical pneumonitis, followed in 24 to 48 hours by a secondary bacterial infection. Fortunately, the use of nonparticulate antacids (eg, sodium citrate), regional anesthesia, and rapid sequence induction of general anesthesia with cricoid pressure have dramatically reduced the incidence of aspiration-related maternal mortality (ACOG, 1996). Other causes of aspiration pneumonia include anything that may diminish consciousness, such as seizures and drug or alcohol abuse. Delayed gastric emptying, decreased esophageal sphincter tone, and elevated intragastric pressure are normal physiologic changes in the gastrointestinal tract during pregnancy that predispose a woman to aspiration. Acute symptoms of aspiration include cough, significant bronchospasm, and hypoxia. Signs of infection begin 6 to 24 hours after aspiration and include tachypnea, tachycardia, hypotension, and frothy pulmonary edema (Rodrigues & Niederman, 1992). Mechanical ventilation may be necessary and difficult. Superimposed bacterial infection must be identified and treated promptly to minimize significant perinatal morbidity and mortality.

Viral Pneumonia

Influenza, varicella, and measles viruses are associated with significant morbidity for pregnancy women with pneumonia. The most common viral pneumonia is influenza, typically type A. Type A influenza attacks the lung parenchyma and causes edema, hemorrhage, and hyaline membrane formation. Acute onset of malaise, headache, high fever, cough, and myalgias are associated symptoms. During pregnancy, fulminant respiratory failure may develop requiring extended mechanical ventilation. Varicella pneumonia may be more common and more virulent in pregnancy than in nonpregnant patients. Smoking may also be a risk factor for the development of this type of pneumonia, which usually occurs in the third trimester (Rodrigues & Niederman, 1992). Varicella pneumonia typically presents with fever, dyspnea, tachypnea, cough, pleuritic chest pain, and hemoptysis within 2 to 7 days of the vesicular rash. Chest radiographs shows a diffuse miliary or nodular pattern (ACOG, 1996). It is not uncommon to see rapid progression to hypoxia and respiratory failure. In addition to maternal complications, intrauterine infection occurs in up to 26% of cases varicella pneumonia (Rodrigues & Niederman, 1992). Congenital varicella syndrome may occur if infection occurs in the first trimester and is characterized by cutaneous scars, limb hypoplasia, chorioretinitis, cortical atrophy, and other anomalies in the neonate (Balducci et al., 1992). Second trimester varicella may result in congenital zoster in some infants. Premature labor and perinatal varicella infection are significant adverse effects that may result from varicella infection during pregnancy. Rubeola during pregnancy may lead to spontaneous abortion and preterm birth. Pneumonia can complicate up to 50% of cases, and bacterial superinfection is also common.

Nursing Assessment

Obtaining a detailed history of the illness and symptoms and a physical examination are essential. All pregnant women should be questioned about immunity to varicella during the first prenatal visit. Susceptible women should be counseled to avoid contact with individuals who have chickenpox. If exposure occurs, varicella-zoster immune globulin (VZIG) should be administered with 96 hours in an attempt to prevent maternal infection (Chapman, 1998). Laboratory and radiologic findings are important to help diagnose the type of pneumonia present. Clinical presentation and laboratory data help to determine whether the pneumonia is classic or atypical. Careful questioning about underlying chronic conditions and prior illness can identify risk factors. A sputum sample with secretions from the lower bronchial tree must be collected for analysis. Blood cultures should be obtained routinely because positive results are highly specific. These specimens assist in identifying the pathogen responsible for the pneumonia. Because a hemoglobin oxygen saturation level below 95% affects the amount of oxygen delivered to the fetus, it must be monitored continuously. Initial arterial blood gases in the pregnant woman with pneumonia usually reflect significant degrees of hypoxia without hypercapnia or acidosis (Maccato, 1991). The nurse must assess each woman closely for symptoms of hypoxia, including irritability and restlessness, tachycardia, hypertension, cool and pale extremities, and decreased urine output. Confusion, disorientation, and loss of consciousness can result if the hypoxia goes untreated.

Nursing Interventions

Regardless of the type of pneumonia, nursing interventions focus on close monitoring, oxygen supplementation, antipyretics, and adequate hydration. Positioning the woman in a semi-Fowler's or high-Fowler's position usually is most comfortable and promotes maximum oxygenation. Oxygen supplementation to maintain O_2 saturation of greater than 95% by pulse oximeter is vital to ensure adequate maternal oxygen delivery to the fetus. The most common method of oxygen administration is 2 to 4 L/min through a nasal cannula. If the woman requires more than 4 L of oxygen to maintain adequate hemoglobin oxygen saturation, the use of a simple or Venturi mask to deliver higher and more specific levels of oxygen is standard. Mechanical ventilation is necessary for women who are unable to maintain a PaO_2 above 60 mm Hg despite high concentrations of inspired oxygen. These women are best cared for in an intensive care setting. Other supportive measures may have some benefit in therapy of the pregnant woman with respiratory insufficiency secondary to pneumonia. For women who are unable to cough effectively, postural drainage and tracheal suctioning can be valuable in mobilizing secretions. The use of incentive spirometry may be helpful as well. The development of preterm labor as a complication of infection may be the result of the response of the uterus to certain mediators of inflammation and infection. Prompt attention to regular uterine contractions and cervical changes is necessary to minimize the risks of preterm birth as a result of significant maternal illness. Conversely, in patients in whom respiratory and cardiovascular status continue to deteriorate despite maximum supportive efforts, birth may be necessary for fetal and maternal survival.

Pharmacologic Therapy

Antimicrobial therapy must be specific to the pathogen present, along with consideration for its safety during pregnancy (Riley, 1997) (Table 8–18). Until identification of the causative organism, symptoms, sputum Gram stain, and chest radiography can direct initial antibiotic use. Ampicillin is administered if *S. pneumoniae* or *H. influenzae* is the suspected pathogen. With an increase in ampicillin-resistant patients, third-generation cephalosporins, erythromycin, and trimethoprim-sulfamethoxazole are other choices for most cases of classic pneumonia (Riley, 1997; Yost, Bloom, Richey, Ramin, & Cunningham, 2000). These antibiotics may be the most appropriate first-line medications for sick patients when there is high probability of resistance. Varicella pneumonia must be treated promptly with acyclovir, with 8 to 10 mg/kg given intravenously every 8 hours to decrease complications and mortality. Patients who receive this medication early in the course of their illness benefit from lower temperatures and respiratory rates and from improved oxygenation without risk to their fetus. Varicella embryopathy may occur as a result of maternal infection, particularly in the first half of pregnancy, with an incidence of 1% to 2% (Chapman, 1998). Varicella of the newborn is a life-threatening illness that may occur when a newborn is delivered within 5 days of the onset of maternal illness

TABLE 8–18 ■ ANTIBIOTIC THERAPY FOR PNEUMONIA PATHOGENS

Pathogen	Ampicillin	Cephalosporin	Erythromycin	Trimethoprim-Sulfamethoxazole
S. pneumoniae	+	+	+	+
H. influenzae	+	+	−	+
M. catarrhalis	−	+	+	+
C. pneumoniae	−	−	+	−
L. pneumophila	−	−	+	−
M. pneumoniae	−	−	+	−
P. carinii	−	−	−	+

or after postbirth exposure to varicella. Susceptible newborns should be given VZIG (Chapman, 1998).

Aspiration pneumonia is best treated with broad-spectrum antimicrobials to cover Gram-negative and Gram-positive bacteria that are usually present. Antiviral agents amantadine and ribavirin have been used in the treatment of influenza pneumonia during pregnancy. Although they have shown teratogenicity in some animal studies, both have been effective in decreasing the severity of illness associated with influenza during pregnancy without adverse effects to humans.

MULTIPLE GESTATION

Significance and Incidence

Multiple gestation occurs in 3% of all pregnancies (American College of Obstetricians and Gynecologists [ACOG], 1998). Multiple gestation is not a complication of pregnancy, but rather a condition that presents an increased risk of morbidity and mortality for the mother and her babies. Although many multiple gestations are uncomplicated, the perinatal team must be alert for potential complications during pregnancy, labor, birth, and the postpartum period.

Natality data from the National Center for Health Statistics (NCHS) reveals a significant increase in the number of multiple births in the United States (Ventura, Martin, Curtin, Mathews, & Park, 2000). In 1998, the number of twins increased from 1997 by 6% to 110,670 births. This was the largest 1-year increase since these data began to be recorded from certificates of live births. Between 1997 and 1998, the number of triplets rose 13% to 6,919 births. In 1998, twins represented 1 in every 36 births, and triplets represented 1 in every 500 births. Since 1980, the twin birth rate has risen 49% (18.9 to 28.1 per 1,000 live births), and the rate of triplet and higher-order multiples has risen 423% (37 to 193.5 per 100,000 live births). From 1980 to 1998, the twin birth rate increased 77% for women 40 to 44 years old and more than 1,000% for women 45 to 49 years old. Over the same period, the triplet birth and higher-order multiples birth rate increased 461% for women in their thirties and almost 15 times for women in their forties. In 1998, 1 in every 6 infants born to women between the ages of 45 and 49 years and one in every 3 infants born to women between the ages of 50 and 54 years was born in a multiple birth.

Approximately 80% of triplets and higher-order multiple gestations are the result of fertility techniques. The trend to delay childbirth among some women has contributed to the increase in the number of multiple births. Older women are likely to have a multiple birth even without the use of fertility therapy (MacDorman & Atkinson, 1999).

According to data from the Maternal and Child Health Bureau, Health Resources and Services Administration, multiple births account for an increasing percentage of all LBW infants, preterm births, and infant mortality (Kogan et al., 2000). Approximately 54% of twins are LBW (<2,500 g), and approximately 55% are born preterm (before 37 completed weeks' gestation). Approximately 14% of twins born preterm are small for gestational age, and approximately 20.5% of twins born at term are small for gestational age. In 1997, the infant mortality rate for triplet and higher-order births was 69%, more than double the rate for twin births (31.5%) and 10 times the rate for singleton births (6.4%). Maternal mortality associated with multiple pregnancy is rare (estimated to be 1 in 3,000 pregnancies). The risk of preterm birth increases with the number of fetuses. For women pregnant with higher-order multiples, it is estimated that each additional fetus decreases the potential for completed weeks of gestation by 3.5 weeks. Nulliparous women pregnant with higher-order multiples are more likely to give birth preterm than women pregnant with higher-order multiples who have previously given birth to a term infant. For higher-order multiple pregnancies, parity appears to increase the length of gestation by approximately 2 weeks. Maternal height is an additional advantage for prolonging pregnancy for higher-order multiples.

Although the high rate of mortality is related to preterm birth, infants born from multiple gestations weighing 1,000 to 2,499 g have a lower mortality rate than singletons, whereas at 500 to 999 g, the mortality rate is similar (Gall, 1998). The singleton mortality rate reaches the lowest point at 40 weeks' gestation and increases after 40 weeks. However, with twins the mortality rate is lowest at 38 weeks and increases steadily from 39 to 42 weeks (Kiely, Kleinman, & Kiely, 1992; Minakami, & Sato, 1996). The growth peak of twins also seems to occur earlier (Luke, 1998). Based on these data, it has been recommended that the gestational age of maturity be lowered to 38 weeks because twins appear to be mature at this time (Kiely, 1998; Luke, 1998; Minikami & Sato, 1996).

IUGR is the second most important factor affecting mortality and morbidity, especially after 30 weeks' gestation. The rate of IUGR is higher for twins than singletons. IUGR is considered to exist when the estimated fetal weight decreases below the 10th percentile for a singleton fetus or in multiple fetuses when there is a 20% difference in the weight of one of the fetuses. The incidence of IUGR is increased in multiple gestation because of increased fetal metabolic demands, placental and cord anomalies, and the increased incidence of maternal complications, such as PIH (Hamilton, Platt, Morin, Usher, & Kramer, 1998). Because of these factors, monochorionic twins with IUGR are more than twice as likely to die in the perinatal period. Conditions other than prematurity and IUGR that have been reported to increase perinatal morbidity and mortality include congenital anomalies, placenta previa, placental abruption, PIH, cord accidents, and malpresentations.

Admissions to NICUs are considered a measure of morbidity and occur for approximately 22.7% of twins, 64.1% of triplets, and 75% of quadruplets. The length of stay averages 12.0 days for twins, 17.4 days for triplets, and 57.8 days for quadruplets (Gall, 1998).

Physiology of Twinning

Zygoticity

Twinning can develop in three ways. Dizygotic (DZ) "fraternal" twins constitute about two thirds of multiples. Monozygotic (MZ) "identical" twins occur in about 25% of multiples. A third type of twinning, called intermediary twinning, half-identical polar body, or monovular-dispermic twinning, has been suggested. In higher-order multiple conceptions, any combination of these mechanisms can occur. Table 8–19 provides the definitions of terms.

Most ovulation-induced pregnancies are DZ, the result of multiple eggs fertilized by separate sperm. Although they develop during the same pregnancy, they are no more genetically alike than any siblings of the same family. Each DZ zygote has a separate placenta, chorion, and amnion, making them dichorionic-diamniotic. Factors that influence the rate of DZ twinning are listed in Display 8–34. Older women (>30 years) are more likely to produce multiple eggs at ovulation. They are equally as likely to have ovulation problems that require treatment with ovulation-induction agents that lead to the production of multiple eggs. The rate of DZ twinning is influenced by race. The incidence is highest among African-American women and lowest among Asian, Hispanic, and Native-American women, although the number of multiples has increased in all races (Ventura et al., 2000). Heredity has an important influence over DZ twinning. The chance of multiples is highest if the mother was a twin. The father's history of twinning is also significant, but only about one half the rate of a positive maternal history. Multiples increase with parity and are about four times as likely in the fourth or fifth birth, regardless of maternal age (Taffel, 1995). There is also an increase of DZ multiples after the cessation of oral contraception.

Monozygotic twinning occurs when one sperm fertilizes one egg. This fertilized egg then divides, resulting in two or more identical zygotes. MZ twinning is thought to be an aberrant occurrence with no known

TABLE 8–19 ■ DEFINITION OF TERMS

Term	Definition
Monozygotic	Identical, formed from one egg and one sperm
Monochorionic	One chorionic membrane
Monoamniotic	One amniotic sac
Dizygotic	Fraternal, formed from two separate eggs and two sperm
Dichorionic	Two chorionic membranes
Diamniotic	Two amniotic sacs

Adapted from Dauphinee, J. D., & Bowers, N. A. (1997). *Nursing management of multiple birth families: Preconception through postpartum* (Nursing Module). White Plains, NY: March of Dimes Birth Defects Foundation.

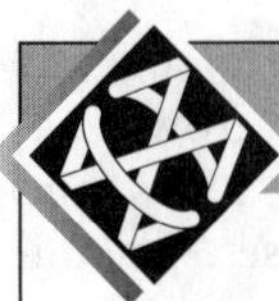

DISPLAY 8–34

Factors Associated With Dizygotic Twinning

- Increased maternal age
- Race
- Heredity
- Higher parity
- Ovulation induction agents or assisted reproductive technologies
- Oral contraception discontinuation

From Dauphinee, J. D., & Bowers, N. A. (1997). *Nursing management of multiple birth families: Preconception through postpartum* (Nursing Modules). White Plains, NY: March of Dimes Birth Defects Foundation.

causes or predisposing factors. The increase in MZ pregnancies may be caused by assisted reproduction. Most MZ multiples are twins, but identical triplets and quadruplets do occur. Because MZ multiples are genetically identical, they are always the same sex. Monozygotic multiples may not be exactly identical in physical appearance because of environmental or nutritional factors. "Mirror twinning" may occur when identical twins have opposite characteristics such as left- and right-handedness or reversed hair patterns. In rare cases, genetic aberrations can result in MZ multiples with different chromosomal patterns or phenotypes. MZ multiples are at higher risk for congenital anomalies and other complications than dizygotic multiples, especially the 1% of MZ multiples who are monoamniotic.

Intermediary twinning, also called "half-identical," polar body, or monovular-dispermic twinning, has been suggested. It is thought that the secondary oocyte divides before fertilization, resulting in two unfertilized yet identical eggs that could be fertilized by two separate sperm. Potentially, the children would have identical maternal but differing paternal chromosomes. It is generally accepted that aging of the oocyte plays a role in this process, but there are limited human data about this phenomenon (Keith, Papiernik, Keith, & Luke, 1995).

Placentation

Multiple gestations have several different placental structures depending on the number of chorions and amnions. Each DZ zygote has a separate chorion and amnion, making them diamniotic-dichorionic with separate circulations. In contrast there can be different placental configurations in MZ multiples. Approximately 30% of MZ pregnancies are diamniotic-dichorionic and have their own circulation (Gall, 1998). Placentas of higher-order multiples conform to these same rules. However, MZ and DZ placentation can occur in the same pregnancy; for example, a triplet pregnancy could consist of two fetuses that are MZ with monochorionic-monoamniotic placentation, and the third fetus could be DZ with its own amnion and chorion.

Placentas that are dichorionic may be separate or fused, which can make it difficult to distinguish whether the fetuses have one placenta or separate fused placentas. When placentas fuse, there can be a discrepancy in infant weights. They may appear to be unequal, but the actual size of the placenta is not as important as the vascular structure and functioning area. Vascular anomalies occur more frequently, and perinatal death caused by placental infarction is twice as common during the birth of the second twin. Because of the dichorionic placenta structure, marginal and velamentous cord insertions occur in 14% of these placentas (Gall, 1998).

When placentas are monochorionic, numerous anastomoses can develop between each placental circulation in three ways: artery to artery, vein to vein, and artery to vein. The first two anastomoses, depending on the size and flow rate, usually cause few problems. However, when an artery to vein anastomoses occurs (usually in the deep circulation), there are significant risks to the fetuses. Artery-to-vein anastomoses are responsible for most of the morbidity and mortality seen in monochorionic-diamonitic twins, including vanishing twin syndrome, fetus papyraceus (ie, fetus retained in the uterus beyond the natural term that has a mummified appearance), and twin-to-twin transfusion (Gall, 1998). The incidence of marginal and velamentous cord insertions in monochorionic placentas is 27%, and single umbilical arteries are common (Benirschke, 1992).

Monochorionic-monoamniotic placentas occur in 2% to 5% of all twin pregnancies (Gall, 1998). These structures have one amniotic sac with at least two umbilical cords, in which velamentous insertion commonly occurs. The fetal loss rate has been reported as high as 50% to 70% because of cord entanglement and knotting, prematurity, congenital anomalies, twin-to-twin transfusion syndrome (TTS), and intertwin locking during birth (Benirschke & Kaufman, 1995; Gall, 1998).

It is important that zygosity and placental structure be determined as early as possible during pregnancy because of the potential complications of multiple pregnancy, especially for those that are MZ. Additional prenatal visits with ultrasound assessment are needed for MZ multiples because of the risk of acardia (ie, congenital absence of the heart), cord entanglement, and conjoined twins. Meticulous identification of each baby after birth with their placenta is essential because determination of zygosity is helpful in evaluating developmental differences and congenital anomalies. It also becomes important if blood transfusions or organ transplantation are necessary. Identification of the type of twinning is important for understanding the occurrence of twinning in future pregnancies, even if the babies were conceived through assisted fertilization. MZ is established when a single chorionic disc is present. DZ and MZ twins can be identified by the babies' blood types, HLA typing, and blood group. Comparison of DNA fingerprinting using placental tissue, cord blood, or infant blood samples is highly accurate in determining zygosity (Dauphinee & Bowers, 1997).

Identification of Multiple Gestation

Medical History

There is an ongoing debate regarding the necessity of early ultrasound in all pregnancies. Routine ultrasound examination during pregnancy is not recommended by ACOG (1998). A detailed history from the woman and her family is important in the identification of multiple gestation, because there is a hereditary tendency to multiple ovulation in DZ twinning. Women who have become pregnant while using fertility drugs (ie, clomiphene citrate or gonadotropins) or after cessation of oral contraceptives should also be screened for multiple gestation. Other indications for multiple gestation screening include African-American race, increased maternal age, and increased parity (>4) with or without increased maternal age. Maternal perceptions of excessive fatigue and increased appetite and weight gain, especially in early pregnancy, have been associated with multiple gestation. Pregnancy discomforts may begin early, and fetal activity may be perceived as increased. Some multiparous women have also reported that this pregnancy "just feels different" than their other pregnancies.

Clinical Assessment

A thorough clinical assessment should establish the need for ultrasound. If the woman's menstrual history is considered accurate, McDonald measurements of fundal height may be helpful in the differential diagnosis of multiple gestation. A uterus that is 2 cm or larger than normal for the gestational age suggests multiple gestation. This increase in uterine growth occurs at about 14 weeks' gestation for twins and sooner when there are more than two fetuses. The initial suspicion of multiple pregnancy commonly is related to finding a larger uterus than would have been expected at the current gestational age. When palpation during the Leopold maneuver demonstrates multiple fetal parts or the presence of more than two fetal poles, the clinician should suspect multiple gestation. Another important finding is auscultation of more than one fetal heart sound, particularly with a difference of 10 beats/min. Anemia that does not respond to the usual treatment with iron and folic acid may be an indicator of multiple gestation, because multiple fetuses require extra iron and folic acid.

Ultrasound

The use of ultrasound is decisive in confirming the diagnosis of multiple gestation in 95% to 100% of cases (Keith et al., 1995). Ultrasound examination can also exclude other causes of an enlarged uterus, such as errors in gestational age, polyhydramnios, fetal macrosomia, fetal malformations, uterine leiomyomas, and ovarian tumors (D'Alton & Mercer, 1990). In addition to confirmation of multiple gestation, ultrasound can be used during multiple gestation to determine placental structure, detect major fetal structural defects, discordance, and assess for twin-to-twin transfusion syndrome. Today, the diagnosis of multiple gestation can be made as early as 6 to 8 weeks by identifying two separate sacs within the uterus. Using abdominal ultrasound, cardiac activity can be identified during the next 2 weeks. Detection of multiple gestation can be made even earlier with vaginal ultrasound (D'Alton & Mercer, 1990). Different fetal parts can readily be observed starting at 16 weeks' gestation; therefore, serial ultrasounds should be initiated to assess fetal growth (Knuppel & Drukker, 1993). Placental structure can and should be identified early, because this assessment becomes more difficult with advanced gestation. With access to care and ultrasound availability, the diagnosis of multiple gestation should be 99% accurate and confirmed before labor begins.

Biochemical Tests

The results of indirect biochemical methods of determining multiple gestation are conflicting. High initial quantitative hCG levels in infertility care are often the earliest indications of multiple gestation. However, hCG may be elevated without multiple gestation;

therefore, ultrasound should be used to make a definitive diagnosis (Knuppel & Drukker, 1993). In twin pregnancy, a maternal serum MSAFP result at 14 to 20 weeks' gestation is 2.5 times higher than for singleton pregnancies (three times higher for triplets and four times higher for quadruplets) (Johnson, Harman, Evans, MacDonald, & Manning, 1990). A MSAFP greater than 4.5 for multiples in an uncomplicated twin gestation is abnormal and requires follow-up (ACOG, 1998).

Psychological Aspects of Diagnosis of Multiple Gestation

The diagnosis of multiple pregnancy can generate a variety of feelings for women and their families. Having more than one baby may be a dream come true, or an additional child may be a burden to the entire family. Revealing the diagnosis of multiple pregnancy should be done with sensitivity to each woman's individual situation. All professionals should use a factual, nonemotional approach initially and gauge their enthusiasm by the woman's response. Most women are shocked by the news, even if they were given advance warning of this possibility. Normal responses of joy, shock, resentment, gratitude, fear, and optimism can all occur together and may continue throughout the pregnancy. Most women adjust to their pregnancy, but they worry about the practical issues of caring for more than one baby after birth.

The perinatal team should assist the patient and her family to understand the risks and potential problems of multiple gestation. The family needs access to information to be prepared for their experience and set reasonable expectations for pregnancy and postpartum. Counseling should focus on self-confidence and development of skills to prepare them for changes (Nys, Colpin, DeMunter, & Vandemeulebroecke, 1998). Because of the risk of first trimester loss of one or all of the fetuses, the parents may want to delay their "multiple" announcement to family and friends until 12 to 13 weeks' gestation.

Depression or anxiety disorders affect more than 25% of mothers and fathers of multiple gestations. Mothers at risk for perinatal depression often have an unsupportive partner or marital distress; adverse life events, such as sexual abuse or fetal or infant death; poor social support; and cognitive influences, such as serious doubts about one's abilities or unrealistic expectations. Other risk factors include a history of depression or drug and alcohol abuse (Leonard, 1998). Fathers who are at higher risk for depression have a history of depression, are unemployed, and have an unsupportive partner or one with perinatal depression (Leonard, 1998). Physical symptoms can be initiated by these psychological problems. Leonard (1998) reported that severe panic attacks in women with multiple gestation could initiate preterm labor and premature rupture of the membranes. Support groups and twin clinics may be helpful in prevention, identification, and treatment of these psychological complications.

Prenatal Education

Historically, multiple birth families were given the same prenatal care as parents of singletons. However, with the dramatic increase in the rate of multiple births in the past two decades, the unique needs of these expectant families are much more apparent (Dauphinee & Bowers, 1997). In a study, only one half of mothers of multiples thought they were sufficiently prepared for their postpartum experience (Nys et al., 1998). They would have liked to have received more information about the medical issues associated with multiple pregnancy, labor, and birth and information about the amount of work involved in parenting multiples. A "twins hot line" to answer questions during the first few postpartum weeks is especially helpful to parents (Malmstrom, Faherty, & Wagner, 1988).

The typical mother of multiple babies is older and has a higher level of education than her counterparts of earlier years (Jewell & Yip, 1995). Many of these women are career oriented and are likely to demand more from their healthcare providers (Dauphinee & Bowers, 1997). Comprehensive prenatal classes for multiples have been very successful, and compared with national statistics, women who have attended such classes are more likely to give birth closer to term with higher birth weights (Mosher, 1994). In addition to education, class members provide an immediate support system. The curriculum for multiple birth classes can supplement standard prenatal education offering tips and practical advice on handling multiple newborns. A visit to the NICU may also be helpful. Women who attend classes are more willing to attempt and succeed at breast-feeding their multiples (Drevets, 1994).

Antepartum Management

Antepartum management of multiple pregnancy should be a collaborative effort of the members of the obstetric healthcare team, including the perinatologist, obstetrician, nurse midwife, registered nurses, advanced practice nurses, perinatal educator, social worker, and dietitian. Couples should be encouraged to contact support groups such as Mothers of Twins' Clubs or The Triplet Connection. Multiple birth families should be given accurate information about the difficulties that they may encounter, how those problems can be handled, and counseling to help them with effective coping skills. When a multiple pregnancy is at exceptionally high risk for complications, such as a quadruplet pregnancy or a monoamniotic twin gestation, families should be given a realistic view of possible outcomes.

The primary clinical objective in the management of multiple gestation is the early detection of pregnancy complications that increase the risk of maternal and fetal morbidity and mortality (ACOG, 1998). Specialized, multidisciplinary twin clinics have been established to provide comprehensive care with rewarding outcomes (Ellings, Newman, Hulsey, Bivins, & Keenan, 1993; Newman & Ellings, 1995; Papiernik, Keith, Oleszczuk, & Cervantes, 1998). These clinics include consistent evaluation of maternal symptoms and cervical status by a single caregiver; comprehensive preterm birth prevention education; individualized modification of maternal activity; nutrition planning; follow-up for missed appointments; and a supportive environment. This type of comprehensive approach to care has resulted in improved perinatal outcomes, including higher mean birth weight, fewer infants who weighed less than 1,200 g, fewer NICU admissions, fewer NICU days, and less perinatal mortality (Papiernik et al., 1998). Prenatal visits are scheduled more frequently than for singleton gestations because of the higher risk of pregnancy complications. In extremely high-risk pregnancies, weekly visits, frequent ultrasound, and NSTs are common. Laboratory assessment and testing would be the same as singleton pregnancies with the additions of a hemoglobin assessment in each trimester because of the high incidence of anemia in multiple pregnancies. An MSAFP multiple marker test should be done between 16 and 20 weeks. Screening for diabetes mellitus should be done at 24 to 28 weeks, unless the patient has a history of gestational diabetes or a family history of the disease; then testing begins at 20 weeks. Serial cervical examinations performed by the same caregiver are also a keystone in the management and detection of preterm labor. Their use has been questioned because of the concern of introducing infection, but Papiernik, Keith, Bouyer, Dreyfus, and Lazar (1989) found that serial examinations result in fewer pregnancies complicated with premature rupture of the membranes and fewer babies with neonatal sepsis. A plan of care for multiple gestation is outlined in Table 8–20. An assessment of fetal movement, uterine contractions, vaginal discharge, and overall sense of well-being should be included at each prenatal visit. A woman's perceptions of her own body and of the well-being of her fetuses play a significant role in the recognition of preterm labor and other complications. Teaching and reinforcing the signs and symptoms of preterm labor and other complications should be a regular part of prenatal visits.

At each visit a psychosocial evaluation should take place so the woman's questions can be answered and to assess how she and her family are coping. The perinatal team can provide positive emotional support throughout pregnancy to help increase a woman's self-confidence and reduce her anxiety. Encouragement about weight gain, positive comments about her appearance, and a "can do" attitude help the woman and family adjust to her body and adapt to the pregnancy. Additional support can also be provided through telephone calls. Women should be encouraged to call with their questions and concerns regarding psychological and physical problems. Regular, frequent, nurse-initiated telephone contacts can also be reassuring and play a significant role in preterm labor identification.

Patients who have conceived through an infertility program may have special needs, including extraordinary expectations for their care. Typically, they have had many months of personal interaction with nurses and physicians who have meticulously monitored their status with weekly visits and ultrasounds. When they graduate to "routine prenatal care," these women naturally expect this level of detailed care to continue and often feel abandoned and apprehensive when their first appointment is delayed or if this personalized care is not provided. It may be appropriate to schedule early prenatal visits at more frequent intervals to help ease the emotional transition into the prenatal care system.

Nutritional Needs

Optimal nutrition and pregnancy weight gain corresponds with improved perinatal outcomes in multiple pregnancy as well as singleton pregnancy. Length of gestation, maternal prepregnant weight, smoking, and gestational weight gain are important factors influencing twin birth weight (Luke & Leurgans, 1996). The maternal physiologic changes in fluid volume, the fetal drain on iron and calcium stores, and overall increased energy needs require a nutritionally sound diet high in calories, carbohydrates, vitamins, and minerals. Supplementation beyond prenatal vitamins should include iron and folic acid. There is a need for additional calcium supplementation when women have been prescribed magnesium sulfate tocolysis and bed rest (Levav, Chan, & Wapner, 1998). Fluids should be en-

TABLE 8–20 ■ PATIENT CARE FOR MULTIPLE GESTATIONS

Test or Study	Antepartum Outpatient	Antepartum Inpatient	Intrapartum	Postpartum
Blood pressure, pulse, and respiration	Each visit	Every 8 hours (more frequently if hypertensive)	Every hour	After birth, then every 15 minutes ×4; then every 30 minutes ×2; then every 8 hours (unless hypertensive, then more frequent BP indicated)
Temperature	Each visit	Every 8 hours	Every 4 hours	After birth, then every 8 hours
Fetal heart rate	Weekly NST starting at 26–28 weeks' gestation (may be earlier with monoamniotic multiples); kick counts	Weekly NST/CST starting at 26–28 weeks' gestation (may be earlier with monoamniotic multiples)	Continuously with electronic fetal monitor (internal and external); if monitor not available, every 15 minutes in the first stage and every 5 minutes in the second stage	
Contractions	Weekly (daily home monitoring may be used), starting at 20 weeks' gestation	Every 8 hours	Continuously with electronic fetal monitor, preferably internal; if monitor not available, every 1 hour by palpation	
Lochia				Fundal checks every 15 minutes ×4; every 30 minutes ×2; every hour until stable; then every 8 hours

(continued)

couraged to prevent dehydration with first-trimester nausea and vomiting and later in pregnancy to reduce the risk of preterm labor. Increasing fluids also reduces the risk of UTIs and constipation. Women who are vegetarians may need additional counseling to ensure adequate intake of proteins and other nutrients.

A balanced diet provides the best source of nutrition, and women expecting twins need at least 2,700 calories each day. Adding 300 calories per fetus per day when there are more than two fetuses is recommended (ACOG, 1998). Frequent nutritional snacks assist in satisfying dietary needs. As pregnancy progresses, small but frequent meals may be easier to digest as the stomach becomes crowded by the uterus. Women who are breast-feeding more than one infant need to supplement their pregnancy diet with additional calories and fluids to maintain an adequate milk supply and fat stores.

In twin pregnancies, low prepregnancy weight and low overall pregnancy weight gain are associated with

TABLE 8–20 ■ PATIENT CARE FOR MULTIPLE GESTATIONS (continued)

Test or Study	Antepartum Outpatient	Antepartum Inpatient	Intrapartum	Postpartum
Laboratory studies				
Hemoglobin	Each visit	Weekly	Admission	First day postpartum
Hemotocrit	Each visit	Weekly	Admission	First day postpartum
50-g glucose challenge	At 20–28 weeks	At 20–28 weeks		PRN
Sonogram	At least one level II sonogram before 24 weeks to rule out major congenital anomalies; serial sonograms for estimated fetal weight every 3 weeks; BPP weekly from 30 weeks			
Assess cervix for changes	After 20 weeks, once each week	After 20 weeks, once each week	PRN	
Assess fundal height	Each visit	Each visit		

BPP = biophysical profiles; CST = contraction stress test; NST = nonstress test.
Adapted from Dauphinee, J. D., & Bowers, N. A. (1997). *Nursing management of multiple birth families: Preconception through postpartum* (Nursing Modules). White Plains, NY: March of Dimes Birth Defects Foundation.

LBW babies (Luke & Leurgans, 1996). ACOG (1998) recommends a weight gain of approximately 1.5 pounds/week for a total of 35 to 45 pounds for the normal-weight woman. Women who are underweight should gain more—about 1.75 pounds/week in the second half of pregnancy (Lantz, Chez, Rodrigues, & Porter, 1996). Women who are overweight may need to gain less, with adequate fetal growth as an indicator of appropriate weight gain. With higher-order multiples, most practitioners usually encourage an additional 10 pounds of maternal weight gain per fetus. Ongoing dietary assessment and counseling by members of the perinatal team is important to help women eat an appropriate diet and gain enough weight. Emotional support may be needed, especially if she is having a difficult time accepting the rapid growth and sometime unpleasant changes in her body and appearance. Women should be reminded that their weight gain is important to the health of their fetuses. Higher infant birth weights and shorter length of newborn stays for twin pregnancies are associated with a higher rate of gain after 24 weeks' gestation (Luke, 1998). Nutritional education should be initiated during pregnancy and supported in the postpartum period to assist with exercise strategies and weight loss.

Antepartum Complications

Fetal Loss

Early detection of multiple gestation assists in the timely identification of complications and assists in the reduction of perinatal morbidity and mortality. The incidence of spontaneous abortions is more common in twin pregnancies than in singleton pregnancies, especially with MZ twins. As the number of fetuses increases, there is a greater risk of spontaneous second trimester abortion. There is a 20% to 30% increase in spontaneous abortions when pregnancy occurs as a result of fertility drugs. There is a lower rate of spontaneous abortion with clomiphene than with hMG and hCG (Schenker, Yarkoni, & Granat, 1981). Several factors account for this higher rate of abortions in multiples, including faulty ova; high levels of estradiol, causing increased motility and placing the conceptus too soon into a poorly prepared endometrium; and luteal-phase deficiency (Schenker, Yarkoni, & Granat, 1981). Earlier diagnosis of twins in women receiving fertility drugs may also have an impact on this higher loss rate.

The rate of twin conception is thought to be 20% to 50% higher than the rate of birth because of the early loss of multifetal gestations (ACOG, 1998; D'Alton & Mercer, 1990). In monochorionic pregnancies, the death of one fetus occurs three times more frequently (D'Alton, Newton, & Cetrulo, 1984; Enbom, 1985; Hanna & Hill, 1984). Bleeding in the first trimester with a resultant singleton pregnancy may be the result of the spontaneous loss of a twin. This phenomenon, called the *vanishing twin,* has been documented by ultrasound and is widely accepted. The prognosis for the remaining fetus or fetuses is good, and serial ultrasounds can confirm continued growth (Landy & Nies, 1995), but the co-twin has a substantial risk for anomalies. Acute hemodynamic changes, including hypotension and subsequent ischemia for the survivor at the time of the co-twin's death, may cause these anomalies (ACOG, 1998; Fusi, McParland, Fisk, Nicolini, & Wigglesworth, 1991; Larroche, Droulle, Delezoide, Narcy, & Nessmann, 1990). Twin embolization syndrome can occur when there are vascular injuries to the surviving monochorionic fetus caused by thrombotic emboli or disseminating intravascular coagulation. In contrast, Keith and colleagues (1995) suggest that the increase of anomalies occur because of an increase incidence of anomalies in multifetal pregnancies.

It has been estimated that 3% to 7% of twin pregnancies that reach the second trimester will lose one or both of the fetuses by the beginning of the third trimester (Grobman & Peaceman, 1998). Although the cause of fetal death in the second trimester may be unknown, several factors occur more frequently in multiple gestation, including congenital anomalies, IUGR, chromosomal abnormalities, and velamentous and marginal insertion of the umbilical cord. Twin-to-twin transfusion can also cause fetal demise in the second or third trimester. When twins are dichorionic, there may be no injury to the second twin, but there is a greater risk of preterm birth (Petersen & Nyholm, 1999).

Two unusual things can happen to a monochorionic fetus when it dies in utero. Fetus-in-fetus is a rare occurrence; one of the fetuses dies and can be found in the body of one of the other fetuses (Yasuda, Mitomori, Mastsuura, & Tanimura, 1985). Others have proposed that these masses are well-differentiated teratomas (Alpers & Harrison, 1985). The other phenomenon is fetus papyraceous, which occurs later in pregnancy when the fetus with bone ossification dies in utero and becomes progressively compressed. Sometimes, they are overlooked because they present as masses of compressed fetal bone incorporated into the placenta. Although rare, large fetus payryracei may cause birth dystocia. As with other losses, when fetus papyraceous occurs, the surviving fetus often has anomalies (Benirschke, 1990). After a fetal loss, the risks for the surviving fetus or fetuses are small, and conservative management is recommended, with aggressive intervention used only when necessary (Burke, 1990; Cattanach, Wedel, White, & Young, 1990). Recommendations for management when caring for women with vanishing twin phenomenon are listed in Display 8–35.

Fetal and Newborn Complications

Because of the higher incidence of anomalies, genetic counseling should be offered to all women with multifetal pregnancies. Dizygotic twins have the same incidence of structural malformations as a singleton pregnancy, but the rate of chromosomal anomalies in DZ twins is double that in singletons (Gall, 1998). Because each DZ fetus comes from a different egg and sperm, the risk of sharing a genetic disorder is not increased. Each DZ twin could have a different chromosomal abnormality, but this is rare (Keith et al., 1995). Monozygotic twins have 2.5 times more structural malformations than DZ twins or singletons (Gall, 1998). Monozygotic twins usually have the same congenital abnormalities (Keith et al., 1995). All multiple fetuses are at increased risk for congenital anomalies, including congenital heart defects, intestinal tract anomalies, neural tube defects, hydrocephaly, some craniofacial defects, skeletal defects, anencephaly, and encephalocele (Gall, 1998).

A unique malformation of MZ multiples is acardia (ie, absence of the heart), which occurs in 1 of 100 MZ births (Keith et al., 1995). The affected fetuses are always of the same sex and are almost always female. Acardia is fatal for the affected fetus, and 10% of the unaffected fetuses have malformations (Schinzel, Smith, & Miller, 1979). Ultrasound assessment is used to identify the acardiac fetus. In some babies with acardia, the kidneys do not function and may cause oligohydramnios. Acardia always occurs with monochorionic placentas and vascular anastomoses that maintain the life of the acardiac fetus before delivery.

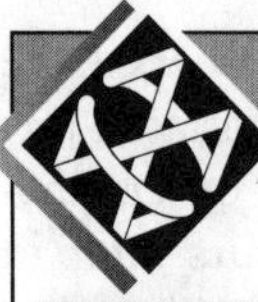

DISPLAY 8–35

Management of the Pregnant Woman With a Vanishing Twin

- Recognize vaginal bleeding as a frequent symptom associated with the vanishing twin phenomenon.
- Provide extensive ultrasonic studies when the loss is in the second trimester to assess the surviving fetus for anomalies. Fetal injury may lead to pregnancy termination.
- Provide continued assessment of the remaining fetus(es) when the loss is late in pregnancy with nonstress tests and biophysical profiles.
- Use serial ultrasound scans to follow the regression of the vanishing process and confirm viability and continued growth of the remaining fetus(es).
- Evaluate the placenta and membranes after delivery to confirm evidence of the vanishing process.
- Systematically evaluate the surviving neonate(s), including neurologic assessment, appropriate intracranial studies, and assessment of the gastrointestinal and renal systems.
- Counsel the parents when anomalies occur, because many of these anomalies do not recur unless the mother is again pregnant with monozygotic twins; however, syndromes unrelated to twinning should be identified.

Adapted from Dauphinee, J. D., & Bowers, N. A. (1997). *Nursing management of multiple birth families: Preconception through postpartum* (Nursing Module). White Plains, NY: March of Dimes Birth Defects Foundation.

Conjoined twins occur in MZ twins because of an incomplete separation of the embryo between days 15 to 17. It is a random event, and therefore the risk of recurrence is negligible (van den Brand, Nijhuis, & van Dongen, 1994). The incidence is about 1 in 500 to 600 twin deliveries (Gall, 1998). Conjoined twins have been reported to occur in triplet and quadruplet pregnancies (Gardeil, Greene, NiScanaill, & Skinner, 1998) Approximately 70% of conjoined twins are female; most are stillborn and premature. The success of surgical separation depends on the degree of shared organs, the absence of major anomalies, and the presence of separate hearts.

TTS is a complication of MZ twins who are monochorionic and monoamniotic or diamniotic (Bajoria, 1998). The incidence of TTS in monochorionic twins is between 10% and 35% (Machin & Keith, 1998). Monochorionic-diamniotic placentas usually have a number of vein-to-vein or artery-to-artery anastomoses in addition to the arteriovenous shunt, which is associated with a higher incidence of TTS. TTS syndrome occurs when the anastomoses result in the shunting of blood from the high-pressure arterial circulation of the donor twin to the low-pressure venous system of the recipient twin. Most monozygotic-monochorionic twins share some vascular connections in their placentas that do not cause complications because they tend to be bi-directional, allowing hemodynamic equilibrium.

The hemodynamic imbalance of TTS causes the recipient fetus to become fluid overloaded while the donor twin becomes hypovolemic. The secondary effect is that the recipient develops organomegaly and polycythemia and suffers from congestive heart failure from circulatory overload (hydropic changes) and cardiomegaly. To compensate for the extra blood volume, the recipient excretes large amounts of urine, causing polyhydramnios (Machin & Keith, 1998). Thrombosis of peripheral vessels may also develop in association with this hypertransfused state. In contrast, the donor becomes growth restricted, anemic, and oliguric from the chronic hypovolemia caused by the shunting of its blood supply (Blickstein, 1990; DeLia, Cruikshank, & Keye, 1990; Gardner, 1993). The twin in this oligohydramnios or anhydramniotic sac may appear to be stuck to the uterine wall on ultrasound examination, even after the mother has been repositioned. This is known as the "stuck twin" syndrome (Reisner et al., 1993). Other conditions, such as fetal anomalies or viral infections, that cause polyhydramnios in one twin and oligohydramnios in the other can also cause the appearance of the stuck twin.

Clinically, a sudden increase in uterine height at approximately the end of the second trimester or the beginning of the third trimester may indicate TTS (Blickstein, 1990). Unequal fetal growth may also be a symptom of TTS, and a differential diagnosis must be made between TTS and other complications. The identification of growth restriction in one fetus is made when the other twin is normal in size and has a normal amount of fluid. A rare condition that should also be excluded is the presence of a normal twin with normal fluid and a larger co-twin who is hydropic and may have anomalies or erythroblastosis. Although the criteria for the diagnosis of TTS are not clear-cut, with minor variations, they include most of the assessments listed in Display 8–36.

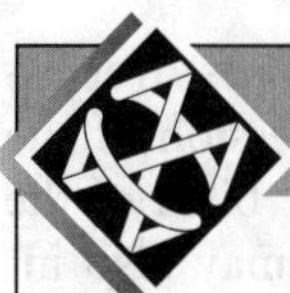

DISPLAY 8–36

Criteria for the Diagnosis of Twin-to-Twin Transfusion Syndrome

- Proven monochorionicity
- Hydramnios or oligohydramnios
- Growth discordance (not always present)
- In the recipient fetus
  - Larger umbilical cord, abdominal circumference, kidneys and bladder with measured polyuria over time
  - Large, hypodynamic heart with tricuspid incompetence
  - Dilated inferior vena cava, ductus venosus, umbilical vein with abnormal flow patterns
  - Abnormal systemic arterial flow patterns
  - Rapid recurrence of hydramnios after amniocentesis
- In the donor fetus
  - Peripheral vascular shutdown with oligohydramnios, abnormal Doppler studies of venous and arterial flows
  - Biophysical improvements after amniocentesis
  - Smaller abdominal circumference with small cord, often velamentously inserted
- Discordant hematocrit and plasma protein levels by cordocentesis (not always present)
- Transfer of intravascularly injected adult red blood cells from donor to recipient
- Temporary paralysis of both twins after intravascular pancuronium infusion of one twin
- Elevated erythropoietin levels in both twins
- Elevated atriopeptin level in recipient twin

Adapted from Machin, G. A., & Keith, L. G. (1998). Can twin-to-twin transfusion syndrome be explained, and how is it treated? *Clinical Obstetrics and Gynecology, 41*(1), 105–113.

Decompression amniocentesis to remove excess fluid from the polyhydramnic sac has been recommenced to decrease the amount of fluid that can cause complications. This procedure has been reported to reduce the mortality rate from 100% to 48% (Machin, & Keith, 1998). Daily ultrasounds are performed to assess fluid volume, and additional fluid is withdrawn if necessary. This therapeutic amniocentesis has even been reported to reverse the TTS (Keith, Papiernik, & Luke, 1991). However there is a risk of uterine decompression that can cause placental abruption, preterm labor, or premature rupture of the membranes.

Measures to reduce the discomfort of polyhydramnios may include an egg-crate mattress, repositioning, relaxation techniques, and tactile stimulation and massage. Pain medication may also be needed to reduce discomfort from the overdistended uterus. Tocolytic agents can be helpful in reducing contractions (Gardner, 1993). Parental education should include the fetal risks and detailed information about treatments such as the recurrent need for amniocentesis.

Two syndromes are related to TTS: twin reversed arterial perfusion (TRAP) and acute perinatal twin transfusion (AperiTTS). TRAP occurs when there are large, direct artery-to-artery and vein-to-vein anastomoses associated with acardia. AperiTTS occurs when the blood in the placental parenchyma drains into the second twin after the clamping of the cord of the first twin and could therefore cause the antepartum donor twin to be born plethoric (Machin, & Keith, 1998). The opposite effect occurs in MZ twins when blood drains into the delivered twin, causing exsanguination and even death of the undelivered twin. Acute neonatal hemodynamic changes can also occur from an acute fetomaternal hemorrhage (Machin & Keith, 1998).

Maternal Complications

Women who have multiple pregnancies are more likely to have a cesarean birth and are at increased risk for the maternal complications listed in Display 8–37. Women with multiple gestation have a two to three times higher incidence of hypertension. The development of hypertension warrants assessment for multiple gestation. Hypertension tends to develop earlier in multiple pregnancies and tends to be more severe than in singleton pregnancies (Cunningham et al., 1997). When women have preeclampsia with a multiple pregnancy, serum uric acid levels are much higher. Serum uric acid levels of 6.3 mg/dL for twins

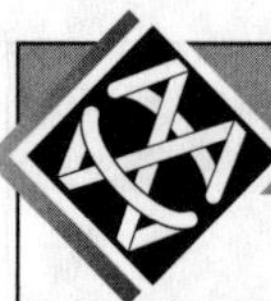

DISPLAY 8–37

Maternal Complications of Multiple Gestations

- Cardiopulmonary
  - Pulmonary edema
  - Complications of tocolysis
  - Pregnancy-induced hypertension
  - Preeclampsia
- Gastrointestinal
  - Acute fatty liver of pregnancy
  - Cholestasis of pregnancy
- Hematologic
  - Anemia
- Obstetric
  - Preterm labor
  - Cervical effacement and dilation
  - Increased incidence of cesarean birth
  - Increased use of tocolysis
  - Antepartum hemorrhage
  - Abruptio placenta
  - Uterine rupture
  - Postpartum hemorrhage
  - Infections
  - Increased hospitalizations
  - Gestational diabetes

Adapted from Gall, S. A. (1998). Ambulatory management of multiple gestation. *Clinical Obstetrics and Gynecology, 41*(3), 564–583.

and 6.8 mg/dL in triplet gestations may be used for the diagnosis of preeclampsia (Hsu, Chung, Lee, Chou, & Copel, 1997)

Polyhydramnios occurs in approximately 12% of multiple pregnancies (Cetrulo, Ingardia, & Sbarra, 1980) when the increased uterine volume of fluid and fetuses may be 10 L and weigh as much as 20 pounds (Knuppel & Drukker, 1993). The overdistention of the uterus is uncomfortable for the mother and contributes to risk of preterm labor, premature rupture of the membranes, and abruptio placentae. Polyhydramnios is associated with an increased rate of fetal gastrointestinal and CNS abnormalities (Knuppel & Drukker, 1993).

Risk of hemorrhage is increased in multiple gestation because of the increased incidence of placental previa, abruptio placentae, and postpartum hemorrhage. The increased incidence of placental previa is caused by the increased mass of the placenta (Keith et al., 1995). The increased rate of abruption may be associated with polyhydramnios, which causes overdistention of the uterus and rapid decompression of the uterus after rupture of the membranes or birth of the first baby. Overdistention of the uterus may also increase contraction frequency, and cause premature rupture of the membranes. Risk of abruptio placentae is also increased with hypertension, which is more prevalent in multiple gestation.

Preterm premature rupture of the membranes (PPROM) occurs in approximately 5% to 15% of twin pregnancies and increases with the number of fetuses. The catalysts for PPROM in multiple gestation includes early cervical ripening, increasing the vulnerability of the fetal membranes; exposure to antepartum hemorrhage; and overdistention caused by polyhydramnios and multiple fetuses (Keith et al., 1995).

Fetal Surveillance

Nonstress Test

Weekly NST can be used as the primary approach for antepartum surveillance in twin gestation. Monoamniotic-monochorionic twins should have biweekly (twice each week) NSTs starting at 28 weeks' gestation (Keith et al., 1995). Weekly NSTs for monochorionic-diamniotic twins should be started at 30 to 32 weeks' gestation. Keith et al. (1995) also suggested that diamniotic-dichorionic twins without other complications could be assessed with weekly NSTs starting at 34 weeks. However if IUGR is identified, it has been recommended that biweekly NSTs be initiated with weekly umbilical Doppler studies. Outcome criteria for NSTs should be the same for multiple gestations as it is for singletons. These criteria can be found in Chapter 7.

Assessment may be difficult because 50% of healthy fetuses exhibit synchrony when their heart rates are recorded simultaneously with a dual channel monitor (Eganhouse & Petersen, 1998). Devoe and Azor (1981) described this phenomenon as similarity in baseline oscillations and the timing and frequency of periodic changes, including accelerations and decelerations. Sometimes, the tracings are so similar that the fetal monitor cannot discriminate between the FHRs. FHR discrimination technology has been developed to alert the practitioner when the dual tracings being received are from the same fetus.

It is important to carefully document which heart rate belongs to which fetus. It may be most appropriate to identify each tracing by the corresponding fetal position. An ultrasound before the NST may be helpful in identifying the position of the fetuses, especially if there are more than two. Once the positions are identified, the fetuses should continue to be referred to in those positions on all documentation. The birth order should be clarified and compared with the NSTs and ultrasounds, especially if complications are expected for a particular fetus.

Biophysical Profile

The BPP is appropriate for multifetal gestations, as well as for singletons. The method and outcome criteria for this test are described in Chapter 7. There are a few things to take into consideration when assessing multiples with BPPs. When the pregnancy is diamniotic, the fluid must be measured in each sac to determine whether it is normal. The definition for polyhydramnios and oligohydramnios is the same for each individual sac as it would be for the sac of a single fetus. When assessing tone, care must be taken to determine the discrete movement and tone of each individual fetus.

Contraction Stress Test

Theoretically, there is increased risk of preterm labor during a contraction stress test, but several studies have established that the test is not likely to cause preterm labor in multiple gestations (Blake et al., 1984; Knuppel, Rattan, Scerbo, & O'Brien, 1985). The contraction stress test is rarely used for follow-up evaluation because the BPP has become more accepted and has fewer potential risks.

Fetal Movement Counting

ACOG (1998) recommends the use of fetal movement counting in multiple pregnancy, but there are limitations in using this technique with more than one fetus, because it may be difficult to distinguish movement of the separate fetuses. Overdistention of the uterus may make it difficult for the mother to feel fetal movements.

Doppler Assessment

Doppler studies assess velocity through vessels using ultrasound technology. Resistance to blood flow is detected in many blood vessels; the most common are the umbilical, middle cerebral, renal, and uterine arteries. The ability to identify the middle cerebral and uterine arteries has been enhanced by color coding (Keith et al., 1995). There are three methods of Doppler velocimetry assessment: the systolic/diastolic (S/D) ratio, resistance index (RI), and pulsatility index (PI). Normal ratios are determined based on gestational age. When the S/D ratios of the umbilical arteries of normal twins pregnancies are compared with singletons at comparable gestational age, they are similar (Keith et al., 1995). When twins have abnormal Doppler readings, there is a higher incidence of stillbirths, structural anomalies, and TTS (Keith et al., 1995). As fetal condition changes, there is a progression from absent flow velocities to reversal of diastolic flow in the weeks proceeding death (Eganhouse & Petersen, 1998). Umbilical artery waveform studies have been shown to predict fetal growth restriction and fetal death (Giles, Trudinger, Cook, & Connelly, 1993).

Amniocentesis

Amniocentesis can be used for assessment in multiple gestation, but there is an increased risk of fetal loss (2.8% to 8.1%) compared with that for a singleton gestation (<1%) (ACOG, 1998; Anderson, Goldberg, & Golbus, 1991; Antsaklis, Gougoulakis, Mesogitis, Papantoniou, & Aravantinos, 1991). Fluid for amniocentesis is collected in much the same way that it is collected in a singleton pregnancy. When twins are MZ, there is no need to obtain fluid from more than one sac (ACOG, 1998). When twins are dizygotic, separate fluid samples from different amniotic sacs are needed for genetic studies and Rh sensitization. Several studies (Sims, Cowan, & Parkinson, 1976; Spellacy, Cruz, Buhi, & Birk, 1977) found that the lecithin-sphingomyelin (L/S) ratios were closely related. The information obtained in one sac is probably a reliable estimate of functional pulmonary maturity for both twins and is even more so if a value of 2.5 or greater is used as the lower limit for lung maturation.

Chorionic Villus Sampling

Chorionic villus sampling (CVS) can be used to collect tissue for genetic diagnosis or diagnosis of multiple gestation. It is collected in the same way that it is collected for singleton pregnancies. Distinct placentas must be identified by ultrasound to identify genetic disorders specific for each fetus. Complications with CVS in twin pregnancies are caused by the inability to obtain an adequate sample and contamination of one sample with tissue from the second (ACOG, 1998).

Ultrasound Surveillance

Sonography has made a significant impact on the early and accurate diagnosis of multiple gestation. After multiple gestation is diagnosed, ultrasound scans should be initiated at 24 weeks' gestation to evaluate fetal growth and development of discordance. If discordance is present, sonograms should be performed weekly (Gall, 1998). When IUGR is present in one or more fetuses below the 10th percentile for gestational age, especially if associated with an abnormal head circumference, fetal surveillance should be initiated and early birth may be necessary (Gall,

1998). Monochorionic twins should have serial ultrasounds every 2 to 3 weeks (Gall, 1998) to assess for TTS and other complications.

Alexander, Kogan, Martin, and Papiernik (1998) demonstrated intrauterine growth patterns for twins and triplets that are significantly different from those for singletons. Significant deviation occurred at 28 weeks for twins and triplets and then widened progressively. However, according to ACOG (1998), there is no clear clinical advantage to the use of twin- or triplet-specific ultrasound growth tables. Evaluation of serial fetal growth should include estimated fetal weight of each fetus and appropriate and concordant interval growth. Luke, Minogue, & Witter (1993) described a flattening of growth patterns at 36 weeks' gestation.

Ethical Considerations for Complications of One Fetus

A clinical and ethical dilemma occurs when one fetus demonstrates a persistent abnormal pattern while the other shows signs of well-being. Careful clinical judgment and assessment of underlying complications can determine the timing of delivery. Knuppel and Drukker (1993) made the following suggestions:

- If one of the fetuses has a nonreactive FHR pattern but shows no late decelerations with uterine contractions, a BPP should be performed and the pregnancy allowed to continue if the BPP demonstrates fetal well-being.
- If one fetus has a persistent nonreactive pattern with late decelerations or a low BPP score, an amniocentesis should be performed; if pulmonary maturity has been achieved, birth should be accomplished by an expeditious and safe method; if the L/S ratio is below 2, administer betamethasone (12 mg intramuscularly in two doses 24 hours apart) and then proceed with birth.

When the fetuses are less than 28 weeks' gestation, the decision may be made to postpone birth as long as the one fetus has a reactive NST and reassuring BPP. This is a difficult decision, because the fetus with the abnormal testing may die in utero, and as that fetus dies, the normal fetus may die as well. However, if the normal twin is delivered electively, it may suffer the consequences and complications of prematurity. Before a birth decision is made, a careful assessment of the nonreactive fetus is necessary to determine if the test results are caused by congenital anomalies incompatible with extrauterine life. When confronted with any of these dilemmas, the parents should be active members with the perinatal team in this decision-making process.

Antenatal Home Care

Although evidence does not support bed rest or decreased activity, most women are relieved to have permission to slow down because of their size, awkwardness, and the physical discomforts of carrying two or more babies. Many women have the responsibility of a job, care of other children, and maintaining a home, and they may not have the financial resources for household help. These women should be encouraged and given permission to decrease activity. They should also be encouraged to call on friends and family for help with child care and household chores (Dauphinee & Bowers, 1997). In some facilities, HUAM is used to monitor contractions in multiple pregnancies, especially for higher-order multiples (see the earlier section on Preterm Labor and Birth).

Hospital Management

Sometimes, hospitalization is necessary for women with multiple gestation because of pregnancy complications such as preterm labor, premature rupture of the membranes, and antepartum bleeding. While in the hospital, the same daily and weekly assessments should continue as if the woman was an outpatient (see Table 8–20). Once stabilized, women are managed at home and may have home care visits. If complications continue, the woman remains in the hospital until birth. The advantages of keeping patients in the hospital are to provide intravenous medications and for of emergent intervention in case of hemorrhage or complications of premature rupture of the membranes such as cord prolapse.

Intrapartum Management

Birth Environment for Multiple Gestation

In the ideal situation, multiple gestation would continue until 40 weeks, but ultimately, the healthcare provider has to weigh the risks and benefits of continuing the pregnancy when complications occur. There are few data about the gestation of twins beyond 40 weeks, but most experts believe birth should be accomplished by that time (ACOG, 1998). Most multiple births occur in a hospital environment because of the high-risk nature of multiple gestation and increased likelihood for cesarean birth of one or more babies. Ideally, birth of triplets and higher-order multiples occur in a tertiary center with a NICU. Antepartum transport to a high-risk perinatal center is recommended for twin pregnancies with complications or patients with higher-order multiples to minimize the risks to mother and babies.

Although many twins are born by cesarean section, there are many women who can safely have a vaginal birth. In some hospitals, vaginal birth of multiples takes place in an operative suite because of the possible necessity of surgical intervention. Even when that is necessary, labor and most of the second stage can occur in a labor, delivery, recovery, and postpartum (LDRP) room; labor, delivery, and recovery (LDR) room; or traditional labor room. Some healthcare providers may even opt for a vaginal birth in the LDRP or LDR as long as there is immediate access to the surgical suite, anesthesia, and ultrasound.

Preparation for birth should be as calm and orderly as possible, and each procedure should be explained to the parents. When possible, the father or other support person should be allowed to remain during all preparations. Assigning one nurse to care for this family provides consistency and facilitates communication, ensuring that their needs and questions are addressed. If complications are anticipated, the neonatologist should meet with the parents to discuss these issues.

If the woman is moved to the surgical suite or traditional delivery room, the expectant parents should be prepared for the appearance of the room. Women are frequently surprised at the large team of personnel that typically attends a multiple birth. Minimizing the noise and lights can help reduce the high-tech atmosphere and keep the focus on the family and their birth. This also helps to establish a calm, orderly atmosphere where even difficult birth can be less hectic and less stressful for all involved.

During some vaginal births, internal version or abdominal fetal guidance may be needed to direct the second baby into position (Display 8–38). The mother should be prepared for the pressure and discomfort that this may cause. She should also be prepared for the possibility of an emergent cesarean birth if the baby does not descend appropriately or if fetal status deteriorates.

After an uncomplicated, term, vaginal birth, there is usually time for the mother to see and hold her first baby before the birth of her second baby. When she prepares for birth of the second twin, the support person can hold their baby, or the baby can be placed under a warmer and positioned in clear view of the mother.

Preterm and emergent birth of multiples causes high stress for both parents and healthcare providers. Preterm labor often accelerates very quickly, with a precipitous birth. Maternal complications or nonreassuring fetal status may also require an unexpected early birth. In these situations, the parents need to understand the reasons for the early birth of their babies. Unfortunately, because of their high levels of emotional stress, they may not grasp all the information or the implications for the health of mother and ba-

DISPLAY 8–38

Considerations for Attempted External Version During Vaginal Birth

- An initial sonographic assessment of the size of each fetus should be made. If twin B is larger than twin A and a great disparity exists, version with attempts at vaginal birth is best avoided.
- Epidural anesthesia is advisable before version to provide abdominal wall relaxation.
- Intact membranes are required for consideration of a version.
- Version should be performed only if immediate cesarean section is available.
- The version should be attempted immediately after or even during the birth of the first twin while the uterus is most relaxed.
- A real-time ultrasound machine should be in the birthing room to accurately determine fetal presentation after the birth of the first twin.
- The fetal heart rate should be monitored continuously thereafter.
- Gentle pressure with the transducer may be used to guide the fetal head into vertex presentation above the birth canal. If this is not successful, external version can be attempted with a forward or a backward roll. The shortest arc between the vertex and the pelvic inlet should be attempted first. Undue force should always be avoided.
- If version to vertex presentation is successful, membranes should then be ruptured, and oxytocin augmentation may be used.
- If the version is unsuccessful, if the fetal heart rate of twin B shows evidence of fetal distress, or if twin B fails to descend after successful version, cesarean birth or breech birth is necessary.

Adapted from Dauphinee, J. D., & Bowers, N. A. (1997). *Nursing management of multiple birth families: Preconception through postpartum* (Nursing Modules). White Plains, NY: March of Dimes Birth Defects Foundation.

bies. Information should be presented simply, clearly, and completely to the family. The family needs reassurance that the well-being of mother and babies is the goal of all involved.

Expectant parents' birth plans may have included a special bath or breast-feeding in the delivery room, taking photographs, or videotaping their babies' birth. Although such plans may need to be modified for a high-risk birth, they do not necessarily have to be canceled. For example, the mother who wants to breast-feed and cannot do so initially because of neonatal complications should be reassured that she can begin pumping breast milk as soon as possible after birth. This gives her a feeling of control and purpose and lessens the risk of postpartum hemorrhage due to poor uterine tone.

Fetal Presentation and Method of Birth

When developing an intrapartum plan of care, fetal presentation is the primary consideration for management of the birth (Fig. 8–7). Twins can present in three combinations: twin A and B vertex (42.5%); twin A vertex and twin B nonvertex (38.4%); and twin A nonvertex (19.1%) (Keith et al., 1995). Malpresentation is common in preterm multiples; 20% of first twins and 30% of second twins present in the breech presentation when they are preterm (Keith et al., 1995). Vaginal birth is recommended when twins are in the vertex-vertex presentation. The best method of birth for nonvertex twins has not been established based on available literature (ACOG,

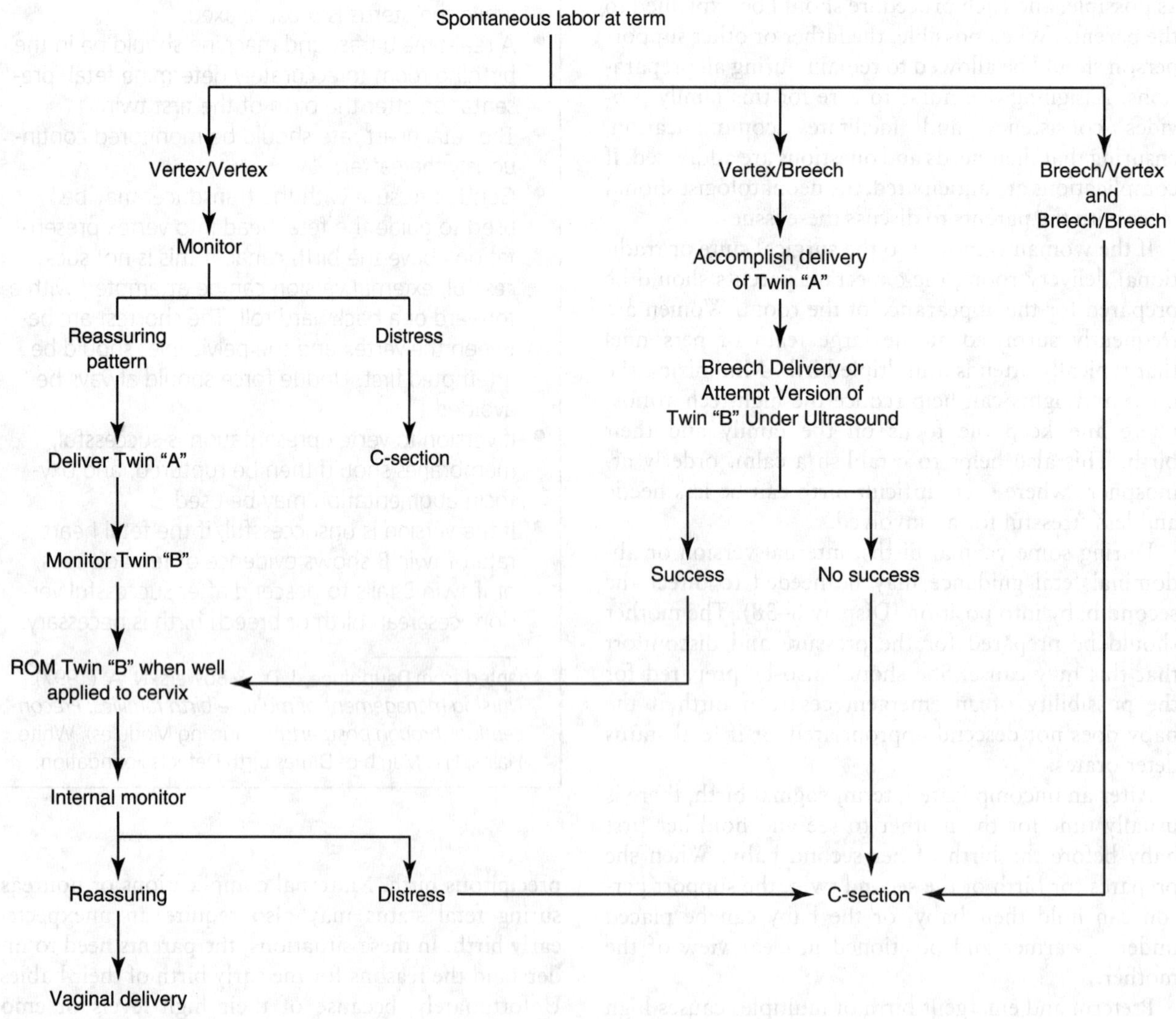

FIGURE 8–7. Management of the birth of twins.

1998). Persistent transverse lie or traumatic and difficult breech birth of the second twin after birth of the first are the most frequently cited reasons for cesarean birth. In the United States, the current management of choice for nonvertex first twin presentation is cesarean birth (ACOG, 1998). Guidelines for the vaginal birth of twins are presented in Display 8–39.

At the onset of labor, if there is any doubt about presentation, an ultrasound examination should be done to assess fetal presentation. Simultaneous EFM using a monitor with external twin capabilities is ideal. If this type of monitor is not available, an alternate option is monitoring the presenting twin with a scalp electrode and the second twin externally. If it is difficult to externally assess both FHRs, artificial rupture of the membranes can be performed with application of the scalp electrode to the first twin, while the second twin continues to be monitored by ultrasound. Some fetal monitors have the capacity to simultaneously monitor triplets externally. If triplets are laboring, the first fetus can be monitored with a spiral electrode on one monitor, and the second and third babies can be assessed with a second dual channel external monitor. The key issue is to initiate a system in which the fetal status of all babies can be continuously assessed during labor.

After the birth of twin A, the vertex of the second twin should be guided into the pelvis. Ultrasound equipment should be immediately available because it may be necessary to assist in guiding the fetus. The FHR of the next baby or babies should be assessed by ultrasound as soon as possible. When the presenting part is accessible and membranes have ruptured, a fetal scalp electrode is applied. When there are no complications and a reassuring FHR, there is no time limit for the birth of the second twin (ACOG, 1998). The average time between the birth of twin A and twin B is 30 minutes (Ellings, Newman, & Bowers, 1998). If labor does not resume within a reasonable amount of time after the birth of the first baby, oxytocin may be used for augmentation of labor if twin B is continually assessed with EFM (ACOG, 1998).

Intervals up to 131 days between the birth of twins have been reported (Bakos, Cederholm, & Kieler, 1998; Mikkelsen, & Hansen, 1996;), but this is uncommon. The success of delaying birth for an extended period after the birth of one fetus has been reported in several studies (Jenkins, Ghidini, & Eglinton, 1997; Kalchbrenner, Weisenborn, Chye, Kaufman, & Losure, 1998; Porreco, Sabin, Heyborne, & Lindsay, 1998). An extended interval between births can be considered when the undelivered fetus has intact membranes. If the first placenta is retained, the cord should be clamped and cut close to the placenta. Although Keith et al. (1995) did not recommend cerclage and tocolysis, later studies demonstrated success with tocolysis and cerclage placement (Kalchbrenner et al., 1998; Porreco et al., 1998). These investigators also recommended the use of broad-spectrum antibiotics.

The method of birth when twin A is vertex and twin B is breech or transverse lie is controversial. Some experts advocate cesarean birth, but others believe vaginal birth can be safely accomplished. There are insufficient and conflicting data in the literature about the management of twins in vertex-breech and vertex-transverse presentations (ACOG, 1998) (Display 8–40). When the presenting twin is not in the vertex presentation, cesarean birth is the recommended method of birth (ACOG, 1998). All monoamniotic twins should be born by cesarean section because of the possibility of interlocking or cord entanglement.

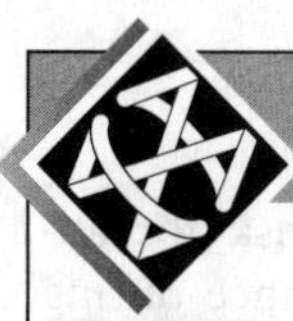

DISPLAY 8–39

Guidelines for Vaginal Birth of Twins

- Two units of crossmatched whole blood should be readily available.
- Intravenous infusion is accomplished with a large-bore catheter.
- Surgical suite should be immediately available.
- An obstetrician experienced in the vaginal birth of twins and an assistant should be present.
- Epidural anesthesia may be the best choice for vaginal birth.
- An anesthesiologist or nurse anesthetist capable of administering general anesthesia for a cesarean birth or intrauterine manipulation should be available.
- A neonatal team for each baby should be present at birth to provide neonatal resuscitation if necessary.

Adapted from Dauphinee, J. D., & Bowers, N. A. (1997). *Nursing management of multiple birth families: Preconception through postpartum* (Nursing Modules). White Plains, NY: March of Dimes Birth Defects Foundation.

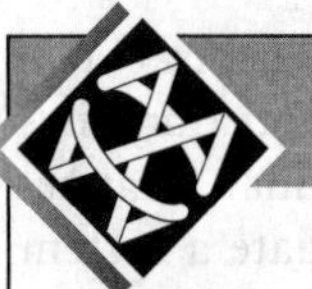

DISPLAY 8–40

Indications for Cesarean Birth When the Second Twin is Breech

- Prematurity with an estimated fetal weight between 800 and 2,500 g
- Footling breech
- Evidence of contracted pelvis
- Hyperextension of the fetal head
- Lack of expertise of the medical staff in vaginal breech delivery
- Nonreassuring fetal heart status

Adapted from Dauphinee, J. D., & Bowers, N. A. (1997). *Nursing management of multiple birth families: Preconception through postpartum* (Nursing Modules). White Plains, NY: March of Dimes Birth Defects Foundation.

Cesarean Birth and Vaginal Birth After Cesarean Delivery

Cesarean birth is recommended for higher-order multiples. However, it has been suggested that experienced physicians with skills in version and breech extraction may be able to offer vaginal birth to parents in some clinical situations (ACOG, 1998). General or epidural anesthesia will probably be needed for this type of birth to obtain abdominal relaxation (Gabbe, Niebyl, & Simpson, 1996). Some institutions have been successful in providing VBAC. According to ACOG (1998), there are insufficient data to assess the safety of VBAC in cases of multiple gestation. There are limited reports about multifetal VBAC (Miller, Mullin, Hou, & Paul, 1996; Strong, Phelan, Ahu, & Sarno, 1989).

Anesthesia Considerations

Choosing analgesic or anesthetic techniques for multifetal labor and birth may be challenging. The perinatal team should discuss the anesthesia management with the woman during pregnancy and again in early labor. Informing the patient and her support person that there may be a need to quickly adapt the plan as changes occur in the labor or birth process helps to prepare them if the plan needs to be altered. These changes may include immediate anesthesia to allow uterine relaxation for version, breech extraction, or cesarean birth (Keith et al., 1995).

Women with multiple pregnancies are at risk for an emergent cesarean birth during labor. It is recommended that they be treated as if a general anesthetic were going to be administered. The plan of care should include intravenous access, withholding liquids and solid food, evaluation of the airway, and provision of an antacid to prevent gastric aspiration syndrome. Epidural anesthesia is the technique of choice because there are usually fewer complications, including less gastric aspiration; fewer narcotic depressant effects, especially for premature infants; and less risk of postpartum hemorrhage. Continuous epidural anesthesia is often the anesthesia of choice for the vaginal birth of twins, because it provides pain relief during labor and birth, offers relaxation for internal version or fetal guidance, and is already in effect in case an operative delivery is needed. Epidural anesthesia may be continued after birth, facilitating pain management and allowing mothers to be more alert in the postpartum recovery period (Keith et al., 1995). General anesthesia has been recommended in some cases of higher-order multiple births to provide additional abdominal relaxation.

Multiple Gestations of More Than Two

Higher-order multiples are at increased risk for adverse outcomes and require more surveillance during pregnancy than twins. Women pregnant with higher-order multiples should avoid household chores, painting or decorating the nursery, sexual intercourse, traveling, and strenuous exercise except for swimming. A 2-hour rest period in the morning, afternoon, and evening is encouraged (Adams, Sholl, Haney, Russell, & Silver, 1998; Papiernik et al., 1998). HUAM may be presecribed for women with cervical changes, preterm labor, or a history of premature birth. Routine surveillance for multiple fetal pregnancies should begin at 30 to 32 weeks unless other complications indicate initiating testing sooner.

The recommended method for birth of triplets has been cesarean section, but data support vaginal delivery for uncomplicated triplet pregnancies without an increase in perinatal morbidity or mortality (Alamia, Royek, Jaekle, & Meyer, 1998; Bakos, 1998; Dommergues, Mahieu-Caputo, & Dumez, 1998). Criteria suggested by Dommergues Mahieu-Caputo, and Dumez (1998) for vaginal birth of triplets are listed in Display 8–41.

Regardless of the method, birth of higher-order multiples should occur in a tertiary care center where there is an NICU and a neonatal team can be available for each baby at birth. Optimal antepartum care

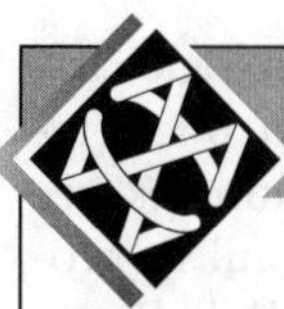

DISPLAY 8–41

Criteria for Vaginal Birth of Triplets

- Noncontracted pelvis
- Vertical lie of first triplet
- Unscarred uterus
- Onset of labor at ≥32 completed weeks of gestation

Adapted from Dommergues, M., Mahieu-Caputo, D., & Dumez, Y. (1998). Is the route of delivery a meaningful issue in triplets and higher order multiples? *Clinical Obstetrics and Gynecology, 41*(1), 25–29.

should be available at the tertiary center or in consultation with the tertiary center to provide early identification and appropriate management of fetal and maternal complications.

Postpartum Complications

Postpartum hemorrhage is the most common complication after the birth of multiple fetuses and is caused by overdistention of the uterus. The frequency of postpartum hemorrhage increases with the use of general anesthesia because of relaxation of the uterus. The reported rate of postpartum hemorrhage is up to 30% after the birth of multiples (Goldman, Dicker, Peleg, & Goldman, 1989). Severe postpartum hemorrhage may necessitate hysterectomy and require blood transfusion. The rate of postpartum infection is increased for triplet and quadruplet pregnancies (Botting et al., 1991)

Postpartum muscle weakness has been reported in women who have been on bed rest for extended periods. Osteoporosis with bilateral stress fractures of the calcanei has been reported with long-term use of $MgSO_4$ and bed rest (Levav et al., 1998). Slower postpartum recovery and postoperative complications such as thromboembolus and respiratory problems may occur because of the woman's slow return to activity (Dauphinee & Bowers, 1997).

Family Adjustments

From the moment of diagnosis, the typical family has many concerns and questions about caring for multiples. Often, they do not foresee the potential difficulties associated with the pregnancy experience itself. Families should be counseled to prepare for lifestyle changes because of the high likelihood of complications and the addition of more than one new baby. Every woman should have contingency plans for household responsibilities and, if appropriate, for child care and job responsibilities. The focus of the perinatal team is necessarily on the mother carrying the multiple fetuses, but fathers need to be included in counseling and decisions. Fathers have responses similar to those of their wives to the announcement of more than one baby. To some, especially those who have undergone infertility treatment, this news can be very exciting and perhaps even expected. Fathers often feel frustrated at their inability to be in control. They focus on potential problems, financial worries, and the health of the mother and fetuses. The father may be concerned as he faces the responsibility of having twice (or more) the number of dependents to support (May, 1994). Fathers need help to reorganize their lives to deal with their increased household and child care responsibilities successfully. Men sometimes are frustrated by the prohibition of sexual intercourse because of pregnancy complications. Intimacy such as cuddling and holding should be encouraged to decrease stress for both parents. Many men are not able to verbalize their feelings to others, and providing a safe, listening ear can be very supportive. These fathers need continued reassurance that their feelings are normal and that they are coping well with their new responsibilities. May (1994) reported that fathers described few sources of personal support and little or no contact with healthcare professionals.

Children in families expecting multiples need the same reassurance as any sibling expecting a baby. More support is needed if complications arise, their mother is hospitalized, or her activity is restricted. Preschool children are especially vulnerable because they may not understand their mother's restrictions, and if she is hospitalized, they may feel abandoned. Older children need reassurance that the family unit is secure and that their mother is safe. When hospitalization occurs, arrangements should be made for children to make regular visits to see their mother, even though the good-byes sometimes are difficult. Maintaining a stable routine for all children, limiting the numbers of strangers and caretakers, and providing individualized attention can reduce the family's stress.

Grandparents may also feel overwhelmed and guilty because they are not helping more. They may feel, especially if they are older, that they are not able to help with two or more active babies and may need guidance in how they can assist the family. When there are older siblings, the grandparents may feel more comfortable caring for these children, which provides a tremendous amount of help for the parents. They may also find that assisting with meals and household chores is easier for them than directly assisting with the babies.

Finances are often a tremendous source of stress for these families. Financial concerns may increase if the mother unexpectedly has to stop working. This situation is amplified if additional child care is also needed. The greatest costs are often associated with the long-term handicaps of a preterm infant, and the family may have no means to support one or more chronically ill children. Even when there are no complications, multiple birth families must plan for the increased day-to-day expenses of caring for more than one baby.

Well Baby Care

Nursery care of uncomplicated multiple babies is similar to a singleton's, with a few modifications. Extreme care should be taken to maintain the exact identities of each baby, especially when the babies are MZ. It is thought that multiple fetuses share a unique womb-sharing experience that allows for supporting each other (co-regulation). This can be continued with the practice of co-bedding (Nyquist & Lutes, 1998). Placing the babies in the same bed replicates the intrauterine environment and allows prenatal interaction to continue, promoting comfort and decreasing stress.

LDRPs have facilitated the ability for parents and their babies to stay together. The mother should be assessed to identify if she feels overwhelmed by having both babies with her at the same time. If hospital staff is unable to give extra assistance to the mother and her babies, it may be helpful for a support person to stay with this new family. The availability of a cot in the room for the father or support person helps the family stay together to care for their babies. Nursing assessments should include evaluation of the mother's interactions with each baby, particularly watching for differences in attachment behaviors.

Neonatal Intensive Care

Most twins and higher-order multiples are born preterm or at a LBW (or both). They encounter the same risks as singleton preterm infants, including respiratory distress syndrome, hypoglycemia, hyperbilirubinemia, anemia, and septicemia. Most higher-order multiples and about one half of twins weigh less than 2,500 g at birth, which is probably the single most important factor associated with the neonatal problems of multiples (Fraser, Picard, & Picard, 1991). Many of these babies need specialized care in a level II or level III nursery. Although physiologic care is similar to the care of singleton infants, there are indications that the emotional needs of multiples are different, and co-bedding has been successful in providing continued emotional contact (DellaPorta, Aforismo, & Butler-O'Hara, 1998). Co-regulation activities that have been observed in preterm twins include moving close, touching, holding, hugging, rooting, sucking on each other, smiling, being awake at the same time, and a decreased need for ambient temperature support. Data from a multicenter study of co-bedding of extremely premature multiples indicates improved health, shorter hospital stays, and decreased costs (Nyquist & Lutes, 1998). Babies should not be in the same bed if one baby has an infection that could be passed on to his or her sibling. When co-bedding is used or the babies are in the NICU, a second Isolette should be set up and available at all times in case an emergency occurs (DellaPorta, et al., 1998). Ideally, one nurse should take care of both babies. If one baby is sicker than the other, it is important to assess for overstimulation of the healthier baby. Parents providing day-to-day care of their babies increases their confidence in parenting and caregiving skills, as well as affirming emotional ties. Nesting rooms, where parents can stay overnight with their babies in the hospital, prepare parents for discharge.

Separation of Infants at Discharge

Frequently, multiple babies cannot be discharged at the same time. Some institutions allow the family and well twin to stay in the hospital without cost to the family. This arrangement is especially appreciated when families live far from the hospital. The hospital may require a release to decrease liability and to be certain that the family understands that no extra services will be provided.

When separation does occur, the parents are often torn between the needs of each baby and are constantly traveling back and forth to the hospital. This is physically and emotionally stressful for the family, especially for the mother who is still recovering from birth. If rooms are not available for parents to stay overnight, "parenting rooms" may be provided for parents to have a place for daytime visits and privacy for breast-feeding. Discharging babies separately may be easier for families with higher-order multiples. When babies go home one or two at a time, the parents can become acquainted with each baby individually before facing the overwhelming tasks of caring for all of the babies together (Dauphinee & Bowers, 1997).

Follow-up Pediatric Care and Neonatal Assessment

Families of preterm and LBW multiples should be referred after discharge to a special infant development clinic where adjunct services such as physical therapy and social services are available. Long-term studies have shown that, although twins were small at birth, their growth is often accelerated in their early years, and by age 8, they are usually on par with their singleton peers (Falkner & Matheny, 1995). Because there is an increased incidence of developmental disability, cerebral palsy, mental retardation, sensory impairments, language delays, learning disability, and attention and behavior problems (Allen & Alexander, 1994), primary care providers should be alert to identify problems as early as possible to obtain appropriate services.

After discharge, it is essential that the parents be allowed to be the babies' primary caretakers. Eager friends and family need to assist with housekeeping, laundry, cooking, grocery shopping, and sibling care and should be allowed to help. Parents find taking care of the babies physically exhausting. The mother's time should be dedicated to feeding her babies and resting. When the babies begin sleeping more consistently, the mother can start taking back more responsibilities.

Breast-feeding

Some mothers of multiples may be unaware that breast-feeding is an option while others are doubtful that they can produce enough milk to meet the needs of two or more babies. Mothers of multiples need the same basic information about breast-feeding as other women. They need information regarding positions for simultaneous feeding, feeding rotation, and milk production. Breast-feeding positions for multiples are pictured in Figure 8–8. The babies can be fed on demand, feeding each one when it demonstrates feeding cues, or fed together, with the mother actively waking the second twin when the first one shows feeding cues. This method of feeding takes less time than feeding the babies individually. Many mothers use a combination of individual and simultaneous feedings. The infants should be rotated so that each can spend a similar amount of time at each breast, maximizing milk production.

Bonding and Individualization

The process of individualization of multiple fetuses begins during pregnancy as expectant parents first see their babies on the ultrasound scan, perhaps as early as 6 or 7 weeks. As the fetuses grow, nurses or ultrasound technicians can help parents visualize fetal positions and movements. Fetal movement may be felt earlier with multiples, and many women learn to differentiate each baby's movements and begin identifying personality traits as early as 21 weeks' gestation. Parents may choose to know the sex of their babies so they can refer to each baby by name.

After birth, the attachment and individualization process continues. At first, the emotional attachment is to the unit or group of babies. To assist the parents with individualizing each baby, they should be encouraged to use the babies' names rather than calling them "the twins" or "the babies." The mother may start to focus on one baby at a time and may seem disinterested in the others. Then she may shift her focus as she gets to know another baby. It is important that the parents are able to experience each baby as an individual, with a unique personality and characteristics; this may be more difficult for MZ babies who look alike.

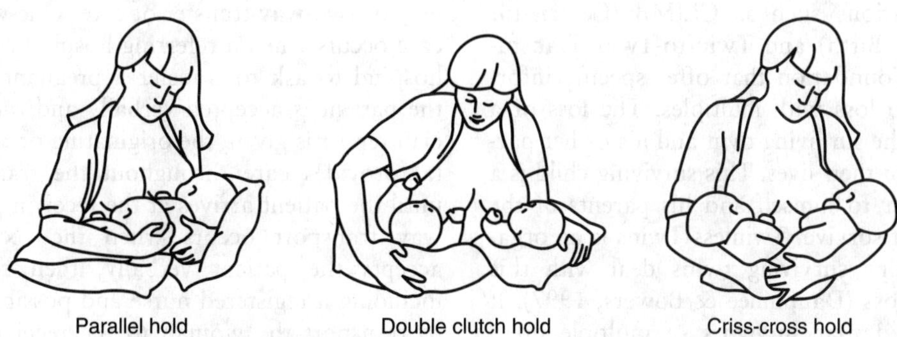

FIGURE 8–8. Breast-feeding positions for mothers of multiples.

Grief with the Death of One or More Infants

In multiple pregnancies, there is a higher rate of early loss, stillborns, and neonatal deaths than in singleton pregnancies. The loss of an entire multiple pregnancy is devastating to parents. When only one fetus of a multifetal pregnancy dies, the emotional tasks are conflicting and cause greater consequences. It is hard for parents to bond to a new baby when they are grieving. This is true not only when one or more babies of a multiple set dies, but is also true for other deaths of other close family members at the time of birth. The parental emotions were well described in an article by Limbo and Wheeler (1986): "We are grieving and loving at the same time. But it's not like pulling and tugging. It's more like ripping and tearing." This imperfect bonding may be further disrupted because the surviving baby may need to stay in the NICU before he or she can come home. The NICU stay adds to the parental concerns about their baby, and they may avoid attachment because they are afraid that this baby may also die. Being given permission to express all of their emotions and preparing them for the continuing contradictions in feelings can assist parents. To help parents with the grieving process, they need to separate their babies and come to terms with their individuality (Limbo & Wheeler, 1986) so that they can grieve for the one who has died and attach to their new baby. Ignoring the death of the baby who died is inappropriate, and statements such as "Well, you still have one baby that lived; you should be grateful" are devastating to parents and increase their emotional conflicts.

No matter how many babies survive, the parents are still parents of multiples, and special memories should be created (Dauphinee & Bowers, 1997). Photographs should be taken with all of the babies together as well as individually. Footprints, handprints, or both of all of the babies can be placed on the same card as well as separately. Other mementos, such as a lock of each baby's hair, should be individually labeled. Families should be given information about support organizations such as CLIMB (Center for Loss in Multiple Birth) and Twin-to-Twin Transfusion Syndrome Foundation that offer specific information related to loss with multiples. The loss of a twin may affect the surviving twin and his or her parents for the rest of their lives. This surviving child is a constant reminder to himself and his parents of the baby that did not survive. Twinless Twins is an organization that helps surviving twins deal with this unique sense of loss (Dauphinee & Bowers, 1997). It has been reported that survivors of multiple pregnancy loss may have a sense of incompleteness and may always feel a longing for the lost fetus.

Multiple Birth Resources and Support Organizations

During pregnancy, birth, and the months after the birth, each family of multiples experiences "a constellation of stresses which jeopardize physical and mental health and family functioning" (Malmstrom & Biale, 1990). These stresses cut across all socioeconomic and educational levels and include increases in child abuse, parental substance abuse, and marital dysfunction, and divorce (Malmstrom & Biale, 1990). Leonard (1998) described three disorders affecting multiple birth families: depression, panic attacks, and obsessive-compulsive disorders. Several studies indicate that there are increased levels of depression, which may be as high as 45% for postpartum depression in mothers of multiples (Coroyer & Casati, 1996). Organizations for multiple birth families provide a supportive environment for parents to network and learn from others. National organizations often offer free brochures and handouts that can be included in packets created especially for the expectant parents of multiples.

MATERNAL TRANSFER

Maternal transfer from a level I or level II institution to a level III institution is an option in the care of pregnant women. Each case is considered individually. Suggested guidelines for transfer of care of the mother are provided in Display 8–42. Before transfer, the severity of the clinical situation and the time and distance to the receiving hospital are considered. Chapter 2 discusses the Federal Emergency Medical Treatment and Labor Act as it applies to maternal transfers.

Maternal transport can be accomplished by a one-way or two-way transfer of care. One-way transfer of care occurs when a referring hospital calls a receiving hospital to ask to transfer a pregnant patient. After the patient is accepted verbally and the initial physician report is given, the originating or referring hospital provides care throughout the transport process until the patient arrives at the receiving facility. Two-way transport occurs when the receiving facility accepts the patient verbally, then sends a team, including a registered nurse and possibly a physician, to transport the woman to the receiving facility. In

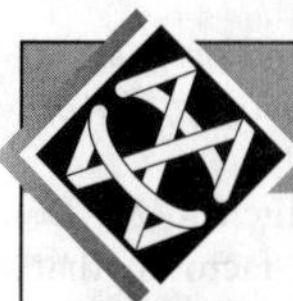

DISPLAY 8-42

Guidelines for Maternal Transfer

FROM A LEVEL I INSTITUTION*

- Labor with cervical change less than 34–36 weeks' gestation
- Preterm premature rupture of membranes (PPROM) less than 34–36 weeks' gestation
- Labor and/or PPROM when dating data are uncertain
- Preterm labor with maternal or fetal complications
- Bleeding less than 34–36 weeks' gestation
- Twin or triplet gestation with contractions or labor less than 34–36 weeks
- Severe preeclampsia
- Eclampsia if maternal condition stabilized
- Intrauterine growth restriction
- Oligohydramnios
- Polyhydramnios (severe or uncertain origin)
- Fetal hydrops
- Fetal anomalies, especially at gestational ages less than 34–36 weeks, that require specialized neonatal intervention (eg, diaphragmatic hernia, oomphalocele, severe neural tube defects)
- Fetal conditions requiring cordocentesis and/or transfusion
- Maternal medical conditions outside of the scope of medical and nursing care available (eg, liver transplant, renal dialysis, severe mitral stenosis, cancer, active lupus, pulmonary embolism)
- Maternal (and possibly fetal) trauma
- Unusual fetal heart dysrhythmia (eg, complete fetal heart block)

FROM A LEVEL II INSTITUTION

- Any fetus requiring long-term ventilatory support as a newborn
- Any fetus requiring neonatal care less than 30–34 weeks' gestation depending on the institution resources
- Maternal complications listed above

*All guidelines assume maternal and fetal stability.

this case, the transferring facility turns over the care and responsibility of the patient once the patient is under transport. Transport is accomplished by a variety of methods, including private ambulance, public rescue vehicles, helicopters, and airplanes.

An accurate, thorough nursing report is a critical element of transfer of care. A photocopy of the original record accompanies the patient. Any nursing or medical action performed en route (eg, vital signs, palpating for contractions) is documented, and a copy is left with the receiving hospital. Many institutions have specific forms for the transfer of obstetric patients. The decision about the necessity of a nurse, physician, or both accompanying the patient in transfer is made in each case. If the nurse feels it inappropriate to transfer a specific patient without a physician present and one has not been provided, the institutional chain of command can provide a method for conflict resolution (see Chapter 2).

Based on an assessment of maternal–fetal status, appropriate equipment is required to ensure patient safety during the transfer process. For the woman with preeclampsia, a nasal airway, Ambu bag, and anticonvulsant and antihypertensive agents should be included. Transport vehicles routinely are stocked with intravenous solutions and emergency equipment. Maternal transfer is less often initiated for women who are bleeding unless the patient is hemodynamically stable (ie, the blood pressure and pulse are within normal limits, and the FHR tracing is reassuring). When transferring women at risk for preterm labor, a birth kit from the originating hospital should be included; the rescue kits on the ambulance are usually minimally stocked. A full birth kit with suction catheters, suction bulb, blankets, and hat for the newborn is necessary. One-quart zip-lock plastic bags are useful to place the newborn in after birth, with the zip-lock closed on either side around the newborn's neck to prevent body heat loss. It is recommended that all patients have at least two infusion lines because attempting to start an intravenous line en route is extremely difficult.

SUMMARY

Perinatal nurses may be challenged by the complications of pregnancy, especially when they occur unexpectedly in the low-risk setting. A thorough knowledge of the nursing care for common perinatal complications, including timely identification and appropriate interventions, is required to ensure optimal outcomes for mothers and babies.

REFERENCES

Hypertensive Disorders

Adams, E. M., & Finlayson, A. (1961). Familial aspects of preeclampsia and hypertension in pregnancy. *Lancet, 2*, 1375–1378.

Ales, K. L., Norton, M. E., & Druzin, M. L. (1989). Early prediction of antepartum hypertension. *Obstetrics and Gynecology, 73*(6), 928–933.

American College of Obstetricians and Gynecologists. (1996). *Management of preeclampsia* (Technical Bulletin No. 219). Washington, DC: Author.

Baird, D. (1977). Epidemiological aspects of hypertensive pregnancy. *Clinical Obstetrics and Gynecology, 4*(3), 531–548.

Barron, W. M. (1991). Hypertension. In W. M. Barron & M. D. Lindheimer (Eds.), *Medical Disorders in Pregnancy* (pp. 1–42). Chicago: Mosby–Year Book.

Barton, J. R., Witlin, A. G., & Sibai, B. M. (1999). Management of mild preeclampsia. *Clinical Obstetrics and Gynecology, 42*(3), 455–469.

Beer, A. E. (1978). Possible immunologic bases of preeclampsia/eclampsia. *Seminars in Perinatology, 2*(1), 39–59.

Belizán, J. M., & Villar, J. (1980). The relationship between calcium intake and edema-proteinuria and hypertension-gestosis: An hypothesis. *American Journal of Clinical Nutrition, 33*(10), 2202.

Branch, D. W., Andres, R., Digre, K. R., Rote, N. S., & Scott, J. R. (1989). The association of antiphospholipid antibodies with severe preeclampsia. *Obstetrics and Gynecology, 73*(4), 541–545.

Branch, D. W. (1990). Antiphospholipid antibodies and pregnancy: Maternal implications. *Seminars in Perinatology, 14*(2), 139–146.

Branch, D. W., Dudley, D. J., LaMarche, S., & Mitchell, M. D. (1992). Sera from preeclamptic patients contain factor(s) that stimulate prostacyclin production by human endothelial cells. *Prostaglandins, Leukotrienes, and Essential Fatty Acids, 45*(3), 191–195.

Branch, D. W., Dudley, D. J., & Mitchell, M. D. (1991). Preliminary evidence for homeostatic mechanism regulating endothelin production in pre-eclampsia [See comments]. *Lancet, 337*(8747), 943–945.

Branch, D. W., Silver, R. M., Blackwell, J. L., Reading, J. C., & Scott, J. R. (1992). Outcome of treated pregnancies in women with antiphospholipid syndrome: An update of the Utah experience. *Obstetrics and Gynecology, 80*(4), 614–620.

Brewer, T. (1974). Metabolic toxemia of late pregnancy in a county prenatal nutrition education project: A preliminary report. *Journal of Reproductive Medicine, 13*(5), 175–176.

Brewer, T. (1976). Role of malnutrition in preeclampsia and eclampsia. *American Journal of Obstetrics and Gynecology, 125*(2), 281.

Brown, M. A., & Buddle, M. L. (1995). Inadequacy of dipstick proteinuria in hypertensive pregnancy. *Australian and New Zealand Journal of Obstetrics and Gynaecology, 35*(4), 366–369.

Butler, N. R., & Alberman, E. D. (1958). *Perinatal problems: Second report of the British Perinatal Mortality Survey*. Edinburgh: ES Livingstone.

Campbell, D. M., MacGillivray, I., & Carr-Hill, R. (1985). Pre-eclampsia in second pregnancy. *British Journal of Obstetrics and Gynaecology, 92*(2), 131–140.

Campbell, J. W. (1985). A possible teratogenic effect of propranolol [Letter]. *New England Journal of Medicine, 313*(8), 518.

Chaudhuri, S. K. (1971). Role of nutrition in the etiology of toxemia of pregnancy. *American Journal of Obstetrics and Gynecology, 110*(1), 46–48.

Chesley, L. C., & Annitto, J. E. (1947). Pregnancy in the patient with hypertensive disease. *American Journal of Obstetrics and Gynecology, 53*, 372–381.

Chesley, L. C., Annitto, J. E., & Cosgrove, R. A. (1968). The familial factor in toxemia of pregnancy. *Obstetrics and Gynecology, 32*(3), 303–311.

Chesley, L. C. (1978). *Hypertensive disorders in pregnancy*. New York: Appleton-Century-Crofts.

Chesley, L. C. (1984). History and epidemiology of preeclampsia-eclampsia. *Clinical Obstetrics and Gynecology, 27*(4), 801–820.

Chesley, L. C., & Cooper, D. W. (1986). Genetics of hypertension in pregnancy: Possible single gene control of pre-eclampsia and eclampsia in the descendants of eclamptic women. *British Journal of Obstetrics and Gynaecology, 93*(9), 898–908.

Chesley, L. C., & Sibai, B. M. (1987). Blood pressure in the midtrimester and future eclampsia. *American Journal of Obstetrics and Gynecology, 157*(5), 1258–1261.

Chez, R., & Sibai, B. M. (1994). Labetalol for intrapartum hypertension. *Contemporary OB/GYN, 39*, 37–38.

Clark, S. L., Cotton, D. B., Hankins, G. D. V., & Phelan, J. P. (Eds.). (1997). *Critical care obstetrics* (3rd ed.). Malden, MS: Blackwell Science.

Crowther, C., Bouwmeester, A. M., & Ashurst, H. M. (1992). Does admission to hospital for bed rest prevent disease progression or improve fetal outcome in pregnancy complicated by nonproteinuric hypertension? *British Journal of Obstetrics and Gynaecology, 99*(1), 13–17.

Cruickshank, D. J., Robertson, A. A., Campbell, D. M., & MacGillivray, I. (1992). Does labetalol influence the development of proteinuria in pregnancy hypertension? A randomised controlled study. *European Journal of Obstetrics Gynaecologic Reproductive Biology, 45*(1), 47–51.

Cunningham, F. G., Cox, S. M., Harstad, T. W., Mason, R. A., & Pritchard, J. A. (1990). Chronic renal disease and pregnancy outcome. *American Journal of Obstetrics and Gynecology, 163*(2), 453–459.

Cunningham, F. G., & Leveno, K. J. (1988). Management of pregnancy-induced hypertension. In P. C. Rubin (Ed.), *Handbook of Hypertension* (Vol. X). Amsterdam: Elsevier Science.

Davies, A. G. (1971). *Geographical epidemiology of the toxemias of pregnancy*. Springfield, IL: Charles C. Thomas.

Davies, A. M., Czaczkes, J. W., Sadovsky, E., Prywes, R., Weiskopt, P., & Stesk, W. (1970). Toxemia of pregnancy in Jerusalem. I. Epidemiological studies of a total community. *Israeli Journal of Medical Science, 6*(2), 253–266.

Dekker, G. A. (1999). Risk factors for preeclampsia. *Clinical Obstetrics and Gynecology, 42*(3), 422–435.

Dekker, G. A., Robillard, P. Y., & Hulsey, T. C. (1998). Immune maladaptation in the etiology of preeclampsia: A review of corroborative epidemiologic studies. *Obstetric and Gynecologic Survey, 53*(6), 377–382.

Dekker, G. A., & Sibai, B. M. (1998). Etiology and pathogenesis of preeclampsia: Current concepts. *American Journal of Obstetrics and Gynecology, 179*(5), 1359–1375.

Dildy, G. A., Phelan, J. P., & Cotton, D. B. (1992). Complications of pregnancy-induced hypertension. In S. L. Clark, D. B. Cotton, G. D. V. Hankins, & J. P. Phelan (Eds.), *Critical care obstetrics* (2nd ed., pp. 251–288). Boston, MA: Blackwell Scientific.

Dizon-Townson, D. S., Major, H., & Ward, K. (1998). A promoter mutation in the tumor necrosis factor alpha gene is not associated with preeclampsia. *Journal of Reproductive Immunology, 38*(1), 55–61.

Dizon-Townson, D. S., Nelson, L. M., Easton, K., & Ward, K. (1996). The factor V Leiden mutation may predispose women to severe preeclampsia. *American Journal of Obstetrics and Gynecology, 175*(4, Pt. 1) 902–905.

Duffus, G. M., & MacGillivray, I. (1968). The incidence of preeclamptic toxaemia in smokers and non-smokers. *Lancet, 1*(7550), 994–995.

Duvekot, J. J., Cheriex, E. C., Pieters, F. A., Menheere, P. P., & Peeters, L. H. (1993). Early pregnancy changes in hemodynamics and volume homeostasis are consecutive adjustments triggered by a primary fall in systemic vascular tone. *American Journal of Obstetrics and Gynecology, 169*(6), 1382–1392.

Easterling, T. R., Benedetti, T. J., Schmucker, B. C., & Millard, S. P. (1990). Maternal hemodynamics in normal and preeclampsia pregnancies: A longitudinal study. *Obstetrics and Gynecology, 76*(6), 1061–1069.

Egerman, R. S., & Sibai, B. M. (1999). HELLP syndrome. *Clinical Obstetrics and Gynecology, 42*(2), 381–389.

Eskenazi, B., Fenster, L., & Sidney, S. (1991). A multivariate analysis of risk factors for preeclampsia. *Journal of the American Medical Association, 266*(2), 237–241.

Fairlie, F. M., & Sibai, B. M. (1993). Hypertensive diseases in pregnancy. In E. A. Reece, J. C. Hobbins, M. J. Mahoney, & R. H. Petrie (Eds.), *Medicine of the fetus and mother*. Philadelphia: J.B. Lippincott.

Feeney, J. G., & Scott, J. S. (1980). Pre-eclampsia and changed paternity. *European Journal of Obstetrics, Gynecology and Reproductive Biology, 11*(1), 35–38.

Felding, C. F. (1969). Obstetric aspects in women with histories of renal disease. *Acta Obstetricia et Gynecologica Scandinavica, 48*(Suppl. 2), 1–43.

Fenakel, K., Fenakel, G., Appelman, Z., Lurie, S., Katz, Z., & Shoham, Z. (1991). Nifedipine in the treatment of severe preeclampsia. *Obstetrics and Gynecology, 77*(3), 331–337.

Fitzgibbon, G. (1922). The relationship of eclampsia to other toxemias of pregnancy. *British Journal of Obstetrics and Gynaecology, 29*, 402.

Friedman, S. A., Schiff, E., Lubarsky, S. L., & Sibai, B. M. (1999). Expectant management of severe preeclampsia remote from term. *Clinical Obstetrics and Gynecology, 42*(3), 470–478.

Friedman, S. A., Taylor, R. N., & Roberts, J. M. (1991). Pathophysiology of preeclampsia. *Clinics in Perinatology, 18*(4), 661–682.

Garner, P. R., D'Alton, M. E., Dudley, D. K., Huard, P., & Hardie, M. (1990). Preeclampsia in diabetic pregnancies. *American Journal of Obstetrics and Gynecology, 163*(2), 505–508.

Gavette, L., & Roberts, J. (1987). Use of mean arterial pressure (MAP-2) to predict pregnancy-induced hypertension in adolescents. *Journal of Nurse-Midwifery, 32*(6), 357–364.

Gilstrap, L. C., 3rd, Cunningham, F. G., & Whalley, P. J. (1978). Management of pregnancy induced hypertension in the nulliparous patient remote from term. *Seminars of Perinatology, 2*(1), 73–81.

Goldberg, G. L., & Craig, C. J. T. (1983). Obstetric complications in adolescent pregnancies. *South African Medical Journal, 64*(22), 863–864.

Goldenberg, R. L., Cliver, S. P., Bronstein, J., Cutter, G. R., Andrews, W. W., & Mennemeyer, S. T. (1994). Bed rest in pregnancy. *Obstetrics and Gynecology, 84*(1), 131–136.

Gonik, B., & Cotton, D. B. (1984). Peripartum colloid osmotic pressure changes: Influence of intravenous hydration. American Journal of *Obstetrics and Gynecology, 150*(1), 90–100.

Grisaru, D., Zwang, E., Peyser, M. R., Lessing, J. B., & Eldor, A. (1997). The procoagulant activity of red blood cells from patients with severe preeclampsia. *American Journal of Obstetrics and Gynecology, 177*(6) 1513–1516.

Gruppo di Studio Iperensione in Gravidanza. (1998). Nifedipine versus expectant management in mild to moderate hypertension in pregnancy. *British Journal of Obstetrics and Gynaecology, 105*(7), 718–722.

Guzick, D. S., Klein, V. R., Tyson, J. E., Lasky, R. E., Gant, N. F., & Rosenfeld, C. R. (1987). Risk factors for the occurrence of pregnancy-induced hypertension. *Clinical and Experimental Hypertension—Part B, Hypertension of Pregnancy, B6*(2), 281–297.

Hays, P. M., Cruikshank, D. P., & Dunn, L. J. (1985). Plasma volume determination in normal and preeclamptic outcomes. *American Journal of Obstetrics and Gynecology, 151*(7), 958–966.

Hoyert, D. L., Kochanek, K. D., & Murphy, S. L. (1999). Deaths: Final data for 1997. *National Vital Statistics Report, 47*(19), 1–104.

Jones, D. C., & Hayslett, J. P. (1996). Outcome of pregnancy in women with moderate or severe renal insufficiency. *The New England Journal of Medicine, 335*(4), 226–232.

Khan, K. S., & Daya, S. (1996). Plasma glucose and pre-eclampsia. *International Journal of Gynaecology and Obstetrics, 53*(2) 111–116.

Kilpatrick, D. C., Liston, W. A., Gibson, F., & Livingstone, J. (1989). Association between susceptibility to pre-eclampsia within families and HLADR4. *Lancet, 2*(8671), 1063–1065.

Kirshon, B., Moise, K. J., Jr., Cotton, D. B., Longmire, S., Jones, M., Tessem, J., & Joyce, T. A., III. (1988). Role of volume expansion in severe pre-eclampsia. *Surgery, Gynecology and Obstetrics, 167*(5), 367–71.

Klonoff-Cohen, H. S., Savitz, D. A., Cefalo, R. C., & McCann, M. F. (1989). An epidemiologic study of contraception and preeclampsia. *Journal of the American Medical Association, 262*(22), 3143–3147.

Kuo, V. S., Loumantakis, G., & Gallery, E. D. (1992). Proteinuria and its assessment in normal and hypertensive pregnancy. *American Journal of Obstetrics and Gynecology, 167*(3), 723–728.

Leduc, L., Wheeler, J. M., Kirshon, B., Mitchell, P., & Cotton, D. B. (1992). Coagulation profile in severe preeclampsia. *Obstetrics and Gynecology, 79*(1), 14–18.

Levine, R., & CPEP Study Group. (1997, January 20–25). *Calcium for preeclampsia prevention (CPEP): A double-blind, placebo-controlled trial in healthy nulliparas.* Paper presented at the Society of Perinatal Obstetricians, 1997 17th Annual Meeting, Anaheim, CA.

Lie, R. T., Rasmussen, S., Brunborg, H., Gjessing, H. K., Lie-Nielsen, E., & Irgens, L. M. (1998). Fetal and maternal contributions to risk of pre-eclampsia: Population based study. *British Medical Journal, 316*(7141), 1343–1347.

Lindoff, C., Ingemarsson, I., Martinsson, G., Segelmark, M., Thysell, H., & Astedt, B. (1997). Preeclampsia is associated with a reduced response to activated protein C. *American Journal of Obstetrics and Gynecology, 176*(2), 457–460.

Liston, W. A., & Kilpatrick, D. C. (1991). Is genetic susceptibility to pre-eclampsia conferred by homozygosity for the same single recessive gene in mother and fetus? *British Journal of Obstetrics and Gynaecology, 98*(11), 1079–1086.

Long, P. A., Abell, D. A., & Beischer, N. A. (1979). Parity and preeclampsia. *Australian and New Zealand Journal of Obstetrics and Gynaecology, 19*(4), 203–206.

Lu, J. Y., Cook, D. L., Javia, J. B., Kirmani, Z. A., Liu, C. C., Makadia, D. N., Makadiam, T. A., Omasayie, O. B., Patel, D. P., Reddy, V. J., Walker, B. W., Williams, C. S., & Chung, R. A. (1981). Intake of vitamins and minerals by pregnant women with selected symptoms. *Journal of the American Dietary Association, 78*(5), 477–482.

Mabie, W. C., Pernoll, M. L., & Biswas, M. K. (1986). Chronic hypertension in pregnancy. *Obstetrics and Gynecology, 67*(2), 197–205.

MacGillivary, I., Rose, G. A., & Rowe, B. (1969). Blood pressure survey in pregnancy. *Clinical Science, 37*(2), 395–407.

Magann, E. F., Martin, J. M., Jr., Isaacs, J. D., Perry, K. G., Jr., Martin, R. W., & Meydrech, E. F. (1993). Immediate postpartum curettage: Accelerated recovery from severe preeclampsia. *Obstetrics and Gynecology, 81*(4), 502–506.

Marcoux, S., Berube, S., Brisson, J., & Fabia, J. (1992). History of migraine and risk of pregnancy-induced hypertension. *Epidemiology, 3*(1), 53–56.

Marx, G. F., Schwalbe, S. S., Cho, E., & Whitty, J. E. (1993). Automatic blood pressure measurements in laboring women: Are they reliable? *American Journal of Obstetrics and Gynecology, 158*(3, Pt. 1), 796–798.

Mathews, D. D., Agarwal, V., & Shuttleworth, T. P. (1980). The effect of rest and ambulation on plasma urea and urate levels in pregnant women with proteinuric hypertension. *British Journal of Obstetrics and Gynaecology, 87*(12), 1095–1098.

Meyer, N. L., Mercer, B. M., Friedman, S. A., & Sibai, B. M. (1994). Urinary dipstick protein: A poor predictor of absent or severe proteinuria. *American Journal of Obstetrics and Gynecology, 170*(1, Pt. 1), 137–141.

Mittendorf, R., Lain, K. Y., Williams, M. A., & Walker, C. K. (1996). Preeclampsia: A nested, case-control study of risk factors and their interactions. *Journal of Reproductive Medicine, 41*(7), 491–496.

Montagu, M. F. A. (1979). *Reproductive development of the female.* (3rd ed.). Littleton, MA: John Wright–PSG Publishing.

Moore, M. P., & Redmon, C. W. (1983). Case-control study of severe pre-eclampsia of early onset. *British Medical Journal, 287*(6392), 580–583.

Moutquin, J. M., Rainville, C., Giroux, L., Raynauld, P., Amyot, G., Bilodeau, R., & Pelland, N. (1985). A prospective study of blood pressure in pregnancy: Prediction of preeclampsia. *American Journal of Obstetrics and Gynecology, 151*(2), 191–196.

Myatt, L., & Miodovnik, M. (1999). Prediction of preeclampsia. *Seminars in Perinatology, 23*(1), 45–57.

Nelson, T. R. (1955). A clinical study of preeclampsia, Parts I and II. *Journal of Obstetrics and Gynaecology in the British Empire,* 64, 48–66.

Ness, R. B., & Roberts, J. M. (1996). Heterogeneous causes constituting the single syndrome of preeclampsia: A hypothesis and its implications [See comments]. *American Journal of Obstetrics and Gynecology, 175*(5), 1365–1370.

O'Brien, J. M., Mercer, B. M., Friedman, S. A., & Sibai, B. M. (1993). Amniotic fluid index in hospitalized hypertensive patients managed expectantly. *Obstetrics and Gynecology, 82*(2), 247–250.

O'Brien, W. F. (1990). Predicting preeclampsia. *Obstetrics and Gynecology, 75*(3, Pt. 1), 445–452.

O'Brien, W. F. (1992). The prediction of preeclampsia. *Clinical Obstetrics and Gynecology, 35*(2), 351–364.

Odendaal, H. J., Pattinson, R. C., Bam, R., Grove, D., & Kotze, T. J. (1990). Aggressive or expectant management for patients with severe preeclampsia between 28–34 weeks' gestation: A randomized controlled trial. *Obstetrics and Gynecology, 76*(6), 1070–1075.

Out, H. J., Bruinse, H. W., Christiaens, G. C., van Vliet, M., de Groot, P. G., Nieuwenhuis, H. K., & Derksen, R. H. (1992). A prospective, controlled multicenter study on the obstetric risks of pregnant women with antiphospholipid antibodies. *American Journal of Obstetrics and Gynecology, 167*(1), 26–32.

Page, E. W., & Christianson, R. (1976). The impact of mean arterial pressure in the middle trimester upon the outcome of pregnancy. American Journal of Obstetrics and Gynecology, 125(6), 740–746.

Page, E. W. (1939). Relation between hydatid moles, relative ischemia of gravid uterus, and the placental origin of eclampsia. *American Journal of Obstetrics and Gynecology, 37,* 291–293.

Pattinson, R. C., Kriegler, E., Odendaal, H. J., Muller, L. M., & Kirsten, G. (1989). Increased placental resistance and late decelerations associated with severe proteinuric hypertension predicts poor fetal outcome. *South African Medical Journal, 75*(5) 211–214.

Phelan, J. P (1991). Fetal considerations in the critically ill obstetric patient. In S. L. Clark, D. B. Cotton, G. D. V. Hankins, & J. P. Phelan (Eds.), *Critical Care Obstetrics* (2nd ed., pp. 634–658). Boston: Blackwell Scientific Publications.

Plouin, P. F., Breart, G., Maillard, F., Papiernik, E., Relier, J. P., & The Labetalol Methyldopa Study Group. (1988). Comparison of antihypertensive efficacy and perinatal safety of labetalol and methyldopa in the treatment of hypertension in pregnancy: A randomized controlled trial. *British Journal of Obstetrics and Gynaecology, 95*(9), 868–876.

Plouin, P. F., Breart, G., Llado, J., Dalle, M., Keller, M. E., Goujon, H., & Berchel, C. (1990). A randomized comparison of early with conservative use of antihypertensive drugs in the management of pregnancy-induced hypertension. *British Journal of Obstetrics and Gynaecology, 97*(2), 134–141.

Redman, C. (1995). Hypertension in pregnancy. In G. Chamberlain (Ed.), *Turnbull's obstetrics* (2nd ed., pp. 441–479). Edinburgh: Churchill Livingstone.

Redman, C. W., Bodmer, J. G., Bodmer, W. F., Beilin, L. J., & Bonnar, J. (1978). HLA antigens in severe pre-eclampsia. *Lancet,* 2(8086), 397–399.

Repke, J. T. (1993). Hypertension and preeclampsia. In T. R. Moore, R. C. Reiter, R. W. Rebar, & V. V. Baker (Eds.), *Gynecology and obstetrics: A longitudinal approach* (pp. 463–477). New York: Churchill Livingstone.

Roberts, J. (1999). Pregnancy-related hypertension. In R. Creasy & R. Resnik (Eds.), *Maternal-fetal medicine* (4th ed., pp. 833–872). Philadelphia: W.B. Saunders.

Roberts, J. M., Taylor, R. N., Friedman, S. A., & Goldfien, A. (1990). New developments in preeclampsia. *Fetal Medicine Review, 2*, 125.

Robillard, P., Hulsey, T. C., Perianin, J., Janky, E., Miri, E. H., & Papiernik, E. (1994). Association of pregnancy-induced hypertension with duration of sexual cohabitation before conception. *Lancet, 344*(8928), 973–975.

Ross, R., Perizweig, W., Taylor, H., McBryde, A., Yates, A., & Kondutyer, A. (1954). A study of certain dietary factors of possible etiologic significance in toxemias of pregnancy. *American Journal of Obstetrics and Gynecology, 351*, 426.

Rotten, W., Sachtleben, M., & Friedman, E. (1959). Migraine and eclampsia. *Obstetrics and Gynecology, 14*, 322–330.

Rubin, P. C., Butters, L., Clark, D. M., Reynolds, B., Sumner, D. J., Steedman, D., Low, R., & Reid, J. L. (1983). Placebo-controlled trial of atenolol in treatment of pregnancy-associated hypertension. *Lancet, 1*(8322), 431–434.

Saftlas, A. F., Olson, D. R., Franks, A. L., Atrash, H. K., & Pokras, R. (1990). Epidemiology of preeclampsia and eclampsia in the United States, 1979–1986. *American Journal of Obstetrics and Gynecology, 163*(2), 460–465.

Schaffir, J. A., Lockwood, C. J., Lapinski, R., Yoon, L., & Alvarez, M. (1995). Incidence of pregnancy-induced hypertension among gestational diabetics. *American Journal of Perinatology, 12*(4) 252–254.

Schiff, E., Friedman, S. A., & Sibai, B. M. (1994). Conservative management of severe preeclampsia remote from term. *Obstetrics and Gynecology, 84*(4), 626–630.

Sibai, B. M. (1990a). Eclampsia VI. Maternal-perinatal outcome in 254 consecutive cases. *American Journal of Obstetrics and Gynecology, 163*(3), 1049–1054.

Sibai, B. M. (1990b). The HELLP syndrome (hemolysis, elevated liver enzymes, and low platelets): Much ado about nothing? [See comments]. *American Journal of Obstetrics and Gynecology, 162*(2), 311–316.

Sibai, B. M. (1990c). Magnesium sulfate is the ideal anticonvulsant in preeclampsia-eclampsia. *American Journal of Obstetrics and Gynecology, 162*(5), 1141–1145.

Sibai, B. M. (1991). Immunologic aspects of preeclampsia. *Clinical Obstetrics and Gynecology, 34*(1), 27–34.

Sibai, B. M. (1996). Treatment of hypertension in pregnant women. *New England Journal of Medicine, 335*(4), 257–265.

Sibai, B. M., Anderson, G. D., Spinnato, J. A., & Shaver, D. C. (1983). Plasma volume findings in patients with mild pregnancy-induced hypertension. *American Journal of Obstetrics and Gynecology, 147*(1), 16–19.

Sibai, B. M., Barton, J. R., Akl, S., Sarinoglu, C., & Mercer, B. M. (1992). A randomized prospective comparison of nifedipine and bed rest versus bed rest alone in the management of preeclampsia remote from term. *American Journal of Obstetrics and Gynecology, 167*(4, Pt. 1), 879–884.

Sibai, B. M., Gonzalez, A. R., Mabie, W. C., & Moretti, M. (1987). A comparison of labetalol plus hospitalization versus hospitalization alone in the management of preeclampsia remote from term. *Obstetrics and Gynecology, 70*(3, Pt. 1), 323–327.

Sibai, B. M., Gordon, T., Thom, E., Caritis, S. N., Klebanoff, M., McNellis, D., Paul, R. H., & National Institute of Child Health and Human Development Network of Maternal-Fetal Medicine Units. (1995). Risk factors for preeclampsia in healthy nulliparous women: A prospective multicenter study. *American Journal of Obstetrics and Gynecology, 172*(2, Pt. 1), 642–648.

Sibai, B. M., Mercer, B. M., Schiff, E., & Friedman, S. A. (1994). Aggressive versus expectant management of severe preeclampsia at 28 to 32 weeks' gestation: A randomized controlled trial. *American Journal of Obstetrics and Gynecology, 171*(3), 818–822.

Siddiqi, T., Rosenn, B., Mimouni, F., Khoury, J., & Miodouink, M. (1991). Hypertension during pregnancy in insulin-dependent diabetic women. *Obstetrics and Gynecology, 77*(4), 514–519.

Simon, P., Fauchet, R., Pilorge, M., Calvez, C., Le Fiblee, B., Cam, G., Ang, K. S., Genctet, B., & Cloup, B. (1988). Association of HLADR4 with the risk of recurrence of pregnancy hypertension. *Kidney International, 25*, S125–S128.

Simpson, K. R., Luppi, C. J., & O'Brien-Abel, N. (1998). Acute fatty liver of pregnancy. *Journal of Perinatal and Neonatal Nursing, 11*(4), 35–44.

Slattery, M. A., Khong, T. Y., Dawkins, R. R., Pridmore, B. R., & Hague, W. M. (1993). Eclampsia in association with partial molar pregnancy and congenital abnormalities. *American Journal of Obstetrics and Gynecology, 169*(6), 1625–1627.

Spellacy, W. N., Miller, S. J., & Winegar, A. (1986). Pregnancy after 40 years of age. *Obstetrics and Gynecology, 68*(4), 452–454.

Taylor, D. J. (1988). Epidemiology of hypertension during pregnancy. In P. C. Rubin (Ed.), *Handbook of hypertension: Hypertension in pregnancy* (pp. 223–240). New York: Elsevier.

Tervila, L., Vartianen, E., Timonen, S., & Kauppinen, M. (1975). The urine-plasma ratio of some proteins in gestosis. *Acta Obstetricia et Gynecologica Scandinavia, 54*(1), 85–88.

The Eclampsia Collaborative Group. (1995). Which anticonvulsant for women with eclampsia? Evidence from the collaborative eclampsia trial. *Lancet, 345*(89623), 1455–1463.

Thompson, S. A., Lyons, T. L., & Makowski, E. L. (1987). Outcomes of twin gestations at the University of Colorado Health Sciences Center, 1973–1983. *Journal of Reproductive Medicine, 32*(5), 328–339.

Thornton, J. G., & Onwude, J. L. (1991). Pre-eclampsia: Discordance among identical twins. *British Medical Journal, 303*(6812), 1241–1242.

Ventura, S. J., Martin, J. A., Curtin, S. C., Mathews, T. J., & Park, M. M. (2000). Births: Final data for 1998. *National Vital Statistics Reports, 48*(3), 1–100.

Villar, M. A., & Sibai, B. M. (1989). Clinical significance of elevated mean arterial blood pressure in second trimester and threshold increase in systolic and diastolic blood pressure during third trimester. *American Journal of Obstetrics and Gynecology, 160*(2), 419–423.

Ward, K., Hata, A., Jeunemaitre, X., Helin, C., Nelson, L., Namikawa, C., Farrington, P. F., Ogasawera, M., Suzumori, K., & Tomoda, S. (1993). A molecular variant of angiotensinogen associated with preeclampsia. *Nature Genetics, 4*(1), 59–61.

Weinstein, L. (1982). Syndrome of hemolysis, elevated liver enzymes, and low platelet count: A severe consequence of hypertension in pregnancy. *American Journal of Obstetrics and Gynecology, 142*(2), 159–167.

Weinstein, L. (1985). Preeclampsia/eclampsia with hemolysis, elevated liver enzymes, and thrombocytopenia. *Obstetrics and Gynecology, 66*(5), 657–660.

White, P. (1935). Pregnancy complicating diabetes. *Surgical Gynecology and Obstetrics, 61*, 324–332.

Yamamoto, T., Takahashi, Y., Geshi, Y., Sasamori, Y., & Mori, H. (1996). Anti-phospholipid antibodies in preeclampsia and their binding ability for placental villous lipid fractions. *Journal of Obstetric and Gynaecologic Research, 22*(3), 275–283.

Zeeman, G. G., Dekker, G. A., van Geijn, H. P., & Kraayenbrink, A. A. (1992). Endothelial function in normal and pre-eclamptic pregnancy: A hypothesis. *European Journal of Obstetric and Gynecologic Reproductive Biology, 43*(2), 113–122.

Bleeding

Abouleish, E., Joumaa, A. B., Lopez, M., & Gupta, D. (1995). *British Journal of Anesthesia, 75*(4), 486–487.

American College of Obstetricians and Gynecologists. (1998a). *Obstetric aspects of trauma management* (Educational Bulletin No. 251). Washington, DC: Author.

American College of Obstetricians and Gynecologists. (1998b). *Postpartum hemorrhage* (Educational Bulletin No. 243). Washington, DC: Author.

American College of Obstetricians and Gynecologists (1999a). *Induction of labor* (Practice Bulletin No. 10). Washington, DC: Author.

American College of Obstetricians and Gynecologists (1999b). *Induction of labor with misoprostol* (Committee Opinion No. 228). Washington, DC: Author.

American College of Obstetricians and Gynecologists. (1999c). *Vaginal birth after previous cesarean delivery* (Educational Bulletin No. 5). Washington, DC: Author.

Ananth, C. V., Savitz, D. A., & Williams, M. A. (1996). Placental abruption and its association with hypertension and prolonged rupture of membranes: A methodologic review and meta-analysis. *Obstetrics and Gynecology, 88*(2), 309–318.

Ananth, C. V., Smulian, J. C., & Vintzileos, A. M. (1997). The association of placenta previa with history of cesarean delivery and abortion: A meta-analysis. *American Journal of Obstetrics and Gynecology, 177*(5), 1071–1078.

Barth, W. H., Jr. (1997). Severe acute asthma in pregnancy. In S. L. Clark, D. B. Cotton, G. D. V. Hankins, & J. P. Phelan (Eds.), Critical care obstetrics (3rd ed., pp. 325–346). Boston: Blackwell Scientific.

Bennett, B. B. (1997). Uterine rupture during induction of labor at term with intravaginal misoprostol. *Obstetrics and Gynecology, 89*(5, Pt. 1), 832–833.

Berg, C. J., Atrash, H. K., Koonin, L. M., & Tucker, M. (1996). Pregnancy-related mortality in the United States, 1987–1990. *Obstetrics and Gynecology,* 88 (2), 161–167.

Blanco, J. D., Collins, M., Willis, D., & Prien, S. (1992). Prostaglandin E_2 gel induction of patients with a prior low transverse cesarean section. *American Journal of Perinatology, 9*(2), 80–83.

Brar, H. S., Greenspoon, J. S., Platt, L. D., & Paul, R. H. (1989). Acute puerperal inversion: New approaches to management. *The Journal of Reproductive Medicine, 34*(2), 173–177.

Centers for Disease Control and Prevention. (1999). State-specific maternal mortality among black and white women—United States, 1987–1996. *Morbidity and Mortality Weekly Report, 48*(23), 492–496.

Chan, C. C., & To, W. W. (1999). Antepartum hemorrhage of unknown origin-what is its clinical significance? *Acta Obstetricia et Gynecologica Scandinavica, 78*(3), 186–190.

Chelmow, D., Andrew, D. E., & Baker, E. R. (1996). Maternal cigarette smoking and placenta previa. *Obstetrics and Gynecology, 87*(5, Pt. 4), 703–706.

Clark, S. L. (1997). Hypovolemic shock. In S. L. Clark, D. B. Cotton, G. D. V. Hankins, & J. P. Phelan (Eds.), *Critical care obstetrics* (3rd ed., pp. 412–422). Boston: Blackwell Scientific.

Clark, S. L. (1999). Placenta previa and abruptio placenta. In R. K. Creasy & R. Resnick (Eds.), *Maternal-fetal medicine* (4th ed., pp. 616–631). Philadelphia: W.B. Saunders.

Clark, S. L., Koonings, P. P., & Phelan, J. P. (1985). Placenta previa/accreta and prior cesarean section. *Obstetrics and Gynecology, 66*(1), 89–92.

Clark, S. L., Greenspoon, J. S., Aldahl, D., & Phelan, J. P. (1986). Severe preeclampsia with persistent oliguria: Management of hemodynamic subsets. *American Journal of Obstetrics and Gynecology, 154*(3), 490–494.

Cunha, M., Bugalho, A., Bique, C., & Bergstrom, S. (1999). Induction of labor by vaginal misoprostol in patients with previous cesarean delivery. *Acta Obstetricia et Gynecologica Scandinavica, 78*(7), 653–654.

Cunningham, F. G., McDonald, P. C., Gant, N. F., Leveno, K. J., Gilstrap, L. C., Hanking, G. D., & Clark, S. L. (1997). *Williams obstetrics* (20th ed.). Stamford, CT: Appleton & Lange.

Curet, M. J., Schermer, C. R., Demarest, G. B., Bieneik, E. J., III, & Curet, L. B. (2000). Predictors of outcome in trauma during pregnancy: Identification of patients who can be monitored for less than 6 hours. *Journal of Trauma, 49*(1), 18–25.

Daddario, J. (1999). Trauma in pregnancy. In L. Mandeville & N. Troiano (Eds.), *High-risk and critical care intrapartum nursing* (2nd ed., pp. 322–352). Philadelphia: J.B. Lippincott.

Dansereau, J., Joshi, A. K., Helewa, M. E., Doran, T. A., Lange, I. R., Luther, E. R., Farine, D., Schulz, M. L., Horbay, G. L., Griffin, P., & Wassenaar, W. (1999). Double-blind comparison of carbetocin versus oxytocin in prevention of uterine atony after cesarean section. *American Journal of Obstetrics and Gynecology, 180*(3, Pt. 1), 670–676.

Dayan, S. S., & Schwalbe, S. S. (1996). The use of small-dose intravenous nitroglycerin in a case of uterine inversion. *Anesthesia and Analgesia 82*(5), 1091–1093

Dubois, J., Garel, L., Grignon, A., Lemay, M., & Leduc, L. (1997). Placenta percreta: Balloon occlusion and embolization of the internal iliac arteries to reduce intraoperative blood losses. *American Journal of Obstetrics and Gynecology, 176*(3), 723–726.

Frederiksen, M. C., Glassenberg, R., & Stika, C. S. (1999). Placenta previa: A 22 year analysis. *Obstetrics and Gynecology, 180*(6, Pt. 1), 1432–1437.

Grubb, D. K., Kjos, S. L., & Paul, R. H. (1996). Latent labor with an unknown uterine scar. *Obstetrics and Gynecology, 88*(3), 351–355.

Gupton, A., Heaman, M., & Ashcroft, T. (1997). Bed rest from the perspective of the high-risk pregnant woman. *Journal of Obstetric, Gynecologic and Neonatal Nursing, 26*(4), 423–430.

Holt, V. L., & Mueller, B. A. (1997). Attempt and success rates for vaginal birth after caesarean section in relation to complications of the previous pregnancy. *Paediatric and Perinatal Epidemiology, 11*(Suppl. 1), S63–S72.

Hudon, L., Belfort, M. A., & Broome, D. R. (1998). Diagnosis and management of placenta percreta: A review. *Obstetrical and Gynecological Survey, 53*(8), 509–517.

Hung, T. H., Shau, W. Y., Hsieh, C. C., Chiu, T. H., Hsu, J. J., & Hsieh, T. T. (1999). Risk factors for placenta accreta. *Obstetrics and Gynecology, 93*(4) 545–550.

Jones, W. K. (2000). *Safe motherhood: Preventing pregnancy-related illness and death.* Washington, DC: National Center for Chronic Disease Prevention and Health Promotion.

Johnson, C., Oriol, N., & Flood, K. (1991). Trial of labor: A study of 110 patients. *Journal of Clinical Anesthesiology, 3*(3), 216–218.

Knab, D. R. (1978). Abruptio placenta: An assessment of the time and method of delivery. *Obstetrics and Gynecology, 52*(5), 625–629.

Kupferminc, M. J., Gull, I., Bar-Am, A., Daniel, Y., Jaffa, A., Shenhav, M., & Lessing, J. B. (1998). Intrauterine irrigation with prostaglandin F2-alpha for management of severe postpartum hemorrhage. *Acta Obstetricia et Gyneclogica Scaninavica, 77*(5), 548–550.

Leung, A. S., Farmer, R., Leung, E. K., Medearis, A. L., & Paul, R. H. (1993). Risk factors associated with uterine rupture during trial of labor after cesarean delivery: A case control study. *American Journal of Obstetrics and Gynecology, 168*(5), 1358–1363.

Love, C. D., & Wallace, E. M. (1996). Pregnancies complicated by placenta praevia: What is appropriate management? *British Journal of Obstetrics and Gynaecology, 103*(9), 864–867.

Lowe, T. W., & Cunningham, F. G. (1990). Placental abruption. *Clinical Obstetrics and Gynecology, 33*(3), 406–413.

Macones, G. A., Sehdev, H. M., Parry, S., Morgan, M. A., & Berlin, J. A. (1997). The association between maternal cocaine use and placenta previa. *American Journal of Obstetrics and Gynecology, 177*(5), 1097–1100.

Mahon, T. R., Chazotte, C., & Cohen, W. R. (1994). Short labor: Characteristics and outcome. *Obstetrics and Gynecology, 84*(1), 47–51.

Maloni, J. H. (1998). *Antepartum bedrest: Case studies, research and nursing care* (Symposia). Washington, DC: Association of Women's Health, Obstetric and Neonatal Nurses.

Menihan, C. A. (1998). Uterine rupture in women attempting a vaginal birth following prior cesarean birth. *Journal of Perinatology 18*(6, Pt. 1) 440–443.

Menihan, C. A. (1999). Clinical practice exchange: The effect of uterine rupture on fetal heart rate patterns. *Journal of Nurse-Midwifery, 44*(1), 40–46.

Miller, D. A., Chollet, J. A., & Goodwin, T. M. (1997). Clinical risk factors for placenta previa-placenta accreta. *American Journal of Obstetrics and Gynecology, 177*(1), 210–214.

Miller, D., Diaz, F., & Paul, R. (1994). Vaginal birth after cesarean: A 10 year experience. *Obstetrics and Gynecology, 84*(2), 255–258.

Norman, M., & Ekman, G. (1992). Preinductive cervical ripening with prostaglandin E_2 in women with one previous cesarean section. *Acta Obstetricia et Gynecologica Scandinavica, 71*(5), 351–355.

O'Brien, W. F. (1993). Puerperal complications. In T. R. Moore, R. C. Reiter, R. W. Rebar, & V. V. Baker (Eds.), *Gynecology and obstetrics: A longitudinal approach* (pp. 637–654). New York: Churchill Livingstone.

Odunsi, K., Bullough, C., Henzel, J., & Polanska, A. (1996). Evaluation of chemical tests for fetal bleeding from vasa previa. *International Journal of Obstetrics and Gynecology, 55*(3), 207–212.

Oyelese, K. O., Turner, M., Lees, C., & Campbell, S. (1999). Vasa previa: An avoidable obstetric tragedy. *Obstetrical and Gynecological Survey, 54*(2), 138–145.

Page, E. W., & Christianson, R. (1976). The impact of mean arterial pressure in the middle trimester upon the outcome of pregnancy. *American Journal of Obstetrics and Gynecology, 125*(6), 740–746.

Pearlman, M. D. (1997). Motor vehicle crashes: Pregnancy loss and preterm labor. *International Journal of Obstetrics and Gynaecology, 57*(2), 127–132.

Plaut, M. M., Schwartz, M. L., & Lubarsky, S. L. (1999). Uterine rupture associated with use of misoprostol in the gravid patient with a previous cesarean section. *American Journal of Obstetrics and Gynecology, 180*(6, Pt. 1), 1535–1542.

Rageth, J. C., Juzi, C., & Grossenbacher, H. (1999). Delivery after previous cesarean: A risk evaluation. *Obstetrics and Gynecology, 93*(3), 332–337.

Rasmussen, S., Irgens, L. M., & Dalaker, K. (1997). The effect on the likelihood of further pregnancy of placental abruption and the rate of its recurrence. *British Journal of Obstetrics and Gynecology, 104*(11), 1292–1295.

Rebarber, A., Odunsi, K., Baumgarten, A., Copel, J., & Sipes, S. (1998). In vitro assessment of fetal contamination of human blood processed through the Cell-Saver 5 (CS5) at cesarean section (C/S). *American Journal of Obstetrics and Gynecology, 178*(Suppl. 1), 80S.

Rebarber, A., Lonser, R., Jackson, S., Copel, J., & Sipes, S. (1998). The safety of intraoperative autologous blood collection and autotransfusion during cesarean section. *American Journal of Obstetrics and Gynecology, 179*(3, Pt. 1), 715–720.

Reis, P. M., Sander, C. M., & Pearlman, M. D. (2000). Abruptio placentae after auto accidents: A case control study. *Journal of Reproductive Medicine, 45*(1), 6–10.

Rosen, M. G., Dickinson, J. C., & Westhoff, C. L. (1991). Vaginal birth after cesarean: A meta-analysis of morbidity and mortality. *Obstetrics and Gynecology, 77*(3), 465–470.

Sciscione, A. C., Nguyen, L., Manley, J. S., Shlossman, P. A., & Colmorgen, G. H. (1998). Uterine rupture during preinduction cervical ripening with misoprostol in a patient with a previous cesarean delivery. *Australian New Zealand Journal of Obstetrics and Gynaecology, 38*(1), 96–97.

Sherer, D. M., & Anyaegbunam, A. (1997). Perinatal ultrasonographic morphologic assessment of the umbilical cord: A review, Part I. *Obstetrical and Gynecological Survey, 52*(8), 506–514.

Shipp, T., Zelop, C., Repke, J., Cohen, A., Caughey, A., & Lieberman, E. (1999). Uterine rupture during a trial of labor comparing a lower segment vertical incision to a lower segment transverse incision. *American Journal of Obstetrics and Gynecology, 180*(Suppl. 1), S112.

Signore, C. C., Sood, A. K., & Richards, D. S. (1998). Second-trimester vaginal bleeding: Correlation of ultrasonographic findings with perinatal outcome. *American Journal of Obstetrics and Gynecology, 178*(2), 336–340.

Simpson, K. R., Luppi, C. J., & O'Brien-Abel, N. (1998). Acute fatty liver of pregnancy. *Journal of Perinatal and Neonatal Nursing, 11*(4), 35–44.

Taipale, P., Hiilesmaa, V., & Ylostalo, P. (1997). Diagnosis of placenta previa by transvaginal sonographic screening as 12–16 weeks in a nonselected population. *Obstetrics and Gynecology, 89*(3), 364–367.

Thorp, J. M., Jr. (1993). Third-trimester bleeding. In T. R. Moore, R. C. Reiter, R. W. Rebar, & V. V. Baker (Eds.), *Gynecology and obstetrics: A longitudinal approach* (pp. 479–485). New York: Churchill Livingstone.

Thorp, J. M., Jr., Wells, S. R., Wiest, H. H., Jeffries, L., & Lyles, E. (1998). First-trimester diagnosis of placenta previa percreta by magnetic resonance imaging. *American Journal of Obstetrics and Gynecology, 178*(3), 616–618.

Veronikis, D. K., & O'Grady, J. P. (1994). What to do-or not to do-for postpartum hemorrhage. *Contemporary OB/GYN, 39*(8), 11–18.

Wheeler, T. C., Anderson, T. L., Kelly, J., & Boehm, F. H. (1996). Placenta previa increta diagnosed at 18 weeks gestation: Report of a case with sonographic and pathologic correlation. *Journal of Reproductive Medicine, 41*(3), 198–200.

Wing, D. A., Lovett, K., & Paul, R. H. (1998). Disruption of prior uterine incision following misoprostol for labor induction in women with previous cesarean delivery. *Obstetrics and Gynecology, 91*(5, Pt. 2), 828–830.

Wing, D. A., & Paul, R. H. (1999). Vaginal birth after cesarean section: Selection and management. *Clinical Obstetrics and Gynecology, 42*(4), 836–848.

Wing, D. A., Paul, R. H., & Millar, L. K. (1996). Management of the symptomatic placenta previa: A randomized, controlled trial of inpatient versus outpatient expectant management. *American Journal of Obstetric and Gynecology, 175*(4, Pt. 1), 806–811.

Witlin, A. G., Saade, G. R., Mattar, F., & Sibai, B. M. (1999). Risk factors for abruptio placentae and eclampsia: Analysis of 445 consecutively managed women with severe preeclampsia and eclampsia. *American Journal of Obstetrics and Gynecology, 180*(6, Pt. 1), 1322–1329.

Zahn, C. M., & Yeomans, E. R. (1990). Postpartum hemorrhage: Placenta accreta, uterine inversion, and puerperal hematomas. *Clinical Obstetrics and Gynecology, 33*(3), 422–431.

Zelop, C., Shipp, T., Cohen, A., Repke, J. T., & Lieberman, E. (2000). Outcomes of trial of labor following previous cesarean beyond the estimated date of delivery. *Obstetrics and Gynecology, 94*(4, Suppl. 1), S79.

Preterm Labor and Birth

Abrams, B., Newman, V., Key, T., & Parker, J. (1989). Maternal weight gain and preterm delivery. *Obstetrics and Gynecology, 74*(4), 577–583.

American Academy of Pediatrics & American College of Obstetricians and Gynecologists. (1997). *Guidelines for perinatal care* (4th ed.). Elk Grove Village, IL: Author.

American College of Obstetricians and Gynecologists. (1995). *Preterm labor* (Technical Bulletin No. 206). Washington, DC: Author.

American College of Obstetricians and Gynecologists. (1996a). *Home uterine activity monitoring* (Committee Opinion No. 172). Washington, DC: Author.

American College of Obstetricians and Gynecologists. (1996b). *Nutrition and women* (Educational Bulletin No. 229). Washington, DC: Author.

American College of Obstetricians and Gynecologists. (1998). *Special problems of multiple gestation* (Educational Bulletin No. 253). Washington, DC: Author.

American College of Obstetricians and Gynecologists. (2000). *Smoking cessation* (Educational Bulletin No. 260). Washington, DC: Author.

Banks, B. A., Cnaan, A., Morgan, M. A., Parer, J. T., Merrill, J. D., Ballard, P. L., Ballard, R. A., & the North American Thyrotropin-Releasing Hormone Study Group. (1999). Multiple courses of antenatal corticosteroids and the outcome of premature neonates. *American Journal of Obstetrics and Gynecology, 181*(3), 709–717.

Basso, O., Olsen, J., Knudsen, L. B., & Christensen, K. (1998). Low birth weight and preterm birth after short interpregnancy intervals. *American Journal of Obstetrics and Gynecology, 178*(2), 259–263.

Besinger, R. E., Niebyl, J. R., Keyes, W. G., & Johnson, T. R. (1991). Randomized comparative trial of indomethacin and ritodrine for the long term treatment of preterm labor. *American Journal of Obstetrics and Gynecology, 164*(4), 981–988.

Brown, H. L., Britton, K. A., Brizendine, E. J., Hiett, A. K., Ingram, D., Turnquest, M. A., Golichowski, A. M., & Abernathy, M. P. (1999). A randomized comparison of home uterine activity monitoring in the outpatient management of women treated for preterm labor. *American Journal of Obstetrics and Gynecology, 180*(4), 798–805.

Brown, H. L., Watkins, K., & Hiett, K. (1996). The impact of the Women, Infants, and Children Food Supplement Program on birth outcome. *American Journal of Obstetrics and Gynecology, 174*(4), 1279–1283.

Carey, J. C., Klebanoff, M. A., Hauth, J. C., Hillier, S. L., Thom, E. A., Ernest, J. M., Heine, R. P., Nugent, R. P., Fischer, M. L., Leveno, K. J., Wapner, R., Varner, M., Trout, W., Moawad, A., Sibai, B. M., Miodovnik, M., Dombrowski, M., O'Sullivan, M. J., Van Dorsten, P., Langer, O., & Roberts, J. (2000). Metronidazole to prevent preterm delivery in pregnant women with asymptomatic bacterial vaginosis. The National Institute of Child Health and Human Development Network of Maternal Fetal Medicine Units. *New England Journal of Medicine, 342*(8), 534–40.

Carmichael, S. L., & Abrams, B. (1997). A critical review of the relationship between gestational weight gain and preterm delivery. *Obstetrics and Gynecology, 89*(5, Pt. 2), 865–873.

Cnattingius, S., Granath, F., Petersson, G., & Harlow, B. L. (1999). The influence of gestational age and smoking habits on the risk of subsequent preterm deliveries. *New England Journal of Medicine 341*(13), 943–948.

Cogswell, M. E., & Yip, R. (1995). The influence of fetal and maternal factors on the distribution of birth weight. *Seminars in Perinatology, 19*(3), 222–240.

Cole, F. S. (2000). Extremely preterm birth: Defining the limits of hope. *New England Journal of Medicine, 343*(6), 429–430.

Collaborative Group on Preterm Birth Prevention (1993). Multicenter randomized controlled trial of a preterm birth prevention program. *American Journal of Obstetrics and Gynecology, 169*(2, Pt. 1) 352–366.

Copper, R. L., Goldenberg, R. L., Das, A., Elder, N., Swain, M., Norman, G., Ramsey, R., Cotroneo, P., Collins, B. A., Johnson, F., Jones, P., Meier, A. M., & the National Institute of Child Health and Human Development Maternal Fetal Medicine Units Network. (1996). The preterm prediction study: Maternal stress is associated with spontaneous preterm birth at less than thirty-five weeks' gestation. *American Journal of Obstetrics and Gynecology, 175*(5), 1286–1292.

Crane, J. M., Van den Hof, M., Armson, B. A., & Liston, R. (1997). Transvaginal ultrasound in the prediction of preterm delivery: Singleton and twin gestations. *Obstetrics and Gynecology, 90*(3), 357–363.

Creasy, R. K., & Merkatz, I. R. (1990). Prevention of preterm birth: A clinical opinion. *Obstetrics and Gynecology, 76*(1, Suppl.), 2S–4S.

Curtin, S. C., & Martin, J. A. (2000). Births: Preliminary data for 1999. *National Vital Statistics Report, 48*(14), 1–24.

Curry, M. A., Perrin, N., & Wall, E. (1998). Effects of abuse on maternal complications and birthweight in adult and adolescent women. *Obstetrics and Gynecology, 92*(4, Pt. 1), 530–534.

Davies, B. L., Stewart, P. J., Sprague, A. E., Niday, P. A., Nimrod, C. A., & Dulberg, C. S. (1998). Education of women about the prevention of preterm birth. *Canadian Journal of Public Health, 89*(4), 260–263.

Dyson, D. C., Danbe, K. H., Bamber, J. A., Crites, Y. M., Field, D. R., Maier, J. A., Newman, L. A., Ray, D. A., Walton, D. L., & Armstrong, M. A. (1998). Monitoring women at risk for preterm labor. *New England Journal of Medicine, 338*(1), 15–19.

Elimian, A., Verma, U., Visintainer, P., & Tejani, N. (2000). Effectiveness of multidose antenatal steroids. *Obstetrics and Gynecology, 95*(1), 34–36.

Ellard, G. A., Johnstone, F. D., Prescott, R. J., Ji-Xian, W., & Jian-Hua, M. (1996). Smoking during pregnancy: The dose dependence of birth weight deficits. *British Journal of Obstetrics and Gynecology, 103*(8), 806–813.

Fiscella, K. (1996). Racial disparity in preterm births: The role of urogenital infections. *Public Health Reports, 111*(2), 104–113.

Freda, M. C., Anderson, H. F., Damus, K., Poust, D., Brustman, L., & Merkatz, I. R. (1990). Lifestyle modification as an intervention for inner city women at risk for preterm birth. *Journal of Advanced Nursing, 15*(3), 364– 372.

Freda, M. C., Damus, K., Andersen, H. F., Brustman, L. E., & Merkatz, I. R. (1990). A "PROPP" for the Bronx: Preterm birth prevention education in the inner city. *Obstetrics and Gynecology, 76*(1, Suppl.), S93–S96.

Freda, M. C., Damus, K., & Merkatz, I. R. (1991). What do pregnant women know about the prevention of preterm birth? *Journal of Obstetric, Gynecologic, and Neonatal Nursing, 20*(2), 140–145.

Freda, M. C., & DeVore, N. (1996). Should intravenous hydration be the first line of defense with threatened preterm labor? A critical review of the literature. *Journal of Perinatology 16*(5), 385–389.

French, N. P., Hagan, R., Evans, S. F., Godfrey, M., & Newnham, J. P. (1999). Repeated antenatal corticosteroids: Size at birth and subsequent development. *American Journal of Obstetrics and Gynecology, 180*(1, Pt 1), 114–121.

Freston, M. S., Young, S., Calhoun, S., Fredericksen, T., Salinger, L., Malchodi, C., & Egan, J. F. (1997). Responses of pregnant women to potential preterm labor symptoms. *Journal of Obstetric, Gynecologic, and Neonatal Nursing, 26*(1), 35–41.

Garcia-Velasco, J. A., & Gonzalez Gonzalez, A. (1998). A prospective, randomized trial of nifedipine vs. ritodrine in threatened preterm labor. *International Journal of Gynecology and Obstetrics, 61*(3), 239–244.

Gibbs, R. S., Romero, R., Hillier, S. L., Eschenbach, D. A., & Sweet, R. L. (1992). A review of premature birth and subclinical infection. *American Journal of Obstetrics and Gynecology, 166*(5), 1515–1528.

Goldenberg, R. L. (1994). The prevention of low birth weight and its sequelae. *Preventative Medicine, 23*(5), 627–631.

Goldenberg, R. L., Cliver, S. P., Bronstein, J., Cutter, G., Andrews, W., & Mennemeyer, S. (1994). Bed rest in pregnancy. *Obstetrics and Gynecology, 84*(1), 131–136.

Goldenberg, R. L., & Rouse, D. J. (1998). Prevention of premature birth. *New England Journal of Medicine, 339*(5), 313–320.

Goldenberg, R. L., & Williams, W. W. (1996). Intrauterine infection and why preterm prevention programs have failed. *American Journal of Public Health, 86*(6), 781–783.

Grimes, D. A., & Shulz, K. F. (1992). Randomized controlled trials of home uterine activity monitoring: A review and critique. *Obstetrics and Gynecology, 79*(1), 137–142.

Groff, J. Y., Mullen, P. D., Mongoven, M., & Burau, K. (1997). Prenatal weight gain patterns and infant birthweight associated with maternal smoking. *Birth, 24*(4), 234–239.

Guinn, D. A., Goepfert, A. R., Owen, J., Wenstrom, K. D., & Hauth, J. C. (1998). Terbutaline pump maintenance therapy for prevention of preterm delivery: A double-blind trial. *American Journal of Obstetrics and Gynecology, 179*(4), 874–878.

Hartmann, K., Thorp, J. M., Jr., McDonald, T. L., Savitz, D. A., & Granados, J. L. (1999). Cervical dimensions and risk of preterm birth: A prospective cohort study. *Obstetrics and Gynecology, 93*(4), 504–509.

Hauth, J. C., Goldenberg, R. L., Andrews, W. W., DuBard, M. B., & Copper, R. L. (1995). Reduced incidence of preterm delivery with metronidazole and erythromycin in women with bacterial vaginosis. *New England Journal of Medicine, 333*(26), 1732–1736.

Hellerstedt, W. L., Himes, J. H., Story, M., Alton, I. R., & Edwards, L. E. (1997), The effects of cigarette smoking and gestational weight change on birth outcomes in obese and normal-weight women. *American Journal of Public Health, 87*(4), 591–596.

Herron, M. A., Katz, M., & Creasy, R. K. (1982). Evaluation of a preterm birth prevention program: A preliminary report. *Obstetrics and Gynecology, 59*(4), 442–446.

Higby, K., Xenakis, E. M., & Pauerstein, C. J. (1993). Do tocolytic agents stop preterm labor? A critical and comprehensive review of efficacy and safety. *American Journal of Obstetrics and Gynecology, 168*(4), 1247–1256.

Hill, W. C., & Lambertz, E. L. (1990). Let's get rid of the term "Braxton-Hicks contractions." *Obstetrics and Gynecology, 75*(4), 709–710.

Hillier, S. L., Nugent, R. P., Eschenbach, D. A., Krohn, M. A., Gibbs, R. S., Martin, D. H., Cotch, M. F., Edelman, R., Pastorek, J. G., 2nd, Rao, A. V., McNellis, D., Regan, J., Carey, J. C., & Klebanoff, M. (1995). Association between bacterial vaginosis and preterm delivery of a low birth-weight infant. *New England Journal of Medicine, 333*(26), 1737–1742.

Hobel, C. J., Ross, M. G., Bemis, R. L., Bragonier, J., Jr., Nessim, S., Sandhu, M., Bear, M., & Mori, B. (1994). The West Los Angeles Preterm Birth Preventions Project I: Program impact on high-risk women. *American Journal of Obstetrics and Gynecology, 170*(1, Pt. 1), 54–62.

How, H. Y., Hughes, S. A., Vogel, R. L., Gall, S. A., Spinnato, J. A. (1995). Oral terbutaline in the outpatient management of preterm labor. *American Journal of Obstetrics and Gynecology, 173*(5), 1518–1522.

Iams, J. D., Johnson, F. F., & Parker, M. (1994). A prospective evaluation of the signs and symptoms of preterm labor. *Obstetrics and Gynecology, 84*(2), 227–230.

Iams, J. D., Stilson, R., Johnson, F. F., Williams, R. H., & Rice, R. (1990). Symptoms that precede preterm labor and preterm premature rupture of the membranes. *American Journal of Obstetrics and Gynecology, 162*(2), 486–490.

Institute of Medicine. (1985). *Preventing low birthweight.* Washington, DC: National Academy Press.

Joffe, G. M., Jacques, D., Bemis-Heys, R., Burton, R., Skram, B., & Shelburne, P. (1999). Impact of the fetal fibronectin assay on admissions for preterm labor. *American Journal of Obstetrics and Gynecology, 180*(3, Pt. 1), 581–586.

Jones, W. K. (2000). *Safe motherhood: Preventing pregnancy-related illness and death.* Washington, DC: National Center for Chronic Disease Prevention and Health Promotion.

Katz, V. L., & Farmer, R. M. (1999). Controversies in tocolytic therapy. *Clinical Obstetrics and Gynecology, 42*(4), 802–819.

Katz, M., Goodyear, K., & Creasy, R. K. (1990). Early signs and symptoms of preterm labor. *American Journal of Obstetrics and Gynecology, 162*(5), 1150–1153.

Katz, M., Gill, P. J., & Newman, R. B. (1986). Detection of preterm labor by ambulatory monitoring of uterine activity: A preliminary report. *Obstetrics and Gynecology, 68*(6), 773–778.

Kogan, M. D., Alexander, G. R., Kotelchuck, M., MacDorman, M. F., Buekens, P., Martin, J. A., & Papiernik, E. (2000). Trends in twin birth outcomes and prenatal care utilization in the United States, 1981–1997. *Journal of the American Medical Association, 284*(3), 335–341.

Lewis, R., Mercer, B. M., Salama, M., Walsh, M. A., & Sibai, B. M. (1996). Oral terbutaline after parenteral tocolysis: A randomized double-blind, placebo-controlled trial. *American Journal of Obstetrics and Gynecology, 175*(4, Pt. 1), 834–837.

Leviton, L. C., Goldenberg, R. L., Baker, C. S., Schwartz, R. M., Freda, M. C., Fish, L. J., Cliver, S. P., Rouse, D. J., Raczynski, J., Chazotte, C., Merkatz, I. R., & Raczynski, J. M. (1999). Methods to encourage the use of antenatal corticosteroid therapy for fetal maturation: A randomized controlled trial. *Journal of the American Medical Association, 281*(1), 46–52.

Lieberman, E., Lang, J. M., Ryan, K. J., Monson, R. R., & Schoenbaum, S. C. (1989). The association of inter-pregnancy interval with small for gestational age births. *Obstetrics and Gynecology, 74*(1), 1–5.

Lockwood, C. J. (1994). Recent advances in elucidating the pathogenesis of preterm delivery, the detection of patients at risk, and preventative therapies. *Current Opinion in Obstetrics and Gynecology, 6*(1), 7–18.

Lockwood, C. J., Senyei, A. E., Desche, M. R., Casal, D., Shah, K. D., Thung, S. N., Jones, L., Deligdisch, L., & Garite, T. J. (1991). Fetal fibronectin in cervical and vaginal secretions as a predictor of preterm delivery. *New England Journal of Medicine, 325*(10), 669–674.

Lopez-Bernal, A., Watson, S. P., Phaneuf, S., & Europe-Finner, G. N. (1993). Biochemistry and physiology of preterm labor and delivery. *Ballieres Clinical Obstetrics and Gynecology, 7*(3), 523–552.

Lowe, J. B., Windsor, R., Balanda, K. P., & Woolby, L. (1997). Smoking relapse prevention methods for pregnant women: A formative evaluation. *American Journal of Health Promotion, 11*(4), 244–246.

Lynam, L. E., & Miller, M. A. (1992). Mothers' and nurses' perceptions of the needs of women experiencing preterm labor. *Journal of Obstetric, Gynecologic, and Neonatal Nursing, 21*(2), 126–136.

MacDorman, M. F., & Atkinson, J. O. (1999). Infant mortality statistics for the 1997 period linked birth/infant death data set. *National Vital Statistics Reports, 47*(23), 1–24.

Macones, G. A., Berlin, M., & Berlin, J. A., (1995). Efficacy of oral beta-agonist maintenance therapy in preterm labor: A meta-analysis. *Obstetrics and Gynecology, 85*(2), 313–317.

Macones, G. A., & Robinson, C. A. (1998). Is there justification for using indomethacin in preterm labor? An analysis of neonatal risks and benefits. *American Journal of Obstetrics and Gynecology, 177*(4), 819–824.

Macones, G. A., Sehdev, H. M., Berlin, M., Morgan, M. A., & Berlin, J. A. (1997). Evidence for magnesium sulfate as a tocolytic agent. *Obstetrical and Gynecological Survey, 52*(10), 652–658.

Main, D., & Gabbe, S. G. (1989). Risk scoring for preterm labor: Where do we go from here? *American Journal of Obstetrics and Gynecology, 157*(4, Pt. 1), 789–793.

Maloni, J. A., Chance, B., Zhang, C., Cohen, A. W., Betts, D., & Gange, S. J. (1993). Physical and psychosocial side effects of antepartum hospital bed rest. *Nursing Research, 42*(4), 197–203.

March of Dimes (1997). *Stat book.* White Plains, NY: March of Dimes Birth Defects Foundation.

McFarlane, J., & Gondolf, E. (1998). Preventing abuse during pregnancy: A clinical protocol. *MCN, The American Journal of Maternal- Child Nursing, 23*(1), 22–27.

Mercer, B. M., & Lewis, R. (1997). Preterm labor and preterm premature rupture of the membranes: Diagnosis and management. *Infectious Disease Clinics of North America, 11*(1), 177–201.

Mittendorf, R., Herschel, M., Williams, M. A., Hibbard, J. U., Moawad, A. H., & Lee, K. S. (1994). Reducing the frequency of low birthweight in the United States. *Obstetrics and Gynecology, 83*(6), 1056–1059.

Monga, M., & Creasy, R. K. (1995). Pharmacologic management of preterm labor. *Seminars in Perinatology, 19*(1), 84–96.

Moore, M. L., Elmore, T., Ketner, M., Wagoner, S., & Walsh, K. (1995). Reduction and cessation of smoking in pregnant women: The effect of a telephone intervention. *Journal of Perinatal Education, 4*(1), 35–39.

Moore, M. L., Meis, P. J., Ernest, J. M., Wells, H. B., Zaccaro, D. J., & Terrell, T. (1998). A randomized trial of nurse intervention to reduce preterm and low birth weight births. *Obstetrics and Gynecology, 91*(5, Pt. 1), 656–661.

Moore, M. L., & Freda, M. C. (1998). Reducing preterm and low birthweight births: Still a nursing challenge. *MCN, The American Journal of Maternal-Child Nursing, 23*(4), 200–209.

Moore, M. L. (1999). Biochemical markers for preterm birth: What is their role in caring for pregnant women? *MCN, The American Journal of Maternal-Child Nursing, 24*(2), 80–86.

Moore, M. L., & Zaccaro, D. J. (2000). Cigarette smoking, low birthweight and preterm births in low income African American women. *Journal of Perinatology 20*(3), 176–80.

Morrison, J. C., Martin, J. N., Jr., Martin, R. W., Gookin, K. S., & Wiser, W. L. (1987). Prevention of preterm birth by ambulatory assessment of uterine activity: A randomized study. *American Journal of Obstetrics and Gynecology, 156*(3), 536–543.

Mozurkewich, E. L., Naglie, G., Krahn, M. D., & Hayashi, R. H. (2000). Predicting preterm birth: A cost effective analysis. *American Journal of Obstetrics and Gynecology, 182*(6), 1589–1598.

Mullen, P. D., Richardson, M. A., Quinn, V. P., & Ershoff, D. H. (1997). Postpartum return to smoking: Who is at risk and when. *American Journal of Health Promotion, 11*(5), 323–330.

National Center for Health Statistics. (1998). Maternal mortality: United States, 1982–1996. *Morbidity and Mortality Weekly Report, 47*(34), 705–707.

National Institutes of Health Consensus Development Panel on the Effect of Corticosteroids for Fetal Lung Maturation and Perinatal Outcomes. (1995). Effect of corticosteroids for fetal maturation on perinatal outcomes. *Journal of the American Medical Association, 273*(5), 413–418.

Nickolson, W. K., Frick, K. D., & Powe, N. R. (2000). Economic burden of hospitalizations for preterm labor in the United States. *Obstetrics and Gynecology, 96*(1), 95–101.

Nightingale, S. L. (1998). Warning on use of terbutaline sulfate for preterm labor: From the food and drug administration. *Journal of the American Medical Association, 279*(1), 9.

Nordentoft, M., Lou, H. C., Hansen, D., Nim, J., Pryds, O., Rubin, P., & Hemmingsen, R. (1996). Intrauterine growth retardation and premature delivery: The influence of maternal smoking and psychological factors. *American Journal of Public Health, 86*(3), 347–354.

O'Campo, P., Davis, M. V., & Gielen, A. C. (1995). Smoking cessation interventions for pregnant women: Review and future directions. *Seminars in Perinatology, 19*(4), 279–285.

O'Connor, A. M., Davies, B. L., Dulberg, C. S., Buhler, P. L., Nadon, C., McBride, B. H., & Benzie, R. J. (1992). Effectiveness of a pregnancy smoking cessation program. *Journal of Obstetric, Gynecologic, and Neonatal Nursing, 21*(5), 385–392.

Papiernik, E. (1989). *Effective prevention of preterm birth: The French experience at Hagenau.* New York: March of Dimes Birth Defects Foundation.

Parker, B., McFarlane, J., & Soeken, K. (1994). Abuse during pregnancy: effects on maternal complications and birthweight in adult and teenage women. *Obstetrics and Gynecology, 84*(3), 323–328.

Patterson, E. T., Douglas, A. B., Patterson, P. M., & Bradle, J. B. (1992). Symptoms of preterm labor and self-diagnostic confusion. *Nursing Research, 41*(6), 367–372.

Ricci, J. M., Hariharan, S., Helfgott, A., Reed, K., & O'Sullivan, M. J. (1991). Oral tocolysis with magnesium chloride: A randomized controlled prospective clinical trial. *American Journal of Obstetrics and Gynecology, 165*(3), 603–610.

Roberts, W. E., & Morrison, J. C. (1998). Has the use of home monitors, fetal fibronectin, and measurement of cervical length helped predict labor and/or prevent preterm delivery in twins? *Clinical Obstetrics and Gynecology, 41*(1), 94–102.

Rust, O. A., Bofill, J. A., Arriola, R. M., Andrews, M. E., & Morrison, J. C. (1996). The clinical efficacy of oral tocolytic therapy. *American Journal of Obstetrics and Gynecology, 175*(4, Pt. 1), 838–842.

Schieve, L. A., Cogswell, M. E., Scanlon, K. S., Perry, G., Ferre, C., Blackmore-Prince, C., Yu, S. M., & Rosenbery, D., for the NMHS Collaborative Working Group. (2000). Pregnancy body mass index and pregnancy weight gain: Associations with preterm birth. *Obstetrics and Gynecology, 96*(2), 194–200.

Sciscione, A. C., Stamilio, D. M., Manley, J. S., Shlossman, P. A., Gorman, R. T., & Colmorgen, G. H. (1998). Tocolysis of preterm contractions does not improve preterm delivery rates or perinatal outcomes. *American Journal of Perinatology, 15*(3), 177–81.

Secker-Walker, R. H., Vacek, P., Flynn, B., & Mead, P. (1997). Smoking in pregnancy, exhaled carbon monoxide and birth weight. *Obstetrics and Gynecology, 89*(5, Pt. 1), 648–653.

Seidman, D. S., Ever-Hadani, P., & Gale, R. (1989). The effect of maternal weight gain in pregnancy on birth weight. *Obstetrics and Gynecology, 74*(2), 240–246.

Simpson, W. J. (1957). A preliminary report on cigarette smoking and the incidence of prematurity. *American Journal of Obstetrics and Gynecology, 73*, 808–815.

St. John, E. B., Nelson, K. G., Cliver, S. P., Bishnoi, R. R., & Goldenberg, R. L. (2000). Cost of neonatal care according to gestational age at birth and survival status. *American Journal of Obstetrics and Gynecology, 182*(1, Pt. 1), 170–175.

Stevenson, D. K., Wright, L. L., Lemons, J. A., Oh, W., Korones, S. B., Papile, L., Bauer, C. R., Stoll, B. J., Tyson, J. E., Shankaran, S., Fanaroff, A. A., Donovan, E. F., Ehrenkranz, R. A., & Verter, J. (1998). Very low birth weight outcomes of the National Institute of Child Health and Human Development Neonatal Research Network: January 1993 through December 1994.

American Journal of Obstetrics and Gynecology, 179(6, Pt. 1), 1632–1639.

U.S. Public Health Service. (1989). *Caring for our future: The content of prenatal care.* Washington, DC: Author.

Valenzuela, G. J., Germain, A., & Foster, T. C. (1993). Physiology of uterine activity in pregnancy. *Current Opinion in Obstetrics and Gynecology, 5*(5), 640–646.

Ventura, S. J., Martin, J. A., Curtin, S. C., Mathews, T. J., & Park, M. M. (2000). Births: Final data for 1998. *National Vital Statistics Report, 48*(3), 1–100.

Viamontes, C. (1996). Pharmacologic intervention in the management of preterm labor: An update. *Journal of Perinatal and Neonatal Nursing, 9*(4), 13–30.

Vitoratos, N., Botsis, D., Girigoriou, O., Bettas, P., Papoulias, I., & Zourlas, P. A. (1997). Smoking and preterm labor. *Clinical and Experimental Obstetrics and Gynecology, 24*(4), 220–222.

Wadhwa, P. D., Porto, M.,. Garite, T. J., Chicz-DeMet, A., & Sandman, C. A. (1998). Maternal corticotropin-releasing hormone levels in the early third trimester predict length of gestation in human pregnancy. *American Journal of Obstetrics and Gynecology, 179*(4), 1079–1085.

Wenstrom, K. D., Weiner, C. P., Merrill, D., & Niebyl, J. (1995). A placebo-controlled randomized trial of the terbutaline pump for prevention of preterm delivery. *American Journal of Perinatology, 14*(2), 87–91.

Wisborg, K., Henriksen, T. B., Hedegaard, M., & Secher, N. J. (1996). Smoking during pregnancy and preterm birth. *British Journal of Obstetrics and Gynecology, 103*(8), 800–805.

Wood, N. S., Marlow, N., Costeloe, K., Gibson, A. T., & Wilkinson, A. R. for the EPICure Study Group. (2000). Neurologic and developmental disability after extremely preterm birth. *New England Journal of Medicine, 343*(6), 378–384.

Yost, N. P., Bloom, S. L., Twickler, M. D., & Leveno, K. L. (1999). Pitfalls in ultrasonic cervical length measurement for predicting preterm birth. *Obstetrics and Gynecology, 93*(4), 510–516.

Diabetes

American College of Obstetricians and Gynecologists. (1994). *Diabetes and pregnancy* (Technical Bulletin No. 200). Washington, DC: Author.

American Diabetes Association (1997). Report of the expert committee on the diagnosis and classification of diabetes mellitus. *Diabetes Care, 20*(7), 1183–1197.

American Diabetes Association (1999a). Continuous subcutaneous insulin infusion. *Diabetes Care, 22*(Suppl. 1), S87.

American Diabetes Association (1999b). Diabetes mellitus and exercise. *Diabetes Care, 22*(Suppl. 1), S49–S53.

American Diabetes Association (1999c). Gestational diabetes mellitus. *Diabetes Care, 22*(Suppl. 1), S74–S76.

American Dietetic Association (1993). Position of the American Dietetic Association: Use of nutritive and non-nutritive sweeteners. *Journal of the American Dietetic Association, 93*(7), 816–821.

Atilano, L. C., Lee-Parritz, A., Lieberman, E., Cohen, A. P., & Barbieri, R. L. (1999). Alternative methods of diagnosing gestational diabetes mellitus. *American Journal of Obstetrics and Gynecology, 181*(5, Pt. 1), 1158–1161.

Bartha, J. L., Martinez-Del-Fresno, P., & Comino-Delgado, R. (2000). Gestational diabetes mellitus diagnosed during early pregnancy. *American Journal of Obstetrics and Gynecology, 182*(2), 346–350.

Bevier, W. C., Fischer, R., & Jovanovic, L. (1999). Treatment of women with an abnormal glucose challenge test (but a normal oral glucose tolerance test) decreases the prevalence of macrosomia. *American Journal of Perinatology, 16*(6), 269–275.

Blank, A., Grave, G. D., & Metzger, B. E. (1995). Effects of gestational diabetes on perinatal morbidity reassessed. *Diabetes Care, 18*(1), 127–129.

Bloomgarden, Z. T. (1999). The European association for the study of diabetes annual meeting, 1998: Type 1 diabetes. *Diabetes Care, 22*(9), 1578–1583.

Boden, G. (1996). Fuel metabolism in pregnancy and gestational diabetes mellitus. *Obstetrics and Gynecology Clinics of North America, 23*(1), 1–10.

Bouhanick, B., Biquard, F., Hadjadj, S., & Roques, M. (2000). Does treatment with antenatal glucocorticoids for the risk of premature delivery contribute to ketoacidosis in pregnant women with diabetes who receive continuous subcutaneous insulin infusion (CSII)? *Archives in Internal Medicine, 160(2), 242–243.*

Boyd, K. L., Ross, E. K., & Sherman, S. J. (1995). Jelly beans as an alternative to a cola beverage containing 50 grams of glucose. *American Journal of Obstetrics and Gynecology, 173*(6), 1889–1892.

Buchanan, T. A., & Kitzmiller, J. L. (1994). Metabolic interactions of diabetes and pregnancy. *Annual Review of Medicine, 45,* 245–260.

Butte, N. F. (2000). Carbohydrate and lipid metabolism in pregnancy: Normal compared with gestational diabetes mellitus. *American Journal of Clinical Nutrition, 71*(Suppl. 5), S1256–S1261.

Carpenter, M. W. (2000). The role of exercise in pregnant women with diabetes mellitus. *Clinical Obstetrics and Gynecology, 43*(1), 56–64.

Carpenter, M. W., & Coustan, D. R. (1982). Criteria for screening tests for gestational diabetes. *American Journal of Obstetrics and Gynecology, 144*(7), 768–773.

Centers for Disease Control and Prevention. (1998). Diabetes during pregnancy-United States, 1993–1995. *Morbidity and Mortality Weekly Report, 47*(20), 408–414.

Chauhan, S. P., & Perry, K. G., Jr. (1995). Management of diabetic ketoacidosis in the obstetric patient. *Obstetrics and Gynecology Clinics of North America, 22*(1), 143–155.

Conway, D. L., & Langer, O. (1999). Effects of new criteria for type 2 diabetes on the rate of postpartum glucose intolerance in women with gestational diabetes. *American Journal of Obstetrics and Gynecology, 81*(3), 610–614.

Cordero, L., & Landon, M. B. (1993). Infant of the diabetic mother. *Clinics in Perinatology, 20*(3), 635–648.

Cullen, M. T., Reece, E. A., Homko, C. J., & Sivan, E. (1996). The changing presentations of diabetic ketoacidosis during pregnancy. *American Journal of Perinatology, 13*(7), 449–451.

Davidson, M. B., & Schwartz, S. (1998). Hyperglycemia. In M. M. Funnell (Ed.), *A core curriculum for diabetes education* (pp. 415–438). Chicago: American Association of Diabetes Educators.

Engelgau, M. M., Herman, W. H., Smith, P. J., German, R. R., & Aubert, R. E. (1995). The epidemiology of diabetes and pregnancy in the U.S., 1988. *Diabetes Care, 18*(7), 1029–1033.

Entrekin, K., Work, B., & Owen, J. (1998). Does a high carbohydrate preparatory diet affect the 3-hour oral glucose tolerance test in pregnancy? *Journal of Maternal-Fetal Medicine, 7*(2), 68–71.

Gabbe, S. G. (2000). New concepts and applications in the use of the insulin pump during pregnancy. *Journal of Maternal Fetal Medicine, 9*(1), 42–45.

Garner, P. (1995). Type 1 diabetes mellitus and pregnancy. *Lancet, 346*(8968), 157–159.

Hagay, Z. J. (1994). Diabetic ketoacidosis in pregnancy: Etiology, pathophysiology, and management. *Clinical Obstetrics and Gynecology, 37*(1), 39–49.

Hagay, Z. J., & Reece, E. A. (1992). Diabetes mellitus in pregnancy. In E. A. Reece, J. C. Hobbins, M. J. Mahoney, & R. H. Petrie (Eds.), *Medicine of the fetus and mother* (pp. 982–1020). Philadelphia: J.B. Lippincott.

Hagay, Z., & Weissman, A. (1996). Management of diabetic pregnancy complicated by coronary artery disease and neuropathy. *Obstetrics and Gynecology Clinics of North America, 23*(1), 205–220.

Harris, M. I., Flegal, K. M., Cowie, C. C. Eberhardt, M. S., Goldstein, D. E., Little, R. R., Wiedmeyer, H. M., & Byrd-Holt, D. D. (1998). Prevalence of diabetes, impaired fasting glucose, and impaired glucose tolerance in U.S. adults. *Diabetes Care, 21*(4), 518–524.

Harvey, M. G. (1992). Diabetic ketoacidosis during pregnancy. *Journal of Perinatal and Neonatal Nursing, 6*(1), 1–13.

Hirsch, I. B., McGill, J. B., Cryer, P. E., & White, P. F. (1991). Perioperative management of surgical patients with diabetes mellitus. *Anesthesiology, 74*(2), 346–359.

Homko, C. J. (1998). Gestational diabetes: A screening and management update. *Advance for Nurse Practitioners, 6*(12), 59–61, 63.

Homko, C. J., & Khandelwal, M. (1996). Glucose monitoring and insulin therapy during pregnancy. *Obstetrics and Gynecology Clinics of North America, 23*(1), 47–74.

Jornsay, D. L. (1998). Continuous subcutaneous insulin infusion (CSII) therapy during pregnancy. *Diabetes Spectrum, 11*(1), 26–32, 51.

Jovanovic, L. (2000). Role of diet and insulin treatment of diabetes in pregnancy. *Clinical Obstetrics and Gynecology, 43*(1), 46–55.

Jovanovic-Peterson, L., & Peterson, C. M. (1996). Rationale for prevention and treatment of glucose mediated macrosomia: A protocol for gestational diabetes. *Endocrine Practice,* 2, 118–119.

Jovanovic, L., Ilic, S., Pettitt, D. J., Hugo, K., Gutierrez, M., Bowsher, R. R., and Bastyr, E. J. (1999). Metabolic and immunologic effects of insulin Lispro in gestation diabetes. *Diabetes Care, 22*(9), 1422–1427.

Kendrick, J. M. (1997). *Diabetes in pregnancy* (Nursing Module). White Plains, NY: March of Dimes Birth Defects Foundation.

Kendrick, J. M. (1999). Diabetes mellitus in pregnancy. In L. K. Mandeville & N. H. Troiano (Eds.), *High risk and critical care intrapartum nursing* (pp. 224–254). Philadelphia: Lippincott Williams & Wilkins.

Kent, L. A., Gill, G. V., & Williams, G. (1994). Mortality and outcome of patients with brittle diabetes and recurrent ketoacidosis. *Lancet, 344*(8925), 778–781.

Kilvert, J. A., Nicholson, H. O., & Wright, A. D. (1993). Ketoacidosis in diabetic pregnancy. *Diabetic Medicine, 10*(3), 278–281.

Kitabchi, A. E., Young, R., Sacks, H. I., & Morris, L. (1979). Diabetic ketoacidosis: Reappraisal of therapeutic approach. *Annual Review of Medicine, 30*, 339–357.

Kjos, S. L. (2000). Postpartum care of women with diabetes. *Clinical Obstetrics and Gynecology, 43*(1), 75–86.

Klein, B. E., Moss, S. E., & Klein, R. (1990). Effect of pregnancy on progression of diabetic retinopathy. *Diabetes Care, 13*(1), 34–40.

Kousta, E., Lawrence, N. J., Penny, A., Millauer, B. A., Robinson, S., Dornhorst, A., de Swiet, M., Steer, P. J., Grenfell, A., Mather, H. M., Johnston, D. G., & McCarthy, M. I. (1999). Implications of new diagnostic criteria for abnormal glucose homeostasis in women with previous gestational diabetes. *Diabetes Care, 22*(6), 933–937.

Lamar, M. E., Kuehl, T. J., Cooney, A. T., Gayle, L. J., Holleman, S., & Allen, S. R. (1999). Jelly beans as an alternative to a fifty-gram glucose beverage for gestational diabetes screening. *American Journal of Obstetrics and Gynecology, 181*(5, Pt. 1), 1154–1157.

Landon, M. B. (2000). Obstetric management of pregnancies complicated by diabetes mellitus. *Clinical Obstetrics and Gynecology, 43*(1), 65–74.

Langer, O. (2000). Management of gestational diabetes. *Clinical Obstetrics and Gynecology, 43*(1), 106–115.

Langer, O., & Mazze, R. S. (1986). Diabetes in pregnancy: Evaluating self-monitoring performance and glycemic control with memory-based reflectance meters. *American Journal of Obstetrics and Gynecology, 155*(3), 635–637.

Langer, O., Brustman, L., Anyaegbunam, A., & Mazze, R. (1987). The significance of one abnormal glucose tolerance test value on adverse outcome in pregnancy. *American Journal of Obstetrics and Gynecology, 157*(3), 758–763.

Langer, O., Rodriguez, D. A., Xenakis, E. M., McFarland, M. B., Berkus, M. D., & Arrendondo, F. (1994). Intensified versus conventional management of gestational diabetes. *American Journal of Obstetrics and Gynecology, 170*(4), 1036–1046, discussion 1046–1047.

Lesser, K. B., & Carpenter, M. W. (1994). Metabolic changes associated with normal pregnancy and pregnancy complicated by diabetes mellitus. *Seminars in Perinatology, 18*(5), 399–406.

Macleod, A. F., Smith, S. A., Sonksen, P. H., & Lowy, C. (1990). The problem of autonomic neuropathy in diabetic pregnancy. *Diabetic Medicine, 7*(1), 80–82.

Major, C. A., de Veciana, M., Weeks, J., & Morgan, M. A. (1998). Recurrence of gestational diabetes: Who is at risk? *American Journal of Obstetrics and Gynecology, 179*(4), 1038–1042.

Mazze, R. S., Shamoon, H., Pasmantier, R., Lucido, D., Murphy, J., Hartmann, K., Kuykendall, V., & Lopatin, W. (1984). Reliability of blood-glucose monitoring by patients with diabetes mellitus. *American Journal of Medicine, 77*(2), 211–217.

McElvy, S. S., Miodovnik, M., Rosenn, B., Khoury, J. C., Siddiqi, T., Dignan, P. S., & Tsang, R. C. (2000). A focused preconceptional and early pregnancy program in women with type 1 diabetes reduces perinatal mortality and malformation rates to general population levels. *Journal of Maternal-Fetal Medicine, 9*(1), 14–20.

Metzger, B. E., & Coustan, D. R. (1998). Summary and recommendations of the Fourth International Workshop-Conference on Gestational Diabetes Mellitus: The Organizing Committee. *Diabetes Care, 21*(Suppl. 2), B161–B169.

Miller, E. H. (1994). Metabolic management of diabetes in pregnancy. *Seminars in Perinatology, 18*(5), 414–431.

Moore, T. R. (1999). Diabetes in pregnancy. In R. K. Creasy & R. Resnik (Eds.), *Maternal-fetal medicine: Principles and practice* (4th ed., pp. 964–995). Philadelphia: W.B. Saunders.

Moses, R. G. (1986). Assessment of reliability of patients performing SMBG with a portable reflectance meter with memory capacity (M-Glucometer). *Diabetes Care, 9*(6), 670–671.

Neiger, R., & Coustan, D. R.(1991). The role of repeat glucose tolerance tests in the diagnosis of gestational diabetes. *American Journal of Obstetrics and Gynecology, 165*(4, Pt. 1), 787–790.

Neiger, R., & Kendrick, J. (1994). Obstetric management of diabetes in pregnancy. *Seminars in Perinatology, 18*(5), 432–450.

Persson, B., & Hanson, U. (1996). Fetal size at birth in relation to quality of blood glucose control in pregnancies complicated by pregestational diabetes mellitus. *British Journal of Obstetrics and Gynaecology, 103*(5), 427–433.

Perucchini, D., Fischer, U., Spinas, G. A., Huch, R., Huch, A., & Lehmann, R. (1999). Using fasting plasma glucose concentrations to screen for gestational diabetes mellitus: Prospective population based study. *British Medical Journal, 319*(7213), 812–815.

Raychaudhuri, K., & Maresh, M. J. (2000). Glycemic control throughout pregnancy and fetal growth in insulin-dependent diabetes. *Obstetrics and Gynecology, 95*(2), 190–194.

Reece, E. A., & Homko, C. J. (1994). Infant of the diabetic mother. *Seminars in Perinatology, 18*(5), 459–469.

Reece, E. A., & Homko, C. J. (2000). Why do diabetic women deliver malformed infants? *Clinical Obstetrics and Gynecology, 43*(1), 32–45.

Reece, E. A., Homko, C. J., & Hagay, Z. (1995). When the pregnancy is complicated by diabetes. *Contemporary OB/GYN, 40*(7), 43–61.

Reece, E. A., Homko, C. J., & Hagay, Z. (1996). Diabetic retinopathy in pregnancy. *Obstetrics and Gynecology Clinics of North America, 23*(1), 161–171.

Rey, E., Attie, C., & Bonin, A. (1999). The effects of first-trimester diabetes control on the incidence of macrosomia. *American Journal of Obstetrics and Gynecology, 181*(1), 202–206.

Rosenn, B. M., & Miodovnik, M. (2000). Medical complications of diabetes mellitus in pregnancy. *Clinical Obstetrics and Gynecology, 43*(1), 17–31.

Schaefer, U. M., Songster, G., Xiang, A., Berkowitz, K., Buchanan, T. A., & Kjos, S. L. (1997). Congenital malformations in offspring of women with hyperglycemia first detected during pregnancy. *American Journal of Obstetrics and Gynecology, 177*(5), 1165–1171.

Shivvers, S. A., & Lucas, M. J. (1999). Gestational diabetes: Is the 50-g screening result > or = 200 mg/dL diagnostic? *Journal of Reproductive Medicine, 44*(8), 685–688.

Tyrala, E. E. (1996). The infant of the diabetic mother. *Obstetric and Gynecology Clinics of North America, 23*(1), 221–241.

Uvena-Celebrezze, J., & Catalano, P. M. (2000). The infant of the woman with gestational diabetes mellitus. *Clinical Obstetrics and Gynecology, 43*(1), 127–139.

White, P. (1949). Pregnancy complicating diabetes. *American Journal of Medicine, 7*, 609.

Whiteman, V. E., Homko, C. J., & Reece, E. A. (1996). Management of hypoglycemia and diabetic ketoacidosis in pregnancy. *Obstetrics and Gynecology Clinics of North America, 23*(1), 87–107.

Wiznitzer, A., & Reece, E. A. (1999). Assessment and management of pregnancy complicated by pregestational diabetes mellitus. *Pediatric Annals, 28*(9), 605–613.

Cardiac Disease

American College of Obstetricians and Gynecologists. (1992). *Cardiac disease in pregnancy* (Technical Bulletin No. 168). Washington, DC: Author.

Autore, C., Brauneis, S., Apponi, R., Commisso, C., Pinto, G., & Fedele, F. (1999). Epidural anesthesia for cesarean section in patients with hypertrophic cardiomyopathy: A report of three cases. *Anesthesiology, 90*(4), 1205–1207.

Bestetti, R. B. (1989). Cardiac involvement in the acquired immune deficiency syndrome. *International Journal of Cardiology, 22*(2), 143–146.

Bruce, I. N., Urowitz, M. B., Gladman, D. D., & Hallet, D. C. (1999). Natural history of hypercholesterolemia in systemic lupus erythematosus. *Journal of Rheumatology, 26*(10), 2137–2143.

Chan, W. S., & Ray, J. G. (1999). Low molecular weight heparin use during pregnancy: Issues of safety and practicality. *Obstetrical and Gynecological Survey, 54*(10), 649–654.

Clark, S. L. (1991). Structural cardiac disease in pregnancy. In S. L. Clark, G. D. V. Hankins, D. B. Cotton, & J. P. Phelans (Eds.), *Critical care obstetrics* (2nd ed.). Boston: Blackwell Scientific.

Criteria Committee of the New York Heart Association. (1979). *Nomenclature and criteria for diagnosis of diseases of the heart and great vessels* (8th ed.). New York: New York Heart Association.

Cunningham, F. G., Pritchard, J. A., Hankins, G. D. V., Anderson, P. L., Lucas, M. J., & Armstrong, K. F. (1986). Peripartum heart failure: Idiopathic cardiomyopathy or compounding cardiovascular events? *Obstetrics and Gynecology, 67*(2), 157–168.

DeAngelis, R. (1985). The cardiovascular system. In J. G. Alspach & S. M. Williams (Eds.), *Core curriculum for critical care nursing* (3rd ed., pp. 101–118). Philadelphia: W.B. Saunders.

deSwiet, M. (1993). Maternal mortality from heart disease in pregnancy. *British Heart Journal, 69*(6), 524.

Elkayam, U., Ostrzega, E., Shotan, A., & Mehra, A. (1995). Cardiovascular problems in pregnant women with the Marfan syndrome. *Annals of Internal Medicine 123*(2), 117–122.

Felblinger, D. M., & Akers, M. C. (1998). Marfan's syndrome in pregnancy: Implications for advanced practice nurses. *AACN Clinical Issues, 9*(4), 563–568.

Gianopoulos, J. G. (1989). Cardiac disease in pregnancy. *Medical Clinics of North America, 73*(3), 639–651.

Ginsberg, J. S., & Hirsh, J. (1995). Use of antithrombotic agents during pregnancy. *Chest, 108* (4, Suppl.), 305S–311S.

Hansen, J. P. (1986). Older maternal age in pregnancy outcome: A review of the literature. *Obstetrical and Gynecological Survey, 41*(11), 726–742.

Hoffman, J. I. (1995). Incidence of congenital heart disease: II. Perinatal incidence. *Pediatric Cardiology, 16*(4), 155–165.

Hogberg, U., Innala, E., & Sandstrom, A. (1994). Maternal mortality in Sweden, 1980–1988. *Obstetrics and Gynecology, 84*(2), 240–244.

Homans, D. C. (1985). Peripartum cardiomyopathy. *New England Journal of Medicine, 312*(23), 1432–1437.

Hsieh, T. T., Chen, K. C., Soong, J. H. (1993). Outcome of pregnancy in patient with organic heart disease in Taiwan. *Asia Oceania Journal of Obstetrics and Gynecology, 19*(1), 21–27.

Landon, M. B. (1996). Cardiac and pulmonary disease. In S. G. Gabbe, J. R. Niebyl, & H. L. Simpson (Eds.), *Obstetrics: Normal and problem pregnancies* (3rd ed., pp. 997–1024). New York: Churchill Livingstone.

Luppi, C. J. (1999). Cardiopulmonary resuscitation in pregnancy. In L. K. Mandeville & N. H. Trioano (Eds.), *High risk intrapartum and critical care nursing* (2nd ed., pp. 353–379). Philadelphia: Lippincott Williams & Wilkins.

Mabie, W. C., & Freire, C. V. (1995). Sudden chest pain and cardiac emergencies in the obstetric patient. *Obstetric and Gynecology Clinics of North America, 22*(1), 19–37.

Marx, G. F., Schwalbe, S. S., Cho, E., & Whitty, J. E. (1993). Automated blood pressure measurements in laboring women: Are they reliable? *American Journal of Obstetrics and Gynecology, 168*(3, Pt. 1), 796–798.

Mayet, J., Steer, P., & Somerville, J. (1998). Marfan syndrome, aortic dilatation, and pregnancy. *Obstetrics and Gynecology, 92*(4, Pt. 2), 713.

McMinn, T. R., Jr., & Ross, J., Jr. (1995). Hereditary dilated cardiomyopathy. *Clinical Cardiology, 18*(1), 7–15.

Meschengieser, S. S., Fondevila, C. G., Santarelli, M. T., & Lassari, M. A. (2000). Anticoagulation in pregnant women with mechanical heart valve prostheses. *Heart, 82*(1), 23–26.

Patton, D. E., Lee, W., Cotton, D. B., Miller, J., Carpenter, R. J., Jr., Huhta, J., & Hankins, G. (1990). Cyanotic maternal heart disease in pregnancy. *Obstetrical and Gynecological Survey, 45*(9), 594–600.

Pearson, G. D., Veille, J. C., Rahimtoola, S., Hsia, J., Oakley, C. M., Hosenpud, J. D., Ansari, A., & Baughman, K. L. (2000). Peripartum cardiomyopathy: National Heart, Lung, and Blood Institute and Office of Rare Diseases (National Institutes of Health) workshop recommendations and review. *Journal of the American Medical Association, 283*(9), 1183–1188.

Pierce, J. A., Price, B. O., & Joyce, J. W. (1963). Familiar occurrence of postpartal heart failure. *Archives of Internal Medicine, 111*, 651–655.

Ralston, D. H., Shnider, S. M., & DeLorimier, A. A. (1974). Effects of equipotent ephedrine, metaraminol, mephentermine and methoxamine on uterine blood flow in the pregnant ewe. *Anesthesiology, 40*(4), 354–370.

Ratnoff, O. D., & Kaufman, R. (1982). Arterial thrombosis in oral contraceptive users. *Archives of Internal Medicine, 142*(3), 447–448.

Rerkpattanapipat, P., Wongpraparut, N., Jacods, L. E., & Kotler, M. N. (2000). Cardiac manifestations of acquired immunodeficiency syndrome. *Archives of Internal Medicine, 160*(5), 602–608.

Rochat, R. W., Koonin, L. M., Atrash, H. K. Jewett, J. F., & the Maternal Mortality Collaborative. (1988). Maternal mortality in the United States: Report from the Maternal Mortality Collaborative. *Obstetrics and Gynecology, 72*(1), 91–97.

Shabetai, R. (1999). Cardiac diseases. In R. K. Creasy & R. Resnik (Eds.), *Maternal-fetal medicine* (4th ed., pp. 793–819). Philadelphia: W.B. Saunders.

Shnider, S. M., DeLorimier, A. A., Holl, J. W., Chapler, F. K., & Morishima, H. O. (1968). Vasopressors in obstetrics: Correction of fetal acidosis with ephedrine during spinal hypotension. *American Journal of Obstetrics and Gynecology, 102*(7), 911–919.

Simon, A., Sadovshy, E., Aboulafia, Y., Ohel, G., & Zajicek, G. (1986). Fetal activity in pregnancies complicated by rheumatic heart disease. *Journal of Perinatal Medicine, 14*(5), 331–334.

Sullivan, J. M., & Ramanathan, K. B. (1985). Management of medical problems in pregnancy: Severe cardiac disease. *New England Journal of Medicine, 313*(5), 304–309.

Weis, M., & von Scheidt, W. (2000). Coronary artery disease in the transplanted heart. *Annual Review of Medicine, 51*, 81–100.

Weitz, J. I. (1997). Low molecular weight heparins. *New England Journal of Medicine, 337*(10), 688–698.

Pulmonary Complications

Alexander, S., Dodds, L., & Armson, B. A. (1998). Perinatal outcomes in women with asthma during pregnancy. *Obstetrics and Gynecology, 92*(3), 435–440.

American College of Obstetricians and Gynecologists. (1996). *Pulmonary disease in pregnancy* (Technical Bulletin No. 224). Washington, DC: Author.

Balducci, J., Rodis, J. F., Rosengren, S., Vintezileos, A. M., Spivey, G., & Vosselles, C. (1992). Pregnancy outcome following first-trimester varicella infection. *Obstetrics and Gynecology, 79*(1), 5–6.

Baren, J. M. Henneman, P. L., & Lewis, R. J. (1996). Primary varicella in adults: Pneumonia, pregnancy and hospital admission. *Annals of Emergency Medicine, 28*(2), 165–169.

Berkowitz, K., & LaSala, A. (1990). Risk factors associated with the increasing prevalence of pneumonia during pregnancy. *American Journal of Obstetrics and Gynecology, 163*(3), 981–985.

Briggs, G. G., Freeman, R. K., & Yaffe, S. J. (1998). *Drugs in Pregnancy and lactation* (5th ed.). Baltimore: Williams & Wilkins.

Brown, M. A., & Halonen, M. (1999). Perinatal events in the development of asthma. *Current Opinion in Pulmonary Medicine, 5*(1), 4–9.

Chapman, S. J. (1998). Varicella in pregnancy. *Seminars in Perinatology, 22*(4), 339–346.

Chandra, P. C., Patel, H., Schiavello, H. J., & Briggs, S. L. (1998). Successful pregnancy outcome after complicated varicella pneumonia. *Obstetrics and Gynecology, 92*(4, Pt. 2), 680–682.

Clark, S. L. (1993). Asthma in pregnancy: National Asthma Education Program Working Group on Asthma and Pregnancy. National Institutes of Health, National Heart, Lung and Blood Institute. *Obstetrics and Gynecology, 82*(6), 1036–1040.

Coleman, M. T., & Rund, D. A. (1997). Nonobstetric conditions causing hypoxia during pregnancy: Asthma and epilepsy. *American Journal of Obstetrics and Gynecology, 177*(1), 1–7.

Cousins, L. (1999). Fetal oxygenation, assessment of fetal well-being, and obstetric management of the pregnant patient with asthma. *Journal of Allergy and Clinical Immunology, 103*(2, Pt. 2), S343–S349.

Cydulka, R. K., Emerman, C. L., Schreiber, D., Molander, K. H., Woodruff, P. G., & Camargo, C. A., Jr. (1999). Acute asthma among pregnant women presenting to the emergency department. *American Journal of Respiratory and Critical Care Medicine, 160*(3), 887–892.

Dombrowski, M. P. (1997). Pharmacologic therapy of asthma during pregnancy. *Obstetrics and Gynecology Clinics of North America, 24*(3), 559–574.

Dykewicz, M. S. (1992). Allergen immunotherapy for the patient with asthma. *Immunology and Allergy Clinics of North America, 12*, 125.

Goodrum, L. A. (1997). Pneumonia in pregnancy. *Seminars in Perinatology, 21*(4), 276–283.

Grant, A. (1996). Varicella infection and toxoplasmosis in pregnancy. *Journal of Perinatal and Neonatal Nursing, 10*(2), 17–29.

Greenberger, P. A. (1992). Asthma in pregnancy. *Clinics in Chest Medicine, 3*(4), 597–605.

Huff, R. W. (1989). Asthma in pregnancy. *Medical Clinics of North America, 73*(3), 653–660.

Juniper, E. F., & Newhouse, M. T. (1993). Effect of pregnancy on asthma: A systematic review and meta-analysis. In M. Schatz, R. S. Zeiger, & H. C. Claman (Eds.), *Asthma and immunological diseases in pregnancy and early infancy*. New York: Marcel Dekker.

Kallen, B., Rydhstroem, H., & Aberg, A. (2000). Asthma during pregnancy: A population based study. *European Journal of Epidemiology, 16*(2), 167–171.

Kerstjens, J. A. M., Brand, P. L. P., Hughes, M. D., Robinson, N. J., Postma, D. S., Sluiter, H. J., Bleeckes, E. R., Dekhuijzen, P. N., DeJong, P. M., & the Dutch Chronic Non-Specific Lung Disease Study Group (1992). A comparison of bronchodilator therapy with or without inhaled corticosteroid therapy for obstructive airways disease. *New England Journal of Medicine, 327*(20), 1413–1419.

Kurinczuk, J. J., Parsons, D. E., Dawes, V., & Burton, P. R. (1999). The relationship between smoking and asthma. *Women and Health, 29*(3), 31–47.

Mabie, W. C. Asthma in pregnancy (1996). *Clinical Obstetrics and Gynecology, 39*(1), 56–69.

Mabie, W. C., Barton, J. R., Wasserstrum, N., & Sabai, B. M. (1992). Clinical observations on asthma in pregnancy. *Journal of Maternal Fetal Medicine, 1*(1), 45–50.

Maccato, M. L. (1991). Respiratory insufficiency due to pneumonia in pregnancy. *Obstetrics and Gynecology Clinics of North America, 18*(2), 289–299.

Maccato, M. L. (1989). Pneumonia and pulmonary tuberculosis in pregnancy. *Obstetrics and Gynecology Clinics of North America, 16*(2), 417–430.

Madinger, N. E. Greenspoon, J. S., & Ellrodt, A. G. (1989). Pneumonia during pregnancy: Has modern technology improved maternal and fetal outcome? *American Journal of Obstetrics and Gynecology, 161*(3), 657–662.

Mays, M., & Leiner, S. (1995). Asthma: A comprehensive review. *Journal of Nurse-Midwifery, 40*(3), 256–268.

Minerbi-Codish, I., Fraser, D., Avnun, L., Glezerman, M., & Heimer, D. (1998). Influence of asthma in pregnancy on labor and the newborn. *Respiration, 65*(20), 130–135.

Moore-Gillon, J. (1994). Asthma in pregnancy. *British Journal of Obstetrics and Gynaecology, 101*(8), 658–660.

Munn, M. B., Groome, L. J., Atterbury, J. L., Baker, S. L., & Hoff, C. (1999). Pneumonia as a complication of pregnancy. *Journal of Maternal-Fetal Medicine, 8*(4), 151–154.

National Heart, Lung, and Blood Institute National Asthma Education Program Working Group on Asthma and Pregnancy. (1993). *Management of asthma during pregnancy* (NIH Pub. No. 93-3279). Washington, DC: Department of Health and Human Services.

Neu, H. C., & Sabath, L. D. (1993). Criteria for selecting oral antibiotic therapy for common acquired pneumonia. *Infectious Medicine, 10*(Suppl. 2), 33S.

Nolan, T. E., & Hankins, G. D. V. (1995). Acute pulmonary dysfunction and distress. *Obstetrics and Gynecology Clinics of North America, 22*(1), 39–54.

Perlow, J. H., Montgomery, D., Morgan, M. A., Towers, C. V., & Porto, M. (1992). Severity of asthma and perinatal outcome. *American Journal of Obstetrics and Gynecology, 167*(4, Pt. 1), 963–967.

Rigby, F. B., & Pastorek, J. G., III. (1996). Pneumonia during pregnancy. *Clinical Obstetrics and Gynecology, 39*(1), 107–119.

Riley, L. (1997). Pneumonia and tuberculosis in pregnancy. *Infectious Disease Clinics of North America, 11*(1), 119–133.

Rodrigues, J., & Niederman, M. S. (1992). Pneumonia complicating pregnancy. *Clinics in Chest Medicine, 13*(4), 679–691.

Schatz, M. (1992). Asthma during pregnancy: Interrelationships and management. *Annals of Allergy, 68*(2), 123–133.

Schatz, M. (1999). Interrelationships between asthma and pregnancy: A literature review. *Journal of Allergy and Clinical Immunology, 103*(2, Pt. 2), S330–S336.

Shatz, M., Zeiger, R. S., Harden, K., Hoffman, C. C., Chilingar, L., & Petitti, D. (1997). The safety of asthma and allergy medications during pregnancy. *Journal of Allergy and Clinical Immunology, 100*(3), 301–306.

Scheffer, A. L.(1991). Guidelines for the diagnosis and management of asthma (National Heart, Lung, and Blood Institute, National Asthma Education Program, Expert Panel Report). *Journal of Allergy and Clinical Immunology, 88*(3, Pt. 2), 425–534.

Terr, A. I. (1998). Asthma and reproductive medicine. *Obstetrical and Gynecological Survey, 53*(11), 699–701.

Witlin, A. G. (1997). Asthma in pregnancy. *Seminars in Perinatology, 21*(4), 284–297.

Yost, N. P., Bloom, S. L., Richey, S. D., Ramin, S. M., & Cunningham, F. G. (2000). An appraisal of treatment guidelines for Antepartum community-acquired pneumonia. *American Journal of Obstetrics and Gynecology, 183*(1), 131, 135.

Multiple Gestation

Adams, D. M., Sholl, J. S., Haney, E. I., Russell, T. L., & Silver, R. K. (1998). Perinatal outcome associated with outpatient management of triplet pregnancy. *American Journal of Obstetrics and Gynecology, 178*(4), 843–847.

Alamia, V., Royek, A. B., Jaekle, R. K., & Meyer, B. A. (1998). Preliminary experience with a prospective protocol for planned vaginal delivery of triplet gestations. *American Journal of Obstetrics and Gynecology, 179*(5), 1133–1135.

Alexander, G. R., Kogan, M., Martin, J., & Papiernik, E. (1998). What are fetal growth patterns of singletons, twins, and triplets in the United States? *Clinical Obstetrics and Gynecology, 41*(1), 115–125.

Allen, M. C., & Alexander, G. R. (1994). Screening for cerebral palsy in preterm infants: Delay criteria for motor milestone attainment. *Journal of Perinatology, 14*(3), 190–193.

Alpers, C. E., & Harrison, M. R. (1985). Fetus in fetu associated with an undescended testis. *Pediatric Pathology, 4*(1–2), 37–46.

American College of Obstetricians and Gynecologists. (1998). *Special problems of multiple gestation* (Educational Bulletin No. 253). Washington, DC: Author.

Anderson, R. L., Goldberg, J. D., & Golbus, M. S. (1991). Prenatal diagnosis in multiple gestations: 20 years experience with amniocentesis. *Prenatal Diagnosis, 11*(4), 263–270.

Antsaklis, A., Gougoulakis, A., Mesogitis, S., Papantoniou, N., & Aravantinos, D. (1991). Invasive techniques for fetal diagnosis in multiple pregnancy. *International Journal of Gynaecology and Obstetrics, 34*(4), 309–314.

Bajoria, R. (1998). Abundant vascular anastomoses in monoamniotic versus diamniotic monochorionic placentas. *American Journal of Obstetrics and Gynecology, 179*(3, Pt. 1), 788–793.

Bakos, O. (1998). Birth in triplet pregnancies. Vaginal delivery—How often is it possible? *Acta Obstetricia et Gynecologica Scandinavica, 77*(8), 845–848.

Bakos, O., Cederholm, M., & Kieler, H. (1998). Very prolonged membrane rupture and delayed delivery of the second twin. *Fetal Diagnosis and Therapy, 13*(3), 147–149.

Benirschke, K. (1990). The placenta in twin gestation. *Clinics in Obstetrics and Gynecology, 33*(1), 18–31.

Benirschke, K. (1992). The contribution of placenta anastomoses to perinatal twin damage. *Human Pathology, 23*(12), 1319–1320.

Benirschke, K., & Kaufmann, P. (1995). *Multiple pregnancy: Pathology of the human placentas* (3rd ed.; 636–753). New York: Springer-Verlag.

Blake, G. D., Knuppel, R. A., Ingardia, C. J., Lake, M., Aumann, G., & Hanson, M. (1984). Evaluation of nonstress fetal heart rate testing in multiple gestations. *Obstetrics and Gynecology, 63*(4), 528–532.

Blickstein, I. (1990). The twin-twin transfusion syndrome. *Obstetrics and Gynecology, 76*(4), 714–722.

Burke, M. S. (1990). Single fetal demise in twin gestation. *Clinics in Obstetrics and Gynecology, 33*(1), 69–78.

Cattanach, S. A., Wedel, M., White, S., & Young, M. (1990). Single intrauterine fetal death in a suspected monozygotic twin pregnancy. *Australian and New Zealand Journal of Obstetrics and Gynaecology, 30*(2), 137–140.

Cetrulo, C. L., Ingardia, C. J., & Sbarra, A. J. (1980). Management of multiple gestation. *Clinics in Obstetrics and Gynecology, 23*(2), 533–548.

Cunningham, F. G., MacDonald, P. C., Grant, N. F., Leveno, K. J., Gilstrap, L. C., Hankins, G. D., & Clark, S. L. (1997). *Williams obstetrics* (20th ed.). Stamford, CT: Appleton & Lange.

D'Alton, M. E., & Mercer, B. M. (1990). Antepartum management of twin gestation: Ultrasound. *Clinical Obstetrics and Gynecology, 33*(1), 42–51.

D'Alton, M. E., Newton, E. R., & Cetrulo, C. L. (1984). Intrauterine fetal demise in multiple gestation. *Acta Geneticae Medicae et Gemellolgiae, 33*(1), 43–49.

Dauphinee, J. D., & Bowers, N. A. (1997). *Nursing management of multiple birth families: Preconception through postpartum.* (Nursing Module) White Plains, NY: March of Dimes Birth Defects Foundation.

DeLia, J. E., Cruikshank, D. W., & Keye, W. R. (1990). Fetoscopic neodymium: YAG laser occlusion of placental vessels in severe twin-twin transfusion syndrome. *Obstetrics and Gynecology, 75*(6), 1046–1053.

DellaPorta, K., Aforismo, D., & Butler-O'Hara, M. (1998). Cobedding of twins in the neonatal intensive care unit. *Pediatric Nursing, 24*(6), 529–531.

Devoe, L. D., & Azor, H. (1981). Simultaneous nonstress fetal heart rate testing in twin pregnancy. *Obstetrics and Gynecology, 58*(4), 450–455.

Dommergues, M., Mahieu-Caputo, D., & Dumez, Y. (1998). Is the route of delivery a meaningful issue in triplets and higher order multiples? *Clinical Obstetrics and Gynecology, 41*(1), 24–29.

Drevets, B. (1994). Twins and more: Meeting the special needs of prospective parents of mulitples. *Childbirth Instructor Magazine, 4*(3), 30–33.

Eganhouse, D. J., & Petersen, L. A. (1998). Fetal surveillance in multifetal pregnancy. *Journal of Obstetric, Gynecologic, and Neonatal Nursing, 27*(3), 312–321.

Ellings, J. M., Newman, R. B., & Bowers, N. A. (1998). Intrapartum care for women with multiple pregnancy. *Journal of Obstetric, Gynecologic, and Neonatal Nursing, 27*(4), 466–472.

Ellings, J. M., Newman, R. B., Hulsey, T. C., Bivins, H. A., & Keenan, A. (1993). Reduction in very low birth weight deliveries and perinatal mortality in a specialized, multidisciplinary twin clinic. *Obstetrics and Gynecology, 81*(3), 387–391.

Enbom, J. A. (1985). Twin pregnancy with intrauterine death of one twin. *American Journal Obstetrics and Gynecology, 152*(4), 424–429.

Falkner, F., & Matheny, A. P. (1995). The long-term development of twins: Anthropometric factors and cognition. In: L. G. Keith, E. Papiernik, D. M. Keith, & B. Luke, (Eds.), *Multiple pregnancy: Epidemiology, gestation and perinatal outcome.* New York: Parthenon Publishing.

Fraser, D., Picard, R., & Picard, E. (1991). Factors associated with neonatal problems in twin gestations. *Acta Geneticae Medicae et Gemellolgiae, 40*(2), 193–200.

Fusi, L., McParland, P., Fisk, N., Nicolini, U., & Wigglesworth, J. (1991). Acute twin-twin transfusion: A possible mechanism for brain-damaged survivors after intrauterine death of a monochorionic twin. *Obstetrics and Gynecology, 78*(3, Pt. 2), 517–520.

Gabbe, S. G., Niebyl, J. R., & Simpson, J. L. (Eds.). (1996). *Obstetrics: Normal and problem pregnancies* (3rd ed.). London: Churchill Livingstone.

Gall, S. A. (1998). Ambulatory management of multiple gestation. *Clinical Obstetrics and Gynecology, 41*(3), 564–583.

Gardeil, F., Greene, R., NiScanaill, S., & Skinner, J. (1998). Conjoined twins in a triplet pregnancy. *Obstetrics and Gynecology,* 92(4, Pt. 2), 716.

Gardner, K. (1993). Twin transfusion syndrome. *Journal of Obstetric, Gynecologic, and Neonatal Nursing, 22*(1), 64–71.

Giles, W., Trudinger, B., Cook, C., & Connelly, A. (1993). Placental microvascular changes in twin pregnancy with abnormal umbilical artery waveforms. *Obstetrics and Gynecology, 81*(4), 556–559.

Goldman, G. A., Dicker, D., Peleg, D., & Goldman, J. A. (1989). Is elective cerclage justified in the management of triplet and quadruplet pregnancy? *Australian and New Zealand Journal of Obstetrics and Gynaecology, 29*(1), 9–12.

Grobman, W. A., & Peaceman, A. M. (1998). What are the rates and mechanisms of first and second trimester pregnancy loss in twins? *Clinical Obstetrics and Gynecology, 41*(1), 36–45.

Hamilton, E. F., Platt, R. W., Morin, L., Usher, R., & Kramer, M. (1998). How small is too small in a twin pregnancy? *American Journal of Obstetrics and Gynecology, 179*(Pt. 13), 682–685.

Hanna, J. H., & Hill, J. M. (1984). Single intrauterine fetal demise in multiple gestation. *Obstetrics and Gynecology, 63*(1), 126–130.

Hsu, C. D., Chung, Y. K., Lee, I. K., Chou, K., & Copel, J. A. (1997). Maternal serum uric acid levels in preeclamptic women with multiple gestations. *American Journal of Perinatology, 14*(10), 613–617.

Jenkins, C. B., Ghidini, A., & Eglinton, G. S. (1997). Delayed delivery of the second twin: Watchful waiting or rescue cerclage? *Contemporary OB/GYN, 12*(6), 138–147.

Jewell, S. E., and Yip, R. (1995). Increasing trends in plural births in the United States. *Obstetrics and Gynecology, 85*(2), 229–232.

Johnson, J. M., Harman, C. R., Evans, J. A., MacDonald, K., & Manning, F. A. (1990). Maternal serum alpha fetoprotein in twin pregnancy. *American Journal of Obstetrics and Gynecology, 162*(4), 1020–1025.

Kalchbrenner, M. A., Weisenborn, E. J., Chye, J. K., Kaufman, H. K., & Losure, T. A. (1998). Delayed delivery of multiple gestations: Maternal and neonatal outcomes. *American Journal of Obstetrics and Gynecology, 179*(5), 1145–1149.

Keith, L. G., Papiernik, E., Keith, D. M., & Luke, B. (Eds.). (1995). *Multiple pregnancy: Epidemiology, gestations and perinatal outcome.* New York: The Parthenon Publishing Group.

Keith, L. G., Papiernik, E., & Luke, B. (1991). The costs of multiple pregnancy. *International Journal of Gynaecology and Obstetrics, 36*(2), 109–114.

Kiely, J. L., Kleinman, J. C., Kiely, M. (1992). Triplets and higher-order multiple births. Time trends and infant mortality. *American Journal of Diseases of Children, 146*(7), 862–868.

Kiely, J. L. (1998). What is the population based risk of preterm birth among twins and other multiples? *Clinical Obstetrics and Gynecology, 41*(1), 3–11.

Knuppel, R. A., Rattan, P. K., Scerbo, J. C., & O'Brien, W. F. (1985). Intrauterine fetal death in twins after 32 weeks of gestation. *Obstetrics and Gynecology, 65*(2), 172–175.

Kogan, M. D., Alexander, G. R., Kotelchuck, M., MacDorman, M. F., Buekens, P., Martin, J. A., & Papiernik, E. (2000). Trends in birth outcomes and prenatal care utilization in the United States, 1981–1997. *Journal of the American Medical Association, 284*(3), 335–341.

Landy, H. J., Weiner, S., Corson, S. L., Batzer, F. R., & Bologuese, R. J. (1986). The "vanishing twin": Ultrasonic assessment of fetal disappearance in the first trimester. *American Journal of Obstetrics and Gynecology, 87*(4), 551–555.

Lantz, M. E., Chez, R. A., Rodrigues, A., & Porter, K. B. (1996). Maternal weight gain patterns and birth weight outcome in twin gestation. *Obstetrics and Gynecology, 87*(4), 551–555.

Larroche, J. C., Droulle, P., Delezoide, A. L., Narcy, F., & Nessmann, C. (1990). Brain damage in monozygous twins. *Biology of the Neonate, 57*(5), 261–278.

Leonard, L. G. (1998). Depression and anxiety disorders during multiple pregnancy and parenthood. *Journal of Obstetric, Gynecologic, and Neonatal Nursing, 27*(3), 329–337.

Levav, A. L., Chan, L., & Wapner, R. J. (1998). Long-term magnesium sulfate tocolysis and maternal osteoporosis in a triplet pregnancy: A case report. *American Journal of Perinatology, 15*(1), 43–46.

Limbo, R. K., & Wheeler, S. R. (1986). *When a baby dies: A handbook for healing and helping.* LaCross, WI: LaCross Lutheran Hospital: Resolve Through Sharing.

Luke, B. (1998). What is the influence of maternal weight gain on the fetal growth of twins. *Clinical Obstetrics and Gynecology, 41*(1), 57–64.

Luke, B., & Leurgans, S. (1996). Maternal weight gains in ideal twin outcomes. *Journal of the American Dietetic Association, 96*(2), 178–181.

Luke, B., Minogue, J., & Witter, F. R. (1993). The role of fetal growth restriction and gestational age on length of hospital stay in twin infants. *Obstetrics and Gynecology, 81*(6), 949–953.

MacDorman, M. F., & Atkinson, J. O. (1999). Infant mortality statistics for the 1997 period linked birth/infant death data set. *National Vital Statistics Reports, 47*(23), 1–23.

Machin, G. A., & Keith, L. G. (1998). Can twin-to-twin transfusion syndrome be explained, and how is it treated? *Clinical Obstetrics and Gynecology, 41*(1), 104–113.

Malmstrom, P. M., & Biale, R. (1990). An agenda for meeting the special needs of multiple birth families. *Acta Geneticae Medicae et Gemellolgiae, 39*(4), 507–514.

Malmstrom, P. E., Faherty, T., & Wagner, P. (1988). Essential non-medical perinatal services for multiple birth families. *Acta Geneticae Medicae et Gemellolgiae, 37*(2), 193–198.

May, K. A. (1994). Impact of maternal activity restriction for preterm labor on the expectant father. *Journal of Obstetric, Gynecologic, and Neonatal Nursing, 23*(3), 246–251.

Mikkelsen, A. L., & Hansen, P. K. (1996). Survival of second twin 37 days after abortion of the first. *Acta Obstetricia et Gynecologica Scandinavica, 65*(7), 795–796.

Miller, D. A., Mullin, P., Hou, D., & Paul, R. H. (1996). Vaginal birth after cesarean section in twin gestation. *American Journal of Obstetrics and Gynecology, 175*(1), 194–198.

Minakami, H., & Sato, I. (1996). Reestimating date of delivery in multifetal pregnancies. *Journal of the American Medical Association, 275*(18), 1432–1434.

Mosher, R. C. (1994). Your very own childbirth class! *Twins Magazine, 10*(6), 42–43.

Newman, R. B., & Ellings, J. M. (1995). Antepartum management of the multiple gestation: The case for specialized care. *Seminars in Perinatology, 19*(5), 387–403.

Nyquist, K. H., & Lutes, L. M. (1998). Co-bedding twins: A developmentally supportive care strategy. *Journal of Obstetric, Gynecologic, and Neonatal Nursing, 27*(4), 450–456.

Nys, K., Colpin, H., DeMunter, A., & Vandemeulebroecke, L. (1998). Feelings and the need for information and counseling of expectant parents of twins. *Twin Research, 1*(3), 142–149.

Papiernik, E., Keith, L., Oleszczuk, J. J., & Cervantes, A. (1998). What interventions are useful in reducing the rate of preterm delivery in twins? *Clinical Obstetrics and Gynecology, 41*(1), 12–23.

Petersen, I. R., & Nyholm, H. C. (1999). Multiple pregnancies with single intrauterine demise. Description of twenty-eight pregnancies. *Acta Obstetricia et Gynecologica Scandinavica, 78*(3), 202–206.

Porreco, R. P., Sabin, E. D., Heyborne, K. D., & Lindsay, L. G. (1998). Delayed-interval delivery in multifetal pregnancy. *American Journal of Obstetrics and Gynecology, 178*(1, Pt. 1), 20–23.

Reisner, D. P., Mahony, B. S., Petty, C. N., Nyberg, D. A., Porter, T. F., Zingheim, R. W., Williams, M. A., & Luthy, D. A. (1993). Stuck twin syndrome: Outcome in thirty-seven consecutive cases. *American Journal of Obstetrics and Gynecology, 169*(4), 991–995.

Schenker, J. G., Yarkoni, S., & Granat, M. (1981). Multiple pregnancies following induction of ovulation. *Fertility and Sterility, 35*(2), 105–123.

Schinzel, A. A., Smith, D. W., & Miller, J. R. (1979). Monozygotic twinning and structural defects, *Journal of Pediatrics, 95*(6), 921–930.

Sims, C. D., Cowan, D. B., & Parkinson, C. E. (1976). The lecithin/sphingomyelin (L/S) ratio in twin pregnancies. *British Obstetrics and Gynaecology, 83*(6), 447–451.

Spellacy, W. N., Cruz, A. C., Buhi, W. C., Birk, S. A. (1977). Amniotic fluid L/S ratio in twin gestation. *Obstetrics and Gynecology, 50*(1), 68–70.

Strong, T. H., Phelan, J. P., Ahn, M. O., & Sarno, A. P. (1989). Vaginal birth after cesarean delivery in the twin gestation. *American Journal of Obstetrics and Gynecology, 161*(1), 29–32.

Taffel, S. M., (1995). Demographic trends in twin births: USA. In L. G. Keith, E. Papiernik, D. M. Keith, & B. Luke (Eds.), *Multiple pregnancy: Epidemiology, gestation and perinatal outcome.* New York: Parthenon Publishing Group.

van den Brand, S. F., Nijhuis, J. G., & van Dongen, P. W. (1994). Prenatal ultrasound diagnosis of conjoined twins. *Obstetrics and Gynecology Survey, 49*(9), 656–662.

Ventura, S. J., Martin, J. A., Curtin, S. C., Mathews, T. J., & Park, M. M. (2000). Births: Final data for 1998. *National Vital Statistics Report, 48*(3), 1–100.

Yasuda, Y., Mitomori, T., Mastsuura, A., & Tanimura, T. (1985). Fetus-in-fetu: Report of a case. *Teratology, 31*(3), 337–344.

APPENDIX **8A**

Guidelines for Home Care Management of Selected High-Risk Pregnancy Conditions

GENERAL GUIDELINES

Pregnant women with complications who are in stable condition, generally do well at home with supportive care from family members and friends along with healthcare provider–initiated telephone calls and home visits. For appropriately selected women, being at home avoids the stress and boredom of lengthy hospitalization and allows continued contact and interaction with family members. Successful home care management requires a collaborative effort of the woman, her family, and the healthcare team.

Patient education is a critical component of home care. During the first visit, the woman and her family are provided with information about the importance of adhering to the prescribed treatment plan and prompt notification of the primary care provider of any signs or symptoms indicative of worsening disease. Regular review of these signs and symptoms reinforces the information. Education related to use of any technology or testing methods (eg, daily weights, blood pressure (BP) measurement, urinalysis using the dipstick method, fetal movement counting, uterine activity monitoring, medications) and required documentation are also essential. Written materials provided to the woman and family members reinforce the teaching and serve as a resource when questions arise.

Key points in home care management include the following:

- Willingness of the woman and her family to adhere to the prescribed treatment plan, including activity restriction, fetal movement counting, blood pressure monitoring, daily weights, urinalysis, uterine activity monitoring, medications, and documentation
- Support systems in place to allow for activity restriction, including child care, if appropriate, and meal preparation.
- Telephone service to allow daily phone contact between the woman and perinatal nurse
- Knowledge of when to call the primary care provider and when to go to the hospital
- Support persons should be identified to transport the woman to the hospital if necessary.

GUIDELINES FOR HOME CARE MANAGEMENT OF PREECLAMPSIA

The following diagnostic criteria and considerations are suggested for home care management of women with mild preeclampsia:

- Gestational age ≥20 weeks
- BP <150/100 mm Hg sitting or <140/90 mm Hg in the lateral position
- Proteinuria <100 mg/L on urine dipstick or <1 g/24 hours
- No evidence of the following:
  - Headaches associated with visual disturbances
  - Epigastric pain judged to be related to preeclampsia
  - Marked edema or clonus
  - Pulmonary edema

- Laboratory values: platelets >100,000/mm^3; aspartate aminotransferase (AST) <50 U/L; alanine aminotransferase (ALT) <200 U/L, serum creatinine <1.32 mg/dL or within normal limits
- Ability to use electronic BP equipment

The following parameters should be assessed based on the individual clinical situation. Protocols or physician orders are used to determine thresholds for each parameter:

- BP two to four times per day in the same arm in the same position
- Weight at the same time each day, usually in the morning, preferably on the same scale
- Urine dipstick for protein, using the first voided midstream specimen. A 24-hour urine collection may be ordered weekly.
- Daily to twice-daily fetal movement counts beginning at 24 weeks
- Daily to twice-weekly home visits for comprehensive maternal-fetal assessments, including BP, fundal height, edema, reflexes, fetal heart rate auscultation and nonstress test (NST) after 26 to 28 weeks. Blood samples may be obtained for laboratory analysis. Ultrasound examination of amniotic fluid index may also be performed at home.
- Daily provider-initiated phone contact for assessment of signs and symptoms of PIH and review of BP, urinalysis, fetal movement counting after 24 weeks, weight and activity level, and adherence to prescribed treatment plan
- Weekly office visits for maternal–fetal assessments and laboratory tests

Medications:

- Antihypertensive drugs as ordered
- Low-dose aspirin therapy (60 to 80 mg/day) may be ordered
- Prenatal vitamins and iron

Diet:

- A well-balanced diet is recommended containing at least 60 to 70 g of protein, 1,200 mg of calcium, adequate zinc, sodium (2 to 6 g), magnesium, and 6 to 8 glasses of water each day

Activity:

- Eight or more hours of sleep each night and a rest period midday promote mobilization of edematous fluid back into the intravascular space and enhance renal and placental perfusion. Protocols range from usual activities of daily living to modified bed rest to strict bed rest.

GUIDELINES FOR HOME CARE MANAGEMENT OF ANTEPARTUM BLEEDING

The following diagnostic criteria and considerations are suggested for home care management of women with antepartum bleeding:

- No evidence of active bleeding
- Hematocrit of >30%
- Reassuring fetal heart rate pattern
- No evidence of signs and symptoms of preterm labor
- Home within reasonable distance to hospital (no more than 15 to 20 minutes from hospital)
- Emergency support systems in place for immediate transport to the hospital

The following parameters should be assessed based on the individual clinical situation. Protocols or physician orders are used to determine threshold for each parameter:

- Monitoring of vaginal discharge or bleeding after each urination or bowel movement or more frequently as needed
- Daily fetal movement counts after 24 weeks
- Warning signs of preterm labor should be reviewed and a demonstration of uterine self-palpation provided. The nurse should observe the woman palpate for uterine activity.
- Daily uterine activity assessment by self-palpation or electronic monitor or more frequently if needed (contraction threshold of 3 to 5 per hour)
- Daily to twice-weekly home visits for comprehensive maternal-fetal assessments, including fundal height, auscultation of fetal heart rate and NST after 26 to 28 weeks. Blood may be drawn for a complete blood cell count with a differential cell assessment
- Daily provider-initiated phone contact for assessment of uterine activity, bleeding, fetal movement counting after 24 weeks, activity level, and adherence to prescribed treatment plan

Medications:

- Prenatal vitamins and iron
- Tocolytic agents may be ordered
- Stool softeners may be ordered

Diet:

- Recommendations for the usual well-balanced diet during pregnancy

Activity:

- Most women with antepartum bleeding are restricted to bed rest with commode or bathroom privileges only.

GUIDELINES FOR HOME CARE MANAGEMENT OF PRETERM LABOR

The following diagnostic criteria and considerations are suggested for home care management of women with preterm labor:

- No evidence of preterm labor (<3 to 5 contractions per hour)
- No evidence of intraamniotic infection
- Cervical dilation less than 3 cm

The following parameters should be assessed based on the individual clinical situation. Protocols or physician orders are used to determine thresholds for each parameter:

- Warning signs of preterm labor should be reviewed and a demonstration of uterine self-palpation provided. The nurse should observe the woman palpate for uterine activity.
- At least twice-daily uterine activity assessment by self-palpation or electronic monitor
- Monitoring of vaginal discharge with heightened awareness of signs of spontaneous rupture of membranes
- Assessment for urinary frequency, burning on urination, diarrhea, pelvic heaviness, pelvic pressure, maternal temperature, uterine tenderness, and cramping
- Frequent home visits for comprehensive maternal-fetal assessments, including fundal height measurement, NST, and possibly cervical examinations
- Reinforcement of warning signs of preterm labor and when to the call the primary care provider or come to the hospital
- Daily provider-initiated phone contact for assessment of warning signs of preterm labor, fetal movement counting after 24 weeks, activity level, and adherence to prescribed treatment plan

Medications:

- Tocolytic agents may be ordered
- Prenatal vitamins and iron
- Stool softeners as needed

Diet:

- Recommendations for the usual well-balanced diet during pregnancy
- Increased fluid intake to 6–8 glasses per day
- Include roughage and foods high in calcium
- Increase protein intake

Activity:

- Protocols range from usual activities of daily living to modified bed rest to strict bed rest.
- Range of motion and/or passive exercises may be ordered if bed rest period is extended.

GUIDELINES FOR HOME CARE MANAGEMENT OF DIABETES

The following diagnostic criteria and considerations are suggested for home care management of women with diabetes:

- Patient and family willingness and ability to learn and follow diet, perform blood glucose monitoring, and insulin adjustment and administration if needed
- Family member knowledge of signs and symptoms of severe hypoglycemia and ability to administer glucagon (0.05 mg) subcutaneously if this should occur
- Family member knowledge of how and when to call for emergency assistance
- A safe and clean storage place for insulin and other supplies
- Absence of abnormal laboratory values. Glycemic control can be assessed over time (previous 4–6 weeks) using measurements of glycosylated hemoglobin (HgA_{1c}). Fasting and random blood glucose levels provide information about blood glucose levels at the time of testing.

The following parameters should be assessed based on the individual clinical situation. Protocols or physician orders are used to determine threshold for each parameter:

- Diabetes care should be reviewed with the woman and family, including blood glucose monitoring, urine testing for ketones and glucose, diet, and insulin administration
- Assessment for skill in blood glucose monitoring as ordered, including trouble-shooting equipment problems

- Review of daily log of dietary intake, blood glucose levels, daily weights, and medications
- Assessment for insulin self-injection
- Home or office visit for comprehensive maternal–fetal assessment, including fundal height, review of daily fetal movement counting log (after 24 weeks' gestation), auscultation fetal heart rate or NST one to two times weekly after 26 to 28 weeks
- Sick day care management guidelines should be reviewed with the woman and family to ensure knowledge of how to make adjustments in insulin dosages if needed to offset altered food intake.
- Assessment for development of complications such as preterm labor, pregnancy-induced hypertension (PIH), bleeding, or infection
- Review of record of daily dietary intake, blood glucose levels, urine testing for ketones and glucose, daily weights, and medications
- Review of warning signs to report to primary care provider: hyperglycemia (blood glucose level >200 mg/dL), decreased fetal movement, illness (especially if dietary intake is altered), skin breakdown, visual or neurologic symptoms, and signs of renal involvement

Medications:

- Insulin (as prescribed)
- Prenatal vitamins and iron

Diet:

- Specific American Diabetes Association diet recommended by healthcare provider. Current recommendations for dietary management include 24–30 kcal/kg for normal-weight women, 40 kcal/kg for underweight women, and 24 kcalk/kg for overweight women. These calories should be consumed in three meals and three snacks, comprising <40% carbohydrates, 20% to 25% protein, and 35% to 40% predominately monounsaturated and polyunsaturated fats.

Activity

- Activities of daily living
- Exercise within parameters recommended by the healthcare provider

GUIDELINES FOR HOME CARE MANAGEMENT OF CARDIAC DISEASE

The following diagnostic criteria and considerations are suggested for home care management of women with cardiac disease:

- Disease or condition stability
- Systems in place to support modified activity restriction if ordered
- Emergency transportation arrangements in place
- Family members have completed a class in cardiopulmonary resuscitation.
- For women with parental therapy (heparin), ensure that venous or subcutaneous access can be maintained.

The following parameters should be assessed based on the individual clinical situation. Protocols or physician orders are used to determine thresholds for each parameter:

- Frequency of home visits based on individual clinical situation: daily, two to three times weekly, and weekly (supplemented by provider initiated telephone calls)
- Assessment of maternal cardiovascular and pulmonary status (eg, blood pressure, pulse, heart sounds, respirations, lung sounds, edema)
- Report the following signs and symptoms to the healthcare provider: hypertension, apical pulse rate above 120 beats/min; differences in apical pulse rate and radial pulse rate, increased edema as evidenced by sudden weight gain; puffy hands, face, and feet; dyspnea; adventitious lung sounds
- Review signs of cardiac decompensation (eg, palpitations, cough, generalized edema, feeling of smothering, difficult breathing, chest pain), and emphasize the importance of calling the primary care provider immediately if these should occur.
- Daily to periodic maternal weight assessment, as ordered
- Assessment of fetal status, including auscultation of the fetal heart rate, daily to twice-daily fetal movement counting after 24 weeks, and NSTs after 26 to 28 weeks
- Assessment for development of complications such as preterm labor, PIH, bleeding, or infection

For women on heparin therapy:

- Review administration techniques: site rotation, site cleaning and preparation, use of infusion pump
- Review side effects: nosebleeds, hematuria, bleeding gums, excessive bruising, uticaria
- Collect blood samples for laboratory tests
- Change infusion site every 3 to 4 days

Medications:

- As prescribed and based on the type of cardiac disease (eg, anticoagulants, diuretics, antihypertensives, antiarrhythmics)

- Heparin therapy (if prescribed) may be twice-daily subcutaneous injections or continuous infusion (usually for prophylaxis) or intravenous infusion (usually) for an existing clot
- Stool softeners

Activity:

- Activities of daily living or limited activity such as modified bed rest
- Women with class I and II cardiac disease need 10 hours of sleep each night and a 0.5-hour rest period after meals in a semi-Fowler's position.
- Women with class III and IV cardiac disease probably need modified bed rest.

Diet:

- Well-balanced diet (low salt and fluid restriction may be ordered based on type of cardiac disease)
- If the woman is taking diuretics, decrease the sodium intake and include foods high in potassium (eg, bananas, citrus fruits, whole grains).
- If the woman is on heparin therapy, avoid foods high in vitamin K (eg, raw, dark green, leafy vegetables) that can counteract the effects of heparin. A substitute form of folic acid is needed.

ADAPTED FROM THE FOLLOWING REFERENCES:

Grohar, J. L. (1994). Nursing protocols for antepartum home care. *Journal of Obstetric, Gynecologic and Neonatal Nursing, 23*(8), 687–694.

Lowermilk, D. L., & Grohar, J. L. (1998). *High risk antepartal home care* (Nursing Module). White Plains, NY: March of Dimes Birth Defects Foundation.

Simpson, K. R. (1992). *Protocols for the homecare management of high risk pregnancies.* St. Louis: Healthy Homecomings.

PART 3

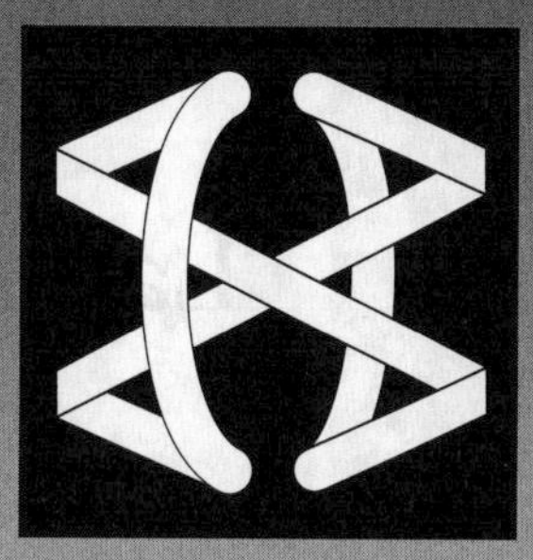

INTRAPARTUM

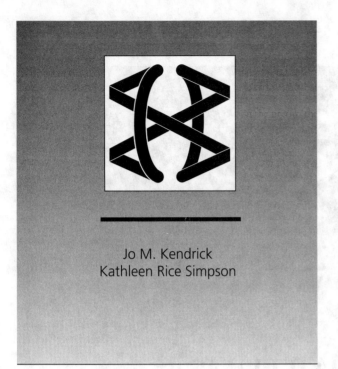

Jo M. Kendrick
Kathleen Rice Simpson

CHAPTER 9

Labor and Birth

Labor and birth are natural processes. Most women do well with support and minimal, selected intervention. Minimal intervention acknowledges that most pregnancies, labors, and births are normal and that intervention creates the potential for iatrogenic maternal–fetal injuries (Knox, Simpson, & Garite, 1999). Interventions should move forward on a continuum from noninvasive to least invasive and from nonpharmacologic to pharmacologic according to the wishes of the woman and at the discretion of healthcare providers based on individual clinical situations. A philosophy of minimal intervention works in the context of a well-designed safety net (ie, ability to intervene when necessary in a clinically timely manner) (Knox et al., 1999).

During the intrapartum period, nurses use knowledge about the physiologic and psychosocial aspects of birth and selected pharmacologic therapies to provide comprehensive care for women and families. This chapter focuses on nursing interventions that facilitate the labor and birth process. The physiology of labor and birth is discussed briefly. Maternal–fetal assessments, influence of maternal positioning on labor progression, and opportunities for supporting family attachment throughout the birth process are described. Clinical interventions, including cervical ripening, labor induction or augmentation, and amnioinfusion, are also presented. Strategies to ensure consistency with perioperative standards of care for cesarean births are included, as well as controversial issues such as fundal pressure, perineal massage, and management of the second stage of labor. The evidence for each of these topics is discussed, with recommendations given for practices that contribute to the best possible outcomes for mothers and babies.

OVERVIEW OF LABOR AND BIRTH

Onset of Labor

Multiple theories have been proposed to explain the biophysiologic factors that initiate labor, but this process is not fully understood. It is likely that a combination of maternal–fetal factors influence labor onset (Display 9–1). The fetus may determine the length of gestation, whereas the mother influences the actual timing of labor and birth (Ulmsten, 1997). A complex series of events must occur during labor and birth that represent a reversal of roles for the uterus and cervix during pregnancy (Simpson & Poole, 1998a). The myometrium, which has remained relatively quiet for many months, must become active, and the cervix, which has functioned to prevent birth, must lose its resistance (Olah & Gee, 1996). Despite extensive research, knowledge about the exact mechanism for spontaneous labor remains incomplete. Most of what is known is from animal studies and in vitro investigations of biopsies obtained from the myometrium and cervix at cesarean birth (Ulmsten, 1997).

The forces of labor are uterine contractions acting on the resistance of the cervix. The uterine walls are flexible, expanding over time until the onset of labor, when the myometrium converts from a quiet state to a highly active, contractile organ. The cervix is composed of connective tissue that remains firmly closed until it is time for labor to begin, and then the cervix undergoes rapid, dramatic changes, including ripening, effacement, and dilation (Ulmsten, 1997). The conditions and processes that result in term labor are regulated by several compounds and biochemical sys-

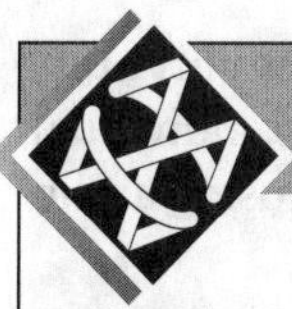

DISPLAY 9–1

Possible Causes of the Onset of Labor

Maternal Factor Theories

Uterine muscles are stretched, causing release of prostaglandin.

Pressure on cervix stimulates nerve plexus, causing release of oxytocin by maternal posterior pituitary gland (the Ferguson reflex).

Oxytocin stimulation in circulating blood increases slowly during pregnancy, rises dramatically during labor, and peaks during second stage. Oxytocin and prostaglandin work together to inhibit calcium binding in muscle cells, raising intracellular calcium and activating contractions .

Estrogen/progesterone ratio change: estrogen excites uterine response, and progesterone quiets uterine response. Decrease of progesterone allows estrogen to stimulate the contractile response of the uterus.

Fetal Factor Theories

Placental aging and deterioration triggers initiation of contractions.

Fetal cortisol concentration, produced by the fetal adrenal glands, rises and acts on the placenta to reduce progesterone formation and increase prostaglandin. Anencephalic fetuses (no adrenal glands) tend to have prolonged gestation.

Prostaglandin, produced by fetal membranes (amnion and chorion) and the decidua, stimulates contractions. When arachidonic acid stored in fetal membranes is released at term, it is converted to prostaglandin.

tems, including progesterone withdrawal and prostaglandin synthesis. Activation of the myometrium requires receptors sites, increased production of prostaglandin, and formation of gap junctions. Gap junctions are specialized protein units located within the cell membrane that connect neighboring cells and provide communication channels (Ulmsten, 1997). The amount of gap junctions and their permeability and performance have a direct influence on myometrial function during labor.

It is theorized that, after the preparation and activation period, the myometrium is ready to be stimulated for contractions. Prostaglandin and oxytocin are the most important biochemical factors in stimulating term myometrial activity (Olah & Gee, 1996). Prostaglandin synthesis during the cervical ripening period also prepares the myometrium to respond to oxytocin. Oxytocin alone cannot induce the formation of gap junctions. The hormone is synthesized by the hypothalamus and then transported to the posterior lobe of the pituitary gland, from where it is released into maternal circulation. The release of oxytocin is caused by breast stimulation, sensory stimulation of the lower genital tract, and cervical stretching (Shyken & Petrie, 1995a). The milk-ejection reflex results from oxytocin released by breast stimulation. Oxytocin released in response to vaginal and cervical stretching results in uterine contractions through Ferguson's reflex. There are differences in reported plasma concentrations of oxytocin during pregnancy and spontaneous labor that can be attributed in part to individual variations among pregnant women and to the methods used to measure levels of oxytocin, but it is generally accepted that, in addition to a tonic baseline release of oxytocin, a pulsatile release action may increase in amplitude and frequency during labor (Brindley & Sokol, 1988).

Two types of oxytocin receptors have been identified and quantified in the human uterus: myometrial and decidual. Both play an important part in the initiation of spontaneous labor and birth. Oxytocin receptors are present in low concentrations until late in the third trimester, during which their numbers increase dramatically. This lack of receptors until late pregnancy probably is the cause for the lack of uterine response to oxytocin other than during the third trimester (Sultatos, 1997). Oxytocin receptors in the myometrium and decidua reach their peak levels at slightly different times during pregnancy and labor. During pregnancy, as the weeks of gestation progress, there is a steady increase in the number of oxytocin receptors in the myometrium (Calderyo-Barcia & Poseiro, 1960). Myometrial receptors are thought to peak in early spontaneous labor and significantly contribute to the initiation of uterine activity (Fuchs, Fuchs, Husslein, & Soloff, 1984). It is likely that the concentration of myometrial receptors plays a dominant role in the uterine response to endogenous and exogenous oxytocin. Oxytocin receptors in the decidua are thought to increase as labor progresses and reach peak levels at birth (Fuchs, Husslein, & Fuchs, 1981). During labor, oxytocin stimulates the production and release of arachidonic acid and prostaglandin $F_{2\alpha}$ by the decidua that has been sensitized to oxytocin, potentiating oxytocin-induced uterine activity (Husslein, Fuchs, & Fuchs, 1981). All oxytocin-receptor site interactions do not result in uterine muscle contraction. Although oxytocin does occupy myometrial and decidual receptor sites during labor, the uterus is not in a constant state of contraction. Labor contractions are rhythmic and coordinated, providing evidence that some smooth muscle cells have their oxytocin receptor sites occupied without stimulating contraction (Sultatos, 1997).

The exact mechanism of muscle cell coordination during labor remains unknown. One theory is that a signal from pacemaker cells, possibly located in the uterine fundus, is transmitted to other myometrial cells by cell-to-cell communication through gap junctions (Sultatos, 1997). Another theory is that, although there is a tonic baseline release of oxytocin from the posterior lobe of the pituitary gland, it is the pulsatile release action that may increase in amplitude and frequency during labor that is responsible for the rhythmic nature of uterine contractions (Brindley & Sokol, 1988). More data are need to confirm or dispute these theories.

During the first stage of spontaneous labor, maternal circulating concentrations of endogenous oxytocin approximate levels that would be achieved with a continuous infusion of exogenous oxytocin at 2 to 4 mU/min (Dawood, Ylikorkala, Trivedi, & Fuchs, 1979). The fetus is thought to secrete oxytocin during labor at a level similar to an infusion of oxytocin at approximately 3 mU/min (Dawood, Wang, Gupta, & Fuchs, 1978). The combined effects of maternal–fetal contributions to maternal plasma oxytocin concentration is equivalent to a range of about 5 to 7 mU/min (Shyken & Petrie, 1995a). Plasma clearance of oxytocin occurs through the maternal kidneys and liver by means of the enzyme oxytocinase, with only a small amount of oxytocin excreted unchanged in the urine. The maternal metabolic clearance rate of oxytocin at term is 19 to 21 mL/kg/min (Zeeman, Kahn-Dawood, & Dawood, 1997).

Because of lack of knowledge about the exact physiology of labor, it is difficult to determine the optimal dosages to be used to correct abnormal labor with artificial pharmacologic compounds. Hyperstimulation with oxytocin and other prostaglandin compounds is often evident during cervical ripening and stimulation of labor and is a result of knowledge gaps in this area. What is known is that each woman has an individual myometrial sensitivity to oxytocin and prostaglandin (Ulsten, 1997).

Premonitory signs such as lightening, urinary frequency, pelvic pressure, changes in vaginal discharge, bloody show, loss of the mucous plug, and irregular contractions are frequently reported several weeks before actual labor begins. Some women also describe changes in sleep patterns and increased energy levels in the final weeks of pregnancy. True labor is characterized by contractions that produce progressive effacement and dilation of the cervix, with fetal descent into the maternal pelvis (Display 9–2).

Duration of Labor

Wide variations in labor progress and duration exist among childbearing women. There is no consensus among perinatal experts on the appropriate length of labor and its relationship to risks of adverse maternal–fetal outcomes. The Friedman curve is still most commonly used in the clinical setting to assess normal progression of labor. Generally, characteristics of most unmedicated labors will be similar in length, progression, cervical changes, and fetal descent, as outlined by Friedman, Niswander, Bayonet-Rivera, & Sachtleben (1966), but it is important to consider that this classic research was done before the significant increase in the use of medications to ripen the cervix and stimulate uterine contractions and the use regional analgesia in the United States and Canada.

Based on available data (Albers, 1999; Albers, Schiff, & Gorwoda, 1996; Cohen, 1977; Menticoglou, Manning, Harman, & Morrison, 1995; Moon, Smith, & Rayburn, 1990), it is likely that previously held arbitrary time frames for the duration of labor (Friedman, 1978; Friedman, Niswander, Bayonet-Rivera, & Sachtleben, 1966; Hellman & Prystowsky, 1952) are no longer valid for all women. Multiple factors, including timing and dosage of epidural analgesia or anesthesia, use of oxytocin or misoprostol, amniotomy, fetal size and position, and maternal psyche, labor positions, and pelvic structure, influence the progress of labor (Malone et al., 1996; Rojansky, Tanos, Reubinoff, Shapira, & Weinstein, 1997; Thorp & Breedlove, 1996). There is a relationship between parity and the type of labor progression variances. Women in labor with their first child are more likely to experience hypertonic uterine dysfunction, primary inertia, or a prolonged latent phase in early labor. During second and subsequent labors, deviations from the Friedman criteria during

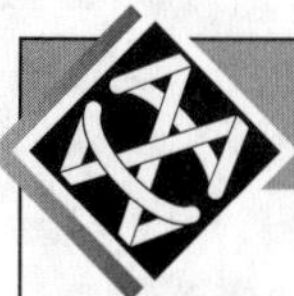

DISPLAY 9–2

Comparison of False and True Labor

FALSE LABOR	TRUE LABOR
Regular contractions	Regular contractions
Decrease in frequency and intensity; longer intervals	Progressive frequency and intensity; closer intervals
Discomfort in lower abdomen and groin	Discomfort begins in back, radiating to the abdomen
Activity has no effect or decreases contractions; disappear with sleep	Activity such as walking increases contractions; continue even when sleeping
No appreciable change in cervix	Progressive effacement and dilation of cervix
Sedation decreases or stops contractions	Sedation does not stop contractions
Show usually not present	Show usually present

active labor, such as hypotonic uterine dysfunction, secondary inertia, and protraction or arrest of the active phase, are more common. Figure 9–1 shows an expected labor pattern and commonly seen deviations.

Although previously it was thought that limiting the second stage of labor to 2 hours was essential to decrease risks of fetal morbidity and mortality (Hellman & Prystowsky, 1952; Wood, Ng, Hounslow, & Benning, 1973), it is now known that waiting beyond 2 hours for the fetus to descend spontaneously is safe. This recommendation was made before the widespread use of continuous electronic fetal monitoring (EFM) and epidural anesthesia (Simpson & Knox, 2001). Based on a substantial body of literature, the arbitrary 2-hour time frame is no longer clinically valid. As long as the fetal heart rate (FHR) is reassuring and there is evidence of fetal descent, there is no risk to the mother or fetus in waiting for spontaneous birth (Albers et al., 1996; Cohen, 1977; Derham, Crowhurst, & Crowther, 1991; Maresh, Choong, & Beard, 1983; Menticoglou et al., 1995; Moon et al., 1990; Paterson, Saunders, & Wadsworth, 1992; Thomson, 1993). Maternal–fetal status and individual clinical situations provide the best data for labor assessment and management.

Stages of Labor and Birth

Labor and birth have traditionally been divided into four stages. The first stage is subdivided into the latent, active, and transition phases of labor. Cervical changes are used in assessing progression through each phase: latent phase, 0 to 3 cm; active phase, 4 to 7 cm; and transition, 8 to 10 cm. A woman having her first baby usually experiences complete cervical effacement before dilation. Increasing effacement usually occurs simultaneously with dilation in multiparous women. Table 9–1 summarizes the stages of labor, including average duration, cervical changes, uterine activity, maternal activity, and physical sensations.

Facilitating Labor and Birth

Nursing care during childbirth includes measures directed toward providing information so the woman knows what to expect. The nurse helps with interpreting physical sensations, encouraging maternal position changes, reinforcing breathing and other relaxation efforts, offering support during the second stage, and providing continued pain management. Attention is also given to the woman's partner or support person and family members in attendance. Every effort should be made to support and encourage those in attendance to assist the woman during labor and to allow as many support persons as the woman desires. Arbitrary rules prohibiting more than one support person during labor and birth are contrary to the philosophy that the birth experience belongs to the woman and her family rather than to those providing clinical care. Although healthcare providers are sometimes inclined to attempt to control this aspect of the birth process using various arguments about safety and convenience, when examined critically, these arguments have little scientific merit. Women should be able to choose who will be with them during this very special and unique life experience (Rouse & MacNeil, 2000). Family-centered care supports the concept that the "family" is defined by the childbearing woman. Families should be free to take still pictures and record video or audio tapes during labor and birth.

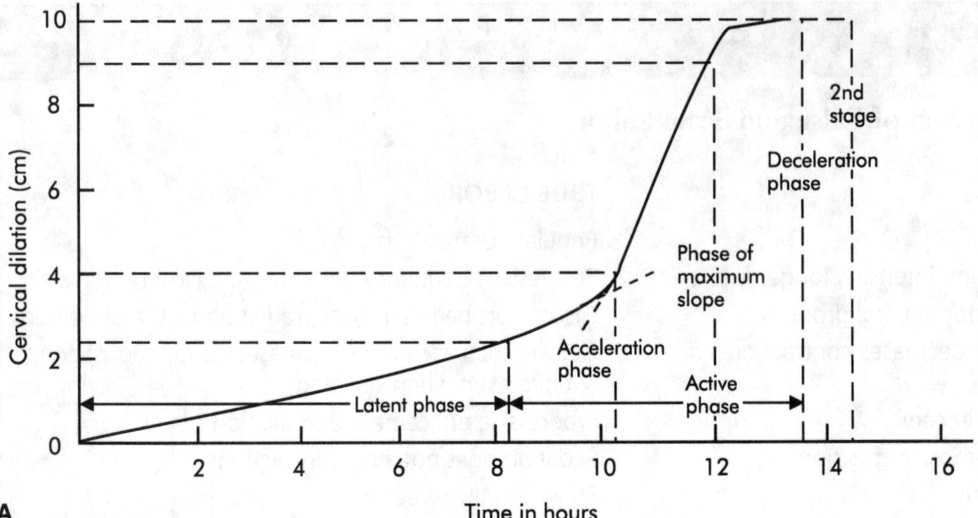

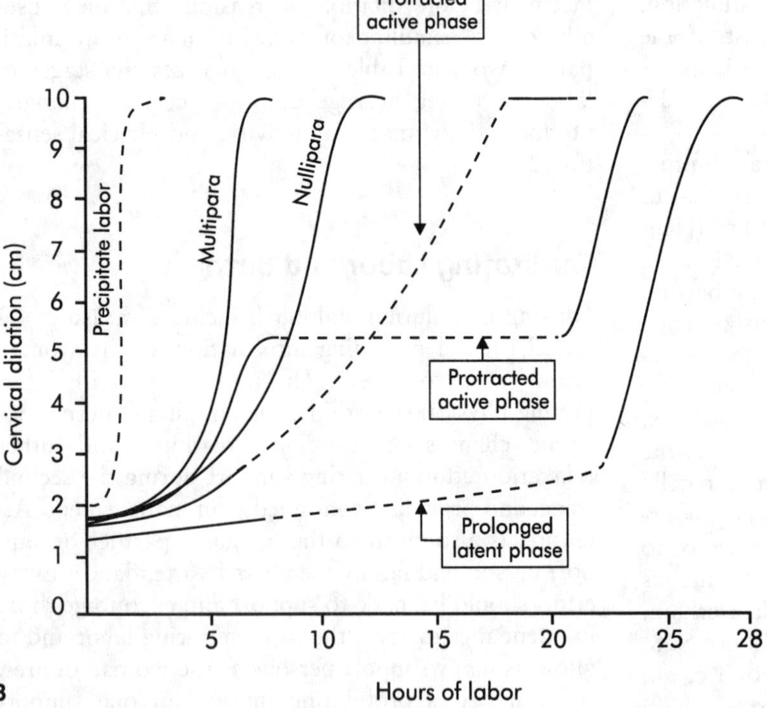

FIGURE 9–1 **(A)** Partogram of a normal labor. **(B)** Major types of deviation from normal progress of labor may be detected by noting dilation of cervix at various intervals after labor begins. If a woman exhibits an abnormal labor pattern, as depicted by broken lines, physician or certified nurse midwife should be notified. (From Bobak, I. M., & Jensen, M. D. [1991]. *Essentials of maternity nursing* [p. 765]. St. Louis, MO: Mosby–Year Book. Copyright 1991 by Mosby–Year Book. Reprinted with permission.)

Policies restricting cameras are in conflict with the philosophy that the birth experience should be, within reason, what the woman and her family desire. Concerns about safety, liability, privacy, and space limitations can be adequately addressed without restrictive policies about visitors and use of cameras during labor and birth if care providers are committed to meeting the needs of childbearing women and their support persons.

Nursing Assessments

Initial Assessment of Maternal–Fetal Status

Major roles of the perinatal nurse caring for laboring women include a thorough admission assessment and ongoing maternal–fetal assessments. Appendix 9A contains a sample intrapartum admission assessment. The focus of this assessment is on prior obstetric history, current pregnancy, labor symptoms, and a history and physical examination emphasizing the respiratory, cardiovascular, gastrointestinal, urinary, and musculoskeletal systems. *Guidelines for Perinatal Care* (American Academy of Pediatrics [AAP] & American College of Obstetricians [ACOG], 1997) provides recommendations for the components of a comprehensive admission assessment for pregnant women.

Pregnant women may come to the hospital's labor and birth unit not only for perinatal care, but also for treatment of any sign or symptom of illness. Any pregnant woman presenting to a hospital for care should, at a minimum, be assessed for the following: FHR, maternal vital signs, and uterine contractions (AAP & ACOG, 1997). The responsible perinatal healthcare provider should be informed promptly of any of the following findings: vaginal bleeding, acute abdominal pain, temperature of 100.4°F or higher, preterm labor, preterm premature rupture of membranes, and hypertension (AAP & ACOG, 1997). When a pregnant woman is evaluated for labor, the following factors should be assessed and recorded: blood pressure (BP), pulse, temperature, frequency and duration of uterine contractions, FHR, clinical estimation of fetal weight, urinary protein and glucose levels, cervical dilatation and effacement unless contraindicated (e.g., placenta previa), fetal presentation and station of the presenting part, status of the membranes, and date and time of the woman's arrival and notification of the provider (AAP & ACOG, 1997).

If the woman has had prenatal care and a recent examination has confirmed the normal progress of pregnancy, her admission evaluation may be limited to an interval history and physical examination directed at the presenting complaint (AAP & ACOG, 1997). Previously identified risk factors should be recorded in the prenatal record. If no new risk factors are found, attention may be focused on the following historic factors: time of onset and frequency of contractions, status of the membranes, presence or absence of bleeding, fetal movement, history of allergies, time, content, and amount of most recent food or fluid ingestion, and use of any medication (AAP & ACOG, 1997).

Pregnant women sometimes come to the hospital before labor is established. They may be experiencing uterine contractions that have not yet resulted in cervical changes, or they may be in very early labor. If a thorough maternal–fetal assessment results in the decision to discharge the woman, it is important to ensure that assessment and discharge processes are consistent with federal regulations according to the Emergency Medical Treatment and Labor Act (EMTALA). Chapter 2 discusses EMTALA and the implications for perinatal services.

The initial interaction during the admission process is used to develop rapport with the woman and her family and to get a sense of their expectations about their birth experience. Ideally, the amount of childbirth preparation and type of pain management anticipated during labor is covered during the admission assessment. A review of preferences for childbirth, including a discussion of options that are available at the institution, works best to facilitate a positive experience. Although some labor nurses have negative feelings about written birth plans, a birth plan can be valuable in helping the nurse meet the couple's expectations and indicates the woman has given considerable thought to how she would like labor and birth to proceed.

Ongoing Assessment of Maternal–Fetal Status

Limited data are available to support prescribed frequencies of maternal–fetal assessments during labor and birth. No prospective study was found in a Medline search about how often to assess the mother and fetus during labor. A reasonable approach to determining frequency of assessment is based on individual clinical situations, guidelines and standards from professional organizations, and unit policies. ACOG recommends that maternal temperature, pulse, respirations, and BP be assessed and recorded at regular intervals during labor or at least every 4 hours (AAP & ACOG, 1997). This frequency may be increased, particularly as active labor progresses according to clinical signs and symptoms.

During the active phase of the first stage of labor, the FHR should be assessed at 30-minute intervals, preferably just after a contraction, and during the second stage of the labor, the FHR should be assessed at 15-minute intervals, unless fetal risk status or response to labor indicates the need for more frequent assessment (AAP & ACOG, 1997). If risk factors are identified on admission or develop during the course of labor, the FHR should be assessed every 15 minutes, preferably just after a contraction, during the active phase of the first stage of labor, and every 5 minutes during the second stage of labor (AAP & ACOG, 1997). These assessments can occur by intermittent auscultation of the FHR or by continuous EFM (AAP & ACOG, 1997). The use of regional analgesia, oxytocin dosage rate, and intervals between increases in the oxytocin dosage rate are additional considerations when determining how often to assess maternal–fetal well-being during labor.

TABLE 9–1 ■ STAGES OF LABOR

Stage	Duration	Contraction Frequency	Contraction Duration	Contraction Intensity	Physical Sensations	Maternal Behavior
First Stage						
Latent, 0–3 cm	Primigravida, 8.6 hr; multigravida, 5.3 hr	3–30 min; may be irregular	30–40 sec	Mild by palpation; 25–40 mm Hg by intrauterine pressure catheter (IUPC)	Menstrual-like cramps; low, dull backache; light bloody show; diarrhea; possible rupture of membranes	Pain controlled fairly well; able to ambulate and talk through most contractions; range of emotions—excited, talkative, and confident versus anxious, withdrawn, and apprehensive
Active, 4–7 cm	Primigravida, 4.6 hr; multigravida, 2.4 hr	2–5 min	40–60 sec	Moderate to strong by palpation; 50–70 mm Hg by IUPC	Increasing discomfort; trembling of thighs and legs; pressure on bladder and rectum; persistent backache with occipitoposterior fetal position	Begins to work at maintaining control during contractions; accepts "coaching" efforts of perinatal staff and support persons; quieter

Guidelines for ongoing labor assessments are described in *Standards and Guidelines for Professional Nursing Practice in the Care of Women and Newborns* (Association of Women's Health, Obstetric, and Neonatal Nurses [AWHONN], 1998), AWHONN's symposium *Cervical Ripening and Induction and Augmentation of Labor* (Simpson & Poole, 1998a), and *Didactic Content and Clinical Skills Verification for Professional Nurse Providers of Basic, High Risk, and Critical Care Intrapartum Nursing* (AWHONN, 1999). *Guidelines for Perinatal Care* (AAP & ACOG, 1997), *Fetal Heart Rate Patterns: Monitoring, Interpretation, and Management* (ACOG, 1995b), *Standards* (Joint Commission on Accreditation of Healthcare Organizations [JCAHO], 2000), perinatal nursing textbooks, and some state board of health publications are other resources that provide guidelines for initial and ongoing nursing assessments of women in labor. Based on these guidelines, each perinatal center develops standards of care related to maternal–fetal assessment. Display 9–3 provides the suggested guidelines for maternal and fetal assessment during a normal, uncomplicated labor. Appendix 9B provides a sample medical record form for documentation during labor.

Although most providers in the United States choose continuous or intermittent EFM, the institution's policy should include guidelines for intermittent auscultation based on the AAP and ACOG (1997) recommendations if electronic monitoring is not the preference of the woman, physician, or certified nurse midwife (CNM). The AWHONN symposium on *Fetal Heart Rate Auscultation* (Feinstein, Sprague, & Trepanier, 2000) provides a comprehensive discussion about technique, rationale, interpretation, and clinical

(text continues on page 308)

TABLE 9–1 ■ STAGES OF LABOR (continued)

Stage	Duration	Contraction Frequency	Contraction Duration	Contraction Intensity	Physical Sensations	Maternal Behavior
Transition, 8–10 cm	Primigravida, 3.6 hr; multigravida, variable	1.5–2 min	60–90 sec	Strong by palpation; 70–90 mm Hg by IUPC	Increased bloody show; urge to push; Increased rectal pressure; membranes may rupture if they have not already	Ambulation difficult with uterine contractions; may be irritable and agitated; self-absorbed and may appear to sleep between contractions; need for support increases; verbalizes feelings of discouragement and doubts her ability to cope
Second Stage						
10 cm to birth	Primigravida, up to 3 hr; multigravida, 0–30 min	2–3 min	40–60 sec	Strong by palpation; 70–100 mm Hg by IUPC	As presenting part descends, urge to push increases; increased rectal and perineal pressure; sensation of burning, tearing, and stretching of vagina and perineum	Excited and eager to push; reluctant, ineffective at pushing
Third Stage						
Birth of the infant to birth of the placenta	5–30 min				Mild uterine contractions; feeling of fullness in vagina as placenta is expelled	Attention is focused on the newborn; feelings of relief

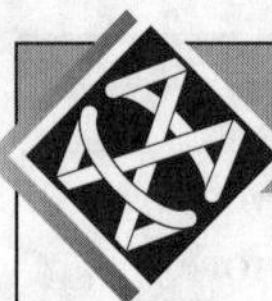

DISPLAY 9–3

Current Guidelines From Professional Organizations for Maternal–Fetal Assessments During Labor and Birth and Maternal–Newborn Assessments During the Immediate Postpartum Period

ASSESSMENTS FOR ANY HOSPITAL ADMISSION OF PREGNANT WOMEN

Pregnant women may come to the hospital's labor and birth unit for obstetric care and for treatment of any sign or symptom of illness. Any pregnant woman presenting to a hospital for care should, at a minimum, be assessed for the following:

- Fetal heart rate
- Maternal vital signs
- Uterine contractions

The responsible obstetric care provider should be informed promptly if any of the following findings are present:

- Vaginal bleeding
- Acute abdominal pain
- Temperature of 100.4° F or higher
- Preterm labor
- Preterm premature rupture of membranes
- Hypertension (AAP & ACOG, 1997)

ASSESSMENTS DURING ADMISSION FOR LABOR PROCESS

When a pregnant woman is evaluated for labor, the following factors should be assessed and recorded:

- Blood pressure, pulse, temperature
- Frequency and duration of uterine contractions
- Fetal heart rate
- Clinical estimation of fetal weight
- Urinary protein and glucose
- Cervical dilatation and effacement, unless contraindicated (eg, placenta previa)
- Fetal presentation and station of the presenting part
- Status of the membranes
- Date and time of the woman's arrival and notification of the provider (AAP & ACOG, 1997)

If the woman has had prenatal care and a recent examination has confirmed the normal progress of pregnancy, her admission evaluation may be limited to an interval history and physical examination directed at the presenting complaint. Previously identified risk factors should be recorded in the prenatal record. If no new risk factors are found, attention may be focused on the following historic factors:

- Time of onset and frequency of contractions
- Status of the membranes
- Presence or absence of bleeding
- Fetal movement
- History of allergies
- Time, content, and amount of most recent food or fluid ingestion
- Use of any medication (AAP & ACOG, 1997)

ASSESSMENTS DURING LABOR AND BIRTH

Maternal Vital Signs

Maternal vital signs should be assessed and recorded at regular intervals, at least every 4 hours. This frequency may be increased, particularly as active labor progresses according to clinical signs and symptoms (AAP & ACOG, 1997)

Fetal Heart Rate

The intensity of fetal heart rate (FHR) monitoring used during labor should be based on risk factors.

In the absence of risk factors, use the following guidelines:

- The standard practice is to evaluate and record the FHR at least every 30 minutes during the active phase of the first stage of labor and at least every 15 minutes during the second stage of labor.

When risk factors are present, use the following guidelines:

- During the active phase of the first stage of labor, if auscultation is used, the FHR should be evaluated and recorded at least every 15 minutes after a uterine contraction. If continuous electronic monitoring is used, the tracing should be evaluated every 15 minutes.
- During the second stage of labor, with auscultation, the FHR should be evaluated and recorded at least every 5 minutes. When electronic monitoring is used, the FHR should also be evaluated at least every 5 minutes (ACOG, 1995b; AAP & ACOG, 1997)

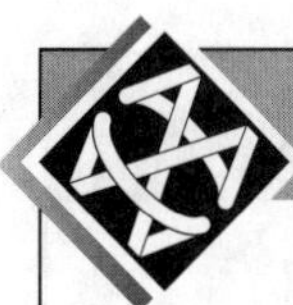

DISPLAY 9–3 (cont.)

Current Guidelines From Professional Organizations for Maternal–Fetal Assessments During Labor and Birth and Maternal–Newborn Assessments During the Immediate Postpartum Period

During oxytocin induction or augmentation, the FHR should be evaluated every 15 minutes during the active phase of the first stage of labor and every 5 minutes during the second stage of labor (AAP & ACOG, 1997).

Evaluation of the FHR should occur at recommended intervals; when electronic fetal monitoring is used to permanently record these data, periodic documentation can be used to summarize FHR status as outlined in institutional protocols. During oxytocin induction or augmentation, at a minimum, document the FHR before every dosage increase (Simpson & Poole [AWHONN], 1998a). If the dosage is maintained at the same rate, a reasonable approach is nursing documentation of the FHR at least every hour during oxytocin administration (Simpson & Poole [AWHONN], 1998a).

Misoprostol should be administered at or near the labor and birth suite, where the FHR can be monitored continuously (ACOG, 1999a).

Cervidil should be administered at or near the labor and birth suite, where the FHR can be monitored continuously while in place and for at least 15 minutes after removal (ACOG, 1999a).

Prepidil should be administered at or near the labor and birth suite, where the FHR can be monitored for at least 30 minutes to 2 hours after placement (ACOG, 1999a).

Uterine Activity and Labor Progress

For women who are at no increased risk for complications, evaluation of the quality of uterine contractions should be sufficient to detect abnormalities in the progress of labor (AAP & ACOG, 1997).

Misoprostol should be administered at or near the labor and birth suite, where uterine activity and the fetal heart rate can be monitored continuously (ACOG, 1999a).

Cervidil should be administered at or near the labor and birth suite, where uterine activity can be monitored continuously while in place and for at least 15 minutes after removal (ACOG, 1999a).

Prepidil should be administered at or near the labor and birth suite, where uterine activity can be monitored for at least 30 minutes to 2 hours after placement (ACOG, 1999a).

During oxytocin induction or augmentation, at a minimum, assess and document characteristics of uterine contractions before every dosage increase (Simpson & Poole [AWHONN], 1998a).

If the dosage is maintained at the same rate, a reasonable approach is nursing assessment and documentation of the characteristics of uterine contractions at least every hour during oxytocin administration (Simpson & Poole [AWHONN], 1998).

Vaginal examinations should be sufficient to detect abnormalities in the progress of labor (AAP & ACOG, 1997) and include assessment of dilatation and effacement of the cervix and station of the fetal presenting part (Simpson & Poole [AWHONN], 1998a).

Additional Parameters During Labor

Assess character and amount of amniotic fluid; clear, bloody, meconium stained, or odor.

Assess character and amount of bloody show or vaginal bleeding.

Assess maternal affect and response to labor.

Assess level of maternal discomfort and effectiveness of pain management or pain relief measures.

Assess labor support person's abilities.

(AAP & ACOG, 1997; Simpson & Poole [AWHONN], 1998a).

During Regional Analgesia/Anesthesia

Women who receive epidural analgesia should be monitored in a manner similar to that used for any patient in labor (ACOG, 1996).

During regional anesthesia for women in labor vital signs and FHR should be monitored and documented by a qualified individual (ASA, 1991).

Maternal vital signs should be monitored at regular intervals by a qualified member of the health-

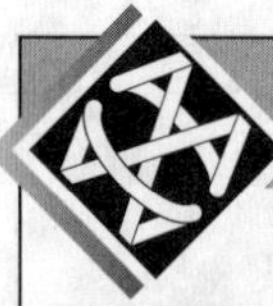

DISPLAY 9–3 (cont.)

Current Guidelines From Professional Organizations for Maternal–Fetal Assessments During Labor and Birth and Maternal–Newborn Assessments During the Immediate Postpartum Period

care team during epidural anesthesia in labor (AAP & ACOG, 1997).

When epidural anesthesia/analgesia is initiated, the nurse monitors maternal vital signs and the fetal heart rate based on each patient's status. The fetal heart rate is assessed before and after the procedure, either intermittently or continuously, and as possible during the procedure. Additional monitoring of the patient is provided during epidural anesthesia/analgesia when the patient's condition warrants. (ASA, 1999; AWHONN, 1998a).

ASSESSMENTS DURING THE IMMEDIATE POSTPARTUM PERIOD

Maternal Assessments

Monitoring of maternal status is dictated in part by the events of the birth process and the complications identified.

During the period of observation immediately after birth, maternal vital signs and additional signs or events should be monitored and recorded as they occur. Maternal blood pressure and pulse should be assessed and recorded immediately after birth and repeated every 15 minutes for the first hour and more frequently if complications are encountered.

The amount of vaginal bleeding should be evaluated often, and the uterine fundus should be identified and massaged and its size and degree of contraction noted (AAP & ACOG, 1997).

Newborn Assessments

Apgar scores should be obtained at 1 minute and 5 minutes after birth and for an extended period until the Apgar score is 7 or greater.

Following an initial evaluation of the newborn's condition, the newborn should be carefully observed during the subsequent stabilization-transition period (the first 6–12 hours after birth). Temperature, heart and respiratory rates, skin color, adequacy of peripheral circulation, type of respiration, level of consciousness, tone, and activity should be monitored and recorded at least once every 30 minutes until the newborn's condition has remained stable for at least 2 hours. (AAP & ACOG, 1997; AWHONN, 1998a).

When determining frequency of maternal–fetal assessments during labor, factors such as stage of labor, maternal–fetal risk status, and institutional policies, procedures, and protocols should be taken into consideration (Simpson & Poole [AWHONN], 1998).

Collaboration between perinatal care providers and reviews of current published guidelines as outlined here can facilitate development of institutional guidelines for practice.

decision-making when using intermittent auscultation during labor.

Maternal–fetal assessment should occur at the bedside by laying hands on the pregnant woman rather than using data obtained from the central monitoring station. Characteristics of FHR patterns are frequently different when obtained by direct observation of the EFM strip at the bedside. Use of automatic BP devices should be avoided because of their inaccuracies during pregnancy and specifically during labor. Use of a mercury BP cuff and stethoscope is the more accurate method of assessing BP in pregnant and laboring women. Automatic BP devices tend to overestimate systolic BP by 4 to 6 mm Hg and underestimate diastolic BP by 10 mm Hg when used for pregnant women (Brown et al., 1994; Franx et al., 1994). Inaccuracies in BP data can lead to inappropriate treatment. For example, a diastolic BP of 95 mm Hg obtained by a nurse using a mercury BP cuff and stethoscope may be recorded as 85 mm Hg by an automatic BP device, and an elevated BP could potentially be missed and not treated appropriately or in a timely manner. In contrast, an underestimated diastolic BP could result in treatment for hypotension after epidural dosage, potentially leading to fetal compromise if a vasopressor is given for hypotension that does not actually exist. Many women report discomfort when automatic BP cuffs are used on a frequent basis during labor.

Standards of care, inaccuracy issues, costs, and patient discomfort should be important considerations in discontinuing routine use of automatic BP devices, cardiac monitors, and pulse oximeters for healthy women during labor. If the woman's clinical condition requires more intensive and frequent monitoring, use of these devices may be appropriate and can provide valuable data about maternal well-being. Data from automatic BP devices can be used for evaluating trends in maternal BP for women who need more intensive and frequent assessment but should be used in the context of what is known about the differences in readings obtained from mercury BP cuffs and a stethoscope compared with these devices.

Evaluation of routine practices for healthy women who desire regional analgesia during labor or are receiving pharmacologic agents to stimulate uterine contractions should be based on available literature and publications from ACOG, AWHONN, and the American Society of Anesthesiologists (ASA). A standards-based protocol contributes to appropriate levels of care according to individual clinical situations while avoiding unnecessary interventions and technology.

There are no standards or guidelines from AWHONN or ACOG about how often BP should be assessed when women are receiving oxytocin, but in many institutions, protocols are in place that require assessments every 15 minutes. These protocols are not based on sound scientific data, and they contribute to the routine use of automatic BP devices during labor because intrapartum nurses find it difficult to manually assess maternal BP every 15 minutes if they are responsible for more than one patient. These protocols have not been shown to contribute to better outcomes during labor. If the nurse-to-patient ratio in labor is more than one to one, the automatic BP device often is activated according to programed intervals while the nurse is not at the bedside. The automatic BP device can be initiated and data recorded during a uterine contraction. Maternal pain and anxiety during the height of a contraction can alter BP. The woman in labor may have repositioned herself while the nurse was out of the room. Maternal positions affect BP. These data are automatically recorded on the EFM strip or manually recorded in the medical record by the nurse when she has time to return to the bedside. BP data obtained by automatic devices are not used in a clinically timely manner and might have been obtained during a uterine contraction or after a maternal position change unknown to the nurse. Retrospective evaluation and documentation of a series of BPs recorded by an automatic BP device while the nurse was out of the room is not consistent with timely assessment during labor.

In many institutions, routine care for healthy women during epidural analgesia includes cardiac monitoring, pulse oximetry, and frequent BP assessment using an automatic BP device. Use of these monitoring devices are not standards of care (AAP & ACOG, 1997; ACOG, 1996; ASA, 1999; AWHONN, 1998) and can lead to increased cost and unnecessary technologic interventions for women without identified risk factors. Unless risk factors have been identified, care of a woman with epidural analgesia may be similar to that of any other woman in labor (ACOG, 1996). Regular assessment of maternal–fetal status should be performed by a qualified healthcare provider during epidural analgesia for labor and birth (ASA, 1999).

Vaginal Examinations

Nurses should develop proficiency in performing vaginal examinations to assess labor progress and determine the need for nursing interventions such as position changes and timing of medication administration. They must first be able to identify situations in which a vaginal examination is required and recognize when a vaginal examination is contraindicated, such as with unexplained vaginal bleeding or with premature rupture of the membranes. Developing clinical proficiency in performing vaginal examinations requires practice and assistance from a knowledgeable preceptor. Women undergoing a vaginal examination should be minimally exposed and should be advised of the necessity of the examination and the findings. The woman should also be positioned on her back with her head slightly elevated. The vaginal examination should be systematic, beginning with assessment of dilation and effacement and then fetal presentation, station, and position. The normal length of the pregravid cervix is 3.5 to 4 cm. The length of the cervix may vary in women who have had cervical surgery such as conization or laser excision procedures.

Assessment of station and position of the fetal head requires more skill. The ischial spines must be identified to assess station in relation to the biparietal diameter of the fetal head. The ischial spines may be identified by pressing in the sidewall of the vagina approximately 1 inch, with the examining fingers at approximately 3 and 9 o'clock, respectively. It is not necessary to identify both spines to assess station. The occiput of the fetal head should be at the level of the ischial spines to be engaged (ie, zero station). The examiner should not be confused by caput formation but instead identify the fetal skull for this assessment. The most difficult determination to make is that of fetal head position: occiput anterior or posterior. The examining nurse must be familiar with the location of the suture lines in the fetal skull, more so than the shape of the anterior or posterior fontanelle, because distortion or overlapping bones alter fontanelle shape. The nurse should first identify the sagittal suture and then slide fingers to a fontanelle and count the number of suture lines extending from it exclusive of the sagittal suture. This can be accomplished by sweeping the examining finger 180 degrees at a right angle to the sagittal suture. The anterior fontanelle has three suture lines extending from it, and the posterior fontanelle has two suture lines. It is unnecessary to palpate the posterior fontanelle to determine position of the fetal head. Determination of the position of the fetal head becomes necessary primarily during the second stage of labor, when descent is slow. Repositioning the woman to a squatting, sidelying, or hands-and-knees position to push may facilitate rotation of the fetal head.

Perineal hygiene is important during periodic vaginal examinations. Attention to clean technique is critical, particularly if membranes are ruptured. Sterile, water-soluble lubricants may be used to decrease discomfort during vaginal examinations, but antiseptics such as povidone-iodine and hexachlorophene should be avoided. These antiseptics have not been shown to decrease infections acquired during the intrapartum period, but they may cause local irritation and are absorbed through maternal mucous membranes (AAP & ACOG, 1997). Lubricants containing these agents and sprays or liquids delivering them directly to the introitus are not recommended for use during labor (AAP & ACOG, 1997).

Leopold Maneuvers

Leopold maneuvers provide a systematic assessment of fetal position and presentation and should be performed before application of EFM as part of the admission assessment. Information obtained while performing these maneuvers supports assessments made during vaginal examinations and assists in determining the best position to locate the FHR (Fig. 9–2). Leopold maneuvers may be difficult with women who are obese, have tense or guarded abdominal muscles, or have polyhydramnios. In these situations, an ultrasound scan may be necessary to determine fetal position and presentation.

Fetal Heart Rate Assessment

Systematic assessment of the FHR by EFM includes determination of the baseline rate, variability, and presence or absence of accelerations or decelerations. Intermittent auscultation of the FHR with a stethoscope or hand-held ultrasound device includes determination of the rate and presence or absence of accelerations or decelerations. If decelerations are identified, further assessment is required to determine the type and duration. Clinical interventions are based on comprehensive assessment of all of the characteristics of the FHR pattern depicted by EFM or noted during auscultation and the individual clinical situation of the mother and fetus, including gestational age and medications administered to the mother. The FHR can be determined by use of the external ultrasound device of the EFM in most situations. If the clinical situation is such that more accurate data are needed about fetal status, an internal fetal scalp electrode (FSE) may be applied. Chapter 10 provides a comprehensive discussion of FHR assessment.

Uterine Activity Assessment

A thorough and accurate assessment of the frequency, duration, and intensity of contractions and the uterine resting tone between contractions is an important component of nursing assessments during labor. An assessment of uterine activity begins with direct palpation. Contraction frequency is measured from the beginning of one contraction to the beginning of the next and is described in minutes. Duration is assessed by the length of the contraction and is described in seconds. Intensity refers to the strength of the contraction and is described as mild, moderate, or strong by palpation or by millimeters of mercury (mm Hg) of intraamniotic pressure with an intrauterine pressure catheter (IUPC). Uterine resting tone is assessed in the absence of contractions or between contractions. By direct palpation, resting tone is described as soft or hard and, by IUPC, in terms of mmHg of intraamniotic pressure.

The external tocodynamometer detects abdominal wall changes during contractions and uterine relaxation. This method provides information about frequency and duration; however, resting tone and intensity must be determined by palpation. Contraction frequency, duration, intensity, and uterine resting tone can be evaluated by palpation and an IUPC. The IUPC is more accurate because direct measurement of intraamniotic pressure is recorded but requires ruptured membranes for insertion. The cervix should be at least 2 to 3 cm dilated before insertion of an IUPC or FSE. As with any procedure, the least invasive approach is preferred unless maternal–fetal status indicates need for more objective data.

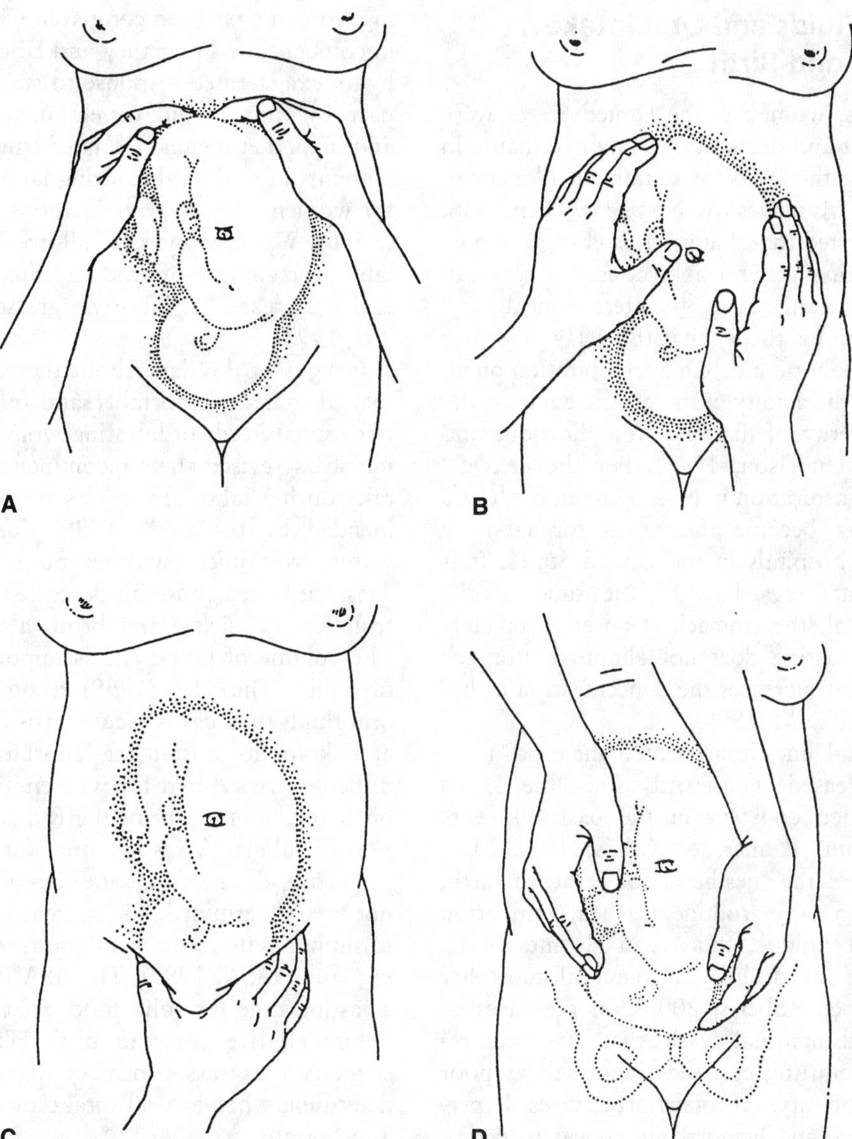

FIGURE 9–2. Leopold Maneuvers. (**A**) First maneuver helps determine fetal presentation or the part of the fetus presenting at the inlet of the pelvis; presentations usually are head or breech. The examiner faces the woman's head and uses the tips of the fingers to palpate the fundus of the uterus. The fetal head feels smooth, globular, and firm and is mobile and ballotts. However, breech presentation feels irregular, rounded, and soft and is less mobile. (**B**) Second maneuver helps to determine fetal position or identifies the relationship of the fetal back and small parts to the front, back, or sides of the maternal pelvis. The examiner continues to face the woman's head and places hands on either side of the uterus. While one hand stabilizes one side of the uterus, the other hand palpates the opposite side of the uterus to determine fetal back or small parts. Then the other side of the uterus is stabilized and palpated to locate the fetal back. The back is a long, smooth, hard plane. The small parts feel irregular and knobby and may be moving. (**C**) Third maneuver helps to determine presenting part. While continuing to face the woman's head, the examiner uses the thumb and fingers of one hand to grasp the woman's lower abdomen at just about the symphysis pubis and notes the contour, size, and consistency of the presenting part. The head feels firm and globular and is mobile if unengaged and immobile if engaged. A breech presentation feels smaller, softer, and irregular. **D**, Fourth maneuver helps to determine fetal attitude or the greatest prominence of the fetal head over the brim of the pelvis. The examiner faces the woman's feet and, using the tips of the first three fingers of each hand, presses deep in the direction of the pelvic inlet. The fingers of one hand will encounter a bony cephalic prominence. If the cephalic prominence is located on the opposite side from the back, it is the infant's brow, and the head is flexed. If the cephalic prominence is located on the same side as the back, it is the occiput, and the head is extended.

Intravenous Fluids and Oral Intake During Labor and Birth

Before the 1940s, women in the United States were encouraged to eat and drink during labor to maintain their stamina for the work of childbirth (American College of Nurse Midwives [ACNM], 1999). In 1946, Mendelson suggested that maternal aspiration of gastric contents during general anesthesia for cesarean birth was a significant cause of maternal morbidity. This was based on his theory that the delay in gastric emptying during labor contributed to aspiration pneumonitis and that the acidity of the gastric contents determined the severity of maternal complications and risk of death (Mendelson, 1946). For the next 50 years, to prevent aspiration in case cesarean birth was necessary, fasting became the norm for laboring women in most hospitals in the United States. It is now known that, regardless of the time of the woman's last meal, the stomach is never completely empty and that fasting does not eliminate stomach contents but rather increases the concentration of hydrochloric acid (ACNM, 1999).

Risks of general anesthesia-related maternal morbidity have decreased significantly since the 1940s but have remained constant in the past 20 years (Hawkins, Koonin, Palmer, & Gibbs, 1997). Decreased use of general anesthesia for cesarean birth, use of cricoid pressure, routine tracheal intubation with improved technique, and use of H_2 antagonists have contributed to decline in maternal mortality (Sommer, Norr, & Roberts, 2000). In the cases of anesthesia-related maternal deaths that have been reported in the literature, complications such as poor physical status, obesity, emergent procedures, hypertension, embolism, and hemorrhage appear to be coexisting factors (ACNM, 1999; Hawkins et al., 1997). Most women in the United States who have a cesarean birth are given regional anesthesia. The case–fatality rate for regional anesthesia between 1985 and 1990 was reported to be 1.9 per million regional anesthetics during cesarean birth (Hawkins et al., 1997). The case–fatality rate for general anesthesia during the same period was 32.2 per million general anesthetics for cesarean birth (Hawkins et al., 1997).

The physiologic requirements for glucose increase during active labor (Wasserstrum, 1992). Fasting depletes the carbohydrates available, and women in labor who are not allowed oral intake may have to metabolize fat for energy (Keppler, 1988). Although there has been limited research about specific nutritional needs during labor, it has been suggested that 50 to 100 calories per hour are needed during active labor (ACNM, 1999). The energy needs of the laboring woman have been compared with those of athletes in competition. Pregnancy and labor are characterized by an exaggerated response to starvation, reflected in part by more rapid development of hypoglycemia and hyperketonemia (Wasserstrum, 1992). Modest amounts of oral intake during labor may be beneficial for women without complications or risks of complications. When women are allowed oral intake during labor, the amount of food and fluids they choose generally decreases as labor progresses (Ludka & Roberts, 1993).

In light of the data about the rarity of anesthesia-related maternal mortality and other evidence about nutritional needs of laboring women, the ASA (1999) members revised their recommendations for oral intake during labor. Examples of clear liquids recommended by the ASA (1999) during labor include water, fruit juices without pulp, carbonated beverages, clear tea, and black coffee. Flavored gelatin, fruit ice, Popsicles, and broth also may be offered. The volume of liquid is less important than the type of liquid. The ASA (1999) recommended restricting oral fluids on a case-by-case basis for women who are at risk for aspiration (eg, morbidly obese, diabetic, difficult airway) and for women at risk for operative birth (eg, nonreassuring FHR patterns, nonprogression of labor). A fasting time for solid food that is predictive of maternal anesthesia complications has not been determined, and there is insufficient evidence to support safe recommendations for solid intake during labor (ASA, 1999). The ASA (1999) recommends a fasting time for solid food of at least 6 to 8 hours before elective cesarean birth. The ACNM (1999) suggests a risk assessment of women in labor should determine whether oral intake of fluids and solids is appropriate.

Each institution should have a policy for oral nutrition in labor that has been developed in collaboration with anesthesia providers. This policy should not arbitrarily restrict oral and solid intake during labor but rather be based on what is known about complications that increase the risk of general anesthesia. Women should be informed about the small, but potentially serious, risks of aspiration related to oral intake during labor (ACNM, 1999). It should be made clear that it is the anesthesia that is the risk, not the oral intake, and that if labor deviates from the normal course, she may be asked to refrain from oral intake (ACNM, 1999).

Normal, healthy women at term have at least 2 L of water stored in their extravascular spaces and have accumulated fat and fluids over the course of the pregnancy (Sleutel & Golden, 1999). A long labor with the woman fasting may deplete those energy resources. Maternal fluid loss occurs with perspiration, use of various breathing techniques, and vomiting. When fasting during labor became the norm after the 1940s, administration of intravenous (IV) fluids became routine practice. Prophylactic IV access was advocated in anticipation of administration of rapid volume expanders and blood products in the case of emergencies that can result in maternal hypovolemia and hemorrhage, such as uterine rupture, abruptio placenta, regional anesthesia complications, and immediate postpartum hemorrhage. Intravenous fluids are thought to increase maternal blood volume with resultant increased blood flow (oxygen) to the placenta. In theory, more oxygen would be available at the placenta site for maternal–fetal exchange. Intravenous fluid boluses are often given during a nonreassuring FHR pattern. However, it is likely that the increase in blood flow to the placenta is partially negated by a decrease in the blood's oxygen-carrying capacity caused by hemodilution with the IV fluid bolus (Sommer et al., 2000).

Administration of IV solutions containing glucose during labor is controversial and probably causes more harm than good (Sleutel & Golden, 1999). In theory, administration of glucose averts maternal hypoglycemia and starvation ketosis, but there is evidence to suggest that IV administration of glucose to the mother can have potentially detrimental effects on fetal status, including increased fetal lactate and decreased fetal pH. If the fetus is hypoxic, relatively small elevations in glucose can lead to lactate acidosis (Wasserstrum, 1992). Intravenous solutions with glucose can cause fetal hyperglycemia and subsequent reactive hypoglycemia, hyperinsulinism, acidosis, jaundice, and transient tachypnea in the newborn after birth (Sleutel & Golden, 1999; Sommer et al., 2000). A bolus of IV solution containing glucose can cause marked maternal hyperglycemia (Wasserstrum, 1992). When the clinical situation is such that a bolus of IV fluids may be necessary to expand plasma volume (eg, initial treatment for preterm labor, before administration of epidural anesthesia, during hypovolemic maternal emergencies), the IV fluids should not contain glucose. Glucose requirements depend on weight, use of anesthesia, phase of labor, fetal status, and other factors, and it is difficult to determine the optimal rate of glucose infusion during labor.

Despite the controversy about glucose administration during labor, lactated Ringer's (L/R) solution and 5% dextrose in lactated Ringer's (D5L/R) are common IV solutions used during labor. Many units alternate these solutions and avoid use of D5L/R when a bolus of IV fluids may be needed. One liter of D5L/R IV solution provides 225 calories (ACNM, 1999). ACOG (1999a) recommends that an isotonic IV solution be used to dilute oxytocin during induction and augmentation of labor. Results of a randomized, controlled trial (RCT) suggest that the usual amount of IV fluids during labor (125 mL/hour) may be insufficient to meet the needs of women and that inadequate hydration during labor may cause complications of labor (Garite, Weeks, & Peters-Phair, 2000). These researchers found that women who received 125 mL/hour of L/R solution had longer labors, more oxytocin, and higher rates of cesarean birth compared with women who received 250 mL/hour of L/R IV fluids. A study of pregnant women comparing different amounts of oral intake considering the same outcome variables would add to what is known about how much and what method of hydration during labor is appropriate.

Individual clinical situations should guide the selection of IV fluids during labor. More data are needed about the appropriate amount and type of IV fluids during labor. This area of intrapartum care has not been well researched, and practice is based on tradition rather than a solid body of evidence. Current resources for guidelines about IV fluids and oral intake during labor include *Practice Guidelines for Obstetrical Anesthesia* (ASA, 1999) and the *Intrapartum Nutrition Clinical Bulletin* (ACNM, 1999).

Maternal Positions During Labor and Birth

Unit culture and patient cultural background often determine the position women assume during labor and childbirth, such as lying down, squatting, sitting, standing, kneeling, or on all fours (Engleman, 1884; Liu, 1989). Recumbency, a Western cultural tradition for the convenience of obstetricians, began when more women were hospitalized for childbirth. This practice gained favor with nurses with the advent of monitoring technology. Even today, maternal position during labor and birth remains controversial and is surrounded by myths. Myths such as women who are not progressing in labor should be confined to bed for electronic monitoring and the lithotomy position is best in the second stage still prevail (Binacuzzo, 1993). Early medical research challenging the recumbent position was ignored (Mengert & Murphy, 1933; Vaughan, 1937). An upright position shortens labor (Liu, 1989). Durations of first- and second-stage labor are shorter for women who labor 30 degrees upright than for those in a flat, recumbent position (Liu, 1989). The second stage of labor is decreased when women are in a squatting position (primiparous women, 23 minutes; multiparous women, 13 minutes); these women have less oxytocin, fewer mechanically assisted births, and fewer and less severe lacerations and episiotomies compared with semirecumbent births (Golay, Vedam, & Sorger, 1993). Sitting on the toilet may be an acceptable and comfortable alternative to squatting for women who are fatigued (Shermer & Raines, 1997). Perineal edema and pelvic congestion can be prevented when using the toilet for first or second stage labor by a position change every 10 to 15 minutes (Shermer & Raines, 1997).

Ambulation during labor has been shown to decrease the rate of operative birth by 50% (Albers et al., 1997). Women who are encouraged to be mobile during labor report greater comfort and ability to tolerate labor and decreased use of analgesia and anesthesia (Bloom et al., 1998; Lupe & Gross, 1986). Although the recent tradition in the United States is confining women in active labor to bed, there is no greater risk of adverse maternal–fetal outcomes when women are encouraged to ambulate during labor (Bloom et al., 1998). If continuous EFM has been selected as the method of fetal assessment during labor, use of EFM by means of telemetry can allow the woman to ambulate while being monitored.

Women are often assisted to hands-and-knees position for certain nonreassuring FHR patterns but returned to a more standard position for birth. Last-minute change of maternal position for birth may be unwarranted, because birth may be just as easily accomplished in a hands-and-knees position (Brunner, Drummond, Meenan, & Gaskin, 1998; Gannon, 1992). Some women may benefit from use of a birth ball for relieving pressure and facilitating a more comfortable position during labor. Figures 9–3 and 9–4 depict positions for labor, using a birthing ball.

It is important to avoid the supine position during labor because of the relationship between lying flat and maternal hypotension and impedance of uteroplacental blood flow. When the woman in labor is supine, the pressure of the uterus against the spine causes compression of the inferior vena cava, aorta, and iliac arteries. If the woman wants to lie down, a left or right lateral position promotes maternal–fetal exchange at the placental level and enhances fetal well-being.

The use of regional anesthesia or analgesia may limit the use of some positions for labor and birth, particularly if there is enough motor blockade to prevent ambulation. Ambulatory epidurals and intrathecal narcotics are becoming more prevalent and are more efficient because they can provide excellent pain management without limiting mobility (Cohen, Yeh, Riley, & Vogel, 2000; Collis, Harding, & Morgan, 1999; Manning, 1996). Using medication dosages that provide an analgesic rather than an anesthetic level of epidural can allow the woman to move about more freely and feel pressure as the fetal head descends (Cohen et al., 2000; Collis et al., 1999; Driver, Popham, Glazebrook, & Palmer, 1996; Olofsson, Ekblom, Ekman-Ordeberg, & Irestedt, 1998). Feeling pressure facilitates spontaneous maternal bearing-down efforts during the second stage of labor. Nurses should be innovative with their use of positioning techniques for women with epidurals to facilitate birth while maintaining maternal safety. If the mother is confined to bed, sitting may still be facilitated by adjusting the birthing bed to a more upright position, dropping the lower section, or by helping the mother sit on the side of the bed with a stool for support (Shermer & Raines, 1997). The use of a bean bag in the bed may also assist with an upright position for women whose epidurals have resulted in decreased motor sensation in the extremities.

Supportive care techniques during labor and interventions to manage the pain most women experience related to labor and birth are covered in Chapter 11.

Nursing Support During the Second Stage of Labor

The second stage of labor begins when the cervix is completely dilated. However, women often begin to have an involuntary urge to push before complete cervical dilation. This urge to push is triggered by the Ferguson reflex as the presenting fetal part stretches pelvic floor muscles (Ferguson, 1941). Stretch receptors are then activated, releasing endogenous oxytocin, supporting the hypotheses that the urge to push depends more on station than dilation (Cosner & deJong, 1993; Noble, 1981). Women report well-defined urges to push that occur before, at, and after complete dilation (McKay, Barrows, & Roberts, 1990). These findings suggest that "when to push" should be individualized to the maternal response rather than labor routines that dictate pushing at complete dilation. The goals during the second stage of labor should be to support, rather than direct, the woman's involuntary pushing efforts leading to movement of the fetus down and out of the pelvis and to minimize the use of the Valsalva maneuver with its associated negative maternal hemodynamic effects and resultant adverse implications for the fetus (AWHONN, 1997).

There are generally two approaches to coaching women during second stage of labor: open- or closed-glottis pushing. The traditional approach is to begin pushing and bearing-down instructions at complete dilation, whether the woman feels the urge to push or not. This technique has been used more frequently since the widespread use of epidural anesthesia, but it has no scientific basis and is known to be harmful to maternal–fetal well-being (Aldrich et al., 1995; Caldeyro-Barcia, 1979; Langer et al., 1997; Thomson, 1993). Typically, women are coached to take a deep breath and hold it for at least 10 seconds while bearing down three to four times during each contraction. Women are instructed not to make a sound and to bring their knees up toward their abdomen with their elbows outstretched while pushing. Many nurses and physicians assist by holding the woman's legs back against her abdomen. These approaches are outdated and physiologically inappropriate.

When the woman takes a deep breath and holds it (ie, closed glottis), the Valsalva maneuver is instituted. This technique increases intrathoracic pressure, impairs blood return from lower extremities, and initially increases and then decreases BP, resulting in a decrease in uteroplacental blood flow. In the newborn, iatrogenic hypoxemia, acidemia, and lower Apgar scores may result. Sustained pushing of 9 to 15 seconds can result in significant decelerations in the FHR (Caldeyro-Barcia et al., 1981) and decreases in fetal oxygen saturation (Aldrich et al., 1995; Langer et al., 1997). There are no data to suggest that aggressively coached closed-glottis pushing results in a clinically significant decrease in the length of the second stage when compared with supportive open-glottis pushing based on the woman's urge to bear down.

Transient and permanent peroneal nerve damage has been reported after prolonged periods of coached pushing with the woman in the supine lithotomy position. When the woman or care provider applies pressure to the peroneal nerve during pushing over a prolonged period, nerve damage resulting in numbness and tingling of the legs, inability to bear weight, and transient loss of feeling can result (Colachis, Pease, & Johnson, 1994; Turbridy & Redmond, 1996). This type of iatrogenic injury can be prevented by encouraging the woman to keep her feet flat on the bed during second stage pushing. Healthcare providers forcibly pushing the woman's legs against her abdomen and placing the woman's legs in stirrups while pushing increases the risks of peroneal nerve damage (Colachis et al., 1994; Turbridy & Redmond, 1996).

The type of pushing and maternal position during pushing have a direct impact on the fetal response to the second stage of labor and newborn transition to extrauterine life. Sustained closed-glottis pushing should be avoided if possible, but if using this technique, some strategies can be used to decrease the impact on fetal well-being. If the fetus is not responding well to coached closed-glottis pushing (ie, take a deep breath and hold it for 10 seconds three or four times during each contraction), the most appropriate intervention is to stop pushing temporarily, assist the woman to a lateral position, and let the fetus recover. If the fetus continues to respond poorly, as evidenced by repetitive variable FHR decelerations or other nonreassuring FHR patterns, and there is a compelling reason to continue pushing, try pushing between alternate contractions while the woman is on her side. It may be necessary to encourage the woman to push with every other contraction or every third contraction to maintain a reassuring FHR pattern. A baseline FHR should be able to be identified between contractions. If the fetus does not tolerate pushing and the woman has an epidural, the passive fetal descent approach works best. Discuss concerns with the physician or CNM if there is pressure or a sense of urgency (unrelated to maternal or fetal status) to get the baby delivered. Evidence suggests that, for women with epidurals, coached pushing does not result in a clinically significant decrease in the length of the second stage (Hansen & Clark, 1996; Mayberry, Hammer, Kelly, True-Driver, & De, 1999). Passive fetal descent results in a similar length of the second stage for women with epidural analgesia or anesthesia compared with the coached closed-glottis pushing approach.

There is no reliable method to know which fetuses can tolerate continued physiologic stress of sustained coached closed-glottis pushing. The FHR pattern therefore must be used as an indicator about how well the fetus is responding. Repetitive variable decelerations during the second stage are associated with respiratory acidemia at birth. Some fetuses may develop metabolic acidemia if this type of pattern continues over a long period. These babies are difficult to resuscitate and may not transition well to extrauterine life.

In contrast, physiologic second-stage management is based on the principles that the second stage of labor is a normal physiologic event and that women should push spontaneously and give birth with minimal intervention (AWHONN, 1997; Cosner & deJong, 1993). Second-stage labor has been divided into two phases. The first is the period from complete dilatation to spontaneous bearing down. The second phase is characterized by vigorous expulsive efforts based on the woman feeling pressure and the urge to push (Roberts & Woolley, 1996). More effective expulsive efforts are associated with delaying pushing until the mother feels the urge to do so.

Women who give birth in an upright position without bearing-down instructions have a shorter labor than women who receive routine bearing-down instructions in upright (26.4 minutes shorter) and recumbent (48.2 minutes shorter) positions (Liu, 1989).

(text continues on page 319)

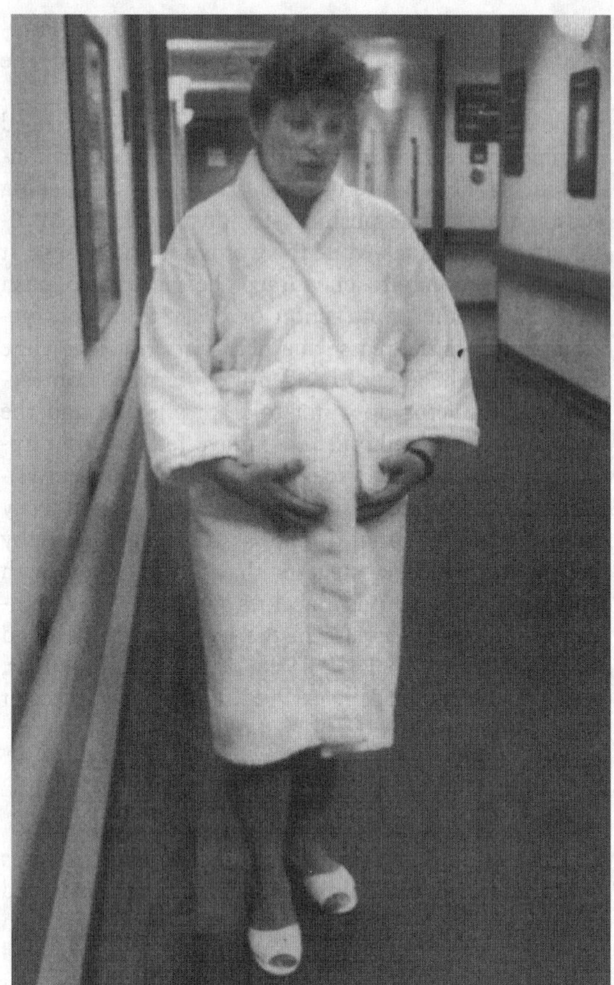

FIGURE 9–3A. Walking

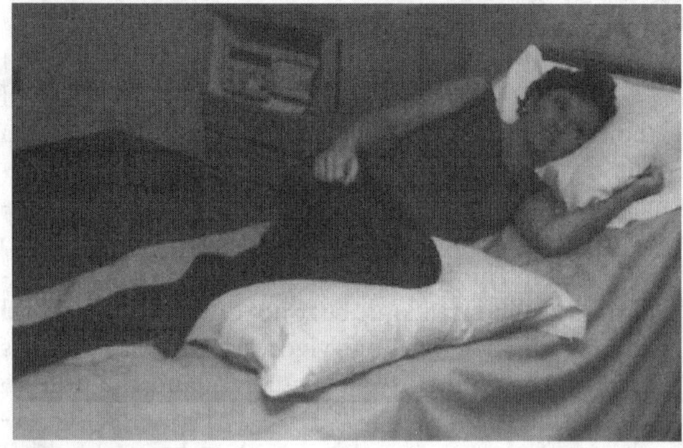

FIGURE 9–3B. Sidelying with pillow support

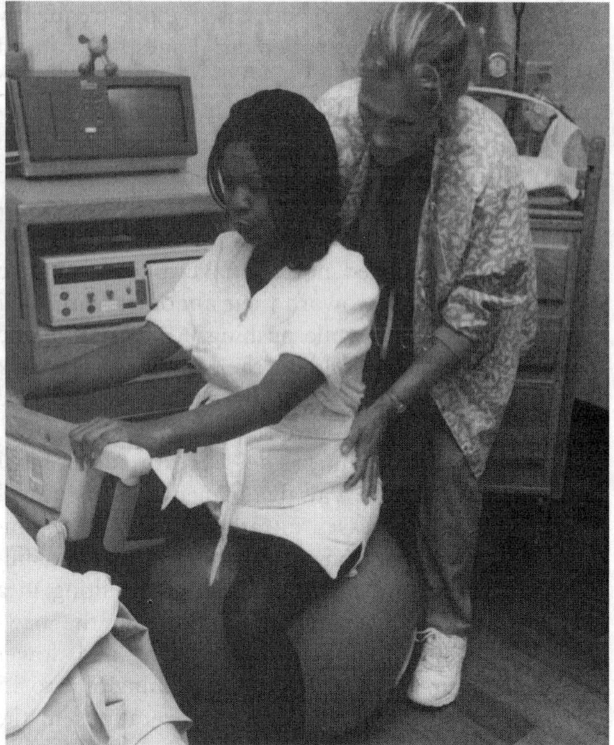

FIGURE 9–3C. Physiologic positions during labor (using birthing ball while sitting)

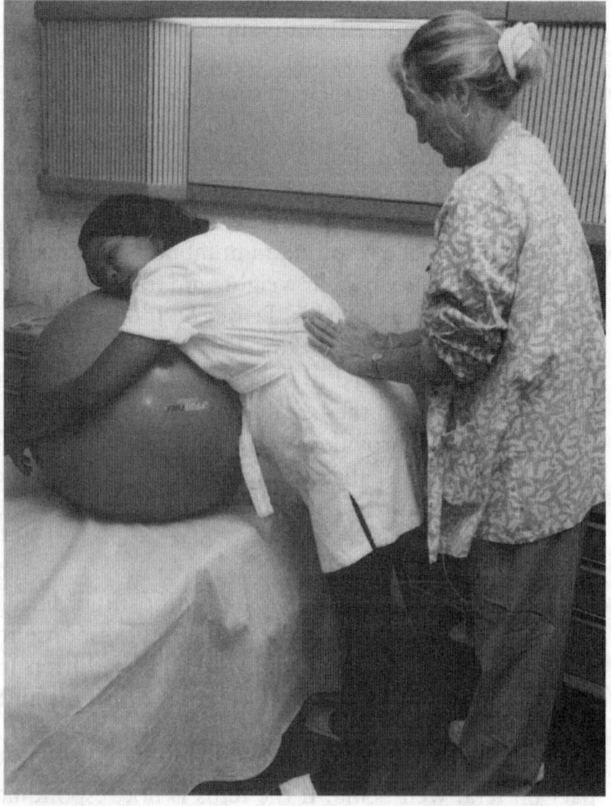

FIGURE 9–3D. Physiologic positions during labor (using birthing ball while standing)

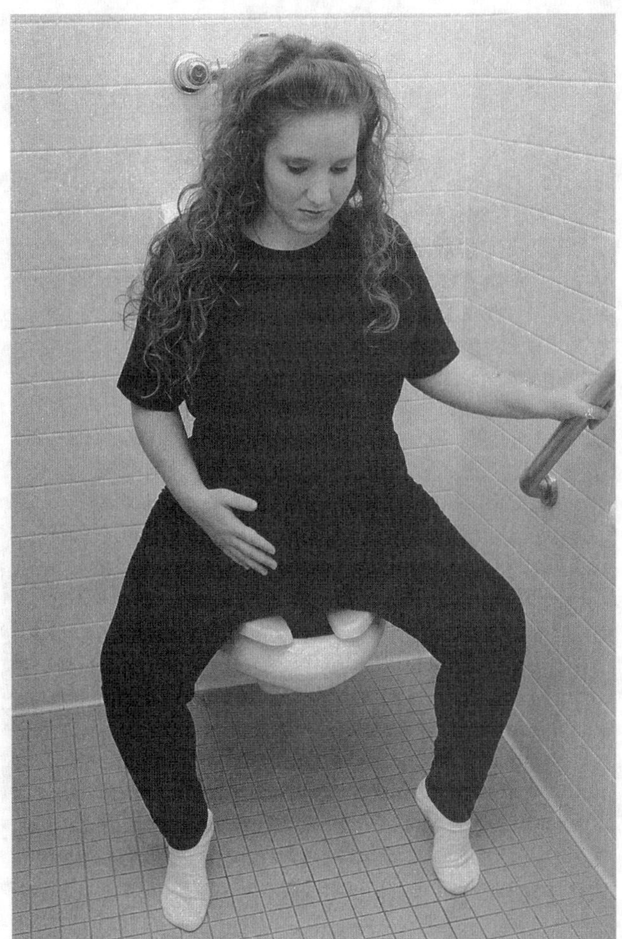

FIGURE 9–3E. Sitting on the toilet

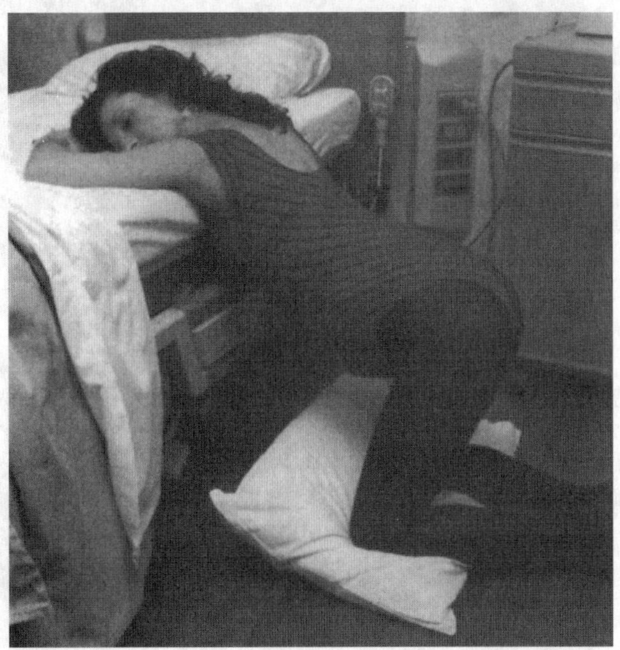

FIGURE 9–3F. Kneeling, chest supported

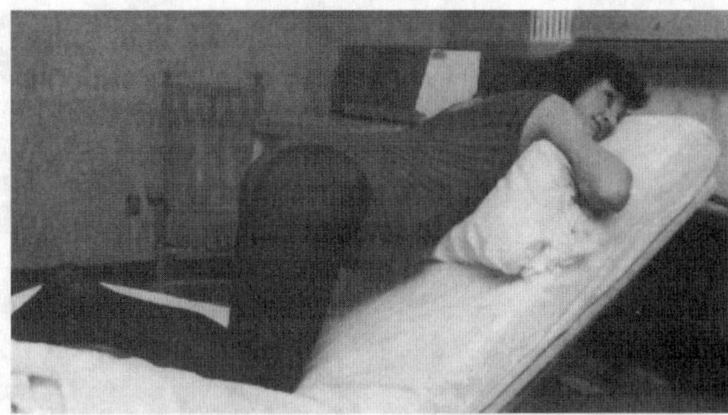

FIGURE 9–3G. Kneeling, chest supported

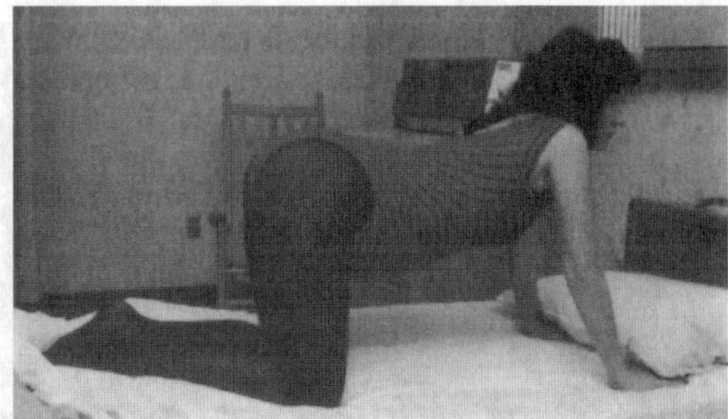

FIGURE 9–3H. Hands and knees

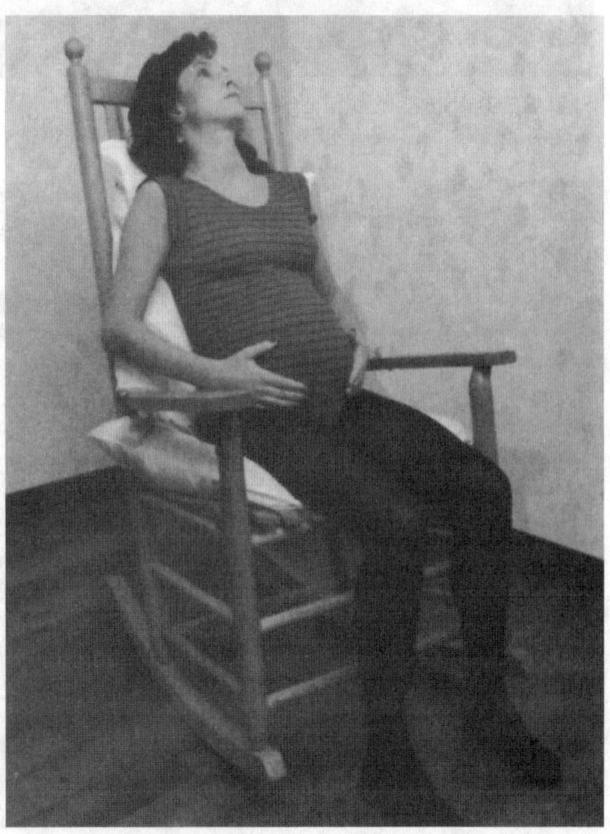

FIGURE 9–3I. Rocking

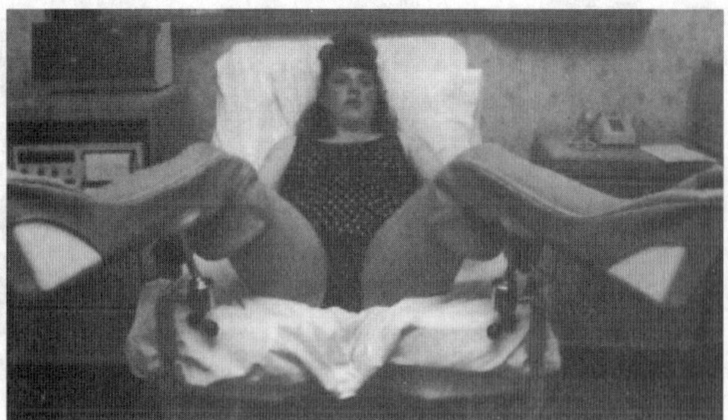

FIGURE 9–4A. Semisitting, stirrup leg supports

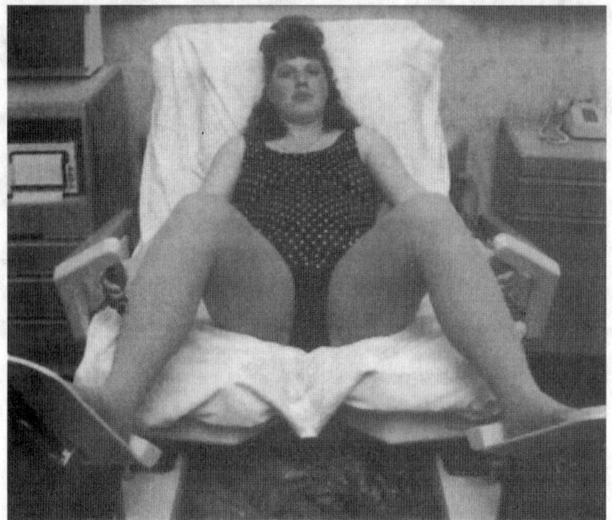

FIGURE 9–4B. Semisitting, feet supported

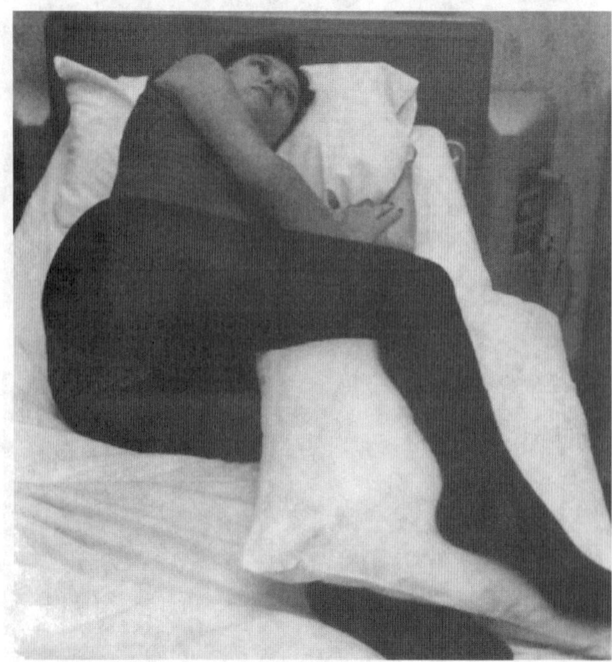

FIGURE 9–4C. Side lying

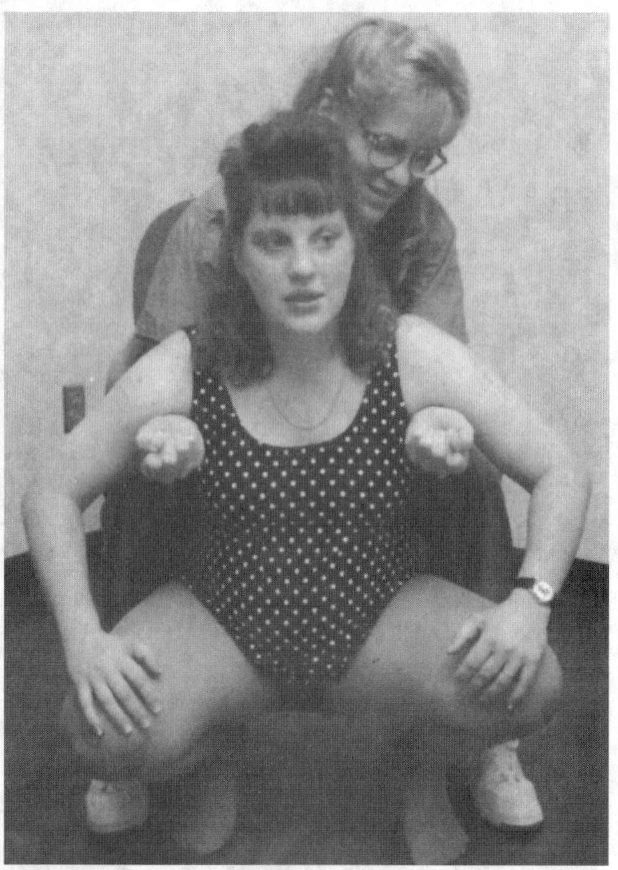

FIGURE 9–4D. Squatting with support

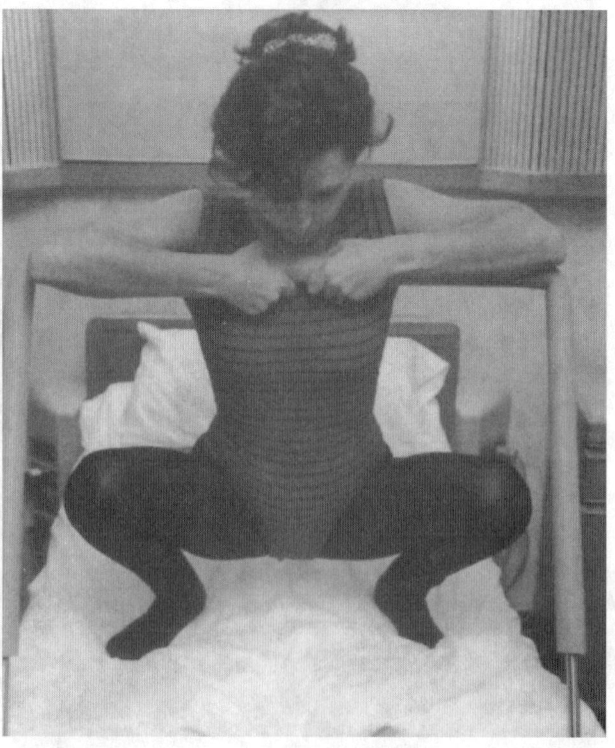

FIGURE 9–4E. Squatting with support bar

Women prefer encouragement and assistance with breathing, relaxation, pushing techniques, and imagery (McKay & Smith, 1993). However, confusion can occur if several caregivers' pushing directions are different or at odds with body sensations (McKay & Smith, 1993). Individualized, consistent coaching (in coordination with the woman's expulsive efforts) that provides necessary instructions, support, and encouragement is important. Figure 9–5 provides an algorithm for physiologic second-stage management. Display 9–4 provides a description with scientific rationale for a more appropriate nursing protocol for managing the second stage of labor (AWHONN, 1997).

With involuntary pushing, women were observed to hold their breath for 6 seconds while bearing down, and they took several breaths between bearing-down efforts (Roberts, Goldstein, Gruener, Maggio, & Mendez-Bauer, 1987). This is in contrast to the traditional second-stage coaching instructions that encourage holding breath for 10 seconds while bearing down and allowing only one quick breath between pushes. Open-glottis or gentle pushing avoids fetal stress, has less impact on uteroplacental blood

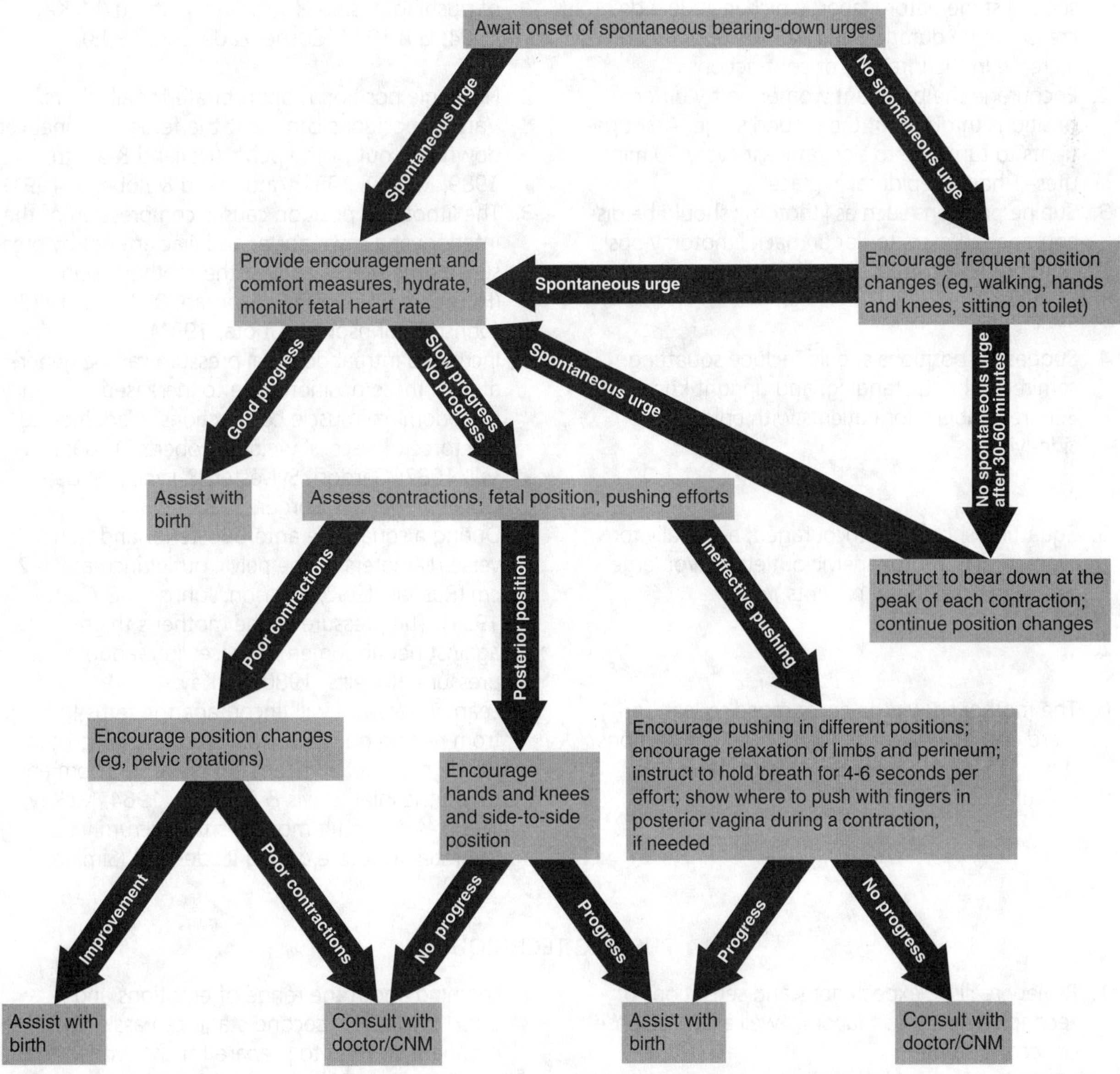

FIGURE 9–5. Flow sheet for second-stage management. (Adapted from Cosner, K. R., & deJong, E. [1993]. Physiologic second-stage labor. *Maternal Child Nursing, 18*[1], 41.)

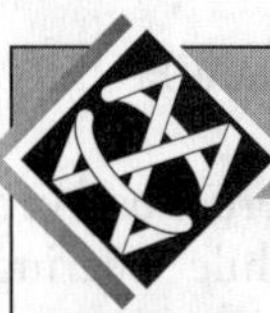

DISPLAY 9–4

AWHONN Second Stage of Labor Nursing Management Protocol

Purpose: To apply research-based knowledge to the clinical practice of management of the second stage of labor. The goals are to assist in promoting the birth of the noncompromised fetus by minimizing negative maternal hemodynamic changes caused by inappropriate positions and pushing techniques and to minimize maternal fatigue.

POSITIONS FOR SECOND STAGE

Practice	*Rationale*
1. All pregnant women should receive information prenatally on the benefits of upright positions for second stage before labor, which include a decrease in the duration and pain of labor as well as increase in the intensity of contractions.	1. Prenatal education can prepare women to take an active role in their labor and encourage practice of pushing positions such as squatting (McKay, 1984; Liu, 1974; Cosner & deJong, 1993).
2. Encourage the pregnant women to try different positions throughout the second stage. Assist patients to turn side to side, at least every 30 minutes–1 hour if epidural in place.	2. No single position is appropriate for all labors. Varying positions can assist the fetus to maneuver down and out of the pelvis (Holland & Smith, 1989; McKay, 1981; Anderhold & Roberts, 1991).
3. Supine positions such as lithotomy should be discouraged. (Refers to flat on back lithotomy position, not a semirecumbent lithotomy position).	3. The lithotomy position causes compression of the inferior vena cava, aorta, and iliac arteries by pressure of the uterus against the mother's spine (Humphrey, Hounslow, Morgan, & Wood, 1973; Johnson, Johnson, & Gupta, 1991).
4. Suggested positions should include squatting, semirecumbent, standing, and upright kneeling. Semirecumbent for patients with epidurals (or side-lying).	4. Increased intraabdominal pressure can be generated in these positions due to increased efficiency of abdominal muscle contractions in addition to the force of visceral weight (Roberts, 1980; Russell, 1982; Gardosi, Sylvester, & Lynch, 1989; Golay, Vedam, & Sorger, 1993).
5. Squatting should be encouraged, especially for women with narrow pelvic outlets and/or large fetuses. (No epidural patients.)	5. During a squat, the anteroposterior and transverse diameters of the pelvic outlet increase 1–2 cm (Russell, 1982; Johnson, Johnson, & Gupta, 1991). The pressure of the mother's thighs against her abdomen increases intraabdominal pressure (Roberts, 1980; McKay, 1984).
6. The mother should be encouraged to lean forward and maintain a pelvic tilt with contractions during the first part of the second stage. (No epidural patients.)	6. Leaning forward will encourage the fetus to keep from resting on the sacral vertebrae, which can misalign the fetus' head and prevent it from entering the inlet (Davis & Renning, 1964; McKay, 1984). A pelvic tilt mobilizes the sacrum, enabling the fetus to rotate during its descent (Simkin, 1982).

PUSHING TECHNIQUE

1. Review realistic expectations and sensations of second stage early in labor as well as at the onset of second stage.	1. Learning about the range of emotions and effort involved in second stage can assist the pregnant woman to prepare for the work and the sensations of second stage (McKay, Barrows, & Roberts, 1990).

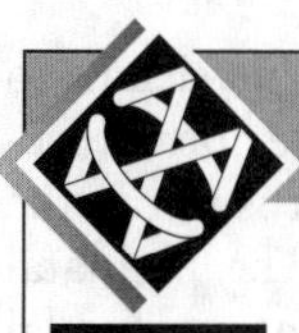

DISPLAY 9–4 (cont.)

AWHONN Second Stage of Labor Nursing Management Protocol

PUSHING TECHNIQUE

Practice	*Rationale*
2. Encourage spontaneous bearing down. If the fetal head has not descended low enough in the pelvis to stimulate Ferguson's reflex (stretch receptors in the pelvic floor), allow the mother to rest until she feels the urge to push.	2. Refraining from instructing a mother to begin pushing before the time she feels the urge to push minimizes maternal fatigue (Benyon, 1957; Roberts, Goldstein, Gruener, Maggio, & Mendez-Bauer, 1987).
3. Consider fetal station and position in addition to dilation in determining a woman's readiness for pushing.	3. Involuntary bearing down may be encouraged if fetal station is favorable (0 to 1+) as well as fetal position (OT to OA), regardless of a cervix that is dilated less than 10 cm (8–9 cm, soft and retracting) (Roberts, Goldstein, Gruener, Maggio, & Mendez-Bauer, 1987).
4. Discourage prolonged maternal breath holding (no more than 6–8 seconds) during pushing (no more than 3 pushing efforts per contraction).	4. Breath holding involves the Valsalva maneuver; increased intrathoracic pressure due to a closed glottis causes a decrease in cardiac output and blood pressure. The fall in pressure causes a decrease in placental perfusion, causing fetal hypoxia (Caldeyro-Barcia, 1979).
5. Support rather than direct the woman's involuntary pushing efforts. These efforts may include grunting, groaning, exhaling during the push, and/or breath holding less than 6 seconds.	5. Spontaneous, involuntary bearing-down efforts match the intensity of each contraction. An open glottis, as seen with grunting and exhale pushing, avoids the Valsalva maneuver and has physiological benefits for both the mother and baby (McKay, Barrows, & Roberts, 1990; Roberts, Goldstein, Grueder, Maggio, & Mendez-Bauer, 1987).
6. Validate normalcy of sensations and sounds the mother is voicing.	6. Mothers and caregivers perceive low-pitched groaning, sighing, and moaning to be sounds of tension release that may assist her in coping with the pain of second stage (McKay & Roberts, 1990).

This protocol does not define a standard of care, nor is it intended to dictate an exclusive course of management. It presents methods and techniques of practice that are currently acceptable and supported by research. The protocol should not be construed as excluding other acceptable methods of handling the second stage of labor or innovations that demonstrably improve the quality of patient care.

flow, allows for perineal relaxation, and is more natural physiologically (AWHONN, 1997; McKay & Roberts, 1985). The woman is more in control and responding to her body's own pushing cues, enhancing maternal confidence and satisfaction with the birth experience. Open-glottis pushing can shorten the length of the second stage of labor compared with closed-glottis (Parnell, Langhoff-Roos, Iversen, & Damgaard, 1993).

Delayed Pushing for Women with Regional Analgesia

When women have regional analgesia or anesthesia, they may not feel the urge to push when they are completely dilated. In this situation, an alternative approach to the second stage is to delay pushing (ie, laboring down) while the fetus descends passively. Various researchers have described success with a protocol allowing nulliparous women to wait 2 hours or until the urge to push and allowing multiparous women 1 hour or until the urge to push (Fraser et al, 2000; Hansen & Clark, 1996; Mayberry et al., 1999). A lateral position facilitates passive fetal descent until the presenting part is low enough to stimulate the Ferguson reflex. There are significantly fewer FHR decelerations when the fetus is allowed to descend spontaneously compared with coached closed-glottis pushing (Hansen & Clark, 1996). The rate of spontaneous vaginal birth is increased and the rate of difficult deliveries is decreased with the laboring-down technique (Fraser et al., 2000). Laboring down is cost effective. The incremental costs per difficult delivery prevented was estimated to be $1,743.06 in a recent study that compared immediate coached pushing at 10 centimeters with delayed pushing until the urge to push was noted for nulliparous women who had epidural anesthesia (Petrou, Coyle & Fraser, 2000) Maternal fatigue is lessened during laboring down compared with immediate pushing when there is no urge to push. Injuries to the structure and function of the pelvic floor are less likely when a passive second stage results in a decreased period of maternal expulsive efforts (Devine, Ostergard, & Noblett, 1999). There are no benefits for the mother and fetus to a policy involving immediate and continued pushing compared with allowing a variable period of rest with spontaneous fetal descent (Hansen & Clark, 1996; Maresh et al., 1983; Mayberry et al., 1999; Vause, Congdon, & Thornton, 1998). Laboring down avoids maternal fatigue and the nonreassuring FHR patterns associated with sustained coached closed-glottis pushing. Allowing maternal rest and passive fetal descent does not result in a clinically significant increase in the duration of the second stage of labor.

Fundal Pressure

Although fundal pressure is still used in some institutions to shorten the second stage of labor, the intensity of the legal climate and lack of scientific data to support fundal pressure as safe for mothers and babies have caused nurses to scrutinize this technique (Kline-Kaye & Miller-Slade, 1990). Because limited data have been published about maternal–fetal injuries related to the use of fundal pressure, it is difficult to accurately quantify the risks to the mother and baby (Simpson & Knox, 2001). The limited data about many known or reported adverse outcomes associated with fundal pressure application during the second stage of labor should not be used to suggest that this practice is acceptable or risk free (Simpson & Knox, 2001). The consequences of not choosing clinical management with the least associated risk become understood only when the rare serious injury occurs (Knox et al., 1999).

Perinatal nurses may feel pressured by physicians to use fundal pressure to shorten an otherwise normal second stage of labor, even when they feel it is not in the best interest of the woman and fetus. The perinatal nurse has the right to refuse to participate in fundal pressure application if uncomfortable with the clinical situation. The potential use of fundal pressure requires well-researched guidelines for practice. These guidelines may contain description of the technique, indications, contraindications, and criteria for medical record documentation, along with suggestions on how to handle clinical disagreements related to fundal pressure that may arise in the clinical setting (Rommal, 1999).

Fundal pressure refers to the application of steady pressure with one hand on the fundus of the uterus at a 30- to 45-degree angle to the maternal spine in the direction of the pelvis (Rommal, 1999) (Fig. 9–6). The pressure is applied in a longitudinal direction with careful avoidance of downward pressure on the maternal spine because of the risk of direct vena cava compression and maternal hypotension (Rommal, 1999).

Fundal pressure may be appropriate in limited clinical situations. For example, fundal pressure is sometimes used to guide the fetal head into the pelvis against the cervix if the fetal station is high when artificial rupture of the membranes is indicated (Maryland State Board of Nursing [MSBON], 1999). Fundal pressure in this situation may decrease the risk of a prolapsed umbilical cord. If the FHR is nonreassuring or difficult to trace electronically or when there is indication for more accurate fetal assessment, some healthcare providers decide to place an internal FSE.

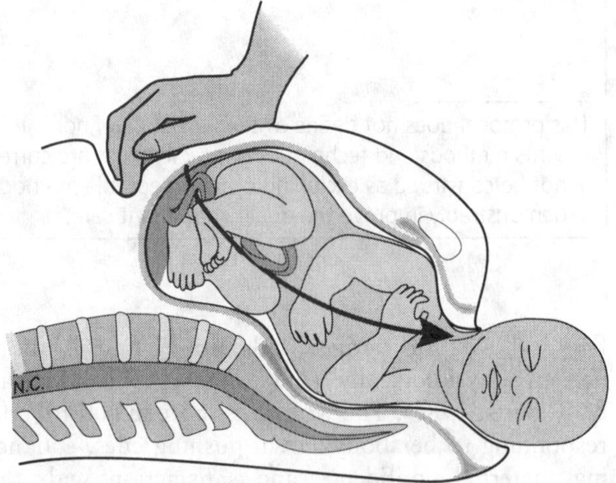

FIGURE 9–6. Fundal pressure. (From Penney, D. S., & Perlis, D. W. [1992]. When to use suprapubic or fundal pressure. *American Journal of Maternal Child Nursing, 17,* 34–36.)

If fetal station is such that application is difficult, gentle fundal pressure may make it easier to apply the FSE. There are situations when the fetal head is crowning, maternal pushing efforts are insufficient to effect birth, and the FHR is nonreassuring, suggesting that an expeditious birth is indicated. In this case, fundal pressure may be the quickest option for birth, but a careful analysis of risks and benefits is required based on the individual clinical situation (Simpson & Knox, 2001). An alternative option is to stop pushing, allow fetal recovery, and proceed with cesarean birth.

Some data suggest that fundal pressure may cause shoulder dystocia if applied concurrently with vacuum extraction. This occurs when the head of a fetus is delivered that would not have descended on its own had fundal pressure and vacuum had not been used (Bahar, 1996; Bofill et al., 1997b). Nesbitt, Gilbert, and Herrchen (1998) found that shoulder dystocia increased 35% to 45% in vacuum- or forceps-assisted births to nondiabetic mothers of infants weighing more than 3,500 g. Hankins (1998) reported a severe lower thoracic spinal cord injury to a fetus with permanent neurologic sequelae when fundal pressure was applied in an attempt to relieve shoulder dystocia. Subgaleal hemorrhage has been reported in cases in which fundal pressure application was combined with vacuum assistance (Simpson & Knox, 2001). This type of fetal injury can result in acute blood loss and shock (Moe & Page, 1999). Excessive fundal pressure can increase fetal intracranial pressure enough to result in significant decreases in cerebral blood flow and nonreassuring FHR patterns (Amiel-Tison, Sureau, & Shnider, 1988). Cord compression and functional alterations in intervillous space blood flow caused by the mechanical forces of fundal pressure compromise fetal status and can lead to fetal hypoxemia and asphyxia (Amiel-Tison et al., 1988).

In addition to an increased risk of fetal injuries, application of fundal pressure increases the risk of injuries to the mother (Simpson & Knox, 2001). Maternal perineal injuries such as third- and fourth-degree lacerations and anal sphincter tears have been associated with the use of fundal pressure (Cosner, 1996; Zetterstrom et al., 1999). Cases of uterine rupture and uterine inversion have also been reported as a result of the use of fundal pressure (Drummond, 1999; Lee, Baggish, & Lashgari, 1978; Rommal, 1996). Other maternal injuries and complications reported include pain, hypotension, respiratory distress, abdominal bruising, fractured ribs, and liver rupture (Simpson & Knox, 2001).

Based on evidence in the literature, case reports, and reviews of malpractice cases that resulted in adverse outcomes, it must be concluded that fundal pressure, used in cases of shoulder dystocia or to shorten the second stage of an otherwise normal labor, presents an increased, although not quantifiable, risk to mothers and babies and to perinatal providers using it (Simpson & Knox, 2001). Each institution should review clinical risk management guidelines provided by their professional liability insurance carrier as part of the process of developing unit guidelines for fundal pressure application (Simpson & Knox, 2001).

Shoulder Dystocia

Shoulder dystocia is an unpredictable obstetric emergency, but there are reasonable steps that nurses can take after shoulder dystocia is identified. A thorough knowledge about what to do if this crisis occurs is essential for perinatal nurses to ensure the best possible outcomes for the woman and fetus (Simpson, 1999). Key nursing interventions include calling for additional help, calm supportive actions, and working in a coordinated fashion with the physician or CNM who is directing the maneuvers to deliver the impacted shoulder (Simpson, 1999). Interventions that have been described in the literature to relieve the impacted shoulder include suprapubic pressure; the McRoberts, Woods, Schwartz-Dixon, Gaskin, and Zavanelli maneuvers; and symphysiotomy (ACOG, 1997) (Figs. 9–7 and 9–8). There is no clear evidence-based order for using these maneuvers (ACOG, 1997). The essential issue is to continue to intervene using an organized, expeditious series of steps until the infant has been delivered (Simpson, 1999). If an injury occurs as a result of shoulder dystocia despite the best efforts of the obstetric providers, it is likely that litigation will follow.

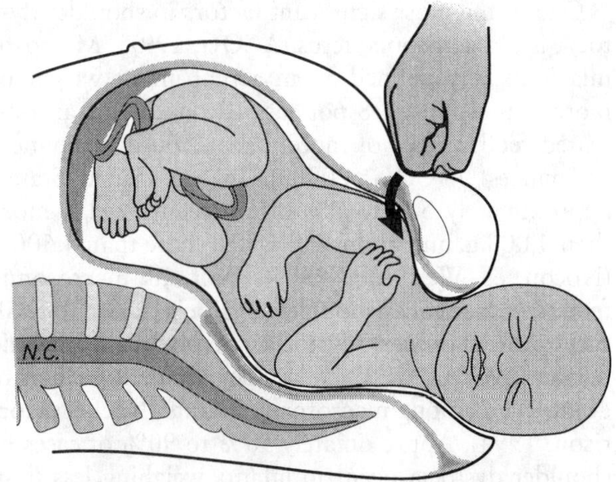

FIGURE 9–7. Suprapubic pressure. (From Penney, D. S., & Perlis, D. W. [1992]. When to use suprapubic or fundal pressure. *American Journal of Maternal Child Nursing, 17,* 34–36.)

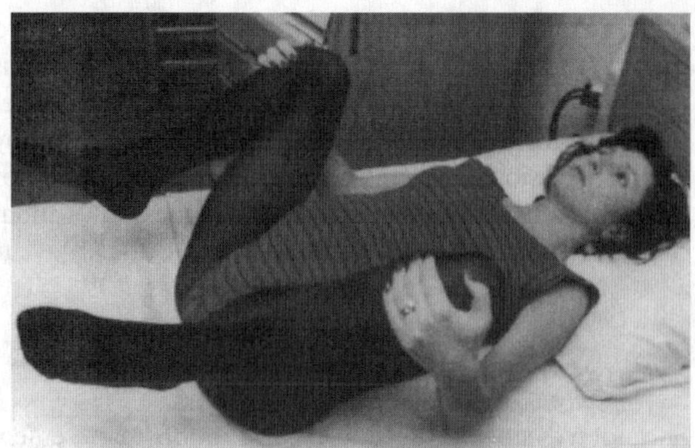

FIGURE 9–8. McRoberts maneuver to facilitate birth with shoulder dystocia.

Numerous risk factors associated with shoulder dystocia have been discussed in the literature, including maternal diabetes, obesity, excessive pregnancy weight gain, abnormal labor progress (including prolonged second stage), disproportionate fetal growth with increased abdominal and chest circumferences, multiparity, male fetus, history of a prior macrosomic infant, history of a prior shoulder dystocia, use of midforceps or vacuum interventions, induction of labor, and macrosomia (ACOG, 2000b, 1997; Bofill et al., 1997b; Bofill et al., 1998; Lewis et al., 1998; Nesbitt, Gilbert, & Herrchen, 1998). However, none of these risk factors individually or in combination can predict shoulder dystocia (ACOG, 1997). The two risk factors most strongly associated with shoulder dystocia are fetal macrosomia and maternal diabetes (ACOG, 1997), but most women with one or more of these risk factors go on to have uncomplicated labor and birth.

One of the most significant factors in shoulder dystocia is a macrosomic fetus (ACOG, 1997). Macrosomia is usually defined as an actual infant weight of more than 4,000 g (8 pounds, 13 ounces) or an estimated fetal weight of more than 4,500 g (9 pounds, 15 ounces) (ACOG, 2000b). In the United States, approximately 5% to 7% of all infants weigh more than 4,000 g, and about 1% weigh more than 4,500 g (Nocon & Weisbrod, 1995). Not all macrosomic fetuses experience shoulder dystocia, and not all cases of shoulder dystocia involve macrosomic fetuses (ACOG, 1997). Shoulder dystocia is a rare event, even among macrosomic infants (Naef & Morrison, 1994). Approximately 50% to 90% of cases of shoulder dystocia occur in infants weighing less than 4,000 g (Naef & Morrison, 1994; Nocon & Weisbrod, 1995). No birth weight category is completely free of risk for shoulder dystocia (Nocon & Weisbrod, 1995). Brachial plexus injuries can occur without shoulder dystocia (ACOG, 1997; Gilbert, Nesbitt, & Danielsen, 1999).

There have been numerous attempts to develop criteria that would accurately diagnose macrosomia before birth, including clinical estimation of fetal weight by abdominal palpation and ultrasonographic parameters. These clinical factors have been statistically associated with shoulder dystocia using retrospective analyses, but none of these factors or criteria has had a high positive predictive value for the individual patient when attempting to predict macrosomia or shoulder dystocia prospectively (ACOG, 2000b, 1993, 1997; Lewis et al., 1998; Naef & Morrison, 1994). The likelihood of an inaccurate prediction of fetal weight increases with the size of the fetus. According to the ACOG (2000b) practice bulletin, *Fetal Macrosomia*, birth weight is underestimated by approximately 0.5 kg (1 pound) or more in 50% of cases in which the fetus is larger than 4,000 g and in as many as 80% of cases in which the fetus is larger than 4,500 g.

Maternal diabetes appears to be consistently related to the risk of shoulder dystocia (ACOG, 1997). Although it is known that women with diabetes tend to have larger infants, there are also anthropometric differences in infants of diabetic mothers that may explain the propensity for shoulder dystocia in this population (McFarland, Trylovich, & Langer, 1998). Macrosomic infants of diabetic mothers tend to have larger shoulder and extremity circumferences, a decreased head-to-shoulder ratio, significantly higher body fat, and thicker upper extremity skinfolds than nondiabetic infants of similar birth weight and birth length (McFarland et al., 1998). The risk of shoulder dystocia for women with diabetes is two to six times greater than for women who do not have diabetes (ACOG, 1997). If the fetus of the woman with diabetes is estimated to exceed 4,250 to 4,500 g, it may be reasonable to plan for cesarean birth (ACOG, 1997). This is a decision made by the CNM or physician in collaboration with the pregnant woman and her family. Individual clinical situations vary, however, and not all women may agree to this course. Macrosomia is relative to maternal pelvic structures and size and to fetal presentation and position. For all practical purposes, shoulder dystocia cannot be predicted with any degree of accuracy (ACOG, 1997; Lewis et al., 1998). The important issue is for perinatal nurses to be aware of maternal–fetal risk factors for individual patients and be prepared if shoulder dystocia occurs.

Shoulder dystocia is diagnosed when gentle traction and episiotomy fails to achieve birth (Gherman, Ouzounian, & Goodwin, 1998). After the diagnosis is made, the nurse assists with maneuvers to disimpact the shoulder under the direction of the physician or CNM (Simpson, 1999). Calmly assisting the woman to the appropriate positions during the maneuvers helps her feel confident that the necessary interventions are being done as quickly as possible by competent healthcare providers (Simpson, 1999).

Fundal pressure should be avoided during shoulder dystocia because it can further impact the fetal shoulder, resulting in an inability to deliver the fetal body as well as contributing to fetal brachial plexus injuries and fractures of the humerus and clavicle (ACOG, 1997; Baskett & Allen, 1995; Gross, Shime, & Farine, 1987). Gross and coworkers (1987) reported a 77% fetal injury rate when fundal pressure was the only maneuver used to relieve shoulder dystocia. Firm suprapubic pressure using the palm of the hand can usually dislodge the impacted shoulder while gentle downward pressure is applied by the physician or CNM. Suprapubic pressure is directed away from the pubic bone to the left or the right side. If suprapubic pressure is not immediately successful, the next approach is usually the McRoberts maneuver (eg, knee-chest position while supine) because it can be accomplished relatively quickly and easily (Gherman et al., 1997).

Some practitioners prefer to use the McRoberts maneuver before suprapubic pressure, because it was previously thought that there was a higher risk of clavicular fracture associated with suprapubic pressure. Later data about obstetric maneuvers for shoulder dystocia suggest this is probably not an accurate assumption (Gherman, Ouzounian, & Goodwin, 1998). The McRoberts maneuver involves hyperflexion of the woman's thighs against her abdomen and can ease delivery of the shoulder by changing the relationship of the maternal pelvis to the lumbar spine. This maneuver may not increase birth canal dimensions, but it does result in flattening of the sacrum relative to the maternal lumbar spine (Gherman, Tramont, Muffley, & Goodwin, 2000). The McRoberts maneuver has been found to reduce potential complications of shoulder dystocia, such as fetal clavicle fractures and brachial plexus stretching, without increasing maternal complications (Baskett & Allen, 1995; Gherman et at., 1997; Gonik, Stringer, & Held, 1983).

As the nurse assists the woman to the McRoberts position, a call for the help of other available nurses and physicians should be considered. If the woman has epidural anesthesia or she is very uncomfortable, another provider may be needed to help support her legs and maintain this position. Suprapubic pressure may be used while the woman is in the McRoberts position. The McRoberts maneuver may not result in disimpaction of the shoulder. Additional maneuvers have been described that can be successful.

There is no clear evidence-based order for use of these maneuvers (ACOG, 1997). The essential issue is to continue to intervene using an organized, expeditious series of steps until the infant has been delivered. Preparations for newborn resuscitation are warranted if additional maneuvers are required after application of suprapubic pressure and the McRoberts maneuver or if several minutes have elapsed since delivery of the fetal head. During shoulder dystocia, the umbilical cord may be partially or completed occluded between the fetal body and maternal pelvis. The normally oxygenated fetus can tolerate several minutes of cord compression without significant adverse effects (Naef & Morrison, 1994). However, most experts believe that more than 5 minutes from delivery of the head to delivery of the body may result in acid-base deterioration in a fetus whose condition was normal before the onset of shoulder dystocia (Benedetti, 1995). If possible, an assessment of fetal status by EFM or hand-held ultrasound devices can provide information about how the fetus is tolerating the interventions. However, time should not be lost attempting to locate the FHR if it is not readily identified. It is better to direct attention to dislodging the fetal shoulder by assisting the woman to the appropriate positions and following the direction of the physician or CNM.

Other maneuvers that have been described include the Woods corkscrew maneuver, the Schwartz-Dixon maneuver, the all-fours or Gaskin maneuver, the Zavanelli maneuver, and symphysiotomy. During the Woods maneuver, the physician or CNM exerts downward pressure on the uterine fundus with one hand while inserting two fingers of the other hand on the anterior aspect of the posterior shoulder and gently rotating clockwise (Nocon, & Weisbrod, 1995). Ideally, this movement delivers the posterior shoulder. With continued synchronized downward pressure on the fundus, two fingers exert gentle counterclockwise pressure upward around the circumference of the pelvic arc to and beyond 12 o'clock, which should unscrew and deliver the remaining shoulder (Nocon and Weisbrod, 1995). This is the only time fundal pressure is appropriate during a disimpaction maneuver. The physician or CNM may direct the nurse to apply fundal pressure during the Woods maneuver, or they may apply fundal pressure themselves.

The Schwartz-Dixon maneuver may be used to deliver the posterior arm, easing delivery of the body. The physician or CNM gently inserts a hand along the curvature of the fetal sacrum, and the fingers follow along the humerus to the antecubital fossa. The fetal forearm is flexed and swept across the chest and face and out the vagina. Ideally, the anterior shoulder slides under the symphysis after the posterior arm is delivered (Nocon & Weisbrod, 1995). There is a risk of fracture of the humerus with this technique. The physician or CNM may need to rotate the baby to achieve delivery using a technique similar to the Woods maneuver.

The all-fours maneuver described by Ina May Gaskin (Bruner et al., 1998) appears to be a rapid, safe, and effective method for reducing shoulder dystocia. For the Gaskin maneuver, the woman is assisted to her hands and knees. The exact mechanism by which this maneuver relieves shoulder dystocia is unknown. However, in a report of 82 consecutive cases of shoulder dystocia, the Gaskin maneuver contributed to a successful vaginal birth in all cases (Bruner et al., 1998). It is possible that the simple act of repositioning may be enough to dislodge the shoulder. An advantage to this position is the ability to continue other maneuvers if the position change does not reduce the shoulder dystocia. The women in this study received no anesthesia for labor or birth. It may be difficult, but not impossible, to assist women with epidural analgesia or anesthesia to this position.

Although performance of a symphysiotomy is described in the literature, most practitioners have not had experience with this procedure (Nocon & Weisbrod, 1995). Risks to the mother include major bladder and urethra damage, long-term pain, and difficulty walking. This procedure is rarely used in the United States (Seeds & Walsh, 1996). Deliberate fracture of the clavicles is also described as a method to reduce shoulder width, but many practitioners find this procedure technically difficult (Nocon & Weisbrod, 1995).

In the event that these or other maneuvers do not result in birth, the physician or CNM may attempt to replace the fetal head into the vagina and proceed with cesarean birth. This is known as the Zavanelli maneuver. It is important that the head be returned to the occipitoanterior or occipitoposterior position and then flexed and slowly pushed back into the birth canal (Nocon & Weisbrod, 1995). A review of 103 published cases of the Zavanelli maneuver from 1985 to 1997 revealed a 92% success rate, with no reports of fetal injuries in those eventually born by cesarean section (Sandberg, 1999). Although this report is probably biased because researchers are more likely to report successful cases in the literature, the success rate is still remarkable for a relatively new procedure for which almost all providers had no previous experience (Sandberg, 1999). If the Zavanelli maneuver is successful, when possible, an assessment of fetal status by EFM or a hand-held ultrasound device is desired while preparing for emergent cesarean birth. Personnel skilled in neonatal resuscitation should be in attendance at the cesarean birth.

After the shoulder has been disimpacted and birth has occurred, the nurse can direct attention to newborn care and assessment. After the newborn and mother are stabilized, documentation about the events surrounding the birth involving shoulder dystocia is possible. Display 9–5 offers suggestions for medical record documentation after birth complicated by shoulder dystocia.

Support and communication with the family is important after birth. The woman and her family probably will be concerned about the condition of the baby and have questions about what occurred. As part of the discussion, the woman should be informed that she is at risk for shoulder dystocia recurrence in subsequent birth (Simpson, 1999).

Perineum Care

Episiotomy is a median or mediolateral incision into the perineum. According to the latest data, episiotomy is performed during approximately 39.5% of births in the United States (Kozak & Lawrence, 1999). This surgical technique has long been thought to permit easier passage of the baby and to decrease risk of perineal trauma. Those who believe routine episiotomy is beneficial cite the following advantages: prevention of perineal tearing, ease of repair when compared with lacerations, reduction in time and the stress of second stage of labor, decreased compression of fetal head (especially for preterm infants), and allowance of easier manipulation during breech or operative vaginal birth. However, the benefits of routine episiotomy have not been demonstrated in any one RCT or by a systematic review of published RCTs between 1966 and 1999 that were designed to evaluate strategies to prevent perineal trauma (Eason & Feldman, 2000; Eason, Labrecque, Wells, & Feldman, 2000). It appears that personal beliefs, education, and experience of the practitioner, rather than evidence, influence clinical judgment about whether to perform an episiotomy (Low, Seng, Murtland, & Oakley, 2000). Based on available data, giving birth over an intact perineum results in less blood loss, less risk of infection, and less perineal pain postpartum (Eason & Feldman, 2000). Methods to prevent perineal trauma during birth include avoidance of episiotomy, avoidance of use of forceps, and slowing birth of the fetal head to allow the perineum time to stretch (Eason & Feldman, 2000).

Episiotomy is often performed when the physician or CNM feels that there is a risk of lacerations of the perineum or vagina during birth. The goal is to protect the perineum and maintain future perineal function and integrity. The use of episiotomy includes significant risks such as increased risk for third- and fourth-degree lacerations (Bansal, Tan, Ecker, Bishop, & Kilpatrick, 1996; Hueston, 1996), anal sphincter injuries (Klein et al., 1994), severe lacerations in subsequent births (Peleg, Kennedy, Merrill, & Zlatnik,

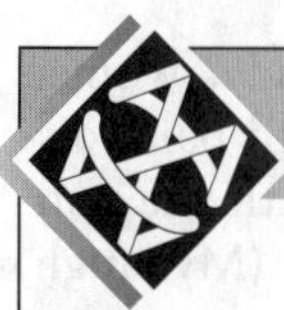

DISPLAY 9–5

Suggestions for Medical Record Documentation After a Birth Complicated by Shoulder Dystocia

- Provide emergent nursing care to the woman and newborn as a first priority.
- A narrative note, summarizing the series of interventions and clinical events with a focus on a logical step-by-step approach to relieving the impacted shoulder and resuscitating the newborn, works best in most situations.
- Avoid documenting a minute-by-minute account of the emergency unless it is absolutely certain that the times included are accurate.
- Attempt to closely approximate the time interval between delivery of fetal head and body.
- Review the electronic fetal monitoring strip, and talk with other providers in attendance to insure most accurate details of clinical circumstances.
- Include fetal assessment data or attempts to obtain data about fetal status during the maneuvers.
- List the order of each maneuver used in clear and precise terms.
- Note that nursing assistance with these maneuvers were under the direction of the physician or certified nurse midwife (CNM).
- If suprapubic pressure was used, make sure it is noted as such to avoid later allegations of fundal pressure.
- If fundal pressure is used during the Woods maneuver or after the shoulder is disimpacted, clearly note when and how it was used.
- Include times for calls for assistance and when other providers arrived.
- Carefully note the condition of the newborn at birth and during the immediate newborn period.
- Describe any resuscitation efforts and those who attended the newborn.
- Make sure that neonatal personnel in attendance understand the difference between suprapubic pressure and fundal pressure to avoid a neonatal note indicating fundal pressure was applied if this is inaccurate.
- If umbilical blood gases were obtained, make sure they become part of the record.
- If a discussion between the physician or CNM and the woman and her family about the shoulder dystocia and subsequent newborn condition occurred after birth, include a note about the content of this conversation and those who were present.
- It may be helpful to compose the note on a separate paper and review it for accuracy before entering these data into the medical record.
- Attempt to document the medical record within a reasonable time after the mother and newborn are stabilized.
- If possible, avoid late entries many hours or days after birth.

From Simpson, K.R. (1999). Shoulder dystocia: Nursing interventions and risk management strategies. *MCN, The American Journal of Maternal Child Nursing, 24*(6), 305–311. Used with permission.

1999), infection, delayed healing (McGuinness, Norr, & Nacion, 1991), increased blood loss (Eason & Feldman, 2000), scarring (Koger, Shatney, Hodge, & McClenathan, 1993), increased pain, sexual dysfunction (Hordnes & Bergsjo, 1993; Klein et al., 1994), and higher costs because of time and suturing. Lacerations of the vagina and perineum are classified according to degree as listed in Display 9–6.

Nursing interventions during labor can have a direct impact on the use and perceived need for episiotomy (Maier & Maloni, 1997). Upright position and open-glottis, gentle pushing that coincide with the woman's natural urges and sensations aid gradual perineal stretching with less pain, avoiding the need for episiotomy and resultant perineal trauma (Devine et al., 1999; Eason, Labrecque, Wells, & Feldman, 2000; Flynn, Franick, Janssen, Hannah, & Klein, 1997). Women who give birth in the lithotomy position are more likely to have an episiotomy than women who give birth in squatting, hands-and-knees, standing, or sitting positions (Rooks, Weatherby, & Ernst, 1992). Passive fetal descent and spontaneous bearing-down efforts compared with directed pushing results in fewer episiotomies and perineal lacerations (Devine et al., 1999; Sampselle, & Hines, 1999).

Other measures that have been proposed to enhance perineal stretching and decrease perineal trauma are the application of warm compresses, gentle perineal mas-

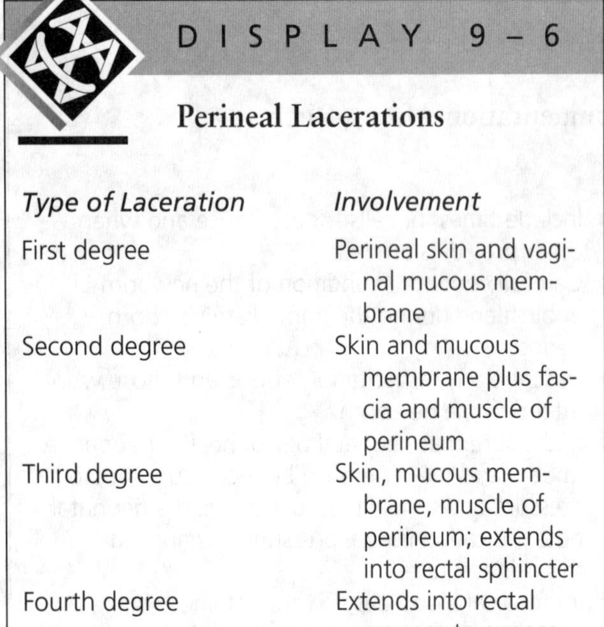

DISPLAY 9–6

Perineal Lacerations

Type of Laceration	*Involvement*
First degree	Perineal skin and vaginal mucous membrane
Second degree	Skin and mucous membrane plus fascia and muscle of perineum
Third degree	Skin, mucous membrane, muscle of perineum; extends into rectal sphincter
Fourth degree	Extends into rectal mucosa to expose lumen of rectum

sage and stretching, and warm oil perineal massage during the second stage of labor. There is no evidence from RCTs that the use of warm compresses and second-stage perineal massage with or without oil decreases the need for episiotomy or decreases the risk of perineal trauma (Eason, Labrecque, Wells, & Feldman, 2000). One study found that perineal massage during the second stage was associated with a greater risk of perineal trauma (Aikens-Murphy & Feinland, 1998), and another study suggested that there was significant disagreement among providers about whether second-stage perineal massage should be used (Stamp, 1997). Without data to suggest benefit, along with limited data to suggest harm, perineal massage during the second stage should be used with caution, if at all, until more evidence is available about risks and benefits. Protection of the perineum immediately before birth by the physician or CNM to allow gradual perineal stretching and to avoid precipitous delivery of the fetal head may be sufficient to decrease the risk of perineal laceration or reduce the extent of the laceration.

Antepartum perineal massage has also been studied as a method to decrease risk of perineal trauma at birth. In these studies, women were taught to use daily perineal massage during the third trimester (Labrecque et al., 1999; Shipman, Boniface, Tefft, & McCloghry, 1997). Limited data exist to support the role of antepartum perineal massage in reducing the rate of episiotomies and perineal trauma (Eason, Labrecque, Wells, & Feldman, 2000; Renfrew, Hannah, Albers, & Floyd, 1998). In one study, women who were taught perineal massage reported pain, discomfort, irritation, fatigue, uneasiness with the concept, and negative physician comments (Mynaugh, 1991). The women who practiced perineal massage also experienced more perineal lacerations than those in the control group (Mynaugh, 1991). In another study, perineal massage was effective in reducing the rate of episiotomy for first-time mothers only (Labrecque et al., 1999). A later study found that perineal massage during pregnancy neither impaired nor substantially protected perineal function at 3 months postpartum (Labrecque, Eason, & Marcoux, 2000). More research is needed to determine whether perineal massage performed by the woman in the weeks before labor and birth is effective in avoiding episiotomy or reducing the extent of lacerations.

EMOTIONAL SUPPORT DURING LABOR AND BIRTH

Impact of the Psyche on Childbirth

The psyche plays a major role in the process of labor and birth. A high level of anxiety has been associated with increased catecholamine secretion that can result in ineffective uterine activity and longer and dysfunctional labor (Lederman, Lederman, Work, & McCann, 1985). Anxiety, uncertainty, loss of control, self-confidence, patterns of coping, support systems, fatigue, optimism, fatalism, and aloneness are some of the psychosocial factors to consider when caring for a women in labor. Previous birth experiences, current support systems, concerns or questions, anxiety or fear, and cultural considerations further contribute to attitudes and expectations for the pregnancy experience.

Women with a history of sexual abuse have unique needs during the intrapartum period. Not all women report or remember sexual abuse. Sensations of labor and birth can mimic physical experiences of the abuse and sometimes cause flashbacks and extreme anxiety. Lack of control and lack of choice are the similarities between sexual trauma and gynecologic procedures (Chalfen, 1993). Pelvic examinations may evoke feelings of depersonalization and powerlessness (Kitzinger, 1990). Nurses caring for women with a history of sexual abuse should have a heightened awareness of potential behavior during labor. The woman may choose to discuss her history of sexual abuse with the nurse. This type of acknowledgment may be a sign of healing and indicate that the woman believes her feelings will be taken seriously (Chalfen,

1993). Not all women will be able to share the history of abuse with the nurse but may exhibit difficulty and anxiety during with pelvic examination. This behavior is a sign of possible previous sexual trauma requiring further exploration. Nurses should help the woman feel empowered to make choices about labor and birth by assuring her that she is in control and that her wishes will be respected. Thorough explanations of all procedures and treatment should be provided and permission obtained before touching the woman. Minimal exposure and talking to the patient during a pelvic examination is vital. Examinations should not be forced. If the woman has not had counseling or is not presently in counseling, a referral would be appropriate.

Fewer perinatal complications, fewer newborns admitted to the neonatal intensive care nursery, and shorter labors result when women have a support person compared with women without support (Klaus, Kennel, Robertson, & Sosa, 1986; Norbeck & Anderson, 1989; Pascoe, 1993). Presence of a support person has also been found to reduce the rate of cesarean births (Klaus, Kennel, McGrath, Robertson, & Hinkley 1988, 1991). There is adequate research to validate significance of promoting support from family members or the coach during the labor and birth experience. Chapter 11 provides a detailed discussion of labor support.

Sibling presence during labor and birth also presents a unique opportunity for nurses to promote family attachment. Parents report that children present at labor and birth show a greater number of mothering and caretaking behaviors than children who were not present (DelGiudice, 1986). Sibling classes to prepare children for the birth experience are imperative. These classes should be age related and include films on childbirth, discussion of maternal behavior and sounds in labor, and reassurance that pain experienced by the mother is temporary. Each child also needs a support person to accompany the child and be familiar with the child's developmental level, so that the child's curiosity and concerns for his or her mother and new brother or sister are answered.

Supporting Family Attachment

Because the family members are introduced to their newborn immediately at birth, explanation of umbilical cord clamping or cutting and inspection of the placenta help them understand the final physiologic separation of the newborn from the mother's life-support system. After stabilization, the nurse can unwrap the newborn and describe normal physical characteristics. Siblings can count fingers and toes. Encouraging interaction with the newborn sets the stage for successful attachment and integration into the family unit. All family members can hold the newborn after birth as desired, and opportunities for photographs should be provided.

CLINICAL INTERVENTIONS FOR WOMEN IN LABOR

Most pregnancies, labors, and births are normal, requiring little or no intervention. However, some women require clinical interventions to optimize outcomes of pregnancies with identified maternal or fetal risk factors. The risk status for the woman and fetus may increase at any time during the pregnancy, labor and birth, or postpartum period. Perinatal nurses must be able to quickly assess and identify changes in maternal–fetal status and adjust nursing care accordingly. For example, nursing management during labor may require intrauterine resuscitation techniques when a nonreassuring FHR occurs, such as maternal position changes, administration of IV fluids, oxygen administration, and discontinuation of oxytocin if infusing. Women who are attempting a trial of labor after a previous cesarean birth may develop signs of uterine rupture requiring prompt identification and immediate interventions. A shoulder dystocia may develop unexpectedly at birth, necessitating ability to work with the physician or CNM to use various maneuvers to disimpact the shoulder. Knowledge of appropriate nursing interventions for common maternal–fetal complications during labor is essential. The nurse must be aware of changes in maternal–fetal status requiring physician or CNM notification.

The next section focuses on the clinical interventions of cervical ripening, induction and augmentation, operative vaginal birth, and amnioinfusion. Implications for nursing care are presented with key points for assessment.

Cervical Ripening and Induction and Augmentation of Labor

Definition of Terms

Cervical ripening is the process of effecting physical softening and distensibility of the cervix in preparation for labor and birth. *Induction* of labor is the stimulation of uterine contractions before spontaneous onset of labor for the purpose of accomplishing vaginal birth. *Augmentation* of labor is the stimulation of ineffective uterine contractions after the spontaneous onset of labor to manage labor dystocia (ACOG, 1995a, 1999a).

Various terminologies and definitions have been used in the literature to describe abnormally excessive uterine activity as a result of pharmacologic agents used for cervical ripening and induction and augmentation of labor. The imprecise and inconsistent use of these terms and definitions has contributed to inaccurate data about the risks and benefits of each agent and the inability to compare adverse effects among agents.

For the purposes of this chapter, one term (hyperstimulation) and one source (ACOG) are used to describe abnormally excessive uterine activity. A clear definition of hyperstimulation is essential because institutional clinical management strategies, policies, and protocols should include interventions that are expected when hyperstimulation is identified. All perinatal healthcare providers in each institution should be aware of clinical criteria established for hyperstimulation and the expected interventions. The ACOG practice bulletin *Induction of Labor* (1999a) defines *hyperstimulation* as a series of single contractions lasting 2 minutes or more or a contraction frequency of 5 or more in 10 minutes. The ACOG technical bulletin *Dystocia and the Augmentation of Labor* (1995a) includes the additional description: contractions of normal duration occurring within 1 minute of each other. Although hyperstimulation of uterine activity can be the result of endogenous maternal oxytocin and prostaglandins, most hyperstimulation is the result of administration of exogenous pharmacologic agents.

Other terms that have been used to describe abnormally excessive uterine activity are tachysystole and hypertonus. There is more variation in the definition and use of these terms than for hyperstimulation, and they are not used in all areas of the United States and Canada. Some practitioners reserve the use of hyperstimulation for a contraction frequency of 5 or more in 10 minutes with evidence that the fetus is not tolerating this contraction pattern, as demonstrated by late decelerations or fetal bradycardia. From the perspective of maternal–fetal safety, a reasonable approach is to avoid prolonged periods of hyperstimulation because they can lead to progressive deterioration in fetal status and nonreassuring FHR patterns. Interventions for hyperstimulation should not be delayed until there is evidence of nonreassuring fetal status.

Incidence

According to the National Center for Health Statistics, in 1998, the most recent year for which natality data are available, approximately 17.8% and 19.2%, respectively, of women who gave birth in the United States had induction and augmentation of labor. These figures represent a 125% (induction) and 75% (augmentation) increase for women at term since 1989, the first year these data began to be routinely collected from certificates of live births (Ventura, Martin, Curtin, Mathews, & Park, 2000).

Indications

Induction of labor has merit as a therapeutic option when the benefits of expeditious birth outweigh the risks of continuing the pregnancy (ACOG, 1999a). Controversy exists in the literature and in clinical practice about the exact nature and intensity of some risks and benefits. Multiple factors influence the decision to induce labor. Not all of the indications are clinical. Display 9–7 provides the criteria, indications, and contraindications for cervical ripening and induction and augmentation of labor (ACOG, 1995a, 1999a).

Although elective induction of labor is at an all-time high in the United States, this procedure is not without risks to the mother and baby. Elective induction of labor for nulliparous women is associated with a risk of cesarean birth twice that for nulliparous women who have spontaneous labor (Maslow & Sweeny, 2000; Yeast, Jones, & Poskin, 1999). Use of pharmacologic agents required for artificial induction of labor increases the risk of complications related to hyperstimulation, nonreassuring FHR patterns and cesarean birth for nonreassuring fetal status, and failure to progress in labor. Women who have an elective induction are at risk for a repeat induction of labor and cesarean birth if the induction is not successful (ACOG, 1999a). Failure to progress, also known as dystocia, is the number one reason for primary cesarean birth in the United States (Ventura et al., 2000). Significant maternal morbidity is associated with cesarean birth (see the Cesarean Birth section). In general, duration of induced labors is longer than that of spontaneous labors. The intrapartum inpatient length of stay is increased when labor is induced compared with that of a woman admitted in spontaneous labor. Intensity of maternal– fetal monitoring is increased during labor induction. These factors lead to increased costs to the institution.

A noted addition to the list of indications in the 1995 ACOG technical bulletin called *Induction of Labor* was "psychosocial indications." Previously, elective induction was not recommended (ACOG, 1991). For many pregnant women at term, the ability to select the most convenient day for birth is an important consideration. Advance planning and prior arrangements can provide reassurance and a sense of control over an otherwise unpredictable process. Factors such as child care for other children, availability of the labor support person or father of the baby,

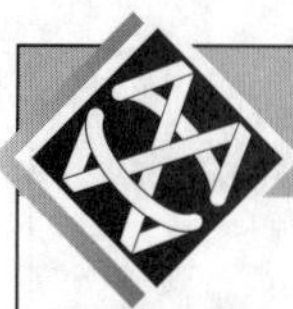

DISPLAY 9–7

Criteria, Indications, and Contraindications for Cervical Ripening and Induction and Augmentation of Labor

CRITERIA TO BE MET BEFORE THE CERVIX IS RIPENED OR LABOR IS INDUCED

- Assessment of gestational age, cervical status, pelvic adequacy, fetal size and fetal presentation
- Consideration of any potential risks to the mother and fetus
- Documentation in the medical record that a discussion was held between the pregnant woman and her healthcare provider about indications, the agents, and methods of labor induction, including the risks, benefits, and alternative approaches and the possible need for repeat induction or cesarean birth
- Personnel familiar with the effects of uterine stimulants on the mother and fetus because uterine hyperstimulation may occur with induction of labor
- Administration of cervical ripening agents at or near the labor and birth suite, where uterine activity and fetal heart rate can be monitored continuously
- Monitoring fetal heart rate and uterine contractions during induction and augmentation as for any high-risk patient in active labor
- A physician capable of performing a cesarean birth readily available

INDICATIONS FOR CERVICAL RIPENING AND INDUCTION OF LABOR

Indications for induction of labor are not absolute but should take into account maternal and fetal conditions, gestational age, cervical status, and other factors. Following are examples of maternal or fetal conditions that may be indications for induction of labor:

- Abruptio placenta
- Chorioamnionitis (intraamniotic infection)
- Fetal demise
- Pregnancy-induced hypertension
- Premature rupture of membranes
- Post term pregnancy
- Maternal medical conditions (eg, diabetes mellitus, renal disease, chronic pulmonary disease, chronic hypertension)
- Fetal compromise (eg, severe fetal growth restriction, isoimmunization)
- Preeclampsia, eclampsia

Labor may also be induced for logistic reasons (eg, risk of rapid labor, distance from the hospital, psychosocial indications). In such circumstances, at least one of the following criteria should be met or fetal lung maturity should be established:

- Fetal heart tones have been documented for 20 weeks by nonelectronic fetoscope or for 30 weeks by Doppler.
- It has been 36 weeks since a positive serum or urine human chorionic gonadotropin pregnancy test was performed by a reliable laboratory.
- An ultrasound measurement of the crown-rump length, obtained at 6 to 12 weeks supports a gestational age of at least 39 weeks.
- An ultrasound at 13 to 20 weeks gestation confirms the gestational age of at least 39 weeks

choice of attending physician on call, avoidance of holidays, maternity leave constraints, and even a federal income tax deduction in the preferred year can enter into the pregnant woman's decision to request an elective induction of labor.

In addition to patient convenience, convenience for the primary healthcare provider is a factor. Although not well documented in the literature or discussed openly in professional forums, a scheduled induction of labor offers some real advantages to the physician and CNM (Simpson & Poole, 1998b). For example, by scheduling several women for an induction of labor on the same day starting early in the morning, patient management can be done concurrently, and most women will give birth by the end of the day. Scheduling labor induction decreases the likelihood that office hours will have to be interrupted and patients rearranged when women go in to spontaneous labor. As the number of patients who have scheduled inductions increase, the number of physician and CNM phone calls and trips to the hospital in the middle of the night and on weekends is likely to decrease. The rates of induction of labor vary widely among physicians, CNMs, and institutions.

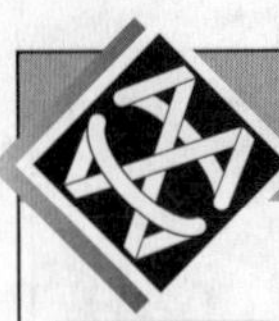

DISPLAY 9–7 (cont.)

Criteria, Indications, and Contraindications for Cervical Ripening and Induction and Augmentation of Labor

determined by clinical history and physical examination.

INDICATIONS FOR AUGMENTATION OF LABOR

Uterine hypocontractility should be augmented only after the maternal pelvis and fetal presentation have been assessed.

- Dystocia
- Uterine hypocontractility

CONTRAINDICATIONS FOR INDUCTION OF LABOR

Generally, the contraindications for labor induction are the same as those for spontaneous labor and vaginal birth. They include but are not limited to the following:

- Vasa previa or complete placenta previa
- Transverse fetal lie
- Umbilical cord prolapse
- Prior transfundal uterine incision

CONTRAINDICATIONS FOR AUGMENTATION OF LABOR

Uterine hypocontractility should be augmented only after the maternal pelvis and fetal presentation have been assessed. Contraindication for augmentation of labor are similar to those for induction of labor and may include but are not limited to the following:

- Placenta or vasa previa
- Umbilical cord presentation
- Prior classic uterine incision
- Active genital herpes infection
- Pelvic structural deformities
- Invasive cervical cancer

OBSTETRIC CONDITIONS THAT MAY REQUIRE SPECIAL ATTENTION

- One or more previous low-transverse cesarean births
- Breech presentation
- Maternal heart disease
- Multifetal pregnancy
- Polyhydramnios
- Presenting part above the pelvic inlet
- Severe hypertension
- Abnormal fetal heart rate patterns not requiring emergency birth

Adapted from American College of Obstetricians and Gynecologists. (1995a). *Dystocia and the augmentation of labor* (Technical Bulletin No. 218). Washington, DC: Author; and from American College of Obstetricians and Gynecologists. (1999a). *Induction of labor* (Practice Bulletin No. 10). Washington, DC: Author.

Risk–Benefit Analysis and Informed Consent

Regardless of physician or CNM preferences, patient psychosocial issues, or clinical indications as factors influencing consideration of labor induction, ACOG (1999a) and JCAHO (2000) recommend a risk-benefit analysis before the procedure and a discussion of the agents, methods, advantages, disadvantages, and alternative approaches with the patient, including the risk of cesarean birth or the possibility of a repeat induction. After this discussion, when the pregnant woman has enough information to participate in the decision-making process, informed consent should be obtained (ACOG, 1999a). Documentation that this discussion has occurred and that the woman has consented to proceed should be included in the medical record.

Although ACOG and JCAHO have long recommended that women having induction of labor be fully informed of indications, risks, and alternative approaches, this is not the usual clinical reality in many perinatal units in the United States. During the initial nursing assessment of many pregnant women who present for elective induction, it is clear that these issues have not been discussed with their primary provider. Although it may not be the nurse's responsibility to provide the required information, it is the nurse's responsibility to ensure that the woman has been given this information by her primary healthcare provider before beginning the procedure (AWHONN, 1998). A unit policy requiring evidence of informed consent before elective cervical ripening and labor induction is initiated is one way to enhance compliance with ACOG (1999a) and JCAHO (2000) recommendations (Simpson & Poole, 1998a). Appendix 9C is a sample form that can be included in the medical record as documentation of informed consent and of indications for cervical ripening and induction of labor.

The Nurse's Role

The nurse providing care for the woman during cervical ripening and induction of labor must be aware of appropriate indications for use, the action of the agent, expected results, and adverse effects of each mechanical method and pharmacologic agent. Before use of any cervical ripening or labor induction agent, maternal status and fetal well-being should be established, and cervical status should be assessed and documented in the medical record (ACOG, 1999a; Simpson & Poole, 1998a). Absence of fetal well-being necessitates direct physician evaluation and written documentation of further clinical management plans (Knox et al., 1999). Indication for preinduction cervical ripening and induction of labor also should be documented. Cervical assessment includes documentation of the Bishop score and the presence or absence of uterine activity. Ongoing maternal–fetal assessments during labor induction are presented in Display 9–3.

Clinical Protocol and Unit Policy Development

Most institutions have policies or protocols in place for cervical ripening and induction and augmentation of labor. Suggestions for key concepts to be included are presented in Display 9–8.

Cervical Status

The most important factor in determining success of induction of labor is cervical status. Cervical status is assessed by using the Bishop pelvic scoring system (Bishop, 1964) (Table 9–2). If the total score is more than 8, the probability of vaginal birth after induction of labor is similar to that of after spontaneous labor (ACOG, 1999). For women at term, a Bishop score of 6 or more may be useful in predicting onset of sponta-

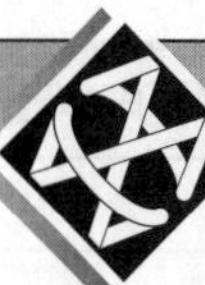

DISPLAY 9–8

Suggestions for Key Concepts of Clinical Protocols and Unit Policies for Cervical Ripening and Induction and Augmentation of Labor

- Criteria for designating patient priority for cervical ripening and induction based on the nature and intensity of the indication that can be used as a framework for decision-making during periods of limited staffing
- Documentation of indication by primary care provider
- Documentation of risk/benefit analysis discussed with pregnant woman by primary healthcare provider and informed decision-making process as recommended by ACOG (1999a) and JCAHO (2000)
- Establishment of maternal–fetal well-being
- Documentation of cervical status
- Method of fetal assessment
- Frequency of maternal–fetal assessments
- Cervical ripening agents to be used
- Initial oxytocin or misoprostol dosage
- Intervals for oxytocin dosage increases and amount of dosage increase
- Interval for misoprostol dosing and amount of misprostol dosage
- Orders for oxytocin and documentation in milliunits per minute (mU/min)
- Titration of oxytocin dosage based on progress of labor and maternal–fetal response
- Dosage of misoprostol based on progress of labor and maternal–fetal status
- Maintenance or decrease in oxytocin dosage if labor is progressing
- Definition of hyperstimulation
- Interventions for hyperstimulation
- Criteria for provider notification
- Interventions for nonreassuring fetal status
- Algorithm or chain of command for clinical disagreements
- Methods for documenting all of the key concepts and interventions outlined in the policy or protocol

Adapted from Simpson, K.R., & Poole, J.H. (1998a). AWHONN Symposium Cervical Ripening and Induction and Augmentation of Labor. Washington, DC: AWHONN.

TABLE 9–2 ■ BISHOP SCORE FOR ASSESSING READINESS FOR INDUCTION

	Assigned Value			
Factor	*0*	*1*	*2*	*3*
Cervical dilation	0	1–2 cm	3–4 cm	5 cm or more
Cervical effacement	0–30%	40–50%	60–70%	80% or more
Fetal station	–3	–2	– 1,0	+1,+2
Cervical consistency	Firm	Moderate	Soft	
Cervical position	Posterior	Midposition	Anterior	

From Bishop, E. H. (1964). Pelvic scoring for elective induction. *Obstetrics and Gynecology, 24,* 266.

neous labor within 7 days (Rozenberg, Goffinet, & Hessabi, 2000). Many mechanical and pharmacologic methods have been used to induce cervical ripening. The ideal ripening agent or procedure should be simple to use, noninvasive, effective within a reasonable period, not stimulate or induce labor during the ripening process, and not increase maternal, fetal, or neonatal morbidity. Unfortunately, the ideal agent or procedure for cervical ripening has not been identified.

Fetal Fibronectin as a Biochemical Marker for Onset of Term Labor and Successful Induction of Labor

The U.S. Food and Drug Administration (FDA) has approved the fetal fibronectin (fFN) assay to assess the likelihood of preterm birth for women who have clinical signs and symptom of preterm labor (Moore, 1999). The information helps in the clinical decision-making process about preterm labor treatment. Evolving data suggest that fFN could be a biochemical marker for impending term labor and successful labor induction (Garite et al., 1996; Rozenberg et al., 2000). Analysis of the published research suggests that a positive fFN assay can predict the likelihood of onset of labor within 3 to 4 days for women at term and can be useful in predicting whether an induction of labor would lead to a vaginal birth (Kiss, Ahner, Hohlagschwandtner, Leitich, & Husslein, 2000). The interval between induction and birth was significantly shorter for women with a positive fFN and unsuccessful induction of labor occurred only in women with fFN-negative cervicovaginal secretions (Kiss et al., 2000). Garite and colleagues (1996) found a positive fFN result predicted shorter labors, easier inductions, and lower cesarean birth rates. Blanch and coworkers (1996) concluded that fFN scoring worked as well as the Bishop score as an index of the ease of which induction of labor could be performed. Kiss (2000) suggested that the presence of fetal fibronectin in the cervicovaginal secretions could be used as a selection criteria for induction of term labor. For women who are at term, information about whether labor and birth were imminent would be helpful in deciding if labor induction was necessary. Waiting a few more days for onset of spontaneous labor would avoid the potential complications of artificial cervical ripening and labor induction. However, the high cost of fFN testing limits clinical application for assessing cervical readiness and success of induction for women at term.

Mechanical Methods of Cervical Ripening

Laminaria Tents

Laminaria tents have been used for cervical ripening for more than a century. Laminaria tents are made from the desiccated stems of cold-water seaweed (*Laminaria digitata* or *L. Japonica*) and appear to act primarily by extracting water from cervical tissues, causing gradual swelling of the seaweed. This swelling applies an expansive radial force to the cervical canal, causing the cervix to expand (Summers, 1997). The action of the laminaria tents causes, active dilatation of the cervix and passive stretching as well (Krammer & O'Brien, 1995). Stretching of the cervix causes local prostaglandin release (Riskin-Mashiah & Wilkins, 1999). Laminaria softens the cervix, changes the Bishop score, and facilitates amniotomy. There is no strong evidence that use of laminaria is associated with a reduced cesarean birth rate or a decrease in the induction-to-delivery interval (Krammer & O'Brien, 1995). Laminaria use does not appear to increase neonatal complications, but it has been associated with an increase in peripartum infections (ACOG, 1999a; Riskin-Mashiah & Wilkins, 1999).

Laminaria stems are 2 to 6 mm in diameter and approximately 60 mm long (Riskin-Mashiah & Wilkins, 1999). When placed in the endocervix for 6 to 12 hours, the diameter of laminaria double to triple without increasing in length (Summers, 1997). If left in place, progressive cervical change continues to occur, even after the laminaria have reached their maximal size. Of the hygroscopic dilators available, laminaria tents produce cervical change more slowly, but they are relatively inexpensive, do not break easily, and more than one laminaria can be placed at one time (Summers, 1997).

Recommended use of laminaria tents should be limited to women with an indication for induction who have little or no cervical effacement. Insertion of laminaria tents should be performed under direct visualization of the cervix using antiseptic technique. Placement of laminaria tents is usually limited to physicians or CNMs. As many laminaria as can be accommodated are placed in the endocervical canal with a long forceps after the cervix is visualized, cleaned, and lubricated with a bacteriostatic cream or jelly. After insertion, the laminaria tents can be held in position with two to four gauze 4 × 4 sponges that have been saturated with a bacteriostatic cream or jelly. The sponges are placed in the upper vagina against the cervix. After placement, documentation should include the number of laminaria tents placed in the cervix and the number of sponges placed in the vagina. Documentation also may include indication for the induction of labor, estimate of gestational age, current cervical status, fetal position, assessment of fetal adequacy, placental location, estimated fetal weight, and how the patient tolerated the procedure. Because the woman is positioned to facilitate placement of the laminaria, care should be taken to minimize the effects of supine hypotension. The woman should be encouraged to assume a lateral position as soon as possible after insertion.

After 6 to 12 hours, the physician or CNM can remove the sponges and examine the cervix. If cervical dilatation is determined to be adequate, the laminaria tents are removed and induction of labor is initiated. If cervical dilatation is determined to be inadequate, the laminaria tents can be removed and fresh tents inserted, or additional laminaria can be placed around those already in position. Regardless of whether the laminaria are removed and replaced or additional laminaria tents are inserted, all laminaria and sponges must be accounted for after their use. Additional nursing assessment and documentation includes notation of the onset of regular painful contractions, maternal fever, rupture of membranes, bleeding, or continuous uterine pain if any of these occur.

Synthetic Hygroscopic Dilators

Synthetic hygroscopic dilators were developed in response to concerns surrounding use of laminaria tents. Because laminaria are natural products, it has been difficult to control their content, consistency of response, and sterility. Two synthetic hygroscopic dilators are in use: Lamicel and Dilapan.

Lamicel (Cabot Medical Corporation, Langhorne, PA) is a polyvinyl alcohol polymer sponge soaked in 450 mg of magnesium sulfate. The cervical effects are the result of osmotic force (Krammer & O'Brien, 1995). After insertion into the endocervical canal, Lamicel absorbs fluid from surrounding tissues, and within 2 to 4 hours, the diameter enlarges threefold to fourfold (Summers, 1997). After Lamicel has enlarged, it becomes a soft, pliable sponge that exerts minimal radial force on the endocervix (Krammer & O'Brien, 1995).

Dilapan (Gynotech, Inc., Lebanon, NJ) is a stable, nontoxic, hydrophilic polymer of polyacrylonitrile, a synthetic dilator that is highly effective in softening an unripe cervix. It enlarges 8 to 10 mm within 2 hours of insertion and enlarges up to 11 to 12 mm within 4 hours (Krammer & O'Brien, 1995). Dilapan is easy to insert, but after insertion, it becomes brittle and may fragment, particularly during removal.

As with the natural laminaria tents, the synthetic hygroscopic dilators are relatively inexpensive, are easy to use, and can produce cervical ripening within a reasonable period. Synthetic hygroscopic dilators can be used safely for women in whom prostaglandin preparations for cervical ripening is relatively contraindicated. Compared with laminaria tents, synthetic hygroscopic dilators tend to swell faster and to a greater extent without an accompanying increase in patient discomfort (Krammer & O'Brien, 1995; Riskin-Mashiah & Wilkins, 1999). Multiple, serial applications within a 24-hour period are possible with the synthetic hygroscopic dilators because of the rapidity of their action. However, the use of multiple devices at one time may be difficult with a highly unfavorable cervix. As with laminaria tents, a physician or CNM inserts hygroscopic dilators. The same nursing assessments and documentation are required for use of synthetic hygroscopic dilators as are for laminaria tents.

Balloon Catheters

Balloon catheters have been used for many years as a means to induce cervical ripening. The balloon catheter is usually a Foley catheter with a 25- to 50-mL balloon that can be passed through an undilated cervix before inflation (Atad, Hallak, Ben-David,

Auslender, & Abramovici, 1997; James, Peedicayil, & Seshadri, 1994; Rouben & Arias, 1993; Summers, 1997). Insertion of a balloon catheter results in gradual cervical dilatation and is associated with minimal patient discomfort. The cervical changes induced by the balloon may also increase uterine activity, augmenting the local effects on the cervix. The mechanism for cervical ripening of the balloon catheter is direct pressure and overstretching of the lower uterine segment and cervix, as well as local secretion of prostaglandins (Riskin-Mashiah & Wilkins, 1999).

The recommended method for placing the balloon catheter through the cervix is under direct visualization. The cervix is prepared in much the same manner as for laminaria insertion. After visualization, the cervix and vagina are sponged with an antiseptic solution, and the physician or CNM passes a Foley catheter into the endocervix above the internal os with a long forceps. After the catheter has been placed, the balloon is inflated with sterile saline, and the catheter is gently withdrawn to the level of the internal cervical os. The catheter can then be secured to the inner aspect of the woman's thigh. Some practitioners administer an extraamniotic saline infusion through the catheter to promote cervical ripening. An infusion of normal saline at 1 mL per minute is infused into the extraamniotic space. This procedure is thought to enhance the mechanical dilation of the cervix by causing irritation of the cervical area and stimulation of the release of prostaglandins. Cervical changes consistent with ripening can usually be seen within 8 to 12 hours after balloon catheter insertion.

Use of an indwelling balloon catheter should be restricted to patients with intact membranes and an unfavorable cervix. Ambulation is appropriate with intermittent fetal assessment. The same precautions and documentation is required as for the other mechanical methods of cervical ripening. Caution should be used if this procedure is used for women with a history of prior cesarean birth or reconstructive uterine surgery. The catheter should be deflated and removed in the presence of rupture of membranes, fever, bleeding, or uterine hyperstimulation. When continuous traction is applied to the catheter the woman may experience vasovagal symptoms. If this occurs, the traction is discontinued (Trofatter, 1992).

Stripping of the Membranes for Cervical Ripening

Stripping, sweeping, or separating the amniotic membranes from the lower uterine segment digitally has been used for many years with various degrees of success. Risks involved with stripping of membranes include bleeding from a low-lying placenta, inadvertent rupture of the membranes with possible umbilical cord prolapse, and infectious morbidity. Pregnant women often report pain and discomfort during the procedure and spotting or bloody vaginal discharge for several hours after membranes have been stripped. Despite the lack of efficacy data, this procedure remains a widely used mechanical method of promoting cervical ripening and induction of labor by physicians and CNMs and other advanced practice perinatal nurses. This procedure is discussed in more detail in the sections on induction of labor.

Pharmacologic Methods of Cervical Ripening

There are various hormonal preparations available to induce cervical ripening. These agents include prostaglandin E_2 preparations (ie, Prepidil and Cervidil) and prostaglandin E_1 (Cytotec). Nurses caring for women receiving any of these agents must be aware that the pharmacologic agents used for cervical ripening may lead to the onset of labor. In the cervix that is unfavorable, cervical softening and thinning are more likely to occur. However, as cervical readiness for labor increases, there is an increased possibility for these agents to initiate labor.

The agents in clinical use for cervical ripening are discussed in the following sections. Display 9–9 summarizes key points about the use of prostaglandin E_2 (Prepidil and Cervidil) for cervical ripening, the use of prostaglandin E_1 (Cytotec) for cervical ripening and induction of labor, and the use of oxytocin for induction and augmentation of labor.

Prostaglandin E_2

Dinoprostone (PGE_2) is one of the most frequently prescribed medications for cervical ripening. The mechanism of action is similar to the natural ripening process, and women often go into spontaneous labor after administration. The successful prostaglandin preparations in use today for cervical ripening produce the desired cervical changes, but all tend to increase myometrial contractility. For this reason, prostaglandins for cervical ripening must be viewed as the first step in labor induction.

In December 1992, the FDA approved the first commercially prepared dinoprostone gel (Prepidil) preparation for cervical ripening for women at or near term who have a medical indication for inducing labor. After introduction of the dinoprostone gel, the FDA approved the use of a dinoprostone vaginal insert (Cervidil) for cervical ripening in 1995.

Prepidil

Prepidil (Upjohn Co., Kalamazoo, MI) was the first commercially available prostaglandin gel approved by the FDA for cervical ripening. It is packaged as a single-dose syringe containing 0.5 mg of dinoprostone (PGE_2) gel in 2.5 mL of a viscous gel composed of colloidal silicon dioxide in triacetin. The syringe is packaged with two soft plastic catheters for intracervical administration. The catheter is shielded to prevent application above the internal cervical os. According to the manufacturer, Prepidil is stable for up to 24 months when stored refrigerated between 2°C and 8°C. Before administration, the gel, which must be kept refrigerated, is brought to room temperature. The process of allowing the gel to attain room temperature should not be forced by using a warm water bath, microwaving, or similar methods because the product is sensitive to heat above 40°C and may be inactivated (Rayburn, Records, & Swanson, 1996).

Placement of Prepidil is performed by a physician or CNM at or near the labor and birth suite, where uterine activity and FHR can be monitored continuously for at least 30 minutes to 2 hours after insertion (ACOG, 1999a). Cervical effacement determines the appropriate catheter tip to use for placement of the gel. If the cervix is not effaced, the 20-mm shielded endocervical catheter is used; the 10-mm catheter is used if the cervix is 50% effaced. The cervix is visualized using a speculum, and then the gel is introduced into the cervical canal just below the level of the internal os.

After placement, ACOG (1999a) recommends that the woman remain recumbent for at least 30 minutes. Positioning of the woman should minimize the risk for hypotension during placement of the gel and for the initial period of bed rest following application. The cervix is reexamined after 6 hours. If there is no response to the initial dose, a repeat dose of 0.5 mg can be applied every 6 hours. The recommended cumulative dose for a 24-hour period is 1.5 mg of dinoprostone (ie, three doses). Previous exposure to PGE_2 attenuates the contractile response to oxytocin (Winkler & Rath, 1999). After the final dose of dinoprostone or after cervical ripening is accomplished, it is recommended that use of IV oxytocin be delayed for at least 6 to 12 hours because the effects of PGE_2 may be heightened with oxytocin (ACOG, 1999a).

Before placement of the gel, the woman should be afebrile, with no vaginal bleeding and without regular contractions. Dinoprostone is rapidly absorbed, with maximum concentrations reported within 15 to 45 minutes; the half-life is approximately 2.5 to 5 minutes (Rayburn et al., 1996). Uterine contractions usually are evident within the first hour and exhibit peak activity in the first 4 hours. After gel application, the plasma concentration increases rapidly within 20 to 30 minutes and remains constantly high for more than 4 hours (Winkler & Rath, 1999). Monitoring of the FHR and uterine activity should continue if regular contractions persist (ACOG, 1999a). If no increase in uterine activity occurs and the FHR is reassuring after the recommended period of observation (30 minutes to 2 hours), continuous monitoring may be discontinued, and the patient may be transferred elsewhere (ACOG, 1999a). In an uncomplicated pregnancy, the woman may be encouraged to ambulate after the initial period of observation. Assessments should focus on uterine activity, monitoring for hyperstimulation and fetal response to therapy. If hyperstimulation occurs, the woman may be placed in a lateral position and tocolytic therapy (0.25 mg of terbutaline given subcutaneously). Irrigation of the cervix and vagina are not beneficial (ACOG, 1999a). The rate of hyperstimulation with Prepidil is approximately 1% to 5% and usually occurs within 1 hour after dosage (ACOG, 1999a).

Dinoprostone use for women with a history of asthma, reactive airway disease, glaucoma, or pulmonary, hepatic, cardiac, or renal disease has been debated. Concern exists about the vascular and pulmonary effects of prostaglandins in inducing maternal compromise. Unlike $PGF_{2\alpha}$, which is a potent bronchoconstrictor, PGE_2 is a bronchodilator and therefore does not cause bronchial constriction, risk of asthma exacerbation, or significant BP changes (ACOG, 1999a).

Cervidil

Cervidil (Forest Pharmaceuticals, St. Louis, MO) contains dinoprostone in a controlled-release vaginal insert. The insert is a thin, flat, rectangular, cross-linked polymer hydrogel that releases dinoprostone (PGE_2) from a 10-mg reservoir at a controlled rate of approximately 0.3 mg/hour in vivo (Forest Pharmaceuticals, 1995; Summers, 1997). The reservoir chip is encased within a pouch of knitted Dacron polyester with a removal cord. The entire system comes preassembled and prepacked in sterile foil packets that are stored at –20°C until immediately before use. The insert does not require warming to room temperature before insertion.

Cervidil may be inserted by perinatal nurse who has demonstrated competence in insertion and if the activity is within the scope of practice as defined by state and provincial regulations. Institutional guidelines for the nurse's role related to Cervidil administration should be established. Cervidil is administered in or near the labor and birth suite, where uterine activity and FHR can be monitored continuously while in place and for at

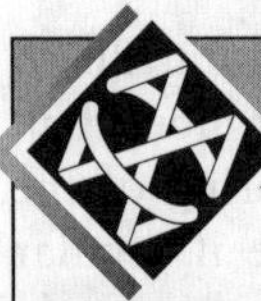

DISPLAY 9–9

Cervical Ripening and Induction Agents

PREPIDIL (PROSTAGLANDIN E_2)

- Food and Drug Administration (FDA) approved in 1992
- 0.5-mg dinoprostone gel package in syringe with two catheters
- If not effaced, 20-mm shielded endocervical catheter
- If ≥50% effaced, 10-mm catheter
- Unstable at room temperature; store in refrigerator (stable up to 2 years when stored at 2°C to 8°C)
- Bring to room temperature just before administration. Do not use warm water bath, microwave, or other methods to speed the process of bringing gel to room temperature, because Prepidil is sensitive to heat and may be inactivated.
- During speculum examination, gel is introduced just below the cervical os.
- Patient stays recumbent for at least 30 minutes.
- If no response, additional 0.5 mg every 6 hours
- Maximum cumulative dose for 24 hours is 1.5 mg of dinoprostone (three doses)
- Half-life of 2.5 to 5 minutes
- Uterine contractions usually within first hour; peak activity within 4 hours
- If needed, oxytocin should be delayed for 6 to 12 hours after last dose because the effects of PGE_2 may be heightened with oxytocin
- Limited research about maternal–fetal assessment techniques other than continuous electronic fetal monitoring (EFM).
- Should administered at or near labor and birth suite, where uterine activity and fetal heart rate can be monitored continuously for a period of 30 minutes to 2 hours after dosage
- Rate of hyperstimulation is approximately 1% to 5%; usually occurs within 1 hour after the gel has been placed
- Cost is $65 to $75 per 0.5-mg dose (ACOG, 1999a; Simpson & Poole, 1998a; Upjohn Company, 1995).

CERVIDIL (PROSTAGLANDIN E_2)

- FDA approved in 1995
- 10-mg dinoprostone in controlled-release vaginal insert with removable cord (0.3 mg/hour released from 10-mg reservoir chip)
- Unstable at room temperature (stable up to 3 years when frozen)
- Keep frozen (–20°C) until immediately before use
- Easy to insert; does not require warming or speculum
- Patient stays supine for 2 hours after insertion, and then may ambulate using EFM telemetry.
- Uterine contractions usually within 5 to 7 hours
- Removal after 12 hours or at onset of labor
- If needed, oxytocin should be delayed at least 30 to 60 minutes after removal of insert.
- No studies without continuous EFM for maternal–fetal assessment
- Should be administered at or near the labor and birth suite, where uterine activity and fetal heart rate can be monitored continuously while in place and for at least 15 minutes after removal
- Rate of hyperstimulation is approximately 5%; usually occurs within 1 hour but may occur up to 9.5 hours after the insert has been placed
- Manufacturer's product insert indicates use is contraindicated in women with history of prior cesarean birth or uterine scar.
- Cost is $165 per insert (ACOG, 1998; 1999a; Forest Pharmaceuticals, 1995; Simpson & Poole, 1998a).

CYTOTEC (MISOPROSTOL [PROSTAGLANDIN E_1])

- Not FDA approved for cervical ripening or labor induction (FDA approved for peptic ulcer prevention)
- Misoprostol is a synthetic PGE_1 analogue used in treatment of peptic ulcers secondary to nonsteroidal antiinflammatory drugs.
- Abortifacient properties well established (400 µg)
- Manufacturer states not to be used for cervical ripening or labor induction
- Available in 100- and 200-µg tablets
- 100-µg tablet not scored (should be prepared by hospital pharmacy)
- Various dosing regimens have been reported: 25 µg (¼ tablet inserted into the posterior vaginal fornix and repeated every 3 to 6 hours, up to 6 doses in 24 hours as needed is the safest approach)

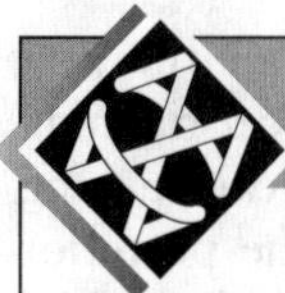

DISPLAY 9–9 (cont.)

Cervical Ripening and Induction Agents

- There are lower rates of uterine hyperstimulation with lower dosages (25 µg versus 50 µg) q 6 hours rather than q 3 hours.
- Redosing is withheld if there are two or more contractions in 10 minutes, adequate cervical ripening is achieved (a Bishop score of 8 or more or the cervix is 80% effaced and 3 cm dilated), the patient enters active labor, or the FHR is nonreassuring.
- The woman should be observed for up to 2 hours after spontaneous rupture of membranes. If cervical condition remains unfavorable, uterine activity is minimal, the FHR is reassuring, and it has been at least 3 hours since the last dose of misoprostol, redosing is permissible.
- If oxytocin is needed, it should not be given until at least 4 hours after the last dose.
- No studies without continuous EFM for maternal-fetal assessment
- Should be administered at or near labor and birth suite, where uterine activity and fetal heart rate can be monitored continuously
- Not recommended for use in women with history of prior cesarean birth or uterine scar
- Not enough data about oral route to recommend oral use at this time
- Cost is $.36 to $1.20 per tablet (ACOG, 1999a; 1999b; Simpson & Poole, 1998a; Wing & Paul, 1999a).

OXYTOCIN

- Only pharmacologic agent approved by the FDA for induction of labor with a live fetus
- Endogenous oxytocin is synthesized by the hypothalamus and then transported to the posterior lobe of the pituitary gland, where it is released into maternal circulation. Release is in response to breast stimulation, sensory stimulation of the lower genital tract, and cervical stretching. Oxytocin released in response to vaginal and cervical stretching results in uterine contractions.
- Synthetic oxytocin is chemically and physiologically identical to endogenous oxytocin.
- Although there are considerable variations in reports of the biologic half-life of oxytocin, the half-life usually is between 7 and 15 minutes.
- Oxytocin concentration and saturation follow first-order kinetics with a progressive, linear, stepwise increase with each increase in the infusion rate (Brindley & Sokol, 1988).
- Three to four half-lives of oxytocin are generally needed to reach a steady-state plasma concentration (Stringer, 1996).
- Uterine response to oxytocin usually occurs within 3 to 5 minutes after intravenous (IV) administration has begun.
- There is an incremental phase of uterine activity when oxytocin is initiated during which contractions progressively increase in frequency and strength, followed by a stable phase, during which time any further increase in oxytocin does not lead to further normal changes in uterine contractions (Dawood, 1995).
- Based on physiologic and pharmacokinetic principles, Seitchik and colleagues (1984) recommended at least a 40-minute interval between oxytocin dosage increases, because the full effect of oxytocin on the uterine response to increases in dosage cannot be evaluated until steady-state concentration has been achieved. Their data suggested that increasing the infusion rate before steady-state concentrations were achieved resulted in laboring women receiving higher doses of oxytocin than were necessary.
- Oxytocin is administered intravenously and is piggybacked into the main line solution at the port most proximal to the venous site.
- There are many variations in the dilution rate. Some protocols suggest adding 10 U of oxytocin to 1,000 mL of an isotonic electrolyte IV solution, resulting in an infusion dosage rate of 1 milliunit (mU) per minute, equalling 6 mL per hour; however other commonly reported dilutions are 20 U of oxytocin to 1,000 mL IV fluids (1 mU/min = 3 mL/hr) and 60 U oxytocin to 1,000 mL of IV fluids (1 mU/min = 1 mL/hr).
- There are no clear advantages for any one dilution rate; the key issues are knowledge of how many milliunits per minute are administered and consistency in clinical practice in each institution.
- To enhance communication among members of the perinatal healthcare team and to avoid confusion, oxytocin administration rates should always be ordered by the physician or certified nurse midwife as mU/min and documented in the medical record as mU/min (ACOG, 1995, 1999a; Simpson & Poole, 1998a).

least 15 minutes after removal (ACOG, 1998b, 1999a). Unlike the transcervical preparations, Cervidil does not require visualization of the cervix for insertion. The insert is placed into the posterior fornix of the vagina with its long axis transverse to the long axis of the vagina. The ribbon end of the retrieval system may be allowed to extrude distally from the vagina or tucked into the vagina. Once placed, Cervidil absorbs moisture, swells, and releases dinoprostone at a controlled rate. The delivery system makes Cervidil relatively simple to insert; it does not require warming and requires only a single digital examination.

Cervidil is removed after 12 hours or when active labor begins (ACOG, 1999a). Regular contractions (3 in 10 minutes lasting 60 seconds or more with moderate patient discomfort) will occur in approximately 25% of women after Cervidil placement (Rayburn, Tassone, & Pearman, 2000). One major advantage of the delivery system of Cervidil is that the system can be easily and quickly removed in the event of uterine hyperstimulation or complications. The rate of hyperstimulation with Cervidil is approximately 5% and usually occurs within 1 hour after dosage but may occur up to 9.5 hours after the insert has been placed (ACOG, 1998b, 1999a). If uterine hyperstimulation occurs, complete reversal of the prostaglandin-induced uterine pattern is usually evident within 15 minutes of insert removal. If needed, terbutaline (0.25 mg) is administered subcutaneously. The manufacturer (Forest Pharmaceuticals, 1995) and ACOG (1999a) recommend a period of 30 to 60 minutes between removal of the system and initiation of oxytocin. Because previous exposure to PGE_2 attenuates the contractile response to oxytocin (Winkler & Rath, 1999), careful maternal–fetal monitoring is warranted when oxytocin is administered after Cervidil has been used for cervical ripening (Raskin, Dachauer, Doeden, & Rayburn, 1999).

Because of the high rate of initiation of regular contractions and the 5% rate of hyperstimulation, Cervidil is not appropriate for outpatient cervical ripening (ACOG, 1998, 1999a; Rayburn et al., 2000). The manufacturer's recommendations include a prior uterine scar as a contraindication for use (Forest Pharmaceuticals, 1995). Risk of uterine rupture when Cervidil is used for women attempting a vaginal birth after a previous cesarean birth has been confirmed by clinical studies (Raskin et al., 1999).

Prostaglandin E_1: Misoprostol

Misoprostol (Cytotec; GD Searle and Company, Chicago, IL) is a synthetic prostaglandin E_1 analogue that has been used for cervical ripening and induction of labor. Misoprostol is FDA approved for the prevention of peptic ulcers but not for cervical ripening or induction of labor. When used for cervical ripening or induction of labor, 25 μg placed in the posterior vaginal fornix should be considered for the initial dose (ACOG, 1999a, 1999b). Higher dosages have been associated with an increased rate of hyperstimulation (ACOG, 1999a, 1999b). Hyperstimulation and nonreassuring FHR changes can be associated with the 25-μg and 50-μg dosages (Blanchette, Nayak, & Eramus, 1999; Kolderup, McLean, Grullon, Safford, & Kilpatrick, 1999; Winkler & Rath, 1999). A systematic review of studies about misoprostol found that the rate of uterine hyperstimulation with and without nonreassuring FHR changes is significantly higher with the use of misoprostol compared with oxytocin (Hofmeyer, Gulmezoglu, & Alfiervic, 1999).

Misoprostol can be repeated every 3 to 6 hours for up to six doses in 24 hours. The 6-hour interval between dosages has been associated with less uterine hyperstimulation than the 3-hour interval (ACOG, 1999a, 1999b). Redosing of misoprostol is withheld if the woman has two or more contractions in 10 minutes, achieves adequate cervical ripening (ie, Bishop score of 8 or more or a cervical effacement of 80% and 3-cm dilation), she enters active labor, or the FHR is nonreassuring (Wing & Paul, 1999a). If the woman's membranes rupture during cervical ripening, she should be observed for up to 2 hours; if her cervical condition remains unfavorable, uterine activity is minimal, the FHR is reassuring, and it has been at least 3 hours since the last dose, redosing of misoprostol is permissible (Wing & Paul, 1999a). According to ACOG (1999a), there are not enough data about maternal–fetal safety to recommend oral use of misoprostol at this time.

Uterine rupture is a complication of use of misoprostol for cervical ripening and labor induction (Hofmeyer et al., 1999; Winkler & Rath, 1999). Wing, Lovett, and Paul (1998) attempted an RCT of women with history of a prior cesarean birth using oxytocin or misoprostol. The study was terminated after two women in the misoprostol group developed a nonreassuring FHR followed by uterine rupture and emergency cesarean birth (Wing et al., 1988). Misoprostol is contraindicated for women with a history of prior uterine surgery or cesarean birth because of risk of uterine rupture (ACOG, 1999a, 1999b).

Misoprostol is available in 100- and 200-μg tablets. The 100-μg tablet is unscored, and there is no assurance that the PGE_1 is uniformly dispersed throughout the tablet. It is possible that one fourth of the tablet may contain more or less than 25 μg of PGE_1. The hospital pharmacist should prepare the tablet in four equal parts before administration of one fourth of the tablet intravaginally (Wing & Paul, 1999a). Individual providers attempting to break the small tablet into four equal parts increases the risk of inaccurate dosage administration.

Those who advocate the use of misoprostol for cervical ripening and induction of labor believe that the low cost, ease of insertion, and quick action are the main advantages. Hyperstimulation, meconium passage, neonatal cord pH below 7.16, low 5-minute Apgar scores, admission to the neonatal intensive care unit, nonreassuring FHR patterns, and a higher rate of cesarean birth related to nonreassuring FHR patterns from hyperstimulation are the most commonly reported adverse effects of misoprostol (ACOG, 1999a, 1999b; Bennett, Butt, Crane, Hutchens, & Young, 1998; Buser, Mora, & Arias, 1997; Farah et al., 1997; Wing & Paul, 1999). These adverse effects can be minimized by using the lowest dose (25 μg) no more than every 3 to 6 hours (ACOG, 1999a, 1999b; Wing & Paul, 1999a). If uterine hyperstimulation and a nonreassuring FHR pattern occur with misoprostol and there is no response to routine corrective measures (ie, maternal repositioning and supplemental oxygen administration), cesarean birth should be considered (ACOG, 1999a). Terbutaline (0.25 mg given subcutaneously) also can be used in an attempt to correct the nonreassuring FHR pattern or the uterine hyperstimulation (ACOG, 1999a; Wing & Paul, 1999a).

If induction or augmentation of labor is required after cervical ripening with misoprostol, some providers use oxytocin. Plasma concentration of misoprostol after vaginal administration of misoprostol rises gradually, attaining peak levels in 1 to 2 hours and declining slowly to an average of 61% of peak level at 4 hours (Zieman, Fong, Benowitz, Banskter, & Darney, 1997). Some women have increased plasma concentrations 4 to 6 hours after vaginal administration (Zieman et al., 1997). There are no recommendations from ACOG in its 1999a practice bulletin *Induction of Labor* and 1999b committee opinion *Induction of Labor with Misoprostol* about the appropriate and safe time interval from the last dose of misoprostol and the initiation of oxytocin. However, in its letter to the FDA (2000a) about the safety of misoprostol, ACOG recommends waiting at least 4 hours after the last dose of misoprostol before using oxytocin to induce or augment labor. ACOG (1999a) recommends at least 3 to 6 hours between doses of misoprostol and includes a cautionary statement that there are lower rates of uterine hyperstimulation with nonreassuring FHR changes with the 6-hour dosage interval compared with the 3-hour dosage interval. ACOG (1999a) also recommends delaying oxytocin for at least 6 to 12 hours after administration of PGE_2 gel because the effect of prostaglandin may be heightened with oxytocin. Misoprostol is a prostaglandin analogue. A reasonable and safe approach is to delay oxytocin administration for induction or augmentation until at least 4 hours after the last dose of misoprostol, based on assessment of uterine activity and fetal status. More data are needed about the safe and effective time intervals between misoprostol cervical ripening and oxytocin augmentation.

Misoprostol can be administered by perinatal nurses, but in most institutions, this practice is deferred to physicians or CNMs. If misoprostol placement is delegated to perinatal nurses, they must have demonstrated competence in insertion and the activity must be within the scope of practice as defined by state and provincial regulations. Institutional guidelines for the nurse's role related to misoprostol administration should be established. Misoprostol is administered in or near the labor and birth suite, where uterine activity and FHR can be monitored continuously (ACOG, 1999a, 1999b).

Mechanical Methods of Induction of Labor

Stripping of the Membranes for Induction of Labor

Digital separation of the chorioamnionic membrane from the wall of the cervix and lower uterine segment during a vaginal examination, commonly referred to as *stripping of the membranes* or *sweeping the membranes*, is sometimes used as a method of labor induction. This procedure is performed by inserting a finger into the internal cervical os and rotating through 360 degrees. Although the exact mechanism of action is not fully understood, there may be a scientific basis for the this technique. Stripping of the membranes is thought to release prostaglandins that are produced locally from the amnion and chorion and the adjacent decidua (Sellers et al., 1980). The amount of prostaglandins released correlates to the area of the membranes stripped (Mitchell et al., 1997) and may also cause release of maternal oxytocin from the posterior pituitary gland (O'Brien & Cefalo, 1996). The best results are seen if the vertex is well applied to the cervix in a term pregnancy. The procedure appears to be most beneficial for women who are pregnant for the first time and have an unripe cervix at term (Krammer & O'Brien, 1995).

Because there has not been much research about stripping membranes compared with waiting for spontaneous labor, the efficacy of the technique remains unknown. The available data are inconsistent, and most studies suffer from small sample size. Several studies of nearly identical design, including randomization, weeks of gestation when the procedure was performed, and outcome measures, produced different results (Berghella, Rogers, & Lescale, 1996; Crane, Bennet, Young, Windrim, & Kravitz, 1997; El-Torkey & Grant, 1992; McColgin et al., 1990). Based on what is known, a decrease in the interval from membrane stripping to spontaneous labor is probably limited to pregnant women at 41 weeks' gestation or more with no increase in adverse maternal–fetal outcomes. More data are needed, including studies with larger sample sizes, to further evaluate efficacy and potential for maternal–fetal complications related to membrane stripping.

Risks of membrane stripping include potential for intraamniotic infection, unplanned rupture of membranes, disruption of an undiagnosed placenta previa, and a precipitous labor and birth (ACOG, 1999a). Stripping of the membranes is contraindicated in women with a history of a low-lying placenta or placenta previa and probably should be avoided in women with a known group β-hemolytic streptococci colonization or infected with *Chlamydia trachomatis* or *Neisseria gonorrhoeae* (Trofatter, 1992). The procedure should also be avoided in women who have had repeated outbreaks of herpes genitalis during the current pregnancy (Trofatter, 1992).

The unpredictable nature of stripping of the membranes and lack of supportive data have prompted some experts to suggest that this procedure should not be used routinely as a method of induction (O'Brien & Cefalo, 1996), but there is no consensus in the literature or in clinical practice about routine membrane stripping. Potential benefits include relative ease of the procedure during routine vaginal examination at term and no costs if done during a scheduled prenatal visit. Probably the greatest potential benefit of membrane stripping is possible avoidance of other methods of induction if successful.

Generally, stripping of the membranes is a procedure reserved for qualified physicians and perinatal nurses in advanced practice roles such as nurse practitioners, clinical nurse specialists and CNMs. Patient education should include expected results from the procedure and possible complications. The woman needs to know to seek medical attention if the membranes rupture, bleeding occurs, there is a decrease in fetal activity, or if she develops a fever, regular contractions begin, or discomfort persists between uterine contractions. Documentation should also include indications for the induction of labor, estimate of gestational age, current cervical status, fetal position, assessment of fetal well-being, placental location, and estimated fetal weight.

Amniotomy

Amniotomy is more frequently used for augmentation when the woman is in active labor, but amniotomy as a method of induction can be successful when the woman has a favorable cervix (Busowski & Parsons, 1995). Amniotomy is particularly successful for multiparous women with cervical dilatation greater than 2 cm. For some women, amniotomy may avoid the need for oxytocin. There have been several reports over the past three decades about the efficacy and safety of amniotomy for labor induction. Most of the research has included oxytocin and other methods of induction in addition to amniotomy. There are few data about amniotomy alone compared with with no intervention. More data are needed about the efficacy of amniotomy alone as a method of induction.

The potential benefit of amniotomy is the possible avoidance of oxytocin if rupture of membranes results in adequate uterine contractions to effect normal labor progress. Risks include the possibility of umbilical cord prolapse, intraamniotic infection, and commitment to labor with an uncertain outcome. Garite, Porto, Carlson, Rumney, & Reimbold (1993) found that elective amniotomy resulted in milder and moderate variable decelerations of the FHR. In a later study of 925 women (Goffinet et al., 1997), amniotomy resulted in an increase in severe variable FHR decelerations and an increase in cesarean birth for nonreassuring fetal status. Unless there is an urgent reason for labor induction, the most reasonable approach is to await sufficient cervical dilatation before rupturing membranes because of the potential risks of umbilical cord prolapse and lack of a solid body of evidence to support efficacy and maternal–fetal outcomes.

Performance of amniotomy is reserved for qualified physicians and CNMs. Amniotomy should not be performed by staff nurses for the convenience of other healthcare providers. Some institutions allow nurses to rupture membranes in rare cases in which the benefits of more data about fetal assessment clearly outweigh the risks associated with the nurse's inability to perform an emergent cesarean birth if prolapse of the umbilical cord occurs. If amniotomy is allowed by the perinatal nurse in these rare cases, an institutional policy, procedure, and protocol that meets the criteria of the scope of nursing practice defined by the state board of nursing should be in place. Application of an internal fetal electrode in the presence of intact amniotic membranes is an amniotomy. Perinatal nurses should defer responsibility for amniotomy to the appropriate healthcare providers. Documentation should include the amount, color, and odor of amniotic fluid; the FHR before amniotomy; and the fetal response after the procedure.

Pharmacologic Methods of Induction of Labor

Oxytocin

Oxytocin is a peptide consisting of nine amino acids and is the only pharmacologic agent approved by the FDA for the induction of labor with a living fetus. Oxytocin circulates in the blood as a free peptide and has a molecular weight of 1,007 daltons (Zeeman et al., 1997). The volume of distribution is estimated to be 305 ± 46 mL/kg; oxytocin is distributed throughout intravascular and extravascular compartments (Zeeman et al., 1997). Although there are considerable variations in reports about the biologic half-life of oxytocin, it is generally agreed that the half-life is between 7 and 15 minutes. Early data based on in vitro studies estimated a plasma half-life of 3 to 4 minutes, but Seitchik, Amico, Robinson, & Castillo (1984) used in vivo methods to study oxytocin pharmacokinetics and found the half-life was probably closer to 10 to 15 minutes.

Oxytocin concentration and saturation follow first-order kinetics, with a progressive, linear, stepwise increase with each increase in the infusion rate (Brindley & Sokol, 1988). Three to four half-lives of oxytocin usually are needed to reach a steady-state plasma concentration (Stringer, 1996). Uterine response to oxytocin usually occurs within 3 to 5 minutes after IV administration has begun. There is an incremental phase of uterine activity when oxytocin is initiated during which contractions progressively increase in frequency and strength, followed by a stable phase, during which any further increase in oxytocin does not lead to further normal changes in uterine contractions (Dawood, 1995).

Based on physiologic and pharmacokinetic principles, Seitchik and colleagues (1984) recommended at least a 40-minute interval between oxytocin dosage increases, because the full effect of oxytocin on the uterine response to increases in dosage cannot be evaluated until a steady-state concentration has been achieved. Their data suggested that increasing the infusion rate before steady-state concentrations were achieved resulted in laboring women receiving higher doses of oxytocin than were necessary. The work of Seitchik & Castillo (1982, 1983) and Seitchik and coworkers (1984) was the basis of oxytocin protocols with intervals in oxytocin dosage increases between 30 and 60 minutes. More data are needed using the most accurate biochemical assessment methods to evaluate the relation between oxytocin infusion rates and uterine activity.

Oxytocin is administered by the IV route and is piggybacked into the mainline solution at the port most proximal to the venous site. There are many variations in the dilution rate. Some protocols suggest adding 10 units of oxytocin to 1,000 mL of an IV isotonic electrolyte solution, resulting in an infusion dosage rate of 1 milliunit (mU) per minute, equalling 6 mL per hour; other commonly reported dilutions are 20 units of oxytocin to 1,000 mL of IV fluids (1 mU/min = 3 mL/hr) and 60 units oxytocin to 1,000 mL of IV fluids (1 mU/min = 1 mL/hr). There are no clear advantages for any one dilution rate; the key issues are knowledge about how many milliunits per minute are administered and consistency in clinical practice in each institution. To enhance communication among members of the perinatal healthcare team and to avoid confusion, oxytocin administration rates should always be ordered by the physician or CNM as milliunits per minute (mU/min) and documented in the medical record as milliunits per minute.

Considerable controversy exists about dosage and rate increase intervals when oxytocin is used for induction of labor. There is no consensus in the literature on the ideal oxytocin dosage regimen, although available data support a lower rate of infusion. Researchers whose opinions are based on the work of Seitchik and colleagues (1984) advocate a *physiologic* approach to oxytocin dosage and rate increase intervals. Others support a *pharmacologic* approach based in part on the results from early studies about more aggressive high-dose oxytocin protocols, sometimes referred to as the active management of labor (AMOL) (O'Driscoll, Foley, & McDonald, 1984; O'Driscoll, Jackson, & Gallagher, 1969). High-dose oxytocin is only one component of the AMOL protocol that is used for augmentation for nulliparous women in active labor.

There have been numerous studies of high-dose oxytocin dosage protocols and shortened oxytocin dosage interval protocols for induction of labor; summary tables of research are provided in AWHONN's symposium *Cervical Ripening and Induction and Augmentation of Labor* (Simpson & Poole, 1998a). Results have varied, but most researchers observed that a decrease in the dosage interval led to more uterine hyperstimulation and nonreassuring FHR patterns. No study demonstrated a clinically significant decrease in the length of labor when using higher dosages or shortened dosage intervals. Higher doses and more frequent increases in dosage rates of oxytocin for induction did not significantly shorten labor but did cause more labor complications in all of the published studies.

A cervical dilation rate of 1 cm/hour in the active phase of labor is an indication that labor is progressing sufficiently and that oxytocin administration is adequate. Traditional definitions of a prolonged latent phase do not apply to induced labor, in which a latent phase exceeding 20 hours is common. High-dose oxytocin and shorter intervals between rate increases tend to have less adverse effects on maternal–fetal status during labor augmentation than during labor induction. This result in part may reflect the fact that, in spontaneous active labor, the unripe cervix is not a significant factor and oxytocin receptor sites are thought to be increased in number and sensitivity.

Other factors that may influence the dose response to oxytocin include maternal body surface area, parity, week of pregnancy duration, and cervical status. Although these factors may be significant, there are no practical predictive models for determining the required oxytocin dosage for successful labor induction. Until more is known about the pharmacokinetics of oxytocin, each pregnant woman receiving oxytocin will continue to represent an individual bioassay.

Research about the effects of uterine contractions and oxytocin-induced uterine hyperstimulation on fetal status has contributed to what is known about how the fetus responds to the physiologic stress of labor induction. McNamara and Johnson (1995) used fetal oxygen saturation monitoring to assess the fetal response to uterine contractions and found that the average fetal oxygen saturation decreases after a contraction. The greatest drop in fetal oxygen saturation is reached about 90 seconds after the contraction, and an additional 90 seconds is required for fetal recovery (McNamara & Johnson, 1995). When uterine hyperstimulation occurs as the result of oxytocin, the same decrease in fetal oxygen saturation occurs, but if the contraction interval is less than 2 minutes, the fetal recovery is incomplete (Johnson, Oudgaarden, Montague, & McNamara, 1994). Using fetal oxygen saturation monitoring, the researchers found that fetal oxygen saturation decreased incrementally after each contraction, resulting in fetal hypoxemia. Recovery to a reassuring fetal oxygen saturation level occurred only after the oxytocin was discontinued (Johnson et al., 1994).

Two reviews of all available data about oxytocin pharmacokinetics and dosage administration protocols were reported by Brindley and Sokol (1988) and by Shyken and Petrie (1995a). Both groups concluded that the evidence supported a low-dose (ie, physiologic) approach to oxytocin administration for labor induction. "The current data overwhelmingly indicate that oxytocin should be started at a low dose (0.5 to 1 mU/min) with a slow arithmetical increase every 30 to 60 minutes" (Brindley & Sokol, 1988, p. 730). According to Brindley and Sokol (1998), the risks of nonreassuring FHR patterns and uterine hyperstimulation were not outweighed by the slight or no decrease in the duration of the interval from induction to birth. Shyken and Petrie (1995a) advocated using the lowest possible doses of oxytocin to effect a clinical response. "Current evidence supports using oxytocin in the physiologic range. Adequate uterine activity will occur in a reasonable amount of time, but without the troublesome uterine hypercontractility" (Shyken & Petrie, 1995a, p. 236). These investigators thought that the low dose and longer intervals for increased dosage ensured sufficient time to reach physiologic steady state and avoided uterine hyperstimulation and the risks of nonreassuring fetal status (Shyken & Petrie, 1995a, 1995b).

Multiple clinical studies and current data based on physiologic and pharmacologic principles have clearly established that 90% of pregnant women at term have successful labor inductions with 6 mU/min or less of oxytocin (Dawood, 1995). Generally, starting doses of 0.5 to 2 mU/min, with increases in 1- to 2-mU/min increments every 30 to 60 minutes, is reasonable. Any shorter interval between dosage increases is associated with a greater risk of hyperstimulation, somewhat shorter duration of labor, and no reduction in the cesarean birth rate.

When uterine hyperstimulation occurs and fetal status is such that oxytocin is discontinued, there are limited data to guide the decision about the timing and dosage of subsequent IV oxytocin administration. A reasonable approach is to use physiologic and pharmacologic principles to determine the most appropriate dosage. If oxytocin has been discontinued for 5 to 10 minutes, the FHR is reassuring, and the contraction frequency, intensity, and duration are normal, it seems reasonable to restart oxytocin at a slightly lower rate of infusion before hyperstimulation. However, if the oxytocin has been discontinued for more than 30 to 40 minutes, most of the exogenous oxytocin has been metabolized, and plasma levels are similar to that of a woman who has not received IV oxytocin. In this clinical situation, it seems reasonable to restart the oxytocin at or near the initial dose that was ordered. There are individual differences in myometrial sensitivity and the response to oxytocin during labor (Ulmsten, 1997). It may be necessary to use a lower dose and increase the interval between dosages because of evidence of the patient's previous sensitivity to the drug (ACOG, 1999a). Nursing responsibility during oxytocin infusion involves careful titration of the drug to the maternal–fetal response. The titration process includes decreasing the dosage rate when contractions are too frequent or fetal status is nonreassuring as well as increasing the dosage rate when uterine activity and progress of labor slows (Clayworth, 2000).

Misoprostol

In addition to cervical ripening, misoprostol is used for induction and augmentation of labor. See the Prostaglandin E_1: Misoprostol section for a full discussion of the agent.

Augmentation of Labor

For some women, labor progresses slower than expected. Some experts use the terms *dystocia* or *failure to progress* to characterize an abnormally long labor, but this diagnosis often is made in error before the woman has entered the active phase of labor and therefore before an adequate trial of labor has been achieved (ACOG, 1995a). Women often have a cesarean birth because of failure to progress in labor, although according to the ACOG (1995a) criteria for the diagnosis of lack of labor of progress, active labor has not begun or labor has not been abnormally long (Gifford et al., 2000). *Cephalopelvic disproportion* is another common term used when labor has not progressed. This condition can rarely be diagnosed with certainty and is usually related to malposition of the fetal head. According to the latest data, dystocia remains the most common reason for primary cesarean birth in the United States, significantly higher than that for nonreassuring fetal status or malpresentation (Gifford et al., 2000; Ventura et al., 2000). ACOG (1995a) recommends two practical classifications for labor abnormalities: slower than normal labor (ie, protraction disorders) and complete cessation of contractions (ie, arrest disorders). These disorders require the woman to be in the active phase of labor; therefore, a prolonged latent phase is not indicative of dystocia, and this diagnosis cannot be made in the latent phase of labor (ACOG, 1995a).

Wide variations in labor progress and duration exist among childbearing women. There is no consensus among perinatal experts on appropriate length of labor and the relationship to risks of adverse maternal–fetal outcomes. Undoubtedly, some believe that there is benefit to decreasing the length of labor, as evidenced by the popularity of AMOL protocols and other high-dose oxytocin protocols in some institutions. It is unclear, however, who benefits most from a shorter labor: the fetus, the mother, the caregivers, the institution, or a combination of all of these parties (Keirse, 1993; Olah & Gee, 1996; Rothman, 1993). Multiple factors, including timing and dosage of regional analgesia, fetal size and position, and maternal pelvic structure, influence progress of labor (ACOG, 1995a). Instead of arbitrary time frames, maternal–fetal status and individual clinical situations provide the best data for labor management.

From a physiologic and pharmacologic standpoint, less oxytocin is needed for labor augmentation than for labor induction, but most studies and clinical protocols report higher doses of oxytocin administration during augmentation of labor (Kierse, 1994). For women in spontaneous active labor, cervical resistance is less than in women who have not yet experienced cervical effacement and dilation. The response to oxytocin seems to depend on preexisting uterine activity and sensitivity rather than the amount of the dose (Brindley & Sokol, 1988). It is unclear why the disparity between scientific evidence and clinical practice occurs. Many of the research studies about labor augmentation in the last decade have focused on variations in the AMOL, which may account for the overrepresentation of studies of high doses of oxytocin in the literature.

Active Management of Labor

Principles of AMOL were developed by O'Driscoll, Jackson, & Gallagher in 1969. These researchers were faced with limited space in their maternity unit in Dublin, Ireland, and an increasing census of women in labor. The protocol was initially implemented as a method of shortening labor and with a goal of achieving more effective use of space and resources. They discovered that this method of augmentation not only shortened labor for most women, but also significantly decreased the cesarean birth rate at their institution (O'Driscoll, Jaskson, & Gallagher, 1970). The protocol was designed to be used for nulliparous women in spontaneous active labor. The Dublin AMOL protocol is precise:

- Candidates include only nulliparous women in spontaneous active labor with a singleton pregnancy, cephalic presentation, and no evidence of fetal compromise.
- To exclude false and prodromal labor, true labor is specifically defined as contractions with bloody show, spontaneous rupture of membranes, or complete (100%) cervical effacement.
- After labor is diagnosed, the woman receives continuous one-to-one labor support from a birth attendant (eg, midwife).
- Amniotomy is performed if membranes are not spontaneously ruptured within 1 hour after labor has been diagnosed.
- If cervical dilation does not progress at least 1 cm each hour, oxytocin augmentation is initiated, beginning at 6 mU/min and increasing by 6

mU/min every 15 minutes until adequate labor is established, to a maximum dose of 40 mU/min.
- Hyperstimulation of uterine activity is defined as more than seven contractions in 15 minutes.

This protocol has been rigorously evaluated using a randomized control trial design in three major U.S. studies with disappointing results (Frigaletto et al., 1995; Lopez-Zeno et al., 1992; Rogers et al., 1997). Although all studies demonstrated a significant difference in length of labor, no study found a significant difference in the cesarean birth rate. All of the studies used protocols very similar to the O'Driscoll protocol.

The logistics of providing nursing care to two women requiring increases in oxytocin every 15 minutes, while accomplishing adequate maternal–fetal assessments and documentation according to published guidelines and standards of care (ACOG, 1995a, 1999a; AAP & ACOG, 1997; Simpson & Poole, 1998a), warrant careful consideration before implementing this type of protocol in clinical practice. The studies demonstrating that this approach was safe for mothers and babies used one-to-one nursing care. The economic and practical implications of providing one nurse to each woman in labor while implementing a high-dose oxytocin protocol seem to outweigh any possible benefits of a slightly shorter labor. The principles of AMOL as a method to decrease cesarean birth rates have not been successful when applied to labor and birth in the United States. A physiologic dosage regimen for labor induction seems to be the best approach for most women because of the risks of higher doses and more frequent intervals for increasing the dose such as uterine hyperstimulation and cesarean birth for nonreassuring fetal status.

Staffing Considerations During Induction and Augmentation of Labor

Scheduled cervical ripening and induction of labor influences nursing staff requirements for labor and birth units. Because induction of labor is likely to occur during the day, resulting in birth in the afternoon, more nurses may be needed during this period than during the late evening or early morning. A record of women who are scheduled for labor induction maintained on the unit is essential to plan staffing and personnel needs based on expected volume. Many units place a limit on the number of scheduled labor inductions that can be performed on any given day to ensure that adequate staff and rooms are available to provide the appropriate level of care. Development of criteria for designating patient priority for induction of labor based on the nature and intensity of the indication can provide a useful decision-making framework in this situation. Ideally, these criteria are developed jointly by physician and nurse members of a unit practice committee. Elective induction of labor may need to be postponed or rescheduled at times, especially if there are not enough resources available. Establishment of a perinatal nurse on-call system may facilitate securing staffing resources as needed in a timely manner.

The appropriate number of qualified professional registered nurses should be in attendance during induction and augmentation of labor (AWHONN, 1998). The current recommendations for the nurse–patient ratio during induction or augmentation of labor is one nurse to two women in labor (AAP & ACOG, 1997; AWHONN, 1998). These recommendations are for women in labor who are healthy and have no significant maternal–fetal complications. Some clinical situations may warrant more intense nursing care during induction or augmentation of labor. Staffing requirements for labor and birth are dynamic, and assessment of the appropriate balance between available resources and patient care needs must be an ongoing process. If a nurse cannot clinically evaluate the effects of the drug at least every 15 minutes or a physician who has privileges to perform a cesarean birth is not readily available, the oxytocin infusion should be discontinued or the initial or subsequent doses of misoprostol delayed until this level of maternal–fetal care can be provided (AAP & ACOG, 1997; ACOG, 1999; Simpson & Poole, 1998a).

Operative Vaginal Birth

The rate of operative vaginal birth has increased over the past 20 years (ACOG, 2000c). However, in the past 10 years, vacuum-assisted births have increased while forceps-assisted births have declined (ACOG, 2000c; Ventura et al., 2000). Approximately 15% of all births include forceps or vacuum devices (Kozak & Lawrence, 1999). The cesarean birth rate is currently 22%; only 63% of births in the United States are spontaneous (Curtin & Martin, 2000). Early research before the 1970s suggested that the risk of fetal morbidity and mortality was higher when the second stage of labor exceeded 2 hours. However, more intensive fetal assessment during labor provides the ability to identify a fetus that may not be tolerating labor well. Thus, the length of the second stage is not in itself an absolute or even strong indication for operative termination of labor (ACOG, 2000c). If other obstetric conditions indicate the need for operative vaginal birth, forceps and vacuum devices can be used. Operative vaginal birth should be performed only by individuals with privileges for these procedures, and in settings in which personnel are readily available to perform a cesarean birth if operative vaginal birth is unsuccessful (ACOG, 2000c).

Persistent efforts to achieve a vaginal birth using different instruments may increase the potential for maternal and fetal injury and often indicates cephalopelvic disproportion. The weight of the evidence appears to be against attempting multiple efforts at operative vaginal birth with different instruments unless there is a compelling and justifiable reason (ACOG, 2000c). The incidence of intracranial hemorrhage is highest in newborns delivered by combined vacuum and forceps, as compared with other methods of delivery (ACOG, 2000c; Towner, Castro, Eby-Wilkens, & Gilbert, 1999). The incidences of other maternal–fetal injuries are increased with combined methods of operative vaginal birth (ACOG, 2000c)

Although sometimes necessary, operative vaginal birth is not without complications for the woman and infant. Among women with operative vaginal birth, there are significant risks for rehospitalization for postpartum hemorrhage, perineal wound infection complications, and pelvic injuries compared with women who had spontaneous vaginal birth (Lydon-Rochelle, Holt, Martin, & Easterling, 2000). The most common reason for rehospitalization for women after operative vaginal birth is perineal wound infection (Lydon-Rochelle et al., 2000). Fetal complications are described in the following sections.

Forceps

Forceps can be used to assist delivery of the fetal head when birth must be facilitated for the health of the mother or fetus. Piper forceps are sometimes used during breech births to assist in delivery of the fetal head after the body has been delivered. According to the latest data, 5.5% of births in the United States involve the use of forceps (Kozak & Lawrence, 1999). Maternal conditions that may necessitate use of forceps are medical complications such as cardiac or pulmonary disease, maternal exhaustion, or high level of regional analgesia that diminishes the woman's expulsive efforts. The fetus may demonstrate signs of compromise, such as bradycardia, marked tachycardia, prolonged and severe variable decelerations, or late decelerations, by means of EFM or FHR auscultation during second-stage labor, suggesting attempts at assisted birth may be warranted.

Forceps should not be considered unless the cervix is completely dilated, membranes are ruptured, the head is engaged, and the woman has adequate anesthesia. The woman's bladder should be emptied before application (Gei & Belfort, 1999; Paluska, 1997). Under very unusual circumstances, such as sudden fetal or maternal compromise, application of forceps above station +2 may be attempted while preparations for an emergent cesarean birth are simultaneously initiated in the event that the forceps maneuver is unsuccessful.

Classification of forceps procedures is given in Table 9–3. All perinatal nurses should be familiar with this classification system so that documentation of the procedure is accurate. Consultation with the provider who applied the forceps before medical record documentation is appropriate to ensure accuracy. The number of forceps applications and attempts with traction are usually documented. Use of forceps are associated with pain, vaginal and cervical lacerations, extension of the episiotomy, perineal

TABLE 9–3 ■ CRITERIA OF FORCEPS DELIVERIES ACCORDING TO STATION AND ROTATION

Types of Procedure	Criteria
Outlet forceps	1. Scalp is visible at the introitus without separating the labia. 2. Fetal skull has reached the pelvic floor. 3. Sagittal suture is in the anteroposterior diameter or right or left occiput anterior or posterior position. 4. Fetal head is at or on the perineum. 5. Rotation does not exceed 45 degrees.
Low forceps	Leading point of the fetal skull is at station ≥ +2 cm and not on the pelvic floor. a. Rotation ≤45 degrees (left or right occiput anterior to occiput anterior, or left or right occiput posterior to occiput posterior) b. Rotation >45 degrees
Midforceps	Station above +2 cm but head engaged
High	Not included in classification

From American College of Obstetricians and Gynecologists. (2000c). *Operative vaginal delivery* (Practice Bulletin No. 17). Washington, DC: Author. Reprinted by permission. Copyright 2000 by American College of Obstetricians and Gynecologists.

wound infection, uterine rupture, bladder trauma, fracture of the coccyx, hemorrhage, increased vaginal bleeding, uterine atony, and anemia (Gei & Belfort, 1999; Lydon-Rochelle et al., 2000). Newborns delivered by forceps should be observed for skin markings, lacerations, bruising, nerve injuries, skull fractures, cephalohematoma, ocular trauma, and intracranial hemorrhage (Gei & Belfort, 1999; ACOG, 2000c). Approximately 2% of newborns delivered by forceps will develop cephalohematoma (ACOG, 2000c). The condition of the mother and newborn at birth should be documented in the medical record.

Vacuum Devices

Some physicians use vacuum extraction in lieu of forceps; the choice usually depends on their education, experience, and hospital privileges. Data indicate that 9.5% of births in the United States involve the use of a vacuum device (Kozak & Lawrence, 1999). Vacuum-assisted birth is usually reserved for fetuses of at least 36 weeks' gestation because of increased risk for intraventricular hemorrhage (ACOG, 2000c).

A vacuum extractor consists of a Silastic cup available in various sizes that has a suction device attached. The cup is placed on the fetal head, and suction is increased gradually until a seal is formed. Delaying episiotomy during vacuum application helps to keep the cup in place. Gentle traction is then applied to deliver the fetal head. Indications and prerequisites for vacuum extraction or for the use of forceps are generally the same, but rotation is not appropriate by vacuum extraction (Bofill, Martin, & Morrison, 1998). Proponents of vacuum extraction feel that its advantages include easier application, less force applied to the fetal head, less anesthesia needed, less maternal soft tissue injury, fewer fetal injuries, and fewer parental concerns (Paluska, 1997).

Complications from vacuum extraction and forceps use depend primarily on the practitioner's skill. Approximately 14% to 16% of fetuses delivered with vacuum extractors develop a cephalohematoma (ACOG, 2000c; Johanson, 1997), but when the duration of vacuum application at maximum pressure exceeds 5 minutes, this incidence increases to 28% (Bofill et al., 1997a). There have been reports of fetal subgaleal hematoma and intracranial hemorrhage after the vacuum extractor has been used. The incidence of subgaleal hematoma after using a vacuum device ranges from 26 to 45 per 1000 vacuum-assisted births (ACOG, 2000c). The FDA issued a warning letter to providers in 1998 alerting them to these risks (ACOG, 1998a; FDA, 1998). Subgaleal hematoma occurs when emissary veins are damaged and blood accumulates in the potential space between the galea aponeurotica (ie, epicranial aponeurosis) and the periosteum of the skull (ie, pericranium). Because the subaponeurotic space has neither containing membranes nor boundaries, the subgaleal hematoma may extend from the orbital ridges to the nape of the neck. This condition is dangerous because of the large potential space for blood accumulation and the possibility of life-threatening hemorrhage (FDA, 1998). Signs and symptoms of subgaleal hematoma include diffuse swelling of the fetal head and evidence of hypovolemic shock (eg, pallor, hypotension, tachycardia, increased respiration rate). These signs and symptoms may be present immediately after birth or may not become clinically apparent until several hours or a few days after birth (FDA, 1998). The swelling is usually diffuse, shifts when the newborn's head is repositioned, and indents easily on palpation. In some cases, the swelling is difficult to distinguish from edema of the scalp. Occasionally, the hypotension and pallor are the dominant signs, but the cranial signs are unremarkable (FDA, 1998).

Intracranial hemorrhage includes subdural, subarachnoid, intraventricular, and intraparenchymal hemorrhage. Signs and symptoms of intracranial hemorrhage include indications of cerebral irritation such as seizures, lethargy, obtundation, apnea, bulging fontanelle, poor feeding, increased irritability, bradycardia, and shock. These signs and symptoms are sometimes delayed until several hours after birth (FDA, 1998). One study found that the rate of intracranial hemorrhage is higher among infants delivered by vacuum extraction, forceps, and cesarean birth after labor than that of infants delivered after spontaneous birth, but that the rate among infants delivered by cesarean section before labor was not higher, suggesting that the common risk factor for intracranial hemorrhage is abnormal labor rather than method of birth (Towner, Castro, Eby-Wilkens, & Gilbert, 1999).

Other potential newborn complications associated with use of vacuum devices include hyperbilirubinemia and retinal hemorrhage (ACOG, 2000c). The higher rate of newborn jaundice associated with vacuums may be related to the higher rate of cephalohematomas (ACOG, 2000c). If torsion is excessive, the vacuum cup can cause scalp lacerations (ACOG, 2000c).

The FDA (1998) recommendations for the use of vacuum devices include: (1) Rocking movements or torque should not be applied to the device; only steady traction in the line of the birth canal should be used. (2) Clinicians caring for the newborn should be alerted that a vacuum device has been used so that they can adequately monitor the newborn for the signs and symptoms of device-related injuries. Nurses who attend a vacuum-assisted birth should make sure that the use of a vacuum is included in documentation on the birth record and the initial newborn assessment and verbally report use of the vacuum to the nurse who will be caring for the newborn.

Maternal complications associated with the use of vacuum devices include pain, vaginal and cervical lacerations, extension of the episiotomy, perineal wound infection, bladder trauma, hemorrhage, increased vaginal bleeding, uterine atony, and anemia (Gei & Belfort, 1999; Lydon-Rochelle et al., 2000). Careful assessment after vacuum-assisted birth is necessary to identify maternal complications and initiate appropriate treatment.

There is a lack of consensus about the number of pulls required to effect birth, the maximum number of cup detachments (ie, pop-offs) that can be tolerated by the fetus, and the total duration of the procedure (ACOG, 2000). However, RCT results suggest that using no more than 600 mmHg of pressure and abandoning the procedure after three pop-offs or 20 minutes' maximum total time of application is consistent with safe care and a decreased risk of fetal injuries (Bofill et al., 1996; Bofill et al., 1998). The manufacturer's recommendations for the vacuum device being used should be followed. The vacuum pressure should not exceed 500 to 600 mmHg, and the pressure should be released as soon as the contraction ends and the woman stops pushing (Brumfield, Gilstrap, O'Grady, Ross, & Schifrin, 1999). As a general guideline, progress in descent should accompany each traction attempt, and no more than three pulls should be attempted (Bofill et al., 1996; Bofill et al., 1998; Brumfield et al., 1999). Traction is used only when the woman is actively pushing.

The vacuum procedure should be timed from the moment of insertion of the cup into the vagina until birth and should not be on the fetal head for longer than 20 to 30 minutes (Bofill et al., 1998; Brumfield et al., 1999). When the cup has been applied at maximum pressure for more than 10 minutes, the rate of fetal injuries increases (Brumfield et al., 1999); although total time of cup application can be 20 to 30 minutes, the time of maximum pressure force should not exceed 10 minutes (Puluska, 1997). As with forceps, there should be a willingness to abandon attempts at a vacuum-assisted birth if satisfactory progress is not made. If the 20- to 30-minute time limit is reached, the vacuum cup is removed, and the procedure is considered a failed vacuum procedure (Bofill et al., 1998). In addition to exceeding the 20- to 30-minute time limit, three pop-offs, evidence of fetal scalp trauma or no descent with appropriate application and traction should warrant abandoning the vacuum procedure (Bofill et al., 1998). A unit policy about the use of vacuum devices and forceps, including a list of those credentialed in these procedures, facilitates safe maternal–fetal care and avoids clinical controversies at the bedside if there is disagreement between healthcare professionals about amount of pressure, length of application, number of pop-offs and pull attempts, and the need to abandon the procedure.

Nurses have a role in educating and reassuring the woman when an assisted vaginal birth is anticipated. Maternal comfort level should be assessed before the application of forceps or vacuum extraction. If a nonreassuring FHR pattern is the indication for the immediate birth, the nurse must be prepared for newborn resuscitation, ensuring that appropriate equipment, supplies, and personnel are available. Nurses should also be aware of potential complications related to use of forceps and vacuums and observe the mother and newborn for associated signs and symptoms. Because some complications may be life threatening for the mother and newborn, prompt identification and initiation of appropriate treatment are necessary. Parents should be prepared and shown any forceps or vacuum-extraction marks on the infant and be reassured that they will disappear in a few days. Complete and accurate medical record documentation is required.

Amnioinfusion

Amnioinfusion is a procedure in which normal saline or lactated Ringer's solution at room temperature is introduced transcervically into the uterus to correct FHR decelerations associated with oligohydramnios or to dilute thickly stained amniotic fluid. The goal is to minimize or prevent adverse fetal effects such as umbilical cord compression and meconium aspiration. There is evidence from well-designed prospective studies that the use of amnioinfusion to resolve variable FHR decelerations is safe and effective (Mino, Puertas, Miranda, & Herruzo, 1999; Miyazaki & Navarez, 1985; Persson-Kjerstadius, Forsgren, & Westgren, 1999). Although most of the studies about amnioinfusion as a preventive therapy for meconium aspiration syndrome have suffered from small sample size and inadequate statistical power to detect a significance in outcomes, there appears to be enough evidence to suggest that amnioinfusion is a safe procedure to dilute thick meconium fluid, decrease incidence of meconium below the vocal cords, and potentially prevent meconium aspiration syndrome (Klingner & Kruse, 1999; Pierce, Gaudier, & Sanchez-Ramos, 2000). Amnioinfusion does not seem to have an effect on the length of labor (Strong, 1997) and appears to be safe for women attempting a vaginal birth after a previous cesarean birth (Ouzounian, Miller, & Paul, 1996).

The amnioinfusion procedure and indications should be explained to the woman and her support persons before initiation. The solutions used for amnioinfusion are usually lactated Ringer's solution or normal saline (Pressman & Blakemore, 1996; Washburne et al., 1996). The initial bolus is usually 250 to 600 mL, which is given over a 15- to 60-minute interval (10 to 15 mL/min) using an infusion pump or gravity flow. During bolus of the infusion and maintenance rate, approximate amount of fluid returning should be noted and recorded to avoid iatrogenic polyhydramnios. Assessment of fluid return can be accomplished by careful observation or by weighing the underpads (ie, 1 mL of fluid equals approximately 1 gram of weight) (Tucker, 2000). If 250 mL have infused with no return, the amnioinfusion is discontinued until the fluid has returned.

A dual-lumen intrauterine catheter is preferred so that estimate of uterine resting tone can be assessed during the infusion; however, similar results can be achieved using two single-lumen, fluid-filled catheters. Uterine resting tone may appear higher than normal during the procedure (25 to 40 mmHg) because the resistance to outflow and turbulence through the tiny holes at the end of the catheter do not allow for accurate recording of uterine resting tone (Tucker, 2000). To accurately assess uterine resting tone, temporarily stop the infusion approximately every 30 minutes. If the uterine resting tone exceeds 20 to 25 mmHg while the infusion is temporarily discontinued for assessment of uterine resting tone, the infusion should be discontinued. When resting tone is below 20 mmHg, the infusion can be resumed. Contraction intensity and frequency should be continually assessed during the procedure. Too much fluid may cause an overdistended uterus and pressure on the diaphragm. This may result in maternal shortness of breath, hypotension, or tachycardia (Tucker, 2000).

Fetal bradycardia may occur if the solution is colder than room temperature or is infused too rapidly (Tucker, 2000). Some providers prefer to warm the solution to body temperature, especially if the fetus is preterm or the flow rate for the bolus exceeds 600 mL/hour. The safest method to warm the solution is by using an electronic fluid warmer. Microwaves and other types of warming techniques should not be used to heat the solution.

When variable FHR decelerations are the indication for amnioinfusion, decelerations usually resolve soon after initiating amnioinfusion. If variable decelerations have not resolved after infusion of 800 to 1,000 mL, the infusion may be discontinued and alternative approaches used (Tucker, 2000). With improvement of decelerations, the physician or CNM may elect to continue the infusion at a lower rate or discontinue the infusion. If discontinued, additional boluses may be given if the decelerations recur or a significant amount of fluid is lost (Schmidt, 1997). If thick meconium fluid is the indication, the amnioinfusion is usually continued until the fluid return is dilute.

CESAREAN BIRTH

Incidence

According to the latest data available from the National Center for Health Statistics, the rate of cesarean birth increased 4% between 1998 and 1999 (21.2% to 22%). This was the third consecutive increase in the cesarean birth rate after declining each year between 1989 and 1996. Despite this increase, the cesarean birth rate in 1999 was still slightly lower than in 1989 (22.8%), the first year these data were available on the birth certificates. The primary cesarean birth rate in 1999 (15.5 per 100 live births to women who had no previous cesarean birth) was 2% higher than in 1998 (14.6). This was the second time this rate increased during the 1989 to 1999 period. The rate of vaginal birth after a previous cesarean birth (VBAC) declined 11% between 1998 and 1999 (from 26.3 to 23.4 per 100 births to women who had a previous cesarean birth). Between 1996 and 1999, the VBAC rate fell 17% after increasing 50% between 1989 (18.9) and 1996 (28.3) (Curtin & Martin, 2000; Ventura et al., 2000). It is possible that the decline in VBAC rates reflect patient and provider concerns about the risk of uterine rupture (ACOG, 1999c).

The most common indications for cesarean birth noted on the birth certificates were maternal medical complications and complications of labor, such as dystocia, breech or malpresentation, cephalopelvic disproportion, and placenta previa (Ventura et al., 2000). Results of one study suggest that cesarean birth is many times performed because of lack of progress in labor when the woman is still in the latent phase of labor or when the second stage of labor is not prolonged (Gifford et al., 2000). Elective induction of labor for nulliparous women is associated with a risk of cesarean birth twice that for nulliparous women who have spontaneous labor (Yeast, Jones, & Poskin, 1999). Women who have cesarean birth have a significantly increased risk of rehospitalization for uterine infection, surgical wound infection, complications from surgical wound, and cardiopulmonary and thromboembolic complications (Lyndon-Rochelle et al., 2000). They are 30 times more likely to have a surgical wound infection than women who have a vaginal birth, but the rate of rehospitalization for wound infection after cesarean birth is relatively low at about 4 cases per 1,000 births (Lydon-Rochelle et al., 2000). The average length of inpatient stay for cesarean birth is 3.8 days, compared with 2.1 days for vaginal birth (Kozak & Lawrence, 1999).

Perioperative Standards and Guidelines for Cesarean Birth

Perioperative perinatal nursing blends the specialties of obstetrics and surgery to provide comprehensive care to women who have a cesarean birth. Perinatal units must maintain the same standards of care as the main hospital surgical suites (OR) and postanesthesia care unit (PACU) (AWHONN, 1998; JCAHO, 2000). Special consideration must be given to incorporating family-centered care (AWHONN, 1998). Obstetric care providers should willingly provide opportunities for those accompanying and supporting the woman giving birth to participate in the process (AAP & ACOG, 1997). To promote safe care, perinatal nurses should receive didactic instruction and participate in a clinical preceptorship for preoperative, intraoperative, and postoperative care as part of a comprehensive orientation to intrapartum nursing. Perioperative assessments and documentation forms used on the perinatal unit should be similar to those used in the main hospital surgical suite PACU. Specific clinical aspects of labor, birth, and fetal status should be included. Display 9–10 contains guidelines for the perioperative cesarean birth.

During the postoperative cesarean birth recovery, the woman should be observed in an appropriately staffed and equipped labor–delivery-recovery (LDR) room or PACU until she has recovered from anesthesia (AAP & ACOG, 1997). After cesarean birth, standards for postanesthesia care on the perinatal unit should not differ from those applied to nonobstetric

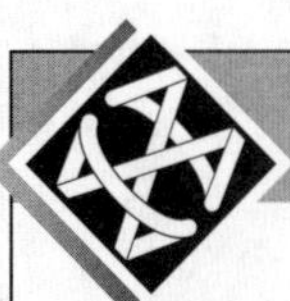

DISPLAY 9–10

Perioperative Cesarean Birth Care

PREOPERATIVE CARE

- Admission assessment comparable to that for all women admitted for labor and birth.
- Obtain a 20- to 30-minute baseline fetal heart rate (FHR) tracing by electronic fetal monitoring (EFM). If the woman is not in active labor and the FHR is reassuring, EFM may be discontinued after this initial assessment.
- Provide a thorough explanation of what to expect in preparation for, during, and after the surgery to the woman and her support person.
- Ensure that the woman has maintained no oral intake (NPO) according to the institutional protocol.
- Initiate intravenous fluids.
- Witness informed consent signature for cesarean birth.
- Obtain surgical laboratory blood specimens if not done prior to admission.
- Shave the abdomen.
- Insert a Foley catheter; note the amount and color of urine; delay until after epidural catheter is placed and dosed if possible.
- Administer preoperative medications according to the physician order.
- If woman is in labor, periodic assessments of maternal–fetal status should continue according to the institutional protocol.
- Transport the woman to the surgical suite or operating room.

INTRAOPERATIVE CARE

- Position the woman on the surgical table with a hip wedge in place.
- If EFM is used, continue monitoring until the abdominal prep is initiated.
- If a fetal scalp electrode is in place, EFM continues until the abdominal prep is completed. The electrode should be removed before birth.
- Prepare abdomen for surgery as per institutional protocol.
- Apply grounding device according to manufacturer's instructions.
- Note maternal vital signs, FHR, condition of the skin before the incision, and the woman's emotional status.
- Assist the support person to a position at the head of the surgical table according to the institutional protocol.
- Ensure that newborn resuscitation equipment is assembled and ready and personnel responsible are in attendance. Responsibility for resuscitation and stabilization of the healthy, full-term newborn differs by institution and could include the circulating nurse, an additional nurse, pediatrician, or neonatal nurse practitioner.
- Perform the duties of a circulating nurse according to the institutional protocol.

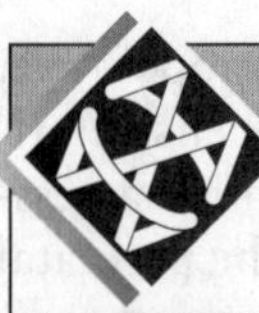

DISPLAY 9–10 (cont.)

Perioperative Cesarean Birth Care

- Ensure that the sponge, needle, and equipment counts are correct according to the institutional protocol.
- Assist with application of abdominal dressing.
- Note maternal and newborn status before transport to the postanesthesia care unit (PACU).
- Assist with transport.

POSTANESTHESIA RECOVERY CARE

- Postoperative assessments are performed according to PACU protocols and should be comparable to care provided in the main hospital PACU.
- Initial and ongoing assessments include review of intraoperative course, including medications and intravenous fluids received:

Respiratory assessment
  Airway patency
  Oxygen needs
  Rate, quality, and depth of respirations
  Auscultation of breath sounds
  Arterial oxygen saturation via pulse oximetry
Circulation assessment
  Blood pressure
  Pulse
  Electrocardiogram
  Color
Level of consciousness
  Orientation
  Response to verbal, tactile, and painful stimulation
Obstetric status
  Uterine fundus position and contraction
  Abdominal dressing
  Maternal–newborn attachment
  Lochia amount and color
  Newborn condition
  Breast-feeding desires
Intake and output
  Intravenous fluids
  Urinary output by Foley catheter
Pain or comfort level
  Patient desires
  Medications given

- Discharge from PACU care occurs after the recovery period and when the woman is stable as determined by PACU discharge criteria.

A scoring system including the following parameters is useful to assess readiness for discharge:
  Level of consciousness
  Neuromuscular activity
  Level of sensation
  Circulation
  Respiration
  Color
(Figure 9–9 provides a sample PACU discharge scoring tool; using this system, the patient's score must be at least 10 before discharge.)
Additional assessment before PACU discharge:
  Vital signs
  Urinary output by Foley catheter
  Uterine fundus position and contraction
  Abdominal dressing
  Intravenous fluids or oral intake
  Pain or comfort level
  Lochia amount and color
  Maternal–newborn attachment
The anesthesia provider is involved in the decision to discharge from PACU care.
If responsibility for care is transferred to another nurse after discharge, a complete report of intraoperative and postanesthesia course is vital.

From Simpson, K.R., & Creehan, P.A. (1996).

surgical patients receiving major anesthesia (AAP & ACOG, 1997; ASA, 1998). A comparable level and type of care that is provided in the main hospital PACU is required for obstetric patients in perinatal units (JCAHO, 2000). When recovery care occurs in an obstetric PACU, the nurse may be able to care for more than one patient, depending on the clinical situation. In settings where the postoperative patient returns to an LDR immediately after surgery, the perinatal nurse remains at the bedside until cardiac monitoring is discontinued and the patient is stable and discharged from postanesthesia care.

The woman should be discharged from the recovery area only at the discretion of and after communication between the attending physician or CNM, anesthesiologist, and certified registered nurse anesthetist in charge (AAP & ACOG, 1997). Perinatal unit guidelines should include postanesthesia discharge criteria as defined in the ASA's (1994) *Standards for Postanesthesia Care.* Postoperative patients may be discharged from postanesthesia care status when the postanesthesia criteria are met. A unit policy should be in place to ensure that a physician is available in the facility, or at least nearby, to manage anesthetic complications and provide cardiopulmonary resuscitation (AAP & ACOG, 1997; ASA, 1998).

A PACU discharge scoring tool (Fig. 9–9) is helpful in conducting a systematic assessment and determining readiness for discharge from postanesthesia care. Displays 9–11 and 9–12 list the critical components of obstetric postanesthesia nursing and necessary equipment. Standards and guidelines for perioperative care are available from the Association of Perioperative Nurses (AORN), the American Society of Perianesthesia Nurses (ASPAN), the American Society of Anesthesiologists (ASA), the American Association of Nurse Anesthetists (AANA), and JCAHO.

Supporting Attachment in Women Experiencing Cesarean Birth

Whether anticipated or unexpected, the need for surgical birth increases the family's anxiety, places additional strain on the maternal–newborn relationship, makes postpartum recovery more difficult for the woman and family, and creates a need for accepting the altered birth experience. Research about women who had planned and unplanned cesarean births suggest that women who give birth by cesarean have special needs for information, presence of the partner throughout cesarean birth, and sustained contact with the newborn (Reichert, Baron, & Fawcett, 1993; Hundley, Miline, Glasener, & Mollison, 1997). An unplanned emergent cesarean birth can result in significant stress for the new mother (Ryding, Wijma, & Wijma, 1997). Continuity in caregivers, choice when possible, and control over specific aspects of care can reduce stress (Hundley et al., 1997). Women having their first baby who had an emergent cesarean birth reported that failure of communication was a major problem that occurred before, during, and after cesarean birth (Hillan, 1992). The father's presence at birth and early contact with the newborn were predicative of self-reported attachment behaviors in

POST ANESTHESIA RECOVERY SCORE			
	CRITERIA	SCORE	DISCHARGE
CONSCIOUSNESS	Fully awake	2	
	Arousable on calling	1	
	Not responding	0	
NEUROMUSCULAR ACTIVITY	Move 4 extremities	2	
	Move 2 extremities	1	
	Move 0 extremities	0	
SENSATION	Normal	2	
	None below pubis	1	
	None below xiphoid	0	
CIRCULATION	B/P 10–20 mmHg ± admission	2	
	B/P 10–50 mmHg ± admission	1	
	B/P >51 mmHg ± admission	0	
RESPIRATION	Deep breathing or cough	2	
	Dyspnea	1	
	Apnea	0	
COLOR	Pink	2	
	Pale, blotchy, jaundiced, other	1	
	Cyanotic	0	
	Total		
Signature:	Date: Time		

FIGURE 9–9. Sample postanesthesia care unit discharge scoring tool.

DISPLAY 9–11

Critical Components of Obstetric Postanesthesia Nursing

1. Women in the obstetric postanesthesia period after major regional or general anesthetic shall receive care equivalent to that available in the surgical postanesthesia care unit (PACU)
2. The anesthesiologist or nurse anesthetist is responsible for determining whether the condition of the woman warrants PACU or routine obstetric postpartum recovery care.
3. If the woman is admitted to obstetric PACU care, surgical PACU standards shall be followed until PACU discharge criteria are met and routine postpartum recovery care ensues.
4. Before patient arrival, the obstetric postanesthesia recovery area shall have required equipment in place. Otherwise, the woman should remain monitored by the anesthesiologist or nurse anesthetist until the recovery area is appropriately equipped to ensure patient safety.
5. A woman transported to the obstetric PACU shall be accompanied by a member of the anesthesia care team, who shall provide a verbal report to the responsible obstetric PACU nurse and remain in the obstetric PACU until the obstetric PACU nurse accepts responsibility for the nursing care of the patient.
6. After the woman is admitted to obstetric PACU care, she shall be continually observed and monitored by methods appropriate to her medical condition. Particular attention should be given to monitoring oxygenation, ventilation, circulation, and temperature. Additional staff may be needed to interact with family members and the newborn infant. After PACU discharge criteria are met, postpartum care should continue per obstetric standards.
7. Each hospital is responsible for developing guidelines, policies, and procedures collaboratively among the obstetric department, anesthesia department, and surgical PACU (eg, assessment criteria, PACU discharge criteria, documentation, malignant hypothermia, crisis management, medications and equipment, staff education and qualifications, staffing requirements).
8. Each hospital shall ensure that advanced cardiac life support (ACLS) care (eg, code team) is readily available at all times. ACLS certification is not required for obstetric nurses providing postanesthesia care. This practice is supported by the Association of Women's Health, Obstetric and Neonatal Nurses Position Statement on Postanesthesia Nursing for Obstetric Patients (1993).
9. For optimal skill development, obstetric postanesthesia education should include didactic and practice components. A period of observation in the surgical PACU is strongly recommended to enhance the obstetric nurse's perspective on recovery room practices.
10. Hospitals in which obstetric postanesthesia patients are consistently recovered in the surgical PACU (eg, some level I obstetric services) may choose to omit this education for their obstetric staff.

From O'Brien-Abel, N., Rink, C., Warner, P., & Nelson, C. (1994). Critical components of obstetric postanesthesia nursing. *Journal of Perinatal and Neonatal Nursing, 8* (3) pp. 4–16. Copyright 1994 by Aspen. Reprinted with permission.

women experiencing cesarean or vaginal births (Fortier, 1988). To facilitate a positive birth experience and attachment to the newborn, ongoing attention should be given to the family members' understanding of cesarean birth, ways to maintain the father or support person's presence throughout the birth experience, and early and sustained contact with the newborn (Fig. 9–10). Encouraging sibling interaction promotes attachment and facilitates integration of the newborn into the family (Fig. 9–11).

Vaginal Birth After Cesarean Birth

The philosophy of "once a cesarean, always a cesarean" has been replaced with encouragement for women who are appropriately selected candidates to attempt a trial of labor after a previous cesarean birth. Published evidence suggests that the benefits of VBAC outweigh the risks in most women with a prior low-transverse cesarean birth and who have no contraindications for vaginal birth, but most of the stud-

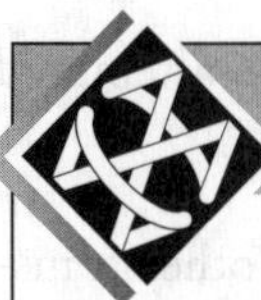

DISPLAY 9–12

Equipment for Obstetric Postanesthesia Care

A. Each postanesthesia recovery bed should have the following:
   1. Oxygen delivery system
   2. Constant and intermittent suction
   3. Blood pressure monitoring equipment
   4. ECG monitoring equipment
   5. Pulse oximeter
   6. Adjustable lighting
   7. Means to ensure patient privacy

B. The obstetric postanesthesia care unit should have the following:
   1. Method to monitor patient temperature
   2. Adult bag-valve-mask and emergency airway supplies
   3. Portable oxygen, suction, and cardiac monitoring equipment for patients requiring such equipment during transport
   4. Method of calling for assistance in emergency situations
   5. Emergency cart:
      a. Supplies for insertion of arterial line, central venous lines, and pulmonary artery catheters
      b. Emergency drugs and equipment
      c. Airway or respiratory equipment
   6. Blanket warmer
   7. Supplies to treat malignant hyperthermic crisis:
      a. Means to deliver 100% oxygen
      b. Dantrolene (Dantrium), 1.0–2.5 mg/kg, up to total of 10.0 mg/kg
      c. Preservative-free, sterile water for reconstitution (60-mL vials)
      d. Mannitol
      e. Sodium bicarbonate
      f. Regular insulin
      g. Cool intravenous fluids and a cooling blanket

From O'Brien-Abel, N., Reinke, C. Warner, P., & Nelson, C. (1994). Critical components of obstetric postanesthesia nursing. *Journal of Perinatal and Neonatal Nursing, 8* (3) pp. 4–16.

ies were done at university or tertiary-level centers with 24-hour in-house physician staff coverage and anesthesia availability (ACOG, 1999c). The evidence for maternal–fetal safety is less well documented in

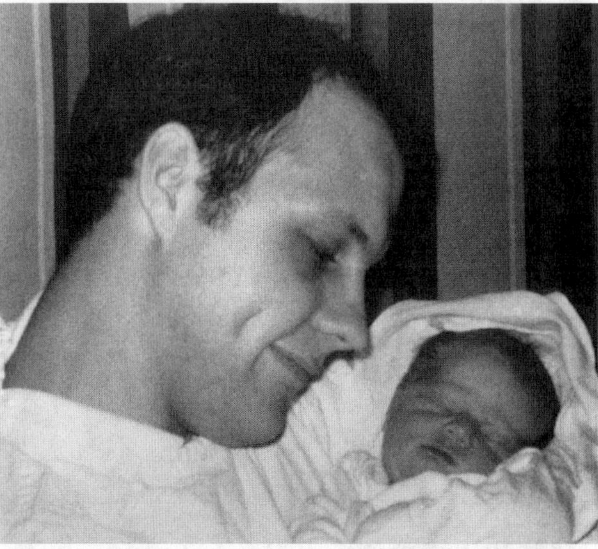

FIGURE 9–10. Promoting father involvement.

smaller community hospitals or institutions where a surgical team (ie, surgeon, anesthesia provider, first assistant, scrub technician or nurse, and circulating nurse) is not available on a 24-hour basis (ACOG, 1999c).

A VBAC is associated with a small but significant risk of uterine rupture with poor maternal–fetal outcomes (ACOG, 1999c; Kirkendall, Jauregui, Kim, & Phelan, 2000). The exact intensity of risk is difficult to determine because of imprecise definitions of uterine rupture and incomplete data about adverse maternal–fetal outcomes in published studies. Uterine rupture and uterine incision dehiscence are sometimes used interchangeably in the literature. Generally, a uterine incision dehiscence is an asymptomatic scar separation or thinning observed at surgery in women with prior low-transverse incision, and it does not result in hemorrhage or other major clinical problems (Depp, 1996). Most researchers define a uterine rupture as any defect that involves the entire uterine wall or is symptomatic and requires operative intervention (Flamm, Goings, Liu, & Wolde-Tsadik, 1994; McMahon, Luther, Bowes, & Olshan, 1996), but some reserve the term uterine rupture for extrusion of fetal parts, the umbilical cord, or the placenta through the uterine scar separation, necessitating emergent operative intervention, or acute maternal bleeding manifested by hypotension or shock (Leung, Leung, & Paul, 1993).

The risk of asymptomatic uterine incision dehiscence is 1.1% to 2.0 % (Miller, Diaz, & Paul, 1994; Phelan, Korst, & Settles, 1998; Rosen, Dickinson, & Westhoff, 1991). The risk of uterine rupture with a prior low-transverse is 0.2% to 1.5% (ACOG,

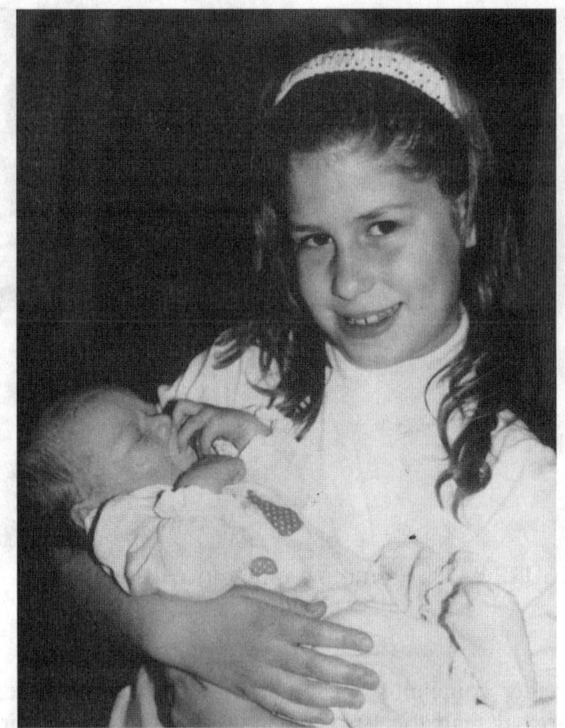

FIGURE 9–11. Promoting sibling attachment.

1999c). The risk of uterine rupture increases with the number of previous incisions. Miller and colleagues (1994) found the risk of uterine rupture nearly tripled for women with a history of more than two prior low-transverse cesarean births compared with the rate for women with one prior cesarean birth (0.06% versus 1.7%). The occurrence of uterine rupture depends on the number, type, and location of the previous incision (ACOG, 1999c; Wing & Paul, 1999b). A thorough discussion between the primary care provider and the woman and her family that includes individual risks and benefits of VBAC is recommended by ACOG (1999c) before a decision about a trial of labor is made.

Selection criteria are used to identify women who are candidates for VBAC (ACOG, 1999c):

- One or two prior low-transverse cesarean births
- Clinically adequate pelvis
- No other uterine scars or previous rupture
- Physician immediately available throughout active labor capable of monitoring labor and performing an emergent cesarean birth
- Availability of anesthesia and surgical team for emergent cesarean birth

Contraindications for a trial of labor include women at high risk for uterine rupture. Circumstances under which a trial of labor should not be attempted are as follows (ACOG, 1999c):

- Prior classic or T-shaped incision or other transfundal uterine surgery
- Contracted pelvis
- Medical or obstetric complication that precludes vaginal birth
- Inability to perform an emergent cesarean birth because of unavailable surgeon, anesthesia provider, sufficient personnel, or facility

Benefits of VBAC include the shorter recovery period and inpatient stay after a vaginal birth and maternal satisfaction. Overall morbidity, mortality, and rehospitalization rates are lower with vaginal births than surgical births (Lydon-Rochelle et al., 2000). There is conflicting evidence from studies with small sample sizes about whether women who have had multiple cesarean sections, unknown uterine scars, breech presentations, twin gestations, postterm pregnancy, and suspected macrosomia should be encouraged to attempt a trial of labor. Until more maternal–fetal data are available, VBAC should not be routinely adopted in these clinical circumstances (ACOG, 1999c).

Waiting for spontaneous labor and thereby avoiding cervical ripening agents and oxytocin appears to significantly decrease the risk of uterine rupture for women attempting VBAC (Holt & Mueller, 1997; Leung, Farmer, Leung, Medearis, & Paul, 1993; Rageth, Juzi, & Grossenbacher, 1999; Zelop, Shipp, Cohen, Repke, & Leiberman, 2000). There are enough data to suggest that prostaglandin E_1 and E_2 and high rates of oxytocin infusion increase the risk for rupture (Blanco, Collins, Willis, & Prien, 1992; Grubb, Kjos, & Paul, 1996; Johnson, Oriol, & Flood, 1991; Norman, & Ekman, 1992; Rosen, Dickinson, & Westhoff, 1991). Because of the significant risk of uterine rupture with the use of misoprostol for cervical ripening or induction (Bennett, 1997; Cunha, Bughalho, Bisque, & Bergstrom, 1999; Plaut, Schwartz, & Lubarsky, 1999; Sciscione, Nguyen, Manley, Shlossman, & Colmorgen, 1998; Wing, Lovett, & Paul, 1998), ACOG (1999a, 1999b) does not recommend misoprostol for women attempting VBAC.

Maternal complications associated with uterine rupture include bladder and ureteral injury, hysterectomy, hemorrhage, hypovolemic shock, anemia, transfusion, bowel laceration, infection, and death (Kirkendall et al., 2000). Complete or partial placental abruption usually occurs concurrently with rupture (84%), and in many cases (60%), the placenta may be at the site of the rupture (Jauregui, Kirkendall, Ahn, & Phelan, 2000). It is possible that the placenta may play a part in uterine rupture, but more data are needed about the relationship between placental implantation or abruption and the process of uterine rupture.

Flamm & Geiger (1997) developed a scoring system to assist in predicting the likelihood of successful vaginal birth for women attempting a trial of labor after a previous cesarean birth. Five maternal factors have been found to be significantly related to likelihood of success: age younger than 40 years, vaginal birth history, reason for first cesarean birth, cervical effacement, and cervical dilation on admission. Younger women, women who have had a prior vaginal birth, women for whom the reason for the first cesarean birth was other than failure to progress, and women who have more favorable cervical status on admission (>75% effacement and <4-cm dilation) are more likely to have a successful trial of labor resulting in a vaginal birth (Flamm & Geiger, 1997).

Some women who labored before their previous cesarean birth may not want to attempt a vaginal birth for fear that they will face a long, uncomfortable labor and still require a cesarean procedure. These concerns and fears must be addressed, and then a joint decision between the woman and her primary healthcare provider is made. According to ACOG (1999c), after appropriate counseling, if the woman who has had a prior cesarean birth does not wish to attempt a trial of labor, a repeat cesarean birth should be performed.

Although decreased costs are often reported to be associated with a trial of labor compared with a cesarean birth, when all factors are considered, this assumption is not always accurate. Higher costs may be incurred by the institution if the woman has a prolonged labor or significant complications or if the newborn has complications necessitating admission to the neonatal intensive care unit (ACOG, 1999c). Women who fail a trial of labor are at greater risk for infection, other morbidity, and rehospitalization (ACOG, 1999c; Clark et al., 2000; Lydon-Rochelle et al., 2000). Major maternal complications such as hemorrhage, uterine rupture, hysterectomy, and operative injury are more likely for women who have a trial of labor compared with women who have a repeat cesarean birth (Clark et al., 2000; McMahon et al., 1996). Infants born by repeat cesarean birth after a failed trial of labor also have a greater risk of infection (Hook, Kiwi, Amini, Fanaroff, & Hack, 1997). The increased costs of more intensive nursing care and physician time are additional factors, but it is difficult to accurately assess the full implications of these variables (ACOG, 1999c). Because VBAC is associated with a small but significant risk of uterine rupture with potentially catastrophic consequences for the infant, costs of acute and long-term care for neurologically injured infants and likely litigation should be considered in a cost–benefit analysis for VBAC (Clark et al., 2000; Kirkendall et al., 2000).

Women undergoing a trial of labor require comprehensive nursing care. The patient and family need additional reassurance and support. Uterine activity and fetal status should be observed closely. Most experts recommend continuous EFM during the trial of labor (ACOG, 1999c). Intravenous access is a reasonable precaution because of the risk of uterine rupture, which would require administration of rapid volume expanders and blood products. The rates of cervical dilation and fetal descent should be assessed frequently and abnormal labor progress reported to the primary care provider. Close attention should be given to any complaints of severe pain in the area of the prior incision. The onset of abdominal pain is classically suprapubic and "stabbing" (Raskin et al., 1999). Epidural anesthesia may be used during a trial of labor because it rarely masks the signs and symptoms of uterine rupture (ACOG, 1999c). Additional maternal clinical signs of uterine rupture include vaginal bleeding, blood-tinged urine, ascending station of the fetal presenting part, and hypovolemia (Mastrobattista, 1999).

Impending rupture may be preceded by increasing uterine hypertonus. Contrary to earlier reports, there is no decrease in uterine tone or cessation of contractions before or during uterine rupture (Leung, Leung et al., 1993; Plaut et al., 1999). The FHR pattern before rupture may reveal variable, late, or prolonged decelerations followed by bradycardia, or fetal bradycardia may have a sudden onset (Leung, Leung, & Paul, 1993; Menihan, 1999). If the uterine rupture is preceded by severe late or variable decelerations, the fetus can tolerate a shorter period of prolonged decelerations (Leung, Leung et al., 1993). Perinatal asphyxia can occur within 10 minutes after the onset of prolonged decelerations resulting from uterine rupture when the prolonged decelerations follow a period of severe late and variable decelerations (Leung, Leung et al., 1993). Significant neonatal morbidity has been reported when the time between onset of prolonged decelerations and birth is equal to or greater than 18 minutes (Leung, Leung et al., 1993). Kirkendall and coworkers (2000) reported a significant risk of brain damage, intrapartum death, and death within 1 year of life for infants who were partially or completely extruded into the maternal abdomen during uterine rupture.

Rupture of the uterus is a perinatal emergency. Maternal–fetal survival depends on prompt identification and surgical intervention. Rapid volume expanders, blood, and blood products should be readily available. A surgeon, surgical team, and anesthesia personnel should be immediately available to perform an emergent cesarean birth. Because uterine rupture can be catastrophic for the woman and fetus, VBAC should not be attempted in institutions not equipped to respond to emergencies with physicians immediately available to provide emergency care (ACOG, 1999c). Policies, procedures, and protocols should be written and evaluated to ensure optimum care for women who are having a trial of labor after a previous cesarean birth. If the primary care provider is a family practitioner or CNM without privileges or ability to perform an emergent cesarean birth, clear policies and protocols should be in place to ensure appropriate and timely surgical coverage in case of maternal complications.

SUMMARY

Nurses who care for women during the intrapartum period require knowledge of the labor process and a thorough understanding of techniques and interventions that enhance safe labor and birth. The woman's desires about her labor and birth experience should guide care. We should consider ourselves supportive guests at the woman's momentous life event rather than routine interventionists. The family and support persons should be integrated into the childbirth process according to the wishes of the woman. A philosophy that labor and birth are normal processes can facilitate appropriate care and avoid unnecessary interventions that can lead to iatrogenic maternal–fetal injuries.

Some of the age-old nursing traditions surrounding birth have not been found to be based on sound scientific evidence. Positioning for labor and birth is evolving from dorsal lithotomy to positions that are more woman and fetus oriented. For most women, fasting during labor is unnecessary to avoid adverse outcomes. Aggressive nurse-coached closed-glottis, second-stage pushing techniques should be abandoned. Routine episiotomy should become a thing of the past. Nurses can influence changes related to routine childbirth practices by keeping abreast of current research in intrapartum nursing and using this knowledge to care for laboring women.

Cervical ripening procedures, labor induction or augmentation, and operative births are necessary interventions for some women to promote optimal maternal and fetal outcome, but the least invasive approach should be the first considered. Nurses must have expertise in perioperative standards for women experiencing cesarean births. An awareness of strategies to resolve clinical conflicts and promote teamwork and collaboration between members of the perinatal team is essential for safe intrapartum care. This chapter has presented an overview of nursing considerations for clinical practice during childbirth. Perinatal care based on national standards and current research can enhance quality outcomes for mothers and babies. The nurse has an important role in facilitating a positive childbirth experience. Attendance at the birth of a healthy newborn and sharing the joy with the new mother constitute one of the most rewarding experiences in perinatal nursing practice.

REFERENCES

Aikens-Murphy, P., & Feinland, J. B. (1998). Perineal outcomes in a home birth setting. *Birth, 25*(4), 226–234.

Albers, L. L. (1999). The duration of labor in healthy women. *Journal of Perinatology, 19*(2), 114–119.

Albers, L. L., Anderson, D., Cragin, L., Daniels, S. M., Hunter, C., Sedler, K. D., & Teaf, D. (1997). The relationship of ambulation in labor to operative delivery. *Journal of Nurse-Midwifery, 42*(1), 4–8.

Albers, L. L., Schiff, M., & Gorwoda, J. G. (1996). The length of active labor in normal pregnancies. *Obstetrics and Gynecology, 87*(3), 355–359.

Aldrich, C. J., D'Antona, D., Spencer, J. A. D., Wyatt, J. S., Peebles, D. M., Delpy, D. T., & Reynolds, E. O. R. (1995). The effect of maternal pushing on cerebral oxygenation and blood volume during the second stage of labour. *British Journal of Obstetrics and Gynaecology, 102*(6), 448–453.

American Academy of Pediatrics, & American College of Obstetricians and Gynecologists. (1997). *Guidelines for perinatal care* (4th ed.). Elk Grove, IL: Author.

American College of Nurse Midwives. (1999). Intrapartum nutrition. (Clinical Bulletin). *Journal of Nurse-Midwifery, 44*(2), 129–134.

American College of Obstetricians and Gynecologists. (1991). *Induction and augmentation of labor* (Technical Bulletin No. 157). Washington, DC: Author.

American College of Obstetricians and Gynecologists. (1993). *Ultrasonography in pregnancy* (Technical Bulletin No. 187). Washington, DC: Author.

American College of Obstetricians and Gynecologists. (1995a). *Dystocia and the augmentation of labor* (Technical Bulletin No. 218). Washington, DC: Author.

American College of Obstetricians and Gynecologists. (1995b). *Fetal heart rate patterns: Monitoring, interpretation, and management* (Technical Bulletin No. 207). Washington, DC: Author.

American College of Obstetricians and Gynecologists. (1996). *Obstetric analgesia and anesthesia* (Technical Bulletin No. 225). Washington, DC: Author.

American College of Obstetricians and Gynecologists. (1997). *Shoulder dystocia* (Practice Pattern No. 7). Washington, DC: Author.

American College of Obstetricians and Gynecologists. (1998a). *Delivery by vacuum extraction* (Committee Opinion No. 208). Washington, DC: Author.

American College of Obstetricians and Gynecologists. (1998b). *Monitoring during induction of labor with dinoprostone* (Committee Opinion No. 209). Washington, DC: Author.

American College of Obstetricians and Gynecologists. (1999a). *Induction of labor* (Practice Bulletin No. 10). Washington, DC: Author.

American College of Obstetricians and Gynecologists. (1999b). *Induction of labor with misoprostol* (Committee Opinion No. 228). Washington, DC: Author.

American College of Obstetricians and Gynecologists. (1999c). *Vaginal birth after previous cesarean delivery* (Practice Bulletin No. 5). Washington, DC: Author.

American College of Obstetricians and Gynecologists. (2000b). *Fetal macrosomia* (Practice Bulletin No. 22). Washington, DC: Author.

American College of Obstetricians and Gynecologists. (2000). *Operative vaginal delivery* (Practice Bulletin No. 17). Washington, DC: Author.

American College of Obstetricians and Gynecologists. (2000a). *ACOG writes FDA on safety of misoprostol.* (ACOG News Release October 27th, 2000). Washington, DC: Author.

American College of Obstetricians and Gynecologists. (2000b). *Fetal macrosomia.* (Practice Bulletin No. 22). Washington, DC: Author.

American College of Obstetricians and Gynecologists. (2000c). *Operative vaginal delivery.* (Practice Bulletin No. 17). Washington, DC: Author

American Society of Anesthesiologists. (1991). *Guidelines for regional anesthesia in obstetrics.* Park Ridge, IL: Author.

American Society of Anesthesiologists. (1994). *Standards for postanesthesia care.* Park Ridge, IL: Author.

American Society of Anesthesiologists. (1999). *Practice Guidelines for Obstetrical Anesthesia.* Park Ridge, IL: Author.

Amiel-Tison, C., Sureau, C., & Shnider, S. M. (1988). Cerebral handicap in full-term neonates related to the mechanical forces of labour. *Baillieres Clinical Obstetrics and Gynaecology, 2*(1), 145–165.

Anderhold, K. J. & Roberts, J. E. (1991). Phases of second stage labor. *Journal of Nurse Midwifery, 36*(15), 267–275.

Association of Women's Health, Obstetric and Neonatal Nurses. (1997). *Second stage labor nursing management protocol.* Washington, DC: Author. Published in Mayberry, L. J., & Strange, L. B. (1997). Strategies for designing a research utilization project for labor and delivery nurses. *Journal of Obstetric, Gynecologic and Neonatal Nurses, 26*(6), 701–708.

Association of Women's Health, Obstetric and Neonatal Nurses. (1998). *Standards and guidelines for professional nursing practice in the care of women and newborns* (5th ed.). Washington, DC: Author.

Association of Women's Health, Obstetric and Neonatal Nurses. (1999). *Didactic content and clinical skills verification for professional nurse providers of basic, high risk, and critical care intrapartum nursing.* Washington, DC: Author.

Atad, J., Hallak, M., Ben-David, Y., Auslender, R., & Abramovici, H. (1997). Ripening and dilation of the unfavourable cervix for induction of labour by a double balloon device: Experience with 250 cases. *British Journal of Obstetrics and Gynaecology, 104*(6), 29–32.

Bahar, A. M. (1996). Risk factors and fetal outcome in cases of shoulder dystocia compared with normal deliveries of a similar birthweight. *British Journal of Obstetrics and Gynaecology, 103*(9), 868–872.

Bansal, R. K., Tan, W. M., Ecker, J. L., Bishop, J. T., & Kilpatrick, S. J. (1996). Is there benefit to episiotomy at spontaneous vaginal delivery? A natural experiment. *American Journal of Obstetrics and Gynecology, 175*(4, Pt. 1), 897–901.

Baskett, T. F., & Allen, A. C. (1995). Perinatal implications of shoulder dystocia. *Obstetrics and Gynecology, 86(1*), 14–17.

Benedetti, T. J. (1995). Shoulder dystocia. *Contemporary OB/GYN, 40*(3), 39–43.

Bennett, B. B. (1997). Uterine rupture during induction of labor at term with intravaginal misoprostol. *Obstetrics and Gynecology, 89*(5, Pt. 1), 832–833.

Bennett, K. A., Butt, K., Crane, J. M. G., Hutchens, D., & Young, D. C. (1998). A masked randomized comparison of oral and vaginal misoprostol for labor induction. *Obstetrics and Gynecology, 92*(4, Pt. 1), 481–486.

Berghella, V., Rogers, R. A., & Lescale, K. (1996). Stripping of membranes as a safe method to reduce prolonged pregnancies. *Obstetrics and Gynecology, 87*(6), 927–931.

Biancuzzo, M. (1993). Six myths of maternal posture during labor. *MCN, The American Journal of Maternal Child Nursing*, 18(5), 264–269.

Bishop, E. H. (1964). Pelvic scoring for elective induction. *Obstetrics and Gynecology, 24*, 266–268.

Blanch, G., Olah, K. S., & Walkinshaw, S. (1996). The presence of fetal fibronectin in the cervicovaginal secretions of women at term—Its role in the assessment of women before labor induction and in the investigation of the physiologic mechanisms of labor. *American Journal of Obstetrics and Gynecology, 174*(1, Pt. 1), 262–266.

Blanchette, H. A., Nayak, S., & Erasmus, S. (1999). Comparison of the safety and efficacy of intravaginal misoprostol (prostaglandin E_1) with those of dinoprostone (prostaglandin E_2) for cervical ripening and induction of labor in a community hospital. *American Journal of Obstetrics and Gynecology, 180*(6, Pt. 1), 1551–1559.

Blanco, J. D., Collins, M., Willis, D., & Prien, S. (1992). Prostaglandin E_2 gel induction of patients with a prior low transverse cesarean section. *American Journal of Perinatology, 9*(2), 80–83.

Bloom, S. L., McIntire, D. D., Kelly, M. A., Beimer, H. L., Burpo, R. H., Garcia, M. A., & Leveno, K. J. (1998). Lack of effect of walking on labor and delivery. *New England Journal of Medicine, 339*(2), 76–79.

Bofill, J. A., Rust, O. A., Schorr, S. J., Brown, R. C., Martin, R. W., Martin, J. N., Jr., & Morrison, J. C. (1996). A randomized prospective trial of the obstetric forceps versus the M-cup vacuum extractor. *American Journal of Obstetrics and Gynecology, 175*(5), 1325–1330.

Bofill, J. A., Rust, O. A., Devidas, M., Roberts, W. E., Morrison, J. C., & Martin, J. N., Jr. (1997a). Neonatal cephalohematoma from vacuum extraction. *Journal of Reproductive Medicine, 42*(9), *565–569.*

Bofill, J. A., Rust, O. A., Devidas, M., Roberts, W. E., Morrison, J. C., & Martin, J. N., Jr. (1997b). Shoulder dystocia and operative vaginal delivery. *Journal of Maternal Fetal Medicine, 6*(4), 220–224.

Bofill, J. A., Martin, J. N., Jr., & Morrison, J. C. (1998). The Mississippi operative vaginal delivery trial: Lessons learned. *Contemporary OB/GYN, 43*(10), 60–79.

Brindley, B. A., & Sokol, R. J. (1988). Induction and augmentation of labor: Basis and methods for practice. *Obstetrical and Gynecological Survey, 43*(12), 730–743.

Brown, M. A., Reiter, L., Smith, B., Buddle, M. L., Morries, R., & Whiteworth, J. A. (1994). Measuring blood pressure in pregnant women: A comparison of direct and indirect methods. *American Journal of Obstetrics and Gynecology, 171*(3), 661–667.

Brumfield, C., Gilstrap, L. C., O'Grady, J. P., Ross, M. G., & Schifrin, B. S. (1999). Cutting your legal risks with vacuum-assisted deliveries. *OBG Management, 3*, 2–6

Bruner, J. P., Drummond, S. B., Meenan, A. L., & Gaskin, I. M. (1998). All-fours maneuver for reducing shoulder dystocia during labor. *Journal of Reproductive Medicine, 43*(5), 439–443.

Buser, D., Mora, G., & Arias, F. (1997). A randomized comparison between misoprostol and dinoprostone for cervical ripening and labor induction in patients with unfavorable cervices. *Obstetrics and Gynecology, 89*(4), 581–585.

Busowski, J. D., & Parson, M. T. (1995). Amniotomy to induce labor. *Clinical Obstetrics and Gynecology, 38*(2), 246–258.

Caldeyro-Barcia, R. (1979). The influence of maternal bearing-down efforts during second stage on fetal well-being. *Birth and the Family Journal, 6*, 71–21.

Caldeyro-Barcia, R., Giussi, G., Storch, E., Poseiro, J. J., Lafrausie, N., Kettenhuber, K., & Ballejo, G. (1981). The bearing down efforts and their effects on fetal heart rate, oxygenation, and acid-base balance. *Journal of Perinatal Medicine, 9*(Suppl. 1), S63–S67.

Chalfen, M. E. (1993). Obstetric-gynecologic care and survivors of childhood sexual abuse. *AWHONN's Clinical Issues in Perinatal and Women's Health Nursing, 4*(2), 191–195.

Clark, S. L., Scott, J. R., Porter, T. F., Schlappy, D. A., McClellan, V., & Burton, D. A. (2000). Is vaginal birth after cesarean delivery less expensive than repeat cesarean delivery? *American Journal of Obstetrics and Gynecology, 182*(2), 599–602.

Clayworth, S. (2000). The nurse's role during oxytocin administration. *MCN, The American Journal of Maternal Child Nursing, 25*(2), 80–84.

Cohen, S. E., Yeh, J. Y., Riley, E. T., & Vogel, T. M. (2000). Walking with labor epidural analgesia: The impact of bupivacaine concentration and a lidocaine-epinephrine test dose. *Anesthesiology, 92*(2), 387–392

Cohen, W. R. (1977). Influence of the duration of second stage labor on perinatal outcome and puerperal morbidity. *Obstetrics and Gynecology, 49*(3), 266–269.

Colachis, S. C., III, Pease, W. S., & Johnson, E. W. (1994). A preventable cause of foot drop during childbirth. *American Journal of Obstetrics and Gynecology, 171*(1), 270–272.

Collis, R. E., Harding, S. A., & Morgan, B. M. (1999). Effect of maternal ambulation on labour with low-dose combined spinal-epidural analgesia. *Anaesthesia, 54*(6), 535–539.

Cosner, K. R. (1996). Use of fundal pressure during second-stage labor: A pilot study. *Journal of Nurse-Midwifery, 41*(4), 334–337.

Cosner, K. R., & deJong, E. (1993). Physiologic second-stage labor. *MCN American Journal of Maternal Child Nursing, 18*(1), 38–43.

Crane, J., Bennett K., Young, D., Windrim, R., & Kravitz, H. (1997). The effectiveness of sweeping membranes at term. A randomized trial. *Obstetrics and Gynecology, 89*(4), 586–590.

Cunha, M., Bugalho, A., Bique, C., & Berstrom, S. (1999). Induction of labor by vaginal misoprostol in patients with previous cesarean delivery. *Acta Obstetricia et Gynecologica Scandinavica, 78*(7), 653–654.

Curtin, S. C. & Martin, J. A. (2000). Births: Preliminary data for 1999. *National Vital Statistics Reports, 48*(14), 1–24.

Davis, J. & Renning, E. L. (1964). The birth canal: Practical applications. *Medical Times, 92*(1), 75–86.

Dawood, M. Y. (1995). Pharmacologic stimulation of uterine contractions. *Seminars in Perinatology, 19*(1), 73–83.

Dawood, M. Y., Wang, C. F., Gupta, R., & Fuchs, F. (1978). Fetal contribution to oxytocin in human labor. *Obstetrics and Gynecology, 52*(2), 205–209.

Dawood, M. Y., Ylikorkala, O., Trivedi, D., & Fuchs, F. (1979). Oxytocin in maternal circulation and amniotic fluid during pregnancy. *Journal of Clinical Endocrinology and Metabolism, 49*(3), 429–434.

DelGiudice, G. T. (1986). The relationship between sibling jealousy and presence at a sibling's birth. *Birth, 13*(4), 250–254.

Depp, R. (1996). Cesarean delivery. In S. Gabbe, J. R. Niebyl, & J. L. Simpson (Eds.), *Obstetrics: Normal and problem pregnancies* (3rd ed., pp. 561–642). New York: Churchill Livingstone.

Derham, R. J., Crowhurst, J., & Crowther, C. (1991). The second stage of labor: Durational dilemmas. *Australian New Zealand Journal of Obstetrics and Gynaecology, 31*(1), 31–36.

Devine, J. B., Ostergard, D. R., & Noblett, K. L. (1999). Long-term complications of the second stage of labor. *Contemporary OB/GYN, 44*(6), 119–126.

Driver, I., Popham, P., Glazebrook, C., & Palmer, C. (1996). Epidural bupivacaine/fentanyl infusions vs intermittent top-ups: A retrospective study of the effects on mode of delivery in primiparous women. *European Journal of Anaesthesiology, 13*(5), 515–520.

Drummond, S. B. (1999). Assessment of the patient in labor. In D. M. Rostant & R. F. Cady (Eds.), *AWHONN's liability issues in perinatal nursing* (pp. 89–103). Philadelphia: Lippincott, Williams & Wilkins.

Eason, E., Labrecque, M., Wells, G., & Feldman, P. (2000). Preventing perineal trauma during childbirth: A systematic review. *Obstetrics and Gynecology, 95*(3), 464–471.

Eason, E., & Feldman, P. (2000). Much ado about a little cut: Is episiotomy worthwhile? *Obstetrics and Gynecology, 95*(4), 616–618.

El-Torkey, M., & Grant, J. M. (1992). Sweeping of the membranes is an effective method of induction of labour in prolonged pregnancy: A report of a randomized trial. *British Journal of Obstetrics and Gynaecology, 99*(6), 455–458.

Engelman, G. J. (1884). *Labor among primitive peoples* (3rd ed.). St. Louis: J.H. Chambers.

Farah, L. A., Sanchez-Ramos, L., Del Valle, G. O., Gaudier, F. L., Delke, I., & Kaunitz, A. M. (1997). Randomized trial of two doses of the prostaglandin E_1 analog misoprostol for labor induction. *American Journal of Obstetrics and Gynecology, 177*(2), 364–369.

Feinstein, N. F., Sprague, A., & Trepanier, M. J. (2000). *Fetal Heart Rate Auscultation* (AWHONN Symposium). Washington, DC: Association of Women's Health, Obstetric and Neonatal Nurses.

Ferguson, J. K. W. (1941). Study of motility of intact uterus at term. Surgery, *Gynecology and Obstetrics, 73*, 359–366.

Flamm, B. L., & Geiger, A. M. (1997). Vaginal birth after cesarean delivery: An admission scoring system. *Obstetrics and Gynecology, 90*(6), 907–910.

Flamm, B. L., Goings, J., Liu, Y., & Wolde-Tsadik, G. (1994). Elective repeat cesarean delivery versus trial of labor: A prospective multicenter study. *Obstetrics and Gynecology, 83*(6), 927–932.

Flynn, P., Franiek, J., Janssen, P., Hannah, W. J., & Klein, M. C. (1997). How can second stage management prevent perineal trauma: Critical review. *Canadian Family Physician, 43*(1), 73–84.

Food and Drug Administration. (1998). *Need for caution when using vacuum assisted delivery devices* (Public Health Advisory). Washington, DC: Author.

Forest Pharmaceuticals, Inc. (1995). *Cervidil prescribing information*. St. Louis: Author.

Fortier, J. C. (1988). The relationship of vaginal and cesarean births to father-infant attachment. *Journal of Obstetric, Gynecologic, and Neonatal Nursing, 17*(2), 128–134.

Franx, A., van der Post, J. A. M., Elfering, I. M., Veerman, D. P., Merkus, H. M. W. M., Boer, K., & van Montfrans, G. A. (1994). Validation of automatic blood pressure recording in pregnancy. *British Journal of Obstetrics and Gynaecology, 101* (10), 66–69.

Fraser, W. D., Marcoux, S., Krauss, I., Douglas, J., Goulet, C. & Boulvain, M. for the PEOPLE (Pushing Early of Pushing Late with Epirdural) Study Group. (2000). Multicenter randomized controlled trial of delayed pushing for nulliparous women in the second stage of labor with continuous epidural analgesia. *American Journal of Obstetrics and Gynecology, 182*(5), 1165–1172.

Friedman, E. A. (1978). *Labor: Clinical evaluation of management* (2nd ed.). New York: Appleton-Century-Crofts.

Friedman, E. A., Niswander, K. R., Bayonet-Rivera, N. P., & Sachtleben, M. R. (1966). Relationship of prelabor evaluation to inducibility and the course of labor. *Obstetrics and Gynecology, 28*(4), 495–501.

Frigoletto, F. D., Jr., Lieberman, E., Lang, J. M., Cohen, A., Barss, V., Ringer, S., & Datta, S. (1995). A clinical trial of active management of labor. *New England Journal of Medicine, 333*(12), 745–750.

Fuchs, A. R., Fuchs, F. Husslein, P., & Soloff, M. S. (1984). Oxytocin receptors in the human uterus during pregnancy and parturition. *American Journal of Obstetrics and Gynecology, 150*(12), 734–741.

Fuchs, A. R., Husslein, P., & Fuchs, F. (1981). Oxytocin and the initiation of human parturition. II: Stimulation of prostaglandin production in the human decidua by oxytocin. *American Journal of Obstetrics and Gynecology, 141*(6), 694–697.

Gannon, J. M. (1992). Delivery on the hands and knees: A case study approach. *Journal of Nurse-Midwifery, 37*(1), 48–52.

Gardosi, J., Sylvester, S. & Lynch, C. B. (1989). Alternative positions in the second stage of labor: A randomized controlled trial. *British Journal of Obstetrics and Gynaecology, 96*(11), 1290–1296.

Garite, T. J., Casal, D., Garcia-Alonso, A., Kreaden, U., Jimenez, G., Ayala, J. A., & Reimbold, T. (1996). Fetal fibronectin: A new tool for the prediction of successful induction of labor. *American Journal of Obstetrics and Gynecology, 175*(6), 1516–1521.

Garite, T. J., Porto, M., Carlson, N. J., Rumney, P. J., & Reimbold, P. A. (1993). The influence of elective amniotomy on fetal heart rate patterns and the course of labor in term patients: A randomized study. *American Journal of Obstetrics and Gynecology, 168*(6, Pt. 1), 1827–1831.

Garite, T. J., Weeks, M. D., & Peters-Phair, K. (2000). A randomized trial on the influence of increased intravenous hydration on the course of nulliparous labor. *American Journal of Obstetrics and Gynecology, 182*(1, Pt. 2), S37.

Gei, A. F., & Belfort, M. A. (1999). Forceps-assisted vaginal delivery. *Obstetrics and Gynecology Clinics of North America, 26*(2), 345–370.

Gherman, R. B., Goodwin, T. M., Souter, I., Neumann, K., Ouzounian, J. G., & Paul, R. H. (1997). The McRoberts' maneuver for the alleviation of shoulder dystocia: How successful is it? *Journal of Obstetrics and Gynecology, 176*(3), 656–661.

Gherman, R. B., Ouzounian, J. G., & Goodwin, T. M. (1998). Obstetric maneuvers for shoulder dystocia and associated fetal morbidity. *American Journal of Obstetrics and Gynecology, 178*(6), 1126–1130.

Gherman, R. B., Tramont, J., Muffley, P., Goodwin, T. M. (2000). Analysis of McRoberts' maneuver by x-ray pelvimetry. *Obstetrics and Gynecology, 95*(1), 43–47.

Gifford, D. S., Morton, S. C., Fiske, M., Keesey, J., Keeler, E., & Kahn, K. L. (2000). Lack of progress as a reason for cesarean. *Obstetrics and Gynecology, 95*(4), 589–595.

Gilbert, W. M., Nesbitt, T. S., & Danielsen, B. (1999). Associated factors in 1611 cases of brachial plexus injury. *Obstetrics and Gynecology, 93*(4), 536–540.

Goffinet, F. Fraser, W., Marcoux, S., Breart, G., Moutquin, J. M., Daris, M., & the Amniotomy Study Group. (1997). Early amniotomy increases the frequency of fetal heart rate abnormalities. *British Journal of Obstetrics and Gynaecology, 104*(5), 548–553.

Golay, J., Vedam, S., & Sorger, L. (1993). The squatting position for the second stage of labor: Effects on labor and on maternal and fetal well being. *Birth, 20*(2), 73–78.

Gonik, B., Stringer, C. A., & Held, B. (1983). An alternate maneuver for management of shoulder dystocia. *American Journal of Obstetrics and Gynecology, 145*(7), 882–884.

Gross, S. J., Shime, J., & Farine, D. (1987). Shoulder dystocia: Predictors and outcome. A five year review. *American Journal of Obstetrics and Gynecology, 156*(2), 334–336.

Grubb, D. K., Kjos, S. L., & Paul, R. H. (1996). Latent labor with an unknown uterine scar. *Obstetrics and Gynecology, 88*(3), 351–355.

Hankins, G. D. (1998). Lower thoracic spinal cord injury: A severe complication of shoulder dystocia. *American Journal of Perinatology, 15*(7), 443–444.

Hansen, S. L., & Clark, S. L. (1996). Rest and descend vs. pushing with epidural anesthesia in the second stage of labor. *American Journal of Obstetrics and Gynecology, 174*(1, Pt. 2), 479.

Hawkins, J. L., Koonin, L. M., Palmer, S. K., & Gibbs, C. P. (1997). Anesthesia-related deaths during obstetric delivery in the United States, 1979–1990. *Anesthesiology, 86*(2), 277–284.

Hellman, L. M., & Prystowsky, H. (1952). Duration of the second stage of labor. *American Journal of Obstetrics and Gynecology, 63*(6), 1223–1233.

Hillan, E. M. (1992). Issues in the delivery of midwifery care. *Journal of Advanced Nursing, 17*(3), 274–278.

Hofmeyer, G. J., Gulmezoglu, A. M., & Alfirevic, Z. (1999). Misoprostol for induction of labour: A systematic review. *British Journal of Obstetrics and Gynaecology, 106*(8), 798–803.

Holt, V. L., & Mueller, B. A. (1997). Attempt and success rates for vaginal birth after caesarean section in relation to complications of the previous pregnancy. *Paediatric and Perinatal Epidemiology, 11*(Suppl. 1), 63–72.

Holland, R. L. & Smith, D. A. (1989). Management of the second stage of labor: A review (Part II). Maternal positioning as it relates to the management of labor is reviewed. *South Dakota Journal of Medicine, 42*(6), 5–8.

Hook, B., Kiwi, R., Amini, S. B., Faranoff, A., & Hack, M. (1997). Neonatal morbidity after elective repeat cesarean section and trial of labor. *Pediatrics, 100*(3, Pt. 1), 348–353.

Hordnes, K., & Bergsjo, P. (1993). Severe lacerations after childbirth. *Acta Obstetricia et Gynecologica Scandinavica, 72*(6), 413–422.

Hueston, W. J. (1996). Factors associated with the use of episiotomy during vaginal delivery. *Obstetrics and Gynecology, 87*(6), 1001–1005.

Humphrey, M., Hounslow, D., Morgan, S. & Wood, C. (1973). The influence of maternal position at birth on the fetus. *Journal of Obstetrics and Gynaecology of the British Commonwealth, 80*(12), 1075–1080.

Hundley, V. A., Milne, J. M., Glazener, C. M. A., & Mollison, J. (1997). Satisfaction and the three C's: Continuity, choice and control: Women's views from a randomised controlled trial of midwife-led care. *British Journal of Obstetrics and Gynaecology, 104*(11), 1273–1280.

Husslein, P., Fuchs, A. R., & Fuchs, F. (1981). Oxytocin and the initiation of human parturition: 1, Prostaglandin release during induction of labor by oxytocin. *American Journal of Obstetrics and Gynecology, 141*(6), 688–693.

James, C., Peedicayil, A., & Seshadri, L. (1994). Use of the Foley catheter as a cervical ripening agent prior to induction of labor. *International Journal of Gynecology and Obstetrics, 47*(3), 229–232.

Jauregui, I., Kirkendall, C., Ahn, M. O., & Phelan, J. (2000). Uterine rupture: A placentally mediated event? *Obstetrics and Gynecology, 95*(4, Suppl. 1), S75.

Johanson, R. (1997). Choice of instrument for vaginal delivery. *Current Opinion in Obstetrics and Gynecology, 9*(6), 361–365.

Johnson, C., Oriol, N., & Flood, K. (1991). Trial of labor: A study of 110 patients. *Journal of Clinical Anesthesiology, 3*(3), 216–218.

Johnson, N., Johnson, V. A., Gupta, J. K. (1991). Maternal positions during labor. *Obstetrical and Gynecological Survey, 46*(7), 428–434.

Johnson, N., van Oudgarrden, E., Montague, I. A., & McNamara, H. (1994). The effect of oxytocin-induced hyperstimulation on fetal oxygen. *British Journal of Obstetrics and Gynaecology, 101*(9), 805–807.

Joint Commission on Accreditation of Healthcare Organizations (2000). *Comprehensive accreditation manual for hospitals.* Oak Park, IL: Author

Keirse, M. J. (1993). A final comment . . . managing the uterus, the woman or whom? *Birth, 20*(3), 159–161.

Keppler, A. B. (1988). The use of intravenous fluids during labor. *Birth, 15*(2), 75–79.

Kirkendall, C., Jauregui, I., Kim, J. O., & Phelan, J. (2000). Catastrophic uterine rupture: Maternal and fetal characteristics. *Obstetrics and Gynecology, 95*(4, Suppl. 1), S74.

Kiss, H., Ahner, R., Hohlagschwandtner, M., Leitich, H., & Husslein, P. (2000). Fetal fibronectin as a predictor of term labor: A literature review. *Acta Obstetricia et Gynecologica Scandinavica, 79*(1), 3–7.

Kitzinger, J. (1990). Recalling the pain . . . medical procedures can bring back memories of sexual violence. *Nursing Times, 86*(3), 38–40.

Klaus, M. H., Kennel, J. H., McGrath, S., Robertson, S. S., & Hinkley, C. (1991). Continuous emotional support during labor in a U.S. hospital: A randomized control trial. *Journal of the American Medical Association, 265*(17), 2197–2201.

Klaus, M. H., Kennel, J. H., McGrath, S., Robertson S. S., & Hinkley, C. (1988). Medical intervention: The effect of social support during labor (The American Pediatric Society and the Society for Pediatric Research, Washington, DC, May 25, 1998). *Pediatric Research, 23*(4, Pt. 2), 211A.

Klaus, M. H., Kennel, J. H., Robertson, S. S., & Sosa, R. (1986). Effects of social support during parturition and maternal and infant morbidity. *British Medical Journal, 293*(6547), 585–587.

Klein, M. C., Gauthier, R. J., Robbins, J. M. , Kaczorowski, J., Jorgensen, S. H., Franco, E., Johnson, B., Waghorn, K., Gelfand, M. M., Guralnick, M. S., Luskey, G., & Joshi, A. (1994). Relationship of episiotomy to perineal trauma and morbidity, sexual dysfunction, and pelvic floor relaxation. *American Journal of Obstetrics and Gynecology, 171*(3), 591–598.

Kline-Kaye, V., & Miller-Slade, D. (1990). The use of fundal pressure during the second stage of labor. *Journal of Obstetric, Gynecologic, and Neonatal Nursing, 19*(6), 511–517.

Klingner, M. C., & Kruse, J. (1999). Meconium aspiration syndrome: Pathophysiology and prevention. *Journal of the American Board of Family Practice, 12*(6), 450–466.

Knox, G. E., Simpson, K. R., & Garite, T. J. (1999). High reliability perinatal units: An approach to the prevention of patient injury and medical malpractice claims. *Journal of Healthcare Risk Management, 19*(2), 24–32.

Koger, K. E., Shatney, C. H., Hodge, K., & McClenathan, J. H. (1993). Surgical scar endometrioma. *Surgery, Gynecology, and Obstetrics, 177*(3), 243–246.

Kolderup, L., McLean, L., Grullon, K., Safford, K., & Kilpatrick, S. J. (1999). Misoprostol is more efficacious for labor induction than prostaglandin E_2, but is it associated with more risk? *American Journal of Obstetrics and Gynecology, 180*(6, Pt. 1), 1543–1550.

Kozak, L. J., & Lawrence, L. (1999). National hospital discharge survey: Annual summary, 1997. *National Center for Health Statistics, Vital Health Statistics, 13*(144), 1–54.

Krammer, J., & O'Brien, W. F. (1995). Mechanical methods of cervical ripening. *Clinical Obstetrics and Gynecology, 38*(2), 280–286.

Labrecque, M., Eason, E., Marcoux, S., Lemieux, F., Pinault, J. J., Feldman, P., & Laperriere, L. (1999). Randomized controlled trial of prevention of perineal trauma by perineal massage during pregnancy. *American Journal of Obstetrics and Gynecology, 180*(3, Pt. 1), 593–600.

Labrecque, M., Eason, E., & Marcoux, S. (2000). Randomized trial of perineal massage during pregnancy: Perineal symptoms three months after delivery. *American Journal of Obstetrics and Gynecology, 182*(1, Pt. 1), 76–80.

Langer, B., Carbonne, B., Goffinet, F., LeGoueff, F., Berkane, N., & Laville, M. (1997). Fetal pulse oximetry and fetal heart rate monitoring during stage II of labour. *European Journal of Obstetrics and Gynecology and Reproductive Biology, 72*(Suppl.), S57–61.

Lederman, R. P., Lederman, E., Work, B., Jr., & McCann, D. S. (1985). Anxiety and epinephrine in multiparous women in labor: Relationship to duration of labor and fetal heart rate pattern. *American Journal of Obstetrics and Gynecology, 153*(8), 870–877.

Lee, W. K., Baggish, M. S., & Lashgari, M. (1978). Acute inversion of the uterus. *Obstetrics and Gynecology, 51*(20), 144–147.

Leung, A. S., Farmer, R., Leung, E. K., Medearis, A. L., & Paul, R. H. (1993). Risk factors associated with uterine rupture during trial of labor after cesarean delivery: A case control study. *American Journal of Obstetrics and Gynecology, 168*(5), 1358–1363.

Leung, A. S., Leung, E. K., & Paul, R. H. (1993). Uterine rupture after previous cesarean delivery: Maternal and fetal consequences. *American Journal of Obstetrics and Gynecology, 169*(4), 945–950.

Lewis, D. F., Edwards, M. S., Asrat, T., Adair, C. D., Brooks, G., & London, S. (1998). Can shoulder dystocia be predicted? Preconceptive and prenatal factors. *Journal of Reproductive Medicine, 43*(8), 654–658.

Liu, Y. C. (1974). Effects of an upright position during labor. *American Journal of Nursing, 74*(12), 2202–2205.

Liu, Y. C. (1989). The effects of the upright position during childbirth. *Image, The Journal of Nursing Scholarship, 21*(1), 14–18.

Lopez-Zeno, J. A., Peaceman, A. M., Adashek, J. A., & Socol, M. L. (1992). A controlled trial of a program for the active management of labor. *New England Journal of Medicine, 326*(7), 450–454.

Low, L. K., Seng, J. S., Murtland, T. L., & Oakley, D. (2000). Clinician-specific episiotomy rates: Impacts on perineal outcomes. *Journal of Nurse-Midwifery and Women's Health, 45*(2), 87–93.

Ludka, L. M., & Roberts, C. C. (1993). Eating and drinking in labor: A literature review. *Journal of Nurse-Midwifery, 38*(4), 199–207.

Lupe, P. J., & Gross, T. L. (1986). Maternal upright posture and mobility in labor: A review. *Obstetrics and Gynecology, 67*(5), 727–734.

Lydon-Rochelle, M., Holt, V. L., Martin, D. P., & Easterling, T. R. (2000). Association between method of delivery and maternal rehospitalization. *Journal of the American Medical Association, 283*(18), 2411–2416.

Maier, J. S., & Maloni, J. A. (1997). Nurse advocacy for selective versus routine episiotomy. *Journal of Obstetrics, Gynecology, and Neonatal Nursing, 26*(2), 155–161.

Malone, F. D., Geary, M., Chelmow, D., Stronge, J. Boylan, P., & D'Alton, M. E. (1996). Prolonged labor in nulliparas: Lessons from the lactive management of labor. *Obstetrics and Gynecology, 88*(2), 211–215.

Manning, J. (1996). Intrathecal narcotic: New approach for labor analgesia. *Journal of Obstetric, Gynecologic, and Neonatal Nursing, 25*(3), 221–224.

Maresh, M., Choong, K. H., & Bread, R. W. (1983). Delayed pushing with lumbar epidural analgesia in labour. *British Journal of Obstetrics and Gynaecology, 90*(7), 623–627.

Maslow, A. S. & Sweeny, A. L. (2000). Elective induction of labor as a risk factor for cesarean delivery among low risk women at term. *Obstetrics and Gynecology, 95*(6, Pt. 1), 917–922.

Mastrobattista, J. M. (1999). Vaginal birth after cesarean delivery. *Obstetrics and Gynecology Clinics of North America, 26*(2), 295–304.

Mayberry, L. J., Hammer, R., Kelly, C., True-Driver, B., & De, A. (1999). Use of delayed pushing with epidural anesthesia: Findings from a randomized controlled trial. *Journal of Perinatology, 19*(1), 26–30.

Maryland State Board of Nursing. (1999). *Registered nurse application of suprapubic and fundal pressure in obstetrical nursing* (Declaratory Ruling 99-3). Baltimore: Author.

McColgin, S. W., Hampton, H. L., McCaul, J. F., Howard, P. R., Andrew, M. E., & Morrison, J. C. (1990). Stripping the membranes at term: Can it safely reduce the incidence of post-term pregnancies? *Obstetrics and Gynecology, 76*(4), 678–680.

McFarland, M. B., Trylovich, C. G., & Langer, O. (1998). Anthropometric differences in macrosomic infants of diabetic and nondiabetic mothers. *Journal of Maternal and Fetal Medicine, 7*(6), 292–295.

McGuinness, M., Norr, K., & Nacion, K. (1991). Comparison between different perineal outcomes on tissue healing. *Journal of Nurse-Midwifery, 36*(3), 192–198.

McKay, S. (1981). Second stage labor: Has tradition replaced safety? *American Journal of Nursing, 81*(5), 1016–1019.

McKay, S. (1984). Squatting: An alternative position for the second stage of labor. *MCN, The American Journal of Maternal Child Nursing, 9*(3), 181–183.

McKay, S., Barrows, T., & Roberts, J. (1990). Women's view of second-stage labor as assessed by interviews and videotapes. *Birth, 17*(4), 192–198.

McKay, S., & Roberts, J. (1985). Second stage labor: What is normal? *Journal of Obstetric, Gynecologic, and Neonatal Nursing, 14*(2), 101–106.

McKay, S. & Roberts, J. (1990). Obstetrics by ear: Maternal and caregiver perceptions of the meaning of maternal sound during second stage of labor. *Journal of Nurse Midwifery, 35*(5), 266–273.

McKay, S., & Smith, S. Y. (1993). What are they talking about? Is something wrong? Information sharing during the second stage of labor. *Birth, 20*(3), 142–147.

McMahon, M. J. (1998). Vaginal birth after cesarean. *Clinical Obstetrics and Gynecology, 41*(2), 369–381.

McMahon, M. J., Luther, E. R., Bowes, W. A., Jr., & Olshan, A. F. (1996). Comparison of a trial of labor with an elective second cesarean section. *New England Journal of Medicine, 353*(10), 689–695.

McNamara, H., & Johnson, N. (1995). The effect of uterine contractions on fetal oxygen saturation. *British Journal of Obstetrics and Gynecology, 102*(8), 644–647.

Mendelson, C. L. (1946). Aspiration of stomach contents into the lungs during obstetric anesthesia. *American Journal of Obstetrics and Gynecology, 52*, 191–205.

Menticoglou, S. M., Manning, F., Harman, C., & Morrison, I. (1995). Perinatal outcome in relation to second-stage duration. *American Journal of Obstetrics and Gynecology, 173*(3, Pt. 1), 906–912.

Menihan, C. A. (1999). The effect of uterine rupture on fetal heart rate patterns. *Journal of Nurse-Midwifery, 44*(1), 40–46.

Mengert, W., & Murphy, D. P. (1933). Intraabdominal pressures created by voluntary muscular effort: Relation to posture in labor. *Surgery and Gynecologic Obstetrics, 57*, 745–751.

Miller, D., Diaz, F., & Paul, R. (1994). Vaginal birth after cesarean: A 10 year experience. *Obstetrics and Gynecology, 84*(2), 255–258.

Mino, M., Puertas, A., Miranda, J. A., & Herruzo, A. J. (1999). Amnioinfusion in term labor with low amniotic fluid due to rupture of membranes: a new indication. *European Journal of Obstetrics, Gynecology, and Reproductive Biology, 82*(1), 29–34.

Mitchell, M. D., Flint, A. P., Bibby, J., Brunt, J., Arnold, J. M., Anderson, A. B., & Turnbull, A. C. (1977). Rapid increases in plasma prostaglandin concentrations after vaginal examinations and amniotomy. *British Medical Journal, 2*(6096), 1183–1185.

Miyazaki, F., & Nevarez, F. (1985). Saline amnioinfusion for relief of repetitive variable decelerations: A prospective randomized study. *American Journal of Obstetrics and Gynecology, 153*(3), 301–306.

Moe, P., & Paige, P. L. (1999). Neurologic disorders. In G. B. Merenstein & S. L. Gardner (Eds.), *Handbook of Neonatal Intensive Care* (pp. 571–603). St. Louis: Mosby.

Moon, J. M., Smith, C. V., & Rayburn, W. F. (1990). Perinatal outcome after a prolonged second stage of labor. *Journal of Reproductive Medicine, 35*(3), 229–231.

Moore, M. L. (1999). Biochemical markers for preterm and birth: What is their role in the care of pregnant women? *MCN, The American Journal of Maternal Child Nursing, 24*(2), 80–86.

Mynaugh, P. A. (1991). A randomized study of two methods of teaching perineal massage: Effects on practice rates, episiotomy rates, and lacerations. *Birth, 18*(3), 153–159.

Naef, R. W., III, & Morrison, J. C. (1994). Guidelines for management of shoulder dystocia. *Journal of Perinatology, 14*(6), 435–441.

Nesbitt, T. S., Gilbert, W. M., & Herrchen, B. (1998). Shoulder dystocia and associated risk factors with macrosomic infants born in California. *American Journal of Obstetrics and Gynecology, 179*(2), 476–480.

Noble, E. (1981). Controversies in maternal effort during labor and delivery. *Journal of Nurse Midwifery, 26*(2), 13–22.

Nocon, J. J., & Weisbrod, L. (1995). Shoulder dystocia. In J. P. O'Grady, M. Gimovsky, & C. J. Mcllhargie (Eds.), *Operative obstetrics*. Baltimore: Williams & Wilkins.

Norbeck, J. S., & Anderson, N. J. (1989). Psychosocial predictors of pregnancy outcomes in low-income black, Hispanic, and white women. *Nursing Research, 38*(4), 204–209.

Norman, M., & Ekman, G. (1992). Preinductive cervical ripening with prostaglandin E_2 in women with one previous cesarean section. *Acta Obstetricia et Gynecologica Scandinaciva, 71*(5), 351–355.

O'Brien-Abel, N., Reinke, C., Warner, P., & Nelson, C. (1994). Obstetric postanesthesia nursing: A staff education program. *Journal of Perinatal and Neonatal Nursing, 8*(3), 17–32.

O'Brien, W. F., & Cefalo, R. C. (1996). Labor and delivery. In S. G. Gabbe, J. R. Niebyl, & J. L. Simpson (Eds.), *Obstetrics: Normal and problem pregnancies* (3rd ed., pp. 371–396). New York: Churchill Livingstone.

O'Driscoll, K., Foley, M., & MacDonald, D. (1984). Active management of labor as an alternative to cesarean section for dystocia. *Obstetrics and Gynecology, 63*(4), 485–490.

O'Driscoll, K., Jackson, R. J., & Gallagher, J. T. (1969). Prevention of prolonged labour. *British Medical Journal, 2*(655), 477–480.

O'Driscoll, K., Jackson, R. J., & Gallagher, J. T. (1970). Active management of labor and cephalopelvic disproportion. *Journal of Obstetrics and Gynaecology of the British Commonwealth, 77*(5), 385–389.

Olah, K. S., & Gee, H. (1996). The active mismanagement of labour. *British Journal of Obstetrics and Gynaecology, 103*(8), 729–731.

Olofsson, C., Ekblom, A., Ekman-Ordeberg, G., & Irestedt, L. (1998). Obstetric outcome following epidural analgesia with bupivacaine-adrenaline 0.25% or bupivacaine 0.125% with sufentanil: A prospective randomized controlled study in 1000 parturients. *Acta Anaesthesiologica Scandinavica, 42*(3), 284– 292.

Ouzounian, J. G., Miller, D. A., & Paul, R. H. (1996). Amnioinfusion in women with previous cesarean births: A preliminary report. *American Journal of Obstetrics and Gynecology, 174*(2), 783–786.

Paluska, S. A. (1997). Vacuum-assisted vaginal delivery. *American Family Physician, 55*(6), 2197–2203.

Parnell, C., Langhoff-Roos, J., Iversen, R., & Damgaard, P. (1993). Pushing method in the expulsive phase of labor: A randomized trial. *Acta Obstetricia et Gynecologica Scandinavica, 72*(1), 31–35.

Pascoe, J. M. (1993). Social support during labor and duration of labor: A community based study. *Public Health Nursing, 10*(2), 97–99.

Paterson, C. M., Saunders, N. S., & Wadsworth, J. (1992). The characteristics of the second stage of labor in 25,069 singleton deliveries in the North West Thames Health Region, 1988. *British Journal of Obstetrics and Gynaecology, 99*(5), 377–380.

Peleg, D., Kennedy, C. M., Merrill, D., & Zlatnik, F. J. (1999). Risk of repetition of a severe perineal laceration. *Obstetrics and Gynecology, 93*(6), 1021–1024.

Penney, D. S., & Perlis, D. W. (1992). Shoulder dystocia: When to use suprapubic or fundal pressure. *MCN, The American Journal of Maternal Child Nursing, 17*(1), 34–36.

Persson-Kjerstadius, N., Forsgren, H., & Westgren, M. (1999). Intrapartum amnioinfusion in women with oligohydramnios: A prospective randomized trial. *Acta Obstetricia et Gynecologica Scandinavica, 78*(2), 116–119.

Petrou, S., Coyle, D., & Fraser, W. D. for the PEOPLE (Pushing Early or Pushing Late with Epidural) Study Group. (2000). Cost-effectiveness of a delayed pushing policy for patients with epidural anesthesia. *American Journal of Obstetrics and Gynecology, 182*(5), 1156–1164.

Phelan, J. P., Korst, L. M., & Settles, D. K. (1998). Uterine activity patterns in uterine rupture: A case-control study. *Obstetrics and Gynecology, 92*(3), 394–397.

Pierce, J., Gaudier, F. L. & Sanchez-Ramos, L. (2000). Intrapartum amnioinfusion for meconium-stained fluid: Meta-analysis of prospective clinical trials. *Obstetrics and Gynecology, 95*(6, Pt. 2)., 1051–1056.

Plaut, M. M., Schwartz, M. L., & Lubarsky, S. L. (1999). Uterine rupture associated with use of misoprostol in the gravid patient with a previous cesarean section. *American Journal of Obstetrics and Gynecology, 180*(6, Pt. 1), 1535–1542.

Pressman, E. K., & Blakemore, K. J. (1996). A prospective randomized trial of two solutions for intrapartum amnioinfusion: Effects on fetal electrolytes, osmolality, and acid-base status. *American Journal of Obstetrics and Gynecology, 175*(4, Pt. 1), 945–949.

Rageth, J. C., Juzi, C., & Grossenbacher, H. (1999). Delivery after previous cesarean: A risk evaluation. *Obstetrics and Gynecology, 93*(3), 332–337.

Raskin, K. S., Dachauer, J. D., Doeden, A. L., & Rayburn, W. F. (1999). Uterine rupture after use of a prostaglandin E_2 insert during vaginal birth after cesarean. *Journal of Reproductive Medicine, 44*(6), 571–574.

Rayburn, W. F., Tassone, S., & Pearman, C. (2000). Is Cervidil appropriate for outpatient cervical ripening? *Obstetrics and Gynecology, 95*(4, Suppl. 1), S63.

Rayburn, W. F., Records, J., & Swanson, K. (1996). Prelabor cervical ripening with prostaglandin E_2 gel and other agents. *Hospital Pharmacist Report, November* (Suppl.), 1–12.

Reichert, J. A., Baron, M., & Fawcett, J. (1993). Changes in attitudes toward cesarean birth. *Journal of Obstetric, Gynecologic, and Neonatal Nursing, 22*(2), 159–167.

Renfrew, M. J., Hannah, W., Albers, L., & Floyd, E. (1998). Practices that minimize trauma to the genital tract in childbirth: A systematic review of the literature. *Birth, 25*(3), 143–160.

Riskin-Mashiah, S., & Wilkins, I. (1999). Cervical ripening. *Obstetrics and Gynecology Clinics of North America, 26*(2), 243–257.

Roberts, J. E., Goldstein, S. A., Gruener, J. S., Maggio, M., & Mendez-Bauer, C. (1987). A descriptive analysis of involuntary bearing-down efforts during the expulsive phase of labor. *Journal of Obstetric, Gynecologic, and Neonatal Nursing, 16*(1), 48–55.

Roberts, J. (1980). Alternative positions for childbirth. Part II: Second stage of labor. *Journal of Nurse Midwifery, 25*(5), 13–19.

Roberts, J., & Woolley, D. (1996). A second look at the second stage of labor. *Journal of Obstetric, Gynecologic, and Neonatal Nursing, 25*(5), 415–423.

Rogers, R., Gilson, G. J., Miller, A. C., Izquierdo, L. E., Curet, L. B., & Qualls, C. R. (1997). Active management of labor: Does it make a difference? *American Journal of Obstetrics and Gynecology, 177*(3), 599–605.

Rojansky, N., Tanos, V., Reubinoff, B., Shapira, S., & Weinstein, D. (1997). Effect of epidural analgesia on duration and outcome of induced labor. *International Journal of Gynaecology and Obstetrics, 56*(3), 237–244.

Rommal, C. (1996). Risk management issues in the perinatal setting. *Journal of Perinatal and Neonatal Nursing, 10*(3), 1–31.

Rommal, C. (1999). *Nursing policy on fundal pressure.* Los Angeles: Farmers Insurance Group, Healthcare Professional Liability Division.

Rooks, J. P., Weatherby, N. L., & Ernst, E. K. (1992). The national birth center study. Intrapartum and immediate postpartum and neonate care, part II. *Journal of Nurse Midwifery, 37*(5), 301–330.

Rosen, M. G., Dickinson, J. C., & Westhoff, C. L. (1991). Vaginal birth after cesarean: A meta-analysis of morbidity and mortality. *Obstetrics and Gynecology, 77*(3), 465–470.

Rothman, B. K. (1993). The active management of physicians. *Birth, 20*(3), 158–159.

Rouben, D., & Arias, F. (1993). A randomized trial of extraamniotic saline infusion plus intracervical Foley catheter balloon versus prostaglandin E_2 vaginal gel for ripening the cervix and inducing labor in patients with unfavorable cervices. *Obstetrics and Gynecology, 82*(2), 290–294.

Rouse, C. L., & MacNeil, J. (2000). Should there be policies to restrict visitors during labor and birth? *MCN, The American Journal of Maternal Child Nursing, 25*(1), 8–9.

Rozenberg, P., Goffinet, F., & Hessabi, M. (2000). Comparison of the Bishop score, ultrasonographically measured cervical length, and fetal fibronectin assay in predicting time until delivery and type of delivery at term. *American Journal of Obstetrics and Gynecology, 182*(1, Pt. 1), 108–113.

Russell, J. G. (1982). The rationale of primitive delivery positions. *British Journal of Obstetrics and Gynaecology, 89*(9), 712–715.

Ryding, E. L., Wijma, B., & Wijma, K. (1997). Posttraumatic stress reactions after emergency cesarean section. *Acta Obstetricia et Gynecologica Scandinavica, 76*(9), 856–861.

Sampselle, C. M., & Hines, S. (1999). Spontaneous pushing during birth: Relationship to perineal outcomes. *Journal of Nurse-Midwifery, 44*(1), 36–39.

Sandberg, E. C. (1999). The Zavanelli maneuver: 12 years of recorded experience. *Obstetrics and Gynecology, 93*(2), 312–317.

Schmidt, J. (1997). Fluid check. Making the case for intrapartum amnioinfusion. *AWHONN Lifelines, 1*(5), 46–51.

Sciscione, A. C., Nguyen, L., Manley, J. S., Shlossman, P. A., & Colmorgen, G. H. (1998). Uterine rupture during preinduction cervical ripening with misoprostol in a patient with a previous cesarean delivery. *Australian and New Zealand Journal of Obstetrics and Gynaecology, 38*(1), 96–97.

Seeds, J. W., & Walsh, M. (1996). Malpresentations. In S. G. Gabbe, J. R. Niebyl, & J. L. Simpson (Eds.), *Obstetrics: Normal and problem pregnancies* (3rd ed., pp. 469–498). New York: Churchill Livingstone.

Seitchik, J., Amico, J., Robinson, A. G., & Castillo, M. (1984). Oxytocin augmentation of dysfunctional labor. IV. Oxytocin pharmacokinetics. *American Journal of Obstetrics and Gynecology, 150*(3), 225–228.

Seitchik, J., & Castillo, M. (1982). Oxytocin augmentation of dysfunctional labor. I. Clinical data. *American Journal of Obstetrics and Gynecology, 144*(8), 899–905.

Seitchik, J., & Castillo, M. (1983). Oxytocin augmentation of dysfunctional labor. III. Multiparous patients. *American Journal of Obstetrics and Gynecology, 145*(7), 777–780.

Sellers, S. M., Hodgson, H. T., Mitchell, M. D., Anderson, A. B., & Turnbull, A. C. (1980). Release of prostaglandins after amniotomy is not mediated by oxytocin. *British Journal of Obstetrics and Gynaecology, 87*(1), 43–46.

Shermer R. H., & Raines, D. A. (1997). Positioning during the second stage of labor: Moving back to basics. *Journal of Obstetric, Gynecologic, and Neonatal Nursing, 26*(6), 727–734.

Shipman, M. K., Boniface, D. R., Tefft, M. E., & McCloghry, F. (1997). Antenatal perineal massage and subsequent perineal outcomes: A randomised controlled trial. *British Journal of Obstetrics and Gynaecology, 104*(7), 787–791.

Shyken, J. M., & Petrie, R. H. (1995a). Oxytocin to induce labor. *Clinical Obstetrics and Gynecology, 38*(2), 232–245.

Shyken, J. M., & Petrie, R. H. (1995b). The use of oxytocin. *Clinics in Perinatology, 22*(4), 907–931.

Simkin, P. (1982). Preparing parents for the second stage. *Birth, 9*(4), 229.

Simpson, K. R. (1999). Shoulder dystocia: Nursing interventions and risk management strategies. *MCN, The American Journal of Maternal Child Nursing, 24*(6), 305–311.

Simpson, K. R., & Knox, G. E. (2001). Fundal pressure during the second stage of labor: Clinical issues and risk management perspectives. *MCN, The American Journal of Maternal Child Nursing, 26*(2), 75–84.

Simpson, K. R., & Poole, J. H. (1998a). *Cervical Ripening, and Induction and Augmentation of Labor* (AWHONN Symposium). Washington, DC: Association of Women's Health, Obstetric and Neonatal Nurses.

Simpson, K. R., & Poole, J. H. (1998b). Labor induction and augmentation: Knowing when and how to assist women in labor. *AWHONN Lifelines 2*(6), 39–42.

Sleutel, M., & Golden, S. S. (1999). Fasting in labor: Relic or requirement. *Journal of Obstetric, Gynecologic and Neonatal Nursing, 28*(5), 507–512.

Sommer, P. A., Norr, K., & Roberts, J. (2000). Clinical decision-making regarding intravenous hydration in normal labor in a birth center setting. *Journal of Midwifery and Women's Health, 45*(2), 114–121.

Stamp, G. E. (1997). Care of the perineum in the second stage of labour: A study of the views and practices of Australian midwives. *Midwifery, 13*(2), 100–104.

Stringer, J. L. (1996). *Basic concepts in pharmacology*. St. Louis: McGraw-Hill.

Strong, T. H., Jr. (1997). The effect of amnioinfusion on the duration of labor. *Obstetrics and Gynecology, 89*(6), 1044–1046.

Summers, L. (1997). Methods of cervical ripening and labor induction. *Journal of Nurse-Midwifery, 42*(2), 71–85.

Sultatos, L. G. (1997). Mechanisms of drugs that affect uterine motility. *Journal of Nurse-Midwifery, 42*(4), 367–370.

Thorp, J. A., & Breedlove, G. (1996). Epidural analgesia in labor: An evaluation of risks and benefits. *Birth, 23*(2), 63–83.

Thomson, A. M. (1993). Pushing techniques in the second stage of labour. *Journal of Advanced Nursing, 18*(2), 171–177.

Towner, D., Castro, M. A., Eby-Wilkens, E., & Gilbert W. M. (1999). Effect of mode of delivery in nulliparous women on neonatal intracranial injury. *New England Journal of Medicine, 341*(23), 1704–1709.

Trofatter, K. F., Jr. (1992). Cervical ripening. *Clinical Obstetrics and Gynecology, 35*(3), 476–486.

Tucker, S. M. (2000). *Pocket guide to fetal monitoring and assessment* (4th ed.). St. Louis: Mosby.

Tubridy, N., & Redmond, J. M. T. (1996). Neurological symptoms attributed to epidural analgesia in labour: An observational study of seven cases. *British Journal of Obstetrics and Gynaecology, 103*(8), 832–833.

Ulmsten, U. (1997). Onset and forces of term labor. *Acta Obstetricia et Gynecologica Scandinavica, 76*(6), 499–514.

Vaughan, K. O. (1937). *Safe childbirth: The three essentials*. London: Ballière, Tindall & Cox.

Vause, S., Congdon, H. M., & Thornton, J. G. (1998). Immediate and delayed pushing in the second stage of labour for nulliparous women with epidural analgesia: A randomized controlled trial. *British Journal of Obstetrics and Gynaecology, 105*(5), 186–188.

Ventura, S. J., Martin, J. A., Curtin, S. C., Mathews, T. J., & Park, M. M. (2000). Births: Final data for 1998. *National Vital Statistics Report, 48*(3), 1–100.

Washburne, J. F., Chauhan, S. P., Magann, E. F., Rhodes, P. G., Naef, R. W., III, & Morrison, J. C. (1996). Neonatal electrolyte response to amnioinfusion with lactated Ringer's solution vs. normal saline. *Journal of Reproductive Medicine, 41*(10), 741–744.

Wasserstrum, N. (1992). Issues in fluid management during labor: General considerations. *Clinical Obstetrics and Gynecology, 35*(3), 505–513.

Wing, D. A., Lovett, K., & Paul, R. H. (1998). Disruption of prior uterine incision following misoprostol for labor induction in women with previous cesarean delivery. *Obstetrics and Gynecology, 91*(5, Pt. 2), 828–830.

Wing, D. A., & Paul, R. H. (1999a). Misoprostol for cervical ripening and labor induction: The clinician's perspective and guide to success. *Contemporary OB/GYN, 44*(4), 46–61.

Wing, D. A., & Paul, R. H. (1999b). Vaginal birth after cesarean section: Selection and management. *Clinical Obstetrics and Gynecology, 42*(4), 836–848.

Winkler, M., & Rath, W. (1999). A risk-benefit assessment of oxytocics in obstetric practice. *Drug Safety, 20*(4), 323–345.

Wood, C., Ng, K., Hounslow, D., & Benning, H. (1973). The influences of differences of birth times upon fetal condition in normal deliveries. *Journal of Obstetrics and Gynaecology of the British Commonwealth, 80*(4), 289–294.

Yeast, J. D., Jones, A., & Poskin, M. (1999). Induction of labor and the relationship to cesarean delivery: A review of 7001 consecutive inductions. *American Journal of Obstetrics and Gynecology, 180*(3, Pt. 1), 628–633.

Zeeman, G. G., Khan-Dawood, F. S., & Dawood, M. Y. (1997). Oxytocin and its receptor in pregnancy and parturition: Current concepts and clinical implications. *Obstetrics and Gynecology, 89*(5, Pt. 1), 873–883.

Zieman, M., Fong, S. K., Benowitz, N. L., Banskter, D., & Darney, P. D. (1997). Absorption kinetics of misoprostol with oral or vaginal administration. *American Journal of Obstetrics and Gynecology, 90*(1), 88–92.

Zelop, C., Shipp, T., Cohen, A., Repke, J. T., & Lieberman, E. (2000). Outcomes of trial of labor following previous cesarean beyond the estimated date of delivery. *Obstetrics and Gynecology, 94*(4, Suppl. 1), S79.

Zetterstrom, J., Lopez, A., Anzen, B., Norman, M., Holmstrom, B., & Mellgren, A. (1999). Anal sphincter tears at vaginal delivery: Risk factors and clinical outcome of primary repair. *Obstetrics and Gynecology, 94*(1), 21–28.

APPENDIX 9A

Admission Assessment

Admission date: ____ / ____ / ____ Time: _______ a.m. / p.m.
Name patient wishes to be addressed by: ______________________ Support person/relationship: ______________________
Arrived by: ☐ Ambulatory ☐ Wheelchair ☐ Cart
Childbirth preparation: ☐ None ☐ Lamaze ☐ Refresher ☐ Cesarean ☐ PCH Instructor ______________________
Reason for admission:
☐ Labor ☐ R/O labor ☐ Induction ☐ Cesarean: ☐ Primary ☐ Repeat ☐ Delivered prior to admission
☐ ROM ☐ Vaginal bleeding ☐ Other ______________________

GRAV	TERM	PREM	ABORTION Spont. Induced:	LIVING	ECTOPIC	MULT. BIRTHS	STILLBORN Term: Prem:	NEONATAL DEATHS: Term: Prem.	LMP	EDC	GEST. IN WEEKS

INITIAL EVALUATION: Vital Signs: Temp ______ Pulse ______ Resp ______ B/P ______
Weight: Present __________ Prepregnant __________ #Gain __________ Height: __________ Wt. Kilos __________
FHT: ______________ ☐ reg. ☐ irreg. Blood Type/Rh ______________
Last Meal: ____ / ____ / ____ at _____ a.m. / p.m. ☐ Fluids ☐ Solids

VAGINAL EXAM
☐ None
☐ Sterile Vaginal Exam
☐ Sterile Speculum
Dilation __________
Effacement __________
CERVIX
☐ Posterior
☐ Midposition
☐ Anterior
CONSISTENCY
☐ Firm
☐ Soft
Station __________
☐ Ballotable

MEMBRANES
☐ Intact
☐ Ruptured
__________ __________
Date Time
☐ Leaking
COLOR
☐ Clear
☐ Bloody
☐ Meconium
☐ Other __________
AMOUNT
☐ Small
☐ Medium
☐ Large
ODOR
☐ Normal
☐ Foul
NITRAZINE
☐ Negative
☐ Positive
☐ Inconclusive

PRESENTATION
☐ NA
☐ Vertex
☐ Brow
☐ Face
☐ Transverse
☐ Indeterminate
☐ Other __________
BREECH
☐ Frank
☐ Complete
☐ Footling

CONTRACTIONS
☐ NA
☐ Absent
☐ Present
____
Date & Time Began
☐ Regular
☐ Irregular
Frequency __________ mins.
Duration __________ secs.
INTENSITY
☐ Mild
☐ Moderate
☐ Strong
☐ Uterus relaxed between contractions

VAGINAL BLEEDING
☐ None
☐ Spotting
☐ Blood show
☐ Frank bleeding
☐ Associated w/ abdominal pain

SPECIAL PROCEDURES
☐ None
☐ NST
☐ OCT
☐ Ultrasound
☐ Amnio.
☐ Biophysical profile
☐ Prenatal Rhogam: Date: __________
☐ Cervical Cultures: Result: __________

____

Fetal Activity: ☐ Present ☐ Diminished ☐ Absent
Prenatal Care: ☐ Yes ☐ No Date began: ____ / ____ / ____
OB Complications/hospitalizations during this pregnancy: ______________________
____
____
____

Type of pain management discussed with M.D.:
____
____
____

PALOS COMMUNITY HOSPITAL
PALOS HEIGHTS, ILLINOIS

ADMISSION ASSESSMENT

P-566
85642
Rev. 11/99

REVIEW OF SYSTEMS:

Skin

Temperature
☐ Warm
☐ Hot
☐ Cool

Turgor
☐ Good
☐ Fair
☐ Poor

Humidity
☐ Dry
☐ Diaphoretic
☐ Clammy

Color
☐ Pink ☐ Flushed
☐ Pale ☐ Cyanotic
☐ Rash ________________
☐ Other ________________

Respiratory
☐ No distress ☐ Dyspnea
☐ Cough ☐ Orthopnea
☐ Dry ☐ Shallow
☐ Productive

Breath Sounds
☐ Clear
☐ Diminished
☐ Equal/bilateral
☐ Unequal
☐ Other ________________

Urinary
☐ Asymptomatic
☐ Urgency
☐ Burning

Protein ____________
Glucose ____________
Ketones ____________

CVAT (if applicable)
Right: ☐ Neg. ☐ Pos.
Left: ☐ Neg ☐ Pos

Cardiovascular
☐ Asymptomatic
☐ Chest pain
☐ Palpitations

Lower extremities
☐ Asymptomatic

Calf Circumference (if applicable)
Right _____cm Left _____cm

Peripheral Pulses (if applicable)
☐ Palpable bilaterally and equal
☐ Other ____________________

☐ Pitting edema
☐ 1 + 2mm ☐ 3 + 6mm
☐ 2 + 4mm ☐ 4 + 8mm

Quantitative edema
☐ 1+ Minimal edema of the pedal & pretibial areas
☐ 2+ Marked edema of the lower extremities
☐ 3+ Edema of the face and hands, lower abdominal wall and sacrum
☐ 4+ Anasarca (Generalized massive edema) & ascites

Homan's Sign
Right: ☐ Neg. ☐ Pos.
Left: ☐ Neg ☐ Pos.

DTR's

Right	Left
_____ + 1	_____ + 1
_____ + 2	_____ + 2
_____ + 3	_____ + 3
_____ + 4	_____ + 4

Musculoskeletal
☐ Asymptomatic
☐ Limitation in ROM ________________
☐ Pain ☐ Weakness
☐ Stiffness ☐ Swelling

Gastrointestinal
☐ Asymptomatic
☐ Nausea
☐ Vomiting
☐ Diarrhea
☐ Constipation
☐ Hemorrhoids

Abdomen
☐ Soft ☐ Gravid ☐ Distended
☐ Hard ☐ Firm

Bowel Sounds (if applicable)
☐ Present
☐ Absent
☐ Hyperactive
☐ Hypoactive

Neurologic
☐ Asymptomatic ☐ Syncope
☐ Headache ☐ Dizziness
☐ Visual disturbance

Behavior
☐ Appropriate/cooperative
☐ Apprehensive
☐ Demanding
☐ Lethargic
☐ Uncooperative
☐ Flat affect

Nutrition Screen
☐ Hyperemesis*
☐ Gestational Diabetes* (admitted during pregnancy not for labor)
☐ Diabetes*

Special diet
☐ Low Sodium* ☐ Vegetarian*
☐ Other* ____________________
☐ History of eating disorder*
☐ WIC/Food stamps* ☐ Substance abuse*
☐ Body Mass Index <19*
☐ Body Mass Index > 29**
☐ Gestational Diabetes** (admitted for Labor)

*** if an indicator is checked, consult Dietary**
**** if an indicator is checked, provide patient w/handouts for Outpatient Nutrition services**

Discharge Planning/Teaching Assessment

Are there any spiritual, emotional, cultural or other needs we can help you with during your stay? ☐ Yes ☐ No
If yes, please specify: ____

Other than information concerning infant care and self care, do you anticipate having any other discharge needs? ☐ Yes ☐ No
If yes, please specify: ____

Referrals will be made to: ☐ None at this time ☐ Social Service ☐ Dietary ☐ Pastoral Care ☐ Other ____________________

Prosthetics: ☐ None ☐ Glasses ☐ Contact lenses: ☐ hard ☐ soft ☐ extended wear ☐ Other ____________________
Dentures: ☐ None ☐ upper ☐ lower ☐ partial ☐ Other ____________________
Orientation: ☐ Call system ☐ Bed controls ☐ Visiting ☐ Smoking ☐ TV ☐ Phone ☐ Single room maternity care ☐ Inpatient classes ☐ Patient Handbook
Feeding Method: ☐ Breast ☐ Bottle

Signature: ____

APPENDIX 9B

Labor Flow Sheet

INTAKE	00	2	4	6	8	10	12	14	16	18	20	22	24
IV													
50cc syringe with 60 units of oxytocin in 1000cc LR													
IV													
PO													
8° TOTAL IN													

OUTPUT	00	2	4	6	8	10	12	14	16	18	20	22	24
Urine/voided													
Urine/catheter													
Emesis													
8° TOTAL OUT													

24° TOTALS	PO INTAKE	IV INTAKE	URINE OUTPUT	OTHER OUTPUT

CERVICAL DILATION Cm (O): 10, 9, 8, 7, 6, 5, 4, 3, 2, 1

STATION (X): −3, −2, −1, 0, +1, +2, +3, +4, +5

Efface-ment

Hour of Labor: 1 2 3 4 5 6 7 8 9 10 11 12 13 14 15 16 17 18 19 20 21

TIME→

PROCEDURES	DATE	TIME	INITIALS
SROM			
AROM by			
Amniotic Fluid	Amount		
	Color		
F.S.E. by			
IUPC by			
Epidural by			
Amnioinfusion			
Other			
IV started			
Needle size/length	Site		
Tolerated well ❑ Yes ❑ No	Labeled ❑ Tubing ❑ Site		

SPECIMEN COLLECTED	
Date/Time	Specimen / Lab Test

INITIALS	SIGNATURE	PRINT NAME

ADDRESSOGRAPH

LABOR FLOW SHEET

ST. JOHN'S MERCY MEDICAL CENTER/ST. LOUIS, MO

Form #422 (Rev. 9/98)

FETAL HEART RATE

BASELINE VARIABILITY
Ab = Absent
Min = ≤ 5 bpm
Mod = 6-25 bpm
Mark = > 25 bpm

PERIODIC PATTERN
L = Late
V = Variable
E = Early
A = Accelerations

* Refer to DAILY NURSES'

PAIN SCALE

1 = None
3 = Mild
5 = Tolerable
7 = Moderate
10 = Severe

CONTRACTIONS

FREQUENCY In Minutes
I = Irregular
Ø = Absent

INTENSITY
M = Mild
Mod = Moderate
S = Strong

MONITOR MODE

E = External
I = Internal
D = Doppler

POSITION

R = Right lateral
L = Left lateral
T = Trendelenberg
SF = Semi Fowlers
C = Chair
HF = High Fowlers

* Indicates further documentation in DAILY NURSES' NOTES

Date / Time														
Temperature														
Pulse														
Respiration														
Blood Pressure														
FHR – Monitor Mode														
FHR – Baseline FHR														
FHR – Baseline Variability														
FHR – Periodic Pattern														
Contractions – Frequency														
Contractions – Duration														
Contractions – Intensity														
Pitocin mu/min.														
Vaginal Exam – Exam by														
Vaginal Exam – Dilatation														
Vaginal Exam – Effacement														
Vaginal Exam – Station														
Position														
Activity														
Response to Labor														
Affect														
Comfort Measures														
Oxygen														
$MgSO_4$ grams/hr														
Pain Assessment														
Initials														

Allergies:

Medication and Patient's Response												
Date/ Time												

RESPONSE TO LABOR

Ø	= Unaware of contractions
T	= Talking through contractions
BW	= Breathing well through contractions
CN	= Coaching necessary to maintain controlled breathing
UP	= Urge to push
PC	= Pushing w/contractions
LD	= Laboring Down

AFFECT

R	= Relaxed
A	= Apprehensive
F	= Fatigued
U	= Uncomfortable

ACTIVITY

S	= Sleeping
TV	= Watching TV
T	= Talking
BP	= On bed pan
BR	= Bathroom
A	= Ambulating
B	= Bedrest

COMFORT MEASURES

R	= Reassurance and encouragement given
P	= Pericare
CP	= Counter pressure
H_2O	= Shower/Tub

Date / Time													
Temperature													
Pulse													
Respiration													
Blood Pressure													
FHR	Monitor Mode												
	Baseline FHR												
	Baseline Variability												
	Periodic Pattern												
Contractions	Frequency												
	Duration												
	Intensity												
Pitocin mu/min.													
Vaginal Exam	Exam by												
	Dilatation												
	Effacement												
	Station												
Position													
Activity													
Response to Labor													
Affect													
Comfort Measures													
Oxygen													
$MgSO_4$ grams/hr													
Pain Assessment													
Initials													

Medication and Patient's Response												
Date/ Time												

QUANTITATIVE DEGREE OF EDEMA
1+ = Minimal edema of the pedal & pretibial areas
2+ = Marked edema of the lower extremities
3+ = Edema of the face and hands, lower abdominal wall & sacrum
4+ = Anasarca (Generalized massive edema) & ascites

DEEP TENDON REFLEXES
4+ = Very brisk or hyperactive, Clonus may be present
3+ = Brisk, somewhat more increased than normal
2+ = Normal
1+ = Hypoactive, depressed
⊖ = Absent

CLONUS
+ = Present/Positive
⊖ = Absent/Negative
Clonus = # of beats

DEGREE OF PITTING EDEMA
1+ = 2 mm
2+ = 4 mm
3+ = 6 mm
4+ = 8 mm

BREATH SOUNDS
E = Equal
Cl = Clear
Rh = Rhonchi
R = Rales
D = Diminished

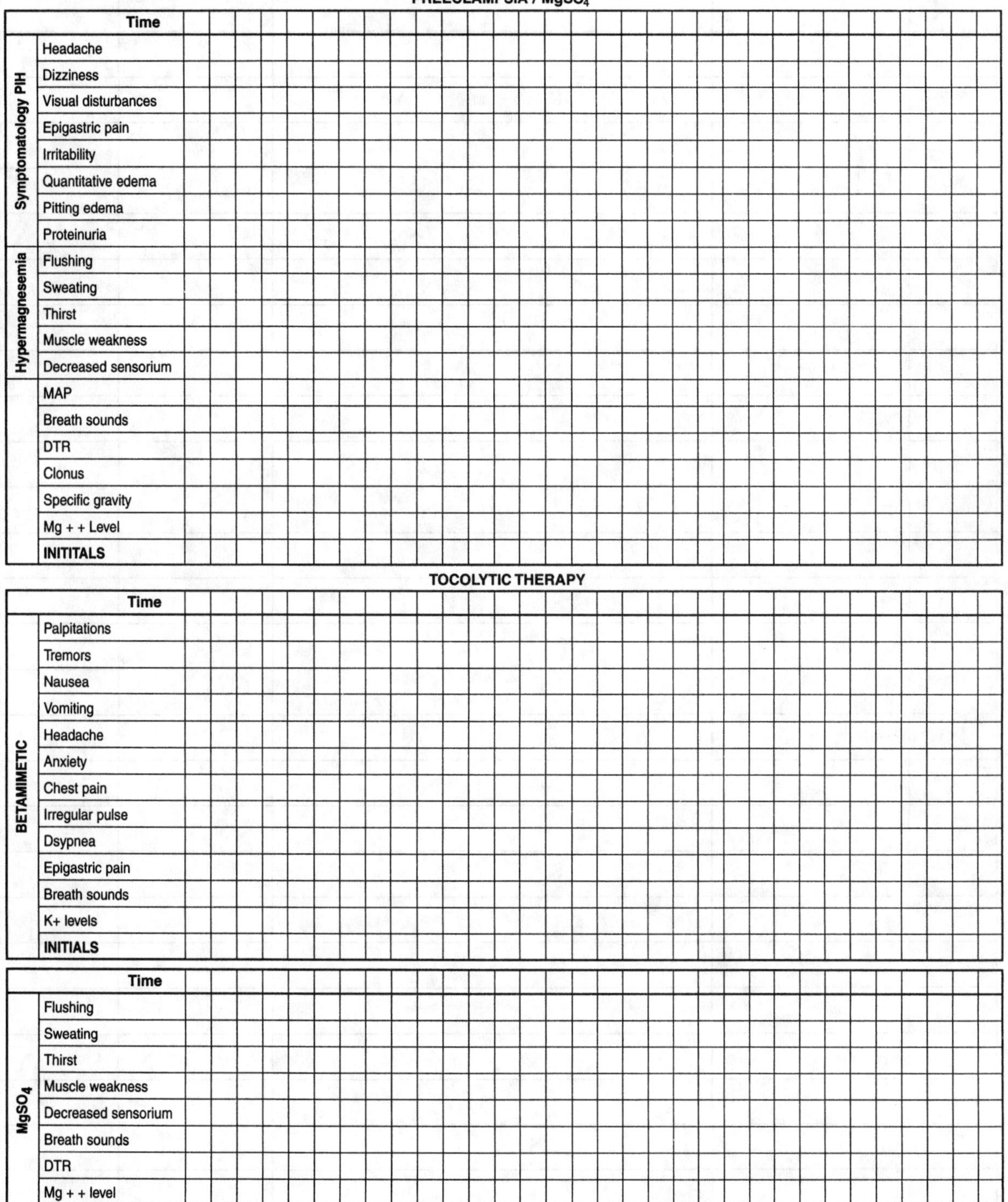

PREECLAMPSIA / $MgSO_4$

	Time																															
Symptomatology PIH	Headache																															
	Dizziness																															
	Visual disturbances																															
	Epigastric pain																															
	Irritability																															
	Quantitative edema																															
	Pitting edema																															
	Proteinuria																															
Hypermagnesemia	Flushing																															
	Sweating																															
	Thirst																															
	Muscle weakness																															
	Decreased sensorium																															
	MAP																															
	Breath sounds																															
	DTR																															
	Clonus																															
	Specific gravity																															
	Mg + + Level																															
	INITITALS																															

TOCOLYTIC THERAPY

	Time																															
BETAMIMETIC	Palpitations																															
	Tremors																															
	Nausea																															
	Vomiting																															
	Headache																															
	Anxiety																															
	Chest pain																															
	Irregular pulse																															
	Dsypnea																															
	Epigastric pain																															
	Breath sounds																															
	K+ levels																															
	INITIALS																															

	Time																															
$MgSO_4$	Flushing																															
	Sweating																															
	Thirst																															
	Muscle weakness																															
	Decreased sensorium																															
	Breath sounds																															
	DTR																															
	Mg + + level																															
	INITIALS																															

Time	Physician	Notified Of	Orders Yes / No	Initials

Date ____________________

Postpartum Observation

Time	Temp	B / P	Pulse	Resp.	Fundus	Lochia	Epis: Dressing	Intake	Output	Initials

POST ANESTHESIA RECOVERY SCORE

	CRITERIA	SCORE	DISCHARGE
CONSCIOUSNESS	Fully awake	2	
	Arousable on calling	1	
	Not responding	0	
NEUROMUSCULAR ACTIVITY	Move 4 extremities	2	
	Move 2 extremities	1	
	Move 0 extremities	0	
SENSATION	Normal	2	
	None below pubis	1	
	None below xiphoid	0	
CIRCULATION	B/P 10-20mmHg ± admission	2	
	B/P 10-50mmHg ± admission	1	
	B/P > 51mmHg ± admission	0	
RESPIRATION	Deep breathing or cough	2	
	Dyspnea	1	
	Apnea	0	
COLOR	Pink	2	
	Pale, blotchy, jaundiced, other	1	
	Cyanotic	0	
	Total		
Signature:	Date: Time		

MEDICATIONS

Time	Drug / Dose / Route	Initials

Transfer to PP Room Notes: Room # ____________

Discharge Nurse ______________________________ Receiving Nurse ______________________________

Transported by: w/c or cart Mobility ____________________________ Time of report ____________________

Birth certificate / papers given ______________ Call light in reach ______________ Side rails up x2 ______________

Care and instructions: Initial if done

Bath; pericare done ______ Tucks applied ________

Ice pack applied: perineum / abdomen Informed re: ask for help up x2 ______

IV site assessed _______ IV dc'd________ Encouraged to TCDB ______

Foley patent and taped to ❑ Left ❑ Right leg Other: ________________

Addressograph

APPENDIX 9 C

Cervical Ripening and Induction of Labor Analysis

CERVICAL RIPENING AND INDUCTION OF LABOR ANALYSIS

Patient Name____ Date______________________

Please place a "P" by primary reason - check all other reasons

A. INDICATIONS BASED ON GESTATION

___40 0/7 wks-40 6/7 wks ___41 0/7 wks-41 6/7 wks ___>42 /0/7 wks Gestational age at start of induction_______

B. INDICATIONS BASED ON FETAL CONDITION (Please complete Fetal Maturity Criteria for indications with an asterisk*)

___Unstable fetal lie*
___Macrosomia*
___Isoimmunization
___Severe intrauterine growth retardation (estimated fetal weight falls below 10th percentile for gestational age)
___Other (list)____
___Fetal demise
___Fetal anomaly (list)______________

C. INDICATIONS BASED ON ANTEPARTAL FETAL TESTING

___Nonreactive nonstress test
___Positive oxytocin challenge stress test
___Positive breast stimulation contraction test
___Biophysical profile score of_____________________
___Other (list)____
___Decreased variability
___Absence of accelerations, nonreactive fetus
___Spontaneous variable or prolonged decelerations

D. INDICATIONS BASED ON MATERNAL CONDITION (Please complete Fetal Maturity Criteria for indications with an asterisk*)

___Cervical dilatation > 4 cms*
___Chorioamnionitis
___Other (list)____
___Pregnancy induced hypertension
___Diabetes mellitus

E. INDICATIONS BASED ON MEMBRANES/AMNIOTIC FLUID STATUS

___Ruptured membranes for_____hours
___Decreased amniotic fluid volume
___Oligohydramnios
___Polyhydramnios

F. INDICATIONS BASED ON LOGISTIC/OTHER FACTORS (Please complete Fetal Maturity Criteria for indications with an asterisk*)

___History of rapid labor*
___Psychosocial (list)*____
___Distance from hospital*

***FETAL MATURITY CRITERIA** (Please complete for indications with an asterisk.)

___Fetal heart tones have been documented for 20 weeks by nonelectronic fetoscope or for 30 weeks by Doppler.
___36 weeks have passed since a positive serum or urine HCG pregnancy test was performed by a reliable method.
___An US measurement of the crown-rump length, obtained at 6-12 weeks, supports a gestational age of 39 weeks or more.
___An US scan, obtained at 13-20 weeks, confirms a gestational age of 39 weeks or more determined by clinic hx and physical exam.

BISHOP SCORE The state of cervix is related to the success of labor induction. When the total cervical score exceeds 8, the likelihood of vaginal birth subsequent to labor induction is similar to that of spontaneous labor. Induction of labor with a poor cervical score has been associated with failure of induction, prolonged labor, and a high cesarean birth rate.

	Factor	0	1	2	3	
Circle	Dilatation	Closed	1-2	3-4	>5	
factors	Effacement	0 - 30%	40 - 50%	60 - 70%	>80%	
present	Station	-3	-2	-1/0	+1/+2	
at start of	Consistency	Firm	Medium	Soft	----	Total score at start
induction	Cervical position	Posterior	Mid-position	Anterior	----	of induction_____

INFORMED CONSENT

I have discussed the indications, methods, agents, risks, benefits and alternative approaches for cervical ripening and/or labor induction including the possibility of repeat induction or cesarean birth with

______________________________ and she has agreed to proceed. ______________________________ Date______________

Patient Name Physician Signature

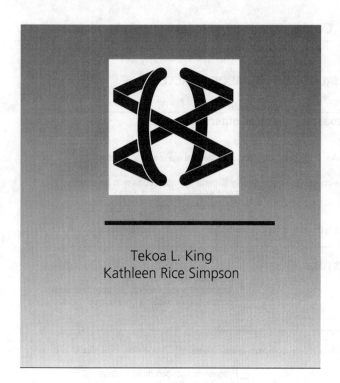

Tekoa L. King
Kathleen Rice Simpson

CHAPTER **10**

Fetal Assessment During Labor

The introduction of electronic fetal monitoring (EFM) in the late 1960s has had far-reaching effects on women's healthcare and the practice of nursing, midwifery, and medicine. Despite debate about advantages and limitations, effects on perinatal morbidity and mortality, and its role in healthcare costs and malpractice litigation, EFM is used in most labor and birth units in the United States and Canada (Curtin & Park, 1999; Parer & King, 1999; Thacker, Stroup, & Peterson, 1995). This chapter discusses the physiologic basis for fetal heart rate (FHR) monitoring, defines FHR patterns, and reviews intrapartum management of characteristic FHR patterns.

HISTORIC PERSPECTIVES

The discovery of fetal heart tones in 1821 marked the beginning of modern obstetric practice (Goodlin, 1979; Sureau, 1996). Jean Alexandre Lejumeau, Vicomte de Kergaradec, used a stethoscope hoping to hear the noise of the water in the uterus. Although he probably was not the first person to identify fetal heart tones, he was the first person astute enough to suggest in print the potential clinical uses for FHR auscultation (Sureau, 1996). In the early 1800s, researchers working independently in Switzerland, Ireland, Germany, France, and the United States described fetal heart tones, and in 1833, the British obstetrician William Kennedy published the first descriptions of "fetal distress" by describing a late deceleration and associating it with poor prognosis (Kennedy, 1833). In 1858, Schwartz of Germany suggested that the FHR be counted often during labor, between and during contractions, to promote improved outcomes. Schwartz described the association between fetal bradycardia and decreased uteroplacental blood flow during contractions. In 1849, Killian proposed forceps-assisted birth for an FHR of less than 100 beats/min or more than 180 beats/min (Goodlin, 1979). Soon after, Winckel described specific FHR criteria to be used for the diagnosis of fetal distress by auscultation (Goodlin, 1979). After invention of the fetoscope in the early 1900s, fetal heart sounds were commonly assessed to document fetal viability during the prenatal period. Winckel's criteria were used in clinical practice until the 1950s, when Hon raised concern about the subjectivity of counting heartbeats during labor.

Although interest in continuous recording of fetal heart tones by various methods dates to the later years of the 19th century, the major development of modern clinical EFM occurred during the 1960s. In 1906, Cramer produced the first electrocardiographic (ECG) recording of the fetal heartbeat (Cramer, 1906). Research using abdominal leads to obtain the fetal ECG continued but remained impractical for clinical use until the mid-1960s, when techniques capable of excluding the maternal ECG from the recording became available. By the 1950s, research on electronic methods of FHR monitoring escalated. In 1958, Hon published the first report of continuous fetal ECG monitoring using a device placed on the maternal abdomen. By the 1960s, Hon, Caldeyro-Barcia, and Hammacher were reporting successful attempts at developing an electronic FHR monitor that could continuously record FHR data (Caldeyro-Barcia, Mendez-Bauer, & Poseiro, 1966; Hammacher, 1969; Hon, 1963). Although many others have contributed to what is known about fetal assessment during labor, EFM as it is used today is largely the result of the work of these three investigators working independently on separate continents. In 1968, the first commercially available electronic fetal monitors were introduced.

Coinciding with the development of EFM technology was the emergence of data that refuted the effectiveness of intermittent auscultation with Delee or Pinard fetoscopes. The Benson, Shubeck, Deutschberger, Weiss, & Berendes (1968) study of more than 24,000 births from the Collaborative Perinatal Project concluded that FHR auscultation during labor was unreliable in determining fetal distress except in extreme cases of terminal bradycardias. Based on this report and rapid technologic advances, intermittent auscultation of the FHR between contractions was rapidly replaced with continuous EFM during the 1970s. Over the next three decades, EFM became the preferred method of fetal surveillance during the intrapartum period in the United States and Canada.

During the 1980s and 1990s, several randomized trials compared intermittent auscultation with continuous EFM (MacDonald, Grant, Sheridan-Pereira, Boylan, & Chalmers, 1985; Thacker et al., 1995; Vintzileos et al., 1993). Disappointingly, EFM did not decrease perinatal mortality or prevent cerebral palsy, and the women in the EFM groups experienced a fourfold increase in operative births (Thacker et al., 1995). The potential reasons why EFM did not demonstrate efficacy in the randomized trials are methodologic flaws, inconsistent criteria and terminology to describe fetal status, and the use of outcome variables for which there were insufficient sample sizes to determine a significant difference between intermittent auscultation and continuous EFM.

The demonstrated increase in cesarean birth rates fueled reexamination of all aspects of EFM use. In 1997, the National Institutes of Child Health and Human Development (NICHD) of the National Institutes of Health (NIH) convened a panel of FHR monitoring experts. This committee proposed detailed, quantitative, standardized definitions of FHR patterns, which can serve as a basis for determining reliability and validity of FHR monitoring (NICHD, 1997).

Clinical reliance on EFM remains high despite the lack of positive results from published research. It is the primary screening technique for the clinical determination of the adequacy of fetal oxygenation during labor (Parer, 1997). This paradox is better understood after a review of the physiology of the fetal heart and its adaptations during labor. The feelings of many clinicians about EFM compared with intermittent auscultation were summarized by Cibils in 1996:

> It is difficult to understand the premise that the intermittent recording (by a crude method) of a given biologic variable [the FHR] will be better to make a clinical decision affecting the mother and fetus than the continuous, precise recording of the same variable.

DEFINITIONS AND APPROPRIATE TERMS DESCRIBING FETAL HEART RATE PATTERNS

Appropriate clinical management of variant FHR patterns depends on the use of standardized definitions that convey accepted meanings among the members of the healthcare team. Adoption of a common language for FHR pattern interpretation and medical record documentation that is mutually agreed on and routinely used by all providers enhances interdisciplinary communication and therefore maternal–fetal safety (Knox, Simpson, & Garite, 1999). Oral communication and written documentation must accurately convey the exact level of concern and record the presumed diagnosis. The chances of miscommunication between care providers, especially during telephone conversations about fetal status, are decreased when everyone is speaking the same language (Simpson & Knox, 2000). Timely intervention during nonreassuring FHR patterns depends on clear communication between providers sharing the care of an individual patient. The NICHD (1997) nomenclature is one method used to describe FHR patterns and is the basis for the pattern descriptions in this chapter (Table 10–1).

Terms such as *stress* and *distress* are vague and lack the precise meaning needed to discriminate levels of concern. In 1998, The American College of Obstetricians and Gynecologists (ACOG) recommended that *nonreassuring fetal status* replace the term *fetal distress*. Another problem is the use of *asphyxia* or *acidosis* when making a presumptive diagnosis of intrapartum hypoxia. Asphyxia means insufficiency or absence of exchange of respiratory gases. The pathologic consequence of asphyxia is injury to the fetal tissues, primarily the brain, with subsequent neurologic impairment. However, asphyxia is a continuum of oxygen deficit that moves from hypoxemia (ie, decreased oxygen content in blood) to acidemia (ie, increased hydrogen ion concentration in blood) to acidemia (ie, increased hydrogen ion concentration in the tissue) (King & Parer, 2000; Parer, 1997). Hypoxemia and acidosis are detectable by pH measurements of fetal scalp blood or umbilical cord blood at birth. These values reveal the acid–base balance within blood but not within tissue and therefore cannot directly reveal the extent or duration of metabolic acidosis or level of asphyxia in tissue. The use of terms such as asphyxia and acidosis in medical record documentation about characteristics of the

TABLE 10–1 ■ FETAL HEART RATE CHARACTERISTICS AND PATTERNS: NICHD (1997) NOMENCLATURE

Term	Definition
Baseline rate	Mean fetal heart rate (FHR) rounded to increments of 5 bpm during a 10-minute segment excluding periodic or episodic changes, periods of marked variability, and segments of baseline that differ by >25 bpm. Duration must be ≥2 minutes.
Bradycardia	Baseline rate of <110 bpm
Tachycardia	Baseline rate of >160 bpm
Variability	Fluctuations in the baseline FHR of two cycles/min or greater
Absent variability	Amplitude from peak to trough undetectable
Minimal variability	Amplitude from peak to trough more than undetectable and ≤5 bpm
Moderate variability	Amplitude from peak to trough 6–25 bpm
Marked variability	Amplitude from peak to trough >25 bpm
Acceleration	Visually apparent abrupt increase (onset to peak is <30 sec) of FHR above baseline. Peak is ≥15 bpm. Duration is ≥15 sec and <2 min. In gestations <32 weeks, peak of 10 bpm and duration of 10 sec is an acceleration.
Prolonged acceleration	Acceleration >2 min and <10 min duration
Early deceleration	Visually apparent gradual decrease (onset to nadir is ≥30 sec) of FHR below baseline. Return to baseline associated with a uterine contraction. Nadir of deceleration occurs at the same time as the peak of the contraction. Generally, the onset, nadir, and recovery of the deceleration occur at the same time as the onset, peak, and recovery of the contraction.
Late deceleration	Visually apparent gradual decrease (onset to nadir is ≥30 sec) of FHR below baseline. Return to baseline associated with a uterine contraction. Nadir of deceleration occurs after the peak of the contraction. Generally, the onset, nadir, and recovery of the deceleration occur after the onset, peak, and recovery of the contraction.
Variable deceleration	Visually apparent abrupt decrease (onset to nadir is <30 sec) in FHR below baseline. Decrease is ≥15 bpm. Duration is ≥15 sec and <2 min.
Prolonged deceleration	Visually apparent abrupt decrease (onset to nadir is <30 sec) in FHR below baseline. Decrease is ≥15 bpm. Duration is ≥2 min but <10 min.

Adapted from National Institute of Child Health and Human Development Research Planning Workshop (1997). Electronic fetal heart rate monitoring: Research guidelines for interpretation. *American Journal of Obstetrics and Gynecology 177*(6), 1385–1390 and *Journal of Obstetric, Gynecologic and Neonatal Nursing*, (1997), 26(6) 635–640.

FHR and fetal or newborn status is inappropriate and confusing. Imprecise and inaccurate terminology used in medical record documentation can be challenging to defend if litigation follows an unpreventable adverse outcome. Documentation of intrapartum events should be descriptive and avoid the use of terms that have diagnostic meaning.

TECHNIQUES OF FETAL HEART RATE MONITORING

Assessment of Uterine Activity

During the intrapartum period, the FHR is interpreted relative to uterine activity. Interpretation of FHR patterns includes complete assessment of four components of the uterine contractions: frequency, duration, and intensity of contractions, and the uterine resting tone between contractions. These assessments can be made by palpation, external tocodynamometer (*tokos* is the Greek word for childbirth), or with an intrauterine pressure catheter (IUPC).

Assessment of uterine activity begins with palpation. Contraction frequency is measured from the beginning of one contraction to the beginning of the next and is described in minutes. Duration is the length of the contraction and is described in seconds. Intensity refers to the strength of the contraction. Intensity is described as mild, moderate, or strong by palpation or in millimeters of mercury (mmHg) if an IUPC is used. Uterine resting tone is assessed in the absence of contractions or between contractions. By direct palpation, resting tone is described as soft or hard (Feinstein & McCartney, 1997), and by IUPC, it is described in terms of mmHg. As with any procedure, the least invasive approach is preferred unless maternal–fetal status indicates a need for more objective data.

Each technique has some limitation. Intensity cannot be determined with a tocodynamometer. The tocodynamometer detects pressure changes from the tightening of the fundus during contractions through the maternal abdomen. This technique gives a fairly accurate reading of the duration and frequency of contractions but is unable to assess intensity or resting tone. With an IUPC, the peak of the contraction as indicated on the fetal monitor tracing depicts the actual strength of the contraction measured in mmHg of pressure within the amnionic fluid. The IUPC is most accurate because direct measurement of intraamniotic pressure is recorded, but it requires ruptured membranes for insertion.

After the frequency, duration, intensity, and resting tone have been determined, the adequacy of uterine activity can be assessed. Normal contraction frequency in the active phase of labor is every 2 to 3 minutes. Some uterine activity patterns are dysfunctional or inadequate for generating progress in labor (Fig. 10–1).

Various definitions of hyperstimulation have been described in the literature. For the purposes of this chapter, *hyperstimulation* is defined as contractions of normal duration occurring within 1 minute of each other, a series of single contractions lasting 2 minutes or more, or a contraction frequency of five or more in 10 minutes (ACOG, 1995a, 1999). Although hyperstimulation can be spontaneous as a result of endogenous maternal oxytocin or prostaglandins, it is more often seen during exogenous stimulation with agents used in cervical ripening and induction and augmentation of labor. Hyperstimulation can cause decreased uteroplacental blood flow and precipitate FHR decelerations. If hyperstimulation occurs during oxytocin administration, the infusion should be decreased or discontinued until the uterine contraction pattern returns to normal to avoid progression to nonreassuring fetal status. If decelerations occur during oxytocin administration and uterine contractions are determined to be too frequent, the infusion should be decreased or discontinued until the FHR decelerations resolve and the uterine contraction pattern returns to normal frequency. After FHR pattern characteristics indicate fetal recovery, resuming the oxytocin at a lower rate of infusion may be the only intervention necessary. If a similar adverse clinical situation occurs with the use of other pharmacologic agents used to ripen the cervix or stimulate contractions that may require repeated dosing (e.g. Cervidil, Prepidil, or misoprostol), the next dose should be delayed until the FHR is reassuring and the uterine contraction pattern returns to normal frequency. *Coupling* or *tripling* refers to a pattern of two or three contractions with little or no interval, followed by a regular interval of 2 to 5 minutes. This is a common pattern early in labor and does not usually initiate FHR responses.

External Doppler Versus Fetal Scalp Electrode

The FHR can be detected with a Doppler ultrasound transducer or fetal electrode. Leopold's maneuvers are used to determine the fetal position before applying the Doppler transducer (see Chapter 9). The Doppler transducer is affixed to the maternal abdomen over the fetal back or chest and transmits a high-frequency ultrasound. A gel is applied to the transducer to help eliminate air between the transducer and maternal abdomen. The ultrasound wave does not conduct to the fetus if there is air between the emission of the wave and the object it is reflecting off. The transducer detects the ultrasound wave that is bounced back off the fetal heart and then counts the FHR by measuring the change in ultrasound wave frequency that occurs when the waveform is reflected off the moving heart (Fig. 10–2).

The monitor counts the time interval between each beat detected, calculates a rate based on that interval and then plots each calculated rate on the paper that is moving at 3 cm/min. The monitor recounts the FHR every one to two beats. Because there is variability in the time interval between each beat in a normally oxygenated fetus, the line produced over time has a jagged appearance that results from the different rates recorded. Early Doppler technology tended to exaggerate the FHR variability, but improvements in technology have resulted in a Doppler recording that sufficiently reflects the true variability in the FHR under observation. Although the Doppler is easy to apply, maternal or fetal movement, uterine contractions, or maternal positions can interrupt a continuous recording.

The direct fetal scalp electrode (FSE) is the most accurate way to assess the FHR but cannot be used unless the cervix is at least 2 to 3 cm dilated and the membranes have ruptured. The electrode has three leads, which detect the PQRST complex. The filter within the electronics of the machine removes all components except the R wave. The R wave then triggers the machine to count; it waits for a second complex, filters all but the R wave, and then calculates how much time elapsed from the first to the second R wave

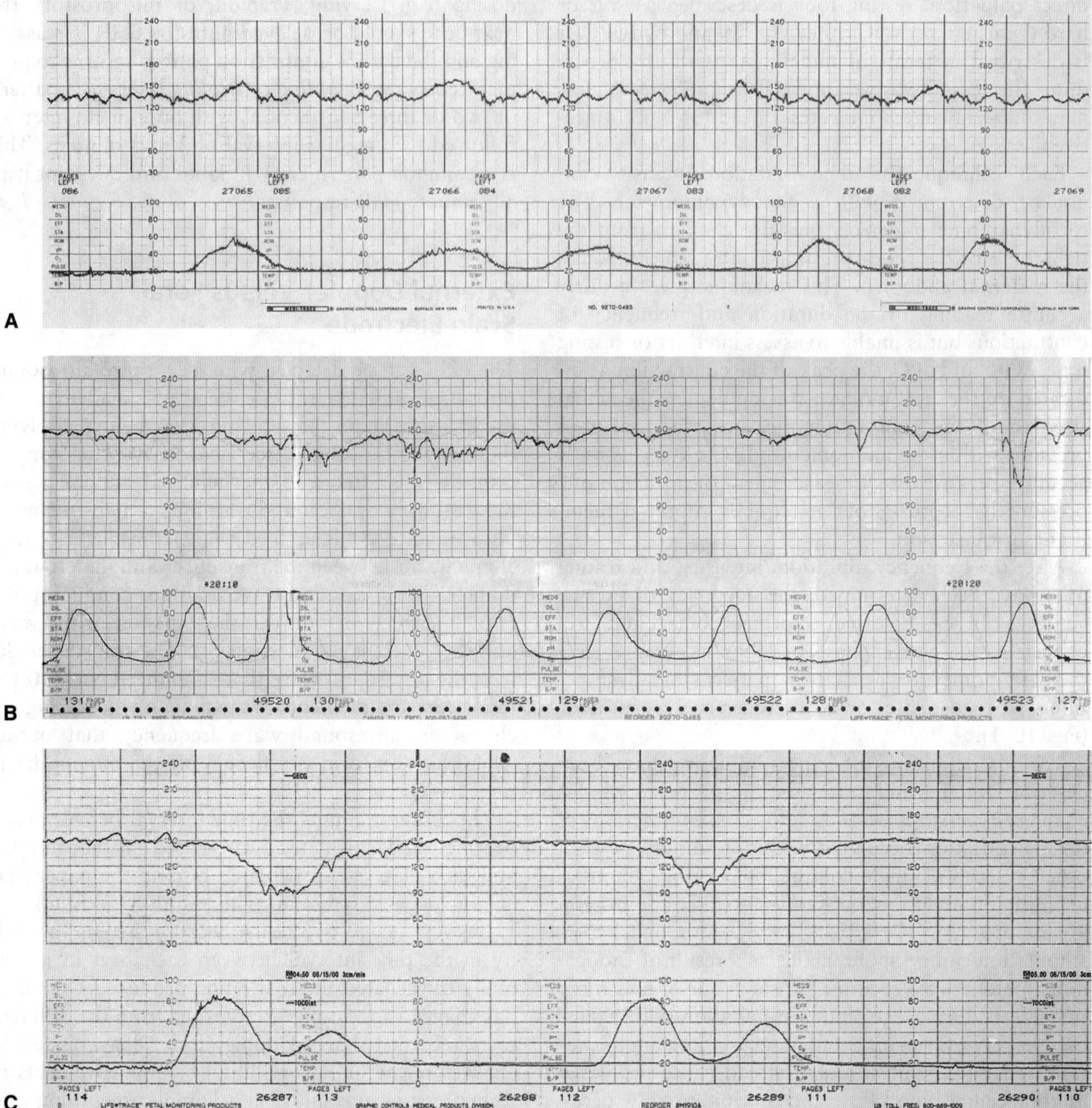

FIGURE 10–1. Three types of uterine contractions. (**A**) Normal contraction frequency, duration and intensity, and uterine resting tone. (**B**) Hyperstimulation of uterine activity. (**C**) Coupling of contractions.

in a fashion similar to the technique used by Doppler machines. The elapsed time between R intervals is converted into beats per minute, and the pen records that rate on the paper. The process repeats itself for every R wave, and the variability that is recorded is slightly, but not significantly, more accurate than the variability that is recorded by Doppler.

Both a Doppler and an FSE can produce FHR recordings that are inadequate for interpretation. Use of EFM during labor requires knowledge of these sources of artifact and solutions for resolution of them. The problem often results from equipment malfunction and can be remedied easily. The most common reasons why FHR tracings do not record accurately, the FHR tracing that is produced, and the solution to the problem are listed in Table 10–2.

Application of an FSE is invasive and increases the risk of maternal–fetal infection. It should be used only when continuous recordings are indicated and are unable to be obtained with external monitoring. If the recording obtained by external EFM is continuous, an FSE is unnecessary to obtain the slightly better display

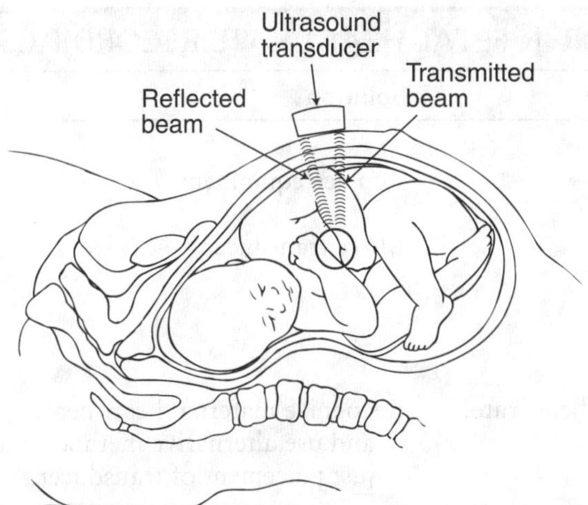

FIGURE 10–2. The Doppler ultrasound device for detecting cardiac activity. The frequency of the reflected beam is changed when it is reflected from a moving structure. (Adapted from Parer, JT. (1997). *Handbook of fetal heart rate monitoring* [2nd ed.]. Philadelphia: W.B. Saunders.)

of FHR variability. Evidence suggests that application of a direct electrode could enhance maternal–fetal transmission of the human immunodeficiency virus (HIV) when used in women who are HIV seropositive (Craven, Steger, & Jarek, 1994; Stein, Handelsman, & Matthews, 2000), and use of an FSE is contraindicated in women who are known to be HIV seropositive (ACOG, 1992). Other relative contraindications to the application of a direct fetal lead include women who have active or chronic hepatitis and those who have herpes simplex virus or other known and non-treated sexually transmitted diseases. Current recommendations are to avoid techniques resulting in a break in the skin when these infectious agents are present (Parer, 1999). Application of a direct fetal lead also may be deferred for women who are known hemophilia carriers when the sex of the fetus is unknown.

Intermittent Auscultation

Before the introduction of Doppler technology, intermittent auscultation of the FHR was done with a Pinard or DeLee stethoscope between contractions. The examiner can obtain baseline rate and ascertain the presence or absence of some decelerations without determination of variability or the type of deceleration with this technique. Auscultation with a non-Doppler stethoscope is no longer common practice in the United States. When the FHR is assessed during labor by an "intermittent auscultation" protocol, usually a hand-held Doppler unit that can detect the FHR during a contraction is used. (Display 10–1). This technique greatly improves the ability to diagnose and name specific FHR patterns.

Current recommendations for using auscultation during the intrapartum period are outlined by the Association of Women's Health, Obstetric and Neonatal Nurses (AWHONN) symposium *Fetal Heart Rate Auscultation* (Feinstein, Sprague, & Trepanier, 2000); the American College of Obstetricians and Gynecologists (ACOG, 1995b) technical bulletin, *Fetal Heart Rate Patterns: Monitoring, Interpretation, and Management*; the Society of Obstetricians and Gynaecologists of Canada (SOGC, 1995) policy statement, *Fetal Health Surveillance in Labour*; and in the *Guidelines for Perinatal Care* (American Academy of Pediatrics [AAP] & ACOG, 1997). In the absence of risk factors, auscultation of the FHR every 30 minutes in the active phase of the first stage of labor and every 15 minutes in the second stage of labor is suggested (AAP & ACOG, 1997). When risk factors have been identified, assessment frequency is increased to every 15 minutes in the active phase of the first stage of labor and every 5 minutes in the second stage (AAP & ACOG, 1997). When auscultation is used as the primary method of fetal surveillance during labor, a 1:1 nurse–fetus ratio is required.

The decision to use intermittent auscultation or EFM rests with the healthcare provider but is made in collaboration with the laboring woman. The decision is based on many factors, including patient history, fetal condition, risk classification, hospital policies and procedures, and the standard of practice. As with EFM, there are benefits and limitations to the use of intermittent auscultation (Display 10–2). Intermittent auscultation and electronic monitoring are effective in fetal evaluation when used appropriately (AAP & ACOG, 1997; ACOG, 1995b; AWHONN, 2000; SOGC, 1995).

PHYSIOLOGIC BASIS FOR FETAL HEART RATE MONITORING

EFM is a technique for fetal assessment based on the premise that the FHR reflects fetal oxygenation. Although an FHR with a normal baseline, moderate variability, and accelerations is a good predictor of a fetus without hypoxemia, the reverse is not true. Variant FHR patterns occur in up to 80% of all fetal heart tracings obtained during labor, but most do not indicate fetal hypoxemia (Berkus, Langer, Samueloff, Xernaxis, & Field, 1999; Goldaber, Gilstrap, Leveno, Dax, & McIntire, 1991; Helwig, Parer, Kilpatrick, & Laros, 1996; Herbst, Wolner-Hanssen, & Ingemars-

TABLE 10–2 ■ SOURCES OF ARTIFACT OR ERROR IN FETAL HEART RATE RECORDINGS

Source of Error	Recording Produced	Solution
Signal Errors		
Faulty leg plate, electrode, or monitor	No recording	Replace equipment
Transducer does not detect fetal heart consistently because of Maternal muscle movements Uterine contractions Maternal positioning	Intermittent recording	Move transducer
Interference by maternal signal	Recording is maternal heart rate.	Recognize maternal heart beat, and use alternative method or adjust placement of transducer.
Limitation of Machinery		
Counting process omits fetal heart rate (FHR) that is >30 bpm different from preceding beat	Dysrhythmia is audible but does not appear on record.	Use fetal electrocardiogram if improved recording needed. Dysrhythmias tend to be regular, and artifact tends to be irregular.
Halving or doubling of audible FHR	Very slow rates may be doubled, and very fast rates (>240 bpm) may be halved.	Auscultate to determine correct rate
Interpretive Errors		
Maternal heart rate recorded Fetal death Electrode on cervix	Rate recorded is equal to maternal pulse.	Compare with maternal pulse.
Scaling error	Two paper speeds are possible on some machines (1 and 3 cm/min). FHR pattern changes at slower speed, exaggerating variability.	Ensure paper speed of 3 ms/min before applying transducers.

Adapted with permission from: Parer J.T. (1997). *Handbook of fetal heart rate monitoring* (2nd ed.). Philadelphia: W.B. Saunders.

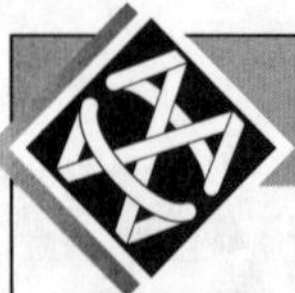

DISPLAY 10–1

Capabilities of Auscultation Devices

Fetoscope

- Detect FHR baseline
- Detect FHR rhythm
- Verify the presence of a dysrhythmia
- Detect increases and decreases from FHR baseline
- Clarify double or half counting by EFM

Doppler

- Detect FHR baseline
- Detect FHR rhythm
- Detect increases and decreases from FHR baseline

EFM, electronic fetal monitoring; FHR, fetal heart rate.

From Association of Women's Health, Obstetric and Neonatal Nurses. (2000). *Symposium on fetal heart rate auscultation* (p. 16). Washington, D.C: Author.

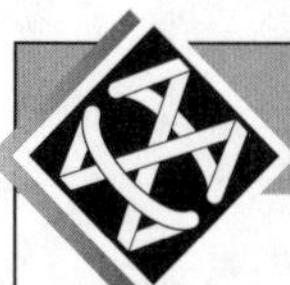

DISPLAY 10–2

Benefits and Limitations of Auscultation

Benefits

- Neonatal outcomes are comparable to those with EFM based on current RCTs.
- Lower cesarean birth rates have been associated with auscultation than with EFM in some RCTs.
- The technique is less invasive.
- Patient's freedom of movement is increased.
- The technology allows for fetal heart assessment if the patient is immersed in water.
- The equipment is less costly than EFM equipment.
- Auscultation is not automatically documented on paper (often a source of debate in legal situations).
- A caregiver must be present at bedside to provide the 1:1 nurse-to-patient ratio that is recommended based on RCTs comparing auscultation and EFM.

Limitations

- Use of a fetoscope may limit the ability to hear the FHR, (eg, in cases of maternal obesity or increased amniotic fluid volume).
- Certain FHR characteristics associated with EFM (eg, variability and types of decelerations, cannot be detected).
- Some patients may feel that auscultation is more intrusive.
- Auscultation is not automatically documented on paper (as EFM is, which is perceived as an important piece of documentation by many practitioners).
- There is a potential need to increase or realign staff to meet the 1:1 nurse-to-patient ratio that is recommended based on RCTs comparing auscultation and EFM.

EFM, electronic fetal monitoring; FHR, fetal heart rate; RCT, randomized clinical trial.
From Association of Women's Health, Obstetric and Neonatal Nurses. (2000). *Symposium on fetal heart rate auscultation* (p. 19). Washington, D.C: Author

son, 1997). Because the high rate of false-positive tracings has many origins and several clinical implications, a working knowledge of FHR physiology can aid clinical interpretation of FHR patterns during labor. The following section reviews oxygen and carbon dioxide transfer in the fetus, intrinsic control of the FHR and the characteristics of the normal FHR.

Maternal Oxygen Status

The fetus depends on well-oxygenated maternal blood flow to the placenta. The hemoglobin concentration or oxygen carrying capacity of maternal blood must be adequate to promote fetal oxygenation. Oxygen tension in maternal arterial blood depends on adequate ventilation and pulmonary integrity and is a determinant of fetal oxygenation (Parer, 1997). Most pregnant women do not have alterations in pulmonary function and do have adequate oxygen saturation. However, maternal conditions such as asthma, congenital heart defects, congestive heart failure, lung disease, seizures, or severe anemia can result in impaired oxygen delivery to the fetus (Parer, 1997).

Uterine, Placental, and Umbilical Blood Flow

At term, approximately 10% to 15% of maternal cardiac output, or 600 to 750 mL of blood volume, perfuses the uterus each minute. Oxygenated blood from the mother is delivered to the intervillous space in the placenta by the uterine arteries. Blood enters the intervillous space under positive arterial pressure from the maximally dilated uterine spiral arterioles, surrounds the villi that fill the intervillous space, and then drains through the uterine veins. Fetal deoxygenated blood is carried to the placental villi by the two umbilical arteries. Maternal–fetal exchange of oxygen and other nutrients occurs in the intervillous space across the membranes that separate fetal and maternal circulations. Oxygen is exchanged through passive diffusion from an area of high concentration (maternal side) to an area of low concentration (fetal side). Other nutrients are exchanged by active transport, facilitated diffusion, and pinocytosis (Fig. 10–3).

Oxygen and carbon dioxide diffuse across membranes rapidly and efficiently. Effective transfer of oxygen and carbon dioxide between the fetal and ma-

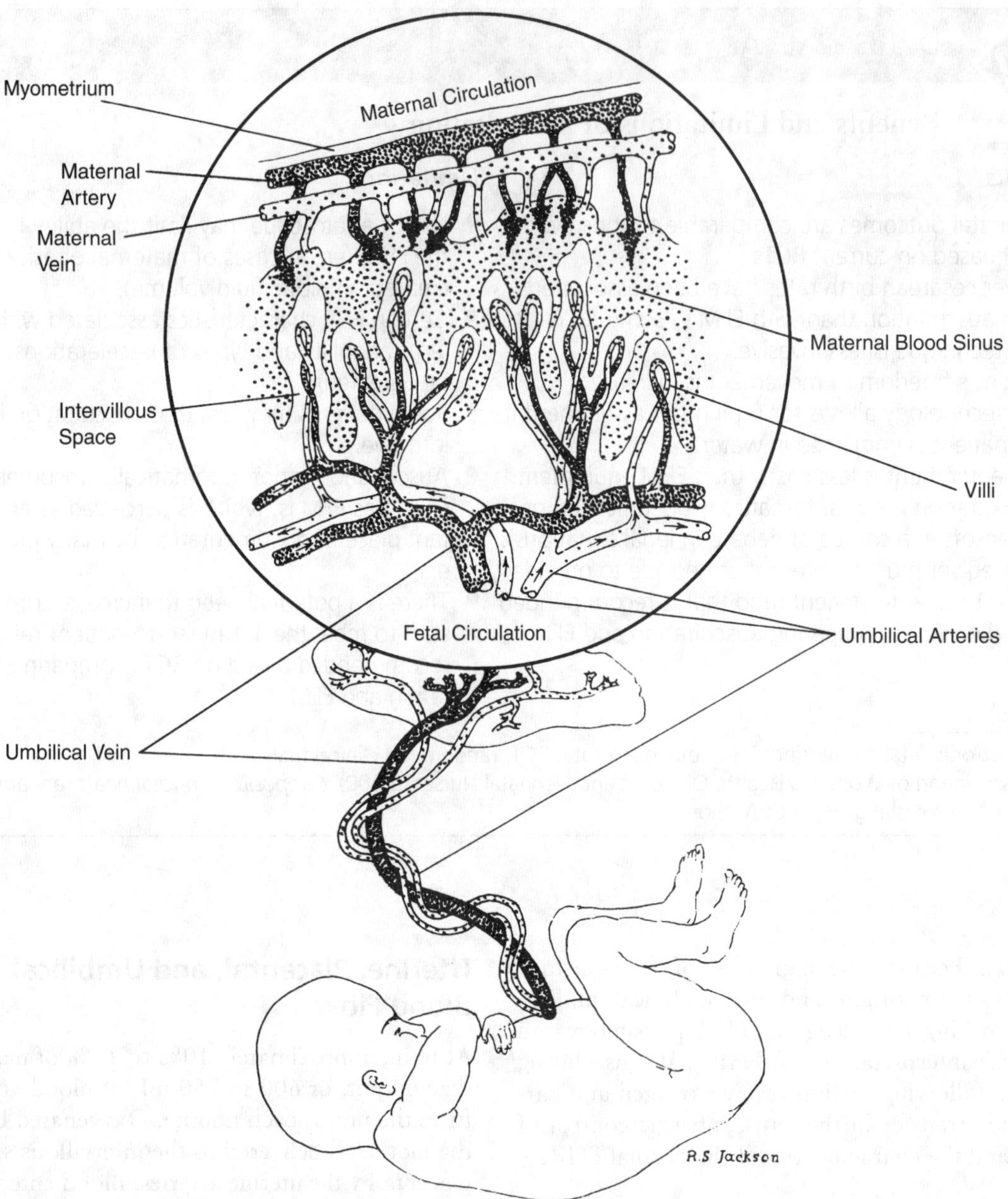

FIGURE 10–3. Maternal-placental-fetal exchange. (From Afriat, C.I. [1989]. *Electronic fetal monitoring.* Rockville, MD: Aspen.)

ternal bloodstreams depends on adequate uterine blood flow, sufficient placental area, and an unconstrained umbilical cord. Uterine blood flow into the intervillous space can be impeded by hypertension (ie, higher pressures decrease the time available for adequate exchange) or hypotension (ie, inadequate perfusion of the intervillous space). A placenta with inadequate diffusing capacity can develop in women who have hypertension or preeclampsia or in those who may have had an in utero infection such as toxoplasmosis. Intrauterine growth restriction may be secondary to decreased placental area or diffusing capacity. Umbilical blood flow is about 360 mL/min, or 120 mL/min/kg, in an undisturbed fetus at term (Gill, Trudinger, Garrett, Kossoff, & Warren, 1981). Umbilical blood flow is most commonly impeded by acute cord compression that can cause partial or, rarely, complete occlusion.

In summary, because poor maternal oxygenation is rare and because oxygen diffuses quite rapidly across most membranes, the significant factors affecting placental exchange of gases and nutrients for the fetus are

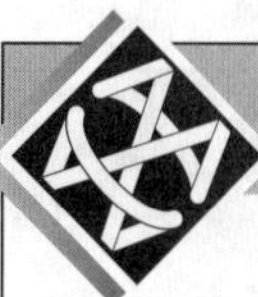

DISPLAY 10–3

Factors Determining Maternal–Fetal Oxygen Transfer

- Intervillous blood flow
- Fetal placenta blood flow
- Oxygen tension in maternal arterial blood
- Oxygen tension in fetal arterial blood
- Oxygen affinity of maternal blood
- Oxygen affinity of fetal blood
- Hemoglobin concentration or oxygen capacity of maternal blood
- Hemoglobin concentration or oxygen capacity of fetal blood
- Maternal and fetal blood pH and partial pressure of carbon dioxide
- Placental diffusing capacity
- Placental vascular geometry
- Ratio of maternal to fetal blood flow in exchanging areas
- Shunting around exchange sites
- Placental oxygen consumption

From Parer, J. T. (1997). *Handbook of fetal heart rate monitoring* (2nd ed.). Philadelphia: W. B. Saunders.

uterine blood flow, umbilical blood flow, and the amount of placental area available for exchange. Display 10–3 lists factors determining maternal–fetal oxygen transfer. The FHR patterns during labor reflect the function of these components of placental function and maternal oxygen status. Before presenting nursing interventions that support these physiologic mechanisms, a review of the physiology of the FHR is in order.

Physiology of the Fetal Heart Rate

Several factors influence the FHR. Interplay among the sympathetic and parasympathetic components of the autonomic nervous system, higher cortical functions in the brain, and chemoreceptors and baroreceptors are reflected in the baseline rate and are in part responsible for the FHR variability seen on the recording from an FHR monitor.

The parasympathetic nervous system influences the heart by means of the vagus nerve. Parasympathetic nerve fibers in the vagus nerve that control heart rate originate in the medulla oblongata of the brain and terminates in the sinoatrial and atrioventricular nodes within the heart. Stimulation of these fibers slow the heart rate by controlling or overriding the intrinsic rate generated within this node (Dalton, Phill, Dawes, & Patrick, 1983). The sympathetic nervous system has fibers that terminate in the muscle of the heart. Stimulation of these nerves causes an increase in heart rate and stroke volume, which then increases cardiac output (Parer, 1999). During gestation, the parasympathetic nervous system matures during the second trimester, and the vagus nerve gradually becomes dominant over sympathetic stimulation, which explains the slow drop in normal baseline rate as the fetus matures.

The vagus nerve is subject to influences from other parts of the central nervous system. The respiratory center is geographically close to the cardioregulatory centers in the medulla oblongata, and the FHR may increase with inspiratory movement and decrease with expiratory movement. Sleep is associated with decreased long-term variability, and gross body movements are associated with accelerations (Dalton et al., 1983; Parer, 1999).

Chemoreceptors and baroreceptors participate in two feedback loops that decrease the heart rate as part of the normal fetal response to transient hypoxemia. Chemoreceptors found in the aortic arch and central nervous system are sensitive to changes in the oxygen and carbon dioxide content of the blood. When uteroplacental blood flow falls below the threshold needed for normal gas exchange, increased carbon dioxide tension in fetal vessels causes the chemoreceptors to stimulate the vagus nerve and slow the FHR. The effect of this bradycardia is decreased cardiac metabolism and a decrease in oxygen

(text continues on page 390)

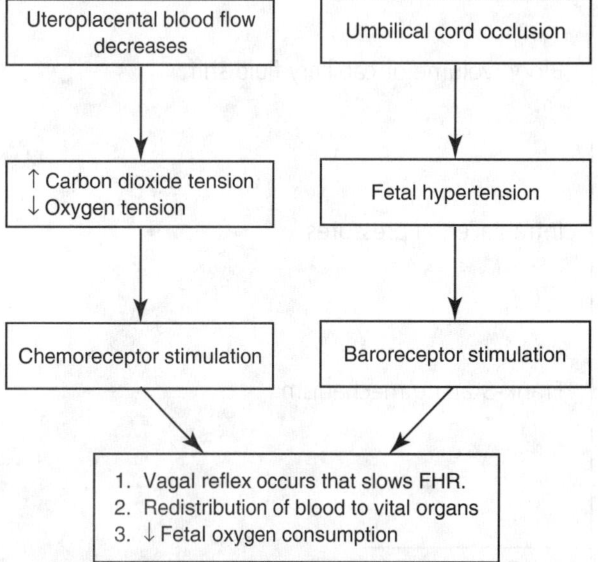

FIGURE 10–4. Fetal response to hypoxemia.

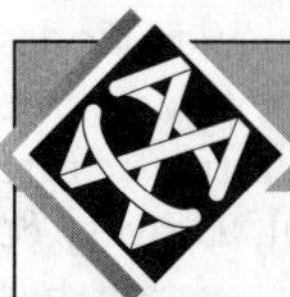

DISPLAY 10-4

Control of the Heart Rate

Factors Regulating Fetal Heart Rate	*Location*
Parasympathetic division of autonomic nervous system	Vagus nerve fibers supply sinoatrial (SA) and atrioventricular (AV) node
Sympathetic division of autonomic nervous system	Nerves widely distributed in myocardium
Baroreceptors	Stretch receptors in aortic arch and carotid sinus at the junction of the internal and external carotid arteries
Chemoreceptors	Peripheral—in carotid and aortic bodies
	Central—in medulla oblongata
Central nervous system	Cerebral cortex
	Hypothalamus
	Medulla oblongata
Hormonal regulation	Adrenal medulla
	Adrenal cortex
	Vasopressin (plasma catecholamine)
Blood volume or capillary fluid shift	Fluid shift between capillaries and interstitial spaces
Intraplacental pressures	Intervillous space
Frank-Starling mechanism	Based on stretching of myocardium by increased inflow of venous blood into right atrium

From Tucker, S.M. (2000). *Fetal monitoring and assessment.* St. Louis: Mosby.

Action	*Effect*
Stimulation causes release of acetylcholine at myoneural synapse	Decreases heart rate Maintains beat-to-beat variability
Stimulation causes release of norepinephrine at synapse	Increases fetal heart rate (FHR) Increases strength of myocardial contraction Increases cardiac output
Responds to increase in blood pressure by stimulating stretch receptors to send impulses by the vagus or glossopharyngeal nerve to the midbrain, producing vagal response and slowing heart activity	Decreases FHR Decreases blood pressure Decreases cardiac output
Responds to a marked peripheral decrease in O_2 and increase in CO_2	Produces bradycardia sometimes with increased variability
Central chemoceptors respond to decreases in O_2 tension and increases in CO_2 tension in blood and/or cerebrospinal fluid	Produces tachycardia and increase in blood pressure with decrease in variability
Responds to fetal movement	Increases variability
Responds to fetal sleep	Decreases variability
Regulates and coordinates autonomic activities (sympathetic and parasympathetic)	
Mediates cardiac and vasomotor reflex center by controlling heart action and blood vessel diameter	Maintains balance between cardioacceleration and cardiodeceleration
Releases epinephrine and norepinephrine with severe fetal hypoxia, producing sympathetic response	Increases FHR Increases strength of myocardial contraction and blood pressure Increases cardiac output
Low fetal blood pressure stimulates release of aldosterone, decreases sodium output, increases water retention, which increases circulating blood volume	Maintains homeostasis of blood volume
Produces vasoconstriction of nonvital vascular beds in the asphyxiated fetus to increase blood pressure	Distributes blood flow to maintain FHR and variability
Responds to elevated blood pressure by causing fluid to move out of capillaries and into interstitial spaces	Decreases blood volume and blood pressure
Responds to low blood pressure by causing fluid to move out of interstitial space into capillaries	Increases blood volume and blood pressure
Fluid shift between fetal and maternal blood is based on osmotic and blood pressure gradients; maternal blood pressure is about 100 mmHg and fetal blood pressure about 55 mmHg; balance is probably maintained by some compensatory factor.	Regulates blood volume and blood pressure
In the adult, the myocardium is stretched by an increased inflow of blood, causing the heart to contract with greater force than before and pump out more blood; the adult then is able to increase cardiac output by increasing heart rate and stroke volume; this mechanism is not well developed in the fetus.	Cardiac output depends on heart rate in the fetus: $\downarrow$ FHR = $\downarrow$ cardiac output $\uparrow$ FHR = $\uparrow$ cardiac output

consumption. Baroreceptors are found in the aortic and carotid arches, where they detect changes in pressure very quickly. When umbilical blood flow is impeded, fetal blood pressure rises, and a very quick reflex occurs by means of the vagus nerve to slow the heart rate rapidly, which decreases blood pressure. In addition to bradycardia, blood is redistributed to vital organs (ie, brain, heart, and adrenal glands) and is shunted away from nonvital organs (ie, gut, spleen, kidneys, and limbs) during fetal hypoxemia (King & Parer, 2000) (Fig. 10–4).

In summary, by means of the vagus nerve, the medulla oblongata cardioregulatory center controls heart rate variability by mediating input from several sources, including the central nervous system, chemoreceptors, baroreceptors, and the respiratory center (Display 10–4).

CHARACTERISTICS OF THE NORMAL FETAL HEART RATE

FHR pattern interpretation involves assessment of five components of the FHR: baseline rate, presence or absence of accelerations, variability, periodic and/or episodic changes, and evolution over time (NICHD, 1997). Baseline changes are those that occur between contractions or in the absence of contractions for more than 10 minutes. Bradycardia and tachycardia are the two alterations in baseline rate of clinical importance. Periodic changes in FHR occur in response to uterine activity. Episodic patterns are not associated with uterine activity and may occur randomly. Early decelerations, late decelerations, prolonged decelerations, and variable decelerations are the periodic or episodic patterns that can develop. Unusual patterns, such as sinusoidal, dysrhythmic, and saltatory patterns, are mentioned briefly. The following sections review characteristics of the normal FHR and the cause and management of the most common periodic and episodic changes.

Baseline Rate

The average baseline heart rate in the normal term fetus before labor is 140 beats/min. The normal range is 110 to 160 beats/min (Feinstein & McCartney, 1997; NICHD, 1997). Early in pregnancy, the FHR is slightly higher. Baseline FHR is determined over a minimum of a 10 minutes. Assessment occurs between contractions and between decelerations or accelerations in the heart rate; therefore, baseline FHR is the FHR in the absence of contractions or periodic changes.

Variability

The FHR of the healthy fetus is displayed as an irregular line on the monitor tracing. These irregularities demonstrate the FHR variability previously described that reflects the slight difference in the time interval between each beat. If all time intervals between heartbeats were identical, the line would be flat or smooth. Baseline FHR variability is defined as fluctuations in the baseline FHR of two cycles per minute or greater. Short-term variability is the beat-to-beat fluctuation in heart rate. Long-term variability is the term used for greater amplitude changes. Clinically, variability is recognized as a unit without deliberately separating short- and long-term components (NICHD, 1997). Table 10–1 lists the criteria for moderate versus minimal or absent variability. Variability is assessed during the baseline of the FHR, not during periodic changes such as decelerations or accelerations.

Accelerations

Accelerations are a visually apparent, abrupt increase (defined as onset of acceleration to peak in less than 30 seconds) in FHR above the baseline (Fig. 10–5). The acme is 15 beats/min above the baseline, and the acceleration lasts at least 15 seconds but less than 2 minutes from the onset to return to baseline. Before 32 weeks' gestation, accelerations are defined as hav-

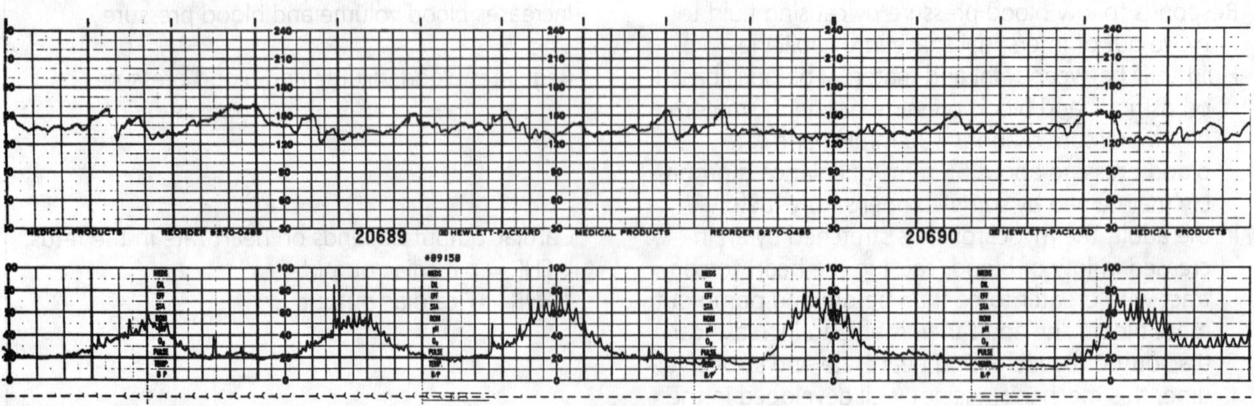

FIGURE 10–5. Accelerations of fetal heart rate.

ing an acme of 10 beats/min above the baseline and duration of 10 seconds. Like moderate variability, the presence of accelerations indicates central oxygenation and predicts the absence of fetal acidosis (Clark, Gimovsky, & Miller, 1984). Accelerations can occur as periodic or episodic changes in the FHR.

In summary, a normal baseline rate with moderate variability, accelerations, and no periodic changes is highly predictive of a well-oxygenated fetus (Berkus et al., 1999; Krebs, Petres, & Dunn, 1981; Krebs, Petres, Dunn, Jordan, & Segreti, 1979; Low, Victory, & Derrick, 1999). There is a close association between the presence of accelerations and normal FHR variability. EFM's greatest contribution to fetal healthcare is the ability to predict normal outcomes. A reassuring fetal tracing virtually ensures that, barring unforeseen acute insults such as abruptio placentae, uterine rupture, or cord prolapse, a well-oxygenated infant will be born.

INTERVENTIONS FOR NONREASSURING FETAL HEART RATE PATTERNS

Before discussing the etiology and management of periodic or episodic changes in the FHR, a review of the interventions used to maximize fetal oxygenation in the presence of variant FHR patterns is warranted.

In utero resuscitation or *physiologic intervention* refers to a series of interventions that includes a change in maternal position, a decrease in uterine activity or uterine contraction frequency, administration of intravenous fluids, and administration of oxygen. None of these techniques has been proven individually or collectively to resolve fetal hypoxemia, and there is no evidence that these techniques can reverse asphyxia. However, these interventions may improve maternal blood flow to the placenta and oxygen delivery to the fetus. If the clinical characteristics of the FHR patterns are thought to represent a serious risk for acidemia, these measures should be initiated only if doing so does not delay the move toward expeditious birth.

Position Change

Changing maternal position alters the relationship between the umbilical cord and fetal parts or the uterine wall and is usually done to minimize or correct cord compression and decrease the frequency of uterine contractions (Clark et al., 1991). Position change can resolve prolonged decelerations and variable decelerations. Position change may also modify late decelerations if the cause of this pattern is decreased uterine blood flow (usually from supine positioning and inferior vena caval compression). The supine position should be avoided in general to prevent compression of the vena cava and supine hypotensive syndrome.

Reduction of Uterine Activity

When uterine contractions are too frequent, there may be insufficient time for blood flow through the intervillous space. If FHR decelerations occur with hyperstimulation, reduction of uterine activity can optimize fetal oxygenation. Reduction of uterine activity can occur by reducing oxytocin dosage or discontinuing oxytocin administration, which decreases contraction frequency, or by having a mother assume the lateral position. The next dose of pharmacologic agents used to ripen the cervix or stimulate contractions should be delayed until uterine activity returns to normal and the FHR is reassuring. Administration of tocolytics is occasionally used as a temporary measure to provide intrauterine resuscitation for a prolonged deceleration or other nonreassuring FHR patterns caused by hyperstimulation. If the pattern does not resolve, preparations for birth are warranted.

Intravenous Fluid Administration

It is believed that administration of fluids maximizes maternal intravascular volume and therefore protects against decreased uteroplacental perfusion. A reduction in uterine blood flow can occur after administration of regional anesthesia because the sympathectomy causes dilation of peripheral vessels, lower peripheral resistance, and a potential drop in uteroplacental blood flow. However, no data suggest that increasing intravenous fluids can positively affect uterine blood flow in a woman who is well hydrated, and fluid administration alone cannot correct fetal hypoxemia. Caution should be used when increasing intravenous fluids. Some clinical situations, such as preeclampsia, preterm labor treated with magnesium sulfate, or preterm labor treated with corticosteroids and β-sympathomimetic drugs, carry an increased risk for pulmonary edema that may necessitate fluid restriction. Oxytocin has an antidiuretic effect, and thus prolonged use of oxytocin can contribute to fluid overload if intravenous fluids are used too liberally. An extreme effect of fluid overload related to excessive use of oxytocin is water intoxication.

Oxygen Administration

No data from randomized, controlled trials show that administering oxygen during labor can improve fetal outcomes. There is evidence that fetal Po_2 increases in the presence of maternal hyperoxia, but the rates of oxygen administration rarely reach the 100% (which must be used with a rebreather mask) level that is required in usual practice (Aldrich, Wyatt, Spencer, Reynolds, & Delpy, 1994; Bartnicki & Saling, 1994; Dildy, Clark, & Loucks, 1994; McNamara, Johnson, & Lilford, 1993). However, administering oxygen is a common practice, has no known adverse effects, and is approved for use for the purpose of improving fetal oxygenation by ACOG (1995a, 1999).

Amnioinfusion

Amnioinfusion has been used to attempt to resolve variable FHR decelerations by correcting umbilical cord compression as a result of oligohydramnios. During amnioinfusion, normal saline or lactated Ringer's solution is introduced transcervically into the uterus by gravity flow or through an infusion pump. Amnioinfusion does significantly resolve patterns of moderate to severe variable decelerations but does not affect late decelerations or patterns with absent variability (Mino, Puerta, Miranda, & Herruzo, 1999; Miyazaki & Nevarez, 1985). Amnioinfusion dilutes thick meconium-stained amniotic fluid, decreases the incidence of meconium below the newborn's vocal cords, and potentially decreases the risk of meconium aspiration syndrome (Klingner & Kruse, 1999; Pierce, Gaudier, & Sanchez-Ramos, 2000). The procedure does not seem to affect the length of labor (Strong, 1997) and appears to be safe for women who are attempting a vaginal birth after a previous cesarean birth (Ouzounian, Miller, & Paul, 1996). Amnioinfusion should be limited to the treatment of moderate to severe variable decelerations or meconium-stained fluid. Careful monitoring and documentation of fluid infused is important to avoid iatrogenic polyhydramnios. Chapter 9 provides a comprehensive discussion of the technique for amnioinfusion.

FETAL HEART RATE PATTERNS

Alterations in the Baseline Rate

Changes in the baseline rate that can occur are tachycardia, with a rate of more than 160 beats/min, or bradycardia, with a rate below 110 beats/min (Feinstein & McCartney, 1997; NICHD, 1997).

Tachycardia

A baseline tachycardia (FHR >160 beats/min for ≥10 minutes) may be caused by fetal conditions such as infection, hypoxemia, anemia, prematurity (<26 to 28 weeks' gestation), cardiac dysrhythmias, and congenital anomalies or by maternal conditions such as fever, dehydration, infection, or medical problems (eg, thyroid disease). β-sympathomimetic drugs such as terbutaline and ritodrine may also cause maternal and fetal tachycardia. Tachycardia represents increased sympathetic tone, decreased parasympathetic autonomic tone, or both. Several causes of tachycardia do not reflect a risk of acidemia; the most common is an elevation in maternal temperature (Table 10–3).

Fetal tachycardia in the presence of chorioamnionitis may result from the maternal fever, may be an indication of fetal infection, or both. Thus, the determination of risk for acidemia in a fetus with tachycardia is especially difficult. Tachycardia with moderate variability in the absence of FHR decelerations rarely represents fetal acidemia (Krebs et al., 1979; Low et al., 1999; Tejani, Mann, Bhakthavathsalan, & Weiss, 1975). In the presence of normal FHR variability and no periodic changes, the tachycardia must be assumed to result from something other than oxygen deprivation in the fetus. Tachycardia is sometimes seen on recovery from asphyxia and probably represents catecholamine activity following sympathetic nervous or adrenal medullary

TABLE 10–3 ■ TACHYCARDIA AND RISK OF FETAL ACIDEMIA

Nonacidemic	Possibly Acidemic	Presumed Acidemia
Tachycardia with moderate or minimal variability; no decelerations	Tachycardia with moderate or minimal variability; mild variable or late decelerations; may develop metabolic acidemia if tachycardia persists	Tachycardia with absent variability; variable or late decelerations
Causes include elevated maternal temperature, fetal dysrhythmia, medications, prematurity	Causes include fetal sepsis	

activity in response to acute nonrepetitive asphyxial stress. Fetal tachycardia without FHR variability signifies a significant risk for fetal acidemia.

Nursing interventions for tachycardia include assessment of maternal temperature and hydration. Elevated maternal temperature is the most common cause of fetal tachycardia in the intrapartum period. Other potential causes may be prematurity and prior medication use. Nursing interventions include notification of the physician or midwife, assisting the woman to a lateral position, an infusion of intravenous fluids, and the administration of oxygen at 8 to 12 L/min by mask. If the fetal tachycardia is associated with absent variability, late decelerations, or variable decelerations, bedside evaluation by a physician is necessary. If maternal fever has been excluded as the cause of the tachycardia, oxytocin infusion should be decreased or discontinued if infusing or the next dose of Cervidil, Prepidil, or misoprostol delayed until fetal status is reassuring. Fetal oxygen saturation monitoring may be initiated.

Bradycardia

A baseline bradycardia (FHR <110 beats/min for ≥10 minutes) may be caused by fetal conditions such as hypoxemia resulting from an acute decrease in oxygen flow to the fetus, vagal stimulation, and rarely, cardiac anomalies or hypothermia. Bradycardias may cause hypoxemia, and they may be the result of hypoxemia. The depth, duration, and presence or absence of variability are critical components in making a clinical association between the bradycardia detected and the presence or absence of fetal hypoxemia (Table 10–4).

A sudden, profound bradycardia is a medical emergency that may signal uterine rupture or placental abruption (Fig. 10–6). This pattern, called *terminal bradycardia,* may precede death in utero if birth does not occur rapidly. The onset of a fetal bradycardia when a woman is laboring after a prior cesarean section should cause concern about the onset of uterine rupture, signaling provider attendance at the bedside and preparation for an emergent cesarean birth. Terminal bradycardias are the most common fetal heart pattern that develops during uterine rupture (Leung, Leung, & Paul, 1993; Menihan, 1998). Leung and colleagues (1993) evaluated the fetal consequences of catastrophic uterine rupture when the diagnosis was made at the onset of a fetal bradycardia. All infants with a previously normal FHR pattern born within 17 minutes after the onset of a prolonged deceleration survived without significant perinatal morbidity (Leung et al., 1993). However, if severe late and variable decelerations are present before the onset of bradycardia, the fetus can tolerate a shorter period of prolonged FHR deceleration, and there is a significantly increased risk for metabolic acidosis (Leung et al., 1993). When severe late and variable decelerations precede the onset of a prolonged deceleration associated with uterine rupture, perinatal asphyxia can occur as soon as 10 minutes after the onset of a prolonged deceleration (Leung et al., 1993). Chapter 9 discusses uterine rupture associated with women attempting a trial of labor after a previous cesarean birth.

Bradycardias that occur during the second stage of labor after a previously normal FHR pattern are much more benign. They may result from increased vagal tone (eg, head compression) (Parer, 1999) or occasionally from umbilical cord occlusion. If the variability remains moderate or minimal and the FHR does not fall below 80 to 90 beats/min, expediting birth is not warranted (Gull et al., 1996).

During a second-stage bradycardia, the woman should be encouraged to push in either lateral position, avoiding the supine position. If possible, she should push with alternating contractions to allow the fetus to gain a few added minutes of improved blood flow. Coaching a laboring woman to push with every other contraction may be difficult if she has no anesthesia, so

TABLE 10–4 ■ BRADYCARDIA AND RISK OF FETAL ACIDEMIA

Nonacidemic	Possibly Acidemic	Presumed Acidemia
Bradycardia <110 bpm and >80 bpm with moderate variability	Bradycardia <80 bpm and >60 bpm with moderate or minimal variability	Bradycardia <60 bpm Second-stage bradycardia that loses variability within first 3 minutes from onset or loses variability for >4 minutes
Causes include idiopathic bradycardia, congenital heart block (50 to 60 bpm)	May develop metabolic acidemia if persists (exception: congenital heart block)	Causes include prolapsed cord, uterine rupture, placental abruption, unexplained sources, congenital heart block (nonacidemic)

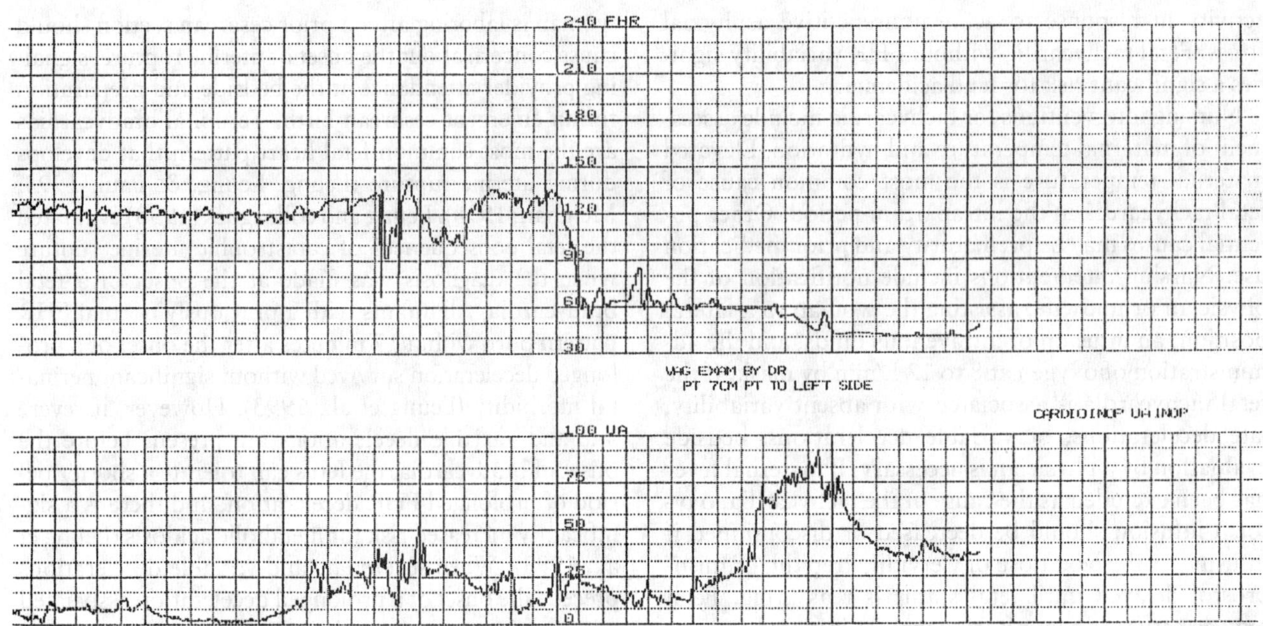

FIGURE 10–6. Terminal bradycardia.

this strategy may only be possible with regional anesthesia in place. If the woman is given a regional anesthetic, another option is to allow the fetus to descend passively with the uterine contractions and without the woman exerting expulsive efforts if the contractions are of sufficient strength. Chapter 9 discusses nursing interventions during the second stage of labor.

Rarely, sustained fetal bradycardia is caused by complete atrioventricular heart block associated with clinical or serologic evidence of maternal collagen vascular disease, especially systemic lupus erythematosus (Hohn & Stanton, 1992). In a fetus with complete atrioventricular heart block, an FHR between 50 and 60 beats/min without variability may be present (Parer, 1997). Interventions during the intrapartum period are usually not warranted; however, the neonatal team should be notified about the impending birth. The newborn may require pacemaker insertion after birth.

Bradycardias may result in hypoxia, and conversely, they may be the result of hypoxia. Studies that have compared the decision to incision times for emergency cesarean section have shown that there are time-dependent relationships among the onset of the bradycardia, the depth of the bradycardia, the presence or absence of variability, and the development of metabolic acidosis (Korhonen & Kariniemi, 1994). If the bradycardia is between 80 and 100 beats/min and variability is maintained, the fetus usually stays well oxygenated centrally and can tolerate these rates for an indefinite time (Gull et al., 1996). Bradycardias with rates of less than 60 beats/min, those associated with late or variable decelerations, and those with minimal or absent variability are most often associated with adverse outcomes (Beard, Filshie, Knight, & Roberts, 1971; Berkus et al., 1999; Dellinger, Boehm, & Crane, 2000; Low et al., 1999).

In the case of a fetal demise, the external ultrasound transducer and the direct fetal electrode can record maternal heart rate, which appears the same as a bradycardic FHR. The external transducer can record maternal heart rate from the aorta, and the direct lead records maternal heart rate, which is conducted through the dead fetal tissue. If there is any question about the origin of a bradycardia, documentation of the maternal pulse should be one of the initial nursing assessments. Other nursing interventions include notification of the physician or midwife with a request for bedside evaluation, assisting the woman to a lateral position, infusion of intravenous fluids, administration of oxygen at 8 to 12 L/min by mask, and discontinuation of oxytocin if infusing. If the bradycardia persists, preparations for an operative birth may be warranted.

Alterations in Variability

FHR variability is described as absent, minimal, moderate, or marked (NICHD, 1997). Moderate variability complexes are the result of the parasympathetic and sympathetic stimuli, fetal states, higher cortical centers, chemoreceptors, baroreceptors, and the cardiac conduction system and therefore reflects adequate cerebral oxygenation more than any other component of the FHR (Parer, 1997). The most common causes of decreased variability not associated with a risk for acidemia are centrally acting drugs such as narcotics,

TABLE 10–5 ■ MINIMAL VARIABILITY AND RISK OF FETAL ACIDOSIS

Nonacidemic	Possibly Acidemic	Presumed Acidemia
Minimal variability: normal baseline rate, no decelerations	Minimal variability with nonrecurrent or mild tachycardia, bradycardia, late decelerations, variable decelerations	Minimal variability with persistent or severe tachycardia, bradycardia, late decelerations, variable decelerations
Causes include narcotics, tranquilizers, $MgSO_4$, barbiturates, anesthetic agents, prematurity, fetal sleep	May develop metabolic acidemia if persistent and/or variability decreases	Causes include metabolic acidemia

tranquilizers, magnesium sulfate, and other analgesics administered to women during labor. Minimal variability is also seen in premature gestations and during fetal sleep cycles (Table 10–5). Minimal variability without concomitant decelerations is almost always unrelated to fetal acidemia (Parer & Livingston, 1990). A fetus with a defective cardiac conduction system, anencephaly, or congenital neurologic deficit may present with minimal or absent variability, and in the case of congenital neurologic impairment, this FHR pattern may represent an asphyxial insult that occurred during the antepartum period (MacLennan, 1999).

Absent variability is seen when a fetus has cerebral asphyxia and therefore experiences loss of fine tuning within the cardioregulatory center in the brain or direct myocardial depression. Loss of variability, especially in the presence of other periodic patterns during labor, is the most sensitive indicator of metabolic acidemia in a fetus (Beard et al., 1971; Clark et al., 1984; Low et al., 1999). Nursing interventions for absent variability include notification of the physician or midwife with a request for bedside evaluation, repositioning the woman to a lateral position, administration of intravenous fluids, and administration of oxygen at 8 to 12 L/min by mask. Oxytocin infusion should be discontinued if infusing or the next dose of pharmacologic agents used to ripen the cervix or stimulate contractions should be delayed until the FHR is reassuring. Fetal stimulation, fetal oxygen saturation monitoring, or both may be initiated. Because absent variability is a hallmark sign of deep central asphyxia, it warrants immediate evaluation when detected (Table 10–6).

Marked variability is less common. Some authors believe marked variability is a fetal response to hypoxia that takes a form different from the usual progression from moderate to minimal and then absent variability (Westgate, Bennet, & Gunn, 1999). The theory is that in this instance parasympathetic stimulation does not predominate over sympathetic stimulation and that the result is larger fluctuations in rate, reflecting the interplay between the factors that increase heart rate (ie, sympathetic stimulation and adrenal release of epinephrine and norepinephrine effects on heart muscle) and those that decrease it (ie, vagal stimulation of the sinoatrial and atrioventricular nodes within the heart). Although some animal and human data support this theory, periods of marked variability do not generally persist, and they are not associated with severe or progressive hypoxia (Parer, 1997; Westgate et al., 1999).

Periodic and Episodic Changes in Fetal Heart Rate

Periodic changes in heart rate are transient changes in rate lasting a few seconds to 1 or 2 minutes, compared with baseline changes in the heart rate, which must last

TABLE 10–6 ■ ABSENT VARIABILITY AND RISK OF FETAL ACIDOSIS

Nonacidemic	Possibly Acidemic	Presumed Acidemia
Intermittent absent variability, normal rate, without deceleration; preceded by periods of moderate variability	Progressive decrease in variability with decelerations	Absent variability with tachycardia, bradycardia, late decelerations, variable decelerations
Causes include idiopathic response	May develop metabolic acidemia if persistent and/or variability decreases	Causes include metabolic acidemia

a minimum of 10 minutes. The four types of FHR decelerations are early, late, variable, and prolonged (Fig. 10–7). Periodic changes in FHR are usually identified and defined within the context of uterine contractions, whereas episodic FHR changes appear to have no relationship to uterine contractions.

Early Decelerations

Early decelerations are presumed to be initiated by fetal head compression. Altered cerebral blood flow causes the decrease in heart rate through a vagal reflex. When the contraction occurs, the fetal head is subjected to pressure, which stimulates the vagus nerve. The heart rate begins to drop at the onset of the contraction, when the head compression begins, and returns to the baseline rate at the end of the contraction, when the head is no longer compressed (Feinstein & McCartney, 1997; NICHD, 1997). Early decelerations mirror the contraction causing them. They are benign decelerations, requiring no intervention or treatment and are not associated with fetal hypoxia or low Apgar scores. The key to assessment of early decelerations is to differentiate them from late decelerations. The presence of variability is important. Vagal stimulation is not caused by hypoxia and does not decrease variability.

Late Decelerations

Late decelerations are defined by NICHD as a "gradual decrease and return to baseline FHR associated with uterine contraction. The deceleration is delayed in timing, with the nadir of the deceleration occurring after the peak of the contraction" (Feinstein & McCartney, 1997; NICHD, 1997). Late decelerations are uniform in shape, symmetrical and smooth.

Originally, all late decelerations were thought to represent uteroplacental insufficiency. Later research has identified an additional mechanism. "Reflex" late decelerations, or late decelerations with retained variability, are neurogenic in origin (Parer, 1999). Early decelerations may be a variant of this pattern, and some believe they are seen more frequently in fetuses in an occiput posterior position and during periods of rapid descent (Fig. 10–8).

When a well-oxygenated fetus experiences a transient reduction in oxygenation during a contraction, chemoreceptors detect the hypoxemia and initiate the vagal bradycardic response. After the contraction recedes, the fetus resumes normal metabolism, and the bradycardia resolves. Because it takes a short time for hypoxemia to develop in this setting, the chemoreceptor reflex occurs as the hypoxemia is detected. The nadir of the deceleration is late relative to the peak of the contraction, because there is a lag in time between the detection of hypoxemia and the FHR response. Early decelerations and reflex late decelerations have retained variability, and neither is associated with significant acidemia.

Late decelerations with concomitant decreased or absent variability possibly result from fetal asphyxia (Beard et al., 1971; Berkus et al., 1999; Clark et al., 1984). This type of periodic change occurs when there is insufficient oxygen for myocardial metabolism or normal cerebral function. These FHR patterns are likely to occur when there is chronic placental insufficiency that cannot support the transient hypoxia episodes that occur during normal labor. Late decelerations with absent variability may evolve after a period of prolonged variable decelerations, bradycardia, tachycardia, or other periodic pattern that with sufficient repetition or duration interrupts normal fetal respiration.

Late decelerations should be evaluated in the context of FHR variability. For example, late decelerations with moderate baseline variability and a stable rate with accelerations warrant less concern than late decelerations in the presence of an abnormal baseline rate, minimal variability, and absence of accelerations. If the FHR pattern had been reassuring before the onset of decelerations, an iatrogenic cause, such as maternal hypotension, frequently can be determined. Obtaining a maternal history to assess risk factors for uteroplacental insufficiency and evaluation of the uterine activity pattern are essential.

Nursing interventions for late decelerations focus on maximizing placental function, improving uteroplacental exchange by maintaining a lateral maternal position, increasing intravenous fluids to correct dehydration or volume depletion, discontinuation of oxytocin, and administration of oxygen at 8 to 12 L/min by mask. The next dose of pharmacologic agents used to ripen the cervix or stimulate contractions should be delayed until uterine activity returns to normal and the FHR is reassuring. The physician or midwife should be notified. If the late decelerations do not resolve after these interventions, a request for bedside evaluation by the physician or midwife is warranted. Iatrogenic insults that may further compromise the placenta, such as hyperstimulation with oxytocin or maternal hypotension due to her supine position, should be avoided. Fetal oxygen saturation monitoring may be initiated.

Variable Decelerations

The most frequently seen FHR deceleration pattern in labor is the variable deceleration. Variable decelerations are a vagal response resulting from umbilical

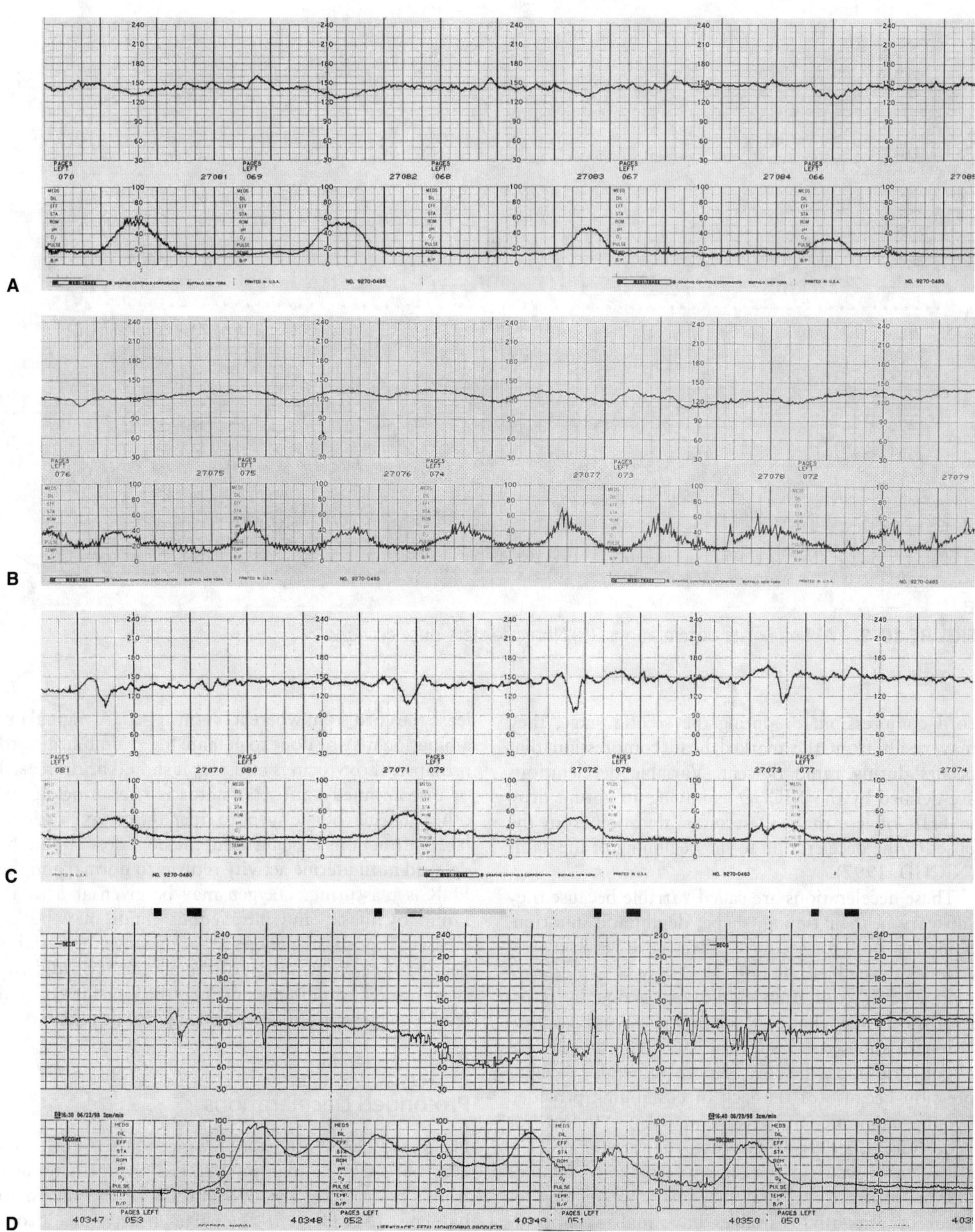

FIGURE 10–7. Four types of FHR decelerations. (**A**) Early. (**B**) Late (**C**) Variable (**D**) Prolonged.

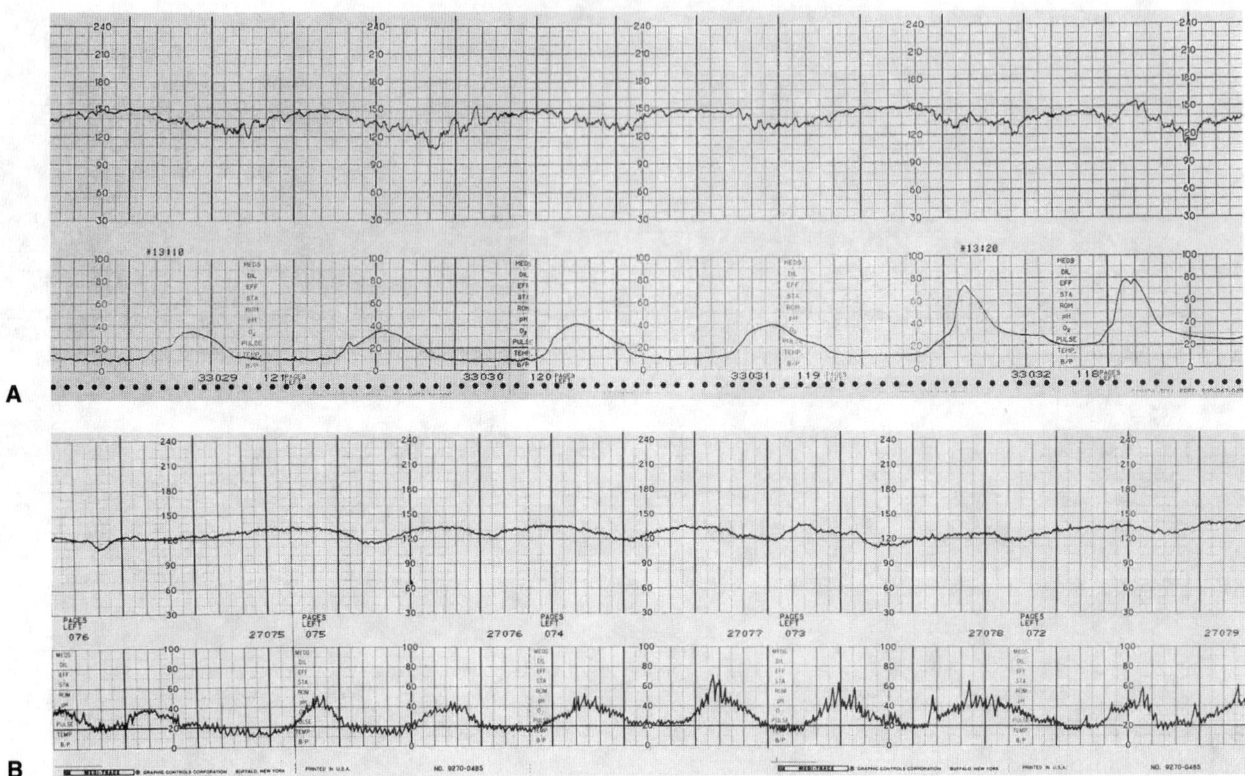

FIGURE 10–8. (**A**) Reflex late decelerations. (**B**) Nonreflex late decelerations.

cord compression, or during the second stage, they may result from the marked head compression that occurs during rapid descent. Variable decelerations are defined by the NICHD as having an abrupt drop in FHR of less than 30 seconds' duration from the onset of the deceleration to the beginning of the nadir (NICHD, 1997).

These decelerations are called variable because they can vary in their timing, shape, depth, and duration. Some last only for seconds; others have very slow recoveries to the baseline rate. They may be caused by a uterine contraction pressing the cord against the fetus, by a short or nuchal cord, or by intense vagal stimulation in the second stage of labor. In the case of oligohydramnios, the cord is more vulnerable to compression because of the lack of cushioning provided by the amniotic fluid (Galvan, Van Mullem, & Broekhuizen, 1989). In this case, the variable decelerations may occur in response to fetal movement or uterine contractions, and they may be frequent or occur occasionally. Variables have multiple appearances in all aspects except one—the initial FHR drop is abrupt.

Nursing interventions to correct variable decelerations focus on alleviating the cord compression and begin with assisting the woman to a lateral position, knee-chest position, or even the supine position to release the cord from where it is entrapped. A vaginal examination may be done to palpate for an umbilical cord prolapse. If oxytocin is infusing, it should be decreased or discontinued until fetal status is reassuring. If another pharmacologic agent to ripen the cervix or stimulate contractions is being used, the next dose should be delayed until uterine activity returns to normal and the FHR is reassuring. Oxygen may be given at 8 to 12 L/min by mask, and intravenous fluids may be increased. If position changes do not resolve the variable decelerations, notification of the physician or midwife is warranted, amnioinfusion may be considered, and fetal oxygen saturation monitoring may be initiated.

Prolonged Decelerations

Prolonged decelerations are changes in the FHR that last more than 2 minutes but less than 10 minutes from the onset of the deceleration to the return to baseline (NICHD, 1997). The heart rate drops abruptly and stays down for several minutes and is usually an isolated occurrence. It may occur in the presence or absence of contractions and may have an abrupt or slow return to the baseline rate. Prolonged decelerations may be the result of an isolated episode of cord compression, maternal hypotension, excessive uterine activity, vagal stimulation, and rarely, maternal seizures or maternal respiratory or cardiac arrest (Feinstein & McCartney, 1997).

During the first stage of labor, transient bradycardias or prolonged decelerations with moderate variability are frequently associated with an occiput posterior position or transverse position and are probably the result of increased vagal tone resulting from pressure on the fetal skull (Freeman, Garite, & Nageotte, 1991). These types of bradycardias also occur when there is a transient decrease in uteroplacental blood flow in a previously well-functioning maternal–fetal unit. This situation sometimes occurs during the administration of regional anesthesia or when the patient is in a supine position. Nonrecurrent, prolonged decelerations that are preceded by and followed with an FHR that has a normal baseline and moderate to minimal variability is not associated with fetal hypoxemia of clinical significance.

Nursing interventions for prolonged decelerations include discontinuation of oxytocin, increasing intravenous fluids, administration of oxygen at 8 to 12 L/min by mask, vaginal examination to exclude a prolapsed cord, and repositioning the woman to remove pressure from the umbilical cord. The next dose of pharmacologic agents used to ripen the cervix or stimulate contractions should be delayed until uterine activity returns to normal and the FHR is reassuring. The physician or midwife should be notified and bedside evaluation requested. A tocolytic agent may also be administered to decrease uterine activity. Fetal oxygen saturation monitoring may be initiated. If a prolonged deceleration occurs during antepartum testing, ultrasound measurement of amniotic fluid volume should be done. The causes and interventions for periodic heart rate changes are listed in Tables 10–7 and 10–8.

Unusual Fetal Heart Rate Patterns

When an unusual tracing is observed from the beginning of electronic monitoring tracing, the possibility of a fetus with a congenital anomaly should be considered. Hydrocephalic and anencephalic fetuses may present with unusual FHR patterns that do not fit any category or definition. If possible, an ultrasound examination may be performed to exclude gross anomalies as the cause of the pattern, although the results of the ultrasound examination may be inconclusive. An anomaly that affects the fetal central nervous system probably affects the variability and the fetal cardiac system's ability to accelerate and decelerate. Unusual decelerations with a flat, fixed rate may be seen.

Sinusoidal Pattern

An unusual pattern type is the sinusoidal tracing. The characteristics include a persistent oscillating pattern, with amplitude of the undulations of approximately 5

TABLE 10–7 ■ CAUSES OF PERIODIC OR EPISODIC FETAL HEART RATE PATTERNS

Early Decelerations	Late Decelerations	Variable Decelerations	Prolonged Decelerations
Head compression	Variability present: head compression or transient decrease in uteroplacental blood flow • Supine positioning • Epidural bolus • Uterine hyperstimulation	Cord compression	Cord compression
Early decelerations may be early form of late deceleration	Variability absent or minimal: uteroplacental insufficiency • Preeclampsia • Maternal smoking • Maternal disease • Diabetes • Collagen disease • Chronic hypertension	Head compression	If associated with moderate variability, may be a transient decrease in uteroplacental blood flow

TABLE 10–8 ■ MANAGEMENT OF VARIANT FETAL HEART RATE PATTERNS

FHR Pattern	Diagnosis	Action
Normal rate, moderate variability, ± accelerations, no periodic or episodic decelerations	The baby is well oxygenated.	None
Normal rate, moderate variability, ± accelerations, mild variant pattern (ie, bradycardia, LD, VD)	The baby is still well oxygenated centrally.	Conservative in utero treatment; expect abolition of variant pattern if cause reversed
Normal rate, moderate variability, ± accelerations, moderate/severe variant pattern (ie, bradycardia, LD, VD)	The baby is still well oxygenated centrally, but the FHR pattern suggests reductions in O_2 that may result in accumulation of fetal O_2 debt.	Conservative in utero treatment, ± amnioinfusion, ± stimulation testing; check ability to deliver rapidly in case pattern worsens
Normal rate, decreasing variability, ± accelerations, moderate/severe variant pattern (ie, bradycardia, LD, VD)	The baby may be on the verge of decompensation.	Operative birth if spontaneous birth remote or if ancillary testing (stimulation and/or blood sampling) supports diagnosis of decompensation. Normal testing results may allow time to await a vaginal birth
Variability absent or minimal, no accelerations, moderate/severe variant patterns (ie, bradycardia, LD, VD)	The baby has evidence of actual or impending damaging asphyxia.	Operative birth; may attempt further evaluation or in utero treatment if it does not unduly delay birth

LD, late decelerations; VD, variable decelerations
Adapted from Parer, J. T., & King T. L. (1999). Whither fetal heart rate monitoring. *Obstetrics, Gynecology and Fertility, 22*(5), 149–192.

to 15 beats/min and a frequency of approximately two to five cycles per minute. In a true sinusoidal pattern, there is a lack of variability, no accelerations, and response to uterine contractions (Feintstein & McCartney, 1997).

The sinusoidal pattern was first identified in the early 1970s during observation of Rh-sensitized fetuses (Rochard et al., 1976). As severe fetal anemia developed, the FHR tracing became persistently rhythmic in an undulating fashion (Fig. 10–9) and remained so. The causes of sinusoidal patterns include maternal–fetal hemorrhage, placental abruption, or fetal anemia, which can be caused by Rh isoimmunization. A sinusoidal pattern caused by anemia will subside when a successful fetal transfusion is performed. A sinusoidal FHR tracing can occur after the maternal administration of some narcotics, especially butorphanol (Stadol). Because this type of sinusoidal tracing resolves as the drug is excreted, it is called a *pseudosinusoidal* or *drug-induced sinusoidal* pattern. The characteristics differ from a true sinusoidal pattern in that there are fewer uniform oscillations, periods of moderate variability, and accelerations. No treatment is indicated.

Saltatory Pattern

The saltatory pattern is characterized by marked increased variability and is defined by an amplitude of greater than 25 beats/min with an oscillatory frequency of more than 6 beats/min for a duration longer than 1 minute (O'Brien-Abel & Benedetti, 1992). This pattern occurs rarely, and although the cause is uncertain, it is believed to result from increased sympathetic stimulation in normally oxygenated fetuses (Parer, 1999). It also may be the result of acute, brief hypoxia in the previously normoxic fetus. Because the fetus with a saltatory pattern is hemodynamically compensated (although it may be mildly hypoxemic), interventions to resolve the pattern such as maternal position change, avoidance of maternal hypotension, avoidance of uterine hyperstimulation, and perhaps administration of oxygen at

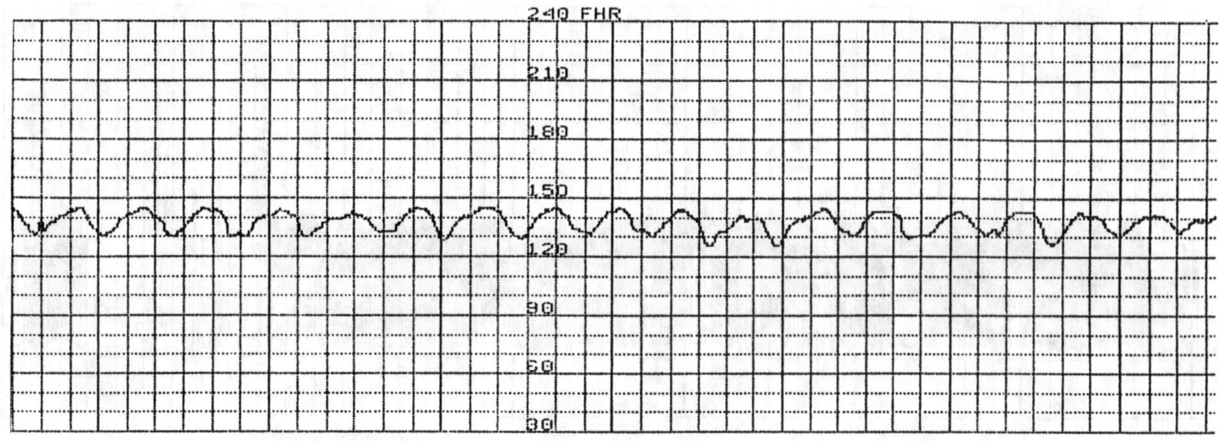

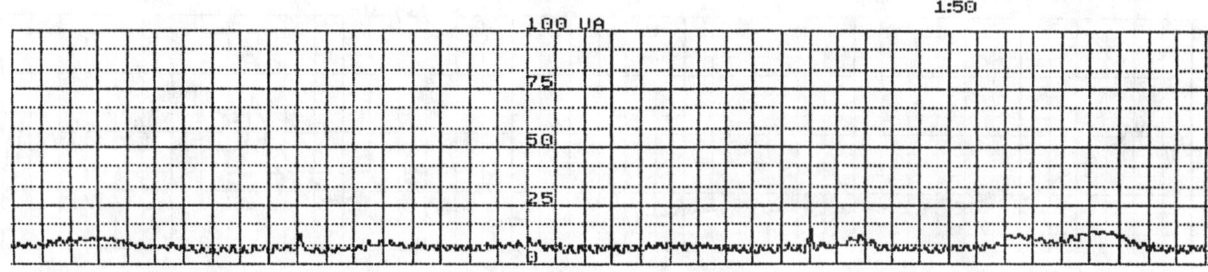

FIGURE 10–9. Sinusoidal fetal heart rate pattern.

8 to 12 L/min by mask are warranted (Parer, 1999). The saltatory pattern is not associated with poor neonatal outcomes (O'Brien-Abel & Benedetti, 1992).

Dysrhythmias

Because the functioning of the electronic fetal monitor is based on its ability to accurately record from one fetal heartbeat to the next, it can detect irregularities of the FHR (Fig. 10–10).

Irregular FHRs, such as premature ventricular contractions (PVCs), PVCs with bigeminy (ie, every other beat is a PVC), premature atrial contractions (PACs), or PACs with bigeminy (ie, every other beat is a PAC), can be recorded accurately with a direct fetal electrode. Irregularities in the FHR have an organized appearance that helps in differentiating them from artifact of the monitoring technology, which appears haphazard. Fetal dysrhythmias such as fetal PVCs and PACs are benign and require no intervention. Assessment of fetal well-being may be difficult in the presence of a dysrhythmia because of the inability to see a consistent baseline or evaluate variability. Auscultating the FHR and listening for the irregularity may verify the presence of a dysrhythmia. The FHR may appear normal on the external heart rate tracing, but if an irregularity is auscultated and a direct electrode applied, the dysrhythmia can be accurately recorded.

Two of the fetal dysrhythmias of concern are supraventricular tachycardia (SVT) and congenital (complete) heart block. In SVT, rates greater than 240 beats/min have been verified by simultaneous auscultation, fetal electrocardiogram, or M-mode ultrasound. The risk to the fetus is congestive heart failure resulting in fetal hydrops and possible fetal death if uncorrected. SVT therefore may require medical intervention with medications (ie, in utero cardioversion) or birth. Approximately 50% to 65% of mothers whose fetuses exhibit congenital heart block have laboratory or clinical evidence of connective tissue disease such as systemic lupus erythematosus. Treatment consists of in utero pharmacologic cardioversion or birth, with placement of a pacemaker after birth (Kleinman, Nehgme, & Copel, 1999).

Most fetal dysrhythmias convert to normal sinus rhythm shortly after birth. After detection of an arrhythmia in utero, ultrasound examination of the fetus to evaluate for fetal or cardiac anomalies is indicated. Fetal echocardiography may also be obtained to further evaluate the fetal heart. In some instances, the neonatal resuscitation team may be requested to attend the birth.

If the heart rate is regular to auscultation but there are unusual excursion tracings on the fetal heart monitor strip, the most likely explanation is that it is artifactual information. Artifact can be caused by the FSE

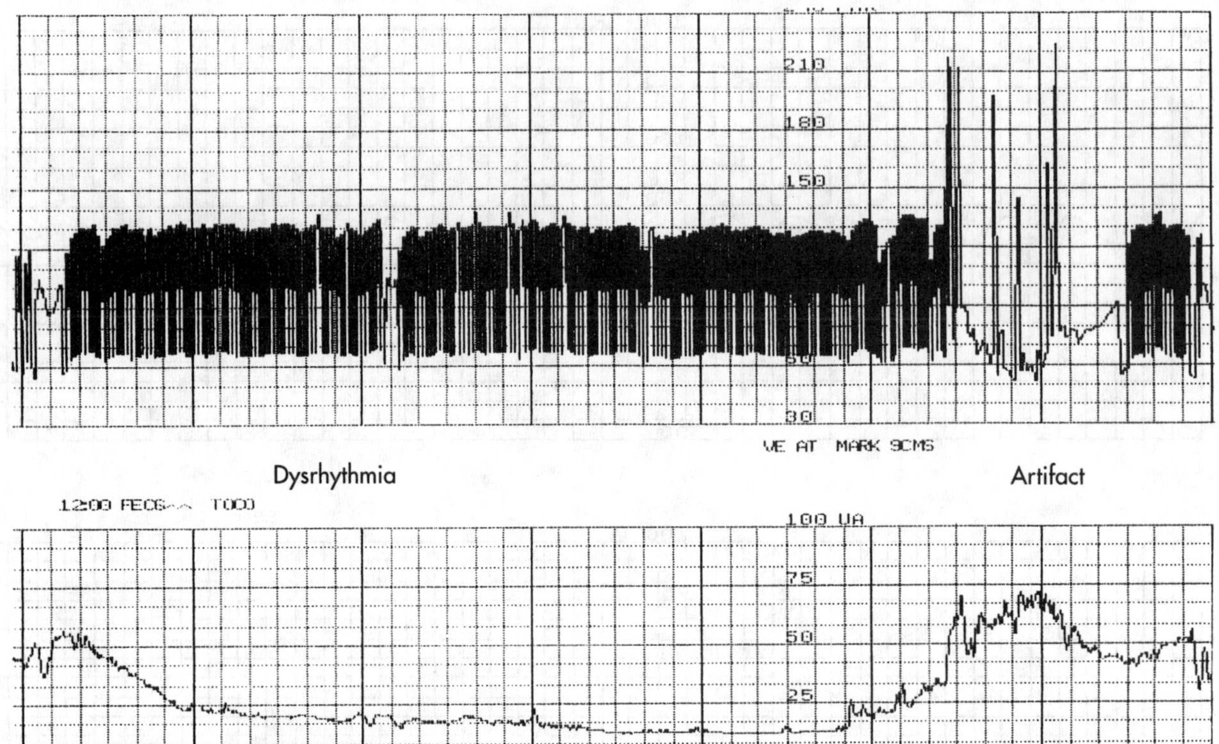

FIGURE 10–10. Dysrhythmia. This tracing demonstrates fetal dysrhythmias and artifact. Note the "randomness" of the artifactual information compared with the "organization" of the dysrhythmias.

having a poor attachment to the fetal presenting part, a broken cable or leg plate, or a machine problem. Attempts to correct the problem can include changing the cable or fetal monitor and replacing the direct electrode (see Table 10–2).

Shoulders and Overshoot

Shoulder and *overshoot* are terms used to describe a short increase in FHR above baseline that occurs just before or just after a deceleration. The term shoulders is usually used to describe an increase in the FHR above baseline before and after a contraction that is associated with moderate variability. These transient rises reflect dominance of the sympathetic nervous system influence over the parasympathetic system as the FHR responds to the cord compression or a transient decrease in oxygenation that caused the deceleration. Shoulders as an isolated finding do not signify fetal hypoxemia and their presence or absence is not clinically indicative of fetal compromise (Parer, 1999).

An overshoot may be used to describe an increase in the FHR of at least 20 beats lasting at least 20 to 30 seconds with absent variability after a variable deceleration (Feinstein & McCartney, 1997). In contrast to shoulders, which appear jagged, overshoots usually occur after the deceleration and are of short duration. Overshoots rise above the baseline after the contraction in a smooth curve with a prolonged return to the baseline. The cause of overshoots is unknown, although they are thought to be an exaggerated compensatory increase in the FHR after a variable deceleration. This type of pattern is unusual and has not been well studied. If repetitive and associated with minimal to absent FHR variability, they may indicate nonreassuring fetal status (Feinstein & McCartney, 1997).

ASSESSMENT OF PATTERN EVOLUTION

In clinical practice, interpretation of the FHR is an ongoing assessment that includes multiple perinatal factors, specific FHR characteristics, and most importantly, evolution of the FHR pattern as labor progresses (Fig. 10–11). A nonreassuring FHR can suddenly develop spontaneously, but the evolution from reassuring to nonreassuring usually follows a typical pattern. FHR patterns that occur during the second stage of labor are a good example of how pattern evolution from moderate to minimal or absent variability reflects an increasing risk of fetal hypoxemia. It is com-

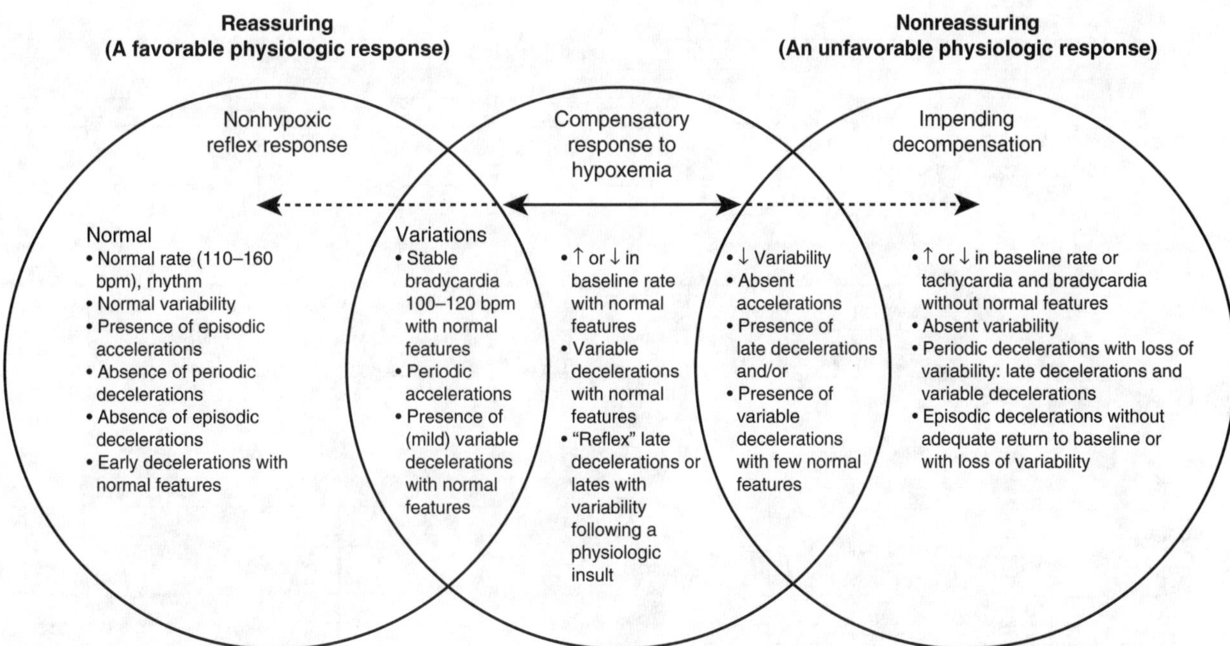

FIGURE 10–11. Alterations of fetal heart rate patterns by physiologic response. (Adapted from AWHONN [1997]. Principles and Practice p. 37).

mon in the second stage of labor for the FHR to develop mild or moderate variable decelerations that become progressively more severe as the fetus descends. In this scenario, if the pattern results from head compression and vagal stimulation during head compression, the FHR maintains variability because the decelerations are not caused by hypoxia. These decelerations can resolve intermittently as the vertex adjusts to pelvic diameters and may resolve completely when the vertex crowns. If the cause of this pattern is cord occlusion that is worsening as the fetus descends, the decelerations may become more severe and develop a concomitant loss of variability as the fetus develops hypoxemia. The provider should assess variable decelerations that evolve into deeper decelerations with tachycardia or loss of variability for emergent birth.

Nursing interventions for variable decelerations in the second stage should include assessment of the pushing technique used. When repetitive variable decelerations during the second stage are associated with coached closed-glottis pushing, the most appropriate approach is to encourage the woman to push with every other or every third contraction. This technique can be attempted for all women but is most effective for women who have regional analgesia. Open-glottis pushing, with the woman bearing down for no more than 6 to 8 seconds, has less effect on fetal status than three or four pushes lasting 10 seconds or more with the woman holding her breath during each contraction (Fig. 10–12). If oxytocin is infusing, a decrease in the dosage or discontinuation of the infusion usually results in contractions that are less frequent. Appropriate nursing management during the second stage of labor can prevent iatrogenic fetal stress and the birth of a depressed baby.

The end-stage mild to moderate bradycardia that retains variability is another version of head compression during rapid descent. If the variability is retained and the rate remains above 80 to 90 beats/min, this pattern should be watched but considered a benign variant. Conversely, a bradycardia pattern that slopes down over several minutes and loses variability within the first 4 minutes of descent is a pattern of evolution that signals fetal decompensation and warrants rapid intervention (Gull et al., 1996).

The nurse should recognize an FHR pattern that precedes death. In any stage of labor, bradycardias that are preceded by a period of late or variable decelerations or a bradycardia that is associated with diminishing variability is associated with metabolic acidosis in the fetus (Beard et al., 1971; Berkus et al., 1999; Clark et al., 1984; Dellinger et al., 2000; Low et al., 1999) (see Fig. 10–6). In either situation, if the problem causing fetal hypoxia is not corrected, the FHR eventually becomes a flat, fixed pattern with no variability before death. Scalp stimulation elicits no response. By auscultation, the examiner can hear a regular rate well within the normal range, providing false reassurance.

In retrospective studies, the investigators reviewed FHR tracings from children with known central ner-

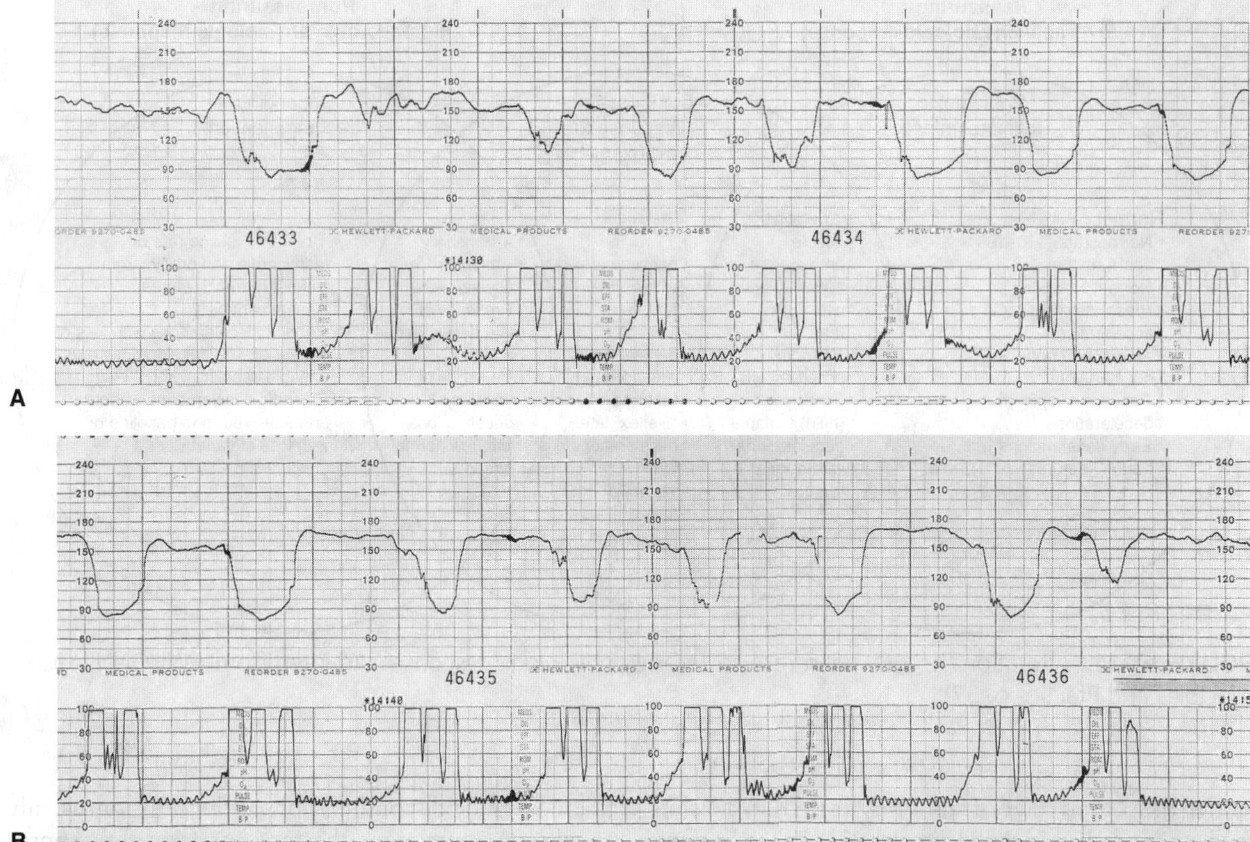

FIGURE 10–12. Iatrogenic nonreassuring fetal heart rate pattern as a result of coached closed-glottis pushing during the second stage of labor.

vous system neurologic impairments. For most of these children, the FHR tracing obtained at admission or that developed during the intrapartum period was a pattern that was persistently nonreactive, had diminished variability, and had FHR decelerations (Phelan & Ahn, 1994). If at first presentation to the hospital or office the FHR tracing is at a persistent rate with decreased variability with or without decelerations and shows no accelerations in response to stimulation, the fetus should be evaluated for acidemia. Although neurologic damage diagnosed at birth is rare, this type of tracing may indicate that neurologic damage has already occurred before admission.

Multiple authors have reviewed the association between FHR patterns and neonatal outcomes. Baseline variability most reliably indicates adequate oxygenation to the brain. A normal baseline rate with moderate variability and absence of periodic or episodic patterns conveys a high level of security that the fetus is well oxygenated and not experiencing asphyxial stress in response to labor progress. Most FHR tracings include some variant pattern, and most of these fetuses are also well oxygenated. The FHR patterns listed in Table 10–9 are those that have consistently

TABLE 10–9 ■ FETAL HEART RATE PATTERNS ASSOCIATED WITH SIGNIFICANT RISK FOR FETAL ACIDEMIA

Absent Variability With	Minimal Variability With
Persistent tachycardia	Tachycardia with variable or late decelerations
Bradycardia <80 bpm	Bradycardia with variable or late decelerations
Recurrent late decelerations	Recurrent late decelerations
Recurrent severe variable decelerations	Recurrent severe variable decelerations
Sinusoidal pattern	Sinusoidal pattern

been associated with fetal acidosis, low Apgar scores, or umbilical artery pH values in the acidotic range. Nurses caring for women during labor should recognize these patterns as ominous and in need of immediate medical consultation.

ANCILLARY TESTS OF FETAL WELL-BEING

Because most variant FHR tracings are not associated with underlying fetal hypoxemia, it is occasionally helpful to employ ancillary testing that can discriminate between the fetus with hypoxemia and the fetus who is centrally well oxygenated. This discrimination can avoid potentially unnecessary interventions if the results of the test are reassuring. Scalp stimulation, fetal scalp blood sampling, and fetal pulse oximetry are the techniques available for this purpose.

Fetal Scalp Stimulation

Fetal scalp stimulation involves placing firm, digital pressure on the fetal scalp during a vaginal examination. In response to scalp stimulation, a well-oxygenated term fetus responds with an acceleration of the FHR that is more than 15 beats/min above the baseline value and that lasts longer than 15 seconds (Fig. 10–13). Research has indicated that this type of acceleration in response to scalp stimulation correlates highly with a fetal blood pH above 7.20 (Clark et al., 1984). The absence of an acceleration does not diagnose acidemia or predict fetal compromise. If the FHR fails to respond to scalp stimulation, a fetal scalp sample for blood gas analysis may be obtained from the presenting part, or fetal oxygen saturation monitoring may be initiated. By performing fetal scalp stimulation when concerned about the well-being of the fetus, the perceived need to use fetal scalp sampling will decrease (Elimian, Figueroa, & Tejani, 1997; Goodwin, Milner-Masterson, & Paul, 1994).

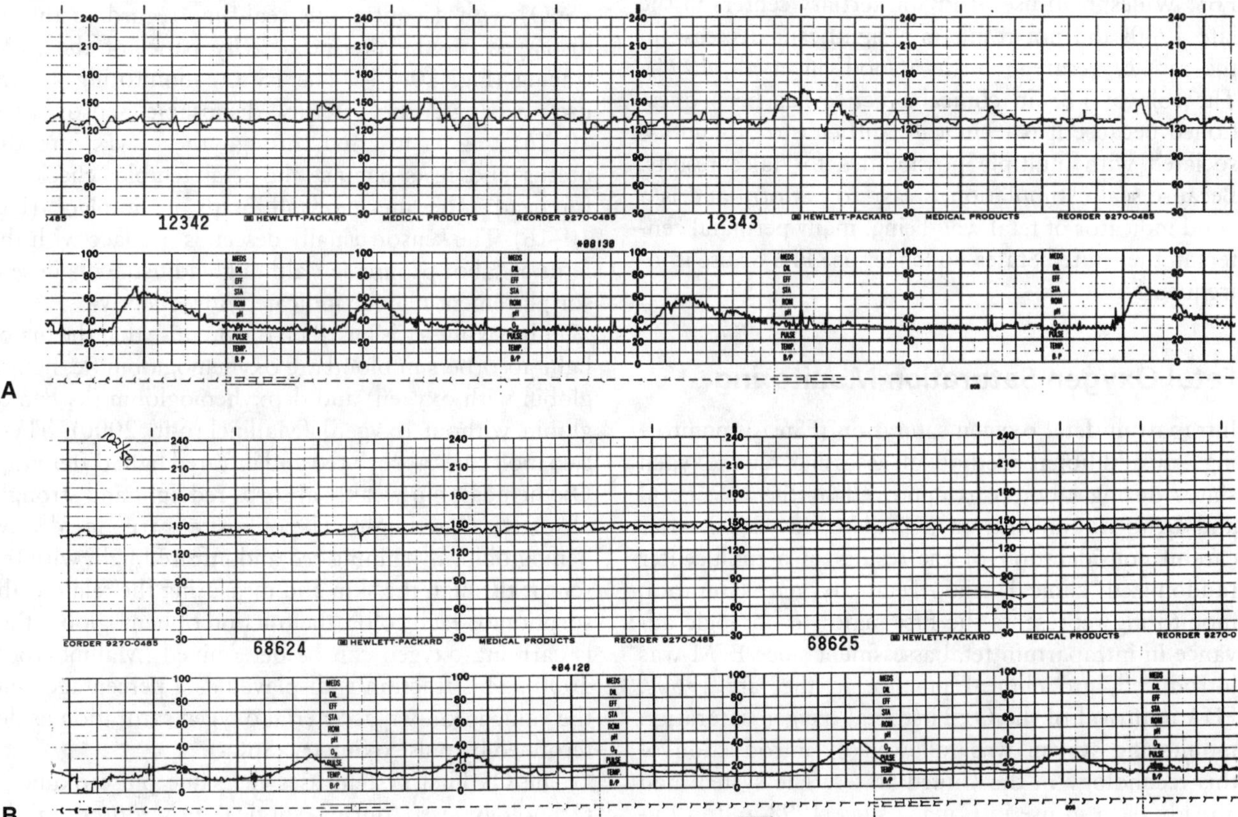

FIGURE 10–13. (A) Accelerations with fetal movement. This tracing was obtained with an external ultrasound transducer. The presence of accelerations indicates a reassuring heart rate pattern. (B) Absence of accelerations. The absence of fetal accelerations may indicate a fetal sleep cycle or the potential of a nonreassuring condition, thus warranting further evaluation.

Fetal Blood Sampling

If the response to fetal scalp stimulation is not reassuring, fetal scalp blood may be obtained for blood gas analysis. The fetal blood gas analysis consists of all of the parameters used in adult blood gas analysis; however, only the pH and base excess typically are used to evaluate fetal status (Mondanlou, 1991). If the pH is less than 7.15 to 7.00 and the base excess is less than −7 to −10, emergent birth is usually instituted.

False-normal and false-abnormal results can occur because of prolonged exposure of the sample to air, protracted sampling time, inadequate temperature control, laboratory technique, timing of sampling relating to contractions, presence of caput succedaneum, or maternal factors such as fever, hypertension, acidemia, or supine position. If a fetal blood sampling (FBS) result seems incongruent with the EFM tracing interpretation, the FBS may be in error and must be repeated. Although FBS provides an adjunct measure to determine fetal status when a nonreassuring FHR is detected, in theory eliminating the need for cesarean birth if the result obtained indicates a well-oxygenated fetus, there has been a trend away from the use of FBS. Widespread use of FBS in tertiary centers in the late 1980s did not result in a significant decrease in the rate of cesarean births (Goodwin et al., 1994). The role of FBS in clinical practice has been questioned because it is technically difficult to do and associated with multiple possibilities for false results. Because scalp stimulation is easy to perform and is a good indicator of fetal well-being, many perinatal centers in the United States no longer use FBS or use it infrequently.

Fetal Oxygen Saturation Monitoring

Intrapartum fetal oxygen saturation ($FSpo_2$) monitoring, an additional method of assessing fetal oxygen status during labor, was approved by the U.S. Food and Drug Administration (FDA) in May 2000, after careful consideration of the results of a multicenter randomized clinical trial. Fetal oxygen saturation monitoring represents the first major technologic advance in intrapartum fetal assessment since EFM was introduced into clinical practice in the late 1960s. FDA approval of the OxiFirst fetal oxygen saturation monitoring system was followed by introduction of this technology in the United States. The system had already been in use in Canada since 1998 and in Europe since 1995. Fetal oxygen saturation monitoring is used with EFM as an adjunct method of assessment when the FHR is nonreassuring or uninterpretable. Results of the randomized clinical trial that led to the FDA approval suggest that $FSpO_2$ monitoring can assist physicians, midwives, and nurses to more accurately assess fetal oxygen status during labor (Garite et al., 2000). These more accurate data can help the practitioner decide whether it is safe for labor to continue or interventions are needed. If the $FSpO_2$ is reassuring (≥30%), unnecessary cesarean births and other procedures such as FBS and operative vaginal birth can be avoided.

The system is to be used for singleton term fetuses (36 weeks or older) in a vertex presentation with a nonreassuring FHR pattern as defined by the randomized clinical trial protocol and found in the *Information for Prescribers* (Mallinckrodt, 2000). Membranes must be ruptured, the cervix dilated at least 2 cm, and the fetus at a −2 station or below. Use is contraindicated in cases of documented or suspected placenta previa, ominous FHR requiring immediate intervention, the need for immediate birth (unrelated to FHR pattern) such as active uterine bleeding, and certain infectious diseases that preclude internal monitoring (ie, active genital herpes, HIV, and hepatitis B and E seropositivity) (Mallinckrodt, 2000).

Fetal oxygen saturation monitoring improves assessment of fetal oxygen status by directly measuring $FSpO_2$ with a continuous real-time recording that is displayed on the uterine activity panel of the EFM tracing (Fig. 10–14). The $FSpO_2$ monitoring system uses a single use, sterile, disposable sensor (Fig. 10–15) that is inserted through the cervix into the uterus and rests against the fetal temple, cheek, or forehead. The uterine wall holds it in place (Fig. 10–16). The sensor usually descends in place with the fetus as labor progresses, although adjustments in sensor placement may be indicated infrequently.

Pulse oximetry is based on the premise that the major light absorbers in blood are oxyhemoglobin (ie, hemoglobin with oxygen) and deoxyhemoglobin (ie, hemoglobin without oxygen) (Mallinckrodt, 2000). These two molecules absorb red and infrared light differently. Oxyhemoglobin weakly absorbs red light and strongly absorbs infrared light. The opposite is true for deoxyhemoglobin. By shining red and infrared light with the sensor through the skin and measuring the relative absorption of each color, the fraction of hemoglobin that is carrying oxygen can be determined (Mallinckrodt, 2000). This fraction is displayed as a percentage, and the value is known as arterial oxygen saturation as determined by pulse oximetry (SpO_2).

The OxiFirst system uses the same pulse oximetry technology used during surgical procedures, in the postanesthesia recovery phase, and for patients for whom there is a concern about oxygen status. In adapting this technology to the fetus, changes in light wavelength and sensor design were required. The

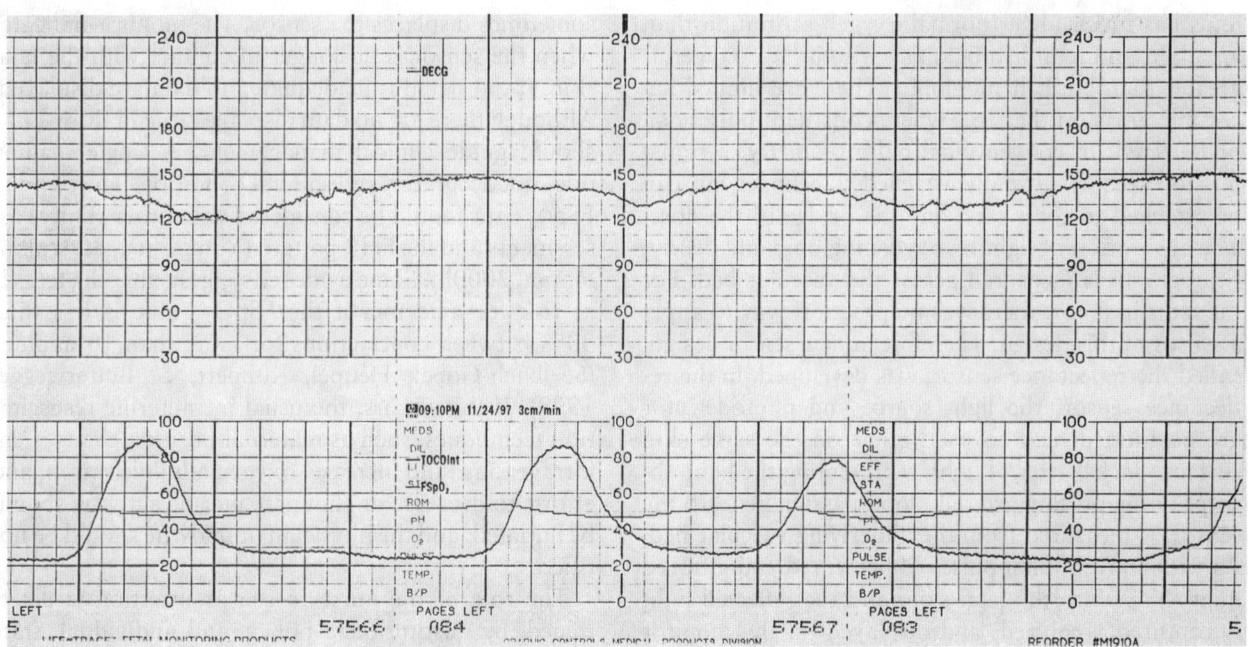

FIGURE 10–14. Fetal oxygen saturation ($FSpO_2$) data displayed on electronic fetal monitoring strip.

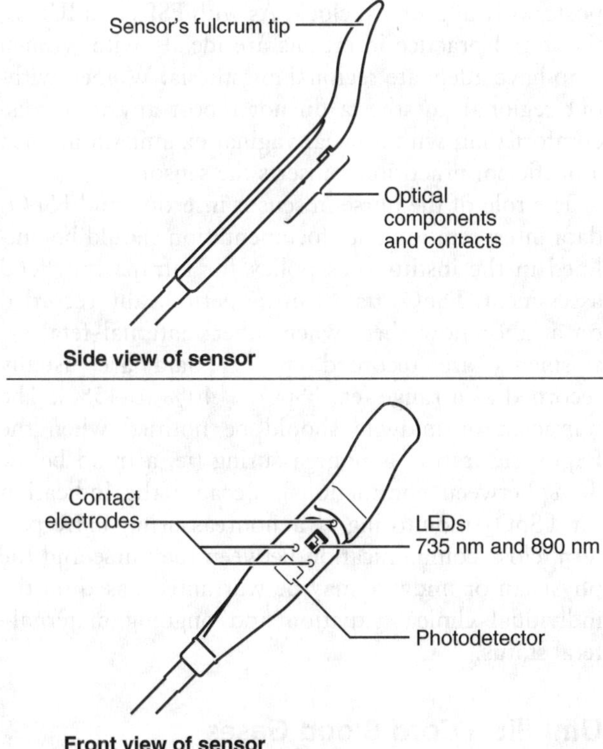

FIGURE 10–15. Fetal oxygen saturation sensor components. (© 2000 Mallinckrodt Inc., St. Louis, MO. All rights reserved.)

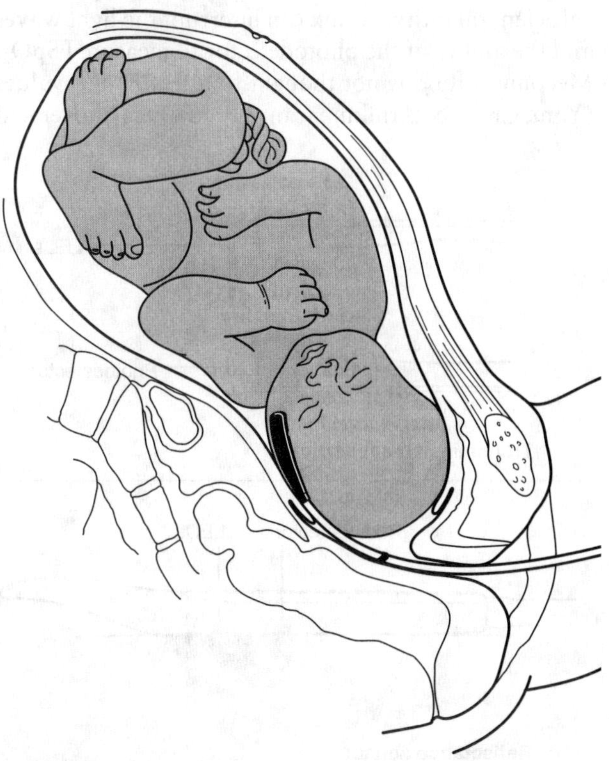

FIGURE 10–16. Fetal oxygen saturation sensor in place. (© 2000 Mallinckrodt Inc., St. Louis, MO. All rights reserved.)

fetus has much lower normal oxygen saturation than an adult, and fetal hemoglobin's affinity for oxygen is greater than adult hemoglobin. There are limited accessible areas on the fetus where consistent pulses can be detected. In conventional pulse oximetry, a transmission sensor is usually attached to a finger but can be attached to toes, ears, and the bridge of the nose. The absorption of light by oxyhemoglobin and deoxyhemoglobin is measured across the vascular bed. For the fetus in labor, there was no practical way to apply a sensor of this design. Therefore, a new sensor design, called the reflectance sensor, was developed. In the reflectance sensor, the light source and photodetector are positioned next to each other on the same skin surface. Backskatter of light, representing the light absorption by pulsing arterial blood passing beneath the sensor, is measured from the underlying vascular bed. As with conventional pulse oximetry, red and infrared light shines into the fetal skin, and the reflected light is captured, analyzed, and displayed on the monitor and on the FHR paper tracing (Fig. 10–17).

The normal $FSpO_2$ for the fetus in labor is 30% to 70%. If the $FSpO_2$ between uterine contractions is 30% or more, the practitioner can be reassured that the fetus is adequately oxygenated. If no $FSpO_2$ data are displayed, the practitioner can attempt to reposition the sensor on the fetal temple, cheek, or forehead. If this is unsuccessful, a new sensor can be inserted. If present in sufficient quantity, vernix can interrupt the light waves and the ability of the photodetector to measure $FSpO_2$. Meconium fluid is not thought to affect $FSpO_2$ values (Yam, Chua, & Arulkumaran, 2000a). Fetal movement sometimes displaces the sensor. The monitor indicates when the sensor is no longer in contact with the fetal skin. If the signal is inadequate, no data are displayed. Although there are no data displayed, the FHR by EFM should guide clinical management. A single reading does not accurately reflect fetal condition. The trend in $FSpo_2$ data should be considered with other clinical assessments and the FHR pattern (Yam, Chua, & Arulkumaran, 2000b). Some evidence suggests that the fetus is at risk for acidemia if the $FSpO_2$ value is less than 30% between contractions for more than 10 minutes (Seelbach-Gobel, Heupel, Kuhnert, & Butterwegge, 1999). If this occurs, the usual intrauterine resuscitation techniques, such as maternal position changes, an intravenous fluid increase, oxygen administration, and efforts to decrease or eliminate uterine activity, should be initiated, and the physician or midwife should be notified.

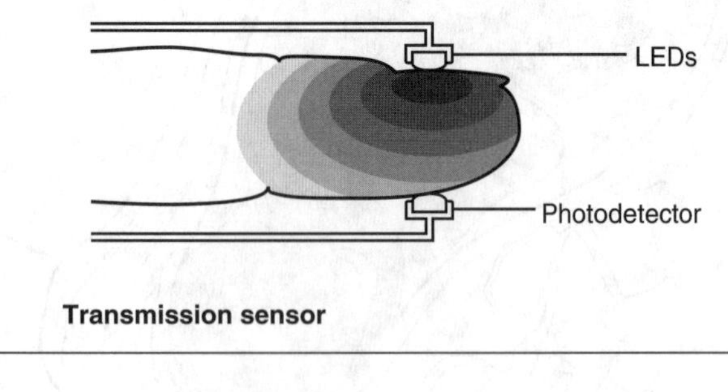

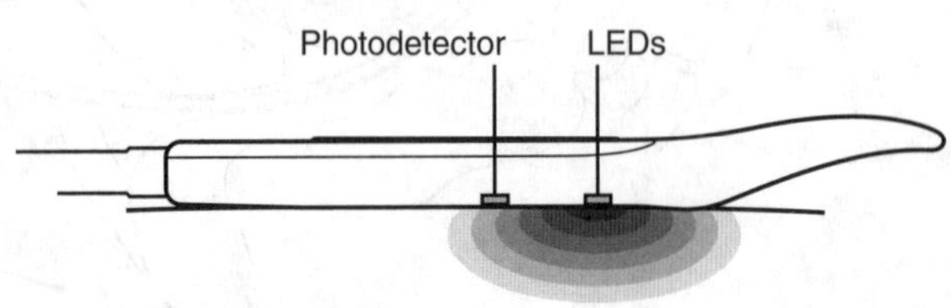

FIGURE 10–17. Reflectance versus transmission fetal oxygen saturation sensors. (© 2000 Mallinckrodt, Inc., St. Louis, MO. All rights reserved.)

The role of the nurse in sensor insertion is determined by institutional policy and individual state boards of nursing (Simpson, 1998). According to the OxiFirst *Information for Prescribers,* clinicians attempting to place sensors should have a mastery of FSE or IUPC insertion before learning fetal oxygen sensor placement (Mallinckrodt, 2000). Sensor insertion is not technically difficult. Proficiency can be achieved after several preceptored practice insertions. Most practitioners find it easier to insert the sensor posteriorly at 5 or 7 o'clock. As with FSEs and IUPCs, the initial practice insertions are ideally with women who have adequate regional anesthesia. Women without regional anesthesia do not report any more discomfort than with a usual vaginal examination when a proficient practitioner inserts the sensor.

The role of the nurse in sensor insertion and $FSpO_2$ data interpretation and documentation should be outlined in the institution's policy for intrapartum fetal assessment. $FSpO_2$ data can be periodically recorded on a labor flow sheet when other maternal–fetal assessments are recorded. $FSpO_2$ data are usually recorded as a range (eg, $FSpO_2$ = 40% to 45%). The physician or midwife should be notified when the $FSpO_2$ saturation is nonreassuring (ie, a trend below 30% between contractions). Because the indication for $FSpO_2$ monitoring is a nonreassuring FHR pattern, close communication between the nurse and the physician or midwife may be warranted based on the individual clinical situation and ongoing maternal–fetal status.

Umbilical Cord Blood Gases

Umbilical cord blood gas determinations at birth provide objective evidence confirming or refuting the presence of intrapartum acidemia. They are not tech-

TABLE 10–10 ■ MEAN BLOOD GAS VALUES IN NONPREGNANT WOMEN VERSUS UMBILICAL ARTERIAL (UA) AND UMBILICAL VENOUS (UV) CORD BLOOD IN FETUSES WITH APGAR SCORE ≥ 7 AT 5 MINUTES

Value	Nonpregnant Women	Pregnant Adults	Term Fetus with Apgar ≥ 7 at 5 Minutes	
			UA	*UV*
PH	7.40	7.40	7.26	7.34
PCO_2	40	34	53	41
PO_2			17	29
Base Excess	0	–4	–4	–3

Adapted from Parer, J.T. (1977). *Handbook of fetal heart rate monitoring* (2nd ed.). Philadelphia: W.B. Saunders.

nically an ancillary method used for the purpose of clinical decision-making during labor but are included here because of the importance this information has in excluding intrapartum asphyxia when the newborn is ill (Thorp, Sampson, Parisi, & Creasy, 1989). In one study, approximately one in four university hospitals surveyed obtained cord samples after all births (Johnson & Riley, 1993). Most centers considered this test to be clinically useful and of assistance in the reduction of medicolegal risks (Johnson & Riley, 1993). According to ACOG (1995c), umbilical cord blood gases are useful for the infant born with low Apgar scores, meconium-stained fluid, and postterm births, as well as in complicated births such as vaginal breech birth or twins.

Umbilical cord gas analysis can diagnose hypoxemia and the presence or absence of metabolic acidosis in blood samples but does not give an indication of the duration of the hypoxemia. Umbilical cord results are an indirect measure of the acid–base status in tissue at the time of birth but do not reveal the duration of the insult or the level of asphyxia in tissue (Table 10–10).

NURSING ASSESSMENT AND MANAGEMENT STRATEGIES

Patient Education about Fetal Heart Rate Monitoring

Preparation for the application of the monitoring equipment requires an explanation of EFM and time for answering the woman's questions. Most women know before labor that some form of EFM may be used. Ideally, objections or concerns regarding EFM have been discussed by the woman and perinatal healthcare provider before admission. However, if the woman does refuse EFM, the nurse should follow institutional procedures for any patient refusing medical treatment. A positive attitude in discussing the rationale for EFM is most effective. One approach is to explain to the woman and support person that the fetal monitor can provide reassurance of fetal well-being. Most women agree to an initial period of EFM to establish fetal well-being. Other options for ongoing fetal assessment include intermittent EFM and intermittent auscultation.

Nursing Assessment of the Fetal Heart Rate

A systematic, organized approach to interpreting FHR patterns prevents misinterpretation and confusion. A deceleration in the middle of the tracing is eye catching and anxiety producing, but it may not be the most important aspect of the tracing. Assessment of the entire FHR tracing, including uterine contractions and all procedures that transpired before the deceleration, is required. Review of the maternal medical record is critical. Assessment should include the following: maternal–fetal risk for uteroplacental insufficiency, administration of regional anesthetic, administration of medications or maternal drug use, and pharmacologic agents used for cervical ripening and labor induction or augmentation.

Physical assessment should include maternal vital signs, hydration status, and position. Maternal fever can cause fetal tachycardia, whereas hypotension can cause fetal bradycardia. Supine positioning can cause bradycardia by means of inferior vena caval compression. Maternal dehydration and ketosis is thought by many to result in minimal variability. Although the mechanism for this effect has never been fully appreciated or tested, women should be well hydrated with adequate blood sugar levels to efficiently complete the work of labor. Chapter 9 addresses oral and intravenous intake during labor.

Experienced perinatal nurses can quickly assess FHR patterns for evidence of fetal well-being. They use a mental checklist (adapted from Simpson, 1997) that includes the following:

- What is the baseline FHR?
- Is it within normal limits for this fetus?
- If not, what clinical factors could be contributing to this baseline rate?
- Is there evidence of baseline variability?
- If not, does external or fetal scalp stimulation elicit an acceleration of the FHR appropriate for gestational age?
- What clinical factors could be contributing to this baseline variability?
- Are there periodic or episodic FHR patterns?
- If so, what are they, and what are the appropriate interventions (if any)?
- Does the FHR pattern suggest a chronic or acute maternal–fetal condition?
- Is uterine activity normal in frequency, duration, intensity, and resting tone?
- What is the relationship between the FHR and uterine activity?
- If the FHR pattern is nonreassuring, do the appropriate interventions resolve the situation?
- If not, are further interventions needed?
- Is the FHR pattern such that notification of the physician or midwife is warranted?

Nurses who are learning the principles of EFM may require more time to complete an assessment of fetal status, but the essential components of a comprehensive assessment remain the same. It is helpful to devise a systematic method for FHR assessment and related appropriate interventions and consistently use that method in clinical practice to enhance optimal maternal–fetal outcomes.

After collecting all pertinent data, the following characteristics of the FHR tracing are interpreted and documented in the medical record: frequency, duration, intensity, and resting tone for uterine activity; baseline rate and variability; presence or absence of accelerations; and presence or absence of periodic or episodic changes (Display 10–5).

Nursing intervention is based first on identification of the precipitating event, if possible, and then interventions should be prioritized based on the level of concern. Eliminating the cause (eg, uterine hyperstimulation, maternal hypotension) or instituting interventions that provide in utero resuscitation may be all that is necessary for the resumption of a reassuring FHR pattern. Conversely, the presence of one of the

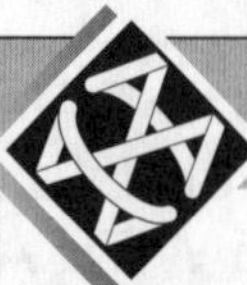

DISPLAY 10–5

Essential Components of Documentation of Fetal Heart Rate Patterns

1. Baseline rate
2. Baseline variability
3. Presence or absence of accelerations
4. Periodic or episodic decelerations
5. Changes in trends of fetal heart rate patterns over time

Adapted from National Institute of Child Health and Human Development Research Planning Workshop. (1997). Electronic fetal heart rate monitoring: Research guidelines for interpretation. *American Journal of Obstetrics and Gynecology 177,* 1385–1390, and *Journal of Obstetric Gynecology and Neonatal Nursing, 26*(6), 635–640.

five FHR patterns listed in Table 10–9 warrants immediate bedside evaluation by a physician who can initiate a cesarean birth. Depending on the clinical situation, an $FSpO_2$ sensor may be placed to determine fetal oxygen status, or there may be a decision for operative birth.

Communication with Primary Providers

It is not unusual for disagreements in the interpretation of FHR patterns to exist among members of the perinatal healthcare team (Beckmann, Van Mullem, Beckmann, & Broekhuizen, 1997; Paneth, Bommarito, & Stricker, 1993; Simpson & Knox, 2000). Intrapartum fetal assessment is one of the most important clinical situations in which nurses, physicians, and midwives need to work together and trust each other's judgment (Fox, Kilpatrick, King, & Parer, 2000; Simpson & Knox, 2000). Much of the communication about ongoing maternal–fetal status during labor occurs while the nurse is at the bedside and the physician is in the office or at home. If the nurse determines that the FHR pattern is nonreassuring, the physician or midwife should be notified. The concerns and observations of the nurse should be described and a clear plan of management collaboratively determined. The general content of this conversation should be documented in the medical record. If the discussion results in a clinical disagreement that cannot be resolved, the nurse should follow institutional policy about resolution of disagreements between providers. This type of policy is usually known as the *chain of command*. Chapter 2 discusses the chain of command.

Physicians, midwives, and nurses are responsible for maintaining competence in FHR pattern interpretation and appropriate interventions based on their interpretation (ACNM, 1997; ACOG, 1995b; AWHONN, 1998, 1999). One way to maintain competence and promote interdisciplinary collaboration is the use of EFM education programs that include physicians, midwives, and nurses together (Simpson, 2001). A group process can be used to review EFM strips, expected responses, appropriate interpretations, and related interventions. Team discussions can lead to an increased knowledge of EFM principles for everyone involved. Developing case studies containing clinical ambiguity is an ideal avenue for clarifying ongoing clinical issues when the interpretations and expectations of all provider groups are not compatible (Simpson, 2001). Educational collaboration among nurses, midwives, and physicians who are jointly responsible for FHR pattern interpretation and clinical interventions enhances collaboration in everyday clinical interactions and promotes maternal–fetal safety (Simpson & Knox, 2000).

ONGOING ISSUES RELATED TO THE USE OF FETAL HEART RATE MONITORING DURING LABOR

Efficacy of Electronic Fetal Heart Rate Monitoring

When EFM was developed and introduced into clinical practice, it was hoped that this technique for fetal assessment would lead to a reduction in the overall incidence of cerebral palsy and intrapartum stillbirth (Simpson & Knox, 2000). This expectation in part reflected the opinion of experts in the 1960s and 1970s that most cases of cerebral palsy and other neurologic morbidity were the result of asphyxia during labor and birth. The randomized trials conducted during the 1980s failed to show a decrease in the incidence of cerebral palsy among infants who were monitored during labor (Shy et al., 1990), but the incidence of cesarean birth and assisted operative birth in the cohorts monitored increased fourfold (Thacker et al., 1995). These results led many to the conclusion that EFM is not efficacious (Freeman, 1990). Later reviews of the methodology used in the randomized trials in combination with newer information on the genesis of cerebral palsy brought to light some of the reasons why FHR monitoring did poorly in the randomized trials that were conducted (Parer & King, 2000). This controversy is unresolved and merits review.

Fetal Heart Rate Monitoring and Cerebral Palsy

EFM has been in wide use for nearly 30 years with no change in the incidence of cerebral palsy (2 cases per 1,000 live births) (Penning & Garite, 1999). The original hope that EFM would predict and therefore prevent fetal asphyxia, which would prevent cerebral palsy, has not come to pass (Simpson & Knox, 2000). Most cases of infant and childhood cerebral palsy are related to prenatal events rather than the labor and birth process. Most cases of cerebral palsy are associated with prematurity, disorders of coagulation, and intrauterine exposure to maternal infections (Grether & Nelson, 1997). Interruption of the oxygen supply to the fetus contributes to approximately 6% of cases of cerebral palsy (Nelson & Grether, 1999), and most experts believe that no more than 2% to 20% of cases of cerebral palsy are caused by intrapartum events (MacDonald, 1996; Nelson, 1988). These wide-ranging estimates are the result of imprecise interpretation of EFM data during labor and of variations in diagnostic classification of the severity and type of cerebral palsy (Lent, 1999). The dramatically improved survival rates of extremely preterm infants have the potential to actually increase the incidence of cerebral palsy and advances in neonatal care may also improve the survival rate of asphyxiated infants of any gestational age. These factors may obscure any effect that EFM has had on the incidence of cerebral palsy. An international panel composed of specialists and researchers in perinatology, neonatology, midwifery, science, and epidemiology reviewed the literature on the causation of cerebral palsy (MacLennan, 1999). The *International Consensus Statement* published by this group lists clinical and biochemical factors that define the criteria that would implicate an acute intrapartum event as the cause of cerebral palsy (Display 10–6).

Specificity, Sensitivity, and Reliability of Electronic Fetal Monitoring

Approximately 30% of fetuses demonstrate a nonreassuring FHR pattern at some time during labor (Garite et al., 2000). However, it is estimated that even the most ominous FHR patterns are associated with at most a 50% to 65% incidence of neonatal depression (Martin, 1998). Overall, EFM can have up to a 99.8% false-positive rate for term fetuses (Nelson, Dambrosia, Ting, & Grether, 1996). Conversely,

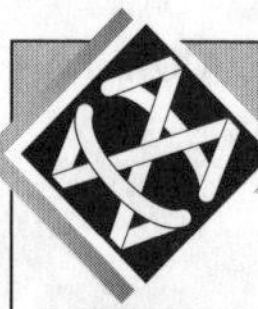

DISPLAY 10–6

Criteria That Define An Acute Intrapartum Hypoxic Event

ESSENTIAL CRITERIA*

1. Evidence of a metabolic acidosis in intrapartum fetal, umbilical arterial cord, or very early neonatal blood samples; pH <7.00 and base deficit ≥12 mmol/L
2. Early onset of severe or moderate neonatal encephalopathy in infants ≥34 weeks' gestation.
3. Cerebral palsy of the spastic quadriplegic or dyskinetic type.

CRITERIA THAT TOGETHER SUGGEST AN INTRAPARTUM TIMING BUT BY THEMSELVES ARE NON-SPECIFIC†

4. A sentinel (signal) hypoxic event occurring immediately before or during labor.
5. A sudden, rapid, and sustained deterioration of the fetal heart rate pattern, usually following the hypoxic sentinel event.
6. Apgar scores of 0–6 for >5 minutes.
7. Early evidence of multisystem involvement.
8. Early imaging evidence of acute cerebral abnormality.

* All three of the essential criteria are necessary before intrapartum hypoxia can be considered the cause of the cerebral palsy.

† If evidence for some of the 4–8 criteria is missing or contradictory, the timing of the neuropathology becomes increasingly in doubt.

Adapted from MacLenan A.H. (1999). *British Medical Journal, 319*(7216), 1016–1017.

when the FHR is reassuring, there is a very high probability (>99.9%) that the fetus is doing well and is adequately oxygenated (Garite et al., 2000). EFM sensitivity (ie, ability to detect a healthy fetus when it is healthy) is high, whereas specificity (ie, ability to detect a compromised fetus when it is compromised and not include healthy fetuses) is low (Simpson & Knox, 2000). The specificity and sensitivity limitations of EFM are related to its inability to directly evaluate fetal oxygen status.

Further complicating the issue is the fact that interobserver and intraobserver reliability in interpreting EFM data is inconsistent (Martin, 1998; Paneth et al., 1993). Not only do experienced clinicians differ in interpretations when evaluating a specific FHR pattern (Chez et al., 1990; Nelson et al., 1996), they disagree with their own interpretation when asked to review the same FHR strip months later (Barrett et al., 1990). This phenomenon particularly affects interpretations suggesting fetal compromise (Simpson & Knox, 2000). Diagnosis of fetal well-being (ie, adequate fetal oxygenation) has much higher interobserver and intraobserver reliability. Communication issues and professional disagreements regarding EFM interpretation are much more likely to occur when attempting to assign a diagnosis of fetal compromise than fetal well-being (Simpson & Knox, 2000).

The differential predictability between specificity and sensitivity and lack of reliability between different providers is the basis of the fundamental issue confounding the use of EFM (Simpson & Knox, 2000). The lack of common understanding by all involved professionals about how FHR monitoring can be relied on when determining fetal status undermines the ability of this technique to guide clinical management (Simpson & Knox, 2000). If the tracing has a normal baseline rate, moderate variability, and no nonreassuring periodic or episodic changes, there is little disagreement about the prediction of fetal well-being. Similarly, patterns with absent variability and bradycardia, tachycardia, variable decelerations, or late decelerations generate significant agreement. These patterns indicate the fetus is at risk for acidosis. However, most FHR patterns are between these two extremes. When different members of the care team are simultaneously making different assumptions concerning EFM data, communication between the involved professionals is compromised (Fox et al., 2000; Simpson & Knox, 2000).

SUMMARY

Monitoring and interpretation of the FHR pattern are critical elements of intrapartum care (Fig. 10–18). The use of standardized terms and definitions must be established and routinely used by all members of the perinatal healthcare team. Knowledge about the physiology underlying specific FHR patterns has increased over time, and nurses, midwives, and physicians must keep abreast of the evolving knowledge to provide the best care for mothers and babies during labor. The use of variability in determining the risk for fetal acidemia is critical. Clinicians caring for women in labor should be able to rapidly identify FHR patterns that truly reflect the absence of fetal acidemia and those that consistently indicate a significant risk for fetal acidemia. If the cesarean birth rate for fetal com-

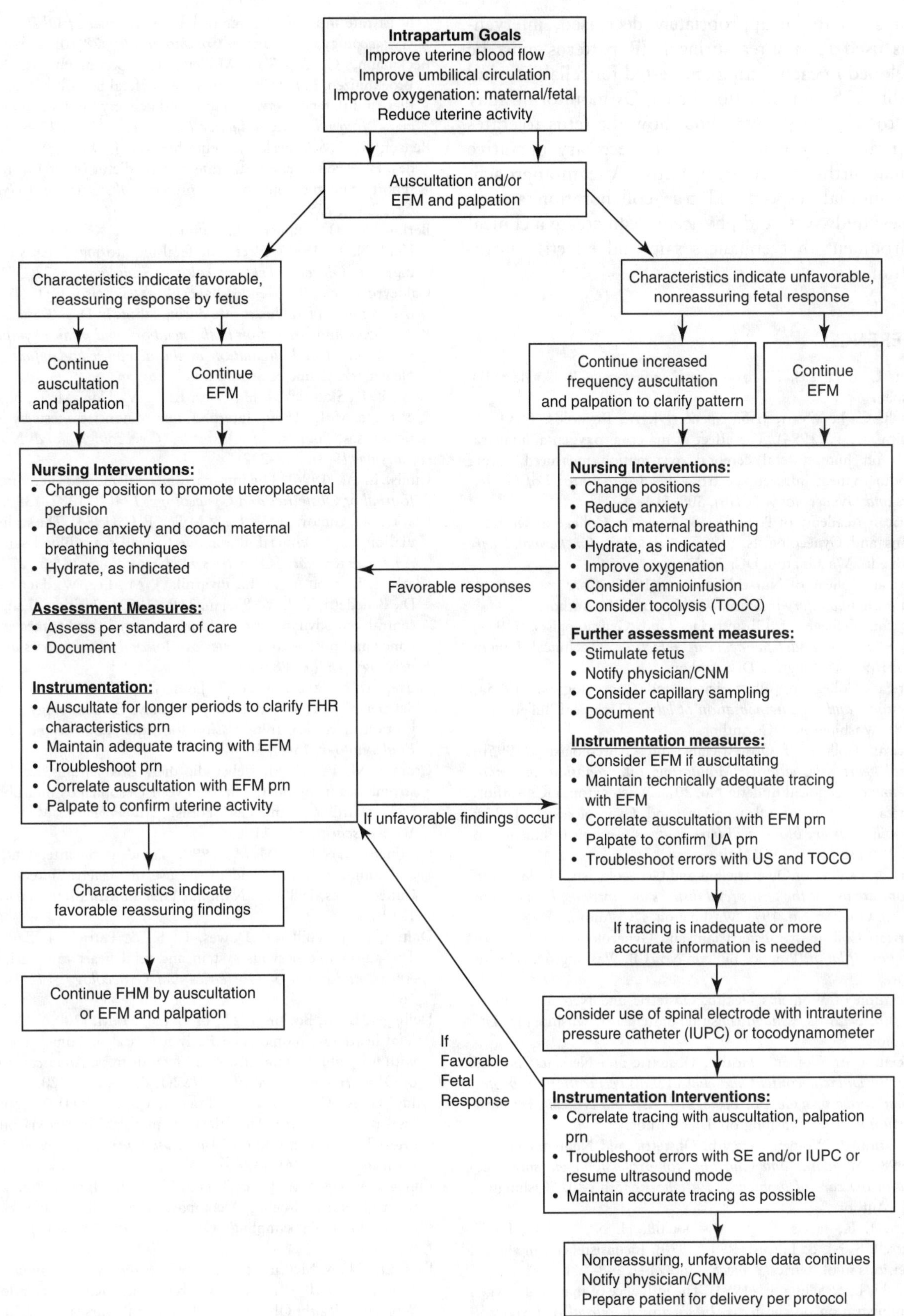

FIGURE 10–18. Decision tree for fetal heart monitoring. CNM, certified nurse midwife; FHR, fetal heart rate; EFM, electronic fetal monitoring; UA, uterine activity; US, ultrasound; SE, scalp electrode.

promise is to be appropriately decreased, interventions used for nonreassuring FHR patterns must be developed in each setting and tested for reliability and validity. The introduction of $FSpO_2$ monitoring may add to what is known about how the fetus tolerates labor and may help decrease unnecessary operative vaginal births and cesarean births. A team approach, with mutual respect and true collaboration among nurses, midwives, and physicians, can create a clinical environment that enhances safe and effective intrapartum care.

REFERENCES

Afriat, C. I. (1989). *Electronic fetal monitoring.* Rockville, MD: Aspen.

Aldrich, C. J., Wyatt, J. S., Spencer, J. A., Reynolds, E. O., & Delpy, D. T. (1994). The effect of maternal oxygen administration on human fetal cerebral oxygenation measured during labour by near infrared spectroscopy. *British Journal of Obstetrics and Gynaecology, 101*(6), 509–513.

American Academy of Pediatrics & American College of Obstetricians and Gynecologists. (1997). *Guidelines for perinatal care* (4th ed.). Washington, DC: Author.

American College of Nurse Midwives. (1997). *Core competencies for basic midwifery practice.* Washington, DC: Author.

American College of Obstetricians and Gynecologists. (1992). *Human immunodeficiency virus infections* (Technical Bulletin No. 169). Washington, DC: Author.

American College of Obstetricians and Gynecologists. (1995a). *Dystocia and the augmentation of labor* (Technical Bulletin No. 218). Washington, DC: Author.

American College of Obstetricians and Gynecologists. (1995b). *Fetal heart rate patterns: Monitoring, interpretation, and management* (Technical Bulletin No. 207). Washington, DC: Author.

American College of Obstetricians and Gynecologists. (1995c). *Umbilical artery blood acid-base analysis* (Technical Bulletin No. 216). Washington, DC: Author.

American College of Obstetricians and Gynecologists. (1998). *Inappropriate use of the terms fetal distress and birth asphyxia* (Committee Opinion No. 197). Washington, DC: Author.

American College of Obstetricians and Gynecologists. (1999). *Induction of labor* (Practice Bulletin No. 10). Washington, DC: Author.

Association of Women's Health, Obstetric and Neonatal Nurses. (2000). *Fetal Assessment* (Position Statement). Washington, DC: Author.

Association of Women's Health, Obstetric and Neonatal Nurses. (1999). *Didactic content and clinical skills verification for professional nurse providers of basic, high risk and critical care intrapartum nursing.* Washington, DC: Author.

Association of Women's Health, Obstetric and Neonatal Nurses. (1998). *Standards and guidelines for professional nursing practice in the care of women and newborns* (5th ed.). Washington, DC: Author.

Barrett, J. F., Jarvis, G. J., MacDonald, H. N., Buchan, P. C., Tyrrell, S. N., & Lilford, R. J. (1990). Inconsistencies in clinical decisions in obstetrics. *Lancet, 336*(8714), 549–551.

Bartnicki, J., & Saling, E. (1994). The influence of maternal oxygen administration on the fetus. *International Journal of Gynaecology and Obstetrics, 45*(2), 87–95.

Beard, R. W., Filshie, G. M., Knight, C. A., & Roberts, G. M. (1971). The significance of the changes in the continuous fetal heart rate in the first stage of labour. *Journal of Obstetrics and Gynaecology of the British Commonwealth, 78*(10), 865–881.

Beckmann, C. A., Van Mullem, C., Beckmann, C. R., & Broekhuizen, F. F. (1997). Interpreting fetal heart rate tracings: Is there a difference between labor and delivery nurses and obstetricians? *Journal of Reproductive Medicine, 42*(10), 647–650.

Benson, R. C., Schubeck, F., Deutschberger, J., Weiss, W., & Berendes, H. (1968). Fetal heart rate as a predictor of fetal distress: A report from the collaborative project. *Obstetrics and Gynecology, 32*(2), 259–266.

Berkus, M. D., Langer, O., Samueloff, A., Xernaxis, E. M., & Field, N. T. (1999). Electronic fetal monitoring: What's reassuring? *Acta Obstetricia et Gynecologica Scandinavica, 78*(1), 15–21.

Caldeyro-Barcia, R., Mendez-Bauer, E., & Poseiro, J. (1966). Control of human fetal heart rate during labor. In D. E. Cassels (Ed.), *The heart and circulation in the newborn and infant: Symposium on the heart and circulation in the newborn and infant* (p. 7). New York: Grune & Stratton.

Chez, B. F., Skurnick, J. H., Chez, R. A., Verklan, M. T., Biggs, S., & Hage, M. L. (1990). Interpretation of nonstress tests by obstetric nurses. *Journal of Obstetric, Gynecologic, and Neonatal Nursing, 19*(3), 227–232.

Cibils, L. A. (1996). On intrapartum fetal monitoring. *American Journal of Obstetrics and Gynecology, 174*(4), 1382–1389.

Clark, S. L., Gimovsky, M. L., & Miller, F. C. (1984). The scalp stimulation test: A clinical alternative to fetal scalp blood sampling. *American Journal of Obstetrics and Gynecology, 148*(3), 274–277.

Clark, S. L., Cotton, D. B., Pivarnik, J. M., Lee, W., Hankins, G. D., Benedetti, T. J., & Phelan, J. P. (1991). Position change and central hemodynamic profile during normal third trimester pregnancy and post partum. *American Journal of Obstetrics and Gynecology, 164*(3), 883–887.

Craven, D. E., Steger, K. A., & Jarek, C. (1994). Human immunodeficiency virus infection in pregnancy: Epidemiology and prevention of vertical transmission. *Infection Control and Hospital Epidemiology, 15*(1), 36–47.

Cramer, M. V. (1906). Ueber die dierkte Ableitung der Akionsstrome des menschlchen hersens vom Oesophagus und uber das Elektrokardiogramm des Fotus. *Muenchener Medizinische Wochenschrift, 53*, 811–813.

Curtin, S. C., & Park, M. M. (1999). Trends in the attendant, place and timing of births, and in the use of obstetric interventions: United States, 1989–97. *National Vital Statistics Reports, 47*(27), 1–12.

Dalton, K. J., Phill, D., Dawes, G. S., & Patrick, J. E. (1983). The autonomic nervous system and fetal heart rate variability. *American Journal of Obstetrics and Gynecology, 146*(4), 456–462.

Dellinger, E. H., Boehm, F. H., & Crane, M. M. (2000). Electronic fetal heart rate monitoring: Early neonatal outcomes associated with normal rate, fetal stress and fetal distress. *American Journal of Obstetrics and Gynecology, 182*(1, Pt. 1), 214–220.

Dildy, G. A., Clark. S. L., & Loucks, C. A. (1994). Intrapartum fetal pulse oximetry: The effects of maternal hyperoxia on fetal arterial oxygen saturation. *American Journal of Obstetrics and Gynecology, 171*(4), 1120–1124.

Elimian, A., Figueroa, R., & Tejani, N. (1997). Intrapartum assessment of fetal well-being: A comparison of scalp stimulation with scalp blood pH sampling. *Obstetrics and Gynecology, 89*(3), 373–376.

Feinstein, N., & McCartney, P. (1997). *Fetal heart rate monitoring: Principles and practices.* Washington, DC: Association of Women's Health, Obstetric, and Neonatal Nurses.

Feinstein, N., Sprague, A., & Trepenier, M. J. (2000). *Fetal Heart Rate Auscultation: Symposium.* Washington, DC: Association of Woman's Health, Obstetric and Gynecologic Nurses.

Fox, M., Kilpatrick, S., King, T., & Parer, J. T. (2000). Fetal heart rate monitoring: Interpretation and collaborative management. *Journal of Midwifery and Women's Health, 45*(6), 498–507.

Freeman, R. (1990). Intrapartum fetal monitoring: A disappointing story. *New England Journal of Medicine, 322*(9), 624–626.

Freeman, R. K., Garite, T. J., & Nageotte, M. P. (1991). *Fetal heart rate monitoring* (2nd ed.). Baltimore: Williams & Wilkins.

Galvan, B. J., Van Mullem, C., & Broekhuizen, F. F. (1989). Using amnioinfusion for the relief of repetitive variable decelerations during labor. *Journal of Obstetric, Gynecologic, and Neonatal Nursing, 18*(3), 222–229.

Garite, T. J., Dildy, G., McNamara, H., Nageotte, M. P., Swedlow, D. B., & the Mallinckrodt (Nellcor) Fetal Oximetry Research Group. (2000). A multicenter randomized trial of fetal pulse oximetry. *American Journal of Obstetrics and Gynecology, 182*(1, Pt. 2), S12.

Gill, R. W., Trudinger, B. J., Garrett, W. J., Kossoff, G., & Warren, P. S. (1981). Fetal umbilical venous blood flow measured in utero by pulsed Doppler and B-mode ultrasound in normal pregnancies. *American Journal of Obstetrics and Gynecology, 139*(6), 720–725.

Goldaber, K. G., Gilstrap, L. C., III, Leveno, K. J., Dax, J. S., & McIntire, D. D. (1991). Pathologic fetal acidemia. *Obstetrics and Gynecology, 78*(6), 1103–1107.

Goodlin, R. C. (1979). History of fetal monitoring. *American Journal of Obstetrics and Gynecology, 133*(3), 323–352.

Goodwin, T. M., Milner-Masterson, L., & Paul, R. H. (1994). Elimination of fetal scalp blood sampling on a large clinical service. *Obstetrics and Gynecology, 83*(6), 971–974.

Grether, J. K., & Nelson, K. B. (1997). Maternal infection and cerebral palsy in infants of normal birth weight. *Journal of the American Medical Association, 278*(3), 207–211.

Gull, I., Jaffa, A. J., Oren, M., Grisaru, D., Peyser, M. R., & Lessing, J. P. (1996). Acid accumulation during end stage bradycardia: How long is too long? *British Journal of Obstetrics and Gynaecology, 103*(11), 1096–1101.

Hammacher, K. (1969). The clinical significance of cardiotocography. In P. Huntingford, K. Huter, & E. Salez (Eds.), *Perinatal Medicine, 1st European Congress, Berlin* (p. 81). New York: Academic Press.

Helwig, J. T., Parer, J. T., Kilpatrick, S. J., & Laros, R. K., Jr. (1996). Umbilical cord blood acid base state: What is normal? *American Journal of Obstetrics and Gynecology, 174*(6), 1807–1814.

Herbst, A., Wolner-Hanssen, P., & Ingelmarsson I. (1997). Risk factors for acidemia at birth. *Obstetrics and Gynecology 90*(1), 125–130.

Hohn, A., & Stanton, R. (1992). The cardiovascular system. In A. A. Fanaroff & R. J. Martin (Eds.), *Neonatal perinatal medicine: Diseases of the fetus and infant* (5th ed., pp. 883–940). St. Louis: Mosby–Year Book.

Hon, E. H. (1958). The electronic evaluation of the fetal heart rate: Preliminary report. *American Journal of Obstetrics and Gynecology, 75*(6), 1215–1230.

Hon, E. (1963). The classification of fetal heart rate. I. A revised working classification. *Obstetrics and Gynecology, 22*, 137–146.

Johnson, J. W., & Riley, W. (1993). Cord blood gas studies: A survey. *Clinical Obstetrics and Gynecology, 36*(1), 99–101.

Kennedy, E. (1833). *Observations of obstetrical auscultation* (p. 311). Dublin: Hodges & Smith.

King, T. L., & Parer, J. T. (2000). The physiology of fetal heart rate patterns and perinatal asphyxia. *Journal of Perinatal and Neonatal Nursing, 14*(3), 20–43.

Kleinman, C. S., Nehgme, R., & Copel, J. A. (1999). Fetal cardiac arrhythmias: Diagnosis and therapy. In R. K. Creasy & R. Resnik (Eds.), *Maternal-fetal medicine* (4th ed., pp. 301–318). Philadelphia: W.B. Saunders.

Klingner, M. C., & Kruse, J. (1999). Meconium aspiration syndrome: Pathophysiology and prevention. *Journal of the American Board of Family Practice, 12*(6), 450–466.

Knox, G. E., Simpson, K. R., & Garite, T. J. (1999). High reliability perinatal units: An approach to the prevention of patient injury and medical malpractice claims. *Journal of Healthcare Risk Management, 19*(2), 24–32.

Korhonen, J., & Kariniemi, V. (1994). Emergency cesarean section: The effect of delay on umbilical arterial gas balance and Apgar scores. *Acta Obstetricia et Gynecologica Scandinavica, 73*(10), 782–786.

Krebs, H. B., Petres, R. E., & Dunn, L. J. (1981). Intrapartum fetal heart rate monitoring. V. Fetal heart rate patterns in the second stage of labor. *American Journal of Obstetrics and Gynecology, 140*(4), 435–439.

Krebs, H. B., Petres, R. E., Dunn, L. J., Jordaan, H. V., & Segreti, A. (1979). Intrapartum fetal heart rate monitoring. I. Classification and prognosis of fetal heart rate patterns. *American Journal of Obstetrics and Gynecology, 133*(7), 762–772.

Lent, M. (1999). The medical and legal risks of the electronic fetal monitor. *Stanford Law Review, 51*(4), 807–837.

Leung, A. S., Leung, E. K., & Paul, R. H. (1993). Uterine rupture after previous cesarean delivery: Maternal and fetal consequences. *American Journal of Obstetrics and Gynecology, 169*(4), 945–950.

Low, J. A., Victory, R., & Derrick, E. J. (1999). Predictive value of electronic fetal monitoring for intrapartum fetal asphyxia with metabolic acidosis. *Obstetrics and Gynecology, 93(2)*, 285–291.

MacDonald, D. (1996). Cerebral palsy and intrapartum fetal monitoring. *New England Journal of Medicine, 334*(6), 659–660.

MacDonald, D., Grant A., Sheridan-Pereira, M., Boylan, P., & Chalmers, I. (1985). The Dublin randomized controlled trial of intrapartum fetal heart rate monitoring. *American Journal of Obstetrics and Gynecology, 152*(5), 524–539.

MacLennan, A. H. (1999). A template for defining a causal relationship between acute intrapartum events and cerebral palsy: International consensus statement. *British Medical Journal, 319*(7216), 1016–1017.

Mallinckrodt. (2000). *OxiFirst information for prescribers*. St. Louis: Author.

Martin C. B., Jr. (1998). Electronic fetal monitoring: A brief summary of its development, problems and prospects. *European Journal of Obstetrics and Gynecology and Reproductive Biology, 78*(2), 133–40.

McNamara, H., Johnson, N., & Lilford, R. (1993). The effect on fetal arteriolar oxygen saturation resulting from giving oxygen to the mother measured by pulse oximetry. *British Journal of Obstetrics and Gynaecology, 100*(5), 446–449.

Menihan, C. A. (1998). Uterine rupture in women attempting a vaginal birth following prior cesarean birth. *Journal of Perinatology, 18*(6, Pt. 1), 440–443.

Mino, M., Puertas, A., Miranda, J. A., & Herruzo, A. J. (1999). Amnioinfusion in term labor with low amniotic fluid due to rupture of the membranes: A new indication. *European Journal of Obstetrics, Gynecology, and Reproductive Biology, 82*(1), 29–34.

Miyazaki, F. S., & Nevarez, F. (1985). Saline amnioinfusion for relief of repetitive variable decelerations: A prospective randomized study. *American Journal of Obstetrics and Gynecology, 153*(3), 301–306.

Mondanlou, H. D. (1991). Uses of biochemical profile of the fetus. *Contemporary Obstetrics and Gynecology, 36*(9), 69–85.

National Institute of Child Health and Human Development Research Planning Workshop. (1997). Electronic fetal heart rate monitoring: Research guidelines for interpretation. *American Journal of Obstetrics and Gynecology 177*(6), 1385–1390, and *Journal of Obstetric Gynecology and Neonatal Nursing, 26*(6), 635–640.

Nelson, K. B. (1988). What proportion of cerebral palsy is related to birth asphyxia? *Journal of Pediatrics, 112*(4), 572–574.

Nelson, K. B., Dambrosia, J. M., Ting, T. Y., & Grether, J. K. (1996). Uncertain value of electronic fetal monitoring in predicting cerebral palsy. *New England Journal of Medicine, 334*(10), 613–618.

Nelson, K. B., & Grether, J. K. (1999). Causes of cerebral palsy. *Current Opinions in Pediatrics, 11*(6), 487–491.

O'Brien-Abel, N. E., & Benedetti, T. J. (1992). Saltatory fetal heart rate pattern. *Journal of Perinatology, 12*(1), 13–17.

Ouzounian, J. G., Miller, D. A., & Paul, R. H. (1996). Amnioinfusion in women with previous cesarean births: A preliminary report. *American Journal of Obstetrics and Gynecology, 174*(2), 783–786.

Paneth, N., Bommarito, M., & Stricker, J. (1993). Electronic fetal monitoring and later outcome. *Clinical and Investigative Medicine, 16*(2), 159–165.

Parer, J. T. (1997). *Handbook of fetal heart rate monitoring* (2nd ed.). Philadelphia: W.B. Saunders.

Parer, J. T. (1999). Fetal heart rate. In R. K. Creasy & R. Resnick (Eds.), *Maternal-fetal medicine* (4th ed., pp. 270–301). Philadelphia: W.B. Saunders.

Parer, J. T., & King, T. L. (2000). Fetal heart rate monitoring: Is it salvageable? *American Journal of Obstetrics and Gynecology 182(4)*, 982–987.

Parer, J. T., & King, T. L. (1999). Whither fetal heart rate monitoring. *Obstetrics, Gynecology and Fertility, 22(5)*, 149–192.

Parer, J. T., & Livingston E. G. (1990). What is fetal distress? *American Journal of Obstetrics and Gynecology 162*(6), 1421–1425; discussion 1427–1475.

Penning, S., & Garite, T. (1999). Management of fetal distress. *Obstetrics and Gynecology Clinics of North America, 26*(2), 259–274.

Phelan, J. P., & Ahn, M. O. (1994). Perinatal observations in forty-eight neurologically impaired term infants. *American Journal of Obstetrics and Gynecology, 171*(2), 424–431.

Pierce, J., Gaudier, F. L., & Sanchez-Ramos, L. (2000). Intrapartum amnioinfusion for meconium-stained fluid: Meta-analysis of prospective clinical trials. *Obstetrics and Gynecology, 95*(6, Pt. 2), 1051–1056.

Rochard, F., Schifrin, B. S., Goupil, F., Legrand, H., Blottiere, J., & Sureau, C. (1976). Nonstressed fetal heart monitoring in the antepartum period. *American Journal of Obstetrics and Gynecology, 126(6)*, 699–706.

Seelbach-Gobel, B., Heupel, M., Kuhnert, M., & Butterwegge, M. (1999). The prediction of fetal acidosis by means of intrapartum fetal pulse oximetry. *American Journal of Obstetrics and Gynecology, 180*(1, Pt. 1), 73–81.

Shy, K. K., Luthy, D. A., Bennett, F. C., Whitfield, M., Larson, E. B., van Belle, G., Hughes, J. P., Wilson, J. A., & Stenchever, M. A. (1990). Effects of electronic fetal heart rate monitoring, as compared with periodic auscultation, on the neurologic development of premature infants. *New England Journal of Medicine, 322*(9), 588–593.

Simpson, K. R. (1997). Electronic fetal heart rate monitoring: A primer for critical care nurses. *AACN Clinical Issues, Advanced Practice in Acute and Critical Care, 8*(4), 516–523.

Simpson, K. R. (1998). Fetal oxygen saturation monitoring during labor. *Journal of Perinatal and Neonatal Nursing, 12*(3), 26–37, 78–79.

Simpson, K. R. (2001). EFM competence validation: The pros and cons of traditional approaches. In C. A. Menihan & E. Zitolli (Eds.), *Evidence-based electronic fetal monitoring interpretation*. Philadelphia: Lippincott, Williams & Wilkins.

Simpson, K. R., & Knox, G. E. (2000). Risk Management and EFM: Decreasing risk of adverse outcomes and liability exposure. *Journal of Perinatal and Neonatal Nursing, 14*(3), 44–58.

Society of Obstetricians and Gynaecologists of Canada. (1995). Fetal health surveillance in labour (policy statement). *Journal of the Society of Obstetricians and Gynaecologists of Canada, 17*(9), 865–901.

Stein, E., Handelsman, E., & Matthews, R. (2000). Reducing perinatal transmission of HIV: Early diagnosis and interventions during pregnancy. *Journal of Midwifery and Women's Health, 45*(2), 122–129.

Strong, T. H., Jr. (1997). The effect of amnioinfusion on the duration of labor. *Obstetrics and Gynecology, 89*(6), 1044–1046.

Sureau, C. (1996). Historical perspectives: Forgotten past, unpredictable future. *Baillieres Clinical Obstetrics and Gynaecology, 10*(2), 167–184.

Tejani, N., Mann, L. I., Bhakthavathsalan, A., & Weiss, R. R. (1975). Correlation of fetal heart rate-uterine contraction patterns with fetal scalp blood pH. *Obstetrics and Gynecology, 46*(4), 392–396.

Thacker, S. B., Stroup, D. F., & Peterson, H. B. (1995). Efficacy and safety of intrapartum electronic fetal monitoring: An update. *Obstetrics and Gynecology, 86*(4, Pt. 1), 613–620.

Thorp, J. A., Sampson, J. E., Parisi, V. M., & Creasy, R. K. (1989). Routine umbilical cord blood gas determinations? *American Journal of Obstetrics and Gynecology, 161*(3), 600–605.

Tucker, S. M. (2000). *Pocket guide to fetal monitoring* (4th ed.). St. Louis: Mosby.

Vintzileos, A. M., Antsaklis, A., Varvarigos, I., Papas, C., Sofatzis, I., & Montgomery, J. T. (1993). A randomized trial of intrapartum electronic fetal heart rate monitoring versus intermittent auscultation. *Obstetrics and Gynecology, 81*(6), 899–907.

Westgate, J. A., Bennet, L., & Gunn, A. J. (1999). Fetal heart rate variability during brief repeated umbilical cord occlusion in near term fetal sheep. *British Journal of Obstetrics and Gynecology 106*(7), 664–671.

Yam, J., Chua, S., & Arulkumaran, S. (2000a). Intrapartum fetal pulse oximetry. Part 1: Principles and technical issues. *Obstetrical and Gynecological Survey, 55*(3), 163–172.

Yam, J., Chua, S., & Arulkumaran, S. (2000b). Intrapartum fetal pulse oximetry. Part 2: Clinical application. *Obstetrical and Gynecological Survey, 55*(3), 173–183.

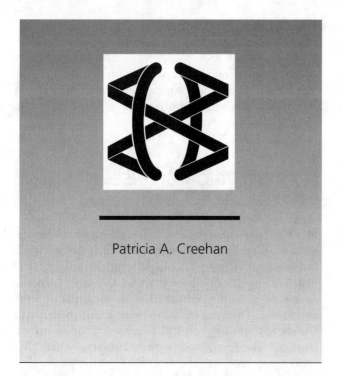

Patricia A. Creehan

CHAPTER 11

Pain Relief and Comfort Measures During Labor

Most pregnant women have concerns about their ability to handle painful contractions during labor. Nearly every woman in labor experiences some degree of discomfort. Perception of pain is highly individual, even when two people experience the same stimuli. An appreciation of each women's unique experience of pain is possible when perinatal nurses understand the physiologic basis of pain, physiologic responses to pain, and psychosocial factors influencing pain perception.

Many women experience intense pain in labor. When the McGill Pain Questionnaire was used to compare reports of intensity of pain for a variety of clinical experiences (eg, chronic back pain, nonterminal cancer pain, phantom limb pain, sprains, fractures), only the pain associated with accidental amputation of a digit and causalgia pain caused more discomfort than labor (Niven & Gijsbers, 1989). In a committee opinion, *Pain Relief During Labor,* the American College of Obstetricians and Gynecologists (ACOG, 2000) acknowledged that labor may result in severe pain for women and that, in the absence of any medical contraindications, pain management should be provided.

During labor, responsibility for managing pain and providing comfort is shared by the laboring woman, nurses, physicians, certified nurse midwives (CNMs), and labor-support persons. Interventions exist along a continuum, from noninvasive to invasive and from nonpharmacologic to pharmacologic. As healthcare professionals move along this continuum, the potential for complications and side effects increases. The goal of pain management during labor is to control pain without interrupting labor or doing harm to the woman or her fetus or newborn.

This chapter discusses the physiologic basis for pain along with the psychosocial factors influencing pain perception. Nonpharmacologic interventions are presented first because, in clinical practice, these are usually used before pharmacologic interventions.

PHYSIOLOGIC BASIS FOR LABOR PAIN

Most pain during childbirth results from normal physiologic events. During the first stage of labor, uterine muscle hypoxia, lactic acid accumulation, cervical and lower uterine segment stretching, traction on ovaries, fallopian tubes, and uterine ligaments, and pressure on the bony pelvis cause afferent pain impulses to be carried along sympathetic nerve fibers entering the neuraxis between the 10th and 12th thoracic and first lumbar spinal segment. During the second stage of labor, distention of pelvic floor muscles, vagina, perineum, and vulva and pressure on the urethra, bladder, and rectum cause afferent pain impulses to be carried along sympathetic nerve fibers entering the neuraxis between the second and fourth sacral spinal segments (Oxone-Foote, 1986). Some women in labor experience continuous low-back pain that is distinct from uterine contractions. This pain may be related to pressure from the fetal occiput on the neural plexus and bony structures of the maternal spine and pelvis.

Labor pain is an example of acute pain. It has a high degree of variability between individuals and at different points in labor. Obstetric factors that contribute to the pain of labor include rate of cervical dilatation, perineal distention, intensity and duration of contractions, and fetal position and size. As pain intensity increases, women experience decreased pain tolerance (Faure, 1991). Sleep deprivation and exhaustion from a long labor may alter the perception of pain (Youngstrom, Baker, & Miller, 1996). Age and parity may also influence an individual's perception of pain (Lowe, 1996). Descriptions of pain during the first and second stage of labor vary (Table 11–1). Some women describe a decrease in intensity during second stage, probably because of maternal focus on pushing. Others experience more painful sensations, possibly because of the position of the fetus descending through the birth canal.

Unique Characteristics of Labor

Unique circumstances of every labor influence the experience of pain. Responsiveness of the cervix to uterine contractions is influenced by prior surgical or diagnostic procedures that compromise the integrity of the cervix. Prior surgical procedures may result in an incompetent cervix and shorter labor or cause scarring and adhesions, resulting in failure to dilate and longer labor. Some medical and nursing procedures are uncomfortable. Interventions such as pharmacologic agents used for induction and augmentation of labor, vaginal examinations performed in the supine position, bed rest, amniotomy, tight external electronic fetal monitor (EFM) belts, and enemas may change the character of labor contractions and increase discomfort. Length of labor does not necessarily correlate directly with a woman's perception of pain. A woman with short labors may experience very intense contractions. Women with a fetus in a persistent posterior position report severe pain during and between uterine contractions.

As duration of intense pain increases, discouragement and fatigue increase, decreasing the woman's ability to cope effectively with contractions. Fatigue may occur with a prolonged latent phase, as experienced by the woman who reports on admission that she has "not slept for 2 days."

PHYSIOLOGIC RESPONSES TO PAIN

In addition to obvious physical discomfort, there are physiologic responses to pain over which women have little control. These physiologic responses may have a negative impact on the fetus and the labor process over time or in the context of other maternal or fetal conditions. Pain during labor may result in anxiety. Unrelieved anxiety causes increased production of cortisol, glucagon, and catecholamines, which increase metabolism and oxygen consumption. Increased levels of catecholamines have been shown to cause uterine hypoperfusion and decreased blood flow to the placenta, resulting in uterine irritability, preterm labor, dystocia, and fetal asphyxia (Britt & Pasero, 1999). Excessive catecholamines influence the labor process by reducing strength, duration, and coordination of uterine contractions, and they influence the fetus, as demonstrated by nonreassuring changes in the fetal heart rate pattern (Lederman, Lederman, Work, & McCann, 1985).

PSYCHOSOCIAL FACTORS INFLUENCING PAIN PERCEPTION

In addition to the physiologic factors that influence the perception of pain, psychosocial factors influence an individual's experience. These factors include labor support, childbirth preparation, and medical and

TABLE 11–1 ■ VERBAL DESCRIPTIONS OF PAIN DURING LABOR AND BIRTH

Sensory	Affective
First Stage of Labor	
Cramping, pulling, aching, heavy, sharp, stabbing, cutting, intermittent, localized, global	Exciting, intense, tiring or exhausting, scary or frightening, bearable or unbearable, distressing, horrible, agonizing, indescribable overwhelming, engulfing
Second Stage of Labor	
Painful pressure, burning, ripping, tearing, piercing, explosive, rending, localized	Exhausting, overwhelming, out-of-body feeling, inner focused or tunnel vision, exciting, horrible, excruciating, terrifying, less intense

nursing interventions, including those that are medically indicated and those that reflect the culture of the organization and individual pain tolerance.

Labor Support

Labor support encompasses provisions for emotional support, comfort measures, information, advocacy, and support for the husband or partner (Simkin, 1995) (Display 11–1). Providing for physical comfort includes offering a variety of nonpharmacologic and pharmacologic interventions. These are discussed at length later in this chapter. Emotional support includes behaviors such as giving praise, encouragement, reassurance, and "being positive"; apearing calm, and confident; assisting with breathing and relaxation; providing explanations about labor progress; identifying ways to include family members in the experience; and treating women with respect (Bryanton, Fraser-Davey, & Sullivan, 1994; Sleutel, 2000). Women identify support, information, interventions, decision-making, control, and pain relief as contributing to a positive labor experience (Lavender, et al., 1999). Labor support should be provided by a registered nurse who understands the physiologic events of labor and has been educated about supportive care in labor. The husband or significant other, family members and friends, or a professional or lay labor-support person (ie, doula or monitrice) may also provide labor support. However, the presence of one or all of these individuals does not decrease the ultimate responsibility of the perinatal nurse.

Quality support, whether offered by a partner, family members, friends, or nursing personnel, has a tremendous impact on a woman's perception of labor. Qualitative research has demonstrated that one of the most significant aspects of the experience of labor for women is the presence of one or more support persons (Lavender et al., 1999). In a meta-analysis of 14 clinical trials, continuous support from nurse, CNM, or lay person decreased use of medication for pain relief, operative vaginal birth, cesarean birth, and 5-minute Apgar scores less than 7 (Hodnett, 2000).

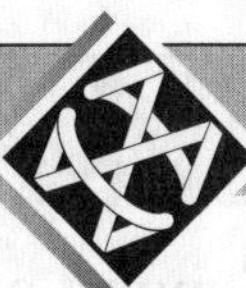

DISPLAY 11–1

Examples of Labor Support

EMOTIONAL SUPPORT

- Companionship
- Eye contact
- Praise
- Distraction
- Affirmation
- Reassurance
- Visualization
- Attention focusing

COMFORT MEASURES

- Reassuring touch
- Holding
- Applications of heat or cold
- Giving ice chips, fluids, food
- Helping with personal hygiene
- Massage
- Hydrotherapy (bath or shower)
- Helping with positioning
- Assisting with ambulation

INFORMATION OR ADVICE

- Providing information
- Offering advice
- Coaching in breathing, relaxation techniques
- Interpreting medical jargon

ADVOCACY

- Supporting the woman's decisions
- Interpreting the woman's wishes to others

SUPPORTING THE HUSBAND OR PARTNER

- Role modeling
- Providing an opportunity for respite
- Encouragement
- Praise

From Simpkin, P. (1995). Reducing pain and enhancing progress in labor: A guide to nonpharmacologic methods for maternity caregivers. *Birth, 22*(3), 161–171.

Registered Nurse

It is the position of the Association of Woman's Health, Obstetric and Neonatal Nurses (AWHONN) that supporting and caring for women during labor is best performed by a registered nurse (Display 11–2). Comprehensive nursing education, clinical patient-management skills, and previous experience make the registered nurse uniquely qualified to provide skilled technical care and complex emotional care women

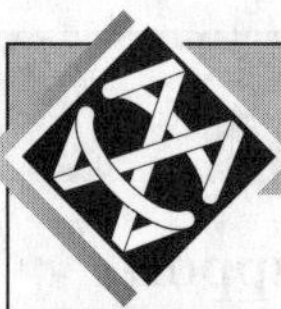

DISPLAY 11–2

Professional Nursing Support of Laboring Women

The Association of Women's Health, Obstetric and Neonatal Nurses (AWHONN) maintains that continuously available labor support by a professional registered nurse is a critical component of achieving improved birth outcomes. The childbirth experience is an intensely physical and emotional event with lifelong implications. AWHONN views labor care and labor support as powerful nursing functions and believes it is incumbent on healthcare facilities to provide an environment that encourages the unique patient–nurse relationship during childbirth. Only the registered nurse combines adequate formal nursing education and clinical patient management skills with experience in providing physical, psychological, and sociocultural care to laboring women.

Because of their comprehensive education and experience, registered nurses are capable of providing highly skilled technical and complex emotional care. The registered nurse facilitates the childbirth process in collaboration with the laboring woman. The nurse's expertise and therapeutic presence influence patient and family satisfaction with the labor and delivery experience. Women who are provided with continuously available support during labor experience improved labor and delivery outcomes compared with those who labor without a skilled support person. Such care can lead to

- Shorter labors
- Decreased use of analgesia or anesthesia
- Decreased operative vaginal delivery or cesarean section
- Decreased need for oxytocin
- Increased satisfaction with the childbirth experience

Professional registered nurses draw on a deep and broad base of nursing knowledge and clinical expertise to provide a level of care and support beyond that of lay personnel. They can effectively implement patient management strategies for low-risk and high-risk patients. The registered nurse can assess, plan, implement, and evaluate an individualized plan of care based on each woman's physical, psychological, and sociocultural needs, including desires and expectations of the laboring process. The support provided by the professional registered nurse should include

- Assessment and management of the physiologic and psychologic processes of labor
- Provision of emotional support and physical comfort measures
- Evaluation of fetal well-being during labor
- Instruction regarding the labor process
- Patient advocacy—the clinical assessment and evaluation that results from collaboration among professional members of the healthcare team
- Role modeling to facilitate family participation during labor and birth
- Direct collaboration with other members of the healthcare team to coordinate patient care

In today's healthcare environment, numerous factors may influence the nurse's ability to provide bedside labor care, including

- Limited number of available experienced registered nurses
- Limited financial resources
- Rigid organizational processes and structures
- Cumbersome documentation requirements
- Decreasing reimbursement by third-party payers in the United States

AWHONN challenges healthcare facilities to continuously evaluate the impact of patient–nurse ratios on resource use, overall operating expenses, patient outcomes, and patient satisfaction. AWHONN also supports evaluation models that can measure the impact a registered professional nurse has on indirect cost savings, such as savings resulting from lower cesarean section rates, shorter labors, and fewer technologic interventions.

AWHONN encourages women and families to request labor support from a professional registered nurse or advanced practice nurse (ie, clinical nurse specialist, certified nurse midwife, or nurse practitioner) for labor and birth.

Studies on professional nursing care for laboring women are in progress. AWHONN supports continued research efforts to document the essential role of professional nursing labor support on maternal–newborn outcomes and the potential financial benefits of such support for the healthcare system.

From Association of Women's Health, Obstetric and Neonatal Nurses. (2000). *Professional nursing support of laboring women.* Washington, DC: Author.

and families need during labor and birth (AWHONN, 2000).

Results of sampled studies in several Canadian hospitals found that perinatal nurses spend very little time in labor support (Gagnon & Waghorn, 1999; McNiven, Hodnett, & O'Brien-Pallas, 1992). Factors that have contributed to individual nurses spending less time with women include increased technology associated with giving birth, increased requests for epidural anesthesia, and institutional staffing patterns. As use of technology has expanded in obstetrics, the perinatal nurse has moved from providing hands-on comfort to monitoring the equipment and relying on pharmacologic interventions. Technology, especially when it is coupled with epidural analgesia or anesthesia, makes it easy for the nurse to focus on machines and assume that, because labor is no longer painful, her presence is not needed. Epidural anesthesia has become more available as women have come to expect this as the standard of care. When staffing patterns require nurses to care for more than one woman in labor, it is impossible to provide continuous one-to-one attention.

No published research supports the positive influence that one-to-one nursing care can have on labor and birth outcomes. In one study, use of one-to-one nursing care, defined as an individual nurse spending up to 90% of her time physically at the bedside and providing physical and emotional support, did not achieve statistically significant results (Gagnon & Waghorn, 1999). There is a larger multicenter, international clinical investigation in progress that should shed light on the effect of one-to-one nursing care.

Husband or Significant Other

Postpartum women report that one of the things contributing to a positive labor experience was the presence of a family member or friend in the room even if "they just sit there" (Lavender et al., 1999). At the time of admission, the laboring woman should identify family members or friends who will act as labor-support persons.

Fathers have an important role in providing physical and emotional support during childbirth. Chapman (1992) described three roles assumed by expectant fathers during labor without epidural analgesia or anesthesia:

Coaches actively assisted their partners during and after labor contractions with breathing and relaxation techniques. Men who assumed the role of coach, led or directed their partners through labor and birth and viewed themselves as managers or directors of the experience.

Teammates assisted their partners throughout the experience of labor and birth by responding to requests for physical or emotional support or both. They sometimes led their partners, but their usual role was that of follower or helper.

Witnesses viewed themselves primarily as companions who were there to provide emotional and moral support. They were present during labor and birth to observe the process and to witness the birth of their child.

These roles were identified by organizing behaviors that partners were observed performing during labor or behaviors women described in interviews after birth. Most men in the study adopted the role of witness rather than teammate or coach (Chapman, 1992).

Chandler and Field (1997) report that witnessing their partners in severe pain caused men to feel helpless and fearful. They became discouraged when the comfort measures they tried did not help their partners. Ultimately, they felt they had failed in their role. These results contrast with the intentions of childbirth educators, who perceive themselves as preparing coaches and teammates for laboring women, and with perinatal nurses, who expect fathers and other family members to take a more active role in labor support.

Men's experience of labor when their partners received epidural analgesia or anesthesia was explored, resulting in the grounded theory called "cruising through labor" (Chapman, 2000) (Display 11–3). During labor, critical experiences for men occurred at two points. In the *holding-out phase* of labor, before making the decision to receive an epidural, men experienced a sense of "losing her." As pain became more severe, women underwent personality changes, becoming frustrated, irritable, exhausted, and panicky. These personality changes may be totally unfamiliar qualities that the men have never seen their partners demonstrate or never demonstrate to the degree that they do in labor. Women also gradually turn inward as they attempt to cope with the pain. Withdrawing into themselves causes women to be unable to communicate their needs and to become unresponsive to their partners' attempts at labor support. Men feel increased levels of anxiety, helplessness, frustration, and emotional pain (Chapman, 2000). These findings are consistent with the work of Somers-Smith (1999), who found that fathers experience childbirth as a stressful event.

The second and most dramatic phase for men sharing the experience of labor is during the *cruising phase.* After the epidural has provided relief from the pain of labor, men describe a sensation of "she's back." The laboring woman again is aware of her surroundings and interacting with those around her. From a man's perspective, labor has gone from a

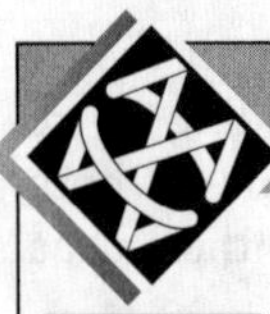

DISPLAY 11–3

Cruising Through Labor: Grounded Theory of the Expectant Father's Epidural Labor Experience

Holding-Out Phase—Onset of labor until the decision is made to receive an epidural. During this phase, couples are seeing how far they can get in labor without needing an epidural or are planning to avoid an epidural.

Surrendering Phase—The point at which the decision is made to receive an epidural, which is described as yielding to the need for an epidural, giving up, feeling they have experienced all the pain they can, and done everything they can to avoid an epidural.

Waiting Phase—The decision has been made and couples are waiting to receive the epidural.

Getting Phase—Period when the epidural was being administered.

Cruising Phase—After the epidural has provided pain relief, the couples' focus changes to rest and enjoyment. Labor has gone from a stressful process to a calm experience. Both may now fall asleep, giving in to the exhaustion they feel as a result of the stress of coping with the pain of labor.

From Chapman, L. L. (2000). Expectant fathers and labor epidurals. *MCN, The American Journal of Maternal Child Nursing, 25* (3), 133–139.

stressful event to a calm experience. Rather than describing their experience in terms of the role they assumed during labor and the frustration and disconnected feelings they had as labor intensified and women's behavior changed (Chapman, 1991, 1992), these men described their experience by the degree of frustration they felt before the epidural and the degree of enjoyment after the epidural (Chapman, 2000). It is important that childbirth educators present this content, discuss this process, and teach men in their classes about the emotions they can expect to witness and experience during labor. Perinatal nurses should remain at the bedside when women are experiencing severe pain. This allows the nurse to provide support to the laboring woman and her partner. According to Chapman (2000), nurses who remained at the bedside, explained what was occurring with the labor, and included the expectant father were viewed by fathers as providing the most support.

Professional or Lay Labor Support Person

There is increased interest in the role of the professional or lay labor-support person, who is present during labor in addition to the perinatal nurse. The movement toward professional or lay labor support is a result of the inability of perinatal nurses to provide women with the support they want during labor and the recognition that husbands or significant others who are usually related to the laboring woman do not always make the best coaches during labor. Traditional childbirth education programs have done a great job training labor-support persons for 30 years. However, the assumption that the husband or significant other makes the best coach may not be accurate (Chapman, 1992). It is important for the father of the baby to be present during the labor and birth, but the presence of a doula may be what the laboring woman needs. Studies involving doulas as the labor-support person have shown significant outcome benefits (Klaus & Kennell, 1997).

Labor-support persons, doulas or monitrices, with a variety of credentials and levels of education, are assisting women and their partners during labor. A monitrice is a registered nurse who performs assessments and provides nursing care in addition to labor support. A doula may be a nurse or lay person who provides nonclinical support including emotional support and physical comfort measures during labor. In a meta-analysis of 11 clinical trials in which continuous support by a doula was compared with traditional intermittent support of a labor and delivery nurse, continuous support was associated with significantly shorter labors; decreased use of analgesia, oxytocin, and forceps; and decreased cesarean births (Scott, Berkowitz, & Klaus, 1999). Women who employed a doula during labor expressed significantly less emotional distress and had higher self-esteem at 4 months postpartum than women who had attended a traditional Lamaze class (Manning-Orenstein, 1998). Doulas of North America (DONA) and Lamaze International offer programs that prepare professionals and lay women to provide labor support. Services of a labor-support person are arranged by the expectant couple before labor.

Childbirth Preparation

There is a relationship between women's expectation of labor and their actual experience of labor (Green, 1993). Women who expect breathing and relaxation techniques to work are more likely to find them helpful. Women who wish to avoid medications can be successful with the help of their support system and perinatal nurses.

The basis of childbirth preparation is the belief that pain during childbirth is a cyclic process (Fig. 11–1). As fear and anxiety heighten, muscle tension increases, inhibiting the effectiveness of contractions, increasing discomfort, and further heightening fear and anxiety. The goal of childbirth education is to interrupt this cycle intellectually with an understanding of what is occurring and physiologically with nonpharmacologic and pharmacologic pain-management strategies. Nonpharmacologic and pharmacologic pain-management strategies provide women with specific techniques they can use to cope with the discomfort of labor, thereby increasing their feelings of control. An awareness of the childbirth preparation and skills that the woman and her partner are prepared to use is helpful when planning nursing support strategies during labor.

Labor admission assessment should include questions related to the type and amount of childbirth preparation (ie, classes, reading, or video tape viewing). As part of the admission assessment, the nurse should ask about the couple's plans for pain management during labor and whether this subject was discussed with the physician or CNM. Asking about their plans and goals validates their efforts to prepare for labor and birth. The nurse should assure them that she understands their goals and that she will do what she can to help them achieve those goals. Nurses have a responsibility whenever possible to facilitate an experience for each couple that matches their expectations. Knowledge and skills learned in childbirth preparation classes are enhanced when the nurse present during labor and birth believes in and actively supports the couple as they apply these principles.

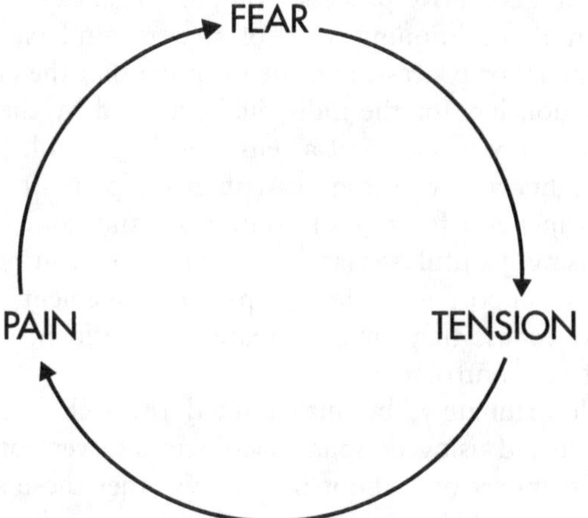

FIGURE 11–1. Fear-tension-pain cycle. (Adapted from Jimenez, S. L. M. [1988]. Supportive pain management strategies. In F. Nichols & S. Humenick [Eds.], *Childbirth education: Practice, research, and theory* (p. 104). Philadelphia: W. B. Saunders.)

Healthcare Environment

Every perinatal unit has a unique approach to caring for laboring women. A culture develops that over time is accepted by most of those working within the department and is a reflection of their values and beliefs. Cultural differences may be as significant as the availability of labor, delivery, recovery, and postpartum rooms (LDRPs) or as subtle as the routine initiation of intravenous fluids on admission. These practices reflect the evolution of intrapartum care within a particular institution. Unit culture extends to treatment of pain and influences the woman's perception of pain. Nurses who value nonpharmacologic approaches to pain management use these techniques in clinical practice.

Pain Tolerance

Pain is a culturally bound phenomenon. When an individual expresses pain, the form that expression takes is related to what her culture has taught her is appropriate. *Pain tolerance* may be defined as the level of stimuli at which the laboring woman asks to have the stimulation stopped. In labor, it is the point at which a woman requests pharmacologic pain relief or increased comfort measures. Descriptive words such as mild, moderate, and severe do not provide a measure of pain tolerance, because laboring women may describe pain as severe but not request pain medication. A woman's pain tolerance or length of time she is able to go without medication may be increased by the use of nonpharmacologic pain management techniques. A uniform system should be adapted by the perinatal department to assess the level of pain.

NONPHARMACOLOGIC PAIN MANAGEMENT STRATEGIES

Nursing expertise in a variety of pain-management strategies is important. Not all nurses believe in or use nonpharmacologic approaches to pain relief when caring for laboring women. Possible reasons are a lack of familiarity with these techniques, routine practices that tend to be pharmacologic, or the fact that caring for a woman with an epidural is less physically and emotionally draining for the nurse than caring for a woman who is planning not to use an epidural. With the increased popularity of epidural anesthesia by healthcare providers and consumers, many nurses new to the specialty have not had the opportunity to learn about or use nonpharmacologic measures. The choice of pain-management strategies by nurses is based on what they have observed to work in practice, are personally comfortable with, or have used during their own labors.

Women choose pain-management strategies based on their previous experience with pain, what they learned in prenatal classes, primary healthcare providers' recommendations, and listening to what worked for family members and friends. Although few randomized, controlled clinical trials exist supporting the effectiveness of specific nonpharmacologic techniques during labor, suggestion and initiation of any of these techniques are within the scope of perinatal nursing practice. For most women, multiple pain-management strategies are necessary during the course of labor. Habituation may occur as the continued use of one technique becomes monotonous or offers insufficient stimuli to interfere with pain perception. As any technique becomes less of a distraction and therefore less effective, perception of pain increases (Bird & Waugaman, 1999).

Perinatal nurses should develop expertise in a variety of pain-management strategies. There are three classifications of nonpharmacologic methods or comfort measures that can be used to decrease or alter painful sensations associated with labor and birth: measures to reduce painful stimuli, methods that activate peripheral sensory receptors and inhibit pain awareness, and cognitive techniques that enhance descending inhibitory neural pathways, thereby reducing a woman's negative psychological reaction to pain (Table 11–2).

Nonpharmacologic pain-management strategies are based on the gate-control theory (Melzack & Wall, 1965). The physiologic processes that contribute to an individual's pain experience provide a theoretical framework that may explain how nonpharmacologic pain-management strategies work (Pasero, Paice, & McCaffery, 1999). The first process is explained by the structure of the central nervous system, which is composed of large and small sensory nerve fibers. Impulses are carried by the spinal cord from the site of the stimuli to the cerebral cortex, where impulses are interpreted. Small, thinly myelinated or unmyelinated fibers transport impulses such as pressure and pain from the uterus, cervix, and pelvic joints. Large, myelinated fibers transport impulses from the skin. Because passage along large fibers occurs more quickly, it is possible for cutaneous stimulation to block or alter painful impulses. Based on this premise, tactile stimulation in the form of touch or massage is often used effectively during labor.

The second process is stimulation of the reticular activating system in the brain stem. The reticular activating system interprets auditory, visual, and painful sensory stimuli. When the cerebral cortex focuses on auditory or visual stimulation, painful stimulation is less able to pass through the "gate." Many forms of distraction are used during labor to decrease pain perception.

TABLE 11–2 ■ NONPHARMACOLOGIC STRATEGIES TO CONTROL PAIN

Technique	Examples
Cutaneous techniques to relieve painful stimuli	Massage Touch Back rub Counterpressure Movement and positioning Application of heat or cold Acupuncture Hydrotherapy Effleurage
Auditory or visual techniques to block the transmission of painful stimuli	Focal point Breathing techniques Attention focusing Distraction Hypnosis Music
Cognitive processes to control the degree to which a sensation is interpreted as painful	Prenatal education Relaxation Labor support Imagery

The third process recognizes the influence of memory and cognitive processes on pain. Past experiences, cultural conditioning, level of anxiety, understanding of the labor process, and the meaning that the current situation has for the individual are used by the cerebral cortex to interpret a sensation as painful. Just as thoughts and emotions can increase pain, they can also increase feelings of confidence and control, decreasing painful sensations. Prenatal education and labor support are effective pain-management strategies because they enhance maternal confidence and a sense of control.

Unfortunately, because limited research has been conducted using nonpharmacologic interventions, little is understood about how or whether these strategies work. It is inaccurate to use terms such as *pain relief* when referring to these interventions. Some interventions may decrease pain, such as positioning, counterpressure, heat and cold, touch, massage, effleurage, and injections of sterile water. Other interventions such as relaxation, imagery, focusing, breathing techniques, and music more likely benefit woman by decreasing anxiety, improving overall mood, and increasing the individual's sense of control in a painful situation (McCaffery & Pasero, 1999).

Cutaneous Pain Relief Techniques

Maternal Position and Movement

Women naturally choose positions of comfort and are more likely to change position during early labor. Modern technology (eg, EFM, intravenous lines, automatic blood pressure monitors, fetal scalp electrodes) may interfere with a woman's ability to find a comfortable position and frequently restrict her to bed. Many nurses and physicians encourage bed rest for labor because it is easier, they feel more in control of the situation, and believe it may be safer for the woman and fetus. However, it is possible to use most of the technology available in obstetrics without maintaining continuous bed rest. An upright position can be accomplished in a recliner, rocking chair, or birthing bed adjusted to a chair position. EFM telemetry units, transducers that can be used in water, or intermittent auscultation of the fetal heart rate can be used to evaluate fetal response to labor while women are out of bed, ambulating, or using hydrotherapy (Bloom et al., 1998).

Women should be encouraged to change their position frequently during labor. Changing position alters the relationship between the fetus and pelvis, and it facilitates fetal positioning and descent. Table 11–3 lists various positions the laboring woman may try

TABLE 11–3 ■ PHYSIOLOGIC POSITIONS AND MOVEMENTS FOR LABOR AND BIRTH

Positions	Contributions of the Position
Standing	Takes advantage of gravity during and between contractions Contractions less painful and more productive Fetus well aligned with angle of pelvis May speed labor if woman has been recumbent May increase urge to push in second stage
Walking	Same as standing, plus movement causes changes in pelvic joints, encouraging rotation and descent
Standing and leaning forward on partner, bed, or birth ball	Same as standing Relieves backache Good position for back rub May be more restful than standing Can be used with electronic fetal monitor (stand by bed)
Slow dancing: mother embraces partner around neck and rests head on his/her chest or shoulder. Partner's arms are around mother's trunk, interlocking fingers at her low back. She drops arms and rests against partner. They sway to music, breathing in same rhythm.	Same as standing Movement causes changes in pelvic joints, encouraging rotation and descent Being embraced by loved one increases sense of well-being Rhythm and music add comfort Partner gives back pressure to relieve back pain
The lunge: mother stands facing forward beside a straight chair and places one foot on chair seat, with knee and foot to side. Bending raised knee and hip, mother lunges sideways repeatedly during a contraction, 5 seconds at a time. She should feel stretch in inner thighs. Lunge in direction of fetal occiput, if known; otherwise in more comfortable direction. Partner secures chair, helps with balance.	Widens one side of pelvis (side toward which she lunges) Encourages rotation of occipitoposterior fetus Can also be done in kneeling position
Sitting upright	Good resting position Some gravity advantage Can be used with electronic fetal monitor

(continued)

TABLE 11–3 ■ PHYSIOLOGIC POSITIONS AND MOVEMENTS FOR LABOR AND BIRTH (continued)

Positions	Contributions of the Position
Sitting on toilet or commode	Same as sitting upright May help relax perineum for effective bearing down
Semisitting	Same as sitting upright Vaginal examination possible Easy position to get into on bed or delivery table
Sitting, rocking in chair	Same as sitting upright Rocking movement may speed labor
Sitting, leaning forward with support	Same as sitting upright Relieves backache Good position for back rub
Hands and knees	Helps relieve backache Assists rotation of baby from occipitoposterior Allows for pelvic rocking and body movements Vaginal examinations possible Takes pressure off hemorrhoids
Kneeling, leaning forward with support on a chair seat, the raised head of the bed, or a birth ball	Same as hands and knees Less strain on wrists and hands
Sidelying	Very good resting position Convenient for many interventions Helps lower elevated blood pressure May promote progress of labor when alternated with walking Rapid second stage Takes pressure off hemorrhoids Easier to relax, between pushing efforts Allows posterior sacral movement in second stage
Squatting	May relieve backache Takes advantage of gravity Widens pelvic outlet Requires less bearing-down effort May enhance rotation and descent in a difficult birth Helpful if mother does not feel an urge to push Allows freedom to shift weight for comfort Mechanical advantage—upper trunk presses fundus
Supported squat: mother leans with back against partner who holds her under the arms and takes all her weight. She stands between contractions	Lengthens mother's trunk, allowing more room for asynclitic fetus to maneuver into position Eliminates restriction of pelvic joint mobility that can be caused by external pressure from bed or chair Gravity advantage
Dangle: partner sits on high bed or counter, feet supported on chairs or footrests, with thighs spread. Mother backs between legs and places flexed arms over thighs. Partner grips woman's sides with thighs. She lowers herself, allowing partner to support her full weight. She stands between contractions.	Same as supported squat, except it is much easier on the partner

From Simkin, P. (1995). Reducing pain and enhancing progress in labor: A guide to nonpharmacologic methods for maternity caregivers. *Birth*, *22*(3), 161–171.

and the benefits of each. Maintaining a horizontal position in labor is associated with decreased blood flow and may increase uterine muscle hypoxia, resulting in the increased perception of pain associated with uterine contractions (Mayberry et al., 2000). Women in an upright position during second stage of labor report less pain than women in a semi-Fowler or semirecumbent position (deJong et al., 1997). Women may initially resist suggestions to change position or may find new positions uncomfortable. When encouraging a woman to change position, the nurse should provide extra support and encouragement and suggest that she remain in the new position through several contractions before deciding whether it is comfortable.

Pillows should be used generously to maintain positions and support extremities. When a sidelying position is used, pillows can be placed behind the back and between the knees. In a semi-Fowler's position, pillows can be placed under knees or arms. Shorter women sitting in a chair may find that a pillow or stool under their feet decreases stretching of leg muscles. Women who labor with the baby's head in an occiput posterior position find that being on their hands and knees relieves back pain.

Localized Pressure to Reduce Back Labor

Interventions can be used by the perinatal nurse or other labor-support person to relieve back labor. These techniques include counterpressure, bilateral hip pressure (eg, double-hip squeeze), and knee press (Simkin, 1995). These maneuvers are performed by applying localized pressure to reduce sacroiliac pain resulting from strain on sacroiliac ligaments caused by mechanisms of labor.

Counterpressure requires application of enough force to meet the intensity of pressure from the fetal occipital bone against the sacrum (Fig. 11–2). Steady pressure from the heel of a support person's hand or another firm object counteracts the strain against the sacroiliac ligaments caused by the fetal occiput (Simkin, 1995). This technique moves the sacrum into normal alignment with the ilium, reducing the pain experienced by laboring women.

Superficial Heat and Cold

The physiologic effects of heat and cold are well accepted, although the exact mechanism of how heat and cold benefit women during labor is not clear (Table 11–4). The benefits of immersion in water during labor are based on the principles of buoyancy, hydrostatic pressure, and heat (Harris, 1999). Buoyancy creates hydrodynamic lift. The loss of gravitational pull allows the body to float. Hydrostatic pressure equalizes the pressure exerted on all parts of the body below the water surface. Together buoyancy and hydrostatic pressure provide greater support and comfort during labor because muscle tension is decreased and pressure is dispersed over the whole body. The transmission of warmth from the heat of the water relaxes muscles that have become tense as a result of stress associated with the discomfort of labor. It is theorized that transmission of temperature sensations

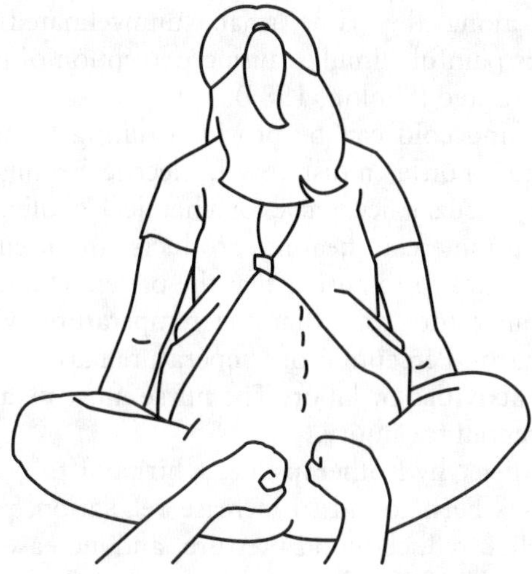

FIGURE 11–2. Firm counterpressure of the fists on the lower back.

TABLE 11–4 ▪ PHYSIOLOGIC EFFECTS OF HEAT AND COLD

Heat	Cold
Increased local blood flow	Decreased local blood flow
Increased local skin and muscle temperature	Decreased local skin and muscle temperature
Increased tissue metabolism	Decreased tissue metabolism
Decreased muscle spasm	Decreased muscle spasm (ie, longer lasting than heat)
Relaxation of tiny muscles in skin (eg, capillaries, hair follicles)	Slowed transmission of impulses over afferent neurons, leading to decreased sensation, numbing effects
Elevated pain threshold	

From Simkin, P. (1995). Reducing pain and enhancing progress in labor: A guide to nonpharmacologic methods for maternity caregivers. *Birth, 22*(3), 161–171.

occurs along the same small, unmyelinated nerve fibers as painful stimuli, causing perception of pain to be interrupted (Simkin, 1989).

Heat and cold can be provided during labor by a hot water bottle, moist towel, electric heating unit, shower, Jacuzzi, ice pack, or chemical cooling unit. When commercial heating products are used, care should be taken to ensure that the patient can tolerate the temperature and that the temperature will not cause harm. Perception of temperature may be altered by the activities of labor. The nurse must be alert to the potential for injury.

Use of jet hydrotherapy (ie, whirlpool tub) during labor has been found to increase relaxation, provide pain relief, reduce blood pressure, and increase diuresis (Church, 1989). When women use a whirlpool tub during labor, they require fewer pharmacologic interventions, have fewer vacuum- and forceps-assisted births, and are more likely to birth over an intact perineum (Aird, Luckas, Buckett, & Bousfield, 1997; Rush et al., 1996).

The point during labor that a woman goes into a tub or whirlpool may influence the ultimate length of labor (Katz, Ryder, Cefalo, Carmichael, & Goolsby, 1990). Hydrostatic pressure from immersion in water causes interstitial fluid to move into the intravascular space, increasing plasma volume and decreasing oxytocin concentration (Katz et al., 1990). Uterine contraction may be slowed or stop completely when use of tub or whirlpool occurs before active labor is established (Simpkin, 1995).

There is no increase in the infection rate when women labor in a tub after rupture of the membranes (Eriksson, Ladfors, Mattsson, & Fall, 1996; Rush et al., 1996; Waldenstrom & Nilsson, 1992). Each perinatal department in conjunction with the organization's infection control department needs to develop a strict protocol for cleaning tubs or whirlpools. Protocols should be based on manufacturers recommendations and the state and local boards of health requirements.

Using a shower may eliminate the potential for infection acquired from a tub or whirlpool. Although the effects of buoyancy and hydrostatic pressure are lacking, there is the benefit of heat. As in a tub or whirlpool, care should be taken to ensure that the water is not too hot and that maternal temperature does not rise to high. Hand-held shower heads can be used to direct the spray of water to where it is most beneficial to the laboring woman. Holding the shower wand allows the expectant father or coach to participate and feel as if he is making his partner more comfortable. Perinatal nurses often share anecdotal reports of women who labored quite successfully for long periods in the shower. Women progress through labor more rapidly and report being more comfortable. Women become so comfortable that it may be difficult to entice them out of the tub or shower.

Hydrotherapy may produce some of the following adverse effects:

- Weakness
- Dizziness
- Nausea
- Maternal or fetal tachycardia
- Maternal hypotension

Side effects usually are related to an increase in body temperature or dehydration, both of which may be prevented by appropriate nursing interventions. Nursing considerations before suggesting the use of hydrotherapy and after implementation of this nursing intervention are listed in Table 11–5. Women may at first be reluctant, embarrassed, or express some inhibition about laboring in a shower or tub; however, they quickly appreciate the relaxing qualities of warm water.

Some women in labor find relief from the application of cold in the form of ice packs, frozen gel packs, cold towels, or other cold objects. A cold washcloth applied to the face or neck is refreshing. Because cold is especially helpful for the relief of musculoskeletal pain, this is an appropriate intervention to suggest when a women experiences back labor. The numbing effect of cold is thought to slow the transmission of impulses over sensory neurons, decreasing the sensation of pain (Simkin, 1995).

Touch and Massage

Studies have shown that, although nurses touch women often during labor, it is mostly for clinical purposes, such as taking a pulse or attaching and inserting devices (McNiven et al., 1992). There is evidence to suggest that nonclinical touch (eg, hand holding, stroking a brow, patting the back) can reduce a woman's systolic blood pressure and pulse rate while increasing her comfort level and ability to cope (McNiven et al., 1992). Perinatal nurses and others providing support during labor use touch consciously and unconsciously throughout labor to communicate their support and presence, to relieve muscle tension, and to decrease the pain of labor. All forms of massage except effleurage are accomplished with moderate pressure, activating large, myelinated nerve fibers. Because habituation can occur, decreasing the beneficial effects of massage, the type of stroke and location should be varied during labor.

TABLE 11–5 ■ PROTOCOL FOR USING A TUB OR SHOWER DURING LABOR

Nursing Intervention	Rationale
Establish fetal and maternal well-being by conducting a thorough assessment before using a tub or shower.	Stable maternal vital signs and reassuring fetal status are necessary before suggesting women labor in a tub or shower.
Use continuous or intermittent fetal monitoring or intermittant auscultation of the fetal heart rate while in the tub or shower.	Frequency of fetal monitoring should be consistent with recognized standards of care and institutional policies and based on the stage of labor.
Encourage oral fluids.	Prevent dehydration.
Maintain water temperature between 96°F and 98°F.	Water temperature above maternal body temperature may cause peripheral vasodilatation and redistribution of blood volume away from the fetus and uterus.
Water in the tub should be as high as possible.	The benefits of buoyancy and hydrostatic pressure are best obtained with the entire body submerged in water.
Using a tub or shower is not contraindicated in the presence of ruptured membranes.	
Contraindications include thick meconium, oxytocin infusion, bleeding or large bloody show, epidural analgesia or anesthesia, and nonreassuring fetal status.	
If an intravenous line or heparin lock is in place it can be covered with plastic.	
Support person or member of the nursing staff should be present at all times. Shower seat should be available in the shower for the laboring woman as well as a seat outside of the shower or tub for their support person.	Warm water may cause dizziness.
Evaluate maternal vital signs according to hospital policy.	When evaluating maternal temperature, keep in mind that core temperature is 0.5–1 degree above oral temperature and that core temperature may more accurately reflect the fetal environmental temperature.

Effleurage

Effleurage is any light massage that glides over the skin but does not cause pressure or movement of deep muscle masses (Tappan, 1978). Effleurage is performed by the laboring woman drawing rhythmic circles or lines with her fingertips on her abdomen or thighs or by a support person using fingertips to gently rub up and down the woman's arm or leg (Fig. 11–3).

Intradermal Injections of Sterile Water

Intradermal injections of sterile water (IISW) to control the pain of labor was first introduced in obstetric literature in the late 1980s. Although this technique is not widely used, it has been reported to relieve the severe, continuous discomfort of back labor that occurs when the fetal occiput is in a posterior position. Back labor is thought to complicate about 30% of labors (Reynolds, 1994).

Four small intradermal injections of 0.1 mL of sterile water are placed over the sacrum of a woman's back, leaving a temporary fluid-filled papule similar to that for a tuberculosis test (Fig. 11–4). Although it is not totally understood how this technique relieves the lower back pain associated with the first stage of labor, some investigators use the gate-control theory as an explanation. Sterile water irritates nerve endings, blocking other painful sensations (Reynolds, 2000).

One hour after women with lower back pain were given IISW, 93% reported the pain disappeared completely (Lytzen, Cederberg, & Moller-Nielsen, 1989). When the effect of IISW was compared with injections of normal saline, women receiving the sterile water re-

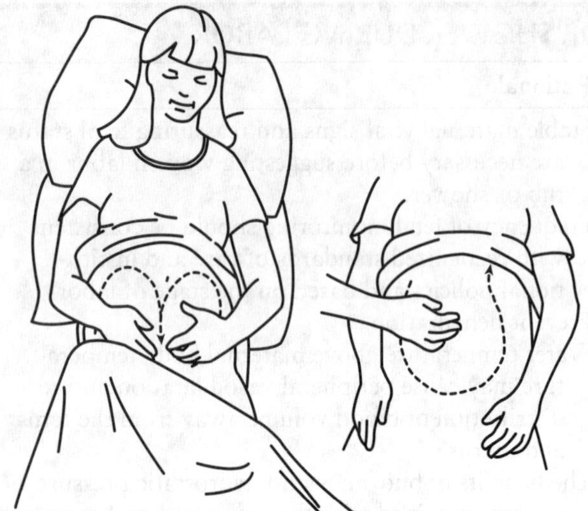

FIGURE 11–3. Effleurage.

ported less pain (Trolle, Moller, Kronborg, & Thomsen, 1991). No difference in the report of pain was found when normal saline injections were compared with sterile water injections. However, the women who received intradermal injections reported less pain than women who did not receive injections, regardless of the type of solution injected (Martensson & Wallin, 1999). When IISW was compared with transcutaneous electrical nerve stimulation (TENS) or standard care such as back massage, whirlpool bath, or position change, women receiving IISW reported less pain than those using TENS or receiving standard care (Labrecque, Nouwen, Bergeron, & Rancourt, 1999). Although the studies included random assignment of participants to a treatment or control group, a major limitation of all studies of TENS and IISW was inadequate sample size to detect significant differences.

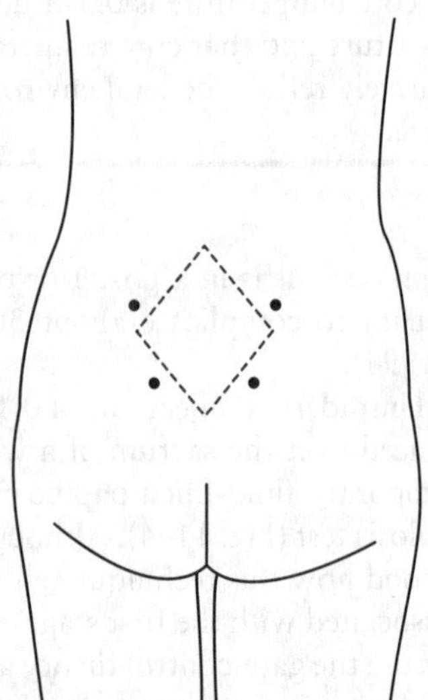

FIGURE 11–4. Location of injection sites in relation to the Michaelis' rhomboid for intradermal injections of sterile water. (From: Martensson, L. & Wallin, G. (1999). Labor pain treated with cutaneous injections of sterile water: A randomized controlled trial. *British Journal of Obstetrics and Gynecology, 106*(7), page 634.)

Pain relief after IISW has been reported to last 1 hour (Labrecque et al., 1999; Martensson & Wallin, 1999) to 3 hours (Lytzen et al., 1989). IISW has several advantages:

- Can be performed by a registered nurse
- Is not a technically difficult procedure
- Provides one more strategy for pain control
- Can be repeated as often as needed

The only side effect associated with the procedure is intense stinging pain at the time of injection that lasts about 30 seconds and a hyperemic zone around the papule that lasts for several hours after injection (Lytzen et al., 1989). The major disadvantage of this intervention is that it is relatively short acting, necessitating repeated injections that women may find displeasing, depending on how uncomfortable it was to receive the intradermal injections.

Cognitive Techniques Altering Pain Perception

Relaxation

Achieving a state of relaxation is the basis of all nonpharmacologic interventions during labor. Women benefit from a state of relaxation because it conserves energy rather than creating fatigue from the prolonged tension of voluntary muscles. Relaxation enhances the effectiveness of nonpharmacologic and pharmacologic pain-management strategies.

Relaxation is a skill and a physical state. In childbirth classes, woman are introduced to the skill of relaxation. How well they learn this skill depends on quality of instruction, the amount of time they practice, and their belief that this technique can be beneficial. Relaxation is as contagious as panic, tension, and feelings of being overwhelmed. Relaxation skills cannot be taught during active labor, but an environment that promotes relaxation can be created by the perinatal nurse (Display 11–4). Women who learn relaxation techniques during childbirth classes benefit from reinforcement and encouragement.

Imagery

Imagery is simple daydreaming. Childbirth educators teach imagery as a skill, encouraging expectant women to focus on pleasant scenes or experiences to increase their level of relaxation. Nurses encourage

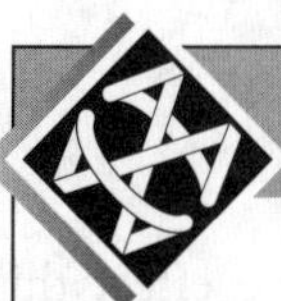

DISPLAY 11–4

Creating a Relaxed Environment During Labor

Control the amount of light, noise, and interruptions.
Maintain an unhurried demeanor.
Use a calm, soft, slow voice.
Recognize the signs of tension:
- Changes in voice
- Frowning
- Clenched fists
- Stiff, straight posture
- Tense arms or legs
- Stiff, raised shoulders

Maintain eye contact.
Use touch or massage if this is acceptable to the woman.
Sit, rather than stand, next to the woman.

women to use imagery by making statements such as "think of the baby moving through the birth canal," "think of the baby moving down and out," and "think about the cervix dilating." Imagery is used to keep women focused and to encourage them to work with their contractions.

Auditory or Visual Techniques to Block Transmission of Pain

Attention Focusing and Distraction

During early labor, distraction is an effective strategy. Distraction is the process by which stimuli from the environment draws a woman's attention away from her pain. Walking in the hallway, sitting in a chair, talking with visitors, watching television, playing cards, and using the telephone keep laboring women occupied. Most women reach a point during labor when they no longer are able to talk comfortably through contractions. Labor is hard work requiring intense concentration to maintain a sense of control. Women are helped to concentrate by focusing on an object in the room or a support person's face or eyes. Attention focusing involves deliberate, intentional activities on the part of the laboring woman. These activities include patterned breathing and visualization or imagery.

Patterned Breathing

Breathing techniques are usually taught in prenatal classes and are used as a distraction during labor to decrease pain and promote relaxation. On admission, the perinatal nurse reviews with the woman and her support person the specific techniques they were taught in prenatal class. If a woman has not attended class, early labor is the time to discuss and practice a slow, controlled breathing pattern.

Most woman are taught to take a deep breath at the beginning of a contraction. This breath ensures oxygen to the mother and baby, signals to people in the room that a contraction is beginning, and stretches and tenses respiratory muscles. Exhaling this breath relaxes respiratory muscles and voluntary muscles. At some point in labor, perinatal nurses may find it necessary to breathe synchronously with a couple through several contractions. Women are encouraged to breathe slowly. However, as labor pain increases, women may need to use a lighter, more accelerated breathing (ie, no more than two times their normal rate). Alternatively, a pant–blow method of breathing may be used in which a woman takes three to four light panting breaths, followed by an exhale (ie, blow). When attempting to control the urge to push, a rapid and shallow breathing pattern may be helpful.

Music

Music is used as a distraction in labor. Familiar music associated with restful or pleasant recollections may be an adjunct to relaxation and imagery. Birthing rooms can be equipped with compact disc or cassette tape players, and women are encouraged to bring their musical preferences. Music creates an atmosphere in the birthing room that also may change the approach of healthcare professionals to laboring women. Perinatal nurses and physicians become more relaxed, slow their activities, and respond with increased respect for the unique personal event in progress (DiFranco, 2000).

During the late 1960s and into the 1980s, several studies were conducted to determine whether music during labor facilitated relaxation and reduced pain. Methodologically, these studies were not well designed, sample sizes were small, and results were inconsistent and contradictory. Wiand (1997) conducted an experimental study using biofeedback modalities to determine whether listening to Baroque or New Age music or to ocean sounds improved relaxation compared with a progressive relaxation exercise. Thirty-six subjects acted as their own controls. Relaxation levels were significantly improved when

Baroque or New Age music or ocean sounds were played compared with progressive relaxation exercise alone. When women use earphones or headsets to listen to music, an auditory sensation is created that is difficult to ignore (Bird & Waugaman, 1999). Women may need to vary the type or style of music and use this technique intermittently to decrease the possibility of habituation.

A major limitation of all nonpharmacologic methods of pain relief in labor is the lack of large, randomized, controlled trials supporting their effectiveness. However, anecdotal reports and expert opinions exist regarding their usefulness. Nurses should encourage women in labor to try a variety of techniques to decrease the discomfort. Ultimately, we must listen to and honor the request of the laboring woman about the effectiveness of nonpharmacologic techniques during her labor.

PHARMACOLOGIC PAIN MANAGEMENT STRATEGIES

The perinatal nurse assesses preferences for pain management on admission and conducts ongoing assessments of factors influencing pain perception throughout labor. There will always be laboring women who need or desire pharmacologic agents. In the absence of any medical contraindications, a woman's request is sufficient medical justification for providing pharmacologic pain relief during labor (ACOG, 2000).

Using pain medications during labor brings with it unique concerns that are not faced in other clinical areas. These include concerns about the effects medications may have on the fetus or newborn, breastfeeding, and the course and outcome of labor. Controversy exists among professionals and consumers about the appropriateness and consequences of relieving labor pain, which is considered by some a normal experience (Cohen, 1997). The decision to use medication should be made in collaboration with the woman and her physician or CNM. Ideally, the laboring woman should clearly understand the benefits and potential maternal–fetal side effects. This information is best introduced during the prenatal period, rather than during the stress of labor.

Pharmacologic pain management is divided into two categories: *analgesia,* which is use of a medication to decrease or alter the normal sensation of pain, and *anesthesia,* which is use of a medication to provide partial or complete loss of sensation with or without loss of consciousness.

Analgesics

Sedatives and Hypnotics

The term *sedative–hypnotic* describes the effect this group of medications has on the individual; it is not a classification of drug. The effects of these drugs are dose related. In low doses, they cause sedation, and higher doses cause a hypnotic effect. Two classifications of drugs used in labor to provide sedative–hypnotic effects are barbiturates and H_1-receptor antagonists (ie, antihistamines).

Barbiturates such as secobarbital sodium (Seconal) and pentobarbital (Nembutal) do not relieve pain. Usually given orally or as an intramuscular injection to induce sleep, in labor, they depress the central nervous system and decrease anxiety (Faucher & Brucker, 2000). Women in prolonged early labor may benefit from a brief period of therapeutic rest or sleep that usually follows administration of barbiturates. After a rest period, there usually is a more coordinated, effective contraction pattern. Because sedatives have a long half-life and cross the placenta, there may also be effects on the neonatal central nervous system such as decreased responsiveness and ability to suck. Use of barbiturates is reserved for early labor, when birth is unlikely for 12 to 24 hours (Huffnagle & Huffnagle, 1999).

H_1-receptor antagonists include promethazine hydrochloride (Phenergan), hydroxyzine hydrochloride (Vistaril), and propiomazine (Largon). These medications are frequently administered with narcotics during labor to relieve anxiety, increase sedation, and decrease nausea and vomiting. They traditionally have been thought to potentiate the effects of narcotics; however, there is no objective evidence to support this belief (Wakefield, 1999). Promethazine hydrochloride is frequently used with meperidine to decrease the nausea and vomiting associated with this drug. Although all H_1-receptor antagonists have a sedative effect on the woman in labor, they do not appear to increase neonatal depression. Routes of administration and side effects are similar for all the medications in this class. Exceptions are promethazine hydrochloride, which can cause respiratory depression, and hydroxyzine, which is limited to intramuscular use.

Parenteral Opioids

Opioids are the drugs most commonly administered parenterally during labor. Drugs in this category bind to one of four receptor sites (ie, mu, kappa, sigma, or delta) on nerve cells located in the brain and spinal cord. Individual drugs have an affinity for one or more receptor sites, which accounts for differences in pharmacodynamics and side effects. Examples are morphine and meperidine, which have a strong affinity for mu receptors, resulting in effective analgesia and dose-dependent respiratory depression. Butorphanol (Stadol) and nalbuphine (Nubaine), with affinity for the kappa and sigma receptors, provide effective analgesia with less respiratory depression. Table 11–6 highlights the most commonly used opioids and their receptor-binding patterns.

Depending on the dose, route of administration, and stage of labor, opioids do not eliminate pain but instead cause a blunting effect, decreasing the perception of pain and allowing women to relax and rest between contractions. Table 11–7 lists the most commonly used opioids in labor and their dose, route of administration, onset of action, time of peak effect, and duration of action. After administration of an opioid during early labor, the frequency and duration of contractions and fetal heart rate variability may decrease (Wakefield, 1999). For this reason, opioids may not be administered until a labor pattern is well established. These medications cause some woman to fall asleep between contractions. Other women experience a short period of decreased uterine activity followed by an increase in uterine activity. Both effects may be the result of decreased anxiety and serum concentrations of catecholamines (Mussell, 1998). If medication administration does result in dozing, coaching by a support person or nurse is important to help the woman anticipate and recognize the beginning of a contraction rather than have her startled awake at the peak of a contraction.

Opioids are administered intravenously or intramuscularly every 3 to 4 hours. When given intravenously, the onset of action is quicker; however, medication effects do not last as long. Intravenous push medications are given slowly during a contraction to decrease transfer of the medication to the fetus. During the peak of a contraction, blood supply to the placenta essentially ceases. Administering the medication at this time allows rapid distribution of the drug and decreased maternal plasma concentration to the placenta when circulation resumes (Spielman, 1987).

Neonatal side effects are related to dosage and timing of administration. Because of the potential for neonatal respiratory depression, the timing of administration relative to birth of the newborn is important. Ideally, birth should occur within 1 hour or after 4 hours following administration (Wakefield, 1999). Kuhnert, Linn, and Kuhnert (1985), in a review of the literature, found that newborn behavioral responses may be altered for several days. Effects include decreased muscle tone and social responsiveness, ineffective suck, problems initiating breast-feeding, and abnormal reflexes. Naloxone hydrochloride (Narcan), a narcotic antagonist, reverses the respiratory depression caused by narcotics. It is administered to the newborn whose mother received an opioid in labor if the newborn fails to breath spontaneously, appears depressed, or requires prolonged resuscitative efforts (American Heart Association & American Academy of Pediatrics [AHA & AAP], 1996).

TABLE 11–6 ■ OPIOIDS AND THEIR RECEPTOR BINDING RELATIONSHIPS

Receptor	Receptor Properties	Medication
Mu	Supraspinal analgesia Respiratory depression Euphoria Physical dependence	Morphine Meperidine Butorphanol (weak) Fentanyl Sufentanil Alfentanil
Kappa	Spinal analgesia Miosis Sedation Slight respiratory depression	Morphine (weak) Butorphanol Nalbuphine
Sigma	Dysphoria Hallucinations Respiratory and vasomotor stimulation May not mediate analgesia	Butorphanol (partial) Nalbuphine Fentanyl (partial)
Delta	Spinal analgesia and smooth muscle relaxation	Morphine (weak) Codeine (weak)

Adapted from Faucher, M.A., & Brucker, M.C. (2000). Intrapartum pain: Parmacologic management. *Journal of Obstetric, Gynecologic, and Neonatal Nursing, 29*(2), 169–180.

TABLE 11–7 ■ NARCOTIC USE IN LABOR

Drug	Dose	Route	Onset of Action (min)	Peak Effect (min)	Duration of Action (h)
Meperidine (Demerol)	50–100 mg	IM	10–20	40–50	2–4
	25–50 mg	IV	3–5	5–10	2–4
Morphine	5–10 mg	IM	10–20	30–60	4–6
	2–5 mg	IV	3–5	20	4–6
Butorphanol (Stadol)	1–3 mg	IM	10–30	30–60	3–4
	0.5–2 mg	IV	1–2	4–5	3–4
Nalbuphine (Nubain)	0.2 mg/kg	IM	15	60	3–6
	0.1–0.2 mg/kg	IV	2–3	30	3–6
Fentanyl (Sublimaze)	50–100 μg	IM	7–15	20–30	1–2
	50–100 μg	IV	1–2	3–5	30–60 min

Adapted from Mussell, S. (1998). Narcotic analgesia during labor and birth: Maternal and newborn effects. *Mother-Baby Journal, 3*(6), 19–23.

Regional Anesthesia

These medications provide almost immediate pain relief at the site of injection or to a large region of the body when injected in the epidural or subarachnoid space.

Local Infiltration

During second stage of labor, a local anesthetic may be injected into the perineum and posterior vagina before performing an episiotomy. This area may be reinjected after delivery of the placenta in preparation for perineal repair.

Pudendal Block

A pudendal block during the second stage of labor anesthetizes the lower vagina, vulva, and perineum. An anesthetic is injected through the lateral vaginal walls into the area of the pudendal nerve (Fig. 11–5). This technique provides adequate anesthesia for vaginal birth, application of outlet forceps, and perineal repair. Because it is possible for a pudendal block to be ineffective, it is frequently combined with local infiltration of the perineum.

Epidural Anesthesia and Analgesia

Of the various pharmacologic methods available, epidural, spinal, and combined spinal-epidural are the most flexible and effective, and they result in the least central nervous system depression of the mother and neonate (ACOG, 2000). Although it is possible for an epidural to be ineffective or only partially effective, most women report effective pain control using this technique (Howell, 2000).

For many years, epidural anesthesia was limited to local anesthetics such as lidocaine (Xylocaine) and chloroprocaine (Nesacaine). These drugs act on nerve fibers as they cross the epidural space, causing sensory blockade. To obtain a therapeutic level of pain relief, the dose of local anesthetic resulted in loss of motor function. This technique also results in a reduced incidence of spontaneous vaginal birth (American Society of Anesthesiologists [ASA], 1999). With the introduction of bupivacaine (Marcaine), practitioners found a longer duration of action, minimal motor blockade, and lack of neonatal neurobehavioral effects (Cohen, 1997). Ropivacaine (Naropin) has properties similar to those of bupivacaine, but this local anesthetic has less cardiotoxic effects, has slightly superior analgesic efficacy, and is associated with a higher incidence of spontaneous delivery (Eddleston et al., 1996).

The goal of pharmacologic pain management during labor is to provide sufficient analgesia effect with as little motor block as possible. With the discovery of spinal cord opioid receptors in the late 1970s and the use of spinal and epidural opioids, pain management in labor was transformed from anesthesia to analgesia. Lower concentrations of local anesthetic (ie, 0.125% or 0.0625% bupivacaine), in combination with narcotics, such as fentanyl (Sublimaze), sufentanil (Sufenta), and alfentanil (Alfenta), result in increased pain relief without significant motor block (ASA, 1999). Epidural narcotics act by crossing the dura into the cerebral spinal fluid and binding to opiate receptors in the dorsal horn of the spinal cord. Adding a narcotic to the local anesthetic lessens the

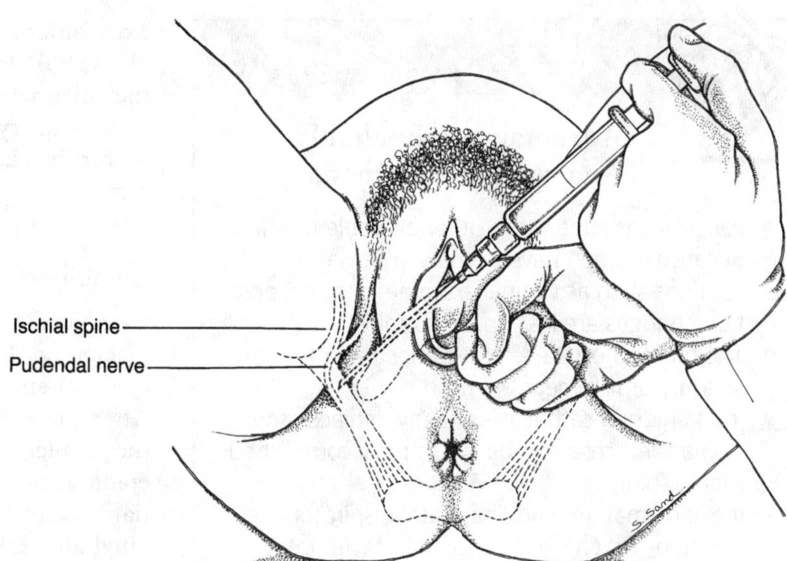

FIGURE 11–5. Procedure for administration of a pudendal block.

risk of toxicity by decreasing the amount of local anesthetic needed, reducing the motor blockade, increasing the duration of pain relief, and improving the quality of pain relief (ASA, 1999). There was no difference in incidence of side effects (ie, nausea and hypotension), increased duration of labor, or adverse neonatal outcomes when epidural local anesthetics with opioids were compared with epidural local anesthetics without opioids (ASA, 1999). Opioid in the epidural infusion causes pruritus that may last approximately 45 minutes after the initial loading dose (Russell & Reynolds, 1996) or continue throughout labor. Adding a small amount of epinephrine with the spinal opioid produces profound pain suppression (Youngstrom et al., 1996).

A meta-analysis of 11 randomized, controlled clinical trials found epidural anesthesia to be associated with longer first and second stages of labor, an increased incidence of fetal malposition, increased use of oxytocin, and increased instrumental vaginal births (Howell, 2000). There is inconsistent evidence in the literature about whether epidural analgesia or anesthesia has a significant effect on the cesarean section rates (Howell, 2000; Thorp & Breedlove, 1996).

The anesthesiologist or certified registered nurse anesthetist (CRNA) is responsible for identifying women with contraindications to the procedure (Display 11–5). During this meeting, the procedure and potential complications are discussed and questions answered. Some institutions provide the opportunity for women to meet with an anesthesia provider before admission. Without this type of preparation, obtaining true informed consent from a woman in active labor is practically impossible. The advantages of spinal or epidural analgesia or anesthesia are outlined in Display 11–6.

Before placement of an epidural catheter, 500 to 1000 mL of intravenous fluid is infused to avoid maternal hypotension (Collis, Harding, & Morgan, 1999). When epidural analgesia or anesthesia is initiated, the fetal heart rate is assessed according to established department guidelines before and after the procedure, intermittently or continuously, and during the procedure if possible; additional monitoring is provided during epidural analgesia or anesthesia when the patient's condition warrants (AWHONN, 1998). Use of epidural analgesia or anesthesia is not contraindicated in the presence of a nonreassuring fetal heart rate pattern (Vincent & Chestnut, 1998). However, it should be used judiciously when nonreassuring fetal heart rate or conditions associated with uteroplacental insufficiency exist (Thorp, 1999). Some practitioners believe that the presence of an epidural catheter permits rapid extension of the block in case cesarean birth for nonreassuring fetal status becomes necessary.

DISPLAY 11–5

Contraindications to Epidural Anesthesia or Analgesia

- Coagulation disorders
- Local infection at the site of injection
- Maternal hypotension and shock
- Nonreassuring fetal heart rate pattern requiring immediate birth

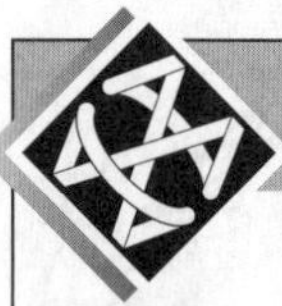

DISPLAY 11–6

Advantages of Epidural Analgesia or Anesthesia

- Pain relief is superior to other available methods.
- Because women have decreased sensation, interventions such as vaginal examinations and position changes are less uncomfortable.
- The method offers effective anesthesia for episiotomy or if forceps are used.
- If an epidural catheter is already in place, anesthesia for a cesarean birth can be accomplished more rapidly.
- It avoids maternal and neonatal respiratory depression, which can be associated with intravenous and intramuscular opioids.

From Vincent, R. D., & Chestnut, D. H. (1998). Epidural analgesia during labor. *American Family Physician, 58*(8), 1785–1792.

Standard Epidural

The epidural catheter is placed in the epidural space between the fourth and fifth lumbar vertebrae. A test dose of a local anesthetic mixed with epinephrine may be injected to determine that the catheter is not in the epidural vein or the subarachnoid space (Fig. 11–6). Injection into an epidural vein causes tachycardia, palpitations, increased blood pressure, numbness of the tongue, metallic taste, lightheadedness, or tinnitus within 2 to 3 minutes. When the anesthesiologist or CRNA is satisfied that the catheter is properly placed, a bolus of anesthetic medication is injected. Traditionally, the medication used was a local anesthetic. Currently, a combination of a long-acting local anesthetic with an opioid (ie, bupivacaine and fentanyl) is used. Combining a local anesthetic with an opioid provides good pain relief with less lower extremity motor block (Russell, Quinlan, & Reynolds, 1995). Depending on the specific medications used, women begin to feel relief in 5 to 10 minutes. A complete block usually occurs in 15 to 20 minutes.

In some women, a test dose may not determine intravascular injection because there is existing maternal tachycardia or because the effects occur too quickly to be observed. For this reason, some practitioners prefer to place a 10-mL anesthetic dose combining bupivacaine, fentanyl, and epinephrine in 5-mL increments through the catheter. If the catheter is positioned correctly, onset of analgesia is approximately 5 minutes, and decreased sensation in lower extremities occurs within 20 minutes (Youngstrom et al., 1996). Inadvertent placement of the catheter in the subarachnoid space causes immediate upper thoracic sensory loss, initiates severe lower extremity motor blockade, and potentially causes respiratory arrest.

Combined Spinal Epidural

Combined spinal epidural (CSE) is performed by first placing a 17- or 18-gauge Tuohy needle in the epidural space using the loss-of-resistance technique. After the needle is positioned in the epidural space, the smaller-gauge spinal needle is placed through the epidural needle into the subarachnoid space. An initial dose of local and opioid analgesia (25 μg of fentanyl and 2.5 mg of bupivacaine) is injected into the subarachnoid space. The spinal needle is removed, and an epidural catheter is threaded through the epidural needle, the needle is removed, and the catheter is taped in place.

Advantages of the CSE are faster onset of pain relief as a result of the intrathecal analgesia or anesthesia, decreased motor blockade, and increased reports of maternal satisfaction. Motor blockade is reduced because the total dose of local analgesia needed is less (Collis, Davies, & Aveling, 1995) as a result of the synergistic effect of opioids and local anesthetics.

Regardless of the technique used, after the catheter is in place, epidural anesthesia or analgesia is administered by intermittent bolus, referred to as "topping-off the epidural," continuous epidural infusion, or patient-controlled epidural analgesia. Advantages of a continuous infusion include a consistent level of pain relief and prevention of hemodynamic changes associated with the repeated occurrence of pain. Continuous flow through the catheter also stabilizes the catheter, decreasing the risk of migration into an epidural vein or through the dura into the subarachnoid space. The continuous infusion may be a local anesthetic alone (0.125% bupivacaine) or a combination of a local and opioid (0.0625% bupivacaine with 2.5 μg/mL of fentanyl or 0.25 μg/mL of sufentanil). Women who receive local anesthetic alone need more medication to obtain satisfactory pain relief than women who receive a combination of local and opioid (Russell & Reynolds, 1996). When a local anesthetic is combined with an opioid, there is less motor block and increased maternal satisfaction with pain management; there is no difference in rate of spontaneous deliveries or perineal pain during second stage labor (Russell & Reynolds, 1996). Women who receive CSE analgesia or anesthesia report significantly more pruritus than women receiving standard epidural (Collis et al., 1995; Nageotte, Larson, Rumney, Sidhu, & Hollen-

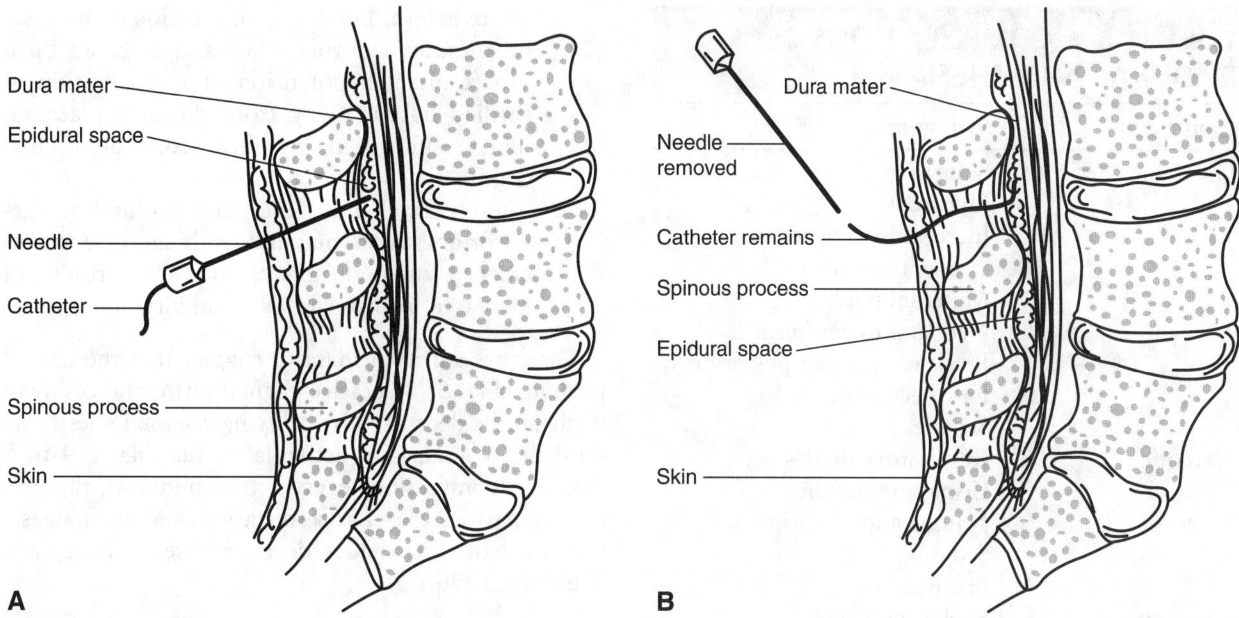

FIGURE 11–6. (**A**) A needle is inserted into the epidural space. (**B**) A catheter is threaded into the epidural space; the needle is then removed. The catheter allows medication to be administered intermittently or continuously to relieve pain during labor and childbirth.

bach, 1997). As cervical dilatation progresses, it may be necessary to increase the rate of continuous infusions or provide a second bolus with a higher concentration of local anesthetic or narcotic.

Walking Epidurals

With the introduction of CSE and reduced motor block during labor, the next logical question became whether it was safe for women to ambulate with regional analgesia in place. Several studies have demonstrated that most women maintain lower limb motor function after CSE analgesia and can safely ambulate (Breen, Shapiro, Glass, Foster-Payne, & Oriol, 1993; Collis et al., 1993, 1995; Shennan, Cooke, Lloyd-Jones, Morgan, & deSwiet, 1995). When the effects of bed rest and ambulation are compared for women receiving CSE, there is no difference in duration of labor, analgesia requirements, mode of delivery, or condition of the baby at the time of birth (Bloom et al., 1998; Collis et al., 1999). Display 11–7 outlines assessment criteria that should be considered before allowing a laboring woman to ambulate while receiving epidural analgesia.

Complications

Disadvantages of epidural anesthesia or analgesia include potential side effects such as longer labor, pruritus, cesarean birth, maternal fever, additional technology added to the birth experience, and before the introduction of the "walking epidural," restriction to bed rest in most institutions. Complications of epidural analgesia or anesthesia and their relation to the type of medication or procedure used are outlined in Table 11–8.

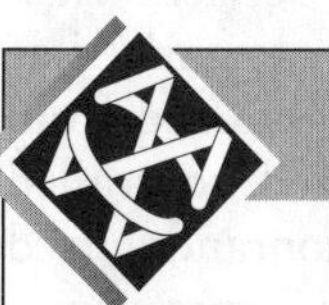

DISPLAY 11–7

Guidelines for Assessing the Ability to Ambulate During Continuous Epidural Analgesia

- Absence of orthostatic hypotension
- Adequate motor strength demonstrated by the ability to perform a standing partial knee bend before ambulating
- Presence of feeling in the plantar surfaces of both feet
- Availability of some person to ambulate with the laboring woman
- Nursing policy prescribing frequency of repeat assessments to determine that the woman can safely ambulate

Youngstrom, P. C., Baker, S. W., & Miller, J. L. (1996). Epidurals redefined in analgesia and anesthesia: A distinction with a difference. *Journal of Obstetric, Gynecologic, and Neonatal Nursing, 25*(4), 350–354.

TABLE 11–8 ■ COMPLICATIONS OF EPIDURAL ANESTHESIA

Cause	Symptom
Local anesthetic	Shivering
	Hypotension
	Increased incidence of operative birth
	Maternal pyrexia
	Neonatal hyperthermia
	Persistent occiput posterior
	Late decelerations
	Seizures
Narcotic	Respiratory depression
	Urinary retention
	Nausea and vomiting
	Sedation
	Pruritus
Result of actual procedure	Backache
	Inadvertent puncture of the dura
	Headache
	Unilateral block
	Migration of the catheter

The latest review of the literature about the effect of epidural analgesia or anesthesia during labor was provided by the United States Preventive Services Task Force (USPSTF, 1997). Best evidence is categorized as level I evidence and includes evidence obtained from at least one properly designed, randomized, controlled trial; level II evidence is derived from nonrandomized or retrospective studies; and level III evidence comes from case reports that lack reliability from the scientific perspective because of their potential for bias (USPSTF, 1997). Using this scheme for classifying evidence, the following conclusions were drawn (Thorp, 1999):

1. There is level I evidence from nulliparous and multiparous populations that epidural analgesia or anesthesia does prolong labor.
2. There is level I evidence that use of epidural analgesia or anesthesia increases requirements for oxytocin augmentation and instrumental birth.
3. There is level I evidence that epidural analgesia or anesthesia is associated with increased incidence of maternal fever, although the mechanism for this effect is not clear.
4. There is conflicting level I evidence about whether epidural analgesia or anesthesia increases the incidence of cesarean birth.
5. There is level I evidence that regional analgesia or anesthesia during labor and cesarean birth can result in hypotension or redistribution of cardiac output away from the uteroplacental unit, resulting in umbilical cord blood acidemia.
6. There is level II evidence that epidural analgesia or anesthesia may indirectly increase the incidence of perineal trauma as a result of increased instrumental vaginal births.

There are sufficient data to suggest that the risk of prolonged labor, operative vaginal birth, and cesarean birth can be decreased by delaying regional anesthesia until the woman is in active labor (ie, dilated 4 to 5 cm, with contractions every 2 to 3 minutes), the presenting part is at least at zero station, and an analgesic rather than anesthetic dose is used (Thorp & Beedlove, 1996).

Intrathecal Analgesia and Anesthesia

The goal of subarachnoid administration of narcotics is to prevent the motor blockade associated with local anesthetics while continuing to provide adequate pain relief during labor. Intrathecal analgesia or anesthesia is a single injection of an opioid that is a slow-onset, long-acting or a rapid-onset, short-acting drug. Morphine has a slow onset of action but is long acting. Morphine is associated with pruritus, nausea, urinary retention, and sedation (Vincent & Chestnut, 1998). Examples of opioids that have a rapid onset of action (5 minutes) but only last about 90 minutes are fentanyl and sufentanil. It is possible to combine a rapid-acting and long-lasting agent in the same injection. Intrathecal analgesia or anesthesia does not provide the flexibility of an epidural, nor does it usually provide pain relief into the second stage of labor.

Nursing Interventions

The AWHONN with the American Association of Nurse Anesthetists (AANA), American Association of Critical Care Nurses (AACN), and Association of Perioperative Registered Nurses (AORN) have prepared a joint position statement providing guidelines for practice for nurses caring for pregnant women receiving anesthesia by catheter techniques (ie, epidural, intrathecal, intrapleural, or peripheral nerve catheters):

- The insertion, initial injection, or initiation of a continuous infusion of epidural catheters for analgesia should be performed only by a qualified, credentialed, licensed anesthesia care provider.

- Rebolus of an epidural catheter includes injection of the catheter or increasing the rate of a continuous infusion. Rebolus should be performed only by a qualified, credentialed, licensed anesthesia care provider.
- A qualified, credentialed, licensed anesthesia care provider must be readily available as defined by institutional policy.
- The registered nurse may monitor the mother and fetus, replace empty infusion syringes or infusion bags with new previously prepared solutions, stop the infusion, and initiate emergency therapeutic measures under protocol if complications arise.
- The registered nurse may remove the catheter from the pregnant or nonpregnant patient when educational criteria have been met and institutional policy and state laws allow. The registered nurse may remove the catheter that has been used for analgesia on receipt of a specific order from a qualified anesthesia or physician provider (AWHONN, 1996).

According to the AANA Position Statement, *Provision of Pain Relief by Medication Administered via Continuous Epidural, Intrathecal, Intrapleural, Peripheral Nerve Catheters or Other Pain Relief Devices* (1995)

> . . . initial injection, reinjection, or continuous infusion of epidural catheters for anesthesia or analgesia for the obstetrical patient in labor should only be performed by a qualified/credentialed anesthesia provider. . . . Obstetrical laboring patients receiving epidural analgesia may be monitored by an obstetrical nurse trained and in accordance with established guidelines provided an anesthesia provider is immediately available as defined by institutional policy. This monitored care should only be done after stabilization of vital signs after either bolus injection or establishment of continuous pump infusion. (AANA, 1995)

Perinatal nurses must be comfortable with the operation of additional technology, be familiar with nursing care during all phases of the procedure, and be able to recognize potential complications. Continuous epidural anesthesia is always delivered through an infusion pump, and continuous EFM is the most frequently used method of fetal assessment. Depending on institutional practice women may also be monitored using a cardiac monitor, pulse oximeter, and automatic blood pressure devices. *Guidelines for Perinatal Care* (AAP & ACOG, 1997) suggest a 1 : 1 nurse-patient ratio for initiating epidural anesthesia.

Published standards and individual state nursing practice acts are inconsistent regarding the role of the nurse in caring for women in labor who receive anesthesia or analgesia and do not provide specific guidelines for how often and what type of monitoring will lead to optimal maternal–fetal outcomes. Controversy exists in the literature and in clinical practice about the frequency of maternal–fetal assessments during epidural anesthesia or analgesia for laboring women. Many perinatal units have policies that require completion of specific aspects of maternal–fetal assessment every 15 to 30 minutes for women with epidurals. There are, however, no published standards of care or practice guidelines from the ASA, AANA, ACOG, or AWHONN that prescribe what the maternal–fetal assessment includes or the specific frequencies for making assessments during epidural infusion for labor and delivery. Existing published standards are general and outlined in Display 11–8. Nursing and medical textbooks may contain suggested protocols and valuable clinical information, but they do not define standards of care. There are no research-based data to demonstrate optimal time intervals for maternal–fetal assessments during epidural infusion. The type and amount of medication used, the level of the block given, and maternal–fetal status should be considered when determining intensity of monitoring. Perinatal nurses, in collaboration with obstetric and anesthesia providers in each institution, must develop protocols that delineate responsibilities and care for women receiving epidural anesthesia or analgesia during labor and delivery.

Table 11–9 contains a sample care plan for intrapartum use of epidural anesthesia or analgesia. Pharmacologic pain-management strategies represent one aspect of intrapartum pain management. They should be used for augmentation, not as a substitute for nonpharmacologic strategies. A woman who has been given intravenous pain medication or received continuous epidural analgesia or anesthesia can still benefit from all of the nonpharmacologic nursing interventions available.

Additional Techniques

Two methods of regional anesthesia, paracervical block and saddle block, were once widely accepted techniques for relief of labor pain. Paracervical block is now rarely used because of the potential for fetal bradycardia caused by rapid absorption of local anesthetic from the paracervical space. Saddle block, an injection of a local anesthetic into the subarachnoid

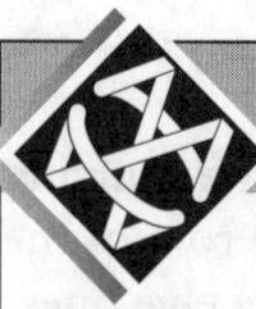

DISPLAY 11–8

Guidelines from Professional Organizations for Maternal–Fetal Assessment Frequencies During Regional Anesthesia or Analgesia

MATERNAL ASSESSMENTS

Guidelines for Perinatal Care (AAP & ACOG, 1997, p. 107)

"When regional anesthesia is administered during labor, the patient's vital signs should be monitored at regular intervals by a qualified member of the health care team."

Standards & Guidelines for Professional Nursing Practice in the Care of Women and Newborns (AWHONN, 1998, p. 33)

"When epidural anesthesia/analgesia is initiated, the nurse monitors maternal vital signs and fetal heart rate based on each patient's status."

"Additional monitoring of the patient is provided during epidural anesthesia/analgesia when the patient's condition warrants."

FETAL ASSESSMENTS

Practice Guidelines for Obstetric Anesthesia (ASA, 1999, p. 5)

"Fetal heart rate should be monitored by a qualified individual before and after administration of regional analgesia for labor. Continuous electronic recording of the fetal heart rate may not be necessary in every clinical setting and may not be possible during placement of a regional anesthetic."

Standards & Guidelines for Professional Nursing Practice in the Care of Women and Newborns (AWHONN, 1998, p. 33)

"When epidural anesthesia/analgesia is initiated the fetal heart rate is assessed before and after the procedure, either intermittently or continuously, and if possible during the procedure."

TABLE 11–9 ■ NURSING CARE: INTRAPARTUM EPIDURAL ANESTHESIA OR ANALGESIA

Nursing Diagnosis	Interventions	Scientific Rationale
Alteration in comfort related to positioning for placement of the epidural catheter	1. Explain procedure and the importance of remaining still during insertion of the catheter. 2. Assist the woman to maintain a sidelying or sitting position. 3. Encourage use of Lamaze breathing techniques during procedure.	Avoid severe spinal flexion because it can decrease the epidural space and increase the possibility of puncturing the dura.
Alteration in comfort related to inadequate level of anesthesia or analgesia	1. Evaluate the effect of the epidural dose. Request that the anesthesiologist/CRNA redose the epidural as necessary, to provide effective pain relief	Promotes spread of medication through epidural space.
	2. If pain continues to be felt on one side of the body, instruct the woman to lie on that side. 3. Assist the woman to change position at least q 1 hr.	Turning avoids continued pressure on one area of the body and decreases the risk of unilateral blocks.

(continued)

TABLE 11–9 ■ NURSING CARE: INTRAPARTUM EPIDURAL ANESTHESIA OR ANALGESIA (continued)

Nursing Diagnosis	Interventions	Scientific Rationale
Potential for maternal injury related to hemodynamic changes	1. Infuse IV bolus of 500–1,000 mL lactated Ringer's or normal saline solution 15–30 min before the procedure	Avoid IV fluids containing glucose. These cause increased insulin production in the fetus and potential hypoglycemia after birth. Avoid rapidly infusing IV fluids into women with cardiac disease or severe preeclampsia without direct measurement of hemodynamic status.
	2. After catheter has been placed, maintain woman in a left lateral tilt.	Because epidural anesthesia causes a sympathetic block and vasodilation, hydration and avoiding the supine position decrease the risk of maternal hypotension, which can result in ulteroplacental insufficiency.
	3. After each injection, monitor blood pressure, pulse, and respirations according to institutional protocol.	
	4. If hypotension occurs, increase IV fluids, maintain uterine displacement, administer oxygen, and administer ephedrine as ordered.	A decrease in systolic blood pressure to <100 mmHg or below 20% from baseline can be corrected by administering ephedrine, 3.0–6.0 mg IV (Parry, Fernandez, Bawa, Poulton, 1998). Ephedrine promotes peripheral vasoconstriction without constricting the umbilical vessels and increases cardiac output.
Potential for maternal injury related to placement of the catheter in the subarachnoid space or toxic response to anesthetic	1. Oxygen and suction are set up and functioning before start of procedure.	
	2. Assess for symptoms of respiratory distress.	
	3. Crash cart with Ambu bag and mask, laryngoscope and blades, and endotracheal tubes immediately available.	
Potential for migration of the catheter out of the epidural space	1. Assess the woman for lack of effect from the anesthetic.	
	2. Evaluate the woman for symptoms such as severe hypotension, motor block (including the upper extremities), and respiratory or cardiac arrest.	These symptoms may indicate migration of the catheter into the subarachnoid space.

(continued)

TABLE 11–9 ■ NURSING CARE: INTRAPARTUM EPIDURAL ANESTHESIA OR ANALGESIA (continued)

Nursing Diagnosis	Interventions	Scientific Rationale
Potential for maternal injury related to late onset of respiratory depression	1. Respiratory rate should continue to be assessed frequently into the postpartum recovery period. When epidural morphine is used, respiratory rates are monitored according to institutional protocol. 2. Administer naloxone if respiratory rate is <10.	Respiratory depression may occur 4–8 hr after the last narcotic dose.
Potential for fetal injury related to hemodynamic changes	1. Obtain a 20–30 min baseline EFM strip before initiation of the epidural, with continuous EFM for the duration of epidural infusion.	Maternal hypotension can decrease uteroplacental blood flow, adversely affecting fetal oxygenation, which is reflected in a nonreassuring FHR pattern.
Alteration in elimination related to decreased sensation of the bladder	1. Encourage the woman to void before the procedure and frequently during the infusion. 2. If the bladder is distended and the woman is unable to void, placement of an indwelling catheter eliminates the need for repeated catheterization.	Naloxone can also be used to reverse this effect on the bladder.
Potential pruritus, related to epidural narcotic administration	1. Assess woman for complaints of itching.	Pruritus is most often seen with the administration of epidural morphine.

CRNA, certified registered nurse–anesthetist;
EFM, electronic fetal monitoring;
FHR, fetal heart rate.

L4–L5 space at the onset of the second stage of labor, is also used infrequently because pain relief is generally so complete that women were unable to push effectively with their contractions, necessitating the application of forceps or a vacuum extractor. Paracervical block and saddle block are uncommon in clinical obstetric practice today because of the popularity of epidural anesthesia.

SUMMARY

The ultimate goal is the birth of a healthy newborn to a healthy mother who is satisfied with her childbirth experience. Performing ongoing assessments, offering a variety of nonpharmacologic comfort measures, supporting women receiving pharmacologic pain management, and recognizing when interventions are no longer effective or complications have developed are basic perinatal nursing practices.

Caring effectively for laboring women requires tremendous energy and commitment. Individual nurses and department managers have a responsibility to examine their own practices and the system as a whole. The challenge is to identify practices that have a positive impact on women's experiences and to respond with flexibility to the opportunity to enhance perinatal nursing care related to pain management during labor and birth.

REFERENCES

Aird, I. A., Luckas, M. J., Buckett, W. M., & Bousfield, P. (1997). Effects of intrapartum hydrotherapy on labor related parameters. *Australian & New Zealand Journal of Obstetrics and Gynecology, 37*(2), 137–142.

American Academy of Pediatrics & American College of Obstetricians and Gynecologists (AAP & ACOG). (1997). *Guidelines for perinatal care* (4th ed.). Elk Grove Village, IL: Author.

American Association of Nurse Anesthetists (AANA). (1995). *Provision of relief by medication administered via continuous epidural, intrathecal, intrapleural, peripheral nerve catheters, or other pain relief devices* (Position Statement). Park Ridge, IL: Author.

American College of Obstetricians and Gynecologists (ACOG). (2000). *Pain relief during labor* (Committee Opinion No. 231), Washington, DC: Author.

American Heart Association & American Academy of Pediatrics (AHA & AAP). (1996). *Textbook of neonatal resuscitation.* Elk Grove Village, IL: American Academy of Pediatrics.

American Society of Anesthesiologists (ASA). (1999). *Practice guidelines for obstetrical anesthesia.* Park Ridge, IL: Author.

Association of Women's Health, Obstetric and Neonatal Nurses (AWHONN). (1996). *Role of the registered nurse (RN) in the management of the patient receiving analgesia by catheter techniques (epidural, intrathecal, intrapleural, or peripheral nerve catheters).* Washington, DC: Author.

Association of Women's Health, Obstetric and Neonatal Nurses (AWHONN). (1998). *Standards and guidelines for professional nursing practice in the care of women and newborns* (5th ed.). Washington, DC: Author.

Association of Women's Health, Obstetric and Neonatal Nurses (AWHONN). (2000). *Professional nursing support of laboring women.* (Policy Statement). Washington, DC: Author.

Bird, I. S., & Waugaman, W. (1999). In S. J. Reeder, L. L. Martin, & D. Koniak (Eds.), *Maternity nursing: Family, newborn, and women's health care* (18th ed., pp. 573–615). Philadelphis: Lippincott Williams & Wilkins.

Bloom, S. L., McIntire, D. D., Kelly, M. A., Beimer, H. L., Burpo, R. H., Garcia, M. A., & Leveno, K. J. (1998). Lack of effect of walking on labor and delivery. *The New England Journal of Medicine, 339*(2), 76–79.

Breen, T. W., Shapiro, T., Glass, B., Foster-Payne, D., & Oriol, N. (1993). Epidural anesthesia for labor in an ambulatory patient. *Anesthesia and Analgesia, 77*(5), 919–924.

Britt, R., & Pasero, C. (1999). Pregnancy, childbirth, postpartum, and breastfeeding. In M. McCaffery & C. Pasero (Eds.), *Pain: Clinical manual* (2nd ed., pp. 608–625). St. Louis: Mosby.

Bryanton, J., Fraser-Davey, H., & Sullivan, P. (1994). Women's perceptions of nursing support during labor. *Journal of Obstetric Gynecologic and Neonatal Nursing, 23*(8), 638–644.

Chandler, S., & Field, P. (1997). Becoming a father: First-time fathers' experience of labor and delivery. *Journal of Nurse-Midwifery, 42*(1), 17–24.

Chapman, L. L. (1991). Searching: Expectant fathers' experience during labor and birth. *Journal of Perinatal and Neonatal Nursing, 4*(4), 21–29.

Chapman, L. L. (1992). Expectant fathers' roles during labor and birth. *Journal of Obstetric, Gynecologic, and Neonatal Nursing, 21*(2), 114–120.

Chapman, L. L. (2000). Expectant fathers and labor epidurals. *MCN, The American Journal of Maternal Child Nursing, 25*(3), 133–139.

Church, L. K. (1989). Water birth: One birthing center's observations. *Journal of Nurse-Midwifery, 34*(4), 165–170.

Collis, R. E., Baxandall, M. L., Srikantharajah, I. D., Edge, G., Kadim, M. Y., & Morgan, B. M. (1993). Combined spinal epidural analgesia with ability to walk throughout labor. *Lancet, 341*(8851), 767–768.

Collis, R. E., Davies, D. W., & Aveling, W. (1995). Randomized comparison of combined spinal-epidural and standard epidural analgesia in labor. *Lancet, 345*(8962), 1413–1416.

Collis, R. E., Harding, S. A., & Morgan, B. M. (1999). Effect of maternal ambulation on labor with low-dose combined spinal-epidural analgesia. *Anaesthesia, 54*(6), 535–539.

Cohen, S. (1997). Strategies for labor pain relief—past, present and future. *ACTA Anaesthesiologica Scandinavia, 110*, 17–21.

DiFranco, J. (2000). Relaxation: Music. In F. Nichols & S. B. Humenick (Eds.), *Childbirth education: Practice, research, and theory* (pp. 201–215). Philadelphia: W.B. Saunders.

deJong, P. R., Johanson, R. B., Baxen, P., Adrians, V. D., vander Westhuisen, S., & Jones, R. W. (1997). Randomized trial comparing the upright and supine positions for the second stage of labor. *British Journal of Obstetrics and Gynecology, 104*(5), 567–571.

Eddleston, J. M., Holland, J. J., Griffin, R. P., Corbett, A., Horsman, E. L., & Reynolds, F. (1996). A double-blind comparison of 0.25% ropivacaine and 0.25% bupivacaine for extradural analgesia in labor. *British Journal of Anaesthesiology, 76*(1), 66–71.

Eriksson, M., Ladfors, L., Mattsson, L. A., & Fall, O. (1996). Warm tub bath during labor: A study of 1385 women with prelabor rupture of the membranes after 34 weeks of gestation. *Acta Obstetricia et Gynecologica Scandinavica, 75*(7), 642–644.

Faucher, M. A., & Brucker, M. C. (2000). Intrapartum pain: Pharmacologic management. *Journal of Obstetric, Gynecologic, and Neonatal Nursing, 29*(2), 169–180.

Faure, E. A. (1991). The pain of parturition. *Seminars in Perinatology, 15*(5), 342–347.

Gagnon, A. J., & Waghorn, K. (1999). One-to-one nurse labor support of nulliparous women stimulated with oxytocin. *Journal of Obstetrics, Gynecology, and Neonatal Nursing, 28*(4), 371–376.

Green, J. (1993). Expectations and experiences of pain in labor: Findings from a large prospective study. *Birth: Issues in Perinatal Care and Education, 20*(2), 65–72.

Harris, K. T. (1999). Hydrotherapy: An alternative method for relieving labor pain. *Mother-Baby Journal, 4*(5), 14–20.

Hodnett, E. (2000). Caregiver support of women during childbirth. *The Cochrane Database Systematic Review,* 2, CD000199.

Howell, C. J. (2000). Epidural versus non-epidural analgesia for pain relief in labour. *The Cochrane Database Systematic Review,* 2, CD000331.

Huffnagle, H. J., & Huffnagle, S. L. (1999). Alternatives to conduction analgesia. In M. C. Norris (Ed.), *Obstetric Anesthesia* (2nd ed., pp. 282). Philadelphia: Lippincott Williams & Wilkins.

Katz, V. L., Ryder, R. M., Cefalo, R. C., Carmichael, S. C., & Goolsby, R. (1990). A comparison of bed rest and immersion for treating the edema of pregnancy. *Obstetrics and Gynecology, 75*(2), 147–151.

Klaus, M. H., & Kennell, J. H. (1997). The doula: An essential ingredient of childbirth rediscovered. *Acta Paediatrica, 86*(10), 1034–1036.

Kuhnert, B. R., Linn, P. L., & Kuhnert, P. M. (1985). Obstetric medication and neonatal behavior. *Clinics in Perinatology, 12*(2), 423–440.

Labrecque, M., Nouwen, A., Bergeron, M., & Rancourt, J. F. (1999). A randomized controlled trial of nonpharmacologic approaches for relief of low back pain during labor. *Journal of Family Practice, 48*(4), 259–230.

Lavender, T., Walkinshaw, S. A., & Walton, I. (1999). A prospective study of women's views of factors contributing to a positive birth experience. *Midwifery, 15*(1), 40–46.

Lederman, R. P., Lederman, E., Work, B., & McCann, D. S. (1985). Anxiety and epinephrine in multiparous women in labor: Relationship to duration of labor and fetal heart rate pattern. *American Journal of Obstetrics and Gynecology, 153*(8), 870–871.

Lowe, N. (1996). The pain and discomfort of labor and birth. *Journal of Obstetric, Gynecologic, and Neonatal Nursing, 25*(1), 82–92.

Lytzen, T., Cederberg, L., & Moller-Nielsen, J. (1989). Relief of low back pain in labor by using intracutaneous nerve stimulation with sterile water papules. *Acta Obstetricia et Gynecologica Scandinavica, 68*(4), 341–343.

Manning-Orenstein, G. (1998). A birth intervention: The therapeutic effects of doula support versus Lamaze preparation on first-time mother's working models of caregiving. *Alternative Therapeutic Health Medicine, 4*(4), 73–81.

Martensson, L., & Wallin, G. (1999). Labor pain treated with cutaneous injections of sterile water: A randomized controlled trial. *British Journal of Obstetrics and Gynecology, 106*(7), 633–637.

Mayberry, L. J., Wood, S. H., Strange, L. B., Lee, L., Heisler, D. R., & Nielsen-Smith, K. (2000). *Second stage labor management: Promotion of evidence-based practice and a collaborative approach to patient care.* (Symposium). Washington, DC: Author.

McCaffery, M., & Paser, C. (1999). Practical nondrug approaches to pain. In M. McCaffery & C. Pasero (Eds.), *Pain: Clinical manual for nursing practice* (2nd ed., pp. 399–427). St Louis: Mosby.

McNiven, P., Hodnett, E., & O'Brien-Pallas, L. L. (1992). Supporting women in labor: a work sampling study of the activities of labor and delivery nurses. *Birth, 91*(1), 3–8.

Melzack, R., & Wall, P. D. (1965). Pain mechanisms: A new theory. *Science, 150*, 971–979.

Mussell, S. (1998). Narcotic analgesia during labor and birth: Maternal and newborn effects. *Mother-Baby Journal, 3*(6), 19–23.

Nageotte, M. P., Larson, D., Rumney, P. J., Sidhu, M., & Hollenbach, K. (1997). Epidural analgesia compared with combined spinal-epidural analgesia during labor in nulliparous women. *New England Journal of Medicine, 337*(24), 1715–1719.

Niven, C. A., & Gijsbers, K. J. (1989). Do low levels of labor pain reflect low sensitivity to noxious stimulation? *Social Science and Medicine, 29*(4), 585–588.

Oxone-Foote, H. (1986). *Human labor and birth* (5th ed.). Norwalk, CT: Appleton-Century-Crofts.

Parry, M. G., Fernando, R., Bawa, G. P. & Poulton, B. B. (1998). Dorsal column function after epidural and spinal blockage: Implications for the safety of walking following low-dose regional analgesia for labor. *Anesthesia, 53*(4), 382–387.

Pasero, C., Paice, J. A., & McCaffery, M. (1999). Basic mechanisms underlying the causes and effects of pain. In M. McCaffery & C. Pasero (Eds.), *Pain: Clinical manual for nursing practice* (2nd ed., pp. 15–34). St Louis: Mosby.

Reynolds, J. L. (1994). Intracutaneous sterile water for back pain in labor. *Canadian Family Physician, 40*, 1785–1788, 1791–1792.

Reynolds, J. L. (2000). Sterile water injections relieve back pain of labor. *Birth, 27*(1), 58–60.

Rush, J., Burlock, S., Lambert, K., Loosley-Millman, M., Hutchison, B., & Enkin, M. (1996). The effects of whirlpool baths in labor: A randomized, controlled trial. *Birth, 23*(3), 136–143.

Russell, R., Quinlan, J., & Reynolds, F. (1995). Motor block during epidural infusions for nulliparous women in labor: A randomized double-blind comparison of plain bupivacaine and low dose bupivacaine with fentanyl. *International Journal of Obstetric Anesthesia, 4*, 82–88.

Russell, R., & Reynolds, F. (1996). Epidural infusion of low-dose bupivacaine and opioid in labor. *Anaesthesia, 51*(3), 266–273.

Scott, K. D., Berkowitz, G., & Klaus, M. (1999). A comparison of intermittent and continuous support during labor: A meta-analysis. *American Journal of Obstetrics and Gynecology, 180*(5), 1054–1059.

Shennan, A., Cooke, V., Lloyd-Jones, F., Morgan, D., & de Swiet, M. (1995). Blood pressure changes during labor and ambulating with combined spinal-epidural analgesia. *British Journal of Obstetric and Gynecology, 102*(3), 192–197.

Simkin, P. (1989). Non-pharmacological methods of pain relief during labor. In I. Chalmers, M. Enkin, & M. J. N. C. Keirse (Eds.), *Effective care in pregnancy and childbirth* (pp. 893–912). Oxford: Oxford University Press.

Simkin, P. (1995). Reducing pain and enhancing progress in labor: A guide to nonpharmacologic methods for maternity caregivers. *Birth, 22*(3), 161–171.

Sleutel, M. R. (2000). Climate, culture, context, or work environment: Organizational factors that influence nursing practice. *Journal of Nursing Administration, 30*(2), 53–58.

Somers-Smith, M. J. (2000). A place for the partner? Expectations and experiences of support during childbirth. *Midwifery, 15*(2), 101–108.

Spielman, F. J. (1987). Systemic analgesics during labor. *Clinical Obstetrics and Gynecology, 30*(3), 495–504.

Tappan, F. (1978). *Healing massage techniques.* Reston, VA: Reston Publishing.

Thorp, J. (1999). Epidural analgesia during labor. *Clinical Obstetrics and Gynecology, 42*(4), 785–801.

Thorp, J. A., & Breedlove, G. (1996). Epidural analgesia in labor: An evaluation of risks and benefits. *Birth, 23*(2), 63–83.

Trolle, B., Moller, M., Kronborg, H., & Thomsen, S. (1991). The effect of sterile water blocks on low back labor pain. *American Journal of Obstetrics and Gynecology, 164*(5, Pt. 1), 1277–1281.

United States Preventive Services Task Force (USPSTF). (1997). *Guide to Clinical Preventive Services.* Baltimore: Williams & Wilkins.

Vincent, R. D., & Chestnut, D. H. (1998). Epidural analgesia during labor. *American Family Physician, 58*(8), 1785–1792.

Wakefield, M. L. (1999). Systemic analgesia: Opioids, ketamine, and inhalational agents. In D. H. Chestnut (Ed.), *Obstetric anesthesia: Principles and practice* (pp. 340–353). St. Louis: Mosby.

Waldenstrom, U., & Nilsson, C. (1992). Warm tub bath after spontaneous rupture of the membranes. *Birth: Issues in Perinatal Care and Education, 19*(2), 57–63.

Wiand, N. E. (1997). Relaxation levels achieved by Lamaze-trained pregnant women listening to music and ocean sound tapes. *The Journal of Perinatal Education, 6*(4), 1–7.

Youngstrom, P. C., Baker, S. W., & Miller, J. L. (1996). Epidurals redefined in analgesia and anesthesia: A distinction with a difference. *Journal of Obstetric, Gynecologic, and Neonatal Nursing, 25*(4), 350–354.

PART 4

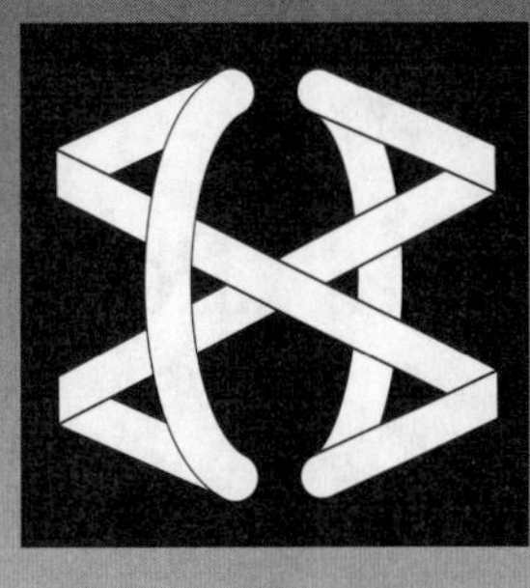

POSTPARTUM

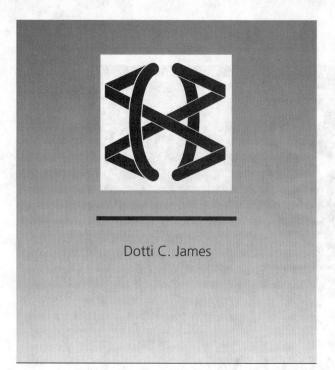

Dotti C. James

CHAPTER 12

Postpartum Care

A woman experiences significant changes in physical and psychosocial status after childbirth. The postpartum period is a time of transition involving physiologic changes, adaptation to the maternal role, and alteration of the family system by the addition of the newborn. Nurses have a unique opportunity to promote and support maternal and family adaptation. Inpatient postpartum care routines are ideally focused on the needs of the mother, newborn, and family rather than on arbitrary rules and unit traditions. Postpartum nursing care should be as individualized and flexible as needed. The perinatal nurse recognizes women and their families as integral members of the healthcare team and encourages them to enter into decision-making processes and planning of care (Association of Women's Health, Obstetric and Neonatal Nurses [AWHONN], 1998). Open visiting and family interaction with the new mother and newborn are supported. The father of the baby and other support persons should be encouraged to be present, according to the desires of the woman, and actively involved in postpartum and newborn care. Family-centered maternity care is based on the philosophy that the physical, social, psychological, and spiritual needs of the family are included in all aspects of the nursing care provided (AWHONN, 1998).

Implementation of family-centered maternity care requires collaboration among childbearing women, families, and healthcare providers. The family is defined by the woman and frequently extends beyond traditional definitions. Cultural beliefs and values of the woman and her family should be respected and accommodated. This chapter begins with a discussion of physiologic changes during the postpartum period and then describes the appropriate nursing assessments and interventions for healthy women and for those with common postpartum complications. Selected topics for patient education are presented. Teaching strategies for new mothers and general maternal–newborn learning needs are included in Chapter 18. Care beyond the inpatient experience is covered in Chapter 19.

ANATOMIC AND PHYSIOLOGIC CHANGES DURING THE POSTPARTUM PERIOD

Uterus

Involution results from a decrease in myometrial cell size, not in the number of myometrial cells. This decrease is the result of ischemia, autolysis, and phagocytosis. Ischemia occurs when the retraction of uterine musculature necessary for hemostasis after placental separation results in decreased blood flow to the uterus. Proteolytic enzymes are released, and macrophages migrate to the uterus, resulting in autolysis or self-digestion and subsequent reduction in myometrial cell size. Some of the excess elastic and fibrous tissue is removed by phagocytosis, but the incomplete process results in a uterus that does not return to its nulliparous size (Burton, 1999; Stables, 1999). Immediately after birth, the uterus weighs approximately 1,000 g (2 lb, 4 oz). As involution occurs, the uterine weight continues to decrease to 500 g (1 week), 300 g (2 weeks), and by 6 weeks postpartum, it weighs 100 g or less. Immediately after delivery, the uterine fundus can be palpated midway between the umbilicus and symphysis pubis. During the first 12 hours after birth, the muscles relax slightly, and the fundus returns to the level of the umbilicus. Beginning on postpartum day 2 or 3, the usual progression of uterine descent into the pelvis is 1 cm/day (Display 12–1).

During the first few days after birth, oxytocin secretion causes strong uterine contractions and a further reduction in size, especially after breast-feeding and in multiparas. Multiparity, multiple gestation, polyhydramnios, and bladder distention can influence uterine size and the progression of uterine involution.

Placental Site and Lochia

The placenta separates spontaneously from the uterus within 15 minutes of birth in 90% of women and within 30 minutes after birth in 95% of women. Separation of the placenta and membranes includes the spongy layer of the endometrium, leaving the decidua basalis in the uterus. This remaining layer reorganizes into basal and superficial layers. The superficial layer becomes necrotic and is sloughed in the lochia, and the basal layer becomes the source of new endometrium. The endometrium is regenerated by 2 to 3 weeks after delivery, except at the site of placental attachment (Cunningham et al., 1997; Stables, 1999). Immediately after delivery of the placenta, the placental site is approximately 8 to 10 cm, and by end of the second week, it is about 3 to 4 cm. Exfoliation, the process of placental site healing, occurs over the first 6 weeks after birth by necrotic sloughing of the infarcted superficial tissues. A reparative process follows in which the endometrium regenerates from the margins and base. This process prevents the formation of a fibrous scar in the decidua. At 7 to 14 days postpartum, the infarcted superficial tissue over the placental site sloughs. At this time, the woman may notice an episode of increased vaginal bleeding, which is usually self-limited. Bleeding lasting more than 1 to 2 hours should be evaluated for late postpartum hemorrhage. Ultrasonography can be useful in determining the presence of retained placental tissue (Creasy & Resnik, 1999).

Lochia is the postpartum uterine discharge. Although lochia varies in amount, the total volume lost usually is 150 to 400 mL. Initially, lochia rubra is reddish and continues 3 to 4 days. Lochia serosa, a pinkish discharge, continues from day 4 to 10. Lochia alba, a yellow-white discharge, follows lochia serosa (Table 12–1). The choice of feeding method for the baby and the use of oral contraceptives do not affect duration of lochia (Burton, 1999; Cunningham et al., 1997).

DISPLAY 12–1

Uterine Involution

Time	*Location of Fundus*
Immediately	At the level of the umbilicus
1–2 hours	Midline, midway between umbilicus and symphysis
12 hours	1 cm above umbilicus
24 hours	1 cm below umbilicus
3 days	3 cm below umbilicus
7 days	Just palpable at symphysis
14 days	Not palpable

Cervix, Vagina, and Pelvic Floor

The cervix and lower uterine segment are thin and flaccid immediately postpartum. Cervical lacerations can occur during any birth; however, women with precipitous labor and operative procedures are at increased risk for lacerations. By the end of the first week, the cervical os narrows to a diameter of 1 cm. The external cervical os remains wider than its pregravid state, and bilateral depressions typically are seen at the site of lacerations. Cervical edema may persist for several months (Cunningham et al., 1997; Steen, 1998; Steen & Cooper, 1997). The vagina and vaginal outlet are smooth walled and may appear bruised early in the puerperium. The apparent bruising, caused by pelvic congestion, disappears quickly after birth. Rugae reappear in the distended vagina by the third week. The voluntary muscles and supports of the pelvic floor gradually regain tone during the first 6 weeks postpartum. These changes occur in response to the reduced amount of circulating progesterone. For some women, vaginal tone may be improved by perineal tightening exercises, such as Kegel exercises (Carroli, Belizan, & Stamp, 1999; Maier & Maloni, 1997; Parsons, 1998; Sampselle, Miller, & Rossie, 1997). In the lactating woman, the hypoestrogenic state resulting from ovarian suppression may cause the vagina to appear pale and without rugae. This may result in dyspareunia.

Ovarian Function and Return of Menses

Although the return of menses and ovulation vary, the first menstrual period usually occurs within 7 to 9 weeks postpartum in nonnursing mothers. There are great variations in the return of menses for women

TABLE 12–1 ■ TYPES OF LOCHIA

Characteristic	Rubra	Serosa	Alba
Normal color	Red	Pink, brown tinged	Yellowish-white
Normal duration	1 to 3 days	3 to 10 days	10 to 14 days, but not abnormal to last longer
Normal discharge	Bloody with clots; fleshing odor; increased flow on standing or breast-feeding or during physical activity	Serosanguineous (blood and mucus) consistency; fleshy odor	Mostly mucus, no strong odor
Abnormal discharge	Foul smell; numerous and/or large clots; quickly saturated perineal pad	Foul smell; quickly saturated perineal pad	Foul smell; saturated perineal pad; reappearance of pink or red lochia; discharge lasts far too long (>4 weeks)

From Compendium of Postpartum Care. (1996). Washington, DC: AWHONN (Association of Women's Health, Obstetric, and Neonatal Nurses), 1.11

who are nursing because of depressed estrogen levels. In nursing mothers, menstruation usually returns between months 2 and 18.

Estrogen and progesterone levels decrease suddenly after placental delivery. For the first 2 to 3 weeks after birth, there is minimal gonadotropin activity, possibly because of a transient pituitary insensitivity to luteinizing hormone-releasing factor. As sensitivity returns, hormonal function returns to normal levels. The first menstrual cycle is usually anovulatory, but 25% of women may ovulate before menstruation. The mean for the return of ovulation is 10 weeks postpartum for women who are not lactating and approximately 17 weeks postpartum for women who are breast-feeding. The delay in the resumption of menses in lactating women in part may result from elevated prolactin levels (Creasy & Resnik, 1999; Cunningham et al., 1997; Stables, 1999).

Metabolic Changes

Prolactin, a pituitary hormone, is responsible for stimulating and sustaining lactation. Like estrogen and progesterone, prolactin levels decrease with placental delivery, although they remain elevated over nonpregnant levels. The decrease in estrogen and progesterone stimulate the anterior pituitary to produce prolactin. Between the third and fourth week postpartum, the prolactin level returns to normal in women who formula-feed their infants. For those who breast-feed, prolactin levels increase with each nursing episode (Creasy & Resnik, 1999).

Thyroid function returns to prepregnant levels within 4 to 6 weeks after birth. Because immunosuppression is a normal physiologic consequence of pregnancy, there is an increased risk of developing transient autoimmune thyroiditis, followed by hypothyroidism. This depression of thyroid function may cause depression, carelessness, and impairment of memory and concentration. There is a slightly increased risk of recurrence of autoimmune hypothyroidism or hyperthyroidism postpartum (Creasy & Resnik, 1999; Cunningham et al., 1997).

Low levels of placental lactogen, estrogen, cortisol, growth hormone, and the placental enzyme, insulinase, reduce their anti-insulin effect in the early puerperium. This results in lower glucose levels for women during this period and a reduction in insulin requirements for insulin-dependent diabetic women (Cunningham et al., 1997). Breast-feeding may precipitate hypoglycemic episodes in women with insulin-dependent diabetes. Women with gestational diabetes often have normal glucose levels immediately postpartum. Nutritional needs must be reassessed during this period. The basal metabolic rate increases 20% to 25% during pregnancy because of fetal metabolic activity. The basal metabolic rate remains elevated for 7 to 14 days after giving birth.

The first 2 hours postpartum, plasma renin and angiotensin II levels (involved in blood pressure maintenance) fall to normal, nonpregnant levels and then rise again and remain elevated for up to 14 days (Creasy & Resnik, 1999). Blood pressure should remain stable during the postpartum period, but lowered vascular resistance in the pelvis may result in orthostatic hypotension when a woman moves from a supine to a sitting position. An increase in blood pressure of 30 mmHg systolic or 15 mmHg diastolic, especially if accompanied by headaches or visual changes, may indicate postpartum preeclampsia and should be evaluated (Creasy & Resnik, 1999; Stables, 1999).

Kidneys and Bladder

Mild proteinuria (1+) may exist for 1 to 2 days after birth in 40% to 50% of women. Nonpathology can be assumed only in the absence of the symptoms of infection or preeclampsia. (Atterbury, Groome, Hoff, & Yarnell, 1998) If a urine specimen is necessary, it should be obtained through catheterization or as a clean-catch maneuver. These methods avoid contamination by protein-laden lochia (Varney, 1997). Glycosuria of pregnancy disappears, and creatinine clearance is usually normal by 1 week postpartum. Pregnancy-induced hypotonia and dilation of the ureters and renal pelves return to the prepregnant state by 8 weeks postpartum. The catabolic process of involution causes an increase of the blood urea nitrogen. By the end of the first week postpartum, the blood urea nitrogen level rises to values of 20 mg/dL, compared with 15 mg/dL in the late third trimester (Creasy & Resnik, 1999; Cunningham et al., 1997; Stables, 1999). Glomerular filtration rate, renal blood flow, and plasma creatinine return to normal levels by 6 weeks postpartum.

Labor may result in displacement of the urinary bladder and stretching of the urethra. Other factors that interfere with normal micturition include the numbing effect of anesthesia and the temporary neural dysfunction of the traumatized bladder These may cause decreased sensitivity. As a result, overdistention and incomplete emptying may occur. Signs of bladder distention include uterine atony reflected in increased lochia, displacement of the uterus to the right and significantly above the umbilicus, decreased urine output compared with oral and intravenous intake, and a "soft fullness," sometimes with a palpable margin, in the suprapubic area. Women may report an urge but inability to urinate. Spontaneous voiding, however, should resume by 6 to 8 hours after birth, and bladder tone usually returns to normal levels 5 to 7 days later. Each voiding should be at least 150 mL. Edema, hyperemia, and submucous extravasation of blood are frequently evident in the bladder postpartum (Creasy & Resnick, 1999; Cunningham et al., 1997). The effects of trauma from labor on the bladder and urethra diminish during the first 24 hours, unless a urinary tract infection is present.

Avoid rapid emptying of the bladder if catheterization is performed. No more than 800 mL of urine should be removed at one time. This can avoid a precipitous drop in intraabdominal pressure, which may result in splenetic engorgement and hypotension.

Stress Incontinence

Many women report transient stress incontinence during the first 6 weeks postpartum. Persistent stress incontinence may result from operative birth, a large baby, and perineal tissue damage. The influences of obstetric factors diminish over 3 months. The length of the second stage of labor, infant head size, birth weight, and episiotomy correlate with the development of postpartum stress incontinence (Foldspang, Mommsen, & Djurhuus, 1999; Wall, 1999). Impairment of muscle function near and surrounding the urethra is an underlying cause of stress incontinence. Prompt catheterization for urinary retention during the postpartum can prevent urinary difficulties (Cunningham et al., 1997). Knowledge about clinical factors implicated in stress incontinence allows anticipatory guidance and interventions for women at risk.

Fluid Balance and Electrolytes

The physiologic reversal of the extracellular or interstitial fluid accumulated during a normal pregnancy begins during the immediate postpartum period. Diuresis begins within 12 hours of delivery and continues up to 5 days. Diuresis occurs in response to the decrease in estrogen that stimulated fluid retention during pregnancy, the reduction of venous pressure in the lower half of the body, and the decrease in residual hypervolemia (Cunningham, et al., 1997). Urine output may be 3,000 mL or more each day. Additional fluid is lost through increased perspiration. Diuresis results in a decrease in body weight of 2 to 3 kg. Electrolyte levels return to nonpregnant homeostasis by 21 days or earlier. Fluid loss is greater in women who have experienced preeclampsia or eclampsia. By the third postpartum day, resolution of the vasoconstriction and additional extracellular fluid of pregnancy-induced hypertension contribute to significant expansion of the vascular volume (Cunningham et al., 1997).

Neurologic Changes

Discomfort and fatigue are common concerns after birth. Afterpains or painful uterine contractions during the first 2 to 3 days after delivery; discomfort associated with episiotomy, incisions, lacerations, or tears; muscle aches; and breast engorgement may contribute to a woman's discomfort during the postpartum period. Neurologic changes related to anesthesia and analgesia are transient and, if present, require attention to ensure the woman's safety. Deep tendon reflexes remain normal. Sleep disturbances contributing to fatigue are related to discomfort and the demands of newborn care. The presence of children or a lack of social support may limit the time available for rest. Natural or pharmacologic comfort measures should be offered. Psychosocial support is necessary, and referral to home-care nursing may be appropriate.

The carpal tunnel syndrome that results from compression of the median nerve by the physiologic edema of pregnancy is relieved by postpartum diuresis. Headaches may result from fluid shifts in the first week after birth, leakage of cerebrospinal fluid into the extradural space during spinal anesthesia, fluid and electrolyte imbalance, pregnancy-induced hypertension, or stress. Assessment of the quality and location of the headache and of the vital signs is necessary. Interventions such as environmental control of lighting, noise levels, and visitors, and administration of analgesic medications may be effective for nonpathologic headaches. Postpartum eclampsia (ie, seizures beginning more than 48 hours and less than 4 weeks after birth) is often preceded by severe headache or visual disturbances. Women may have a postpartum eclamptic seizure without a prenatal diagnosis of preeclampsia or hypertension. Because women may experience prodromal signs and symptoms after discharge from the hospital, information should be provided about these subjective signs and symptoms, which include a severe and persistent occipital headache, scotomata (ie, spots before the eyes), blurred vision, photophobia, and epigastric or right upper quadrant pain. Women should be encouraged to notify their primary healthcare provider if any of these symptoms develop to facilitate immediate evaluation.

Hemodynamic Changes

Changes in the cardiovascular system occur early in the postpartum period, with a variable rate of return to baseline levels that ranges from 6 to 12 weeks. Blood volume changes occur rapidly. Autotransfusion occurs as a result of elimination of blood flow to the placenta. The blood flow of 500 to 750 mL per minute, formerly flowing to the uteroplacental unit, is diverted to maternal systemic venous circulation immediately after birth. The blood loss with an uncomplicated vaginal delivery is approximately 500 mL and 1,000 mL, or more with a cesarean section birth. Plasma volume is diminished by approximately 1,000 mL as a result of blood loss and diuresis. By the third day postpartum, blood volume has decreased 16% from peak pregnancy levels and returns to nearly prepregnant levels by 1 to 2 weeks postpartum.

Cardiac output after birth depends on use and choice of anesthesia or analgesia, mode of delivery, blood loss, and maternal position. Cardiac output peaks immediately after birth to approximately 80% above the prelabor value in women who have received only local anesthesia. After reaching a maximum value at 10 to 15 minutes after birth, cardiac output begins to decline, reaching prelabor values approximately 1 hour postpartum, although it remains elevated for 48 hours after birth (Creasy & Resnick, 1999). It returns to prepregnant levels by 2 to 3 weeks after birth. Because the heart rate is stable or slightly decreased, the cardiac output is most likely caused by an increased stroke volume from venous return. Cesarean birth before labor onset avoids the hemodynamic effect of contractions but not the rise in cardiac output immediately postpartum. It is thought that epidural anesthesia during labor moderates the increase in cardiac output after birth by decreasing pain and anxiety (Creasy & Resnik, 1999; Cunningham et al., 1997).

The pulse rate remains stable or decreases slightly after birth. If the pulse rate is above 100, the woman should be assessed for infection or delayed postpartum hemorrhage. Some women may exhibit puerperal bradycardia, with a pulse rate of 40 to 50 beats/min. No conclusive proof has been given for this phenomenon. Orthostatic hypotension may occur when a woman sits up from a reclining position. Preeclampsia should be suspected if blood pressure values increase by 30 mmHg systolic or 15 mmHg diastolic.

Hematologic and Liver Changes

The decrease in plasma volume is greater than the loss of red blood cells after birth, causing an increase in the hematocrit between day 3 and 7. The hematocrit returns to normal levels 4 to 8 weeks later as red blood cells reach the end of their normal life span (Creasy & Resnik, 1999; Cunningham et al., 1997). In assessing postpartum laboratory values, a 1-g decrease in hemoglobin levels or 2-point decrease in the hematocrit value reflects a 500-mL blood loss. During the first 48 hours after birth, the physiologic reversal of the extracellular fluid accumulated during a normal pregnancy and intravenous fluids given during labor make accurate blood loss assessment difficult, because hemodilution occurs as this fluid enters the vascular system. This phenomenon is seen even in women who have lost 20% of their circulating blood volume during birth. Hemoconcentration may occur with minimal blood loss if a woman has preexisting polycythemia (Creasy & Resnik, 1999; Cunningham et al., 1997; Varney, 1997).

Normal serum iron levels are regained by the second week postpartum. A relative erythrocytosis is seen in women who have received iron supplementation during pregnancy and had an average blood loss during the birth process. In the absence of iron supplementation, iron deficiency develops in most women (Creasy & Resnik, 1999; Cunningham et al., 1997). The serum ferritin level correlates closely with the body's iron stores and is predictive of iron deficiency anemia (Creasy & Resnik, 1999; Cunningham, et. al., 1997). Changes in blood coagulation factors remain for variable periods postpartum. Plasma fibrinogen levels and sedimentation rate levels remain elevated for at least the first week.

Leukocytosis from the stress of labor and birth is seen in the postpartum period. A nonpathologic white blood cell (WBC) count may reach 25,000 to 30,000/μL, with the increase predominantly consisting of granulocytes. Relative lymphopenia (ie, lymphocyte deficiency) and absolute eosinopenia (ie, decreased eosinophils) may also be seen. This phenomenon, coupled with the increase in the sedimentation rate, may confuse the interpretation or assessment of infections during this period. Pathology should be suspected and further evaluation is indicated when the WBCs increase 30% over a 6-hour period (Creasy & Resnik, 1999; Cunningham et al., 1997; Varney, 1997).

The alterations in liver enzymes and lipids that occurred in response to increased estrogen levels and hemodilution during pregnancy are reversed and returned to normal levels within 3 weeks postpartum. Elevated levels of free fatty acids, cholesterol, triglycerides, and lipoproteins seen during pregnancy return to normal levels within 10 days. Alkaline phosphatase, derived from the placenta, liver, and bone during pregnancy, may remain elevated for 6 weeks. The previously atonic gallbladder demonstrates increased contractility as progesterone levels decrease (Creasy & Resnik, 1999; Cunningham et al., 1997; Varney, 1997).

Respiratory and Acid-Base Changes

The respiratory system quickly returns to its prepregnant state after the birth of the baby. These changes result from the decrease in progesterone levels, the decrease in intraabdominal pressure that accompanies emptying of the uterus, and the increased excursion of the diaphragm. This reduction of diaphragmatic pressure results in the immediate return of chest wall compliance to normal levels and partially relieves the dyspnea experienced during pregnancy. Residual volume (ie, amount of air remaining in the lung after maximum expiration) and tidal volume (ie, volume of air inhaled and exhaled during each breath) normalize soon after birth; the expiratory reserve volume (ie, maximum amount of air that can be exhaled), however, may remain in the abnormal range for several months. Vital capacity, inspiratory capacity, and maximum breathing capacity decrease after birth. The response to exercise may therefore be affected in the early postpartum weeks (Creasy & Resnik, 1999; Cunningham et al., 1997).

Length and severity of the second stage of labor appear to contribute to an "oxygen debt" (ie, extra oxygen required after strenuous exercise) that extends into the immediate postpartum period (Creasy & Resnik, 1999; Cunningham et al., 1997). The basal metabolic rate remains elevated for 7 to 14 days into the postpartum period and is attributable to mild anemia, lactation, and psychologic factors.

As progesterone levels fall, the $Paco_2$ rises to the normal prepregnant values (35 to 40 mmHg) within the first 2 days after birth. During the postpartum period, the Pao_2 should be normal at 95% or higher. Normal levels of pH and base excess gradually return by approximately 3 weeks postpartum.

Skin, Muscle, and Weight Changes

Overdistention of the abdominal wall as a result of pregnancy can rupture collagen fibers of the dermis, resulting in striae, which can occur also on the breasts, buttocks, and thighs. Striae eventually become irregular white lines. Diastasis (ie, separation) of the rectus muscles is common, and usually is reapproximated by the late postpartum period. Evidence of diastasis can be assessed by asking the woman to lift her head while lying in a supine position. If diastasis has occurred, a tentlike protrusion in the lower abdomen is noticeable. Abdominal binders are not recommended, and mild exercise to restore tone may be started after 1 to 2 weeks. The joint instability that occurred during pregnancy may not resolve until 6 to 8 weeks postpartum.

A woman loses an average of 12 pounds (5.5 kg) at birth. Additional weight is lost between 2 weeks and 6 months postpartum, especially if the woman is breastfeeding (Cunningham et al., 1997; Varney, 1997). Women who choose formula feeding can expect a 0.5 to 1 kg/week loss when eating a balanced diet containing slightly fewer calories than their usual daily expenditure. Weight loss occurs more rapidly in women of lower parity, age, and prepregnancy weight.

Gastrointestinal Changes

After birth, there is a decrease in gastrointestinal muscle tone and motility. When these changes are coupled with relaxation of abdominal muscles, gaseous distention can occur during the first 2 to 3 days postpartum. Decreased motility can result in postpartum ileus. Constipation may result from hemorrhoids, perineal trauma, dehydration, pain, fear of having a bowel movement, immobility, and medication (eg, magnesium sulfate antenatally for tocolysis, iron supplementation, codeine for pain, anesthetics during labor or surgery). Constipation can be minimized by encouraging the woman to drink adequate fluids and eat foods high in fiber. Hemorrhoids that develop during pregnancy may increase in size during labor and result in significant discomfort during the postpartum period. If the woman has hemorrhoids, suggesting warm or cold sitz baths and applying topical anesthetics can decrease discomfort. Stool softeners and laxatives are sometimes given. Bowel movements typically resume 2 to 3 days after birth, and normal bowel elimination patterns resume by 2 weeks postpartum.

Hernias and Anal Sphincter Damage

Genital hernias (eg, cystocele, rectocele, uterine prolapse, enterocele) may occur because of overstretching or tearing of the muscles or fascia during birth. Controversy exists regarding the use of episiotomy. Some practitioners recommend minimizing the use of midline episiotomy and using mediolateral episiotomy when the risk for extension is increased (eg, macrosomia, shallow perineal body, operative vaginal birth), but there is little supportive evidence for that practice (Eason, Labrecque, Wells, & Feldman, 2000). Episiotomy does not always prevent third- or fourth-degree lacerations and can increase the likelihood of perineal trauma (Eason et al., 2000). Risk factors for lacerations include nulliparity, second-stage labor arrest, persistent occiput posterior positions, forceps assistance, and use of vacuum extractors. Chapter 9 discusses episiotomy.

Obstetric trauma such as injury to the sphincter muscle or damage to the innervation of the pelvic floor is a leading cause of anal incontinence in healthy women (Toglia, 1996). One half of women with third-degree tears experience anal incontinence. Disturbances in bowel function (ie, fecal urgency and anal incontinence of stool and flatus) from mechanical or neurologic injury to the anal sphincter during vaginal birth may also be the result of damage from the large size of the baby's head in relation to the vaginal opening. Women who experience a third- or fourth-degree perineal laceration report a greater incidence of incontinence of flatus than those without anal sphincter rupture. Women with a long second stage of labor, a large newborn, or both have the greatest risk of nerve damage (Bick, 1998; Cunningham et al., 1997).

Embarrassment may prevent women from reporting symptoms of anal sphincter damage. Symptoms may disappear or worsen with time. An accurate history is helpful so that women with major sphincter defects can be offered a cesarean birth when appropriate. Aging, menopause, progression of neuropathy, and effects of subsequent births may contribute to long-term sphincter weakness.

Fluid and Nutritional Needs

After vaginal birth, there are no dietary restrictions for women without underlying medical conditions or pregnancy-induced complications. Oral fluids or intravenous fluid administration helps restore the balance altered by fluid loss during the labor and birth process. Women should be encouraged to drink 3,000 mL of water and other liquids every 24 hours. Encourage healthy food choices with respect for ethnic and cultural preferences. Snack trays should be available for women who give birth when regular food service is unavailable. After cesarean birth, women usually receive clear liquids until bowel sounds are present and then advance to solid foods. For each 20 calories of breast milk produced, the woman must consume an additional 30 calories. This results in a dietary increase of 500 to 1,000 calories each day for women who are maintaining body weight (Creasy & Resnik, 1999). By 6 weeks postpartum, decreased pressure and distortion of the stomach from the gravid uterus and the normalization of lower esophageal sphincter pressure and tone resolves the heartburn experienced by many pregnant women.

POSTPARTUM NURSING CARE

During the immediate postpartum period, the perinatal nurse focuses on maternal and newborn stabilization and recovery from the birth process. Maternal–newborn attachment and breast-feeding (if the woman desires) should be promoted and encouraged. Nursing assessments and interventions should occur concurrently with activities celebrating the joy of childbirth and welcoming the new baby into the family. Family and visitor interactions, including holding the new baby and taking video and still pictures of the first hours of life, should be supported as much as possible based on the condition of the mother and newborn. Every effort should be made to accommodate the wishes of the woman and her family.

When regional analgesia or anesthesia or general anesthesia has been used for vaginal or cesarean birth, the woman should be observed in an appropriately staffed and equipped labor-delivery-recovery room or postanesthesia care unit until she has recovered from the anesthetic (American Academy of Pediatrics & American College of Obstetricians and Gynecologists [AAP & ACOG], 1997; American Society of Anesthesiologists [ASA], 1999). The woman should be discharged from postanesthesia care only at the discretion of and after communication among the attending physician or a certified nurse midwife, anesthesiologist, and certified registered nurse anesthetist (AAP & ACOG, 1997; ASA, 1999).

According to the wishes and condition of the woman, during the inpatient stay, she and the newborn should be kept together as much as possible. Most perinatal units have models of care that support maternal–newborn attachment. Mother–baby or couplet care in which one nurse is responsible for both patients facilitates optimal interaction between the mother and baby and coordination of appropriate nursing assessments and interventions. Opportunities for rest for the new mother should be promoted, although this may be challenging for the nurse because of the number of congratulatory telephone calls and visitors and because of the unit routines that interrupt sleep. Nursing care should be planned so that necessary interventions and medication administration (if needed) can be grouped together, minimizing the need to wake the woman during daytime naps or during the night. A plan for rest designed collaboratively with the new mother and her family works well. Ambulation as soon as the mother feels able should be encouraged, but the woman should be instructed not to get out of bed on her own without assistance the first time after birth (AAP & ACOG, 1997). In the absence of complications or surgical recovery, a regular diet should be resumed as soon as the woman desires. Education for the new mother and her family about maternal postpartum care and newborn care should focus on easing the transition from hospital to home.

Immediate Postpartum Period

During the immediate postpartum period, maternal blood pressure and pulse should be monitored at least every 15 minutes for the first hour or more often as indicated (AAP & ACOG, 1997). Most institutions have protocols that include comprehensive maternal assessments at least every 15 minutes for the first hour, then every 30 minutes for 1 hour, and then every 4 hours (or more frequently if complications are present) for 12 to 24 hours. If the mother is stable, some institutions defer the 4-hour assessments after the first 12 hours when the mother is sleeping. There are no data from prospective clinical trials to determine how often maternal status should be assessed during the postpartum period to promote safety and optimal outcomes. Each institution should develop protocols that are reasonable and based on the condition of the mother. A sample medical form for documentation of the immediate postpartum assessment is included in Chapter 9 (see Appendix 9B). The following clinical parameters are included in a comprehensive assessment during the immediate postpartum period:

- Assess blood pressure and pulse (AAP & ACOG, 1997).
- Assess the uterine fundus for tone and position. Uterine massage is indicated if the uterus is not firmly contracted. Support the lower uterine segment during massage to prevent uterine prolapse or inversion (Fig. 12–1). Uterine inversion is an obstetric emergency associated with hemorrhage and shock.

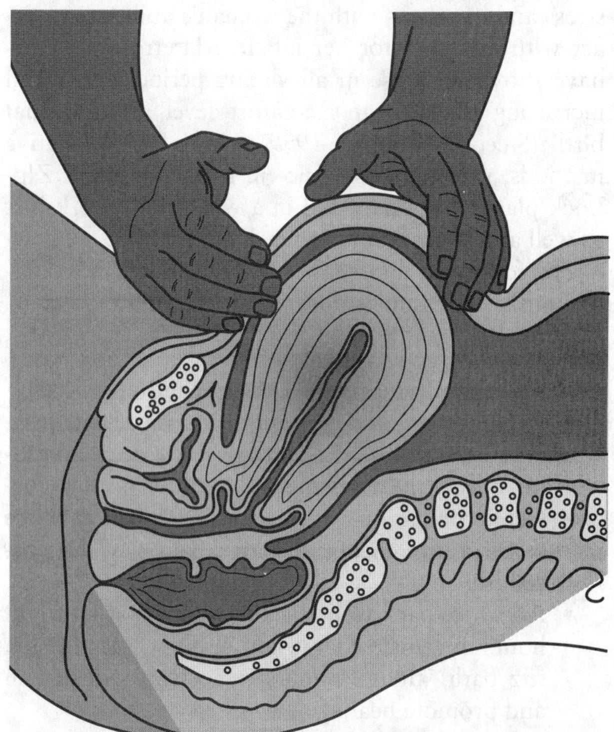

FIGURE 12–1. Fundal massage. The nurse uses two hands for fundal massage. One hand anchors the lower uterine segment just above the symphysis. The other gently massages the fundal area.

- Assess the amount of lochia on perineal pad and under buttocks.
- Assess the condition of the perineum.
- Assess the condition of episiotomy after assisting the woman into lateral position with upper leg flexed; use the acronym REEDA (*r*edness, *e*dema, *e*cchymosis, *d*ischarge, *a*pproximation of edges of episiotomy) to guide assessment.
- Assess the temperature at least every 4 hours (AAP & ACOG, 1997).
- Decisions about postanesthesia status and readiness for discharge from the recovery area are made at the discretion of the attending physician, nurse midwife, anesthesiologist, or certified registered nurse anesthetist (AAP & ACOG, 1997; ASA, 1999).

Pain Management

Pain during the postpartum period may be caused by the episiotomy, lacerations, perineal trauma, incisions, uterine contractions after birth, hemorrhoids, breast engorgement, and nipple tenderness. Nursing assessments, such as fundal assessment, may also result in discomfort. Some strategies can reduce the level of discomfort. After cesarean birth, pain may be related to the incision and intestinal gas. Pain causes stress and interferes with the woman's ability to interact with and care for her infant. Maternity gel pads have shown promise in alleviating perineal pain and increasing the woman's comfort level after vaginal birth (Steen & Cooper, 1999). However, alternative methods, such as crushed ice in freezer-strength Zip-Lock plastic bags wrapped in a washcloth, work just as well at less cost (Simpson & Knox, 1999).

The following interventions are included in a comprehensive assessment during the immediate postpartum period:

- Ask about type and severity of pain.
- Explain rationale for uterine massage and periodic assessments. Encourage slow, deep breathing during the assessment.
- Gentle palpation with warm hands can enhance comfort and encourage participation in the procedure.
- Apply ice pack to perineum during first 24 to 48 hours to reduce edema and apply moist heat (ie, sitz bath) after 24 hours to increase circulation and promote healing.
- Administer analgesic medication as ordered.
- Women who have experienced cesarean birth may or may not require uterine massage to stimulate uterine contraction. If lochia indicates excessive bleeding, combine palpation and pain-management measures. If pain management is inadequate, additional pain medication, reassurance, and comfort measures may be helpful after necessary procedures.
- Gas pains can be relieved by ambulation, rocking in a rocking chair, and avoiding gas-forming foods and carbonated beverages.

Psychosocial Status

Ongoing assessment of the psychosocial status should be personalized during the postpartum period to promote the development of healthy mother–infant relationships and maternal confidence (AAP & ACOG, 1997).

The following interventions are included in a comprehensive assessment during the immediate postpartum period:

- Determine the level of emotional lability and level of social support.
- Identify actual and potential sources of support.
- Assess the fatigue level.
- Ascertain educational needs and the level of confidence.
- Assess the teaching needs based on an interview and observation (see Chapter 17).
- Use interactions with mothers as potential teaching moments.
- Use assessment of the fundus as an opportunity to provide information about involution.
- During perineal care, explain cleaning the vulva from front to back to avoid contamination, changing the pad at least four times each day or after each voiding or bowel movement, and washing hands before and after changing pads.
- Use bathing of the newborn at mother's bedside as an opportunity to discuss basic techniques of newborn care such as feeding, clothing, holding, and safety.
- Assess the interaction with the newborn and attachment behaviors.
- Note whether the mother looks directly at the infant and maintains eye contact (ie, en face position).
- Note whether the mother touches and talks to the infant.
- Note whether the mother interprets the infant's behaviors positively.
- Provide an early opportunity to hold infant after birth, and keep the infant with the parents as much as possible.
- Ensure flexibility in visiting policies and opportunities for privacy.
- Demonstrate acceptance of expression of maternal feelings and reinforce parenting behaviors.

- Be a role model for infant-care activities.
- Assist parents in interpreting infant cues.
- Offer appropriate educational materials (ie, consider age, educational level, and resources).
- Identify risk factors for parenting (ie, lack of economic or psychosocial resources) and assist in obtaining appropriate referrals and assistance.

Physical Status

Physical assessment is an essential component of comprehensive nursing care during the postpartum period. Changes in the breasts, uterus, lochia, bladder, abdomen, perineum, legs, and feet should be assessed periodically and appropriate nursing interventions initiated as needed. A sample medical record form for documentation of ongoing postpartum assessments is included in Appendix 12A.

The following interventions are included in a comprehensive assessment during the immediate postpartum period:

- Assess breasts for redness, pain, engorgement, and if nursing, correct latch-on and removal of the newborn from the breast.
- Assess the uterus and lochia as described previously.
- Note any foul-smelling lochia.
- Assess the bladder for fullness before and after voiding.
- Measure amount of the first void (repeat if an insufficient amount).
- Assess for burning, frequency, and flank tenderness.
- Assess the abdomen for muscle tone, and check the incision site if applicable.
- Assess bowel sounds in all four quadrants.
- Assess the perineum, labia, and anus for edema, redness, pain, bruising, and hematoma.
- Assess the episiotomy or abdominal incision for approximation and drainage.
- Assess for the presence, size, and condition of hemorrhoids.
- Assess dietary intake and elimination patterns.
- Assess legs and feet for edema and varicosities.
- Assess for the Homan's sign (ie, positive if the woman reports pain in calf muscles when the foot is dorsiflexed), and measure the width of the calf if thrombophlebitis is suspected.
- Assess activity tolerance.
- Assess the comfort level and response to pain medication.
- Assess breath sounds if the woman has received magnesium sulfate, other tocolytics, or oxytocin; has been on bed rest; has an infection; or had a multiple birth (ie, greater risk for pulmonary edema, especially if the patient received large amounts of intravenous therapy). Use the acronym BUBBLERS (*b*reasts, *u*terus, *b*ladder, *b*owel, *l*ochia, *e*pisiotomy or incision, emotional *r*esponse, Homans *s*ign) to guide this assessment.

COMPLICATIONS DURING THE POSTPARTUM PERIOD

Postpartum Hemorrhage

Postpartum hemorrhage occurs in about 5% to 6% of women who have a vaginal birth (Cunningham et al., 1997; Stables, 1999). It can occur early (≤24 hours) or late (>24 hours and <6 weeks after birth). Display 12–2 lists the factors associated with postpartum hemorrhage. The term *postpartum hemorrhage* is a description of an event, not a diagnosis (Cunningham et al., 1997). Bleeding during the postpartum period is overestimated and underestimated by as much as 50% (ACOG, 1998; Luegenbiehl, 1997). Postpartum hemorrhage has traditionally been defined as blood loss of 500 mL or more after completion of the third stage of labor or as more than 1,000 mL during a cesarean birth. *Hemorrhage* is defined objectively as a decrease in the hematocrit of 10% between admission and the postpartum period or as the need for blood cell transfusion (ACOG, 1998). The hemoglobin value decreases 1 to 1.5 g/dL and the hematocrit decreases 2% to 4% for each 500 mL of blood loss (Cunningham et al., 1997).

The greatest risk for early postpartum hemorrhage is during the first hour after birth, because large venous areas are exposed after placental separation. According to the ASA (1999), the following resources should be available in the event of an obstetric hemorrhagic emergency: large-bore intravenous catheters, intravenous fluid warmer, forced-air body warmer, blood blank, equipment for infusing intravenous fluids or blood products rapidly, such as hand-squeezed fluid chambers, hand-inflated pressure bags, and automatic infusion devices. Maintaining uterine contraction by using fundal massage and intravenous oxytocin administration (20 units per liter) reduces the incidence of hemorrhage from uterine atony (AAP & ACOG, 1997; Creasy & Resnik, 1999; Scott, 1998). Late postpartum bleeding most commonly occurs between days 6 and 14.

There are some preexisting risk factors for postpartum hemorrhage:

- High parity
- Previous postpartum hemorrhage

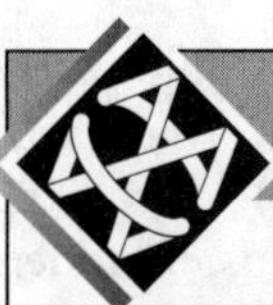

DISPLAY 12-2

Factors Associated with Postpartum Hemorrhage

EARLY POSTPARTUM HEMORRHAGE

Uterine atony (most common)
History of uterine atony or postpartum hemorrhage
Trauma, lacerations, or hematoma of cervix and/or birth canal
Precipitous labor and birth
Difficult third stage (ie, use of aggressive fundal manipulation or cord traction)
Operative vaginal birth (eg, use of forceps or vacuum)
Cesarean birth
Uterine overdistention (eg, large infant, multiple gestation, polyhydramnios)
Multiparity
Sepsis
Retained placenta
Placenta accreta
Coagulopathies
Uterine rupture
Uterine inversion
Drugs (large dosages of oxytocin, magnesium sulfate, beta-adrenergic tocolytic agents; diazoxide [potent antihypertensive agent]; calcium channel blockers, such as nifedipine; and halothane [anesthetic agent]

LATE POSTPARTUM HEMORRHAGE

Infection
Subinvolution
Retained placenta

From American Academy of Pediatrics & American College of Obstetricians and Gynecologists. (1997). *Guidelines for Perinatal Care* (4th ed.). Washington, DC: Author, and from Creasy, R.K., & Resnik, R. (1999). *Maternal-fetal medicine: Principles and practice* (4th ed.). Philadelphia: W.B. Saunders.

- Previous uterine surgery
- Coagulation defects or medical disorders of clotting

The current pregnancy also may have risk factors for hemorrhage:

- Antepartum hemorrhage
- Uterine overdistention (ie, macrosomia, multiple gestation, or polyhydramnios)
- Chorioamnionitis or intraamniotic infection
- Placental abnormality (eg, succenturiate lobe, placenta previa, placenta accreta, abruptio placenta, hydatidiform mole)
- Fetal death

Some risk factors for hemorrhage are associated with labor and birth:

- Rapid or prolonged labor
- Use of tocolytic or halogenated anesthetic agents
- Large episiotomy
- Operative vaginal birth
- Cesarean birth
- Abnormally located or attached placenta
- Inversion of uterus

The following interventions are included in a comprehensive assessment during the postpartum period:

- Assess blood loss.
- Weigh peripads or Chux dressing (1 g = 1 mL); keep a gram scale in the unit.
- Assess excessive bleeding, which is defined as one perineal pad saturated within 15 minutes.
- Look for severe loss that may occur with steady, slow seepage.
- Check vital signs at least every 15 minutes.
- Mean arterial pressure (MAP), which is the mean blood pressure (BP) in arterial circulation, should be assessed because the first blood pressure response to hypovolemia may be a pulse pressure decreased to 30 mmHg or less (Cunningham et al., 1997). MAP in nonpregnant women is normally 86.4 ± 7.5 mmHg, with a slightly higher value for pregnant women (Creasy & Resnick, 1999). MAP can be calculated with this formula:
  MAP = systolic BP + 2 (diastolic BP)/3.
- Check for tachypnea and tachycardia, which may occur while the blood pressure is constant or slightly lowered.
- Assess for shock. Normal vital signs do not mean that the woman is not in shock. Traditional signs of hypovolemic shock are not evident until 15% to 20% of the total blood volume is lost (Creasy & Resnik, 1999). The initial response of vasoconstriction shunts blood to vital organs to maintain their function and viability.
- Maintain accurate measurements of intake and output.
- Ensure large-bore (14-, 16-, or 18-gauge) needle intravenous access.

- Use lactated Ringer's solution or plasma expanders to counteract hypovolemia (ie, produce at least 30 mL/hour of urine output and hematocrit values of 30%) (Cunningham et al., 1997).
- Packed red blood cells should be typed and crossmatched (AAP & ACOG, 1997).
- Transfusion can be withheld with adequate urine output and no appreciable postural hypotension or tachycardia (AAP & ACOG, 1997).
- Deficits in clotting factors may necessitate cryoprecipitate (ie, for fibrinogen deficiency) or fresh-frozen plasma (ie, for decreased levels of clotting factors) (AAP & ACOG, 1997).
- Plan for care and assessment to ensure early recognition of hemorrhage.
- Use correct uterine massage to avoid ligament damage and potential uterine inversion (see Fig. 12–1). Place one hand pointing toward the woman's head with thumb resting on one side of the uterus and fingers along the other side. Use other hand to massage with *only the force needed to effect contraction or expulsion of clots.* Overaggressive uterine massage may tire muscle fibers and contribute to further atony.
- Early recognition minimizes blood loss and potential sequelae such as anemia, puerperal infection, thromboembolism, and necrosis of the anterior pituitary (ie, Sheehan's syndrome).
- Anticipate pain management needs for fundal massage and uterotonic medications for treatment of hemorrhage (Display 12–3).
- Draw blood for hemoglobin and hematocrit (compare with admission), type and crossmatch, coagulation studies (ie, fibrinogen, prothrombin time, partial thromboplastin time, fibrin split products, and fibrin degradation products), and blood chemistry. Arterial blood may be drawn for blood gas determinations. Urine should be sent to the laboratory as indicated.
- Insert a Foley catheter to empty the bladder and allow accurate measurement of output.
- Administer intravenous fluids.
- Administer prescribed drugs; labor and birth units should have available intravenous infusion of oxytocin, 15-α-methyl-prostaglandin $F_{2\alpha}$, and ergot alkaloids (AAP & ACOG, 1997):

Oxytocin	10–40 units in 500–1000 lactated Ringer's solution at 50 mU/minute
Methylergonovine maleate	0.2 mg IM q 2–4 hours (× 5 dose maximum) 0.2 mg PO q 6–12 hours IV administration not recommended
Ergonovine maleate	0.2 mg IM q 2–4 hours (× 5 dose maximum) 0.2 mg PO q 6–12 hours IV administration not recommended
15-α-methyl-prostaglandin $F_{2\alpha}$	IM 250 μm 15–90 minutes (× 5 dose maximum) Physician may administer by intramyometrial route

- Apply pulse oximeter and administer oxygen according to the protocol. This is usually accomplished with a nonrebreathing face mask at 10 to 12 L/min.
- Continuous electrocardiographic monitoring may be indicated for hypotension, continuous bleeding, tachycardia, or shock.
- Elevate the legs to a 20- to 30-degree angle to increase venous return.
- Provide emotional support and explanations for the woman and her family.

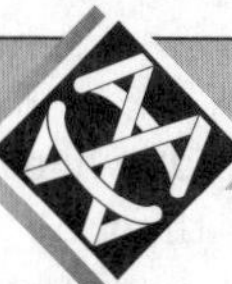

DISPLAY 12–3

Management of Postpartum Hemorrhage

Goals: stop hemorrhage, correct hypovolemia, and return of hemostasis
Identification of risk factors
Early recognition and treatment of hemorrhage
Treatment of underlying cause of hemorrhage

MEDICAL SURGICAL MANAGEMENT

Medications
- Oxytocin
- Ergot
- Prostaglandins

Fundal massage
Bladder management
Mast trousers
Bimanual compression
Uterine packing
Curretage
Ligation of blood vessels (uterine, ovarian, hypogastric arteries)
Arterial embolization
Umbrella pack

Postpartum Infections

A puerperal infection should be suspected when a woman has an oral temperature higher than 38°C (100.4°F) on two occasions that are 6 hours apart during the first 10 days postpartum, exclusive of the first 24 hours. The nursery should be notified of these findings, although the newborn need not be separated from the mother (AAP & ACOG, 1997; Baker, Luce, Chenoweth, & Friedman, 1995; Creasy & Resnik, 1999; Cunningham et al., 1997).

Endometritis

Postpartum endometritis occurs in 1% to 3% of vaginal births and 10% to 50% of cesarean births (Baker et al., 1995; Creasy & Resnick, 1999; Cunningham et al., 1997; Ernest & Mead, 1998). Postpartum uterine infections, called *endometritis* (ie, inflammation of endometrium), *endomyometritis* (ie, inflammation of endometrium and myometrium), or *endomyoparametritis* (ie, inflammation of endometrium and parametrial tissue), are the most commonly identified causes of puerperal morbidity. One of the most effective methods of prevention of infection is handwashing.

The most common cause of uterine infection tends to be polymicrobial, including aerobic and anaerobic organisms that have ascended to the uterus from the lower genital tract. Isolated organisms include streptococci A and B, enterococci, *Staphylococcus aureus, Gardnerella vaginalis, Escherichia coli, Enterobacter, Proteus mirabilis, Klebsiella, Bacteroides* species, *Peptostreptococcus* species, *Ureaplasma urealyticum, Mycoplasma hominis*, and *Chlamydia trachomatis. C. trachomatis* has been specifically associated with late-onset postpartum endometritis (Creasy & Resnik, 1999; Cunningham et al., 1997).

Other causes of postpartum infection include wound and urinary tract infections, pneumonia (usually related to general anesthesia), mastitis, pelvic thrombophlebitis, and necrotizing fasciitis, an uncommon but serious localized infection of the deep soft tissues.

Endometritis is associated with certain risk factors:

- Operative birth, prolonged labor or rupture of membranes, use of invasive procedures (eg, internal monitoring, amnioinfusion)
- Fetal scalp sampling or multiple pelvic examinations
- Excessive blood loss
- Pyelonephritis or diabetes
- Socioeconomic and nutritional factors compromising host defense mechanisms
- Anemia and systemic illness
- Smoking

The following findings and interventions are included in a comprehensive assessment:

- Fever occurring about the third postnatal day is the most important finding.
- Detection of tachycardia (rise of 10 beats/min for every 1°C)
- Determine possible causes of malaise.
- Assess lower abdominal pain.
- Assess uterine tenderness on palpation (extending laterally) and slight abdominal distention.
- Determine cause of foul-smelling lochia (if organism is anaerobic).
- Obtain urinalysis to exclude urinary tract infections (UTIs).
- Assess leukocytosis (WBC count >20,000/mm^3 with increased neutrophils or polymorphonuclear leukocytes).
- Blood cultures are positive in about 10% of women.
- Endometrial cultures may have limited value because of cervicovaginal contamination of the specimen, but they may provide useful information if the woman does not respond to initial antibiotic therapy (Creasy & Resnik, 1999; Cunningham et al., 1997; Stables, 1999; Varney, 1997).
- Parenteral broad-spectrum antibiotic therapy is promptly initiated when postpartum endometritis is diagnosed. Treatment continues until the woman has been afebrile for 48 hours. A common treatment regimen is a combination of clindamycin and gentamicin, with ampicillin added in refractory cases.
- Women usually respond rapidly (48 to 72 hours) to antibiotic therapy. Occasional complications include pelvic abscesses, septic pelvic thrombophlebitis, persistent fever, and retained infected placenta (AAP & ACOG, 1997).
- Increase fluid intake, and encourage adequate nutrition.
  - Encourage intake of a minimum of 6 to 8 glasses (1,500 to 2,000 mL) of water, milk, or juices; 3,000 mL is the preferred amount.
  - Encourage intake of at least 1,800 to 2,000 calories daily if lactating, and 1,500 calories if not lactating.
  - Encourage the woman to eat a varied diet, with representation of foods from all food groups, that is high in protein and vitamin C to promote wound healing.

- Ensure adequate output (30 mL/hour) because renal toxicity can occur with antibiotic therapy.
- Provide comfort through meeting the woman's personal hygiene needs. Cool compresses, linen changes, massage, and positioning may enhance comfort.
- Assess vital signs every 4 hours or every 2 hours if her temperature is elevated.
- Use a semi-Fowler position, ambulation, or both to promote uterine drainage.
- Administer oxytocics as ordered to promote uterine contraction and drainage.
- Observe for signs of septic shock: tachycardia (>120 beats), hypotension, tachypnea, changes in sensorium, and decreased urine output (ie, oliguria) (Cunningham et al., 1997; Varney, 1997). If septic shock develops, increase the frequency of obtaining vital signs and other assessments, depending on the clinical situation.

Wound Infections

Wound infections can be classified as early onset (within 48 hours) or late onset (within 6 to 8 days). Early-onset wound infections are usually treated with antibiotic therapy and excision of necrotic tissue. Late-onset infections are treated with incision and drainage, and they may not require antibiotics unless there is extensive cellulitis (Creasy & Resnik, 1999; Cunningham et al., 1997). Wound infections are associated with certain risk factors:

- History of chorioamnionitis or intraamniotic infection
- Hemorrhage or anemia
- Obesity
- Underlying medical problems such as diabetes and malnutrition
- Multiple vaginal examinations
- Corticosteroid therapy
- Immunosuppression
- Advancing age
- Malnutrition

The following findings and interventions are included in a comprehensive assessment:

- Observe for wound erythema, swelling, tenderness, and purulent discharge.
- Assess for localized pain and dysuria.
- Assess vital signs.
- Check for a low-grade temperature (101°F or 38.3°C).
- Acute cases may exhibit sudden chills and spikes in temperature to 40°C (104°F).
- The pulse usually is less than 100 beats/min.
- Cultures are performed as ordered.
- Assist with drainage, irrigation, and occasionally, débridement procedures.
- Sitz baths are used for cleaning and promotion of increased circulation to the affected area.
- The wound may be packed. Treatment is directed toward cleaning the wound and promoting granulation.
- Change dressings and dispose appropriately of soiled dressings. Dressings may be continued after discharge.
- Ensure frequent changes of peripads.
- Ensure pain management and appropriate administration of analgesia.
- Ensure adequate room ventilation before dressing changes.
- Continued hospitalization or readmission may be required.
- Provide explanations during this stressful period.
- Offer reassurance and encouragement.
- Encourage frequent visits by the family to help reduce anxiety.
- Assist breast-feeding women with pumping or lactation suppression.
- Administer antibiotic therapy as ordered (may be continued after discharge).
- Make referrals for postpartum follow-up visits by home care nurses.
- Reduce anxiety and the incidence of rehospitalization by early identification and treatment of infections.

Necrotizing Fasciitis

A severe wound infection (usually polymicrobial) may be characterized by severe tissue necrosis, erythema, discharge, and severe pain. Necrotizing fasciitis is characterized by partial liquefaction of fascia adjacent to an incision. Secondary healing may take 6 to 12 weeks (Creasy & Resnik, 1999; Cunningham et al., 1997). Necrotizing fasciitis is associated with certain risk factors:

- Diabetes
- Obesity
- Hypertension

The following findings and interventions are included in a comprehensive assessment:

- Wound status (eg, erythema, discharge)
- Pain

- Administration of broad-spectrum antibiotics, as ordered
- Surgical débridement

Mastitis

Congestive or infectious mastitis is more commonly seen in primigravidas and nursing mothers. Symptoms usually appear between the third and fourth week after birth and are typically unilateral. Nipple trauma has been implicated in the development of mastitis. Trauma from incorrect latch-on or removal of the newborn from the breast permits the introduction of organisms from the newborn into the mother's breast. *S. aureus* is the most common causative organism. Administration of penicillinase-resistant antibiotics such as dicloxacillin for 10 days is recommended.

If a breast abscess develops, incision and drainage may be indicated. The decision to continue breast-feeding should be made jointly by the woman and the healthcare provider. If breast-feeding is delayed while purulent drainage continues, the woman may need assistance with breast pumping to reestablish lactation. If advised to discontinue breast-feeding, emotional support, reassurance, and comfort measures are important. Lactation consultant referral is indicated as a preventive or treatment measure when these services are available.

Mastitis is associated with certain risk factors:

- Infrequent breast-feeding
- Incomplete breast emptying
- Plugged milk duct
- Cracked and bleeding nipples

The following findings and interventions are included in a comprehensive assessment:

- Assess fever and chills.
- Assess localized tenderness and a palpable, hard, reddened mass.
- Assess for tachycardia.
- Assess for purulent discharge.
- Offer education about preventive measures (eg, handwashing, breast cleanliness, frequent breast-pad changes, exposure of the nipples to air, and correct infant latch-on and removal from the breast).
- Obtain a culture of the breast milk before initiating antibiotic therapy, if ordered.
- The infection usually resolves within 24 to 48 hours of antibiotic therapy.
- Suggest comfort measures, including warm or cold compresses, wearing a supportive bra, and analgesia as ordered.
- Offer education about completing the full regimen of antibiotic therapy.
- Encourage an increase in fluid intake from 2 to 2.5 L/day.
- Massage, positioning the newborn in the direction of the site, and frequent breast-feeding promote milk flow.
- Assist with the use of a breast pump or manual expression if indicated (Creasy & Resnik, 1999; Cunningham et al., 1997; Stables, 1999; Varney, 1997).

Urinary Tract Infections

UTIs are the most common medical complication occurring during pregnancy. They may be asymptomatic (eg, bacteriuria) or symptomatic (eg, cystitis, acute pyelonephritis). Asymptomatic UTIs occur in 6% of pregnant women. Diagnosis and treatment of bacteriuria can prevent the development of pyelonephritis, which places the fetus at increased risk for preterm birth or low birth weight (Cunningham et al., 1997). Urinary tract infections are associated with certain risk factors:

- A shorter urethra in women than men
- Contamination of the urethra with pathogenic bacteria from vagina and rectum
- High probability that women do not completely empty bladders
- Movement of bacteria into bladder during sexual intercourse
- Pregnancy-related changes (eg, decreased ureteric muscle tone and activity from progesterone and pressure of gravid uterus, resulting in lower rate of urine passing through urinary collecting system)
- Urinary catheterization, frequent pelvic examinations, epidural anesthesia, genital tract injury, and cesarean birth

Asymptomatic Bacteriuria

The following findings and interventions are included in a comprehensive assessment of asymptomatic bacteriuria:

- Evaluate urinalysis for bacteriuria (presence of 10^5 or more bacterial colonies per milliliter of urine on two consecutive, clean-catch, midstream voided specimens).
- *E. coli* is cultured in 60% to 90% of cases.

- Other pathogens include *Proteus mirabilis, Klebsiella pneumoniae,* group B β-hemolytic streptococci, and *Staphylococcus saprophyticus.*
- Educate woman about the importance of repeat urinalysis to determine the effectiveness of antibiotics.
- Risk is associated with sickle cell trait, lower socioeconomic status, increased parity, and reduced availability of medical care.
- Administer or educate the woman to take antibiotics as ordered to eliminate bacteria in urine.
- Ampicillin and cephalosporins are used (no significant risk to the fetus); antibiotics are administered for 7 days.
- If continuous antimicrobial therapy is required, typically use a single daily dose of nitrofurantoin, preferably after the evening meal.

Pyelonephritis and Cystitis

The following findings and interventions are included in a comprehensive assessment of pyelonephritis and cystitis:

- Obtain a urinalysis to detect untreated, asymptomatic bacteriuria.
- The woman with untreated bacteriuria is at high risk for pyelonephritis.
- Bacterial growth may produce more than 100,000 colonies/mL.
- The specimen may contain increased WBCs, protein, or blood.
- The most common bacteria found are are *E. coli* (80%), *Klebsiella, Enterobacter,* and *Proteus.*
- A cephalosporin is the first choice for single-agent therapy.
    - Assess for symptoms of cystitis.
    - Assess for urinary urgency, frequency, and dysuria.
    - Assess for suprapubic pain without fever or tenderness at the costovertebral angle.
    - Assess for gross hematuria.
- Assess for symptoms of pyelonephritis.
    - Assess for shaking chills, fever, tachycardia, flank pain, nausea, and vomiting.
    - Assess for urinary frequency, urgency, dysuria, and costovertebral angle tenderness.
- Endotoxin-mediated tissue damage may occur in pregnant women (Miller & Cox, 1997).
- Administer antibiotics as ordered.
- Short courses (1 to 3 weeks) of sulfonamides, ampicillin, or nitrofurantoin are recommended for pyelonephritis.
- A 7-day course of antibiotics is recommended for acute cystitis in pregnant women.
- Monitor intake and output.
- Maintain adequate hydration (at least 3,000 mL/day) with water and cranberry juice.
- Measure urinary output for adequacy (at least 30 mL/hour).
- Administer antipyretics, antispasmodics, or urinary analgesics (Pyridium) and antiemetics as ordered.
- Encourage rest.
- Monitor vital signs every 4 hours.
- Educate the woman about monitoring temperature, bladder function, appearance of urine, importance of completing antibiotic therapy, proper perineal care (eg, wiping front to back), wearing cotton underwear, adequate hydration, and balanced nutrition.

If readmission for treatment of a UTI is necessary, reassurance and family support are essential. Separation from the newborn is distressing to the mother and child. If the woman has been breast-feeding, interventions such as pumping and newborn visits can help to maintain lactation after antibiotic therapy has been initiated. If breast-feeding is temporarily contraindicated, the nurse can provide emotional support and offer strategies to maintain lactation (eg, breast pump) until breast-feeding can be resumed (Creasy & Resnik, 1999; Cunningham et al., 1997; Stables, 1999; Varney, 1997).

Thrombophlebitis and Thromboembolism

Thrombophlebitis (ie, inflammation of a vein after formation of a thrombus) is classified as superficial or deep. Superficial thrombophlebitis involves the superficial veins of the saphenous system. Deep vein thrombophlebitis affects the veins of the calf, thigh, or pelvis. Stasis is the most significant predisposing event to the development of deep vein thrombosis. Diagnosis of thrombophlebitis is based on objective and subjective signs and symptoms. Septic pelvic thrombophlebitis is a condition more common in women after a cesarean birth and occurs with infections of the reproductive tract. Ascending infection within the venous system results in thrombophlebitis. This condition should be suspected when the infection does not respond to antibiotics and is accompanied by abdominal or flank pain and guarding on the second or third postpartum day.

A more serious complication occurs when a thrombus forms in any of the dilated pelvic veins. Accompanied by thrombophlebitis, these formations can be a source of potentially fatal pulmonary emboli. In those cases, the clot becomes friable, and the pieces detach from the vessel wall and travel through the heart into the pulmonary circulation. Pulmonary embolism should be treated as a life-threatening event; interruption of blood flow to the pulmonary bed can result in cardiovascular collapse and death (Creasy & Resnik, 1999; Cunningham et al., 1997; Falter, 1997; Olson & Nunnelee, 1998; Stables, 1999; Varney, 1997).

Thrombophlebitis and thromboembolism are associated with certain risk factors:

- Normal changes in coagulation status during pregnancy
- History of thromboembolic disease or varicosities
- Increased parity
- Obesity
- Advanced maternal age (≥30 years)
- Immobility associated with antepartum bed rest
- Use of forceps
- Cesarean birth
- Blood vessel and tissue trauma
- Prolonged labor with multiple pelvic examinations
- Sepsis

Thrombus formation can be prevented by instituting certain measures:

- Early ambulation or leg exercises for women on bed rest
- Education about correct posture
- Avoiding crossing legs
- Avoiding extreme flexion of legs at the groin
- Positioning without pressure on the backs of knees
- Use of support hose by women with a history of thrombophlebitis
- Padding of pressure points during birth while in the lithotomy position

Thrombophlebitis

The following findings and interventions are included in a comprehensive assessment of thrombophlebitis:

- Evaluate the woman's physical status.
- A superficial vein (usually varicose) is reddened, hard, and tender.
- Apply a supportive bandage or antiembolic support stockings.
- Apply a soothing agent (ie, glycerin and ichthol) (Ball, 1996).
- Apply warm packs to the affected area.
- Slightly elevate the involved leg.
- Permit ambulation as indicated and ordered.
- Perform serial measurements of the circumferences of the calves; a circumference difference of more than 2 cm is classified as leg swelling.
- Monitor vital signs every 4 hours; there may be a slight increase in temperature.
- Compare pulses in both extremities, which may reveal decreased venous flow to the affected area.
- Evaluate for the Homan's sign bilaterally every 8 hours. A positive sign is pain in the calf when the foot is passively dorsiflexed.
- Heparin anticoagulation therapy may be ordered.
- Nursing interventions for deep vein thrombosis include all of the previously described care measures plus the following:
  - Bed rest until swelling is reduced and anticoagulation therapy is effective
  - Anticoagulation therapy with intravenous heparin, followed by oral warfarin
  - Maintenance of activated partial thromboplastin time that is prolonged by 1.5 to 2 times laboratory control value (Cunningham et al., 1997)
  - Follow dosing regimens (Cunningham et al., 1997):
    - 5,000-U bolus of heparin and then continuous infusion to a total 24,000 to 32,000 U/day
    - Intermittent intravenous injections of 5,000 U every 4 hours or 7,500 U every 6 hours
    - Subcutaneous heparin at dose of 10,000 U every 8 hours or 20,000 U every 12 hours
  - Monitor coagulation laboratory values.
  - Carefully assess unusual bleeding. Heavy vaginal bleeding, generalized petechiae, bleeding from the mucous membranes, hematuria, or oozing from venipuncture sites should be reported to the physician. The heparin antidote protamine sulfate should be readily available.
- Educate and prepare women for diagnostic testing:
  - Physical assessments look for muscle pain, palpable deep linear cord, tenderness, swelling, a positive Homans sign, and dilated superficial veins.
  - Doppler ultrasonography provides more sensitivity and is more specific for the diagnosis of popliteal and femoral vein thrombosis than for calf vein thrombosis. It can evaluate venous flow and possible occlusion.
  - Venography is a more specific test, but it is invasive, expensive, and difficult to interpret. Contrast material may cause chemical phlebitis.
  - Impedance plethysmography has had little research to support its efficacy during pregnancy, but coupled with ultrasound, the reliability increases. A thigh cuff is inflated, resulting in temporary occlusion of venous re-

turn. Release results in a rapid decrease in volume as blood drains proximally. Volume changes are detected by measurement of electrical resistance in the calf.

Blood studies can determine the formation of intravascular fibrin; results are positive in cases of thrombosis. Results are also positive in presence of hematomas or inflammatory exudates containing fibrin.

Septic Pelvic Thrombophlebitis

The following findings and interventions are included in a comprehensive assessment of septic pelvic thrombophlebitis:

- Assess the woman for physical symptoms:
  - Fever and tachycardia
  - Spiking fever persisting despite antibiotic therapy
  - Abdominal and flank pain (paralytic ileus may develop)
- Prepare and support the woman during examination (ie, parametrial mass found on bimanual examination).
- Obtain appropriate laboratory testing:
  - Complete blood count
  - Blood chemistry
  - Coagulation profile
  - Chest radiography, computed tomography, magnetic resonance imaging
- Administer medications as ordered:
  - Heparin regimen initiated with diagnosis
  - Coumarin agent substituted and continued for total course of anticoagulation of 3 to 6 weeks

Pulmonary Embolism

The following findings and interventions are included in a comprehensive assessment of pulmonary embolism:

- The most common signs are dyspnea, chest pain, hemoptysis, and abdominal pain.
- The most serious signs are sudden collapse, cyanosis, and hypotension.
- Prepare the woman for diagnostic testing:
  - Ventilation-perfusion scan
  - Blood gas studies
  - Radiography
  - Pulmonary angiography
- Elevate the head of the bed to facilitate breathing.
- Administer oxygen 8 to 10 L/min using a tight face mask; use pulse oximetry.
- Maintain the PaO_2 at 70 mm Hg.
- Monitor arterial blood gases.
- Frequently assess vital signs.
- Provide for intravenous fluids (ie, pulmonary artery catheter may be placed).
- Administer salt-poor or hypertonic intravenous fluids, as ordered.
- Administer medications as ordered to counteract symptoms:
  - Medium dose of intravenous heparin (continued subcutaneous heparin or oral anticoagulant therapy for 6 months)
  - Total daily heparin dose of 30,000 to 40,000 U (Cunningham et al., 1997)
  - Dopamine to maintain blood pressure
  - Morphine for analgesia
- Maintain adequate staffing:
  - Staff who have completed an Advanced Cardiac Life Support course should be available for full resuscitation support, if needed. Ideally, care should be provided in an obstetric intensive care unit (OB-ICU), but in many institutions, care occurs in a medical-surgical ICU.
  - Collaboration between the ICU staff and perinatal staff is essential. Maternal transport should be considered if the level of care and supportive staff necessary is unavailable.

Although most women have a normal postpartum course, complications can occur. Comprehensive, frequent nursing assessments contribute to early identification and prompt treatment. Collaboration between the perinatal nurse and the primary healthcare provider is essential. Display 12–4 lists the clinical signs and symptoms suggesting postpartum complications that warrant communication with the primary healthcare provider.

INDIVIDUALIZING CARE FOR WOMEN WITH SPECIAL NEEDS

Cesarean Birth

The cesarean birth rate in the United States in 1999 (the last year for which data are available) was 22% (Curtin & Martin, 2000). With a cesarean birth, there is a risk of lowered self-esteem related to a failure to achieve a vaginal birth. Some women report negative reactions to the birth experience related to lack of control and lack of knowledge (Fowles, 1998). The desired outcome of the birth is for each couple to verbalize a positive birth experience and to feel happiness and excitement about a healthy baby. Nurses can assist in achieving this outcome for women

DISPLAY 12–4

Clinical Signs and Symptoms to Report to the Primary Healthcare Provider

- Uterine atony or large or excessive clots; passage of placental tissue
- Excessive bleeding
- Continued bleeding in the presence of a firm uterus (suggests lacerations)
- Perineal pain greater than expected (suggests hematoma)
- Foul-smelling lochia (suggests endometritis)
- Temperature elevated to >100°F (38°C) (suggests dehydration in first 24 hours; after 24 hours, suggests infection, such as thrombophlebitis or systemic infection)
- Bladder distention and/or inability to void
- Diminished urinary output (<30 mL/hour)
- Enlarging hematomas
- Restlessness; pallor of skin or mucous membranes; cool, clammy skin; tachycardia; thready pulse; fearfulness; vertigo; shaking; visual disturbances; (symptoms of shock)
- Pain, redness, warmth, firm area in the calf area (although pain may be absent in deep vein thrombosis)
- Dyspnea, tachypnea, tachycardia, chest pain, cough, apprehension, hemoptysis, change in skin or mucous membrane color (paleness and/or cyanosis): symptoms of pulmonary embolism or amniotic embolism

experiencing a cesarean birth by involving the couple as much as possible in the decision-making process, keeping the couple informed, supporting the coach and family, encouraging verbalization, and providing reassurance that a cesarean birth is not a failure.

Nurses caring for women after a cesarean birth should stress that the woman is a new mother with the same needs as other new mothers and also requires supportive postoperative care. The woman who has experienced a cesarean birth usually has increased levels of fatigue, activity intolerance, and incisional pain. Discharge after cesarean birth typically occurs by the third postoperative day, compared with the second postpartum day after vaginal births (Curtin & Kozak, 1998). Chapter 9 provides a full discussion of cesarean birth.

Antepartum Bed Rest and Postpartum Recovery

The postpartum effects of bed rest have received little attention in the obstetric nursing and medical literature. Despite lack of evidence to support bed rest therapy as contributing to positive outcomes, it has been prescribed routinely for women with high-risk pregnancies. Women with bleeding, preterm labor, and pregnancy-induced hypertension are frequently encouraged to maintain modified or strict bed rest in the hope of prolonging the pregnancy. It has been estimated that up to 18.2% of pregnant women in the United States who give birth after 20 weeks have been prescribed at least 1 week of bed rest at some time during their pregnancy (Goldenberg et al., 1994). Some research suggests that modified rest at home, rather than strict bed rest, is an acceptable form of treatment for pregnancy-induced hypertension (Sibai, 1996).

Complete bed rest causes physiologic and psychosocial changes, including cardiovascular deconditioning; muscle loss, especially in the gastrocnemius muscle (used in ambulation); diuresis with fluid, electrolyte, and weight loss; bone demineralization; increased heart rate and blood coagulation; heartburn and reflux; constipation; glucose intolerance; and sensory disturbances, including depression, fatigue, and inability to concentrate (Maloni et al., 1993). Isometric and isotonic conditioning exercises, Kegel exercises, pelvic tilts, and range-of-motion exercises can be used during hospitalization for the woman on bed rest. Deep breathing and coughing are added to exercise abdominal muscles and promote venous return.

After birth, the woman requires additional time, support, and education to prepare for safe and progressive levels of activity (Maloni, 1998). Postpartum recovery may be prolonged. Ambulation after prolonged bed rest requires the continued presence of the perinatal nurse. Women should be alerted to the possibility of weakness, dizziness, shortness of breath, and muscle soreness and be reassured that these are normal physiologic consequences of prolonged bed rest that will reverse over time after resumption of normal activity (Maloni et al., 1993).

POSTPARTUM LEARNING NEEDS ASSESSMENT AND EDUCATION

Planning for education during the postpartum period begins as soon as possible after inpatient admission. Ideally, women have had opportunities during the prenatal period to learn about postpartum and newborn care, but this may not be true for all pregnant women because of access to care issues, complications of pregnancy, unavailability of resources, or lack of knowledge about existing programs. During shortened hospital stays, there are limited opportunities for assessment and education of new mothers. Access, availability, and acceptability must be considered when providing postpartum education. All available resources may not be able to be integrated within the shortened admission period. Closed-circuit educational television and printed materials collaboratively developed by obstetric and pediatric professionals can help new parents. Individual and group educational sessions held regularly during the postpartum period are beneficial. Newborn care, normal infant behaviors, and expected maternal physical and psychological changes should be included in the educational plans for each mother. New mothers should be aware of available community and healthcare resources (AAP & ACOG, 1997; Grullon & Grimes, 1997). Chapter 18 provides a comprehensive discussion of maternal–newborn learning needs assessment and teaching strategies.

SELECTED POSTPARTUM TEACHING TOPICS

Pelvic-Floor Exercises

Patient education should include pelvic muscle exercises according to the institutional protocol. Kegel exercises help the woman to regain muscle tone lost as pelvic tissues are stretched. Research suggests that 25% of women who learn Kegel exercises perform them incorrectly and may increase their risk of later incontinence (Sampselle & Miller, 1996). Each contraction should be held at least 10 seconds, with a 10-second or longer rest between contractions for muscular recovery. Women with third- or fourth-degree lacerations, a long second stage of labor, a large newborn, or a combination of these factors should be taught to report potential anal sphincter symptoms, such as incontinence of flatus or stool, to the primary healthcare provider.

Postpartum Exercise

Exercise may begin soon after birth with simple exercises such as arm raises, leg rolls, and buttock lifts. After cesarean birth, abdominal exercises should be postponed for 4 weeks. Exercise benefits the mood, self-image, and energy level and improves or maintains muscular endurance, strength, and tone. Women who exercise vigorously demonstrated better scores on measures of postpartum adaptation and were more likely to engage in social activities, hobbies, and entertainment. More active women retained significantly less weight (Sampselle, 1999).

Discharge instructions should include written information regarding activity, rest, and exercise for women who have given birth vaginally or by cesarean. Women should be instructed to listen to their bodies and avoid fatigue and pain. An educational poster entitled "Exercise During Pregnancy and the Postnatal Period" is available from the American College of Obstetricians and Gynecologists (ACOG, 1998). Other commercial videotapes, books, and pamphlets are available as well.

Sexuality

Sexuality is one of the least understood and most superficially discussed topics by healthcare providers during a woman's postpartum experience. Sexuality encompasses physical capacity for sexual arousal and pleasure (ie, libido), personalized and shared social meanings attached to sexual behavior, and formation of sexual and gender identities. Sexuality and gender attitudes and behaviors carry profound significance for women and men in every society. Sexuality is a vital component of physical and emotional well-being for men and women. Display 12–5 lists the factors contributing to decline in sexual interest during the postpartum period (Jones, Lehr, & Hewell, 1997; Smith, 1996).

Nurses must assume responsibility for anticipatory guidance, reassurance, and counseling or referral. Research about dyspareunia (ie, painful intercourse) suggests some nontraditional forms of therapy, such as

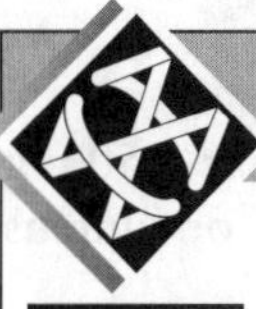

DISPLAY 12–5

Factors Contributing to a Decline in Sexual Interest or Activity During the Postpartum Period

- Fatigue
- Fear of not hearing the infant
- Emotional distress on a continuum from baby blues to postpartum depression
- Adjustments to role change
- Hormonal changes
- Physical discomfort related to changes of vulva, vagina, perineum, and breasts
- Breast-feeding
- Decreased sense of attractiveness

acupuncture (Tureanu & Tureanu, 1997) and ultrasound (Hay-Smith, 1999) may be helpful. Information about sexuality can be provided to the couple prenatally and after birth. Knowledge about normal physiologic and emotional changes allows the couple to discuss coping mechanisms and alternate means of maintaining intimacy during this challenging period. Education about sexuality during the postpartum period should include the following information:

- Sexual intercourse may be resumed approximately 3 to 4 weeks after the birth.
- Partners should avoid intercourse until vaginal bleeding has stopped.
- A water-soluble gel may be necessary for additional lubrication.

Contraception

The women's choice and use of postpartum contraception is influenced by the infant feeding method and the involution process. Ideally, the primary healthcare provider and perinatal nurse discuss the choice, use, advantages, and disadvantages of a variety of contraceptive methods with both partners. Consideration of the couple's needs and preferences is important when selecting a contraceptive method that is acceptable and effective for their unique situation. This approach allows sharing of responsibility, an opportunity to discuss advantages and disadvantages of methods, clarification of misconceptions, and discussion of prevention of sexually transmitted diseases (STDs). Information about contraception should include effectiveness, acceptability, and safety. The available options for women and their partners are described in the following sections.

DEPO-PROVERA

- Injections are given four times each year (150 mg given intramuscularly in the deltoid or gluteus maximus).
- The effectiveness rate is 99.7%.
- Advantages include long-lasting action, unimpaired lactation, and independence from coitus.
- Disadvantages include prolonged amenorrhea or uterine bleeding, weight gain, increased risk of venous thrombosis and thromboembolism, no STD protection, need for continued injections, fluid retention or edema, abdominal discomfort, and glucose intolerance.

NORPLANT

- The subdermal implant is inserted surgically and provides up to 5 years of contraception.
- The effectiveness rate is 99%.
- Advantages include long-lasting and reversible action.
- Disadvantages include menstrual irregularities, need for surgical removal, headaches, weight gain, breast pain, nervousness, nausea, skin changes, vertigo, no STD protection, and raised area on the arm.

ORAL CONTRACEPTIVES—COMBINED ESTROGEN–PROGESTIN

- Dosage is one pill each day.
- The effectiveness rate is 96.8%.
- Advantages include coitus-independent; decreased menstrual blood loss; decreased incidence of dysmenorrhea and premenstrual syndrome; reduction in endometrial adenocarcinoma, ovarian cancer, and benign breast disease; improvement in acne; protection against development of functional ovarian cysts; and decreased risk of ectopic pregnancy (Hatcher & Guillebaud, 1998; Speroff & Darney, 1996).
- Disadvantages include contraindications for women with a history of thromboembolic disorders, cerebrovascular or coronary artery disease, breast cancer, estrogen-dependent tumors, pregnancy, impaired liver function or tumors, hypertension, or diabetes of 20 years' duration and for women who smoke (if older than 35 years), are lactating, or have had a period of immobilization (Hatcher & Guillebaud, 1998; Speroff & Darney, 1996). The drug can cause libido changes, breast tenderness, weight gain, nausea, and a delay in return of fertility.

ORAL CONTRACEPTIVES—PROGESTIN-ONLY

- Dosage is one pill each day.
- The effectiveness rate is 95%.
- In addition to the advantages of oral contraceptives listed previously, lactation is not impaired by this formulation, which is less likely to cause cardiovascular complications, headaches, or hypertension.
- In addition to the disadvantages of oral contraceptives listed previously, drug interactions are more likely, and irregular bleeding, amenorrhea, and functional ovarian cysts can occur. The pill must be taken at same time each day.

BARRIER METHODS

- Device must be used at the time of sexual act.

- The effectiveness rate is 78% to 86%, depending on the device.
- Advantages include prevention of pregnancy, STDs, or both (used in combination with spermicides to achieve maximal protection); newer male condoms have various lengths, shapes, and adhesives.
- Tactylon (approved by the Food and Drug Administration [FDA] in 1991) is a hypoallergenic, synthetic polymer that is impervious to sperm and virus and is not degraded by oxidation or oil-based lubricants; it is used in male and female condoms.
- Reality vaginal pouch (approved by the FDA in 1992) is a female condom with two rings connected by a polyurethane sheath. The inner ring is fitted like a diaphragm; the outer ring protects the vulva and prevents slipping. It has a 15% failure rate.
- A diaphragm covers the cervix and requires fitting by healthcare professional. Its effectiveness is increased with the use of spermicide. It must be refitted after weight loss or gain greater than 22 kg and after birth. It has an 18% failure rate.
- A male condom is a latex or synthetic sheath placed over the erect penis before coitus. It must be applied before penile-vulvar contact and removed before the penis becomes flaccid (ie, risk of sperm leakage at withdrawal). It has a 12% failure rate.

CHEMICAL METHODS (SPERMICIDAL CREAMS, JELLIES, FOAMS, SUPPOSITORIES, AND VAGINAL FILM CONTAINING NONOXYNOL 9)

- Agent must be used at the time of the sex act.
- The effectiveness rate is 50% to 95%.
- Advantages include ease of application, safety, low cost, no prescription required, and help in lubrication.
- Disadvantages include a maximum effect that lasts no longer than 1 hour, required reapplication for repeat intercourse, possibility of an allergic response or irritation, and messiness.

INTRAUTERINE DEVICES (IUD)

- No action is required at time of intercourse.
- Two types are approved for use in United States: Progestasert, which is T shaped with a progesterone reservoir in the stem and must be replaced yearly, and Copper T380, which is T shaped, wrapped with copper, and effective for 8 years.
- The effectiveness rate is 97% to 98%.
- Advantages include use for postpartum and breast-feeding women, long-term and continuous use requiring minimal effort, and no continual expense.
- Disadvantages include contraindications for women with a history of pelvic inflammatory disease or STDs, need for professional insertion, and generation of cramping, pain, and bleeding, which should be evaluated.

POSTPARTUM TUBAL LIGATION/ VASECTOMY (STERILIZATION)

- It requires no additional effort after surgical procedure.
- The effectiveness rate is 99.5% (female) to 99.9% (male).
- Advantages include no need for additional contraception (should be considered permanent although reversal is technically possible).
- Its disadvantage is no STD protection.
- Before surgery, appropriate counseling is necessary regarding risks of failure, surgical risks, and potential psychosocial reactions to the procedure. A signed consent form according to institutional protocol is required.

NATURAL FAMILY PLANNING

- It relies on fertility awareness, observations, and abstinence during the fertile portion of a woman's menstrual cycle.
- It requires an understanding of the changes occurring in a woman's ovulatory cycle.
- The fertile period is calculated with a set formula, basal body temperature, cervical mucus assessment, symptothermal techniques (ie, combines body temperature and cervical mucus assessment), or over-the-counter ovulation test kit (ie, Creighton Model, Billings method, or Sympto Thermal).
- Advantages include a couple-centered method, low cost, lack of harm to fertility, no side effects, usefulness in diagnosing gynecologic disorders and infertility, and use in achieving pregnancy when desired.
- Disadvantages include no STD protection, difficult application during irregular cycles postpartum, need to begin charting 3 weeks after birth, and ovulation possibly occurring before the first postpartum menses (Hilgers & Stanford, 1998).

WOMEN'S PERSPECTIVES ON THE TRANSITION TO PARENTHOOD

Fatigue

The 6 weeks after giving birth are a time of change and adjustment for the woman and the family. Fatigue during the first 2 weeks postpartum is a significant problem for all women (Elek, Hudson, & Fleck, 1997). There is no significant difference in the level of fatigue between the first and third month after birth, although the severity of fatigue remained significantly higher at 3 months postpartum than prepregnancy values (Lee & Zaffke, 1999). Fatigue affects emotional adjustment and adaptation to the maternal role, and it may cause feelings of inadequacy in meeting the needs of other family members and in assuming household responsibilities. Perceptions of fatigue are not related to employment, parity, and family variables (Lee & Zaffke, 1999).

Anticipatory guidance in identifying rest opportunities and organizing new responsibilities and tasks is important for the new mother. Education about the causes of fatigue and possible community and family resources enables the new mother to assume control and promotes problem-solving behaviors. Together, the nurse and woman can develop strategies for requesting help with newborn care, household chores, and sibling care. Listing daily and weekly tasks provides an organizational framework and may serve as a readily available wish list that can be used when family and friends offer to help. Identification of family members and friends available to help provides an initial supportive structure for the new family.

Additional Stressors

In addition to fatigue, several stressors have been identified as contributing to adaptation difficulties in the postpartum period. These stressors include physical changes and complications, role adaptation conflicts, newborn needs, relationship changes, and possibly the return to the workplace and selecting a child care setting.

Postpartum Blues and Depression

Transient emotional disturbances or "baby blues" occur in approximately 50% of women about 3 to 6 days postpartum. These mood disturbances last several days. Insomnia, weepiness, depression, anxiety, poor concentration, irritability, and affective lability may be exhibited (Cunningham et al., 1997).

More severe depressive episodes, with an onset between 2 to 3 months, develop in approximately 8% to 15% of women (Cunningham et al., 1997). The practice of early discharge results in the depression occurring at home. Home visits by skilled perinatal nurses should include an assessment of the psychological adaptation of the new mother. Talking with the woman in a familiar, comfortable environment about the stresses and challenges of new motherhood provides opportunities for early interventions, such as counseling, referrals to support services, and pharmacologic assistance. Postpartum assessment of maternal mental status and adjustment should be a standard part of postpartum clinical nursing assessments (Horowitz & Damato, 1999). If perinatal care providers are knowledgeable about the woman's psychological well-being, early identification of these disorders is made, and crises may be prevented. Chapter 6 discusses postpartum psychological issues.

FAMILY TRANSITION TO PARENTHOOD

After birth, the woman experiences psychological changes as well as physiologic reversal of the physical changes of pregnancy. For the woman, adoption of a maternal role begins during pregnancy as she develops an attachment to the fetus. This role evolution continues postpartum with the birth separation of the mother–infant pair, or polarization (Rubin, 1977). As the mother develops her style of parenting, she considers her behavior in relation to the infant and notices familial characteristics in the infant. These changes in the mother are referred to as maternal role attainment (Mercer, 1995). Mercer identified four stages in this process: anticipatory, formal, informal, and personal. The anticipatory stage, occurring during pregnancy, involves the observation of role models for mothering behaviors. During the formal stage, the new mother tries to perform infant care tasks as expected by others. The mother begins to make personal choices about mothering during the informal stage and attains comfort with the role during the personal stage. The final stages, informal and formal, correspond to the taking-in and taking-hold stages identified by Rubin (1961). During the taking-in phase (first 24 hours or longer), the woman relives the birth experience, clarifies her understanding of the experience, and focuses on food and sleep. The taking-hold phase (second to fourth day) centers on concern with bodily functions, and the woman focuses on regaining control over her life and succeeding in infant-care responsibilities. Rubin (1961) includes the letting-go phase to describe the new mother's letting go of who she was and full participation in the mothering role. Nurses can foster success in these processes by meeting the woman's needs during each stage and providing a supportive environment for listening and educating the new mother.

Paternal satisfaction with the birth experience and its associated stresses influences marital happiness and family life (Rogers & White, 1998). For most women, being comfortable as a mother occurs during the first 3 to 10 months after birth. Nursing assessments about the quality of parenting behaviors during the postpartum period can guide the educational plan for the new couple. Display 12–6 lists adaptive and maladaptive parenting behaviors. Evidence of maladaptive parenting behaviors should prompt nursing communication with the primary healthcare provider and appropriate referral.

Nurses caring for women and families during the postpartum period must consider their cultural expectations and norms when planning care. This requires an open-minded and creative approach. Knowledge about various traditions and services within ethnic groups avoids duplication of these services and en-

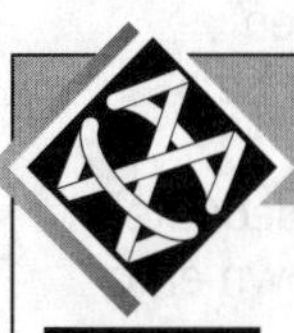

DISPLAY 12–6

Adaptive and Maladaptive Parenting Behaviors

Behavior	*Adaptive*	*Maladaptive*
Feeding	Provides an appropriate amount and type of food	Makes inappropriate types or inadequate amounts of food available
	Burps the child both during and after feeding	Does not burp the baby, although she or he knows it is necessary to do so
	Prepares the meal appropriately	Prepares the meal inappropriately
	Feeds the infant regularly and as frequently as necessary	Rushes or delays feeding the child
Rest	Provides a quiet and relaxed environment for the resting baby	Does not provide a quiet and relaxed environment
	Schedules rest periods	Does not schedule rest periods
Stimulating and caring for infant	Speaks to the child and makes other appropriate sounds	Speaks aggressively or not at all to the infant
	Provides tactile stimulation at a variety of times and not only when the baby is hungry or in danger	Plays aggressively with the baby or does not touch her or him
	Provides age-appropriate toys	Provides inappropriate toys
	Positions infant comfortably while holding the child	Does not hold the baby or ignores child's discomfort when being held
	The baby seems satisfied with the way it is being handled.	The baby seems frustrated with the way it is handled.
	Sees that the baby is dry, warm, and not hungry	Does not care for the baby who is hungry, cold, or soiled
	Exhibits initiative in trying to find how to deal with the baby's problems	Lacks initiative and does not try to meet the baby's needs

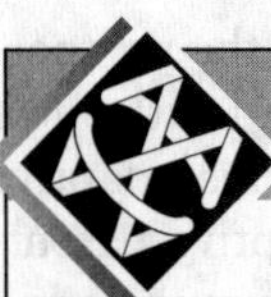

DISPLAY 12–6 (cont.)

Adaptive and Maladaptive Parenting Behaviors

Behavior	*Adaptive*	*Maladaptive*
Self-perception or emotional state of parent	Usually maintains a realistic perception of and realistic expectations for the baby	Develops distorted perceptions of and unrealistic expectations for the baby
	Exhibits a realistic perception of her or his own mothering and fathering abilities	Holds unrealistic expectations of her or his own parenting abilities
	Shows some interest in understanding and/or discussing the childbirth	Is unable or unwilling to discuss the childbirth
	Exhibits friendly or neutral behavior with other children	Exhibits hostility or aggression toward other children
	Appears generally satisfied to be a parent	Appears dissatisfied to be a parent
	Is able or willing to turn to other people for social support when necessary	Is unable to provide adequately for relaxation and own emotional needs
		Is isolated and without adequate social support
		Is depressed

From Compendium of Postpartum Care, (1996). Washington, DC: AWHONN (Association of Women's Health, Obstetric, and Neonatal Nurses), 1.39

courages a collaborative approach to providing these women with a positive and satisfying birth experience (Mayberry, Affonso, Shibuya, & Clemmons, 1999).

The changes that occur within the family are not limited to the woman. The family, however it is defined, experiences changes in structure and process. Parents adapt to these changes more easily when they are involved with a support network. This network may include family, friends, and institutional components. New parents often report a change in their immediate social network. This change typically involves increased contact with other new parents or with families facing similar challenges. For new parents living without immediate access to family, referral to support groups sponsored by hospitals or community centers may provide an opening into a circle of new parents and friends. New parents may place increased importance on family and the traditions they include. For other couples, increased familial contacts may result in an increased level of stress as the new family attempts to meet the external demands placed on them by enthusiastic or demanding family members. If the new mother decides not to return to a work environment outside the home, she may face the challenge of redefining herself as a mother.

Nurses caring for families during this time can provide anticipatory guidance about possible areas of stress and options for stress reduction. Providing this information in a written format enables the couple to review the information as situations develop.

SUMMARY

The postpartum period is a time of transition and change for the new mother and her family. Physiologic and psychologic changes occur immediately and over time, necessitating careful planning to meet the needs of the new family. Timely, frequent assessments and appropriate interventions require clinical skills and adequate knowledge about these processes. Supportive care that includes education for the woman and her family about what to expect in the first few weeks facilitates the transition from the inpatient setting to home. Being present during this period is a responsibility and a privilege that can affect society as a whole, one family at a time.

REFERENCES

American Academy of Pediatrics & American College of Obstetricians and Gynecologists. (1997). *Guidelines for Perinatal Care* (4th ed.). Washington, DC: Author.

American College of Obstetricians and Gynecologists (ACOG). (1998). *Postpartum hemorrhage* (Educational Bulletin No. 243) Washington, DC: Author.

American Society of Anesthesiologists. (1999). *Practice Guidelines for Obstetrical Anesthesia*. Park Ridge, IL: Author.

Association of Women's Health, Obstetric and Neonatal Nurses. (1996). *Compendium of postpartum care*. Washington, DC: Author.

Association of Women's Health, Obstetric and Neonatal Nurses. (1998). *Standards and guidelines for professional nursing practice in the care of women and newborns* (5th ed.). Washington, DC: Author.

Atterbury, J. L., Groome, L. J., Hoff, C., & Yarnell, J. A. (1998). Clinical presentation of women readmitted with postpartum severe preeclampsia or eclampsia. *Journal of Obstetric, Gynecologic, and Neonatal Nursing, 27*(2), 134–141.

Baker, C., Luce, J., Chenoweth, C., & Friedman, C. (1995). Comparison of case-finding methodologies for endometritis after cesarean section. *American Journal of Infection Control, 23*(1), 27–33.

Ball, J. A. (1996). Complications of the puerperium. In V. R. Bennett & L. K. Brown (Eds.), *Myles textbook for midwives* (12th ed.). Edinburgh: Churchill Livingstone.

Bick, D. (1998). Hurt by birth: A review of outcomes that matter in pregnancy and childbirth. *Practising Midwife, 1*(5), 26–28.

Burton, J. (1999). When your patient is postpartum: Are you confident in your skills? *American Journal of Nursing, 99*(2), 64–70.

Carroli, G., Belizan, J., & Stamp, G. (1999). Episiotomy for vaginal birth. [on-line]. *The Cochrane Library, 3*, 9. Available: .

Creasy, R. K., & Resnik, R. (1999). *Maternal-fetal medicine: Principles and practice* (4th ed.). Philadelphia: W.B. Saunders.

Cunningham, F. G., MacDonald, P., Gant, N., Leveno, K., Gilstrap, L., Hankins, G. D., & Clark, S. L. (1997). The puerperium. In *Williams obstetrics* (20th ed.). Norwalk, CT: Appleton & Lange.

Curtin, S., & Kozak, I. (1998). Decline in U.S. cesarean delivery rate appears to stall. *Birth, 25*(4), 259–262.

Curtin, S. C. & Martin, J. A. (2000). Births: Preliminary data for 1999. *National Vital Statistics Reports, 48*(14), 1–24.

Eason, E., Labrecque, M., Wells, G., & Feldman, P. (2000). Preventing perineal trauma during childbirth: A systematic review. *Obstetrics and Gynecology, 95*(3), 464–471.

Elek, S. M., Hudson, D. B., & Fleck, M. O. (1997). Expectant parents' experience with fatigue and sleep during pregnancy. *Birth, 24*(1), 49–54.

Ernest, J. M., & Mead, P. B. (1998). Protocols: Ob-gyn infection, postpartum endometritis. *Contemporary OB/GYN, 43*(1), 33–34.

Falter, H. J. (1997). Deep vein thrombosis in pregnancy and the puerperium: A comprehensive review. *Journal of Vascular Nursing, 15*(2), 58–62.

Foldspang, A., Mommsen, S., & Djurhuus, J. C. (1999). Prevalent urinary incontinence as a correlate of pregnancy, vaginal childbirth, and obstetric techniques. *American Journal of Public Health, 89*(2), 209–212.

Fowles, E. R. (1998). Labor concerns of women two months after delivery. *Birth, 25*(4), 235–240.

Goldenberg, R. L., Cliver, S. P., Bronstein, J., Cutter, G., Andrews, W., & Mennenmeyer, S. (1994). Bed rest in pregnancy. *Obstetrics and Gynecology, 84*(1), 131–136.

Grullon, K. E., & Grimes, D. A. (1997). The safety of early postpartum discharge: A review and critique. *Obstetrics and Gynecology, 90*(5), 860–865.

Gulmezoglu, A. M. (1999). Prostaglandins for management of the third stage of labour. *The Cochrane Library, 4*, 11. Available: .

Hatcher, R., & Guillebaud, J. (1998). The pill: Combined oral contraceptives. In R. Hatcher et al. (Eds.), *Contraceptive Technology* (17th ed.). New York: Ardent Media.

Hay-Smith, E. J. (1999). Therapeutic ultrasound for postpartum perineal pain and dyspareunia. [On-line]. *The Cochrane Library, 3*, 9. Available: .

Hilgers, T., & Stanford, J. (1998). The Creighton Model Napro Education Model for avoiding pregnancy: Use and effectiveness. *Journal of Reproductive Medicine, 43*(6), 495–502.

Horowitz, J. A., & Damato, E. G. (1999). Mothers' perceptions of postpartum stress and satisfaction. *Journal of Obstetric, Gynecologic, and Neonatal Nursing, 28*(6), 595–605.

Jones, K. D., Lehr, S. T., & Hewell, S. W. (1997). Dyspareunia: Three case reports. *Journal of Obstetric, Gynecologic, and Neonatal Nursing, 28*(2), 183–192.

Lee, K. A., & Zaffke, M. E. (1999). Longitudinal change in fatigue and energy during pregnancy and the postpartum period. *Journal of Obstetric, Gynecologic, and Neonatal Nursing, 26*(1), 19–23.

Luegenbiehl, D. L. (1997). Improving visual estimation of blood volume on peripads. *MCN, The American Journal of Maternal Child Nursing, 22*(6), 294–298.

Maier, J. S., & Maloni, J. A. (1997). Nurse advocacy for selective versus routine episiotomy. *Journal of Obstetric, Gynecologic, and Neonatal Nursing, 26*(2), 155–161.

Maloni, J. A. (1998). *Antepartum bedrest: Case studies, research and nursing care* (Symposium). Washington, DC: Association of Women's Health, Obstetric and Neonatal Nurses.

Maloni, J. A., Chance, B., Zhang, C., Cohen, A. W., Betts, D., & Gange, S. J. (1993). Physical and psychosocial effects of antepartum hospital bed rest. *Nursing Research, 42*(4), 197–203.

Mayberry, L. J., Affonso, D. D., Shibuya, J., & Clemmens, D. (1999). Integrating cultural values, beliefs, and customs into pregnancy and postpartum care: Lessons learned from a Hawaiian public health nursing project. *Journal of Perinatal and Neonatal Nursing, 13*(1), 15–26.

Mercer, R. T. (1995). *Becoming a mother*. New York: Springer.

Miller, L. K., & Cox, S. M. (1997). Urinary tract infections complicating pregnancy. *Infectious Disease Clinics of North America, 11*(1), 13–26.

Olson, H. F., & Nunnelee, J. D. (1998). Incidence of thrombosis in pregnancy and postpartum: A retrospective review in a large private hospital. *Journal of Vascular Nursing, 16*(4), 84–86.

Parsons, C. (1998). Damage to the pelvic floor: Causes, prevention, and treatment. *Practicing midwife, 1*(2), 14–16.

Rogers, S. J., & White, L. K. (1998). Satisfaction with parenting: The role of marital happiness, family structure, and parents' gender. *Journal of Marriage and the Family, 60*, 293–308.

Rubin, R. (1961). Puerperal change. *Nursing Outlook, 9*, 753.

Rubin, R. (1977). Binding-in in the postpartum period. *Maternal-Child Nursing Journal, 6*, 67–75.

Sampselle, C. (1999). Physical activity and postpartum well-being. *Journal of Obstetric, Gynecologic, and Neonatal Nursing, 28*(1), 41–49.

Sampselle, C., & Miller, C. (1996). Pelvic muscle exercises: Effective patient teaching. *The Female Patient, 21*(5), 29–36.

Sampselle, C. M., Miller, C., & Rossie, D. (1997). Perineal massage: Further support of protective perineal effect. *Journal of Perinatal Education, 6*(2), 1–5.

Scott, M. (1998). Three keys to avoiding postpartum hemorrhage. *Midwifery Today, 48*, 23–24.

Sibai, B. (1996). Hypertension in pregnancy. In S. Gabbe, J. Niebyl, & J. Simpson (Eds.), *Obstetrics: Normal and problem pregnancies* (3rd ed.). New York: Churchill Livingstone.

Simpson, K. R., & Knox, G. E. (1999). Strategies for developing an evidence-based approach to perinatal care. *MCN The American Journal of Maternal Child Nursing, 24*(3), 122–132.

Smith, J. (1996). Psychology: Sexuality and sexual problems after childbirth. *Modern Midwife, 6*(10), 16–19.

Speroff, L., & Darney, P. (1996). *A clinical guide for contraception* (2nd ed.). Baltimore: Williams & Wilkins.

Stables, D. (1999). *Physiology in childbearing with anatomy and related biosciences*. London: Bailliere Tindall.

Steen, M. (1998). Perineal trauma: How do we evaluate its severity? *Midirs Midwifery Digest, 8*(2), 228–230.

Steen, M., & Cooper, K. (1997). A tool for assessing perineal trauma. *Journal of Wound Care, 6*(9), 432–436.

Steen, M., & Cooper, K. (1999). A new device for the treatment of perineal wounds . . . maternity gel pad. *Journal of Wound Care, 8*(2), 87–90.

Toglia, M. (1996). Anal incontinence: An underrecognized, undertreated problem. *The Female Patient, 21*(1), 17–30.

Tureanu, V., & Tureanu, L. (1997). Acupuncture in sexual dysfunction: Dyspareunia and vaginismus. *Clinical Bulletin of Myofascial Therapy, 2*(1), 25–33.

Varney, H. (1997). *Varney's midwifery* (3rd ed.). Boston: Jones & Bartlett.

Walder, J. (1997). Clinical: Misoprostol: Preventing postpartum haemorrhage. *Modern Midwife, 7*(9), 23–27.

Wall, L. L. (1999). Birth trauma and the pelvic floor: Lessons from the developing world. *Journal of Women's Health, 8*(2), 149–155.

APPENDIX 12A

Daily Postpartum Assessments and Interventions

DAILY POSTPARTUM ASSESSMENTS & INTERVENTIONS

* Indicates further documentation in Integrated Progress Notes.																
	DATE															
	TIME															
SKIN	COLOR Normal, Pale, Cyanotic, Flushed															
	TEMPERATURE Warm, Hot, Cool															
	HUMIDITY Dry, Moist, Clammy, DIA =Diaphoretic															
	IV/CONDITION OF SITE Patent, Occluded, △=Changed, D/C=Discontinued (indicate time) ✓ = No signs of infection * = Refer to Progress Notes (may have signs of infection or infiltration)															
BREASTS	CONDITION Soft, Filling, Full, Engorged, Red, Pain,															
	NIPPLES Normal, Red, Pain, Cracked, Inverted															
UTERUS	HEIGHT U/U = At Umbilicus (measure in finger breaths) FB/U — Above U/FB— Below															
	POSITION Midline, Right of Umbilicus, Left of Umbilicus															
	CONSISTENCY Firm, Boggy, FM = Firm with Massage															
LOCHIA	COLOR Rubra, Serosa, Alba															
	AMOUNT 0 = no flow, Scant, Small, Moderate, Heavy, Clots (larger than quarters)															
	ODOR + = Present 0 = Absent/Normal															
PERINEUM	CONDITION Intact, Ecchymosis, Hematoma, Puffy, Edema, Clean															
	EPISIOTOMY N = Clean, dry, intact, Separated, Edema, Red															
	HEMORRHOIDS + = Present, Edematous, Thrombosed, Soft, Painful															
CESAREAN SECTION	ABDOMEN Soft, Distended															
	BOWEL SOUNDS Normal, ↑ = Hyperactive, ↓ = Hypoactive, O = Absent, Flatus															
	INCISION Normal (clean, dry, intact), Edema, Red, Drainage, Separated, Unseen															
	DRESSING Dry & Intact, △ = Changed, No Dressing															
	SUTURES/STAPLES REMOVED = ✓															
	BREATH SOUNDS Equal, Unequal, Clear, Congested WI = Wheezing on Inspiration WE = Wheezing on Expiration Rales, Rhonchi															
	POSITIONING Left, Right, Supine, Prone, Self, Fowlers															

Palos Community Hospital, Palos Heights, IL.

	DATE															
	TIME															
CARDIO-VASCULAR	EDEMA 1+ Minimal edema of the pedal & pretibial areas 2+ Marked edema of the lower extremities and hands 3+ Edema of the face and hands, lower abdominal wall & sacrum. 4+ Anasarca (Generalized massive edema) & ascites															
	CALF TENDERNESS + = Present (indicate R or L), 0 = Absent															
	HOMAN'S SIGN 0 = Negative + = Positive (indicate R or L)															
LOC/ SEDATION	Alert, Confused, Lethargic, Oriented, Sleeping, Nonresponsive, Arousable															
EMOTIONAL STATUS	Calm, Apprehensive, Anxious, Hostile, Depressed, Labile, Flat Affect															
TREATMENTS	K-PAD Back, Incision, Legs, Other															
	Abdominal binder = ✓															
	Supportive Bra, Breast Binder															
	Breast Pump (hand) (electric) ✓ each time pumping occurs.															
	Breast Shells															
	Ice to Perineum = ✓															
	Sitz = ✓ (check each time used)															
	Inflatable Cushion = ✓															
ACTIVITY	Bed, Chair, Dangle, Ambulatory, BR = Bathroom BRA = Bathroom w/assistance															
HYGIENE	Complete, Partial, Shower Foley Care, Pericare															
DIET	APPETITE NPO, Good, Fair, Poor															
	TYPE General, Clear Liquids, Full Liquids, Soft, Other															
ELIMINATION	STOOLS Formed, Semisolid, Liquid															
	URINATION Void, Straight Cath															
	FOLEY Patent, Irrigated, Changed, D/C = Discontinued (indicate time)															
	SS Enema, Fleets, Suppository															
SAFETY	SIDERAILS ↕ = Up, ↕ = Down (indicate #)															
	CALL LIGHT + = ✓															
	I.D. BAND + = ✓															
INITIALS																

Palos Community Hospital, Palos Heights, IL.

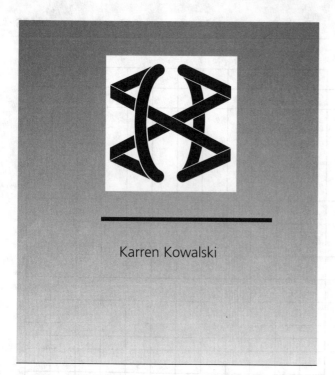

Karren Kowalski

CHAPTER 13

Perinatal Loss and Bereavement

Any death can initiate a grief response. In one sense, each person grieves for his or her own death. Humans function in relationships with the belief that there is always more time: time to correct misunderstandings, time to love someone, time to hold them, and time to communicate innermost thoughts and feelings (Lattanzi, 1983). Perinatal death is unique because it is out of sequence, outside the normal life cycle. It is a reminder of human vulnerability.

Although American culture has focused on the successful pursuit of happiness and the American dream, death in Western culture has become equated with failure. Losses are somehow translated into road blocks and obstacles; they are not to be discussed. This cultural shift has influenced all aspects of daily living, particularly the reproductive cycle that deals with birth and death.

The study of loss and bereavement is an evolving process. In the 1960s and 1970s, loss and bereavement were confined to a medical model. The model had multiple psychopathologic categories to which a particular patient could be assigned. Professionals did not understand that healing often comes from within, that families have choices, or that societal normative behavior might cause problems in the bereavement process. It was more acceptable to diagnose and refer for therapy than to acknowledge the pain and be with the patient in that pain.

Many professionals have yet to differentiate between supportive caring for the bereaved and "fixing" people and situations. Consequently, when a death occurs, some nurses view the event as a personal and professional failure. Their professional image is called into question. A sense of failure is magnified if any aspect of the medical or nursing care was questioned or in error. Nurses may manufacture a reason using "what if" scenarios. For example, what if the nurse had called the physician an hour earlier. This chapter explores experiences of death, loss, and bereavement related to women, their families, reproduction, and nursing care. Loss and bereavement are studied from perspectives of phenomenology, psychology, sociology, ontology, and spirituality.

THE PHENOMENOLOGY OF LOSS

When perinatal loss occurs, women are especially vulnerable. Not only do they experience psychological trauma, but they must also cope with physiologic changes (Association of Women's Health, Obstetric and Neonatal Nurses [AWHONN], 1998). The initial phase of the bereavement response is denial. This is followed by an adjustment phase in which there is developing awareness, characterized by the parents feeling helpless, hopeless, and anxious. They are sad, and they experience severe psychological pain, anger, and guilt. Frequently, extended periods of chronic bereavement occur in which parents function in adaptive or maladaptive ways. In extreme maladaptive instances, the family becomes dysfunctional. They may experience a failed marriage, unemployment, and separation from friends and relatives. It is extremely difficult for them to live each day with what can be perceived as failure. Display 13–1 offers a more detailed description of the stages of bereavement.

Losses take many different forms; they may be anticipated or unexpected, instant or gradual, traumatic

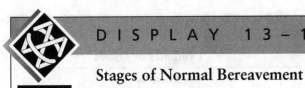

DISPLAY 13–1

Stages of Normal Bereavement

Shock and denial: Period lasting 72 hours or longer during which the individual believes that she is experiencing a bad dream and that she will wake up and everything will be okay.

Disintegration: A general downward spiral or sense of disintegration that overlaps with grief work. Families describe the process as being "on a roller coaster." Any time they begin to feel better physically or emotionally, they feel guilty about feeling better. During this time, bereaved families, particularly the parents of stillborns and newborns who die, seem quite surprised at the depth of their feelings. The mothers feel a strong sense of responsibility and guilt. Fathers may appear to deal with their feelings more quickly by focusing on their careers or work.

Reintegration: A sense of continuity and reintegration is established as the bereaved gradually relinquish parts of their relationship with the deceased. They reestablish their definition of the meaning of life separately from the deceased child. Grief is mastered not by ceasing to care for the dead, but by abstracting the essence of the relationship and reintegrating it to fit a future in which the deceased will not share. Reintegration is more difficult in perinatal losses because these losses are complicated by two additional aspects, loss of creation and loss of a dream.

or nontraumatic. The classic work of Peretz (1970b) identifies four key types of loss: loss of a significant person, loss of some aspect of self, loss of an external object, and loss through stages of growth and development. These losses, how they occur, and examples are given in Table 13–1. Two additional categories have been identified during the reproductive cycle: loss of a dream and loss of creation (Arnold & Gemma, 1994; Kowalski, 1987; Robinson, Baker, & Nackerud, 1999).

Loss of a Dream

Because of the complete dependency of the growing fetus and the newborn on the parents, a unique attachment or bond may be created. Although it is too early for the developing fetus to really demonstrate personality, the parents focus their hopes, dreams, and aspirations on the child he or she will become. When a newborn dies, these hopes and dreams are extinguished. The parents experience a sadness for what might have been (Arnold & Gemma, 1994). As each life transition occurs, as each developmental stage progresses (eg, the first day of school, obtaining a driver's license, graduation from high school, marriage), parents may again grieve their loss and the inability to share such life experience with the child.

Loss of Creation

An artist whose painting is vandalized or destroyed suffers great anguish over loss of control and powerlessness to protect his or her creation. Likewise, human beings create children. This creation is an extension of themselves. Often, the parents invest time, energy, and emotions in the creation of this new life. It is nurtured in the woman's body. As it progresses from embryo to fetus to newborn, it is continually with the mother, a part of her yet separate. When this creation dies, she experiences an event over which she has no control, a process she cannot stop. The narcissistic blow to her self-image can be terrible (Kowalski, 1987). The father may feel loss of control because he is unable to protect his spouse or to provide whatever could have saved the child, and he is alarmed by his partner's distress.

Perceptions of Loss

Peretz (1970a) emphasized that any loss is simultaneously a reality and a perceptual or symbolic event. Objects, persons, or relationships perceived to be of value are mourned. Even perceptual or symbolic events can produce intense reactions. For example, some women who experience a cesarean birth rather than a vaginal birth react to this process as a loss. They perceive that they have lost the experience they desired. Somehow they have failed in actualizing this event called childbearing, and they grieve about this loss or assault to their self-esteem. In contrast, women who experience a perinatal loss would give anything to have been able to deliver a live, healthy newborn, even by cesarean birth. Consequently, grieving about a cesarean birth is incomprehensible to them. Likewise, in spontaneous or even therapeutic abortion, the perception of the pregnancy and the event greatly influence the emotional response (Williams, 2000). Patients and care providers choose how a given event is perceived based on their past experience.

TABLE 13–1 ■ TYPES OF LOSS

Loss	How Losses Occur	Examples of Losses
Loss of significant person	Death Separation Rejection Divorce	Fetal demise Stillbirth Neonatal death Maternal death Relinquishment for adoption
Loss of some aspect of self	Loss of the mental image an individual has of herself. Ideas and feelings about self-attractiveness, normalcy, ability to be loved or body functioning	Structural losses such as hysterectomy or mastectomy Infants with anomalies Functional losses such as infertility or complications of pregnancy
Loss of external objects	Loss of possessions (ie, material objects, money, property)	Loss of a child as a possession ("our child") Loss or giving up of associated objects (ie, furniture, clothes, toys)
Loss of stages of growth and development	Naturally occurring developmental loss as the person progresses through the stages or phases of life	Children lose or relinquish the breast for solid food Adults relinquish the "single life" when they form long-term relationships or marry Couples give up being a dyad to form a family

Perinatal Loss

Perinatal loss can be divided into two major types: death of the fetus or newborn or birth of a less than perfect child. Because the perinatal period represents the total embryonic, fetal, and neonatal life span and because there is greater danger to life during this period than at any other time during the life cycle, adverse outcomes can be expected. A variety of situations of perinatal loss are discussed in this chapter: miscarriage, stillbirth, neonatal death, anomalies or the "less than perfect" newborn, relinquishment for adoption, infertility, and ectopic pregnancy.

Miscarriage

During the past two decades, knowledge has increased about the experience of a miscarriage or spontaneous abortion. Previously viewed as an insignificant event, we know now that the grief experienced by these women may be especially challenging. Unlike when other deaths occur, at the time of a miscarriage, there is little talk of the event, society quickly negates that the event occurred, and there is the absence of a visible social network. The rituals that surround death normally are not present for a miscarriage. This lack of acknowledgment of the event may delay the grief process for some women (Stritzinger, Robinson, & Stewart, 1999).

Women who have experienced a miscarriage need several forms of support:

- Acknowledgment of the reality of the pregnancy and the death of a baby
- Appropriate and sensitive medical intervention
- Recognition of their concern about being able to produce a normal, healthy child (Hutti, 1992)

It is clear that parents, particularly women, respond to miscarriage with intense emotional reactions. A year after a miscarriage, women demonstrate more signs of stress and depression than the general population (Stritzinger et al., 1999). They express a lowered self-concept and loss of self-esteem associated with feeling that their body has betrayed them and wondering if it will ever function properly. This is especially common when health professionals are unable to provide couples with a clear reason or explanation for why the miscarriage occurred. The effect of a miscarriage continues into subsequent pregnancies. When these women have a subsequent pregnancy, they experience more anxiety and depression at 6 months than pregnant women without a previous miscarriage (Statham & Green, 1994).

Stillbirth and Newborn Death

Death occurring before the onset of labor is referred to as fetal death or stillbirth. Neonatal death occurs in the period from birth to 28 days of life. Before the diagnosis of a fetal death, parents often have knowledge that something is not right. There may be no fetal movement, or medical tests may show adverse results. These indications provide time for *anticipatory grief*, when the parents begin the bereavement process before the event. Anticipatory grief also occurs during the period when the newborn is critically ill. There are many commonalities in stillborn and newborn losses. One key difference, however, relates to the length of time the neonate lives. If the fetus dies before birth, the woman is often the only person who has bonded to the child. In contrast, if the neonate survives several days, people other than the mother have an opportunity to become attached to the newborn. The father, grandparents, and other family members may also feel a tremendous loss.

The "Less Than Perfect" Newborn

Bereavement is not limited to death or pregnancy loss. Considerable time and energy are invested in pregnancy and birth. When discrepancies occur between reality and the idealized perfect birth experience, a sense of loss arises. There are also instances when the pregnancy results in a less than perfect newborn. In these situations, parents did not produce the term or perfectly formed newborn they had expected. When a newborn is seriously ill, parents grieve the loss of the fantasized perfect newborn, creating difficulties in the attachment process. Parents have difficulty attaching to a newborn until there is evidence that the newborn will survive. Nurses must understand this process and support parents in their emotional work of bonding to a sick newborn. A similar process may occur when a newborn has anomalies.

It is not uncommon for parents to have definite ideas and fantasies about the preferred sex of their child. For example, the ideal middle-class American family consists of one boy and one girl. In some ethnic groups, it is essential to produce male children. When a child of the "wrong" sex is born, parents may need time to adjust to the idea. Some parents become permanently estranged from the child, creating significant psychological problems. When professionals become aware that the sex of the child is a critical issue, they need to create possibilities in which parents become involved in the birth and care taking. Although parents should always be encouraged to be involved in the process, it is even more critical in this situation. Parent involvement with the process needs to include positive feedback about how great a job they did. By demonstrating her acceptance, a nurse can promote attitudinal changes toward acceptance of the child. Not all situations can be corrected, but most can be improved.

Relinquishment for Adoption

Placing a newborn for adoption involves issues of loss and bereavement. This process, called *relinquishment*, contains aspects of the general bereavement process and of chronic sorrow. Women need to be assured that their newborn is healthy. Nurses should be nonjudgmental and convey an understanding that this decision takes great courage and love and is based on the best interest of the child. Appropriate nursing care during this period allows women to sort through their feelings and find meaning in the relinquishment of their newborn.

Infertility

Infertility is defined as the inability to achieve pregnancy after a year of regular sexual relations or the inability of pregnancy to culminate in a live birth (Mosher & Pratt, 1991). More than a million couples seek treatment annually. There are two types of infertility: organic infertility with a specific physiologic cause and functional infertility with no identified cause. Display 13–2 lists common experiences of infertile couples. Couples that are unable to have a healthy biologic child experience losses that are deeply painful. These losses include loss of a biologic heir (ie, connection to eternity); the experiences of pregnancy, birth, and nurturing; sex-role identity, and self-esteem (Hirsch & Hirsch, 1995). The outcomes of infertility include social isolation and stress on social and marital relationships. Nurses can intervene to support couples in working through these issues.

Ectopic Pregnancy

Ectopic pregnancy is an example of multiple losses occurring in a single event. Ectopic pregnancy, implantation in a site other than the endometrium, occurs in 19.7 of 1,000 pregnancies (Pisarska & Carson, 1999). This 2% incidence may still underestimate total number because of lack of reporting of cases managed as outpatients or in the physician's office. The most common symptoms include abdominal pain and irregular vaginal bleeding. Because these symptoms occur in the early weeks of pregnancy, the mother may not even

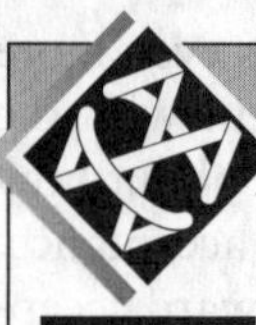

DISPLAY 13–2

Common Experiences of Infertile Couples

- Infertility as a central focus for role identity, especially for women
- Feelings of loss of control
- Feelings of defectiveness and reduced competence
- Loss of status and ambiguity as a couple, a sense of social stigma
- Stress on the marital and sexual relationship
- Strained relationships with health care providers

Greil, A.L. (1997). Infertility and psychological distress: A critical review of the literature. *Social Science & Medicine, 54*(11), 679–704.

realize she is pregnant. This can enhance the shock, denial, and pain. The first type of loss in this situation is the loss of the pregnancy itself. Even though it is an early loss, when the pregnancy was planned and greatly desired, the loss is significant and the subsequent grief can be quite devastating. The second loss is possible loss of fertility. Although there are medical interventions and not all ectopic pregnancies require surgery, there is still the possibility of damage or loss of the fallopian tube and a threat to the ability to conceive in the future. This combination of losses and the "stacking" effect can be extremely difficult for the mother. Her body has definitely failed her.

PSYCHOLOGICAL PERSPECTIVE OF GRIEF

Historic Development of the Understanding of Grief

Psychological explanations of grief originated in the work of Freud (1937) and his classic paper, "Mourning and Melancholia." He emphasized the painful psychological processes involved in relinquishing a loved person or object. Freud was most interested in the pathologic clinical manifestations or aberrations of the grief process.

It was another 15 years before Lindemann (1994) described patterns of "normal" bereavement. He was convinced that pathologic grief was merely an exaggeration or distortion of the normal bereavement process. To recognize the pathology, it is imperative to know the normal process. Lindemann identified the acute phase of bereavement, which he called *acute grief work*. His conclusions, based on extensive interviews and treatment of bereaved individuals, resulted in the grief behaviors listed in Table 13–2. These are the behaviors that nurses witness frequently in families whose loved ones die. Professionals have long attempted to protect patients from the pain of bereavement, primarily as a way to protect themselves. Lindemann (1994) was the first person to identify that the "no tears, stiff upper lip" approach was an aberration of the normal bereavement process.

According to Maris (1974), grief work does not necessarily focus on the loss of the loved one. He believed the fundamental crisis of grief comes from the loss of self rather than the loss of others. It is as though the bereaved mourn their own deaths. The loss of a key person in one's life translates as a loss of structure that has held the survivor's life together. Consequently, a person's life purpose is in question, and the individual feels helpless. A comprehensive review of bereavement literature can be found in the reference list (Benoliel, 1997).

Types of Grief

Anticipatory Grief

Lindemann (1994) also was the first to identify anticipatory grief as a process in families of the terminally ill. During the terminal illness of one family member, others were observed to be depressed, feel concern for the ill family member, and rehearse the death in an attempt to adjust to the consequences. Their hope was that, at the time of the actual death, they might not exhibit acute grief work behaviors because they had been moving in and out of these behaviors throughout the duration of the illness. Anticipatory grief may occur in several situations:

- In threatened abortion during early pregnancy
- When there is a diagnosis of a fetal condition incompatible with life
- As a result of selective pregnancy reduction
- In situations of voluntary termination of the pregnancy
- When a newborn is born prematurely or becomes critically ill

Some parents may appear to experience less grief when a newborn dies because of their anticipatory grief work before the actual death. Families need to be helped to understand what they are experiencing and be supported in their grief work throughout the process.

TABLE 13–2 ■ NURSING CARE IN ACUTE GRIEF WORK

Acute Symptom	Manifestations of Symptom	Nursing Care
Somatic distress	Intense sadness Tears and sobbing Questioning "why did this happen" Loss of appetite Sighing respirations Exhaustion Sleep loss	Do not give sleeping or anxiety medications (these only delay acute grief work and "numb" the emotions until after discharge so that professionals are not available to help). Listen and provide comfort. Answer as many questions as possible. Be truthful; saying "I don't know" is appropriate.
Preoccupation with image of the deceased	Desire of parents to see and hold newborn and have family members also see and hold him	Show infants to parents and family, even the earliest gestations Provide mementos and pictures to make experiences real.
Guilt	Search through the pregnancy for evidence of failure to do "the right thing" to have prevented the loss Parents look for negligence, exaggerate minor omissions or search for standards of care that may have been violated. The father may feel he did not provide for or protect the mother.	Assure parents these feelings are normal. Help parents anticipate they will have feelings of guilt. Support parents to identify ideas that have no basis in realistic fact.
Irritability or anger	Express a desire to be left alone when friends or relatives make an effort to maintain relationships Anger focused on healthcare professionals who are seen as "responsible" or not helpful enough Anger at relationships or systems seen as impersonal or dehumanizing Anger at God	Listen Do not personalize the behavior; realize it is driven by grief. Apologize for problems, misunderstandings, or inability of personnel to meet parents needs. Offer family the opportunity to talk with a spiritual counselor.
Inability to maintain organized patterns of activity	Common tasks undertaken as if only going through the motions. Simple tasks require enormous energy Bereaved mother at home alone, has difficulty structuring time and accomplishing common tasks (i.e., mean preparation, shopping) Difficulty concentrating on specific tasks	Provide bereavement education and information. Focus on normalcy of parents and family members' experience. Recommend support group composed of bereaved parents. Recommend books for bereaved parents when they are able to concentrate on reading.

Chronic Sorrow

Parents and other close family members experience chronic sorrow throughout the lifetime of a child with physical or mental handicaps. Chronic sorrow can also occur when a child has a less obvious problem such as a learning disability (Teel, 1996). Chronic sorrow refers to the understandable and nonneurotic response to a painful tragedy (Olshansky, 1966). Grief and sorrow occurs after the realization that the child has a chronic illness or will be permanently disabled. Parents fear for the child's future, grieve the lifelong dependency the child has on them and other siblings, and acknowledge the extraordinary stress caregiving has on the entire family system (Krafft & Krafft, 1998).

Chronic sorrow is recurring episodes of sadness in response to specific life events or internal thoughts and memories (Lindgren, Burke, Hainsworth, & Eakes, 1992). Chronic sorrow, unlike acute grief, has no end; it represents a lifetime of losses (Krafft & Krafft, 1998). Parents are reminded every day that they have failed to produce a normal, healthy child. They experience and reexperience grief each time someone talks about their child, during major crises and minor illnesses, in response to intense physical care demands, with growth and developmental challenges, and during ongoing battles with school systems for services their child needs (Kowalski, 1985).

Two phases of chronic sorrow have been identified (Copley & Bodensteiner, 1987). The first phase is characterized by denial and grief as parents struggle to cope and adjust. In the second phase, parents acknowledge and accept the impact their child's condition has and will continue to have on the family. They begin to develop coping mechanisms, acknowledge the permanence of the situation, and understand that adaptations for the child will always be needed (Krafft & Krafft, 1998). Chronic sorrow is unlike pathologic grief because parents of these children continue to function everyday.

Parents experiencing chronic grief need support from other parents and from the professional community. They need accurate and complete information about resources and help in planning realistic coping strategies that encompass the needs of all family members. Display 13–3 lists the nursing interventions used when dealing with families experiencing chronic sorrow.

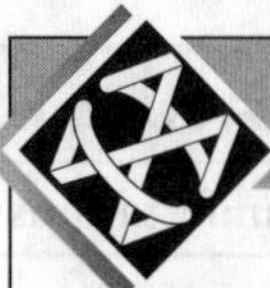

DISPLAY 13–3

Nursing Implications of Chronic Sorrow

- Recognize that the disability or chronic illness of one child affects all family members.
- Demonstrate genuine interest and respect for the child by nonverbal actions toward the child. Address the child by name, and refer to the child by name when talking to parents and other family members.
- Acknowledge that chronic sorrow is an understandable response to the permanent disability or chronic illness of a child.
- Expect periods of sorrow and sadness to occur throughout the lives of all family members, but especially the parents.
- Listen and offer support and encouragement.
- Provide information about the chronic condition and be realistic about anticipated progress or lack of progress.
- Identify written materials, community programs, financial resources, and respite care for these families, because they may not have the stamina to seek this on their own.
- Assess caregiver's ability to recognize the need for and accept assistance and support from other family members, neighbors, friends, and church and community groups.

Krafft, S., & Krafft, L. (1998). Chronic sorrow: Parents' lived experience. *Holistic Nursing Practice, 13*(1), 59–67.

Grief Resolution

One of the false perceptions about the grief experience of parents is that they will reach a point of resolution. When bereaved parents are asked about the issue of resolution, they are quick to tell any listener that there is no resolution. Their loss only becomes "less all-consuming." Some parents report that they will never forget their baby but that the acute pain lessens with time. Although some professionals refer to a concept called *grief resolution,* there is little evidence in the literature to validate such a phenomenon. Resolved implies completion or coming to an end. The bereaved may reestablish normal patterns of daily living. However, they never forget their baby. Many parents, 20, 30, or even 40 years later, talk about their newborn as though the event happened yesterday.

Some women conceive soon after the loss, whereas others choose to wait several months or even question ever getting pregnant again. When women have great difficulty in conceiving after a perinatal loss, it is possible that they are not able to withdraw emotional investment in the lost child (Kowalski, 1987). Events such as anniversary dates, visits from old friends, or the chance discovery of old photographs may awaken feelings of grief and sadness. When women who had experienced a newborn death were interviewed 18 months to 3 years later, they reported believing that their feelings of loss would always be present (Kowalski, 1984). Peppers and Knapp (1980) called this *shadow grief,* a burden parents have for the rest of their lives if they have not received proper psychological interventions. Kowalski (1984) denies that what she calls *bittersweet grief* is a burden. She found that parents had no wish to relinquish the sadness and longing. Parents found a certain bittersweet pleasure in the memories and the few occasions they found to talk about the newborn. With the love and support of family and friends, parents who have coped well still experience this gentle sadness, embrace it, and know how very special it is to always love this newborn who may not have been born alive or whose life was brief.

Duration of Normal Grief

It is difficult to predict the length, duration, or depth of the bereavement process because it depends on many factors:

- Relationship of the couple
- Level of attachment and investment in the fetus or newborn
- Circumstances surrounding the death
- Support of family, friends, and professionals
- Internal resources of the individual

The process is highly individualized and differs with each family. According to Pincus (1974), there could be no norm for grief or for adaptation, just as there is no time limit imposed on the process. Consequently, it is inappropriate for parents to be labeled or placed in categories according to their progress through the grieving process. The inability to cope with life is the only valid indication of pathologic grief (Pincus, 1974). Pathologic labels should not be attached to the experience of grief because of the tremendous amount of work that must occur during this period. Completing the work of grieving, which includes positive growth outcomes, creation of a durable story or picture of the newborn, reconstructing the meaning of the newborn in ongoing life, and emergence of different roles and identities in the couple, takes time (Stroebe & Schut, 1999). Grief requires time for healing. Persons whose behaviors seem to be "unique" often find it very difficult to conform to society's strict and unhelpful definition of bereavement behavior. Table 13–2 lists the symptoms associated with acute grief work.

The wide variations in the definition of "normal" can be further exacerbated by the unusual circumstance of multiple and varied types of losses experienced within a specific time frame (often 1 year). This includes losses from a multiple gestation and is likely to include other deaths within the family or close friendship network. It can include other types of losses such as losing a job or being involved in a natural disaster. When losses multiply within a brief period or are stacked one on another, there is inadequate time to accomplish the grief work for one event before the next insult. This makes the coping process in subsequent losses that much more difficult, and it can even appear "pathologic." The intense feelings, the search for understanding, and the answer to "Why me?" complicate and confuse the process, making the grief work that much more difficult. These multiple losses must be identified in the nursing assessment so that appropriate interventions are created from an informed database.

SOCIOLOGIC PERSPECTIVE OF BEREAVEMENT

Rites of Passage

Transitions in human lives are acknowledged and celebrated. Society focuses attention on important events through the use of symbols and rituals referred to as *rites of passage.* Rites of passage prescribe what gifts are given, what words are spoken, and what behaviors are exhibited. The rites of greatest interest in perinatal care are those of pregnancy, birth, and death.

The rites of passage for pregnancy benefit parents and their relationship to the social group. Rites of passage such as christening, dedication of newborns, and ritual circumcisions may be performed even though parents and family members are not particularly religious. These rituals symbolize acceptance into the social group. The funeral ceremony is also a rite of passage. It is personal in its focus and societal in its consequences. The body is disposed of and the bereaved are helped through their personal shock and social reorientation. The entire societal group is provided with a method of readjusting, after the loss of a member. In effect, funeral rites tie people together through mutual support and comfort. The experience is shared, and a bond is enhanced among members of the social network.

When death occurs near the time of birth but before the community's initiation or recognition of this new life, society has not recognized the new life, and there is little recognition of the newborn's death. Many bereaved individuals in Western societies must accomplish transitions surrounding death alone, with only private symbols to assist them (Kowalski, 1984;

Parkes, 1970). A significant problem in Western society is the factor of time. The transition from bereavement to resumption of normal life in the case of perinatal loss often lasts only a couple of weeks. Friends and family may no longer ask about the welfare of the bereaved couple or demonstrate a willingness to talk about the deceased fetus or newborn.

When grief work is done without the support of the social network, it can be so painful that the individual feels that she is losing contact with reality. Support that is provided to the bereaved person is the key measure of a society's attitude about death (Stevenson, 1980). In Western societies, isolation from and lack of involvement with the bereaved are major problems. Most of the focus on grieving has been the individual's internal experience, coping with death in isolation (Stroebe & Schut, 1999).

Bereaved parents need emotional support from family and members of their social network. They need assurance that their feelings are understood and normal. If the network is to be supportive, there must be congruency in perception of the loss. For example, when no one within the network has had a newborn die or knows anyone who has, the network may be unable to provide the needed support. When members of the social network are confronted with a situation for which they have no prior experience, they often inquire within the network to discover if others have experience. Parents with strong religious beliefs may also seek comfort from their religious community, in which there is congruency and agreement in the understanding of the event.

As bereaved parents search for someone with common experience, new social relationships often occur. For example, a healthcare professional may recommend parents to a support group, or parents may search out such groups through newspaper articles or a contact from a support group member. Although more research is needed to determine what motivates the bereaved to come into groups of strangers to talk about their experience, this may occur because existing networks of the bereaved couple refuse to support the necessary healing process. It has been speculated that failure to receive appropriate support results in pathologic avoidance of the intense emotions of acute grief. Consequently, establishment of new contacts within a social network can be positive and healthy and can facilitate integration of the loss experience into a bereaved couple's lives.

Mourning

Mourning behaviors may have an evolutionary function that ensures group cohesiveness in species for which social bonding is necessary for survival. Averill (1975) indicated that the pain of separation from the social network creates stress that leads to efforts to reconnect with the network. Social acts that encourage people to reconnect were described by Darwin (1864). He observed that the outward signs of adult grief, such as facial expressions of sadness and crying, resemble the behavior of an abandoned child trying to attract the mother's attention. Just as a mother is attracted by this behavior in a child, members of a social network are attracted to bereaved persons who demonstrate sadness and crying. Consequently, the social actions that result from this attraction serve to reinforce the social group and bond its members together.

SPIRITUAL PERSPECTIVE OF BEREAVEMENT

There is variety in the spiritual perspective of bereavement. It is critical to have congruency between the grieving parents and their social network. In fundamental religious groups, in which spiritual convictions are congruent between the bereaved couple and their primary social network, the bereaved parents progress through the process in a constructive way. Many spiritual and religious systems also support the concept of an afterlife that holds the hope and the possibility of being reunited with the deceased.

Other spiritual belief systems hold possibilities for grieving families. An example of such a system is demonstrated by Dr. Steven Sunderland, who works with grieving children at Fernside Center (Warrick, 1993). Sunderland studied and uses teachings in Native American spirituality. Many Native Americans (eg, the Ojibwa elders in Canada) describe a source of healing within each person. Sunderland uses these spiritual belief systems to provide techniques for expressing fear and loss. The premise of this approach is based in Native American spirituality that posits that everyone has "medicine." Inside of every person is a healing energy that is always available and accessible. Because of these spiritual components, Sunderland perceives a grief counselor as a friend whose function is to remind the bereaved of the good in his or her own heart and to help that person bring it forth. Sunderland opens meetings with a prayer for the release of healing energy. He then asks participants and group members to consider whatever can bring them out of their pain. This kind of spiritual approach is all-encompassing, more so than many of the more structured religious doctrines in this country. What makes this most empowering is the suggestion that all of us can choose how we proceed through our life experiences.

ONTOLOGIC PERSPECTIVE OF BEREAVEMENT

An ontologic approach believes that human beings create their own reality and that reality is defined as "what is." Ontology is the science of being. *Being* is the quality or state of having existence, something that actually is. It is required of beings that they are "in the present moment" and that they spend time in the present without judgment but focused on possibilities.

Much of the science of being focuses on people's choices. We choose our responses to any given situation; this includes perinatal loss and bereavement. Most professionals have seen families who spiral downward because of their negative attitude, whereas other families choose to create as positive an approach to the tragedy as they can. In working with the bereaved from an ontologic perspective, the helper can educate about choices, about reality, about acceptance, about pain and suffering, and about forgiveness of self and others.

Such a bereavement support model, based on an ontology model, exists in Reno, Nevada, and Display 13–4 provides a course outline. This program goes a step beyond support. Healthcare professionals observe some people remaining stuck in their suffering, anger, and acting-out behavior. For those who are willing, support can be given to move lives forward. Classes in the bereavement support model in Reno are limited to 8 participants in the children's group and 15 in the adult group. Adult classes meet for 2 hours, and the children's group meets for 1.5 hours. The focus is on using the bereavement process as a facilitative event to promote personal growth in one's life.

Although bereavement groups do not work for everyone, they are exceedingly helpful for many. Research is needed to determine who may benefit most from support groups and what the actual outcomes are for those who participate.

NURSING MANAGEMENT

The professional nurse is the ideal person to plan and facilitate interventions for patients experiencing a perinatal loss. The nurse can assume a leadership role in educating other healthcare professionals and ancillary personnel who may come in contact with these families (AWHONN, 1998). The nurse has usually been with the patient and family for a significant period during the crisis period, and she or he knows the particulars of the situation and has had the opportunity to observe and make an ongoing assessment of the patient and family. The patient and family may feel close to the nurses. In the case of a stillbirth, for example, they remember how the nurses wrapped and held the baby, how respectful they were, how they supported family members to see and hold the baby, that they took pictures, and that they expressed their concern and disappointment. They also remember when nurses' actions were not so helpful. They remember the nurse who rushed from the room and abandoned them without answers to their questions, the nurse who attempted to console them or "fix" the situation with empty platitudes, and the nurse who could not take time to listen to their "story."

A desire to fix things, so prevalent in the nursing profession, can originate from a genuine desire to alleviate pain and suffering. It can also emanate from a desire to alleviate one's own discomfort about situations beyond personal control. It is essential for the nurse to explore her or his own attitudes and feelings about death and mourning in order to to care for these families. Fixing things often gains approval for the fixer. Whatever the motivating factor, in instances of perinatal loss and bereavement, the only thing that will "fix it" is for the baby to be alive and healthy. Because this is impossible, it is essential to support parents through the bereavement experience. Actions are useless unless the nurse is willing to share herself or himself with the bereaved parents at a deep, interpersonal level.

Nursing Assessment

A general assessment of the individual's emotional state includes recognition and identification of behaviors associated with acute grief. Additional assessments include the following:

- Whether the pregnancy was planned and desired
- Presence of and strength derived from a religious belief system
- Presence of supportive family and friends
- Size and types of connections within a social network
- Whether the individual or family has experienced other losses in the past 12 to 24 months
- Opportunity for and length of anticipatory grief period

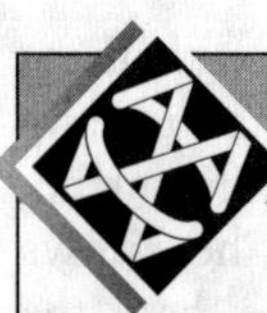

DISPLAY 13–4

Course Outline for Bereavement Support Group

Class 1	Introduction that includes sharing about each other. Discussion of a concept called *acceptance.* Understanding that the participants are in a process. The process requires work. It is not easy, and they will be in it until they decide not to be. These concepts in some form or another are reviewed each week. A distinction is made between pain and suffering. • Suffering: getting stuck in an emotion and having that emotion dominate your life • Pain: being in the process and suddenly becoming tearful The concept of judgment is discussed. Participants are discouraged from judging themselves or others.
Class 2	The focus is on shock and denial about the loss and the processes involved. Discussion focuses on what it was like at the time of the event and how each participant might still be experiencing denial.
Class 3 and 4	The focus is on anger. For example, there is a homework assignment in which participants are asked to define what anger is for them, what loss is to them, and to examine the interrelationships between the two. Participants are asked to observe how they express anger, do they do it in healthy ways? In the fourth class, examples are given of ways to deal with anger appropriately. Vocal and physical methods of reaching past the anger to the pain are explored.
Class 5	Guilt. A distinction is made between shame and guilt. The "could haves," "should haves," and "would haves" are discussed.
Class 6	Depression. The occurrence of depression is acknowledged, and the distinction between clinical depression and the depression occurring as part of the bereavement process are reviewed. The concept of accepting depression and its benefit rather than resisting is presented. It can be looked at as a "time out."
Class 7	Powerlessness. The group looks at what parts of their experience had them feel most out of control. Ways to empower themselves are then discussed.
Class 8	The last class is a summary and closing that includes reconstruction and review. The participants look at the progress made in 8 weeks and examine aspects that are easier for them now. They also look at a life without the deceased person.

From Higgins, P. Reno Bereavement Support Group.

Interventions

After careful assessment of the parents' needs and strengths, the next step is establishing priorities and nursing interventions. Physical comfort and physical support measures are necessary through the pregnancy and birth experience. Psychological support is given by the nursing staff with support for the processes through which the woman and her family are proceeding. The more families know, the better they are able to cope. The Guideline for Providing Care to the Family Experiencing Perinatal Loss and Fetal Death (AWHONN, 1998) suggests that the nurse can support grieving parents and other family members by

- Permitting the woman to make decisions about whether she will stay on the perinatal unit
- Communicating with family members that the nurse is willing to discuss the topic of death, validating rather than minimizing the reality of the pregnancy loss
- Encouraging family members and friends to be available to the parents, waiving hospital visita-

tion rules, educating them about the emotional responses of bereaved parents, and providing them with suggestions about how they can support the parents
- Ensuring that the parents receive some follow-up help after discharge, which may include telephone calls, information about support groups, home visits, or referrals for counseling

Support can be given by allowing the parents to see and hold the dead newborn and to make photographs if they so desire (Riches & Dawson, 1998). However, they should not be forced into situations they desire to avoid. Mementos of the child help in the grieving process. Allowing the parents to know that they can make choices is also beneficial. It may be helpful for the nurse to discuss with the parents how they plan to inform other family members, other children, or friends. Follow-up care should be planned carefully so that the parents are not forgotten or lost in the system. Table 13–3 lists the nursing goals and interventions used when caring for grieving families.

TABLE 13–3 ■ NURSING INTERVENTIONS FOR GRIEVING FAMILIES

Goals	Purpose	Action
Provide psychological support.	To develop a relationship of trust	Be warm and caring. Listen attentively. Exhibit unconditional positive regard. Allow for expression of positive and negative feelings. Support expression of positive and negative feelings. Respond truthfully. Keep parents informed. Minimize number of care givers to promote continuity of care.
Keep families together.	To access knowledge and beliefs about perinatal loss To evaluate congruency of beliefs between parents and other family members To determine existence of support from family and friends	Teach about bereavement process. Answer questions truthfully. Provide follow-up by hospital staff or public health nurse after discharge (ie, phone calls, home visits).
Provide all family members the opportunity to see and hold the newborn.	To create a memory so that a clear connection is made to the family	Offer the mother the option of choosing infant clothes as recognition of important mothering developmental task. Encourage but do not force parent to see and hold the newborn. Describe newborn's appearance before showing Gently bathe newborn before showing. Dress the newborn; offer mother the chance to choose the clothing. Stay with the parents at least initially while the newborn is with them. Show all newborns, even those with anomalies.

(continued)

TABLE 13–3 ■ NURSING INTERVENTIONS FOR GRIEVING FAMILIES (continued)

Goals	Purpose	Action
		Identify family characteristics that connect the newborn to the family. Determine if there are other family members who parents would like to have the opportunity see and hold the newborn, and facilitate this.
Provide photographs and other mementos.	To facilitate integration of the experience into the parent's life	Have Polaroid camera available to take instant photos. Include in the photograph anything that touched the newborn. Use 35-mm camera or commercial hospital photo service to take photos; some commercial baby picture services will provide these free. Take photo of newborn being held by parents. Save mementos in a permanent file if parents say they do not want them; most will claim them within 12 months. Give parents the usual hospital keepsakes (eg, ID bracelet, footprint record, lock of hair) and anything that may have come in contact with the newborn (eg, clothes, blanket, comb).
Provide choices.	To give parents a sense of some control over a situation that feels out of control	Identify choices and options: what hospital unit family wants to stay on, funeral and/or memorial service; who will see and hold newborn; choice to bathe and dress newborn with the RN's assistance.
Participate in hospital paper work.	To prepare parents for decision they will be asked to make	Discuss autopsy. Give death certificate information, including name. Discuss funeral arrangements and memorial service. Because these events happen rarely, have a resource book on the unit to guide personnel working with these families.
Assist parents to develop a plan for how they will tell other siblings.	To support parents in thinking through how they want to tell their other children	Encourage parents to be open and direct with children. Discourage phrases like "the baby went to sleep" or "God took the baby."

(continued)

TABLE 13–3 ■ NURSING INTERVENTIONS FOR GRIEVING FAMILIES (continued)

Goals	Purpose	Action
		Encourage parents to acknowledge with other children feelings of sadness and fear (ie, baby will be missed just as other child would be missed). Help parent place and express the death within the family's religious beliefs. Assure other children they in no way caused the baby's death.
Provide bereavement education.	To teach families about the grief process and normalize their current and future experiences	Identify phases of grief process. Provide list of area parent support groups. Discuss the emotional roller coaster. Assure parents that it is not uncommon for grief work to last 12 months or more. Help parents see that they can choose how they respond to the event (ie, suggest book on grief process). Alert parent to the thoughtless things people will say to them.
Provide for follow-up care.	To ensure ongoing assessment and support after hospital discharge	Schedule physician visits for last appointment of the day so mother can ask questions and can avoid pregnant women and newborns. Ask to go to the office on a gynecologic day; be sure to inform office staff of newborn death when making an appointment. If a support group is available at the office or clinic, try to schedule appointment to coincide. Use all available resources (eg, chaplain, social worker). Provide follow-up phone call or home visit. Prepare parents that final autopsy results may take several weeks.
Prepare for subsequent pregnancy.	To provide information parents need to consider when they begin to think about future attempts to conceive	Suggest parents wait 6 months to attempt conception. Discuss mother's need for emotional healing before conception; this helps future pregnancies to be viewed as normal as possible.

Support Groups

Because of the dichotomy between the reality of the parental experience and the societal behavior of family and friends, parents often feel a need to find support elsewhere. Consequently, in the past 15 years, groups focusing specifically on bereavement support have sprung up across the United States. Examples include hospital-based support groups, Compassionate Friends, community-based grief institutes, and Resolve Through Sharing. Parents find in these groups a supportive social network.

Two distinct types of support groups exist. One is an ongoing group, in which bereaved parents may enter or leave at will. The second type is a structured group, in which a specific number of formal classes are conducted. There are also a variety of structures within the groups. These less formal groups can be facilitated by parents or professionals. If professionals are involved, the groups can be informal and focus on facilitation or formal and focus on therapeutic interventions. In the early days of bereavement support, there was much more focus on informal groups with professionals as facilitators rather than therapists. Originally, the more informal support group participants worked very hard to improve the way healthcare was provided for bereaved parents. They produced pamphlets about issues confronting the newly bereaved, attended hospital physician and nurse staff meetings to educate professionals about the process of bereavement, and distributed information to the community.

HEALING THE HEALER

It takes great stamina and personal peace of mind to care for families experiencing perinatal loss. Nurses who find themselves working with grieving families on a regular basis need to increase their knowledge of the grief process, seek help from skilled colleagues, strive to develop strong communication skills, and recognize their own needs for personal support (Gardner, 1999). Frequently, healthcare professionals are reminded of their own future demise and of losses in their lives. Feelings of sadness and grief over personal and professional losses are often repressed. Nurses and other healthcare professionals often do what society suggests: they "get on with their lives." When losses go unacknowledged and the grief process is denied, losses begin to stack one on top of the other. Consequently, when some nurses are confronted with death, their unacknowledged feelings of failure and their own unprocessed and unacknowledged losses rise to the conscience level. When this happens, the nurse may feel out of control, tearful, and focused on issues of self. Such feelings contribute to the levels of stress that create "burn out," which results in nurses leaving particular units, types of practice, or even the profession. Nurses are not unique in these feelings and responses. Family members and friends of the grieving parents are often in similar positions.

In the process of healing themselves, professionals begin at their own level of awareness of past losses and past behavior. Usually, they make conscious decisions to add value to their own lives and to the lives of bereaved parents by focusing on growth and functioning at a higher level. Professionals commit time and energy to reading, learning, and acknowledging their own processes of loss and bereavement, as well as acquiring skills and tools to better support the bereaved. In acquiring such skills, they provide support to colleagues by demonstrating role-modeling behavior with the bereaved. Expert nurses help novice nurses and physicians to understand their own feelings and how to work with parents. Novice nurses should not be expected to work with these complex situations without prior mentored experience, direction, and role models. It is sometimes necessary for nurses to "take a break." Every perinatal nurse must recognize when he or she needs to ask to be exempt from caring for these families. At the same time, they are responsible for ensuring that qualified persons do assume responsibility for the care of these families.

Professionals can gain more experience and understanding by attending workshops on bereavement support and death and dying. Grief institutes and other relevant workshops and learning experiences focused on adult growth and development can also help. Additional insights into human behavior can support new attitudes and belief systems about involvement with the bereaved. The skills needed to assess and understand families in these crisis situations should be part of the areas of nursing competence used for performance evaluation. Nurses working in complex bereavement situations in pediatric intensive care, neonatal intensive care, and high-risk obstetrics can also be helped by skilled members of the chaplain corps, social work, or psychiatric department. This kind of support for the nursing staff allows them to increase their capacity for compassionate care.

SUMMARY

Providing compassionate care to patients and their families during perinatal loss requires patience, understanding of self and others, and a willingness to examine each painful episode while learning and growing from the experience. These painful events are an opportunity to make a difference for women and families. The nurse, who is the pivotal care provider and the person who spends the most time with the family, is the ideal person to plan, organize, coordinate, and provide care to grieving families. The more nurses understand the many perspectives of loss and bereavement and the more nurses understand their own behavior, the more effective they will be for themselves, their patients, and their peers. When nurses intervene using knowledge and skills gleaned from the perspectives of psychology, sociology, spirituality and ontology, parents feel cared for, understood, and supported.

REFERENCES

Arnold, J., & Gemma, P. (1994). *A child dies: A portrait of family grief.* Philadelphia: The Charles Press Publishers.

Association of Women's Health, Obstetric & Neonatal Nurses. (1998). *Standards and guidelines for professional nursing practice in the care of women and newborns* (5th ed., pp. 20–22). Washington, DC: Author.

Averill, J. (1975). *Grief: Its nature and experience.* Chapel Hill, NC: Health Sciences.

Benoliel, J. Q. (1997). Loss and bereavement: Perspectives, theories, challenges. *Canadian Journal of Nursing Research, 29*(4), 11–20.

Copley, M. F., & Bodensteiner, J. B. (1987). Chronic sorrow in families of disabled children. *Journal of Child Neurology, 2*(1), 67–70.

Darwin, C. (1864). *A concordance to Darwin's: The expression of the emotions in man and animals.* Barret, NY: Cornell University.

Freud, S. (1937). Mourning and melancholia. In *The standard edition of the complete psychological works of Sigmund Freud* (Vol. 14). London: Hogarth.

Gardner, J. M. (1999). Perinatal death: Uncovering the needs of midwives and nurses and exploring helpful interventions in the United States, England, and Japan. *The Journal of Transcultural Nursing, 10*(2), 120–130.

Greil, A. L. (1997). Infertility and psychological distress: A critical review of the literature. *Social Science and Medicine, 54*(11), 679–704.

Hirsch, A. M., & Hirsch, S. M. (1995). The long-term psychosocial effects of infertility. *Journal of Obstetrics, Gynecological and Neonatal Nursing, 24*(6), 517–522.

Hutti, M. H. (1992). Parents' perceptions of the miscarriage experience. *Death Studies, 16,* 401–415.

Kowalski, K. (1984). *Perinatal death: An ethnomethodological study of factors influencing parental bereavement.* Unpublished doctoral dissertation, University of Colorado, Boulder.

Kowalski, K. (1985). The impact of chronic grief. *American Journal of Nursing, 85*(4), 398–399.

Kowalski, K. (1987). Perinatal loss and bereavement. In L. Sonstegard, K. Kowalski, & B. Jennings (Eds.), *Women's health: Crisis and illness in child bearing.* Orlando, FL: Grune & Stratton.

Krafft, S., & Krafft, L. (1998). Chronic sorrow: Parents' lived experience. *Holistic Nursing Practice, 13*(1), 59–67.

Lattanzi, M. E. (1983). Professional stress: Adaptation, coping and meaning. In J. C. Hansen & T. T. Frantz (Eds.), *Death and grief in the family.* Rockville, MD: Aspen Systems.

Lindemann, E. (1994). Symptomatology and management of acute grief. *American Journal of Psychiatry, 151*(6, Suppl.), 155–160.

Lindgren, C. L., Burke, M. L., Hainsworth, M. A., & Eakes, G. G. (1992). Chronic sorrow: A lifespan concept. *Scholarly Inquiry for Nursing Practice, 6*(1), 27–40.

Maris, P. (1974). *Loss and change.* New York: Pantheon.

Mosher, W. D., & Pratt, W. F. (1991). Fecundity and infertility in the United States: Incidence and trends. *Fertility and Sterility, 56*(2), 192–193.

Olshansky, S. (1966). Parent responses to a mentally defective child. *Mental Retardation, 4*(4), 21–23.

Parkes, C. M. (1970). The first year of bereavement: A longitudinal study of the reaction of London widows to the death of their husbands. *Psychiatry, 33*(4), 444–467.

Peppers, L. G., & Knapp, R. S. (1980). *Motherhood and mourning: Perinatal death.* New York: Praeger.

Peretz, D. (1970a). Development, object-relationships and loss. In B. Schoenberg, A. C. Karr, D. Peretz, & A. H. Kutscher (Eds.), *Loss and grief: Psychological management in medical practice.* New York: Columbia University Press.

Peretz, D. (1970b). Reaction to loss. In B. Schoenberg, A. C. Karr, D. Peretz, & A. H. Kutscher (Eds.), *Loss and grief: Psychological management in medical practice.* New York: Columbia University Press.

Pincus, L. (1974). *Death and the family: The importance of mourning.* New York: Pantheon.

Pisarska, M. D., & Carson, S. A. (1999). Ectopic pregnancy. In J. R. Scott, P. J. DiSaia, C. B. Hammond & W. N. Spellacy (Eds.), *Danforth's obstetrics and gynecology* (8th ed., pp. 155–172). Philadelphia: Lippincott, Williams & Wilkins.

Riches, G., & Dawson, P. (1998). Lost children, living memories: The role of photographs in processes of grief and adjustment among bereaved parents. *Death Studies, 22*(2), 121–140.

Robinson, M., Baker, L., & Nackerud, L. (1999). The relationship of attachment theory and perinatal loss. *Death Studies, 23*(3), 257–270.

Statham, H., & Green, J. M. (1994). The effects of miscarriage and other unsuccessful pregnancies on feelings early in a subsequent pregnancy. *Journal of Reproductive and Infant Psychology, 12,* 45–54.

Stevenson, K. M. (1980). *Parental utilization and perceptions of helpful social networks following a sudden infant death.* Unpublished doctoral dissertation, University of Washington, Seattle.

Stritzinger, R. M., Robinson, G. E., & Stewart, D. E. (1999). Parameters of grieving in spontaneous abortion. *International Journal of Psychiatry in Medicine, 29*(2), 235–249.

Stroebe, M., & Schut, H. (1999). The dual process model of coping with bereavement: Rationale and description. *Death Studies, 23*(3), 197–224.

Teel, C. S. (1991). Chronic sorrow: Analysis of the concept. *Journal of Advanced Nursing, 16*(11), 1311–1319.

Warrick, C. (1993). Healing Native American spirituality helps kids deal with grief: Interview with Steve Sunderland. *Cincinnati Post, March 16,* 1B.

Williams, G. (2000). Grief after elective abortion. *AWHONN Lifelines, 4*(2), 37–40.

PART 5

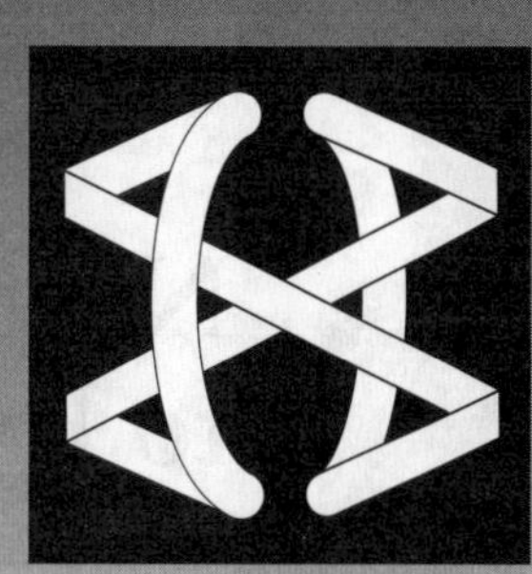

THE NEWBORN

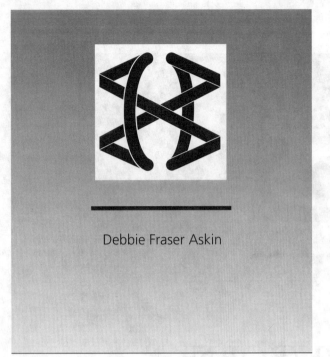

Debbie Fraser Askin

CHAPTER 14

Newborn Adaptation to Extrauterine Life

Transition from fetal to newborn life is a critical period involving diverse physiologic changes. Hemodynamic and thermoregulatory mechanisms promote successful adaptation to the extrauterine environment. This chapter focuses on the maternal history influencing adaptation and physiologic changes during the early newborn period. Nursing assessment and interventions during transition, such as resuscitative needs and interventions facilitating maternal–newborn attachment, also are presented.

INFLUENCE OF MATERNAL HISTORY

Maternal medical and obstetric conditions influence newborn adaptation to extrauterine life. A thorough review of the mother's prenatal and intrapartum history is essential to identify factors with the potential to compromise successful transition. Table 14–1 lists the maternal risk factors and associated fetal and neonatal complications. In addition to identification of current pregnancy complications, it is important to review the obstetric history. Conditions that predispose the newborn to risk may recur in subsequent pregnancies (Display 14–1). Intrapartum risk factors may also influence adaptation (Table 14–2).

Intrapartum fetal assessment provides important data about the fetal response to labor. Electronic fetal heart rate (FHR) monitoring or intermittent auscultation provides documentation of fetal well-being. Requisite perinatal nursing skills include knowledge of the physiologic basis for monitoring, an understanding of FHR patterns, and the initiation of appropriate nursing interventions based on data from the monitor or from auscultation. The FHR reflects the fetal response to labor. The perinatal nurse focuses on discriminating between reassuring and nonreassuring patterns. If the FHR pattern is nonreassuring, intrauterine resuscitation procedures such as maternal position change, oxygen therapy, and intravenous fluids are initiated. Oxytocin should be decreased or discontinued if infusing, or the next dose of Prepidil, Cervidil, or Cytotec should be delayed. Safe passage through the labor and birth process sets the stage for successful transition to extrauterine life.

PHYSIOLOGIC CHANGES DURING TRANSITION

The respiratory, cardiovascular, thermoregulatory, and immunologic systems undergo significant physiologic changes and adaptations during transition from fetal to neonatal life. Successful transition requires a complex interaction between these systems.

Respiratory Adaptations

Critical to the neonate's transition to extrauterine life is the establishment of respiration as lungs become the organ of gas exchange after separation from maternal uteroplacental circulation. Initiation of breathing is a complex phenomena that depends on chemical and sensory stimulation of the respiratory center in the brain and mechanical stimulation of the lung. Pulmonary blood flow, surfactant production, and respiratory musculature also influence respiratory adaptation to extrauterine life. Establishment of inde-

TABLE 14–1 ■ MATERNAL RISK FACTORS AND POTENTIAL FETAL AND NEONATAL COMPLICATIONS

Risk Factors	Potential Complications
Maternal Substance Abuse	
Drug addiction	Small for gestational age (SGA); neonatal abstinence syndrome; neonatal human immunodeficiency virus (HIV)
Alcoholism	Fetal alcohol syndrome
Smoking	SGA; polycythemia
Maternal nutritional status	
Maternal weight <100 lb	SGA
Maternal weight >200 lb	SGA; large for gestational age (LGA)
Maternal Medical Complication	
Hereditary CNS disorders	Inherited central nervous system (CNS) disorder
Seizure disorders requiring medication	Congenital anomalies (e.g., result of medication [Dilantin] use)
Chronic hypertension	Intrauterine growth restriction (IUGR); asphyxia; SGA
Congenital heart disease with congestive heart failure	Preterm birth; inherited cardiac defects
Anemia <10 g	Preterm birth; low birth weight
Sickle cell disease	IUGR; fetal demise
Hemoglobinopathies	IUGR; inherited hemoglobinopathies
Idiopathic thrombocytopenic purpura (ITP)	Transient ITP
Chronic glomerulonephritis, renal insufficiency	IUGR; SGA; preterm birth; asphyxia
Recurrent urinary tract infection	Preterm birth
Uterine malformation	Preterm birth; fetal malposition
Cervical incompetence	Preterm birth
Diabetes	LGA; hypoglycemia & hypocalcemia; anomalies; respiratory distress syndrome
Thyroid disease	Hypothyroidism; CNS defects; hyperthyroidism; goiter
Current Pregnancy Complications	
Pregnancy induced hypertension	IUGR; SGA
TORCH infections	IUGR; SGA; active infection; anomalies
Sexually transmitted diseases	Ophthalmia neonatorum; congenital syphilis
Hepatitis	Hepatitis
AIDS or HIV seropositive	Neonatal HIV
Multiple gestation	Preterm birth; asphyxia; IUGR; SGA
Fetal malposition	Prolapsed cord; asphyxia; birth trauma
Rh sensitization	Erythroblastosis fetalis
Prolonged pregnancy	Postmaturity; meconium aspiration; IUGR; asphyxia
Intraamniotic infection	Newborn sepsis; preterm birth
Group B streptococcal infection	Newborn sepsis; preterm birth

pendent breathing and oxygen–carbon dioxide exchange depends on these physiologic factors.

Chemical Stimuli

The fetus during labor and birth experiences mild, transitory physiologic stress. This normal response occurs because of a temporary interruption in umbilical blood flow during uterine contractions and ultimately when the umbilical cord is clamped. Decreased oxygen concentration, increased carbon dioxide concentration, and a decrease in pH stimulate fetal aortic and carotid chemoreceptors, triggering the respiratory center in the medulla to initiate respiration (Nelson, 1999).

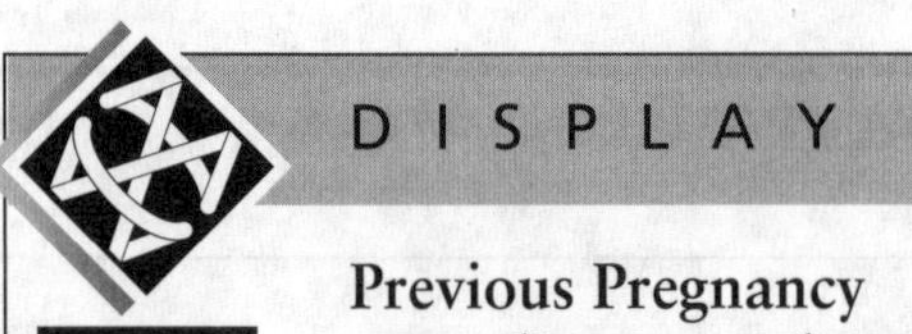

DISPLAY 14–1

Previous Pregnancy Complications That May Recur in Subsequent Pregnancies

Fetal loss beyond 28 weeks' gestation
Preterm birth
Abnormal fetal position or presentation
Bleeding in second or third trimester
Rh sensitization
Fetal compromise of unknown origin
Birth of newborn with anomalies
Birth of newborn weighing more than 10 lb
Birth of postterm newborn
Neonatal death

Mechanical Stimulation

In utero, the fetal lungs are filled with fluid. Mechanical compression of the chest during vaginal birth forces approximately one third of this fluid out of fetal lungs. As the chest is delivered through the birth canal, it reexpands, creating negative pressure and drawing air into the lungs. This passive inspiration of air replaces fluid that previously filled the alveoli. Further expansion and distribution of air throughout the alveoli occurs when the newborn cries. Crying creates a positive intrathoracic pressure that keeps alveoli open and forces the remaining fetal lung fluid into pulmonary capillaries and the lymphatic circulation.

Sensory Stimuli

The newborn is exposed to numerous tactile, visual, auditory, and olfactory stimuli during and immediately after birth. Tactile stimulation begins in utero as the fetus experiences uterine contractions and descent through the pelvis and birth canal. Stimulation to initiate breathing continues after birth as the neonate is exposed to stimuli such as light, sound, touch, smell, and pain. Vigorously drying the newborn immediately after birth is a significant tactile stimulation.

Contributing Factors

Maturation of Alveoli

Newborn lungs contain approximately 50 million alveoli. These terminal air sacs grow in size and number, reaching approximately 300 million during childhood and early adult years (Hanson & Corbet, 1998). Structural characteristics of alveoli unique to the newborn period influence oxygenation and carbon dioxide transport. During the newborn period, the small size and limited number of alveoli decrease the alveolar surface area available for gas exchange.

Pulmonary Blood Flow

In utero, the placenta is the organ of gas exchange for the fetus. Oxygenated blood is delivered from the placenta through the umbilical vein, through the ductus venosus into the inferior vena cava, and ultimately to the right side of the fetal heart. Oxygenated blood is diverted away from pulmonary circulation in utero and instead flows through the foramen ovale and ductus arteriosus to the fetal body.

The fluid-filled lungs of the fetus create a state of alveolar hypoxia. Fetal pulmonary arterioles, which are very sensitive to oxygen, have thick musculature because of low oxygen tension in utero (Loper, 1997). This results in constriction of pulmonary arterioles, which causes increased pulmonary vascular resistance (PVR) and decreased pulmonary blood flow. After birth, pulmonary blood flow is established as PVR decreases with normal changes in arterial PO_2, alveolar PO_2, acid–base status, and absence of vasoactive substances such as prostaglandin and bradykinin. After the onset of breathing, fluid in the lungs is replaced by air. Because oxygen is a potent vasodilator, pulmonary vasodilatation occurs. Adequate pulmonary blood flow is crucial for newborn gas exchange.

Surfactant Production

Pulmonary surfactant is necessary to maintain expanded alveoli. Surfactant lowers surface tension, preventing alveolar collapse during inspiration and expiration. By approximately 34 to 36 weeks' gestation, there is adequate surfactant production to support respiration and protect against development of respiratory distress syndrome (Hagedorn, Gardner, & Abman, 1998). Surfactant deficiency results in atelectasis and requires greater than normal breathing efforts. Oxygen and metabolic needs increase as the newborn must use more energy to maintain respirations. Preterm newborns are at high risk for surfactant deficiency, which may significantly jeopardize respiratory adaptation to extrauterine life.

Respiratory Musculature

Intercostal muscles support the rib cage and assist with inspiration by creating negative intrathoracic pressure. Intercostal muscles may not be fully devel-

TABLE 14–2 ■ INTRAPARTUM RISK FACTORS AND POTENTIAL FETAL AND NEONATAL COMPLICATIONS

Risk Factors	Potential Complications
Umbilical Cord	
Prolapsed umbilical cord	Asphyxia
True knot in cord	Asphyxia
Velamentous insertion	Intrauterine blood loss; shock; anemia
Vasa previa	Intrauterine blood loss; shock; anemia
Rupture or tearing of cord	Blood loss; shock; anemia
Membranes	
Premature rupture of membranes	Infection; respiratory distress syndrome; prolapsed cord; asphyxia
Prolonged rupture of membranes	Infection
Amnionitis	Infection
Amniotic Fluid	
Oligohydramnios	Congenital anomalies
Polyhydramnios	Congenital anomalies; prolapsed cord
Meconium-stained fluid	Asphyxia; meconium aspiration syndrome
Placenta	
Placenta previa	Preterm birth; asphyxia
Abruptio placenta	Preterm birth; asphyxia
Placental insufficiency	Intrauterine growth restriction; small for gestational age; asphyxia
Abnormal Fetal Presentations	
Breech birth	Asphyxia; birth injuries (CNS, skeletal)
Face or brow presentation	Asphyxia; facial trauma
Transverse lie	Asphyxia; birth injuries; cesarean birth; umbilical cord prolapse
Birth Complications	
Forceps-assisted birth	CNS trauma; cephalhematoma; asphyxia; facial trauma
Vacuum extraction	Cephalhematoma
Manual version or extraction	Asphyxia; birth trauma; prolapsed cord
Shoulder dystocia	Asphyxia; brachial plexus injury; fractured clavicle
Precipitous birth	Asphyxia; birth trauma (CNS)
Undiagnosed multiple gestation	Asphyxia; birth trauma
Administration of Drugs	
Oxytocin	Complications of uterine hyperstimulation (asphyxia)
Magnesium sulfate	Hypermagnesemia; CNS depression
Analgesics	CNS and respiratory depression
Anesthetics	CNS and respiratory depression; bradycardia

oped at birth, increasing risk of respiratory compromise by increasing breathing effort.

Cardiovascular Adaptations

Transition from fetal to neonatal circulation is a major cardiovascular change and occurs simultaneously with respiratory system adaptation. To appreciate hemodynamic changes, an understanding of structural and blood-flow differences between fetal and neonatal circulation is necessary. Figure 14–1 illustrates fetal circulation. Also influencing the cardiovascular system are physiologic changes in the vasculature. Decreased PVR, resulting in increased pulmonary blood flow, and increased systemic vascular resistance (SVR) control cardiovascular changes.

Fetal Circulation

In utero, oxygenated blood flows to the fetus from the placenta through the umbilical vein. Although a small amount of oxygenated blood is delivered to the liver,

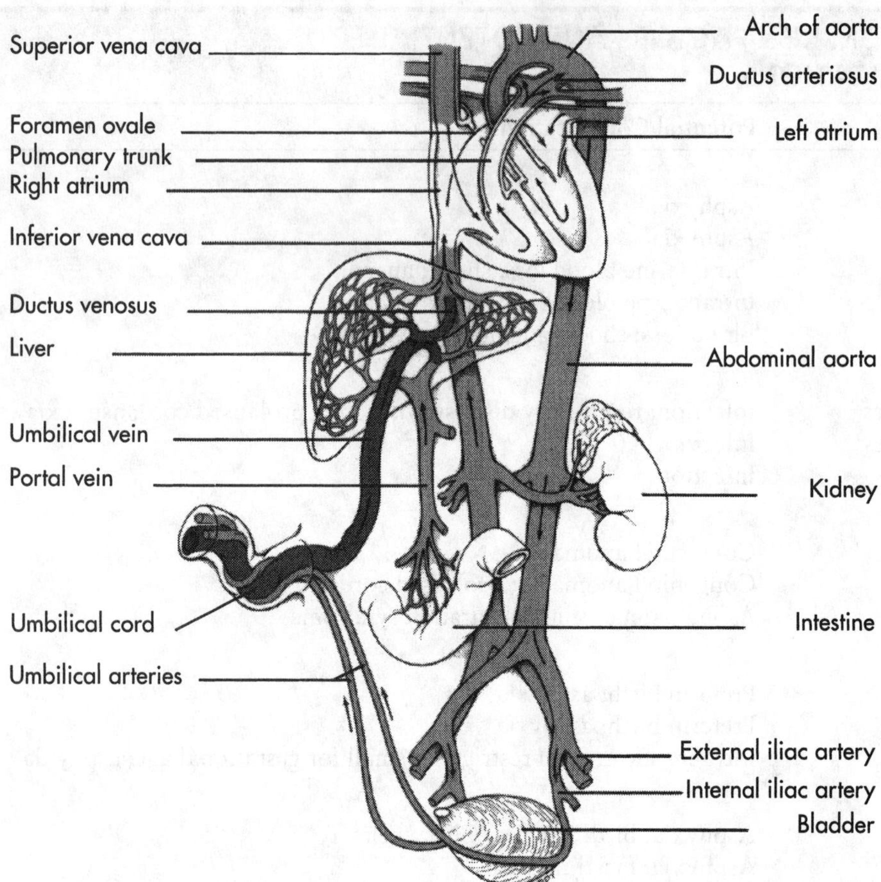

FIGURE 14–1. Fetal circulation.

most blood bypasses the hepatic system through the ductus venosus. The ductus venosus is a vascular structure that forms a connection between the umbilical vein and the inferior vena cava. Oxygenated blood from the vena cava enters the right atrium, and most of it is directed through the foramen ovale to the left atrium, then to the left ventricle, and on to the aorta. The foramen ovale is a flaplike structure between the right and left atria. Blood flows through the foramen ovale because pressure in the right atrium is greater than the left atrium because of the high PVR.

The superior vena cava drains deoxygenated blood from the head and upper extremities into the right atrium, where it mixes with oxygenated blood. A small amount of blood in the right atrium is directed into the right ventricle and pulmonary artery. This blood circulates to lung tissue to meet metabolic needs. Because of the high PVR in fetal lungs, most of the blood in the right atrium is diverted through the ductus arteriosus, a vascular connection between the pulmonary artery and the aorta. This mixture of oxygenated and deoxygenated blood continues through the descending aorta and eventually drains back to the placenta through the umbilical arteries.

Neonatal Circulation

During fetal life, the placenta is an organ of low vascular resistance. Clamping the umbilical cord at birth eliminates the placenta as a reservoir for blood, causing a rise in blood pressure and SVR. Blood returns to the heart through the inferior and superior vena cavae. It enters the right atrium to the right ventricle and travels through the pulmonary artery to the pulmonary vascular bed. Oxygenated blood returns through pulmonary veins to the left atrium, the left ventricle, and through the aorta to systemic circulation. For successful transition from fetal to newborn circulation, structures specific to fetal circulation must cease functioning.

At birth, when the pulmonary vascular bed dilates, there is increased blood flow to the lungs, and pressure in the right atrium falls. The increased pulmonary venous return to the left atrium and less blood flow into the right atrium causes the left atrial pressure to exceed the pressure in the right atrium, resulting in functional closure of the foramen ovale (Loper, 1997; Sansoucie & Cavaliere, 1997). After closure, blood is directed from the right atrium to the right ventricle, rather than through the foramen ovale.

In utero, shunting of blood from the pulmonary artery through the ductus arteriosus to the aorta occurs as a result of high PVR. After birth, SVR rises and PVR falls, causing a reversal of blood flow through the ductus. The major contributing factor to closure of the ductus arteriosus is sensitivity to rising arterial oxygen concentrations in the blood (Bloom, 1996). As the PaO_2 level increases after birth, the ductus arteriosus begins to constrict. In utero, elevated prostaglandin levels helped maintain ductal patency. Removal of the placenta decreases prostaglandin levels, further influencing closure (McCollum, 1998).

Constriction of the ductus arteriosus is a gradual process, permitting bidirectional shunting of blood after birth. PVR may be higher than the SVR, allowing some degree of right-to-left shunting, until the SVR rises above PVR and blood flow is directed left to right. In healthy, term newborns, right-to-left shunting can persist for up to 12 hours of life; however, 82% of these newborns have a closed or closing ductus arteriosus by 48 hours of life (Sansoucie & Cavaliere, 1997). Permanent anatomic closure of the ductus arteriosus occurs within 3 weeks to 3 months of age. Any clinical situation that causes hypoxia, with pulmonary vasoconstriction and subsequent increased PVR, potentiates right-to-left shunting (Lott, 1998).

When the umbilical cord is clamped, blood flow through the umbilical vein to the ductus venosus ceases. Systemic venous blood flow is then directed through the portal system for hepatic circulation. Umbilical vessels constrict, with functional closure occurring immediately. Fibrous infiltration leading to anatomic closure occurs at about 1 to 2 weeks of life (Lott, 1998).

Relationship Between Respiratory and Cardiovascular Adaptation

Successful initiation of respirations and transition from fetal to neonatal circulation is essential to maintain life after birth. Conditions that lead to sustained elevated PVR such as hypoxia, acidosis, sepsis, or congenital heart defects can interrupt the normal sequence of events. Closure of fetal shunts depends on oxygenation and pressure changes within the cardiovascular system. Shunt closure occurs only if PVR drops with the onset of respiration and subsequent oxygenation. The pulmonary vascular bed is very reactive to low oxygen levels. If the neonate experiences significant hypoxia, PVR with resultant decreased pulmonary blood flow and right-to-left shunting across the foramen ovale and ductus arteriosus may occur. These events potentiate a state of hypoxia as deoxygenated blood bypasses the lungs through the patent fetal shunts to be mixed with oxygenated blood entering the systemic circulation. A vicious cycle known as persistent pulmonary hypertension of the newborn (PPHN) results, necessitating aggressive cardiorespiratory support.

Thermoregulation

The newborn's ability to maintain temperature control after birth is limited by external environmental factors and internal physiologic processes. Characteristics of newborns that predispose them to heat loss include a large body surface area in relation to body mass and a limited amount of subcutaneous fat. Newborns attempt to regulate body temperature by nonshivering thermogenesis, increased metabolic rate, and increased muscle activity. Peripheral vasoconstriction also decreases heat loss to the skin surface. Mechanisms of heat loss, including evaporation, conduction, convection, and radiation, play an integral part in newborn adaptation to extrauterine life. Nursing care is critical in supporting thermoregulation through ongoing assessments and environmental interventions to decrease heat loss.

Mechanisms of Heat Production

Nonshivering Thermogenesis

Newborns generate heat through nonshivering thermogenesis. Heat is produced by metabolism of brown fat, a unique process present only in newborns. This highly vascular adipose tissue is located in the neck, scapula, axilla, mediastinum, and around kidneys and adrenal glands. Production of brown fat begins around 26 to 28 weeks' gestation and continues for 3 to 5 weeks after birth (Konrad & Norton, 1998; Noerr, 1997). When exposed to cold stress, thermal receptors in skin transmit messages to the central nervous system, activating the sympathetic nervous system and triggering metabolism of brown fat (Amlung, 1998). Preterm newborns, with smaller stores of brown fat, have decreased ability to generate heat. Instead, they rely on increased oxygen consumption and muscle activity to increase metabolic rate and produce heat (Roncoli & Medoff-Cooper, 1992).

Voluntary Muscle Activity

Heat produced through voluntary muscle activity is minimal in the newborn. Flexion of the extremities and maintaining a fetal position decreases heat loss to the environment. Term newborns have the ability to maintain this flexed posture, whereas preterm and compromised newborns may lack the muscle tone for this posturing, making them more vulnerable to cold stress (Amlung, 1998).

Mechanisms of Heat Loss

Evaporation

Evaporation and heat loss occur as water (ie, amniotic fluid) on skin is converted to a vapor. Drying the newborn immediately after birth and removing wet blankets decreases evaporative losses and prevents further cooling of the skin. The amount of insensible water loss from the skin is inversely related to gestational age. Skin of a preterm newborn is more susceptible to evaporative losses, because the keratin layer of the skin has not matured. Absence or greater permeability of this skin layer allows increased heat loss (Blake & Murray, 1998). The larger the surface area, the greater are the evaporative losses, and the more heat is lost. Because the newborn's head is the largest surface area of the body, covering the head with a knit cap after birth when not under the radiant warmer greatly conserves heat. Under radiant heat, the cap prevents the heat from reaching the newborn and may contribute to cold stress. Adding humidity to the environment may also decrease evaporative heat loss.

Conduction

Conductive heat loss occurs when two solid objects of different temperatures come in contact. Heat loss occurs if the newborn is placed in direct contact with a cold scale, mattress, x-ray plate, or blanket. Mechanisms for preventing conductive heat loss in the birthing room and immediately after birth include using a preheated radiant warmer, using warm blankets for drying, and covering scales and x-ray plates with warm blankets. Preheating the radiant warmer is necessary, because it may take 15 to 30 minutes to warm the mattress.

Providing skin-to-skin contact between mother and newborn after birth helps prevent conductive heat loss and enhances maternal–newborn attachment. Newborns who experience extended periods of skin-to-skin contact beginning soon after birth demonstrate heart rates, respiratory rates, and oxygen saturation levels within normal limits (Ludington-Hoe et al., 1993). Preterm newborns provided with opportunities for skin-to-skin contact with their mothers maintained their temperature, demonstrated normal vital signs, had increased episodes of deep sleep and alert inactivity, cried less, had no increase in infection rates, and had greater weight gain, longer breast-feeding periods, and earlier discharge (Gale & VandenBerg, 1998).

Convection

Convection is the transfer of heat from a solid object to surrounding air. Heat is lost from newborn skin as cooler air passes over it. Convection heat loss depends on the amount of exposed skin surface, temperature of air, and amount of air turbulence created by drafts. Interventions that prevent convection heat loss in the newborn include clothing, eliminating source of drafts, and when necessary, providing heated, humidified oxygen through a face mask or hood (Noerr, 1997).

Radiation

Radiation heat loss occurs when heat is transferred between two objects not in contact with each other. The newborn loses heat by radiation to nearby cooler surfaces such as those of the crib, Isolette, windows, or other objects. Some of the more common and efficient methods for preventing radiant heat loss are use of a radiant warmer after birth, moving the crib or Isolette away from a cold window, and use of a heat shield inside an incubator (for small, preterm newborns), creating an additional warmer barrier between skin and incubator wall.

Effects of Cold Stress

Thermal management of the newborn during the first few hours of life is critical to prevent detrimental effects of cold stress and hypothermia. Table 14–3 summarizes nursing interventions that support the newborn and prevent cold stress. Because heat production requires oxygen consumption and glucose use, persistent hypothermia may deplete these stores, leading to metabolic acidosis, hypoglycemia, decreased surfactant production, increased caloric requirements, and if chronic, impaired weight gain (Noerr, 1997). This process is illustrated in Figure 14–2.

Immune System Adaptation

Newborns are vulnerable to infection because of their immature immune system and lack of exposure to organisms. Neonates depend on passive immunity acquired from their mother transplacentally through active transport of IgG during the third trimester (Cole, 1998). Preterm newborns are at greater risk for infection because they may not have received this passive immunity and because their immune mechanisms are overall more immature (Lott & Kenner, 1998).

TABLE 14–3 ■ MECHANISMS OF HEAT LOSS AND NURSING INTERVENTIONS THAT PREVENT COLD STRESS

Type of Heat Loss	Nursing Interventions
Evaporation	Dry infant thoroughly Remove wet linen Place knit cap on infant's head when not under radiant warmer Bathe infant under radiant heat source after temperature stabilizes
Convection	Move infant away from drafts, open windows, vents, and traffic patterns When necessary, use humidified, warmed oxygen Avoid using ceiling fans in birthing room Move infant in prewarmed transport Isolette
Conduction	Preheat radiant warmer Place infant skin-to-skin with mother Use warmed blanket Warm stethoscope and your hands Place cover between newborn and metal scale or x-ray plate
Radiation	Place stabilizing unit on an interior wall of the birthing room (away from cold windows) Preheat radiant warmer or transport Isolette

Immunity is conferred through immunoglobulins, antibodies secreted by lymphocytes and plasma cells. There are three main classes of immunoglobulins responsible for immunity: IgG, IgA, and IgM. Because of their small molecular size, only IgG antibodies are capable of crossing the placenta. Maternally transmitted IgG provides protection for the newborn against bacterial and viral infections for which the mother already has antibodies (eg, diphtheria, tetanus, smallpox, measles, mumps, poliomyelitis).

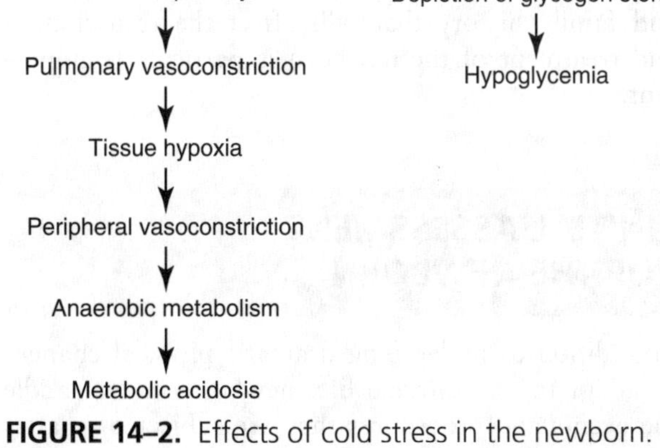

Cold
↓
Activation of Nonshivering Thermogenesis (Metabolism of Brown Fat)
↓
Increased oxygen consumption → Increased respiratory rate → Pulmonary vasoconstriction → Tissue hypoxia → Peripheral vasoconstriction → Anaerobic metabolism → Metabolic acidosis

Increased glucose use → Depletion of glycogen stores → Hypoglycemia

FIGURE 14–2. Effects of cold stress in the newborn.

IgM and IgA immunoglobulins do not cross the placenta. If elevated levels of IgM are found in the newborn, it may indicate the presence of an intrauterine infection such as one of the TORCH agents (ie, *Toxoplasma gondii* [toxoplasmosis]; other agents such as *Treponema pallidum* [syphilis], varicella virus, human immunodeficiency virus, and *Chlamydia*; rubella virus; cytomegalovirus; and herpesvirus). IgA, found in colostrum, is thought to contribute to passive immunity for newborns who are breast-fed (Riordan, 1998).

Immature leukocyte function in the newborn inhibits the ability to destroy pathogens. Deficiency in response prevents mature processes of chemotaxis (ie, movement of leukocytes toward site of infection), opsonization (ie, altering or preparing the cells for ingestion), and phagocytosis (ie, ingestion of cells) from occurring. Low levels of immunoglobulins and complement components (ie, plasma proteins that assist the immune system) leaves newborns, especially preterm newborns, vulnerable to infection (Lott & Kenner, 1998).

Lymphocytes are responsible for the specific response in the immune system that involves antibody production. When lymphocytes are exposed to pathogens, they become sensitized to them. If repeated exposure occurs, lymphocytes will attempt to destroy the pathogen. Because newborns lack exposure to most common organisms, any action by lymphocytes is delayed.

Weak newborn defenses against infection make it imperative for the perinatal nurse and anyone coming in contact with newborns to follow careful handwashing practices and to use aseptic technique. Promoting skin integrity is essential for preventing neonatal infections. Newborn skin is thin and delicate, making it susceptible to alterations in integrity. Fetal scalp electrodes, fetal scalp pH sampling, and skin abrasions create portals for the entry of organisms. Umbilical cord and circumcision sites are also potential sites of infection.

Preterm newborns, with even more fragile skin, are at a greater risk for infection. Invasive procedures, performed during the early hours after birth, further challenge the immune system. Treatments such as vitamin K injection, suctioning, and heel-stick blood samples predispose newborns to infection if proper aseptic technique is not maintained.

STABILIZATION AND RESUSCITATION OF THE NEWBORN

Although most births result in a healthy newborn able to make the transition to extrauterine life without difficulty, perinatal nurses must anticipate and prepare for complications. This includes ensuring immediate availability of functioning resuscitation equipment and knowledge of equipment operation. An International Liaison Committee on Resuscitation (ILCOR) and the American Academy of Pediatrics (AAP) recommend that someone trained in neonatal resuscitation be available for all births (ILCOR, 1999). Display 14–2 identifies equipment that should be available in every birthing room.

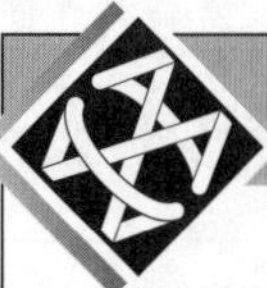

DISPLAY 14–2

Equipment Needed For Neonatal Resuscitation

- Clock with second hand
- Preheated radiant warmer
- Warmed blankets
- Neonatal stethoscope
- Bulb syringe
- Mechanical suction with manometer
- Oxygen source, flowmeter, tubing
- Resuscitation bag capable of delivering 100% oxygen and pressure gauge
- Face masks (newborn and preemie size)
- Laryngoscope with size 0 and 1 blades (extra batteries and bulbs)
- Endotracheal tubes (sizes 2.5 mm, 3.0 mm, 3.5 mm, and 4.0 mm)
- Suction catheters (sizes 5 Fr, 8 Fr, and 10 Fr)
- Meconium aspirator device
- 8 Fr feeding tube
- Syringes (sizes 1, 3, 5, 10, and 20 mL)
- Cord clamp
- Tape
- Resuscitative drugs
  - Epinephrine 1:10,000 concentration
  - Sodium bicarbonate (4.2%)
  - Naloxone hydrochloride (1 mg/mL or 0.4 mg/mL)
  - Volume expanders
    - 5% Albumin
    - Normal saline solution
    - Lactated Ringer's solution

The Neonatal Resuscitation program developed by the American Heart Association and the AAP (AHA & AAP, 2000) has become the standard for educating healthcare providers involved in newborn stabilization. Assessments and interventions during newborn resuscitation are clearly outlined in an algorithm. Figure 14–3 illustrates steps used to evaluate and establish airway, breathing, and circulation as a basis for stabilization of the newborn immediately after birth. Although most newborns respond successfully to oral suctioning and tactile stimulation, 5% to 10% may require additional interventions, including ventilation by bag and mask or endotracheal intubation, chest compressions, and administration of resuscitative medications (ILCOR, 1999).

Good communication among health team members is essential in anticipating and preparing for high-risk births. Communicating the details of the maternal and family history that will affect the resuscitation and treatment of the newborn is particularly important.

INITIAL ASSESSMENT OF THE NEWBORN

In addition to undergoing dramatic physical changes to adapt to extrauterine life, newborns must handle the events and procedures they are subjected to after

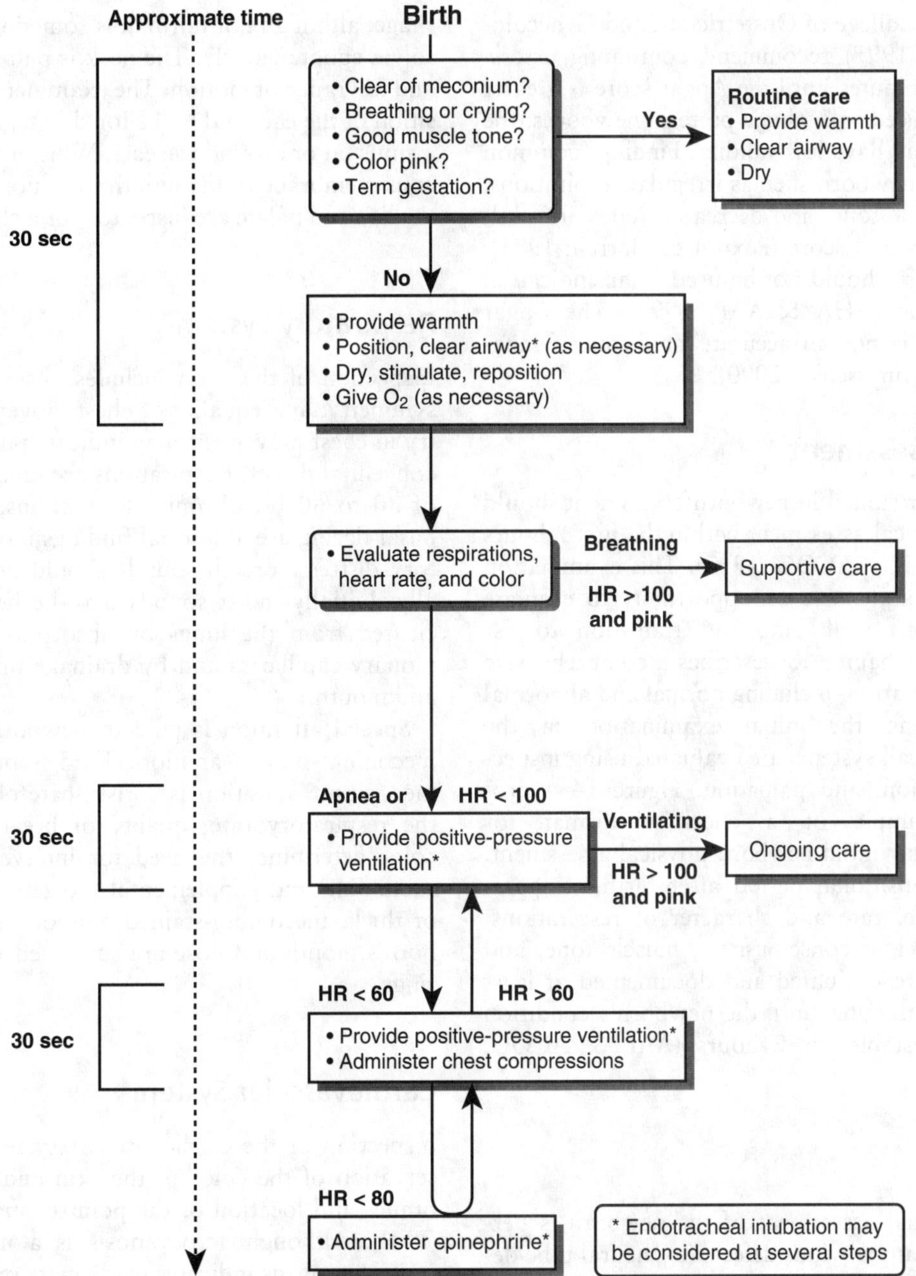

FIGURE 14–3. Resuscitation in the birthing room. (Adapted from American Heart Association and American Academy of Pediatrics (2000). *Textbook of neonatal resuscitation.* (4th ed., pp. 6–9), Elk Grove, IL: American Academy of Pediatrics.)

birth. After airway, breathing, and circulation have been established, a thorough assessment of the newborn is performed. This assessment includes Apgar scoring, evaluation of vital signs, physical examination, and measurements. Ideally, all aspects of transitional assessments are performed in the presence of parents in the birthing room. Only if significant maternal or newborn complications occur are parents and newborns separated.

Apgar Score

The Apgar score was introduced in 1952 by Dr. Virginia Apgar, an anesthesiologist. It provides a simple method to evaluate the condition of the newborn at 1 and 5 minutes after life (Apgar, 1966). Five assessment criteria (ie, heart rate, respiratory rate, muscle tone, reflex irritability, and color) are scored from 0 to 2. The highest total possible score is 10. The AAP and American College of Obstetricians and Gynecologists (ACOG, 1997) recommend continuing assessment every 5 minutes until the Apgar score is greater than 7. When used to evaluate preterm newborns, the Apgar score may have less validity. Findings common in the preterm newborn such as irregular respirations, decreased muscle tone, and decreased reflex irritability affect the overall score (Paxton & Harrell, 1991). The Apgar score should not be used as an indication for resuscitation (AHA & AAP, 1994). The Apgar score by itself is not an accurate predictor of long-term outcome (Juretschke, 2000).

Physical Assessment

A care provider skilled in newborn assessment should perform a physical assessment within the first 2 hours after birth (AAP & ACOG, 1997). This examination gives the perinatal nurse an opportunity to evaluate overall newborn well-being and transition to extrauterine life. Chapter 15 describes a comprehensive physical examination, including normal and abnormal findings. During the initial examination in the birthing room, all systems are evaluated using inspection, auscultation, and palpation. Figure 14–4 provides an example of a checklist format for documenting the initial newborn physical assessment. During the transitional period after birth, temperature, heart rate, rate and character of respirations, skin color, level of consciousness, muscle tone, and activity level are evaluated and documented at least once every 30 minutes until the newborn's condition has remained stable for 2 hours (AAP & ACOG, 1997).

Skin

An overall visual assessment of the newborn is performed noting any obvious defects (eg, neural tube defects, abdominal wall defects, extra digits) or trauma (eg, bruising, petechiae, puncture wound from fetal scalp electrode). Skin is observed for color, texture, birthmarks, rashes, and meconium staining. The newborn's back is inspected, noting a closed vertebral column or presence of abnormalities, such as masses and dimple or tuft of hair at the base of the spine.

Head and Neck

Symmetry of the head and face is noted, as well as the presence of molding, caput succedaneum, and bruising. Fontanelles are palpated. Although it is not uncommon for eyelids to be edematous, drainage from the eye is not normal during this period. Subconjunctival hemorrhage, although not normal, is sometimes seen and resolves spontaneously. The neck is palpated for masses and full range of motion. The examiner assesses the position of the ears and looks for skin tags or evidence of a sinus on or around the ears. While assessing the mucous membrane of the mouth for a normal pink color, the lips and palate are inspected for a cleft.

Respiratory System

Inspection of the chest includes observing the shape, symmetry, and equality of chest movement. Asymmetry in chest movement may indicate pneumothorax or congenital defect. Respirations are unlabored at a rate of 30 to 60 breaths/min. Retractions, grunting, and nasal flaring are abnormal findings indicating respiratory distress. Breath sounds should be equal bilaterally. Initially moist sounds may be heard as fluid is cleared from the lungs by absorption through pulmonary capillaries and by drainage through the nose and mouth.

Special attention is paid to newborns when thick, meconium-stained amniotic fluid is present. Because meconium aspiration is a risk, careful assessment of the respiratory rate, quality of breath sounds, and color determines the need for interventions such as suctioning and supplemental oxygen. In the absence of thick, meconium-stained amniotic fluid, the newborn's mouth and nose are suctioned with a bulb syringe.

Cardiovascular System

Inspection of the cardiovascular system includes observation of the color of the skin and mucous membranes and location of the point of maximal impulse (PMI). Although acrocyanosis is a normal finding, central cyanosis indicates inadequate oxygenation and the need for supplemental oxygen. Heart rate, rhythm, and normal heart sounds and murmurs are best identified when auscultated using a newborn stethoscope.

Cardiovascular assessment also includes palpation for the presence and equality of femoral pulses. Pulses should be equal and nonbounding. Bounding pulses may indicate patent ductus arteriosus, whereas absent or decreased pulses may occur with coarctation of the aorta (Vargo, 1996). Depending on the condition of the newborn, a baseline blood pressure may be recorded. Taking the blood pressure in all four extremities is usually reserved for a newborn showing signs of distress. Routine blood pressure screening for newborns in the absence of risk factors and without

INITIAL ASSESSMENT

DOB ______ Initial Bath: ______ (Time/Initials) Length: ______ cm. ______ in.

TIME ______ Triple Dye to Cord ______ (Time/Initials) Head: ______ cm. ______ in.

TRANSITIONAL CARE ADMINISTERED IN: Infant Removed from Radiant Warmer: Chest: ______ cm. ______ in.

☐ LDRP ☐ Special Care Nursery Date: ______ Time: ______ Abdomen: ______ cm. ______ in.

Weight: ____ gms. lbs. ____ oz. ____

Time	Radiant Warmer Temp	Temp	Pulse	Resp.	Breath Sounds	B/P	Color	Activity	Muscle Tone	SILVERMAN Upper Chest	Lower Chest	Xiphoid	Flare	Grunt	Total	Chest PT	Initials

COLOR: Pink, Pale, Dusky, Jaundiced, Plethoric, Mottled, Cyanosis, Acrocyanosis

✓ = chest PT

MUSCLE TONE: Normal flexion, Flaccidity, Spasticity

ACTIVITY: Active, Active With Stimulation, Quiet, alert, Irritable, Lethargic, Hyperactive, Tremors, Sleeping

BREATH SOUNDS: Equal, Rales, Clear, Diminished, Rhonchi

SKIN
____ Pink ____ Acrocyanosis
____ Central cyanosis ____ Dusky
____ Pale ____ Plethoric
____ Mottled ____ Jaundice
____ Abrasions ______
____ Birthmarks ______
____ Dry ____ Meconium stained
____ Ecchymosis ______
____ Lacerations ______
____ Milia ____ Peeling
____ Mongolian spots ______
____ Petechiae ____ Pustules
____ Rash ______
____ Skin tags ______
____ Vesicles ______

CHEST
____ Symmetrical ____ Asymmetrical
____ Barrel chest
____ Breast engorgement
____ Supranummary nipples
____ Breast discharge

RESPIRATIONS
____ Normal ____ Labored
____ Apnea ____ Grunting
Length ______

BREATH SOUNDS
____ Equal ____ Clear
____ Rales ____ Rhonchi

CLAVICLES
____ Straight ____ Smooth
____ Crepitus ____ Rt ____ Lt

REFLEXES
____ Moro ____ Suck ____ Grasp

CRY
____ Normal ____ Weak ____ Shrill
____ No cry, quiet, alert

HEAD
____ Symmetrical ____ Molding
____ Caput ______
____ Cephalohematoma ____ Lt ____ Rt
____ Forcep marks ______
____ Fontanels normal ______

FACE
____ Symmetrical ____ Asymmetrical

EYES
____ Clear ____ Discharge
____ Lid edema
____ Subconjunctival hemmorhage

NECK
____ Full ROM ____ Limited ROM

HEART
____ Regular ____ Irregular
____ Murmur ____ Abnormal PMI
Location: ______

FEMORAL PULSES
____ Equal ____ Unequal

EXTREMITIES
____ Symmetrical ____ Asymmetrical
____ Normal ROM ____ Limited ROM
____ Hipclicks ____ Rt ____ Lt
____ Polydactylism ____ Syndactylism
____ Abnormal foot position

FEMALE GENITALIA
____ Normal ____ Discharge
____ Vaginal skin tag

MALE GENITALIA
____ Normal
____ Epispadias
____ Hypospadias
____ Undecended testicle
____ Rt ____ Lt
____ Hydrocele

EARS
____ Normal ____ Low set
____ Sinus ____ Skin tags

NOSE
____ Normal ____ Discharge

MOUTH
____ Clear

MUCOUS MEMBRANE
____ Pink ____ Cyanosis ____ Thrush
____ Cleft palate ____ Cleft lip
____ Hard ____ Soft

CORD
____ 3 vessels ____ 2 vessels
____ Meconium stained

ABDOMEN
____ Symmetrical ____ Asymmetrical
____ Flat ____ Scaphold
____ Rounded ____ Distended
____ Soft ____ Hard

BOWEL SOUNDS
____ Present ____ Absent

RECTUM
____ Patent

SPINE
____ Closed vertebral column
____ Asymmetry ____ Mass
____ Dimple ____ Tuft of hair

Initials ______ Date/Time ______

PALOS COMMUNITY HOSPITAL
PALOS HEIGHTS, ILLINOIS

P-768
91480
Rev. 6/94

NEWBORN CARE RECORD

FIGURE 14–4. Documentation of initial newborn assessment.

complications is no longer recommended by the AAP (1993).

Abdomen

The examiner assesses the shape, symmetry, and consistency of the abdomen. The umbilical cord stump is inspected for the presence of three vessels (ie, two arteries and one vein). The umbilical cord of a newborn exposed to meconium in utero for an extended period has a yellowish-brown discoloration. The abdomen is auscultated to detect bowel sounds.

Musculoskeletal System

Extremities are assessed for symmetry, range of motion, and the presence of extra or missing digits. While moving the newborn's arm, clavicles are palpated for crepitus, which may indicate a fracture. The newborn's hips are evaluated for "clicks," which may indicate dislocation. Normal muscle tone is noted during this part of the examination and while evaluating the Apgar score.

Genitalia

The presence of normal male or female genitalia is evaluated. Male newborns are assessed for location of the urethral meatus and presence of a hydrocele. The scrotum is palpated to detect the testes.

Neurologic System

A complete neurologic assessment is usually reserved for newborns that are born with or develop complications. A brief neurologic assessment is performed by evaluating reflexes such as Moro, grasp, and suck.

PROCEDURES PERFORMED IN THE BIRTHING ROOM

In addition to ongoing physical assessments of the newborn, procedures such as newborn identification, instillation of eye prophylaxis, administration of vitamin K, and cord care are performed soon after birth. Ideally, each perinatal unit develops policies and procedures outlining expected newborn care. *Guidelines for Perinatal Care* (AAP & ACOG, 1997) is a resource for developing unit standards.

Newborn Identification

One of the first procedures after birth is newborn identification. Perinatal nurses must be meticulous when recording the identification band number and applying identification bands to mothers and newborns (AAP & ACOG, 1997). Some hospitals use a four-band system that includes a band for the support person or father of the newborn in addition to the band for the mother and two bands for the newborn, with one placed on an ankle and one on a wrist. Newborn footprinting and fingerprinting are not adequate methods of identification (AAP & ACOG, 1997). Some hospitals have abandoned these practices altogether, whereas others continue to do footprinting and fingerprinting but give the prints to the parents as a birth souvenir.

According to the National Center for Missing and Exploited Children (NCMEC, 2000), newborn abductions from hospital facilities decreased 55% between 1991 and 1998 (Table 14–4). In 1999, there were no reports of newborns abducted from hospitals. This was the first year since NCMEC began tracking in 1983 that there was not a single report of a newborn abduction from a U.S. hospital. In 2000, there was at least one newborn abduction reported. NCMEC credits the reduction in newborn abductions from hospital facilities to the prevention training program, Safeguard Their Tomorrows, developed by NCMEC in cooperation with Mead Johnson Nutritionals and the Association of Women's Health, Obstetric and Neonatal Nurses (NCMEC, 2000). This educational program includes a videotape, proactive measures healthcare agencies can take to prevent abduction, abductor profiles, case studies, statistics, safety measures for parents, and instructions for creating a crisis response plan in each hospital. NCMEC also has guidelines that healthcare professionals can use to identify and eliminate the risk of newborn abduction within their facilities.

TABLE 14–4 ■ NUMBER OF NEWBORNS ABDUCTED FROM U.S. HOSPITALS

Period	Number of Abductions
1983–1995	89
1996	4
1997	1
1998	5
1999	0

From National Center for Missing and Exploited Children (NCMEC). (2000). Infant abduction from hospitals reduced by prevention training. Washington, DC: Author.

Newborn safety and security, including unit visiting policies, should be discussed with parents and family members. Parents should be made aware of what the hospital is doing to ensure the safety of every newborn and should understand what they can do to increase safety. An important part of any newborn security program is a discussion with the parents, including directions not to leave their newborn unattended and information about identification of caregivers who may transport the newborn to and from the nursery or other hospital department. Display 14–3 is an example of a form that can be used to review safety issues with parents. Ideally, one copy goes to the parents and a second to the medical record as documentation that this discussion occurred.

The efficacy of electronic newborn security systems in preventing newborn abductions remains controversial. The security programs described previously may be equally effective and much less expensive than electronic systems. No one method is superior; the key issue is that there must be some systematic newborn safety program in place known to the parents and

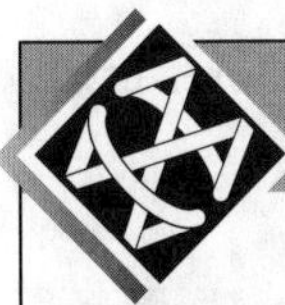

DISPLAY 14–3

Infant Safety Information

We, the nursing staff, welcome you to Palos Community Hospital and hope your family's stay here is a safe and pleasurable experience. During your stay, we ask for your cooperation to ensure your infant's safety.

1. If you are feeling weak, faint, or unsteady on your feet, do not lift your baby. Instead, call for assistance from the nurse.
2. Our birthing beds are narrower than your bed at home. We suggest that you place your baby in the crib when you become drowsy, plan on sleeping, or are using the bathroom. Please call a nurse if you need help. Never leave your newborn alone on your bed.
3. Never leave your baby alone in your room. If you walk in the halls or take a shower, please have a family member watch him or her or return your baby to the nursery.
4. Always keep an eye and hand on your infant when he or she is out of the crib.
5. When walking in the corridor, your baby should be in the crib and the crib flat.
6. Newborns possess some immunity from infections, but we still must protect them. Please ask your visitors to leave if they have any of the following: cold, diarrhea, sore that has a discharge, or contagious disease.
7. The only personnel that should be handling your baby or taking him or her from your room are employees wearing Palos Community Hospital scrubs and a picture ID tag. If you don't know the staff person, call for your nurse to help you.
8. Please call the nurse any time a situation arises with your baby that you do not feel comfortable with. We wish to give you as much teaching and information as possible to make your transition to parenthood as easy as possible.
9. Based on careful evaluation of existing data indicating an association between sudden infant death syndrome (SIDS) and prone (tummy-lying) sleeping position for infants, the American Academy of Pediatrics recommends that normal infants, when being put down for sleep, be positioned on their side or back. It should be stressed that the actual risk of SIDS for an infant placed on his or her stomach is still extremely low.
10. If your new baby's siblings visit, please keep a watchful eye on them so that they do not get hurt.

I understand the above information:

Date: ____________________ Mother's Signature: ____________________

Date: ____________________ *Significant Other: ____________________

If available at the time of admission.

PALOS COMMUNITY HOSPITAL
PALOS HEIGHTS, ILLINOIS

INFANT SAFETY INFORMATION

P-407
85345 White - Chart Yellow = Patient

perinatal healthcare providers to decrease the risk of newborn abduction. Nothing replaces vigilance on the part of parents, perinatal nurses, and other hospital employees.

Vitamin K

The most important cause of a bleeding syndrome in an otherwise healthy newborn is hemorrhagic disease caused by vitamin K deficiency (Johnson, Rodden, & Collins, 1998). During the first week of life, newborns are at risk for bleeding disorders because of an immature liver that is unable to produce several coagulation factors and a sterile gastrointestinal tract that has not begun producing vitamin K. Consumption of breast milk and formula causes colonization of bacteria in the gastrointestinal tract, which is necessary for vitamin K production. Vitamin K stimulates the liver to synthesize coagulation factors II, VII, IX, and X (Shaw, 1998). A single dose of 0.5 mg for newborns weighing less than 1.5 kg and 1 mg for newborns weighing more than 1.5 kg is administered intramuscularly within the first hour of life (AAP & ACOG, 1997).

Eye Prophylaxis

Most states in the United States mandate that every newborn receives prophylaxis against eye infections. Erythromycin ointment is the drug of choice because of its effectiveness against gonococcal and chlamydial infections. Some evidence suggests that when the pregnant woman has received ongoing prenatal care and been screened for sexually transmitted diseases, the decision to use eye prophylaxis can be left up to parents (Bell, Grayston, Krohn, & Kronmal, 1993). After the agent for prophylaxis is chosen, care should be taken to instill the ointment throughout the conjunctival sac. Excessive medication can be wiped away with a sterile cotton ball 1 minute after instillation (AAP & ACOG, 1997).

Umbilical Cord Care

The umbilical cord is examined for the presence of two arteries and a vein. Because a moist cord is vulnerable to pathogens, measures should be taken to promote drying of the cord, including exposing the cord to air. Although no method of cord care has been shown to prevent bacterial colonization, many institutions use alcohol, triple dye, or another antimicrobial agent. Research has shown that use of sterile water or air drying results in cords separating more quickly than those treated with alcohol (Dores et al., 1998; Medves & O'Brien, 1997).

PROMOTING FAMILY–NEWBORN ATTACHMENT

After addressing physiologic adaptation to extrauterine life, the focus of nursing interventions is psychological adaptation. Perinatal nurses are in a position to promote early maternal–newborn attachment. Early and extended contact between mother and newborn facilitates development of a positive relationship (Reeder, Martin, & Koniak-Griffin, 1997). The perinatal nurse assists in the attachment process by encouraging parents to see, touch, and hold their newborn. Providing uninterrupted time for them to be together gives parents the opportunity to recognize and identify unique behavioral and physical characteristics of their newborn.

Practices used to promote attachment usually do not interfere with transition to extrauterine life. The perinatal nurse can make a positive contribution to enhancing the attachment process by modifying practices that separate mothers and newborns immediately after birth. Newborn treatments can be done within the birthing room, decreasing separation time between the mother and newborn. The mother may immediately hold the newborn if the newborn is dried and covered with a warm blanket. The newborn could also be placed skin-to-skin with the mother. If both are covered with a blanket, neonatal thermoregulation is not interrupted. Application of ophthalmic antibiotics may safely occur within the first hour of life, enhancing maternal–newborn eye contact (AAP & ACOG, 1997). Providing the opportunity to breastfeed soon after birth supports the attachment process. Breast-feeding is more than a feeding method; it is an intimate relationship between a mother and her newborn (Hall, Ellerbee, & Newberry, 1997). Early suckling and opportunities for uninterrupted contact between mother and newborn increases breast-feeding duration (Hall, Ellerbee, & Newberry, 1997; International Lactation Consultant Association, 1999).

EXPOSURE TO GROUP B BETA-HEMOLYTIC STREPTOCOCCUS

Infection with group B streptococci (GBS) is the leading cause of neonatal sepsis (Hager et al., 2000; McCracken, 1973). It is estimated that 15% to 30% of women are GBS carriers (AAP Committee on Infectious Diseases and Committee on Fetus and Newborn, 1997). Before the use of prophylactic intrapartum antibiotics, newborns who survived GBS disease experienced developmental disabilities, mental retardation, and hearing and vision loss (Schrag et al., 2000). Pregnant women may be asymptomatic or experience urinary tract infections and amnionitis.

The incidence of early-onset GBS infection is 0.6 cases per 1,000 live births when prenatal screening and a program of intrapartum antibiotic prophylaxis are in place. This represents a 65% decrease in neonatal infections between 1993 and 1998 (Schrag et al., 2000). Early-onset GBS infection can occur in the first 7 days of life but most commonly manifests in the first 24 hours after delivery. Early-onset infection presents as bacteremia, meningitis, or pneumonia. The mortality rate associated with each of these presentations is 4% (Schrag et al., 2000). Risk factors for the development of GBS infection include gestational age less than 37 weeks, rupture of membranes more than 18 hours before birth, intrapartum fever of 38°C (99.4°F) or higher, a previous GBS-infected newborn, and GBS bacteriuria during pregnancy (Hager et al., 2000). Although it is unclear why, rates of GBS infection are higher among African American women than any other ethnic or racial groups. Intrapartum antibiotic treatment of women colonized with GBS appears to reduce neonatal infection (Smaill, 2000).

Late-onset GBS infections occur between 1 week and 3 months of age. Sixty-three percent of these newborns develop bacteremia, 24% develop meningitis, and 2% develop pneumonia; the mortality rate for late-onset GBS is 2.8% (Schrag et al., 2000).

The American Academy of Pediatrics Committee on Infectious Diseases and Committee on the Fetus and Newborn (1997) published guidelines for the prevention of early-onset group B streptococcal infection that offer clinicians a choice of strategies for the management of GBS in pregnancy. Pregnant women may be screened at 35 to 37 weeks' gestation using a combined vaginal–rectal swab and offered treatment with penicillin in labor if the swab is positive. When screening during pregnancy is not carried out or the results are unknown, women with risk factors for GBS are given antibiotics during labor (Fig. 14–5). There are no guidelines for the treatment of women having elective cesarean birth. Vertical transmission in this population is low, and antibiotic chemoprophylaxis is thought to be unnecessary (Hagar et al., 2000).

The assessment and care of a newborn after birth should be based on knowledge of maternal risk factors for GBS sepsis, maternal GBS status if known, and the timing and number of doses of antibiotic administered during labor. After delivery, it is important to evaluate the newborn for signs and symptoms of infection, including respiratory distress, apnea, tachy-

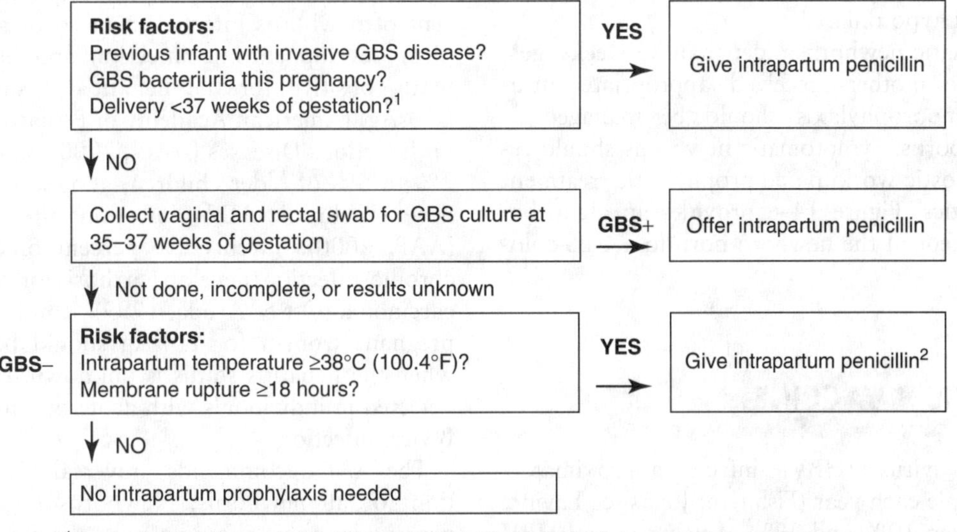
Risk factors:
Previous infant with invasive GBS disease?
GBS bacteriuria this pregnancy?
Delivery <37 weeks of gestation?¹
YES
Give intrapartum penicillin
NO
Collect vaginal and rectal swab for GBS culture at 35–37 weeks of gestation
GBS+
Offer intrapartum penicillin
Not done, incomplete, or results unknown
GBS–
Risk factors:
Intrapartum temperature ≥38°C (100.4°F)?
Membrane rupture ≥18 hours?
YES
Give intrapartum penicillin²
NO
No intrapartum prophylaxis needed
¹No prophylaxis is needed if culture result at 35–37 weeks is known to be negative.
²Broad-spectrum antibiotics may be considered at the discretion of the physician, based on clinical indications.

FIGURE 14–5. Prevention strategy for early-onset group B streptococcus disease, using prenatal culture screening at 35 to 37 weeks of gestation. (From American Academy of Pediatrics Committee on Infectious Diseases and Committee on Fetus and Newborn [1997]. Revised guidelines for prevention of early onset group B streptococcal [GBS] infection. *Pediatrics* 99[3], 489–496.)

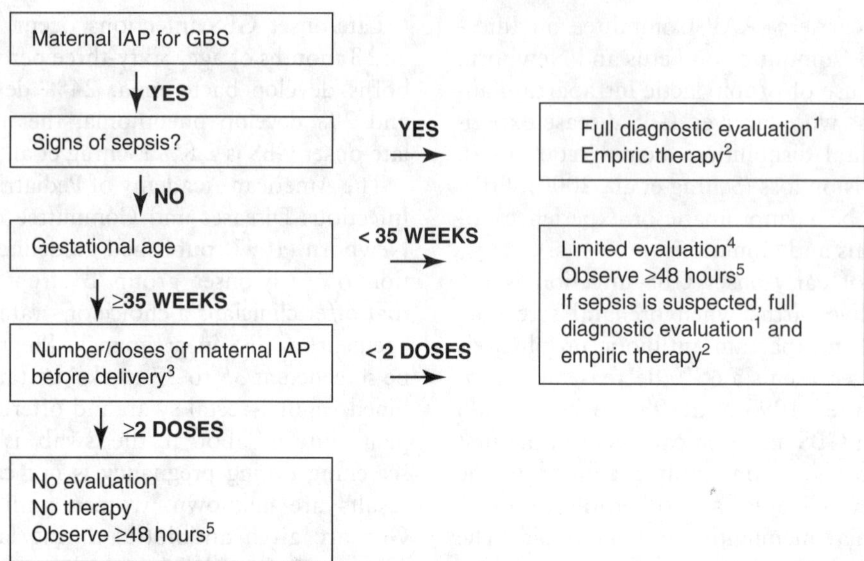

[1] Includes complete blood count (CBC) and differential, blood culture, and chest radiograph if respiratory symptoms. A lumbar puncture is performed at the discretion of the physician.
[2] Duration of therapy will vary depending on results of blood culture and cerebrospinal fluid findings (if obtained), as well as on the clinical course of the infant. *If* laboratory results and clinical course are unremarkable, duration may be as short as 48–72 hours.
[3] Applies to penicillin or ampicillin chemoprophylaxis.
[4] CBC and differential, blood culture.
[5] Does *not* allow early discharge.

FIGURE 14–6. Management of a neonate born to a mother who received intrapartum antimicrobial prophylaxis (IAP) for prevention of early-onset group B streptococcal disease. (From American Academy of Pediatrics Committee on Infectious Diseases and Committee on Fetus and Newborn [1997]. Revised guidelines for prevention of early onset group B streptococcal [GBS] infection. *Pediatrics, 99*[3], 489–496.)

cardia, hypotension, pallor, temperature instability, lethargy, and hypotonia.

Asymptomatic newborns older than 35 weeks' gestation whose mothers received appropriate intrapartum chemoprophylaxis should be managed as healthy newborns. Symptomatic newborns should receive a diagnostic workup and prophylactic treatment with antibiotics. Figure 14–6 provides an algorithm for management of the newborn born to a GBS-colonized mother.

HEPATITIS B VACCINE

Hepatitis B virus (HBV) infects approximately 300,000 people each year (Fishman, Jonas, & Lavine, 1996). Between 10% and 20% of new cases of HBV infection in the United States occur in the pediatric and adolescent populations (Ott & Aruda, 1999). The spectrum of HBV infection ranges from asymptomatic seroconversion through general malaise, anorexia, nausea, and jaundice to fetal hepatitis. Development of a chronic infection is inversely proportional to the age at which the infection was acquired. Ninety percent of newborns infected in utero or at the time of birth develop chronic infection and become persistently positive for the hepatitis B surface antigen (HBsAg) (American Academy of Pediatrics Committee on Infectious Diseases [AAP], 2000). In contrast, only 2% to 6% of older children, adolescents, and adults develop chronic HBV infection after acute illness (AAP, 2000). Twenty-five percent of children with chronic infection develop cirrhosis or hepatocellular carcinoma (Ott & Aruda, 1999). Routine screening of pregnant women for HBsAg should be carried out when the hepatitis status is unknown. HBsAg can be detected in individuals with acute or chronic hepatitis B viral infection.

The AAP recommends universal HBV immunization for all newborns. Newborns born to HBsAg-negative mothers should receive the first dose of vaccine by 2 months of age, with the second dose 1 to 2 months later and the third dose by 6 to 18 months of age. An alternative schedule of vaccinations gives the HBV vaccine at 2, 4, and 6 months of age concurrently with other childhood vaccines (AAP, 2000; AAP & ACOG, 1997). Babies born to HBsAg-positive mothers should receive one dose of hepatitis vaccine within 12 hours of birth, and hepatitis immunoglobulin (HBIG) should be given concurrently at a different site (AAP, 2000). HBIG provides temporary protection in postexposure situations, and HBV vaccine provides long-term protection. Newborns born to women with unknown HBsAg status should receive the first dose of HBV vaccine within 12 hours of birth (AAP, 2000). Because the vaccine is highly effective in preventing infection in this population, further prophylaxis with HBIG can be delayed up to 7 days while awaiting maternal laboratory results.

SUMMARY

Most newborns need minimal support to make the transition to extrauterine life. Diverse and complex system adaptations make it a critical time for newborns. Strong desires to interact with their newborn make this a significant time for parents. The perinatal nurse must be knowledgeable about normal physiologic changes during the period of newborn transition from extrauterine life. Caring for newborns during this time requires the ability to recognize alterations from normal and becoming proficient at the skills necessary for conducting a newborn resuscitation.

REFERENCES

American Academy of Pediatrics & American College of Obstetricians and Gynecologists (AAP & ACOG). (1997). *Guidelines for perinatal care* (4th ed.). Elk Grove Village, IL: American Academy of Pediatrics.

American Academy of Pediatrics Committee on Fetus and Newborn. (1993). Routine evaluation of blood pressure, hematocrit, and glucose in newborns. *Pediatrics, 92*(3), 474–476.

American Academy of Pediatrics Committee on Infectious Diseases (2000). *2000 Red Book* (25th ed.). Elk Grove Village, IL: Author.

American Academy of Pediatrics Committee on Infectious Diseases and Committee on Fetus and Newborn. (1997). Revised guidelines for prevention of early-onset group B streptococcal (GBS) infection. *Pediatrics, 99*(3), 489–496.

American Heart Association & American Academy of Pediatrics (AHA & AAP). (2000). *Textbook of Neonatal Resuscitation.* (4th ed). Elk Grove Village, IL: American Heart Association.

Amlung, S. R. (1998). Neonatal thermoregulation. In C. Kenner, J. W. Lott, & A. A. Flandermeyer (Eds.), *Comprehensive neonatal nursing: A physiologic perspective* (2nd ed., pp. 207–220). Philadelphia: W.B. Saunders.

Apgar, V. (1966). The newborn Apgar scoring system: Reflections and advice. *Pediatric Clinics of North America, 13*(3), 645–650.

Beachy, P., & Deacon, J. (1992). Preventing neonatal kidnapping. *Journal of Obstetric, Gynecologic, and Neonatal Nursing, 21*(1), 12–16.

Bell, T. A., Grayston, J. T., Krohn, M. A., & Kronmal, R. A. (1993). Randomized trial of silver nitrate, erythromycin, and no eye prophylaxis for the prevention of conjunctivitis among newborns not at risk for gonococcal ophthalmitis. *Pediatrics, 92*(6), 755–760.

Blake, W. W., & Murray, J. A. (1998). Heat balance. In G. B. Merenstein & S. L. Gardner (Eds.), *Handbook of neonatal intensive care* (4th ed., pp. 100–115). St. Louis: Mosby–Year Book.

Bloom, R. S. (1996). Delivery room resuscitation of the newborn. In A. A. Fanaroff, & R. J. Martin (Eds.). *Neonatal perinatal medicine: Diseases of the fetus & newborn* (5th ed., pp. 301–324). St. Louis: Mosby–Year Book.

Cole, F. S. (1998). Immunology. In H. W. Taeusch & R. A. Ballard (Eds.), *Avery's diseases of the newborn* (7th ed., pp. 435–452). Philadelphia: W.B. Saunders.

Dore, S., Buchan, D., Coulas, S., Hamber, L., Stewart, M., Cowan, D., & Jamieson, L. (1998). Alcohol versus natural drying for newborn cord care. *Journal of Obstetric, Gynecologic, and Neonatal Nursing, 27*(6), 621–627.

Fishman, L. N., Jonas, M. M., & Lavine, J. E. (1996). Update on viral hepatitis in children. *Pediatric Clinics of North America, 43*(1), 57–74.

Gale, G., & VandenBerg, K. A. (1998). Kangaroo care. *Neonatal Network, 17*(5), 69–71.

Hagedorn, M. I., Gardner, S. L., & Abman, S. H. (1998). Respiratory diseases. In G. B. Merenstein & S. L. Gardner (Eds.), *Handbook of neonatal intensive care* (4th ed., pp. 437–499). St. Louis: Mosby–Year Book.

Hager, W. D., Schuchat, A., Gibbs, R., Sweet, R., Mead, P., & Larsen, J. W. (2000). Prevention of perinatal group B streptococcal infection: Current controversies. *Obstetrics and Gynecology, 96*(1), 141–145.

Hall, M. S., Ellerbee, S. M., & Newberry, R. (1997). Timeline for breastfeeding: The first month. *Mother-Baby Journal, 2*(1), 19–26.

Hanson, T., & Corbet, A. (1998). Lung development and function. In H. W. Taeusch & R. A. Ballard (Eds.), *Avery's diseases of the newborn* (7th ed., pp. 541–551). Philadelphia: W.B. Saunders.

International Lactation Consultant Association. (1999). *Evidence-based guidelines for breast-feeding management during the first 14 days.* Raleigh, NC: Author.

International Liaison Committee on Resuscitation (ILCOR). (1999). An advisory statement from the Pediatric Working Group of the International Liaison Committee on Resuscitation. *Pediatrics, 103*(4), 56.

Johnson, M. M., Rodden, D. J., & Collins, S. (1998). Newborn hematology. In G. B. Merenstein & S. L. Gardner (Eds.), *Handbook of neonatal intensive care* (4th ed., pp. 367–392). St. Louis: Mosby–Year Book.

Juretschke, L. J. (2000). Apgar scoring: Its use and meaning for today's newborn. *Neonatal Network, 19*(1), 17–19.

Konrad, C., & Norton, J. (1998). Newborn temperature regulation: Challenges for mother baby nurses. *Mother-Baby Journal, 3*(4), 12–16.

Loper, D. L. (1997). Physiologic principles of the respiratory system. In D. A. Askin (Ed.), *Acute respiratory care of the newborn.* (2nd ed., pp. 1–30). Petaluma, CA: NICU INK.

Lott, J. W., & Kenner, C. (1998). Assessment and management of immunologic dysfunction. In C. Kenner, J. W. Lott, & A. A. Flandermeyer (Eds.), *Comprehensive neonatal nursing: A physiologic perspective* (2nd ed., pp. 496–519). Philadelphia: W.B. Saunders.

Lott, J. W. (1998). Assessment and management of cardiovascular dysfunction. In C. Kenner, J. W. Lott, & A. A. Flandermeyer (Eds.), *Comprehensive neonatal nursing: A physiologic perspective* (2nd ed., pp. 306–335). Philadelphia: W.B. Saunders.

Ludington-Hoe, S. M., Anderson, G. C., Hollingsead, A., Argote, L. A., Medellin, G., & Rey, H. (1993). Skin-to-skin contact beginning in the delivery room for Colombian mothers and their preterm infants. *Journal of Human Lactation, 9*(4), 241–242.

McCollum, L. (1998). Resuscitation and stabilization of the neonate. In C. Kenner, J. W. Lott, & A. A. Flandermeyer (Eds.), *Comprehensive neonatal nursing: A physiologic perspective* (2nd ed., pp. 190–206). Philadelphia: W.B. Saunders.

McCracken, G. H. (1973). Group B streptococcus: The new challenge in neonatal infections. *Journal of Pediatrics, 82*(4), 703–706.

Medves, J. M., & O'Brien, B. A. (1997). Cleaning solutions and bacterial colonization in promoting healing and early separation of the umbilical cord in healthy newborns. *Canadian Journal of Public Health, 88*(6), 380–382.

Nelson, N. (1999). Onset of respiration. In G. B. Avery, M. A. Fletcher, & M. G. MacDonald (Eds.), *Neonatology: Pathophysiology and management of the newborn* (5th ed., pp. 257–278). Philadelphia: Lippincott Williams & Wilkins.

National Center for Missing and Exploited Children (NCMEC). (2000). *Infant abduction from hospitals reduced by prevention training*. Washington, DC: Author.

Noerr, B. (1997). Keeping the newborn warm: Understanding thermoregulation. *Mother-Baby Journal, 2*(5), 6–12.

Ott, M. J., & Ardua, J. (1999). Hepatitis B vaccine. *Journal of Pediatric Health Care, 12*(5), 211–216.

Paxton, J. M., & Harrell, H. (1991). Delivery room management of the asphyxiated neonate. *NAACOG's Clinical Issues in Perinatal and Women's Health Nursing, 2*(1), 35–47.

Reeder, S. J., Martin, L. L., & Koniak-Griffin, D. (1997). Immediate care of the newborn. In S. J. Reeder, L. L. Martin, & D. Koniak-Griffin. *Maternity nursing* (19th ed., pp. 617–634). Philadelphia: Lippincott-Raven.

Riordan, J. (1998). The biologic specificity of breastmilk. In J. Riordan & K. G. Auerbach (Eds.), *Breast-feeding and human lactation* (2nd ed., pp. 105–134).

Roncoli, M., & Medoff-Cooper, B. (1992). Thermoregulation in low-birth-weight infants. *NAACOG's Clinical Issues in Perinatal and Women's Health Nursing, 3*(1), 25–33.

Sansoucie, D. A., & Cavaliere, T. A. (1997). Transition from fetal to extrauterine circulation. *Neonatal Network, 16*(2), 5–12.

Schrag, S. J., Zywicki, S., Farley, M. M., Reingold, A. L., Harrison, L. H., Lefkowitz, L. B., Hadler, J. L., Danila, R., Cieslak, P. R., & Schuchat, A. (2000). Group B streptococcal disease in the era of intrapartum antibiotic prophylaxis. *New England Journal of Medicine, 342*(1), 15–20.

Shaw, N. (1998). Assessment and management of hematologic dysfunction. In C. Kenner, J. W. Lott, & A. A. Flandermeyer (Eds.), *Comprehensive neonatal nursing: A physiologic perspective* (2nd ed., pp. 520–563). Philadelphia: W.B. Saunders.

Smaill, F. (2000). Intrapartum antibiotics for group B streptococcal colonization. *Cochrane Database* (2), CD000115.

Vargo, L. (1996). Cardiovascular assessment of the newborn. In E. P. Tappero, & M. E. Honeyfield (Eds.), *Physical Assessment of the Newborn* (2nd ed., pp. 77–92). Petaluma, CA: NICU INK.

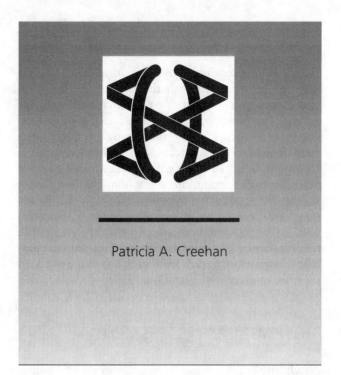

Patricia A. Creehan

CHAPTER 15

Newborn Physical Assessment

Perinatal nurses frequently perform the first head-to-toe physical assessment of the newborn. Ideally, this examination occurs in the presence of the parents. Conducting the examination while parents observe allows the nurse to use this time to identify and discuss normal newborn characteristics and note variations. It also provides an opportunity for parents to ask questions about the newborn's physical appearance and condition. The focus of this chapter is the physical assessment and findings that the perinatal nurse may observe during the time the newborn is in the hospital or birthing center. Home care nurses may also find the information pertinent during early postpartum home visits. Although some references are made to preterm newborns, that subject is not the intended focus of this chapter. It is also assumed that the reader has basic knowledge of physical assessment skills and terminology. Normal findings and common variations for each body system are identified in the text. Tables describe pathologic findings and their causes.

Physical assessment skills of inspection, palpation, and auscultation are used throughout the examination. When performing a physical assessment, the following equipment should be available: scale, tape measure, tongue blades, stethoscope with a neonatal diaphragm, and ophthalmoscope. The initial physical assessment may be conducted with the infant under a radiant warmer or in an open crib. Regardless of the location, attention should be given to avoiding cold stress. Adequate lighting is essential.

The sequence in which the nurse conducts the physical assessment is a matter of personal preference and depends on the cooperation of the newborn. Although we discuss the newborn assessment as a sequential examination covering one system at a time, some nurses conduct the examination in a cephalocaudal fashion, some prefer to examine the newborn system by system, and others evaluate multiple systems simultaneously.

The physical assessment usually begins by observing breathing pattern, overall skin color, general state or level of alertness, posture, and muscle tone. The newborn's *state* refers to general level of alertness and is a reflection of a group of characteristics that occur together. In the newborn, these characteristics include body activity, eye movement, facial movements, breathing pattern, and level of response to internal and external stimuli (Pearson, 1999). Understanding the differences in state provides information about how the newborn will respond to the nurse or parents and about the condition of the newborn's health, and it has implications for the education of parents. Appendix 15A describes newborn states, deep sleep, light sleep, drowsy, quiet alert, active alert, and crying and the implications these states have for caregivers.

The newborn is weighed and measured. Infants usually lose 10% of their birth weight during the first few days of life. Figure 15–1 illustrates the technique for obtaining accurate measurements. Head circumference is 32 to 38 cm (13 to 15 inches), and chest circumference is 30 to 36 cm (12 to 14 inches). As a general rule, head circumference is 2 cm greater than chest circumference. Abdominal circumference is not routinely recorded. The term newborn's length is 45 to 55 cm (18 to 22 inches).

GESTATIONAL AGE ASSESSMENT

The American Academy of Pediatrics (AAP) and American College of Obstetricians and Gynecologists (ACOG) recommend that the gestational age of all

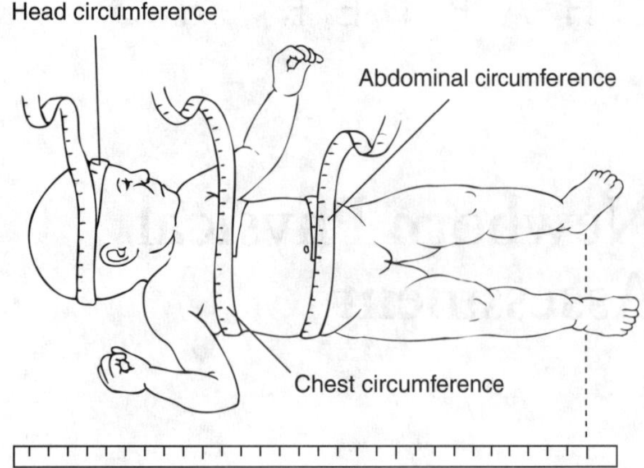

FIGURE 15–1. Newborn measurements. Adapted from Wong, D. L. (Ed.) (1997). *Whaley & Wong's nursing care of infants and children* (6th ed., p. 139). St. Louis, MO: Mosby–Year Book.

newborns be determined after birth (AAP & ACOG, 1997). A gestational age assessment, evaluating physical and neuromuscular characteristics, is usually performed as part of the initial physical examination. Although some perinatal centers make gestational age assessment of all newborns a routine practice, other institutions have established criteria for performing gestational age assessment such as birth weight less than 2,500 g or more than 4,082 g, suspected intrauterine growth restriction, gestation less than 37 weeks, and cesarean birth. Identifying newborns who are preterm, term, or postterm and those who are small for gestational age (SGA), appropriate for gestational age (AGA), or large for gestational age (LGA) increases the likelihood of early identification and timely interventions for potential complications related to birth weight and gestational age during the immediate newborn period. Measures of gestational age are based on differences in physical and neurologic maturity at different gestational ages.

The original tool, the Dubowitz Scoring System, contained 20 items combining neurologic and physical parameters that successfully estimated gestational age in infants older than 34 weeks (Dubowitz, Dubowitz, & Goldberg, 1970). Today, most institutions use the Ballard Maturational Score (BMS) (Ballard, Novak, & Driver, 1979). The original BMS contained 12 items based on the Dubowitz Scoring System. As more low-birth-weight infants were born and survived the initial neonatal period, an instrument that could accurately measure their gestational age was needed. In 1991, the BMS was reevaluated and expanded resulting in the development of a New Ballard Score (Fig. 15–2). Criteria were broadened to provide greater accuracy when evaluating extremely premature neonates (Ballard et al., 1991).

The BMS is conducted by comparing the characteristics of the newborn with the pictures on the form and assigning a number for each characteristic. Appendix 15B describes each characteristic evaluated. Controversy exists about the timing of this assessment. The BMS is most accurate if performed between 10 and 36 hours of age, except for newborns younger than 26 weeks' gestation, for whom the assessment should be conducted within the first 12 hours (Gagliardi, Brambilla, Bruno, Martinelli, & Console, 1993). The examination is separated into two parts: neuromuscular maturity assessment and physical maturity assessment. Scores from both sections are added together to determine gestational age.

INTEGUMENT ASSESSMENT

Newborn skin is assessed using inspection and palpation. Color, birth marks, rashes, skin lesions, texture, and turgor are noted. At birth, newborns are covered with vernix, an odorless, white, cheesy, protective coating produced by sebaceous glands. Vernix develops during the third trimester. The amount seen on the newborn increases with gestational age during the third trimester. At about 37 weeks, the amount of vernix begins to decrease, and at term, it is present only in the creases of the arms, legs, and neck.

Color

Skin color reflects general health. Color is best observed when the newborn is quiet. At birth, color ranges from pale to plethoric, depending on hematocrit and blood flow to the skin. Skin pigmentation depends on ethnic origin and deepens over time. Caucasian newborns have pinkish red skin tones a few hours after birth, and African American newborns have a reddish brown skin color. Hispanic and Asian newborns have an olive or yellow skin tone. Changes in skin color may be the first sign of illness such as sepsis, cardiopulmonary disorders, or hematologic diseases. Variations in skin color indicating illness are more difficult to evaluate in African American and Asian newborns.

Generalized cyanosis may be seen at the time of birth as the newborn transitions from fetal circulation. Whiffs of oxygen applied by a face mask for a short period should quickly help correct this situation if the cause is not underlying pathology. Acrocyanosis, the blue discoloration of newborn hands and feet, is seen in the first 24 to 48 hours of life. Usually a benign condition, it is related to poor peripheral circulation and tends to worsen if the newborn be-

Neuromuscular Maturity

	-1	0	1	2	3	4	5
Posture							
Square Window (wrist)	>90°	90°	60°	45°	30°	0°	
Arm Recoil		180°	140°-180°	110°-140°	90°-110°	<90°	
Popliteal Angle	180°	160°	140°	120°	100°	90°	<90°
Scarf Sign							
Heel to Ear							

Physical Maturity

Skin	sticky friable transparent	gelatinous red, translucent	smooth pink, visible veins	superficial peeling &/or rash few veins	cracking pale areas rare veins	parchment deep cracking no vessels	leathery cracked wrinkled
Lanugo	none	sparse	abundant	thinning	bald areas	mostly bald	
Plantar Surface	heel-toe 40-50 mm:-1 < 40 mm:-2	>50mm no crease	faint red marks	anterior transverse crease only	creases ant. 2/3	creases over entire sole	
Breast	imperceptible	barely perceptilble	flat areola no bud	slippled areola 1-2mm bud	raised areola 3-4mm bud	full areola 5-10 mm bud	
Eye/Ear	lids fused loosely:-1 tightly:-2	lids open pinna flat stays folded	sl. curved pinna; soft; slow recoil	well-curved pinna: soft but ready recoil	formed & firm instant recoil	thick cartillage ear stiff	
Genitals male	scrotum flat, smooth	scrotum empty faint rugae	testes in upper canal rare rugae	testes descending few rugae	testes down good rugae	testes pendulous deep rugae	
Genitals female	clitoris prominent labia flat	prominent clitoris small labia minora	prominent clitoris enlarging minora	majora & minora equally prominent	majora large minora small	majora cover clitoris & minora	

Maturity Rating

score	weeks
-10	20
-5	22
-0	24
5	26
10	28
15	30
20	32
25	34
30	36
35	38
40	40
45	42
50	44

FIGURE 15–2. Gestational age assessment. (From Ballard, J. L., Khoury, J. C., Wedig, K., Ellers-Walsman, B. L., & Lipp, R. [1991]. New Ballard Score, expanded to include extremely premature infants. *Journal of Pediatrics, 119*(3), 417–423.)

comes chilled. Persistent generalized or circumoral cyanosis (surrounding the mouth) may indicate the presence of a pathologic condition and should be reported to the physician or nurse practitioner.

Jaundice

Jaundice, a bright yellow or orange discoloration of the skin, results from deposits of unconjugated bilirubin. Sixty percent of term newborns and 80% of preterm newborns develop jaundice during the first 3 to 4 days of life (Stoll & Kliegman, 2000). Jaundice results from the inability of the newborn's liver to conjugate bilirubin. A mildly elevated indirect bilirubin level is considered normal in the first few days of life. An elevated direct bilirubin level that may occur as early as 24 hours of life is never normal and suggests some pathology involving the liver. The skin color change associated with an elevated direct bilirubin is greenish or muddy yellow (Ulshen, 2000). Jaundice progresses in a cephalocaudal fashion on the head and face, progressing downward to the truck and extremities and then to the sclera of the eye. When gentle pressure is applied to skin over cartilage or a bony prominence, skin blanches to a yellow hue on the face when bilirubin levels are 5 mg/dL, on the abdomen when levels are 15 mg/dL, and on the soles of the feet when levels reach 20 mg/dL (Stoll & Kliegman, 2000). Newborns with a positive Coombs' test result almost certainly develop jaundice. In dark-skinned newborns, jaundice is more easily observed in the sclera and buccal mucosa.

Bruising

Ecchymosis may occur over the head or buttocks if forceps or a vacuum extractor was applied or after a breech or face presentation. Petechiae are common over the presenting part, especially when there has been a rapid descent during second stage of labor. Bruising may also result from a tight nuchal cord or a cord wrapped tightly around the upper body.

Variations Related to Vasomotor Instability

Cutis marmorata, mottling, or a lacelike pattern on the skin is a vasomotor response to chilling, stress, or overstimulation. Parents should be aware that this may continue after discharge. The harlequin sign occurs when some newborns are positioned on their sides. The dependent side of the body becomes pink, and the upper half of the body is pale. The color change lasts 1 to 30 minutes and disappears gradually when the infant is placed on the abdomen or back (Witt, 1996).

Hemangiomas

Hemangiomas are vascular skin lesions composed of dilated blood vessels. Present at birth or within the first 8 weeks of life in 8% to 12% of newborns, hemangiomas are more likely to occur in females than males (Morelli, 1996).

Nevus Vasculosus

Nevus vasculosus, also called strawberry hemangioma, is an elevated red lesion that can occur anywhere on the body. Present at birth or developing soon after, this lesion acquired its name from the characteristic rough texture. Strawberry hemangiomas increase in size for up to 2 years and spontaneously regress over several years. Usually, no treatment is required unless the lesion bleeds, becomes infected, or interferes with breathing or eating.

Cavernous Hemangiomas

Cavernous hemangioma is a soft, compressible swelling (Fig. 15–3). These lesions are always manifest at birth but may be small and not very obvious, appearing as a blue discoloration under normal skin. As they swell and increase in size, they become more obvious and deeper red. Cavernous hemangiomas are frequently located on the head but can be found anywhere on the body and may extend deeply into skeletal muscle, joint, or bones (Brown, Friedman, & Levy, 1998). They increase in size between 6 and 12 months. Some disappear spontaneously in early childhood, but others require a multidisciplinary medical team approach to their management.

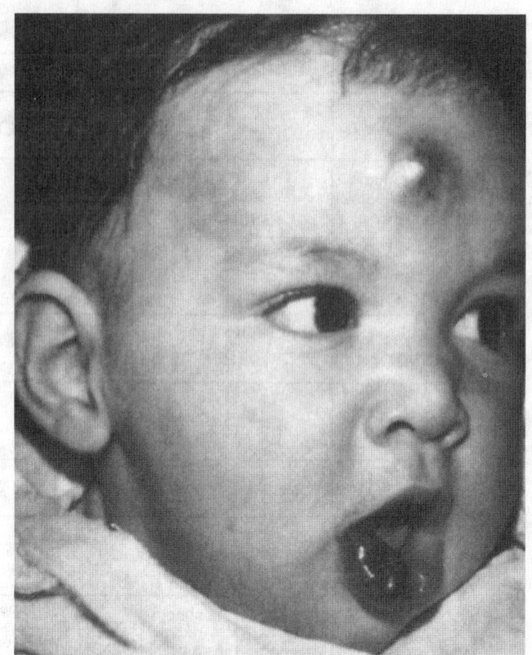

FIGURE 15–3. Hemangioma of the forehead and lip.

Port Wine Stain

Port wine stains (nevus flammeus) are present at birth in 0.3% to 1% of newborns (Hartley & Rasmussen, 1990). Color varies from pink in Caucasian infants to black or deep purple in newborns of African American descent. Most often seen on the head and neck, port wine stains have discrete borders, do not blanch when pressure is applied, and do not lighten as the child ages (Darmstadt, 2000). These lesions are generally benign unless they occur along the trigeminal nerve root, in which case they may be associated with glaucoma or retinal detachment, or in the lumbosacral region, where they may be associated with spinal abnormalities (Brown et al., 1998). Certain types of lasers effectively remove port wine stains and can be used safely on infants.

Nevus Simplex

Nevus simplex, also called stork bite, is a pink, macular lesion. This lesion blanches with pressure and becomes darker when the newborn cries. Lesions may last 1 to 2 years or persist into adulthood. Nevus simplex lesions are most often seen at the back of the neck, on the forehead, on eyelids, on the bridge of the nose, and over the base of the occipital bones. It is the most common lesion seen during the newborn period and may occur on as many as 50% of newborns (Esterly, 1996).

Mongolian Spots

Mongolian spots are blue-gray lesions resembling a bruise and are most often seen over the sacrum and flanks but may be present on the posterior thighs, legs, back, and shoulders (Fig. 15–4). They occur in more than 80% of African American, Native American, East Indian, and Asian newborns and less than 10% of Caucasian newborns (Darmstadt, 2000). They are caused by infiltration of melanin-forming cells into the dermal skin layer rather than the epidermis. Mongolian spots may persist into early childhood but usually fade.

Erythema Toxicum

Erythema toxicum, also called newborn rash, is benign and appears at about 24 to 48 hours of age in approximately 50% of term newborn infants (Darmstadt, 2000). In preterm infants, the rash may not develop for several days or weeks. Erythema toxicum is composed of small, yellow papules surrounded by an erythematous area. The rash continues to appear and disappear over various parts of the body for several days. Most commonly seen on the face, trunk, and limbs, erythema toxicum may continue to appear up to 3 months of age (Witt, 1996).

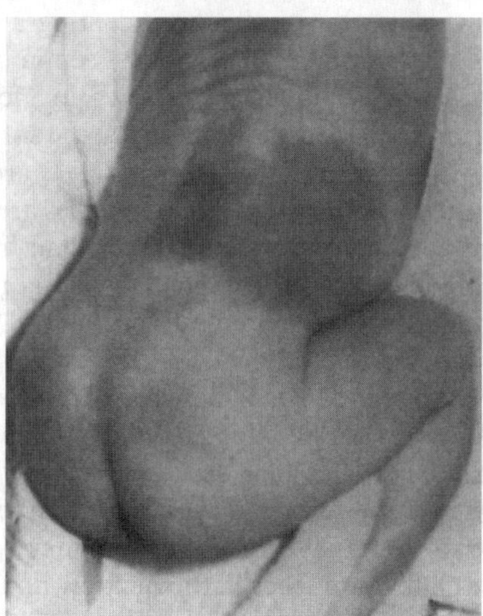

FIGURE 15–4. Mongolian spots.

Milia

Milia, clogged sebaceous glands, appears as tiny, white papules present at birth over the chin, cheeks, forehead, and fleshy area of the nose. They disappear during the first 2 weeks of life.

Texture

Skin is evaluated for texture and the presence of lanugo during the physical examination and as part of the gestational age assessment. Texture ranges from smooth to superficial peeling. Shortly after birth, most term newborns have dry, flaky skin. Peeling, leathery skin with deep cracks indicates postmaturity. Lanugo, a fine, downy hair that covers the body, begins to develop around 20 weeks' gestation (Witt, 1999). It is seen in abundance on premature infants and rarely on infants greater than 42 weeks' gestation. At term, lanugo is confined to the shoulders, ears, and forehead.

Turgor

Skin turgor is the natural rebound elasticity of the skin. It can be assessed anywhere on the body by pinching the skin between the examiners thumb and index finger and then quickly releasing it. Skin turgor is best assessed on the abdomen. Healthy, elastic tissue rapidly resumes its normal position without creases or tenting. Skin that remains tented indicates poor hydration and nutritional status. Table 15–1 identifies skin findings during the physical assessment that are abnormal and their related pathology.

HEAD ASSESSMENT

The newborn head is examined using inspection and palpation and assessed for size, shape, and symmetry. The head of a term, AGA newborn has an occipital-frontal circumference of 32 to 38 cm (12.5 to 14.5 inches). To measure the newborn's head, a tape measure is placed just above the eyebrows and continues around to the occipital prominence at the back of the skull (see Fig. 15–1). Vaginal birth may cause the cranial bones to overlap (ie, molding) as the fetus descends through the birth canal, giving the head an elongated, asymmetric appearance (Fig. 15–5). The overlapping cranial bones can be palpated along the suture lines. Molding may last several days and cause the head circumference to be smaller immediately after birth. The circumference returns to normal within 2 to 3 days after birth. Newborns delivered by cesarean section or in breech position have a more rounded, symmetric head.

TABLE 15–1 ■ INTEGUMENT

Assessment	Pathology
Pallor	Anemia Asphyxia Shock Sepsis Twin-to-twin transfusion Cardiac disease
Central cyanosis	Sepsis Persistent pulmonary hypertension Neurologic disease Congenital heart disease Respiratory disorder
Plethora	Polycythemia
Gray color	Sepsis
Jaundice within 24 hours of birth	Liver disease Blood incompatibilities Sepsis Maternal ingestion of drugs (eg, aspirin)
Generalized petechiae	Clotting disorders Sepsis
Pustules	*Staphylococcus* Beta-hemolytic *Streptococcus* Varicella
Greenish, yellow vernix	Meconium staining Hemolytic disease
Generalized edema	Erythroblastosis fetalis Renal failure Turner syndrome
"Blueberry muffin" spots (purpura)	Congenital viral infection
Multiple tan or light brown macules (café au lait spots)	Neurofibromatosis

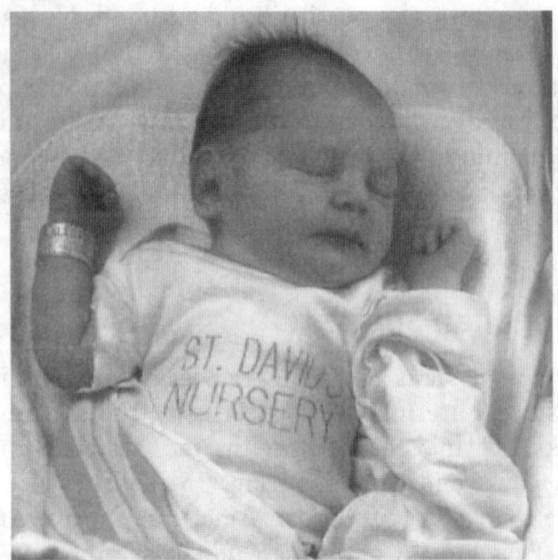

FIGURE 15–5. Molding. (From Pillitteri, A. [1999]. *Maternal and child health nursing* [3rd ed., p. 626]. Philadelphia: Lippincott, Williams & Wilkins.)

Caput succedaneum, edema under the scalp, is caused by pressure over the presenting part of the newborn's head against the cervix during labor. Caput feels soft and spongy, crosses suture lines, and resolves within a few days. Figure 15–6 compares caput succedaneum and cephalhematoma, an abnormal condition further addressed in Table 15–2.

The newborn's head is palpated for the presence of all suture lines (Fig. 15–7). Suture lines feel like soft depressions between the cranial bones. If instead a ridge of bone is felt, the examiner should determine whether it is the result of molding or premature closure of the suture. Normal mobility of the cranial bones is determined by placing each thumb on opposite sides of the suture and alternately pushing in slightly on each side. Lack of mobility of cranial bones indicates premature closure of the sutures (ie, craniosynostosis). The incidence of craniosynostosis is 1 case per 2,000 births (Haslem, 2000). Craniosynostosis leads to an abnormally shaped head as the contents of the cranium enlarges and the cranial bones fail to enlarge. This abnormally shaped head may be apparent at birth or later in infancy.

The skull is palpated for masses and assessed for craniotabes. Craniotabes is a softening of cranial bones caused by pressure of the fetal skull against the bony pelvis. When pressure is exerted with the examiner's fingers at the margins of the parietal or occipital bones, a popping sensation similar to indenting a Ping-Pong ball is felt. Craniotabes is primarily seen in breech presentations and usually disappears within a few weeks.

Anterior and posterior fontanelles, the soft membranous coverings where two sutures meet, are palpated and measured (see Fig. 15–7). Fontanelles are measured diagonally from bone to bone rather than from suture to suture. The anterior fontanelle is diamond shaped, measuring 4 to 5 cm, and closes around 18 months of age. The posterior fontanelle is triangular, measuring 0.5 to 1 cm, and closes between 2 and 4 months. Fontanelles are best palpated when the newborn is quiet. The area is soft, is depressed slightly, and may bulge with crying. Arterial pulsations may be felt over the anterior fontanelle. Molding may make it impossible to palpate fontanelles in the first few hours of life.

The scalp is examined for distribution, amount, and texture of hair. Hair is silky and may be straight,

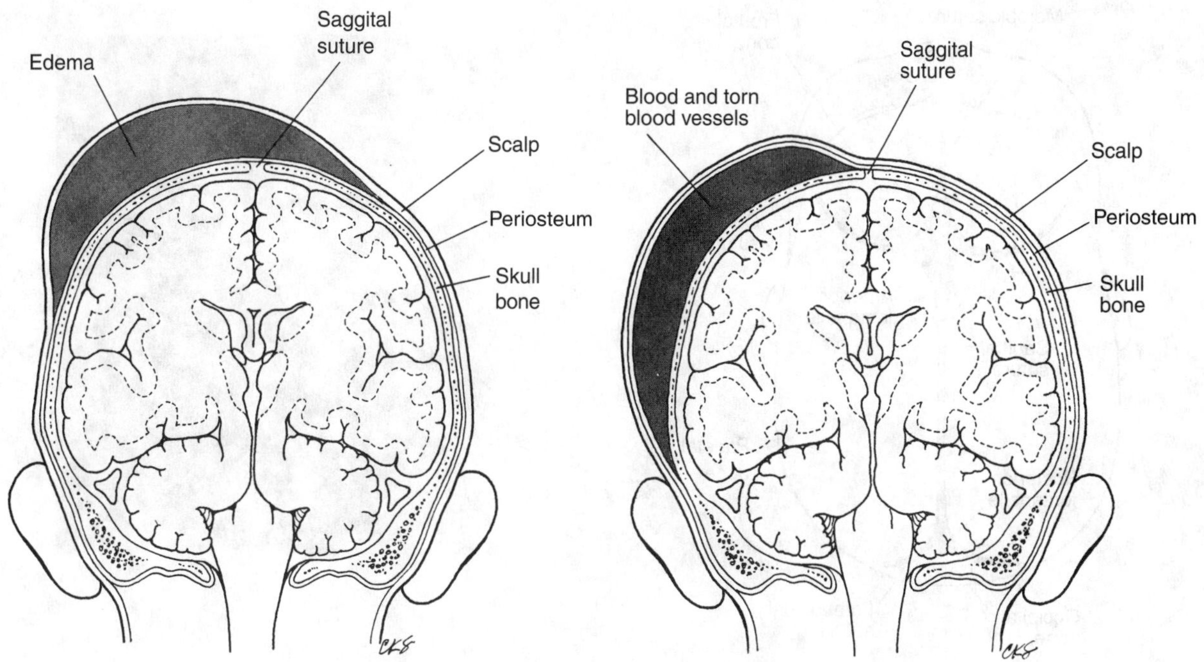

FIGURE 15–6. Comparison of caput succedaneum (*left*) and cephalhematoma (*right*).

TABLE 15–2 ■ HEAD

Assessment	Pathology
The following assessments may indicate increased intracranial pressure: Sutures separated more than 1 cm Bulging, tense fontanelle Head circumference greater than 90th percentile for gestational age	Hydrocephalus Hypothyroidism Tumor Meningitis
Head circumference below 10th percentile for gestational age	Genetic disorder Congenital infection Maternal drug or alcohol ingestion
Depressed fontanelle	Dehydration
Cephalhematoma: swelling due to bleeding between periosteum and skull bone; does not cross suture line; may not be evident until 1 day after birth and take several weeks to resolve (see Fig. 15–6)	Head trauma during birth
Texture of hair is fine, woolly, sparse, coarse, brittle	Prematurity Endocrine disorder Genetic disorder
Increased quantity of hair, low-set hairline	Genetic disorder
Limited forward growth of the skull; skull appears broad	Brachycephaly (fused coronal suture)
Limited lateral growth of the skull; skull appears long and narrow	Saphocephaly (fused sagittal suture)
Collection of fluid in the scalp that crosses suture lines, feels firm, is less pitting than caput, may extend into the neck (Hernandez & Hernandez, 1999).	Subgaleal hematoma

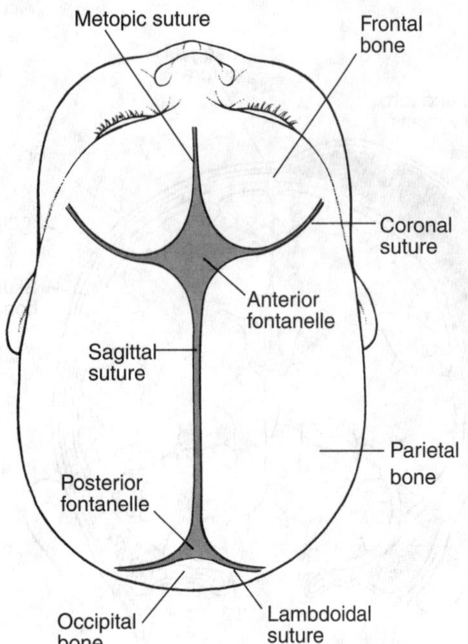

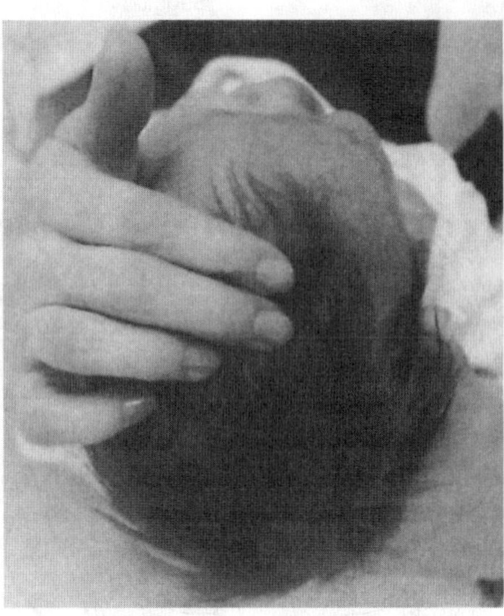

FIGURE 15–7. Palpating the fontanelles.

curly, or kinky, depending on ethnic origin. Bruising, lacerations, and bleeding are frequently seen as the result of the application of a scalp electrode or vacuum extractor. Table 15–2 identifies findings during the physical assessment of the head that are abnormal and their related pathology.

EYE ASSESSMENT

The newborn's eyes are assessed using inspection and an ophthalmoscope. This can be done early in the examination as part of the assessment of the head or whenever the newborn spontaneously opens his eyes. Eyes should be symmetric in size and shape. Lids may be edematous and puffy at birth. The distance between the eyes, measured from the inner canthus of each, is 1.5 to 2.5 cm (Hernandez & Hernandez, 1999). Eyes spaced closer (ie, hypotelorism) or further apart (ie, hypertelorism) may be a variation of normal or associated with other anomalies. Eyes with small palpebral fissures (ie, eye openings) may also be normal or associated with other anomalies.

The colors of eye structures are observed. The iris is usually slate gray, brown, or dark blue. Eye color becomes permanent at about 6 months of age. The normally blue-white sclera may contain subconjunctival hemorrhages, the result of ruptured capillaries during the birth process. Subconjunctival hemorrhages usually resolve within a week. A yellow sclera indicates hyperbilirubinemia. If silver nitrate is used as prophylaxis against ophthalmia neonatorum, the conjunctiva may appear inflamed. Erythromycin ointment usually does not cause this complication.

Tears are usually absent in the newborn until the lacrimal duct becomes fully patent at about 4 to 6 months of age. Prominent epicanthal folds (ie, Mongolian slant) is a normal finding in Asian infants but suggests Down syndrome in other ethnic groups.

Blink reflex, size, and reactivity of pupils are evaluated in a darkened room with a pen light or light from the ophthalmoscope. Pupils are equal and reactive to light (PERL). When a light is shined at an angle toward the eye, the lens should be clear. Presence of and clarity of the red reflex indicates an intact cornea and lens. Lack of a red reflex suggests congenital glaucoma or cataracts. Pale red reflexes are a normal variation in dark-skinned newborns.

Movement of the eye is observed. Strabismus, a cross-eyed appearance, is often seen in newborns because of weak eye musculature and lack of coordination. Nystagmus (ie, constant, rapid, involuntary movement of the eye) may occur and usually disappears by 4 months of age. Newborns are nearsighted at birth and respond to bright or primary colors and to high contrast between colors such as black and white. They see objects clearly 8 to 10 inches in front of them. Table 15–3 identifies findings during the physical assessment of the eye that are abnormal and their related pathology.

TABLE 15–3 ■ EYE

Assessment	Pathology
Persistent purulent discharge	Ophthalmia neonatorum Chlamydia conjunctivitis Blocked lacrimal duct (dacryocystitis)
Blue sclera	Osteogenesis imperfecta
Sclera visible above iris (sunset eyes)	Hydrocephalus
Black or white spots on periphery of iris (Brushfield spots)	Benign or associated with Down syndrome
Pupils not equal, nonreactive, fixed	Neurologic insult
Keyhole-shaped pupil (coloboma)	Usually associated with other anomalies
Mongoloid slant of palpebral fissures (opening between eye lids)	Down syndrome

EAR ASSESSMENT

The newborn ear is assessed by inspection and palpation. External structures are examined for position, consistency of the cartilage, and the presence of abnormal structures. By 38 to 40 weeks' gestation, the pinna is firm and well formed, and incurving exists over two thirds of the ear. The pinna lies on or above an imaginary line drawn from the inner to the outer canthus of the eye back toward the ear (Fig. 15–8). Low-set ears, those that fall below this line, are associated with genetic syndromes. A soft pinna lacking cartilage is seen in premature infants. Temporary asymmetry of the ears can result from intrauterine position. Skin tags (Fig. 15–9) and small pits (Fig. 15–10) located anterior to the ear are usually benign, may be familial, but can also be associated with other malformations or syndromes.

The ear canal is inspected for patency. Use of the otoscope is limited because newborn eustachian tubes contain vernix, mucus, and cellular debris. The ear canals clear spontaneously several days after birth. At this time, the tympanic membrane is visualized by pulling the pinna back and down. The tympanic membrane appears gray-white and highly vascular. If a neonatal infection is suspected, otoscopic examination of the ear is indicated.

Although hearing is well developed at birth, it becomes more acute as the eustachian tubes clear. The newborn responds to high-pitched vocal sounds and the familiar voice of his mother and becomes quiet and relaxed when spoken to in a soft, calm manner. In 1994, the Joint Committee on Infant Hearing (JCIH) proposed that there be universal screening of all newborns for hearing loss as early as possible before 3 months of age and that, when hearing loss is identified through screening, further diagnostic testing be available and interventions begun by 6 months of age (AAP, 1995). The AAP, which held membership in the JCIH, in a separate statement endorsed the implementation of universal newborn hearing screening (UNHS) in any hospital where births occur (AAP, 1999).

The incidence of hearing loss is 1 to 3 cases per 1,000 well newborns and 2 to 4 cases per 1,000 new-

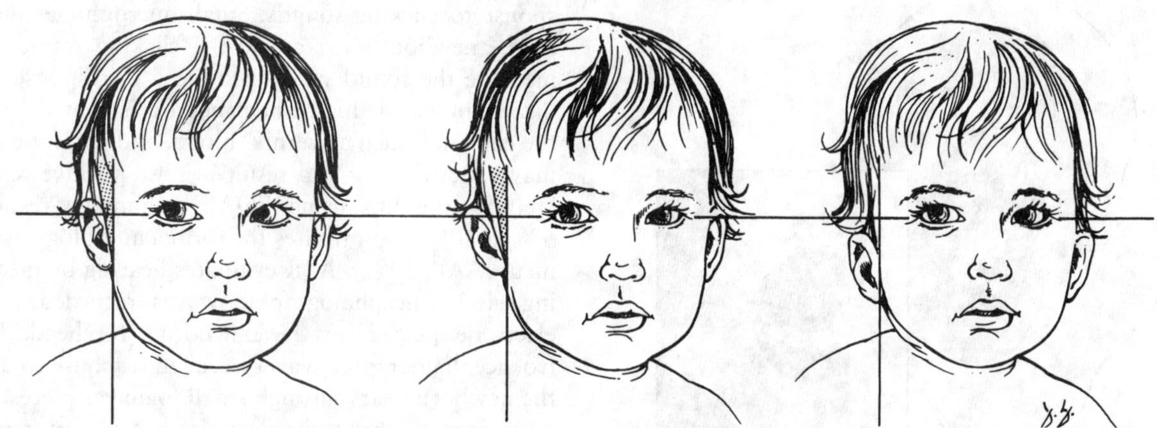

FIGURE 15–8. Normal ear position (*left*). Abnormally angled ear (*middle*). Low-set ears (*right*). (From Reeder, S. J., Martin, L. L., & Koniak-Griffin, D. [1997]. *Maternity nursing: Family, newborn and women's health* [18th ed., p. 706]. Philadelphia: Lippincott-Raven Publishers.)

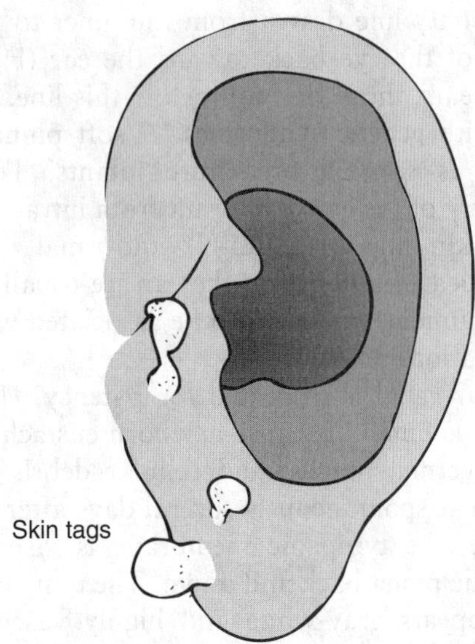

FIGURE 15–9. Preauricular skin tags.

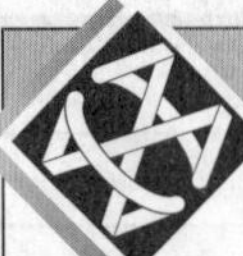
DISPLAY 15–1

Universal Newborn Hearing Screening Program

1. Establish a protocol for screening all newborns, select the screening method, and develop hospital policies and procedures.
2. Provide inservice education and monitor the performance of employees performing universal newborn hearing screening.
3. Provide information to parents regarding screening procedure, cost, potential risks of hearing loss, and benefits of early detection and intervention.
4. Establish a system that provides confidentiality for the parent and newborn, as well as the opportunity for the parents to decline testing.
5. Develop guidelines for documenting the results of screening procedures.
6. Establish mechanisms for communicating results to parents and physicians.

From American Academy of Pediatrics. (1999). Newborn and infant hearing loss: Detection and intervention. *Pediatrics, 103* (2), 527–530.

borns admitted to intensive care nurseries (AAP, 1999). Because early detection and intervention are critical to future speech, language, and cognitive development, many states have enacted legislation requiring UNHS before hospital discharge. Display 15–1 describes the AAP recommendations for hospital-based screening programs. Research indicates that, when newborns are identified before 6 months of age and provided with amplification, their language skills are essentially normal at age 3 years (Mason & Herrmann, 1998; Yoshinaga-Itano, 1999). In programs in which only high-risk newborns are screened (Display 15–2), as many as 50% of newborns with hearing loss may be missed (Mehl & Thomson, 1998).

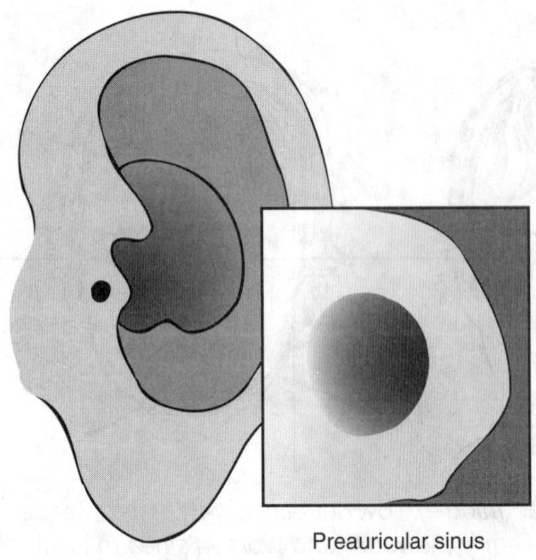

FIGURE 15–10. Preauricular sinus.

Two technologies are available for hearing screening: evoked otoacoustic emissions (EOAE) and auditory brainstem response (ABR). The sensitivity of current technology is at or near 100% (Mehl & Thompson, 1998). These methods are noninvasive, quick, and easy to perform. EOAE evaluates hearing by measuring sound waves in the inner ear. Sound waves are created in the inner ear by the cochlea in response to clicking sounds. Small microphones placed in the newborn's ear create the clicking sounds and measure the sound waves produced in response. The disadvantage of this testing method is that debris in the ear canal such as vernix, blood, and amniotic fluid may effect the test and result in false positive results. UNHS programs using EOAE technology result in 5% to 20% referral rates for formal audiology assessment (AAP, 1999). ABR evaluates hearing by measuring electroencephalographic waves recorded by an electrode placed on the newborn's forehead. Electroencephalographic waves occur in response to clicks the newborn hears through small foam ear pieces. The advantage of this technology is that it is not influenced by debris in the middle or inner ear, and referral rates for formal audiology assessment are less than 3% (AAP, 1999). The challenge to using this technol-

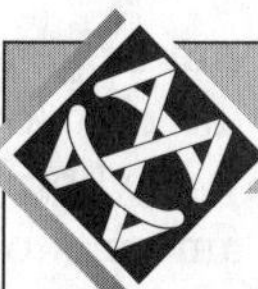

DISPLAY 15-2

Risk Factors for Hearing Loss

- Family history of hereditary childhood sensorineural hearing loss
- In utero infection, such as cytomegalovirus, rubella, syphilis, herpes, or toxoplasmosis.
- Craniofacial anomalies, including infants with morphologic abnormalities of the pinnae and ear canals
- Birth weight less than 1500 g
- Hyperbilirubinemia at a serum level requiring exchange transfusion
- Ototoxic medications, including aminoglycosides used in multiple courses or in combination with loop diuretics
- Bacterial meningitis
- Apgar score of 0–4 at 1 minute or 0–6 at 5 minutes after birth
- Mechanical ventilation lasting 5 days or longer
- Stigmata or other findings associated with a syndrome known to include sensorineural or conductive hearing loss

American Academy of Pediatrics & American College of Obstetricians and Gynecologists (AAP & ACOG). (1997). *Guidelines for perinatal care* (4th ed.). Washington, DC: Author.

ogy is keeping the newborn in a quiet state, preferably sleeping.

Table 15–4 identifies findings during the physical assessment of the ear that are abnormal and their related pathology.

TABLE 15–4 ■ EAR

Assessment	Pathology
Low-set ears	Genetic disorder Kidney abnormality
Poorly formed external ear	Genetic disorder
Small skin tags (see Fig. 15–9)	Familial variation Alteration in normal embryologic development Genetic disorder
Preauricular sinus "pits" located in front of the ear may be closed or extend to the internal ear or brain (see Fig. 15–10)	Familial variation Alteration in normal embryologic development Genetic disorder (brachial-oto-renal syndrome)
Absence of Moro reflex in response to loud noise	Hearing loss

NOSE ASSESSMENT

The newborn's nose is assessed using inspection. The nose should be symmetric and midline but may be misshapen at birth because of the neonate's positioning in utero. If the septum cannot be easily straightened and the nose remains asymmetric, treatment may be required. A flattened or bruised nose may result from passage through the birth canal.

Because newborns primarily breathe through the nose, it is imperative to check the nasal canals for patency. Patency is assessed in one of two ways. A small, soft catheter may be passed down each naris to check for an obstruction, or with the newborn's mouth closed, gentle, alternating pressure is applied on the naris. Assess the newborn's ability to breathe by observing the air passage through the naris not occluded. If the infant exhibits any difficulty in breathing, these finding are reported immediately to a nurse practitioner or physician.

Nasal stuffiness and thin, white mucus is not an uncommon finding immediately after birth. Newborns sneeze to clear the upper respiratory tract. Nasal flaring, widening of the nares, is a compensatory mechanism that decreases upper airway resistance, allowing more air to enter the nasal passages. Nasal flaring is abnormal and one of the first symptoms observed when respiratory distress occurs. Table 15–5 identifies

TABLE 15–5 ■ NOSE

Assessment	Pathology
Flat nasal bridge	Down syndrome
Pink when crying; chest retractions and cyanosis at rest; difficulty feeding	Choanal atresia
Stuffy nose and thin, watery discharge	Neonatal drug withdrawal
"Sniffles" persistent; profuse mucopurulent or bloody discharge (Green, 1998)	Congenital syphilis

findings during the physical assessment of the nose that are abnormal and their related pathology.

MOUTH ASSESSMENT

The newborn mouth is assessed using inspection and palpation. In the sequence of the total examination, this assessment is frequently left until last. If the newborn's mouth is forced open, crying may result, altering aspects of the respiratory or cardiac assessments. The lips are observed for location, color, and symmetry. The mouth should be centrally located along the midline. At rest, the lips appear symmetric. Depending on skin color, the lips are pink or more darkly pigmented. Sucking blisters, centrally located on the upper lip, may be filled with fluid or have the consistency of a callus. Calluses may also be found on the hand as a result of vigorous sucking in utero or after birth. Muscle weakness or facial paralysis is best observed when the infant is sucking or crying; both conditions may be missed altogether if the infant is observed only in a quiet, alert state (Fig. 15–11). Rooting, suck, and gag reflexes are evaluated during this portion of the examination or during feeding.

The mucous membrane and internal structures of the mouth are inspected. If the mouth does not open spontaneously while the newborn cries, it can be gently opened by a downward pressure on the chin or with a pediatric tongue blade. In a healthy newborn, the mucous membrane is pink. Increased amounts of mucus during the first 1 to 2 days of life are removed with a bulb syringe. This is especially common in newborns born by cesarean section, because they do not benefit from compression of the thorax through the birth canal. The tongue is mobile and prominent within the mouth. Occasionally, the frenulum is short, causing a notch at the tip of the tongue. True congenital ankyloglossia (ie, tongue tie) is rare.

Using adequate lighting, the hard and soft palates are examined. The uvula is midline and located at the posterior soft palate. Some practitioners use an index finger to palpate the hard and soft palates for the presence of clefts (Fig. 15–12). Whitish-yellow cysts (ie, Epstein's pearls) containing epithelial cells may be present on the hard palate at birth, but they disappear within a few weeks. Some newborns are born with one or two natal teeth. These immature caps of enamel and dentin have poor root formation and are usually loose. These teeth may be aspirated if dislodged, make breast-feeding difficult, or cause lacerations on the mucosa, lips, or tongue. They are usually removed during the neonatal period. Table 15–6 identifies findings during the physical assessment of the mouth that are abnormal and their related pathology.

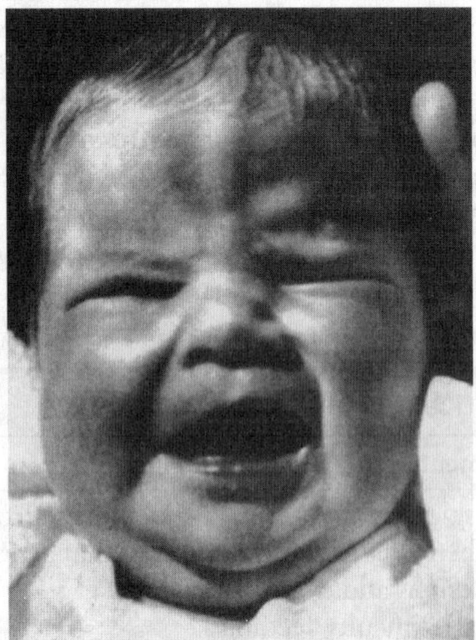

FIGURE 15–11. Facial nerve paralysis. Notice the asymmetry of the mouth during crying. (From Reeder, S. J., Martin, L. L., & Koniak-Griffin, D. [1997]. *Maternity nursing: Family, newborn and women's health* [18th ed., p. 1205]. Philadelphia: Lippincott-Raven Publishers.)

Inspection and palpation are used to assess the neck. The neck is inspected for symmetry and range of motion. Newborns have short, thick necks with multiple skin folds. A predominant fat pad in the back of the neck, redundant skin, and webbing are findings associated with genetic syndromes.

Full range of motion is present at term. The newborn's head should be able to turn completely to face each shoulder. Torticollis, contraction of the neck muscles that pulls the head toward the affected side with the chin pointing toward the opposite shoulder and side, results from injury to the sternocleidomastoid muscle. More common on the right side, this injury may be congenital or occur during the birth process. A small mass at the site of the injury is palpated along the sternocleidomastoid muscle at birth or soon after. Parents are taught to perform stretching exercises to lengthen the muscle, and the newborn is followed by a physical therapist through the first year of life. If the contracture persists after 1 year, surgery may be necessary.

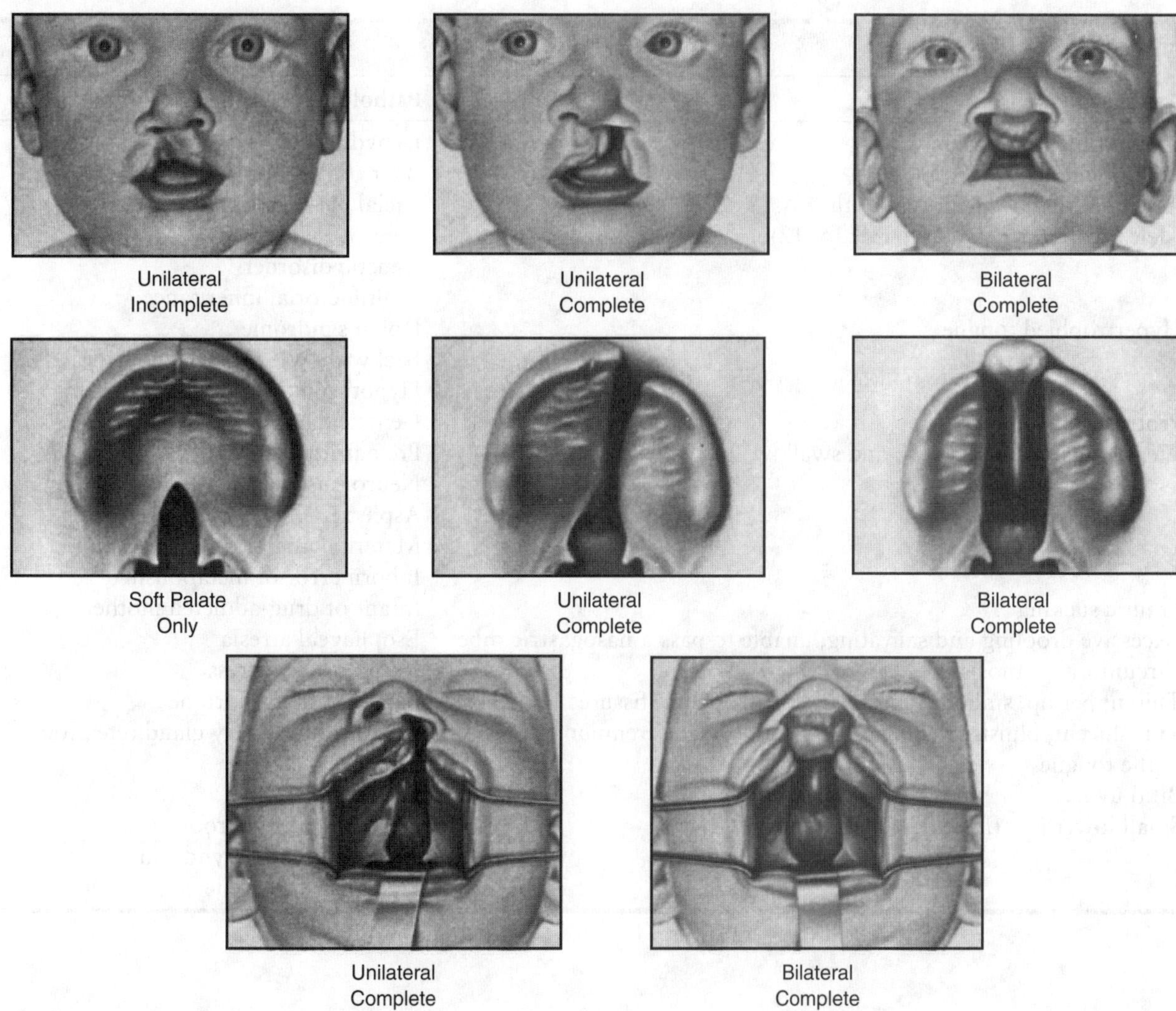

FIGURE 15–12. Cleft lip and cleft palate (Redrawn from drawings by Ross Laboratories). From *Maternity Nursing: Family, Newborn, and Women's Health* (18th ed., p. 1108), by S. J. Reeder, L. L. Martin, and D. Koniak-Griffin, 1997. Philadelphia: Lippincott-Raven Publishers.

Cystic hygroma is one of the most common neck lesions (Fig. 15–13). This particular cystic structure occurs at lymphatic-venous connections, most commonly in the posterior neck (Gallagher, Mahoney, & Gosche, 1999). The lesions vary in size from a few millimeters to large enough to deviate the trachea, cause respiratory distress, or interfere with feeding. A cystic hygroma requires surgical excision.

The neck is palpated along the midline for the trachea and abnormal masses. The thyroid gland is difficult to palpate unless it is enlarged, an unusual finding during the newborn period. A potential for infection exists within all the cystic structures and abnormal sinuses arising around the newborn's neck. Table 15–7 identifies additional findings during the physical assessment of the neck that are abnormal and their related pathology.

CHEST AND LUNG ASSESSMENT

Auscultation and inspection are used to assess the newborn's chest and respiratory status. The newborn's chest is cylindrical. Measured at the nipple line, its circumference is approximately 33 cm or 2 to 3 cm less than the infant's head (see Fig. 15–1). The xiphoid process is sometimes seen as a small protuberant area at the end of the sternum. Respirations are shallow and irregular. Chest movement should be symmetric and not labored. An accurate respiratory rate is obtained by counting for 1 full minute, preferably when the newborn is quiet. Newborns are obligatory nose breathers and have an average respiratory rate of 30 to 60 breaths/min. With each respiration, synchronous abdominal movement occurs. The color

TABLE 15–6 ■ MOUTH

Assessment	Pathology
Mucous membranes dry	Dehydration
Cyanotic mucous membranes	Poor oxygenation
Asymmetric movement of mouth	Facial nerve injury
Cleft lip and/or palate (see Fig. 15–12)	Teratogenic injury
	Genetic disorder
	Multifactorial inheritance
Hypertrophied tongue	Down syndrome
	Beckwith-Wiedmann syndrome
	Hypothryoidism
Protrusion of tongue	Genetic disorder
Weak, uncoordinated suck and swallow	Prematurity
	Neuromuscular disorder
	Asphyxia
	Maternal analgesia during labor
	Inborn error of metabolism
Frantic sucking	Infant of drug-addicted mother
Excessive drooling and salivating; unable to pass a nasogastric tube	Esophageal atresia
Circumoral cyanosis	Respiratory distress
Thin upper lip, smooth philtrum, short palpebral fissures	Fetal alcohol syndrome
Translucent, bluish swelling on either side of the frenulum under the tongue	Mucous or salivary gland retention cyst
Bifid uvula	Genetic disorder
Small lower jaw (micrognathia)	Pierre Robin syndrome
	Treacher Collins syndrome
	De Lange syndrome

of the newborn's skin and mucous membranes is evaluated simultaneously. Presence of cyanosis may be a sign of respiratory distress.

Tachypnea (ie, respiratory rate >60) may be one of the first symptoms of morbidity in the newborn. If tachypnea is present, the respiratory rate may reach 120 breaths/min. The primary healthcare provider should be notified when respiratory rates are increased, and oral feedings should be withheld because of the risk of aspiration.

Other signs of respiratory distress include retractions, nasal flaring, and grunting. Retractions are the drawing inward or shortening of small muscles in the chest wall. Retractions occur when more energy is needed to assist respiratory effort. Retractions are seen between the ribs (intercostal), below the rib cage (subcostal), above the sternum (tracheal tug), below the xiphoid process, and surrounding the clavicles. Flaring of the nares occurs with inspiration. It is a compensatory mechanism used by the newborn in respiratory distress. Flaring of the nares, widens the upper airway, decreasing airway resistance and making breathing easier. Grunting is a sound produced on expiration when air passes through a partially closed glottis. The partially closed glottis is a compensatory mechanism that traps air in the alveoli, increasing the time that gas exchange can occur. Grunting may be audible or heard only with a stethoscope. The Silverman-Anderson Index is a tool used for systematically assessing and documenting newborn respiratory effort and the presence of physical symptoms of respiratory distress (Table 15–8). A score of zero indicates no respiratory distress.

Inspection of the newborn's chest includes placement, shape, and amount of palpable breast tissue. Hypertrophy of breast tissue, with or without secretion of milky fluid, may be present by the second or third day of life because of maternal hormones (Fig. 15–14). This condition lasts approximately 1 week. Supernumerary nipples (ie, accessory nipples) are considered a benign congenital anomaly. They are often seen below and medial to the normal nipples.

Auscultation of the anterior and posterior chest proceeds in an orderly fashion from top to bottom,

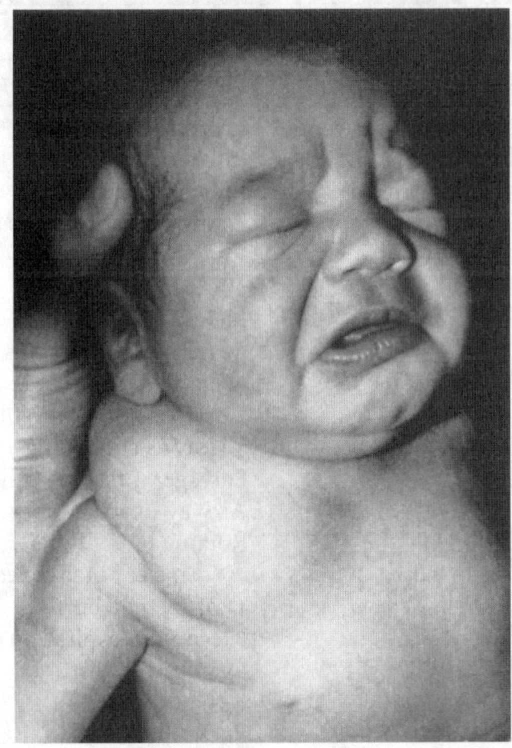

FIGURE 15–13. Cystic hygroma.

TABLE 15–7 ■ NECK

Assessment	Pathology
Multiple skin folds in the lateral, posterior region of the neck (webbing)	Down syndrome Turner syndrome
Enlarged thyroid	Hyperthyroidism Hypothyroidism
Absence of head control	Prematurity Genetic disorder Asphyxia Neuromuscular disorder
Abnormal opening along the anterior surface of the sternocleidomastoid muscle leads to a blind pouch or communicates with deeper structures	Brachial sinus
Mass high in the neck at midline extending to the base of the tongue; often appears after an upper respiratory infection (Darmstadt, 2000)	Thyroglossal duct cyst
Palpable cystic mass may open on to the skin surface or drain into the pharynx (Darmstadt, 2000)	Brachial cleft cyst

comparing from side to side for equality of breath sounds and the presence of abnormal sounds such as grunting and rales. The term *crackles* maybe used in place of the traditional term *rales* for the fine cracking, bubbling, or fine rustling noises heard when air passes fluid. Rhonchi and wheezing are less common in the newborn period. These lower-pitched sounds result from obstruction or narrowing of larger airways.

Newborns have a periodic breathing pattern resulting from the immaturity of their respiratory and central nervous systems. It is common to observe brief pauses in respiratory effort. Pauses lasting 20 seconds or longer and associated with color change or bradycardia are considered apneic periods and should be reported to the primary healthcare provider.

Apnea (ie, pauses in respirations lasting 20 seconds or longer) or other signs of respiratory distress may occur in almost all illnesses in the newborn period. The list of differential diagnoses for respiratory distress and apnea in the newborn is extensive (Table 15–9). Table 15–10 identifies findings during the res-

TABLE 15–8 ■ SILVERMAN-ANDERSON INDEX

Score	Upper Chest	Lower Chest	Xiphoid	Nares	Grunt
0	Chest and abdomen rise together	No intercostal retractions	No xiphoid retractions	No nasal flaring	No expiratory grunt
1	Lag or minimal sinking of upper chest as abdomen rises	Minimal intercostal retractions	Minimal xiphoid retractions	Minimal nasal flaring	Expiratory grunt heard with stethoscope
2	Upper chest and abdomen move as a "see-saw"	Marked intercostal retractions	Marked xiphoid retractions	Marked nasal flaring	Audible expiratory grunt

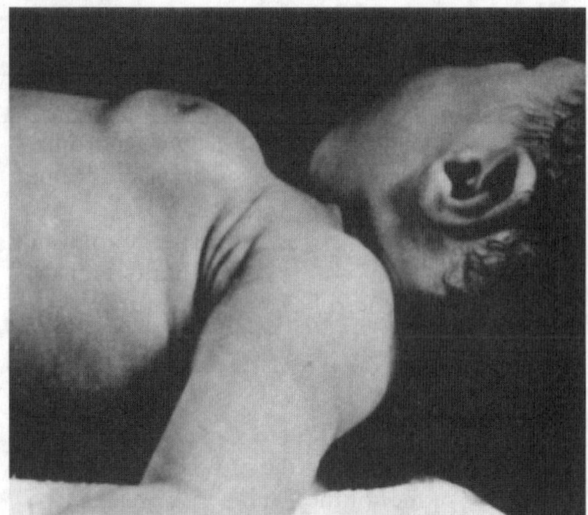

FIGURE 15–14. Neonatal breast hypertrophy.

piratory assessment that are abnormal and their related pathology.

CARDIOVASCULAR SYSTEM ASSESSMENT

The cardiovascular system is assessed using inspection, auscultation, and palpation. The examination begins with inspection of the newborn's color as one indication of oxygenation and perfusion. As the newborn transitions from intrauterine to extrauterine life, skin color changes occur. At birth, the infant may be pale or cyanotic, becoming pink as respirations are established, fetal circulation is reversed, and blood is oxygenated by the lungs and circulated by the strength of the heart muscle.

The precordium (ie, area on the anterior chest to the left of the sternum and above the heart) is inspected and palpated for movement. In a term newborn, very little movement should be observed in this area. The point of maximal impulse (PMI) is normally auscultated or palpated in the third to fourth intercostal space just lateral to the left midclavicular line. Displacement of the PMI can occur with cardiac enlargement, diaphragmatic hernia, dextrocardia, or

TABLE 15–9 ■ DIFFERENTIAL DIAGNOSIS OF RESPIRATORY DISTRESS IN THE NEWBORN

Respiratory	Extrapulmonary
Respiratory distress syndrome	Congenital heart disease
	Patent ductus arteriosus
Transient tachypnea	Metabolic acidosis
Meconium aspiration	Hypoglycemia
Primary pulmonary hypertension	Hypothermia
	Septicemia
Pneumonia	Ventricular hemorrhage
Pulmonary hemorrhage	Edema
	Drugs
Pneumothorax	Trauma
Airway obstruction	Hypovolemia
Diaphragmatic hernia	Twin-to-twin transfusion
Hypoplastic lung	

Adapted from Askin, D. F. (1997). Acute respiratory care of the newborn (p. 32). Petaluma, CA: NICU. INK.

TABLE 15–10 ■ RESPIRATORY SYSTEM

Assessment	Pathology
Cessation of breathing for more than 20 seconds (apnea)	Hypo/hyperthermia Infection Prematurity Respiratory disorders Cardiovascular disorders Neurologic disorders Maternal medications Metabolic disorders Gastroesophageal reflux Vigorous suctioning Passage of feeding tube Airway obstruction
Tachypnea	Retained lung fluid (transient tachypnea of the newborn) Meconium aspiration Respiratory distress syndrome Pneumonia Hyperthermia Pulmonary edema Sepsis Metabolic disorders
Decreased or absent breath sounds	Meconium aspiration Atelectasis Pneumothorax Diaphagmatic hernia Hypoplastic lungs Diaphragmatic hernia
Bowel sounds heard in place of breath sounds	Diaphragmatic hernia

pneumothorax. Increased activity, an active precordium, could indicate patent ductus arteriosus or congestive heart failure in a newborn or occur as a variation of normal in preterm or SGA newborns who are thin and have minimal subcutaneous tissue. Three additional sensations—heave, tap, and thrill—may be felt as the chest is palpated. A heave is a diffuse pulsation that can occur with ventricular volume overload. A tap is a pronounced localized pulsation of the PMI. A thrill is a palpated vibration that is associated with a murmur.

Heart rate and rhythm are best auscultated using the bell and diaphragm of a small neonatal stethoscope while the newborn remains quiet. The stethoscope should be warmed before placement so the newborn is not startled. The apical rate is counted for 1 full minute. The normal heart rate is 120 to 160 beats/min. In deep sleep, the heart rate may be 80 to 110 beats/min but should increase quickly if the newborn is disturbed. Auscultation begins at the mitral area (PMI) and proceeds systematically to the tricuspid, pulmonic, and aortic areas using the diaphragm of the stethoscope. The process is then repeated using the bell of the stethoscope (Fig. 15–15). Heart sounds are louder in infants because of the thin chest wall.

Heart sounds become clearer over the first few hours of life as fetal circulation is reversed. Rapid heart rates often make it difficult to auscultate specific heart sound. The first heart sound, S_1, is traditionally thought to be caused by the closure of the tricuspid and mitral valves as ventricular pressure rises during systole. It is heard best at the apex of the heart, in the fourth intercostal space. S_1 is usually loudest at birth, decreasing in intensity over 24 to 48 hours. The second heart sound, S_2, is thought to be caused by the closure of the pulmonic and aortic valves as the ventricular pressure falls during diastole. Splitting of S_2 with inspiration is common after the first few hours of life. Other forms of splitting may be considered pathologic and a sign of congenital heart disease.

Heart murmurs in newborns are common during the neonatal period. Murmurs are evaluated for loudness or intensity of sound (ie, grade), timing in the cardiac cycle (ie, systolic or diastolic), location of the murmur's maximum intensity, radiation, and pitch or quality of sound. Ninety percent of all murmurs are related to incomplete closure of the ductus arteriosus or foramen ovale and are transient in nature. These murmurs are usually grade 1 or 2 (Display 15–3). Murmurs are best auscultated at the left lower sternal border in the third or fourth interspace. The diaphragm of the stethoscope can detect high-pitched murmurs, whereas the bell is better for detecting low-pitched murmurs.

Peripheral pulses (ie, brachial, radial, femoral, popliteal, and dorsalis pedis) are evaluated for presence, equality, and strength. Femoral pulses may be difficult to palpate but should be present in all infants.

Routine blood pressure screening is not recommended for all newborns (AAP & ACOG, 1997). Evaluating the blood pressure is usually reserved for newborns with signs of distress, persistent murmurs, or abnormal pulses. Blood pressure is measured in all four extremities. Blood pressure varies depending on birth weight (Fig. 15–16), gestational age, cuff size, and state of alertness. An appropriate size of blood pressure cuff is necessary to ensure an accurate measurement. The width of the cuff used should cover no more than 50% to 70% of the length of the extremity being tested, such as 50% to 70% of the length from knee to hip, elbow to shoulder, or ankle to knee (Glass, 1999). At term, the normal blood pressure range is 65 to 95 mm Hg systolic and 30 to 60mm Hg

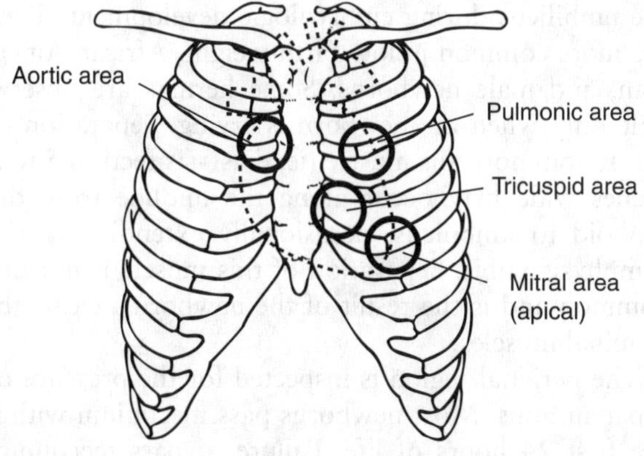

FIGURE 15–15. Ausculatory areas of the heart. (From Tappero, E. P., & Honeyfield, M. E. [Eds.]. [1996]. *Physical assessment of the newborn* [2nd ed., p. 83]. Petaluma, CA: NICU INK.

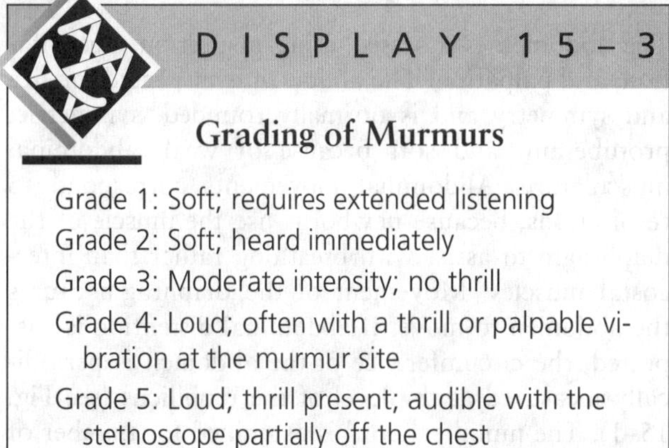

DISPLAY 15–3

Grading of Murmurs

Grade 1: Soft; requires extended listening
Grade 2: Soft; heard immediately
Grade 3: Moderate intensity; no thrill
Grade 4: Loud; often with a thrill or palpable vibration at the murmur site
Grade 5: Loud; thrill present; audible with the stethoscope partially off the chest
Grade 6: Loud; audible with the stethoscope off the chest

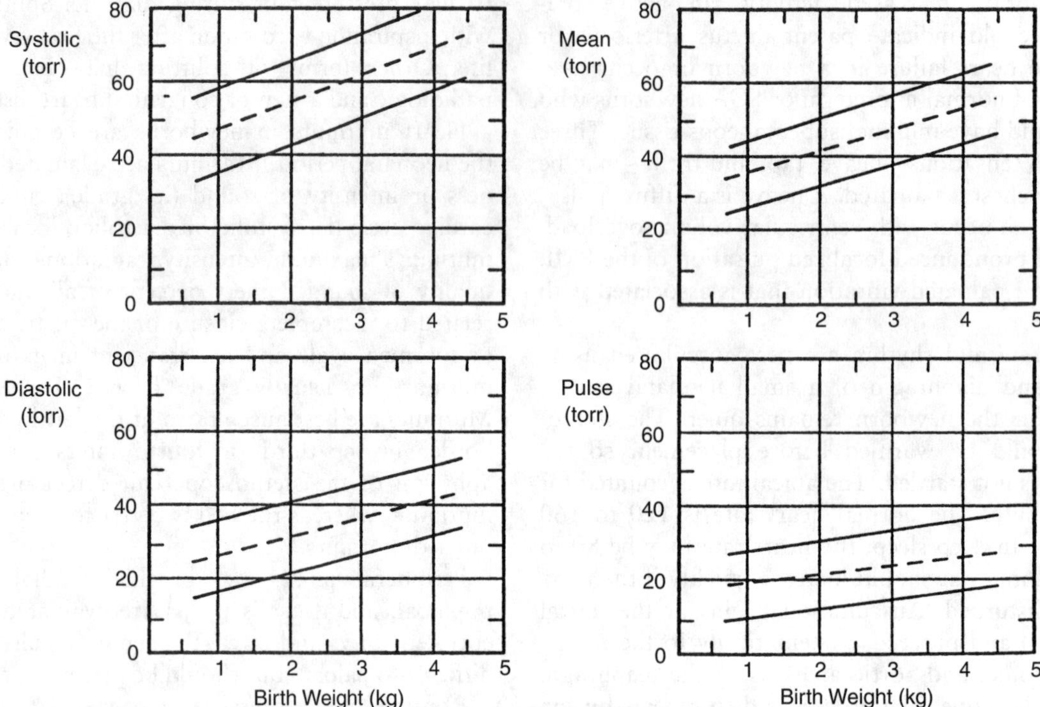

FIGURE 15–16. Normal blood pressure range. Linear regressions (*broken lines*) and 95% confidence limits (*solid lines*) of systolic (*left*) and diastolic (*right*) blood pressure. (Adapted from Tappero, E. P., & Honeyfield, M. E. [Eds.]. [1996]. *Physical assessment of the newborn* [2nd ed., p. 89]. Petaluma, CA: NICU INK, and from Versmold, H. T., Kitterman, J. A., Phibbs, R. H., Gregory, G. A., & Tooley, W. H. [1981]. Aortic blood pressure during the first 12 hours of life in infants 610 to 4220 grams. *Pediatrics, 76*[5], 22.)

diastolic (Hernandez, Zabloudil, & Hernandez, 1999). Blood pressure in the lower extremities is usually higher than in the upper extremities.

Table 15–11 identifies findings during the cardiovascular assessment that are abnormal and their related pathology.

ABDOMINAL ASSESSMENT

The abdomen is assessed using inspection, auscultation, and palpation. The abdomen is inspected for size and symmetry and is normally rounded, symmetric, protuberant, and soft because of weak abdominal musculature. Abdominal movements correspond to respirations, because newborns use the muscle of the diaphragm to assist with breathing rather than intercostal muscles. Movement of the diaphragm causes the abdomen to move. If abdominal distention is suspected, the circumference of the abdomen is periodically measured at the level of the umbilicus (see Fig. 15–1). The umbilical cord is examined for number of vessels, color, and condition. The cord should be opaque to white-blue and contain two arteries and one vein. Variations include a thin, dry cord associated with intrauterine growth restriction or a thick cord seen in LGA newborns. A greenish-yellow discoloration of the cord sometimes occurs with relaxation of the anal sphincter and subsequent passage of meconium. The area surrounding the umbilical cord is observed for masses or the herniation of abdominal contents (Fig. 15–17). Umbilical hernias occur when the intestinal muscle does not close completely around the umbilicus during embryologic development. They are more common in low-birth-weight, African American, and male newborns. Some hernias are observable only when the newborn is crying. Separation of the abdominorectus muscle (ie, diastasis recti) 0.5 to 2 inches wide may occur along the midline from the xiphoid to umbilicus, occasionally extending to the symphysis pubis. Separation of this muscle is not uncommon and is the result of the newborn's weak abdominal muscles.

The perianal region is inspected for the presence of a patent anus. Most newborns pass meconium within the first 24 hours of life. Failure to pass meconium may indicate a gastrointestinal obstruction and necessitates further evaluation.

Bowel sounds are normally present within the first hour of life as the newborn swallows air with crying

TABLE 15–11 ■ CARDIOVASCULAR SYSTEM

Assessment	Pathology
Tachycardia >160 beats/min	Anemia Congestive heart failure Shock or hypovolemia Respiratory distress Supraventricular tachycardia Sepsis Congenital heart anomalies Hyperthermia
Persistent bradycardia <100 beats/min	Congenital heart block Sepsis Asphyxia Hypoxemia Increased intracranial pressure
Persistent murmurs	Persistent fetal circulation Congenital heart defects Peripheral pulmonic stenosis
Muffled heart sounds	Pneumothorax Pneumopericardium Diaphragmatic hernia Pneumomediastinum
Heart sound muffled on left side, loud on right side	Dextrocardia Pnemothorax with mediastinal shift
Decrease in intensity or absence of femoral pulses	Hip dysplasia Coarctation of the aorta
Bounding peripheral pulses; active precordium	Patent ductus arteriosus Fluid overload Congestive heart failure Ventricular septal defect
Difference of blood pressure >20 mm Hg between upper and lower extremities	Coarctation of aorta
Central cyanosis	Congenital heart disease Lung disease Sepsis Persistent pulmonary hypertension Hypertension
Cyanosis that does not improve with 100% oxygen	Congenital heart disease
Cyanosis that worsens with crying	Congenital heart disease

and the sympathetic nervous system stimulates peristalsis. Bowel sounds are auscultated in all four quadrants.

Most perinatal nurses conduct a limited assessment of the abdomen using light palpation for consistency and the presence of masses. A more detailed examination is conducted by the primary healthcare provider. The lower border of the liver is sharp, soft, and palpated in the right upper quadrant 1 to 2 cm below the costal margin. The spleen, located in the left upper quadrant, may be palpable in preterm newborns but rarely in term newborns. The spleen should not be palpated more than 1 cm below the left costal margin (Hernandez & Hernandez, 1999). Kidneys are 4 to 5 cm long and are usually only palpable during the first 6 hours of life. After this time, the bowel and stomach become distended with fluid and air, making this assessment difficult. With the newborn's legs flexed against the abdomen, kidneys are located using deep palpations at the level of the umbilicus, lateral to the midclavicular line. The right kidney may be lower than the left (Fig. 15–18).

Inspection and palpation of the femoral region is conducted during this portion of the examination or as part of the cardiovascular assessment. A soft, com-

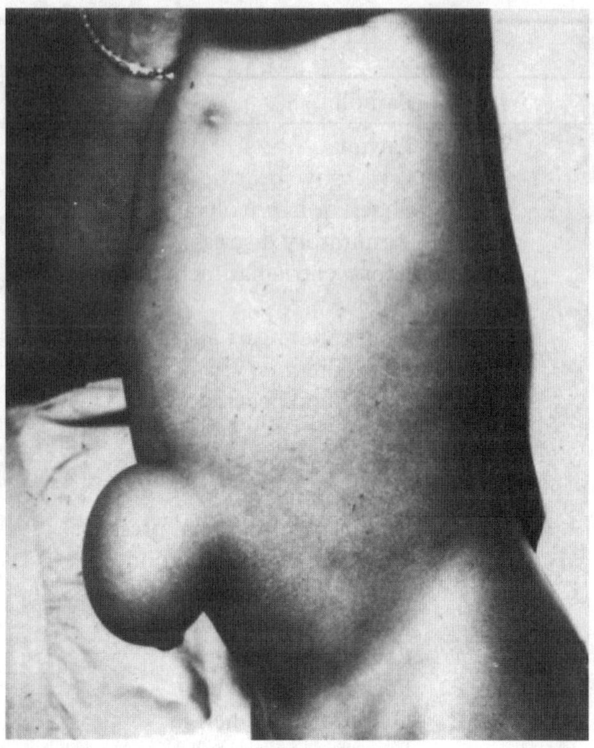

FIGURE 15–17. Umbilical hernia. (Courtesy of Dr. Mark Ravitch.)

pressible swelling in the groin may indicate an inguinal hernia or undescended testes (Fig. 15–19). Bowel sounds can be auscultated in the testis if swelling is caused by herniation of the bowel. Table 15–12 identifies findings during the physical assessment of the abdomen that are abnormal and their related pathology. Figure 15–20 illustrates the prune belly syndrome; this condition is further addressed in Table 15–12.

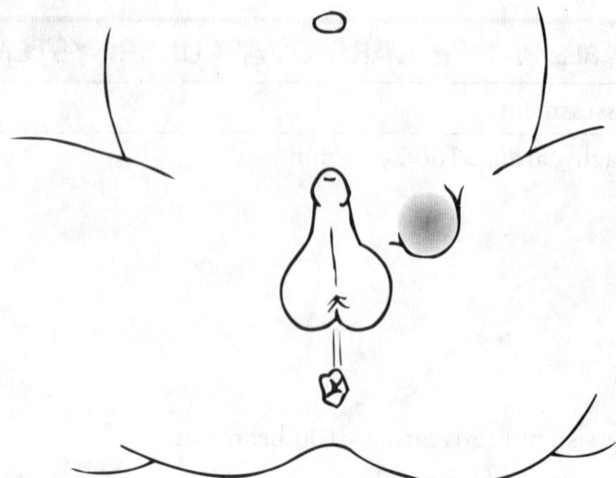

FIGURE 15–19. Left inguinal hernia producing a bulge in the groin of the affected side.

GENITOURINARY SYSTEM ASSESSMENT

The genitourinary system is assessed using inspection and palpation. External genitalia are evaluated as part of the physical examination and gestational age assessment. Newborns should void within 24 hours of birth. A rust-colored stain on the diaper, which in some instances can be flaked off, is a normal variation caused by uric acid crystals in the urine. Bruising and edema of the genitalia and buttocks can occur in newborns who had a breech presentation.

Female Newborns

In term newborns, the clitoris and labia minora are covered by the labia majora. The urinary meatus is lo-

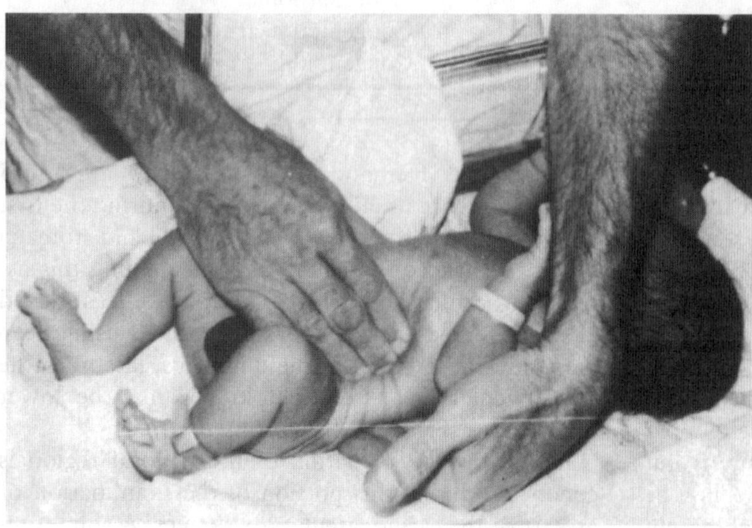

FIGURE 15–18. Examiner demonstrating technique for palpation of the left kidney.

TABLE 15–12 ■ ABDOMEN

Assessment	Pathology
Scaphoid	Diaphragmatic hernia Malnutrition
"Prune belly" flabby, wrinkled abdominal wall (see Fig. 15–20)	Congenital absence of abdominal musculature; associated with other gastrointestinal (GI) or genitourinary (GU) anomalies
Asymmetric abdomen	Abdominal mass GI/GU anomalies
Abdominal distention	GI obstruction Masses Enlargement of abdominal organs Infection (Hernandez & Hernandez, 1999)
Distention in left upper quadrant	Pyloric stenosis Duodenal or jejunal obstruction
Ascites	Hydrops fetalis Viral infections (congenital)
Umbilical cord with one artery and one vein	Associated with GI/GU anomalies
Thin membrane covering herniation of abdominal contents through a defect in the umbilical ring	Omphalocele—associated with other congenital anomalies
Uncovered protrusion of abdominal contents, usually to the right of the umbilicus	Gastroschisis
Red, oozing, or foul-smelling cord	Infection (omphalitis)
Persistently moist umbilicus; clear discharge from umbilical cord stump (Conner, 1996)	Persistent embryologic connection between bladder and umbilicus (patent urachus) or ileum and umbilicus (omphalomesenteric duct)
Failure to pass meconium stool	Imperforate anus Meconium ileus Hirschsprung disease Meconium plug syndrome
Passage of sticky, thick, small plugs of meconium	Meconium ileus Cystic fibrosis
Bruit	Arteriovenous malformation Renal artery stenosis
Partial or complete herniation of the bladder through the abdominal wall	Bladder extrophy results from absence of muscle and connective tissue in the anterior abdominal wall occurring during embryologic development

cated beneath the clitoris. The labia majora and clitoris are enlarged because of maternal hormones circulated to the newborn in utero. In preterm newborns, the labia majora does not cover the labia minora and clitoris. Bruising and swelling of the external genitalia may be present after a vaginal birth.

In some newborns, when the introitus is gently separated, a hymenal tag is seen in the vagina. This tissue, which developed from the hymen and labia minora, disappears in 1 to 2 weeks (Cavaliere, 1996). A white mucous discharge from the vagina is not uncommon during the first week of life. Pseudomenstruation, caused by withdrawal of maternal hormones, is a pink-tinged mucous discharge lasting 2 to 4 weeks.

The labia majora are palpated for masses that could indicate a hernia or ectopic glands. Palpating a suprapubic mass or mass between the labia majora suggests an imperforate hymen. An imperforate hymen causes secretions to pool within the vagina (Fig. 15–21).

Male Newborns

In term male newborns, the external genitalia are observed for a penis, with a mean length of 3.5 cm (Elder, 2000), the urethral opening located on the tip of the glans, and the glans covered by the prepuce or foreskin. The foreskin may need to be retracted slightly to accurately determine the location of the meatus. Circumci-

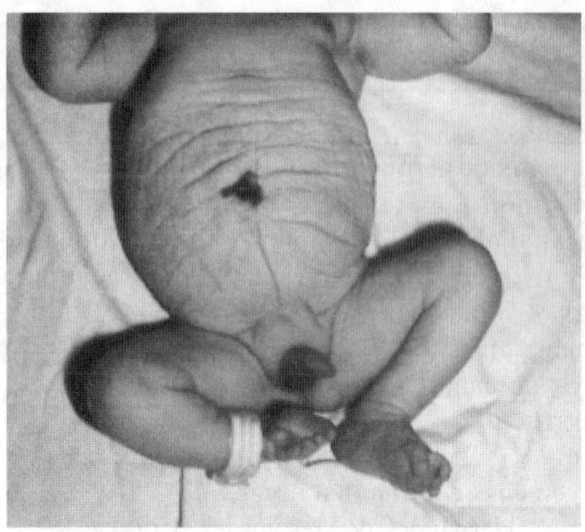

FIGURE 15–20. Prune belly syndrome. (From Pillitteri, A. [1999]. *Maternal and child health nursing* [3rd ed., p. 1352]. Philadelphia: Lippincott, Williams & Wilkins.

sion is delayed when an abnormally located urinary meatus is observed. A physiologic phimosis (ie, inability to retract the prepuce or foreskin) is present at birth. By 3 years of age, the foreskin usually is able to be retracted in 90% of uncircumcised males because adhesions between the prepuce and glans lyse and the distal phimotic ring loosens (Elder, 2000). Small, white cysts filled with epithelial cells may be transiently present on the distal portion of the prepuce. Smegma, a whitish-yellow, cheesy substance from sebaceous glands, collects between the glans and prepuce.

The scrotum is more darkly pigmented than the skin surrounding it. This color variation is especially prominent in African American, Indian, and Hispanic newborns. The scrotum is palpated with the thumb and forefinger for the presence of the testes. Rugae (ie, ridges or creases) begin to appear on the surface of the scrotum around 36 weeks' gestation, and by term, the entire surface of the scrotum is covered. The scrotum may be enlarged because of the effects of maternal hormones. Rugae and a pendulous scrotum usually indicate descent of the testes. Before 28 weeks' gestation, the testes lie within the abdomen. Migration through the inguinal canal to the scrotum occurs as a result of the effect of androgen on the genitofemoral nerves. Stimulation of these nerves causes the gubernaculum testis, a fetal ligament connecting the testes to the scrotum, to move the testes into the scrotum (Ferrer & McKenna, 2000). Undescended testis (ie, cryptorchidism) may be unilateral or bilateral and occurs in about 3% of term newborns and up to 30% of preterm newborns, depending on gestational age (Elder, 2000). Undescended testes are found along the normal path of descent between the abdomen and scrotum, most often below the external inguinal ring but not in the scrotum. They can also be within the inguinal canal or still in the abdomen. If undescended at birth, the testes usually descend by 3 months of age because of the influence of rising androgen levels during infancy. It is possible for one testis or both testes to migrate to an ectopic location, away from the normal path to the scrotum, if the gubernaculum ligament is in an abnormal location. Either or both of the testes can be classified as retractile. A testis is referred to as retractile if, when stimulated by palpation or cold, the cremastic reflex causes it to move to the upper scrotum or as far as the external inguinal ring. This condition differs from the classification of undescended because gentle pressure can bring the testis completely down into the scrotum. To prevent stimulation of the cremastic reflex during examination, the index finger of the examiner's nondominant hand can be used to apply pressure to the inguinal canal to prevent the testis from slipping out of the scrotum. Surgical intervention for undescended or ectopic testes occurs when the child is 6 months to 1 year old.

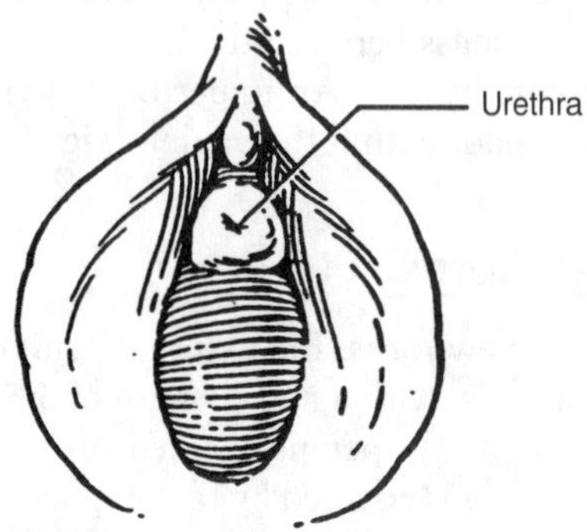

FIGURE 15–21. Imperforate hymen.

An enlarged scrotum is evaluated for the presence of a hydrocele, which is an accumulation of fluid. Fluid accumulates during fetal development when sexual differentiation occurs. This fluid is usually reabsorbed in utero. If a hydrocele is present at birth, it should disappear within 3 months. The ability to transilluminate a hydrocele differentiates it from a solid or blood-filled mass.

Table 15–13 identifies the findings of the physical assessment of male and female newborns that are abnormal and their related pathology.

MUSCULOSKELETAL SYSTEM ASSESSMENT

Inspection and palpation are used to assess the musculoskeletal system. Examination begins by observing the newborn at rest, noting position, symmetry, and

TABLE 15–13 ▪ GENITOURINARY SYSTEM

Assessment	Pathology
Ambiguous genitalia	Genetic disorder
Decreased or no urination within 24 hours of birth	Urinary tract obstruction Potter syndrome Polycystic kidney Hydronephrosis Renal failure
Female	
Urinary meatus near or just inside vagina (hypospadias)	Genitourinary (GU) anomaly
Fecal discharge from vagina	Fistula between rectum and vagina
Male	
Epispadias—meatus on dorsal surface of glans	GU anomaly
Hypospadias—meatus on ventral surface of glans (1 of 250 newborns) (Elder, 2000)	
Scrotal mass which transilluminates	Hydrocele
Scrotal mass which does not transilluminate	Inguinal hernia (see Fig. 15–19)
Testes not palpable in scrotum or inguinal canal	Undescended testes
Red to bluish red scrotal sac; swelling or small mass palpable (Cavaliere, 1996)	Twisting of the testes and spermatic cord (testicular torsion)
Urinary stream not straight; weak urinary stream	Stenosis of the urethral meatus Urinary malformation

presence of abnormal movements. The hands and feet are inspected for the number of digits. Nails are soft and cover the entire nail bed. In a postmature newborn, the nail may extend beyond the fingertips. Newborns exposed to meconium in utero have yellow discoloration of their nails.

Arms and legs are inspected for flexion and symmetry. Extremities should be flexed and move symmetrically through a full range of motion. Clavicles are assessed for fractures that may have occurred during the birth process. This assessment is performed by palpating along the entire length of the clavicle feeling for a mass. The newborn's arm is moved through passive range of motion while the examiner uses her other hand to palpate the newborn's clavicle on that same side. Crepitus, produced when the bone slides against itself, is felt over the clavicle if a fracture exists.

Legs appear slightly bowed with everted feet. A persistent breech presentation in utero may result in abducted hips and extended knees (Fig. 15–22). Positional deformities in the newborn period are often caused by intrauterine positioning and may continue to be present for a few days or weeks. Passive range of motion should correct positional deformities.

The newborn's hips are evaluated for developmental dysplasia. Developmental dysplasia of the hip (DDH) describes the continuum of pathologic hip disorders in the newborn traditionally referred to as congenital dislocation of the hip. This terminology has been adapted by the AAP, American Academy of Orthopeadic Surgeons, and Pediatric Orthopaedic Society of North America (French & Dietz, 1999). When 18,060 newborns were evaluated using physical assessment and ultrasonography at several points during the first 6 weeks of life, the incidence of DDH was 5 cases per 1,000 newborns (Bialik et al., 1999). The exact cause of DDH is unknown. It is probably related to a variety of factors or situations interfering

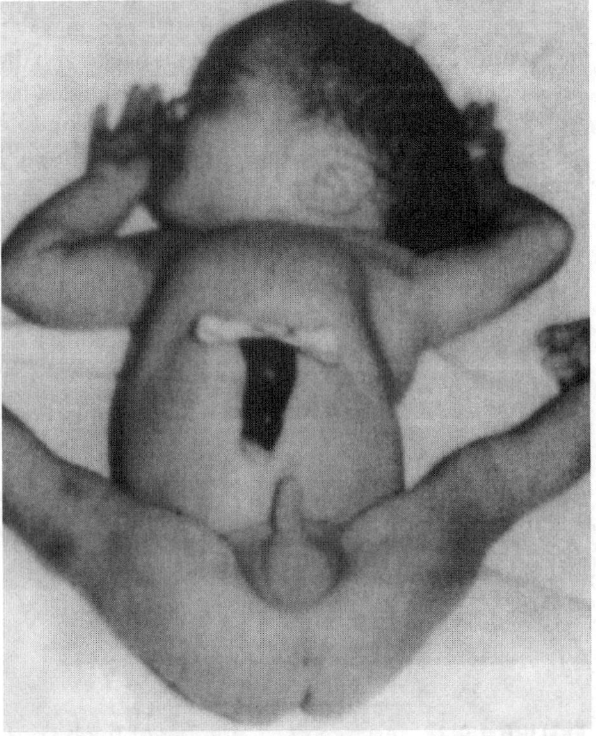

FIGURE 15–22. Result of a persistent breech position in utero. (Courtesy of Dr. David A. Clark, Louisiana State University Medical Center and Wyeth-Ayerst Laboratories, Philadelphia, PA.)

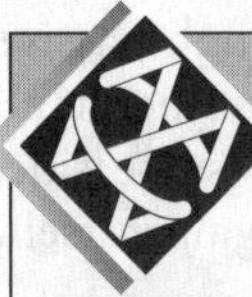

DISPLAY 15-4

Factors Associated with Developmental Dysplasia of the Hip

- Family history of developmental dysplasia of the hip
- Oligohydramnios
- Breech presentation
- Foot deformities
- Primiparity
- Female sex
- Multiple pregnancy

with the normal development of the acetabulum. Failure of the acetabulum to develop eventually allows the bell-shaped femoral head to migrate completely or partially out of normal position. Because of intrauterine position, DDH is more common in the left hip (Tachdjian, 1997). Factors that put newborns at risk for DDH are listed in Display 15–4.

Evaluating the newborn's hips requires the child to be in a quiet state. Crying causes increased muscle tone that could prevent the examiner from identifying an unstable hip. Assessing the newborn for DDH begins with inspection. Position the newborn on his back, with diaper off, hips and knees flexed at 90-degree angles, and feet level (Fig. 15–23). The presence of more skin folds on the medial aspect of the thigh or one knee noticeably lower than the other knee (Galeazzi sign) may indicate the femoral head is dislocated or no longer positioned within the acetabulum.

To further determine the presence of an unstable or dislocated hip, the newborn's hips are put through three maneuvers. With the newborn's hips and knees still flexed at 90-degree angles, the hips are simultaneously abducted gently toward the examination table. Normal hips should abduct almost 90 degrees (ie, thighs resting on the table). This is followed by the Ortolani and Barlow maneuvers. To perform the Ortolani maneuver, the examiner stabilizes one hip while the thigh of the hip being tested is abducted and gently pulled anteriorly. If the hip is dislocated, a palpable and sometimes audible "clunk" will be detected as the femoral head moves over the posterior rim of the acetabulum and back into position (Fig. 15–24). The

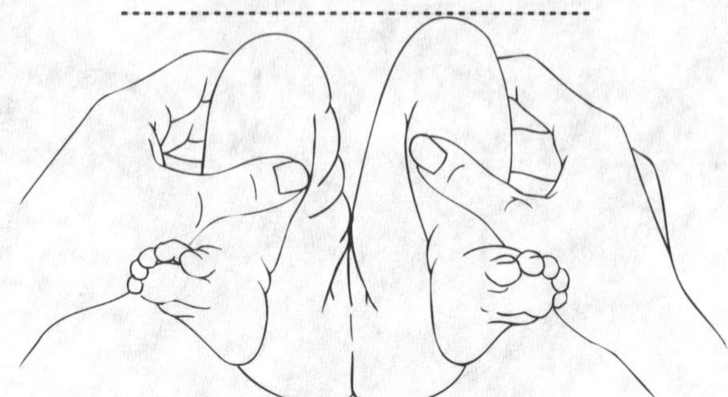

FIGURE 15–23. Asymmetry in number of thigh skin folds and uneven knee level. (Adapted from Ballock, R. T., & Richards, B. S. [1997]. Hip dysplasia: Early diagnosis makes a difference. *Contemporary Pediatrics, 14*[4], 110.)

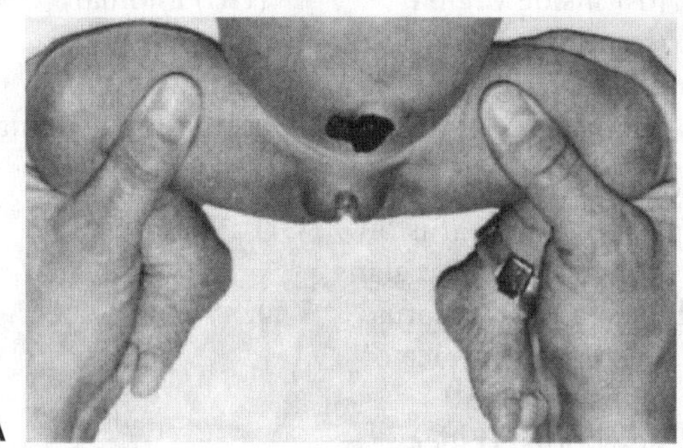

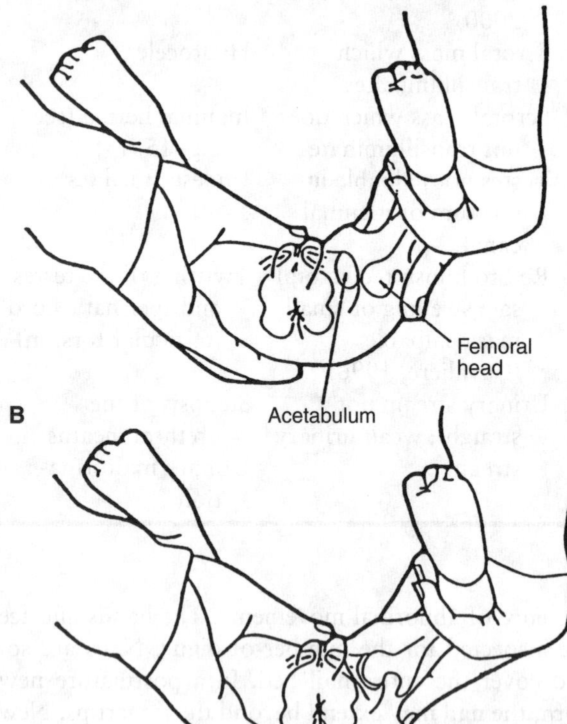

FIGURE 15–24. Ortolani's Maneuver. (**A & B**) With the newborn's legs flexed, the thumb is over the femur and the fingers are on the trocanter. The femur is lifted forward as the thighs are abducted toward the bed. (**C**). A "click" is heard or felt as the head of the femur moves into the acetabulum.

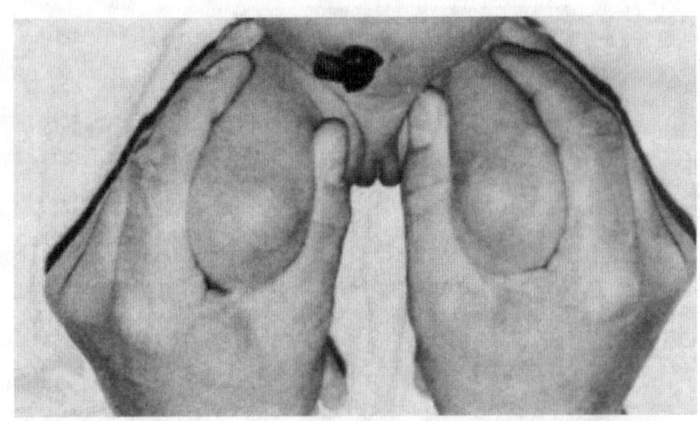

FIGURE 15–25. Barlow maneuver performed by adducting the thighs. If the head of the femur dislocates, it is felt and seen as it suddenly jerks over the acetabulum.

Barlow maneuver is performed by adducting the hip while pushing the thigh posteriorly to determine whether the hip can be dislocated (Fig. 15–25). If the hip is dislocated by this maneuver, it is relocated by performing the Ortolani maneuver. An algorithm for the evaluation of a newborn hip is presented in Figure 15–26.

The continuum of DDH from dysplasia to dislocation is depicted in Figure 15–27. Only about 60% of DDH is identified clinically with initial newborn assessment (Rosenberg, Bialik, Norman, & Blazer, 1998). In combination with ultrasound evaluation when DDH is suspected, identification increases to 90% (Donaldson & Feinstein, 1997; Rosenberg et al., 1998). Because clinical screening techniques cannot

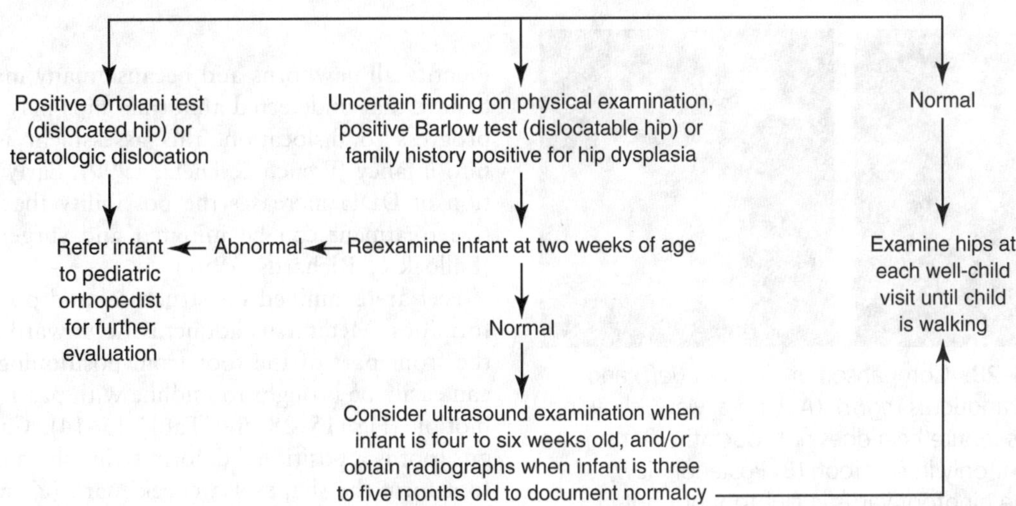

FIGURE 15–26. Algorithm for the evaluation of infants' hips. (From French, L. M. & Dietz, F. R. [1999]. Screening for developmental dysplasia of the hips. *American Family Physician, 60*[1], p. 182.)

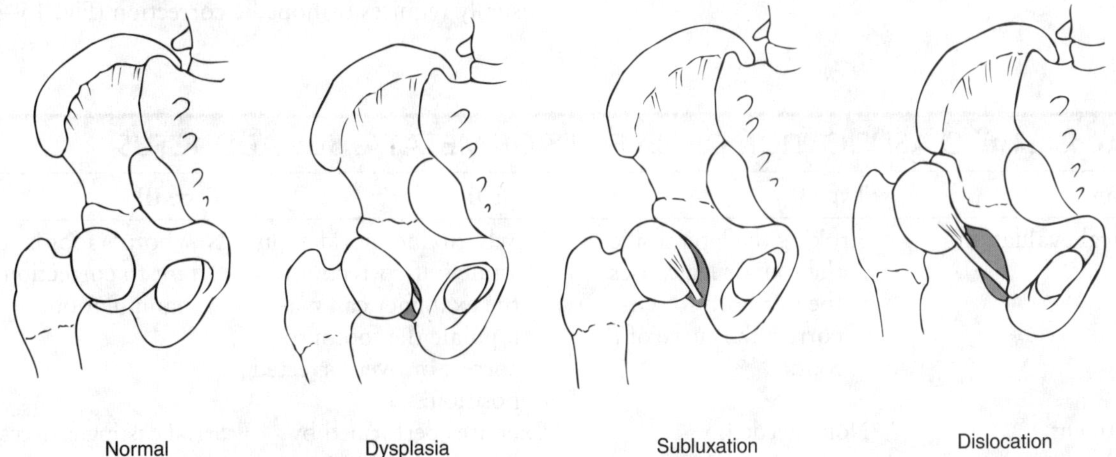

FIGURE 15–27. Relationship of structures in developmental dysplasia of the hip. (Modified from Wong, D. L. [Ed.]. [1997]. *Whaley & Wong's essentials of pediatric nursing* [5th ed., p. 1137]. St. Louis: Mosby.)

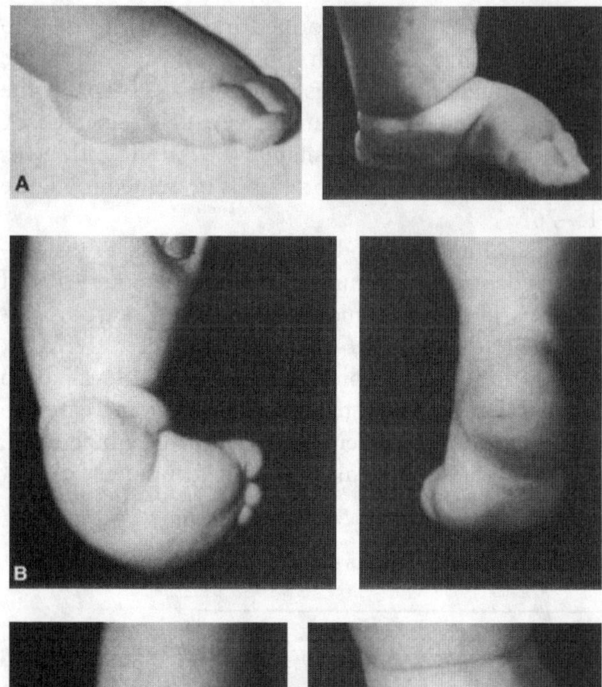

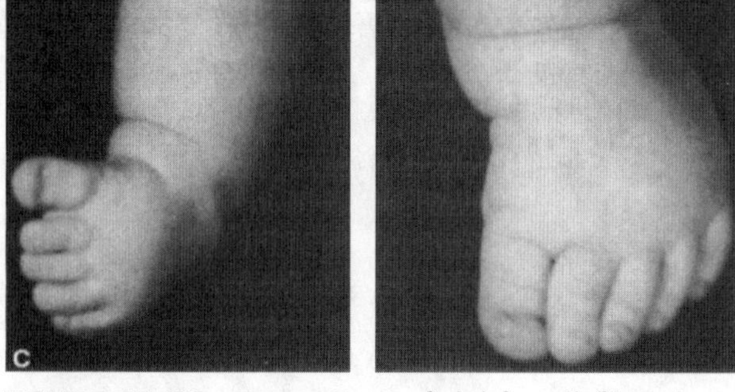

FIGURE 15–28. Comparison of clubfoot (*left*) and metatarsus adductus (*right*). (**A**) Lateral view, showing the equinus (entire heel does not touch the flat surface) present only in clubfoot. (**B**) Posterior view, showing the hindfoot varus in clubfoot but not in metatarsus adductus. (**C**) Anterior view, showing adduction in both feet, with the varus also present in clubfoot.

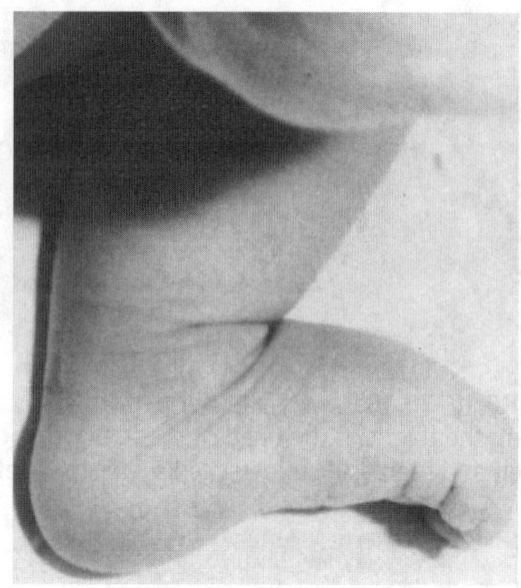

FIGURE 15–29. Talipes calcaneovalgus.

identify all newborns and because many investigators believe that undetected abnormal hips may eventually progress to dislocation, this assessment is repeated into infancy (French & Dietz, 1999). Early identification of DDH increases the possibility that conservative treatment can be initiated and surgery avoided (Ballock & Richards, 1997).

Feet are examined for structural and positional deformities. Metatarsus adductus (ie, inward turning of the front part of the foot from positioning in utero) can easily be brought to midline with passive range of motion (Fig. 15–28 and Table 15–14). Calcaneovalgus foot is a positional deformity in which the leg and foot form the shape of a check mark (✓) rather than an "L." (Fig. 15–29). Conservative treatment such as exercises performed by the parents is usually all that is necessary for correction (Fernbach, 1998). The most serious deformity, clubfoot, has many variations and usually requires orthopedic correction (Fig. 15–30).

TABLE 15–14 ■ CLASSIFICATION OF SEVERITY OF METATARSUS ADDUCTUS

Action	Type I	Type II	Type III
Clinical evaluation	Stroking the lateral side of the foot or leg causes the newborn to self-correct the curve of the foot.	Newborn does not demonstrate self-correction; the examiner can manipulate the foot into a correct or overcorrected position.	Newborn's foot is resistant to correction by manipulation.
Treatment	None needed.	Exercises performed by parents should correct it.	Serial casting is necessary.

Crawford, A. H., & Gabriel, K. R. (1987). Foot and ankle problems. *Orthopedic Clinics of North America, 18* (4), 649–666.

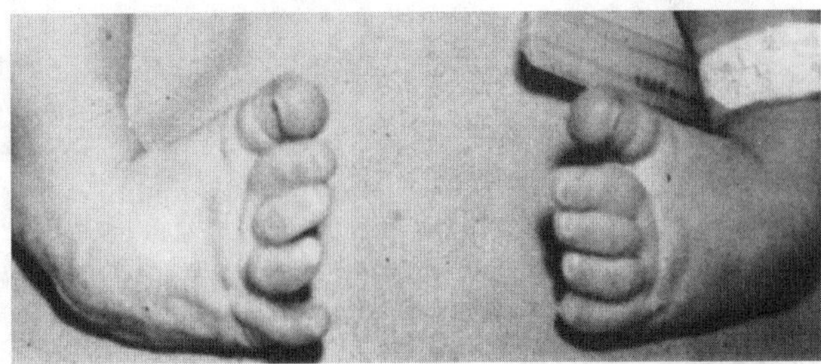

FIGURE 15–30. Clubfoot.

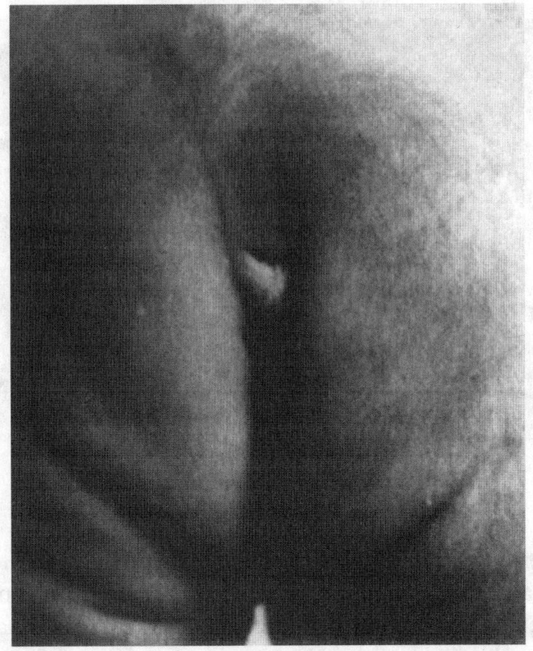

FIGURE 15–32. Pilonidal dimple. (Courtesy of Dr. David A. Clark, Louisiana State University Medical Center and Wyeth-Ayerst Laboratories, Philadelphia, PA.)

In a prone position, the newborn's back is examined for asymmetric gluteal folds indicating the presence of a congenital hip dislocation (Fig. 15–31). During this portion of the examination, the length of the spinal column is palpated for masses and abnormal curvatures. The sacral area is inspected for the presence of a pilonidal dimple (Fig. 15–32), tuft of hair, skin lesion, or increased pigmentation that could indicate pathology. Table 15–15 identifies findings of the musculoskeletal assessment that are abnormal and their related pathology. Figures 15–33 and 15–34 illustrate polydactyly and syndactyly; these conditions are further addressed in Table 15–15.

TABLE 15–15 ■ MUSCULOSKELETAL SYSTEM

Assessment	Pathology
Weak or absent muscle tone	Neurologic disorder Prematurity Genetic disorder
Extra digit (polydactyly) (see Fig. 15–33)	Inherited as dominant trait
Partial or complete fusion of digits, more often in feet than hands (syndactyly) (see Fig. 15–34)	Inherited as dominant trait
Short fingers, incurving of fifth finger, fusion or palmar creases (simian crease), wide space between big toe and second toe	Down syndrome
Jitteriness	Hypoglycemia Hypocalcemia
Arm extended and limp, hand rotated inward, absence of normal movement, absent Moro reflex on affected side	Brachial plexus palsy

NEUROLOGIC ASSESSMENT

Assessment of the central nervous system is integrated throughout the physical examination and includes evaluation of posture, cry, muscle tone, and move-

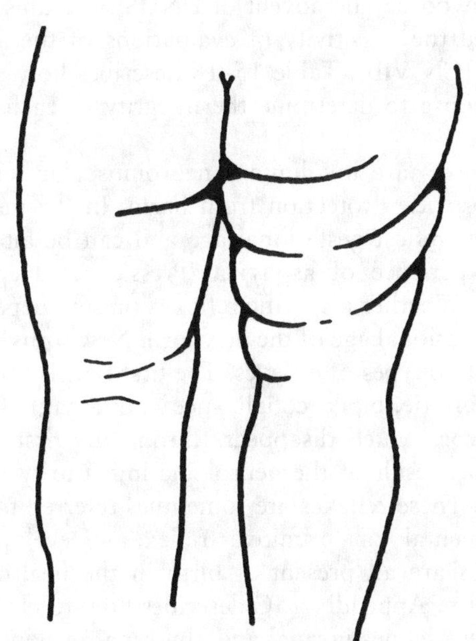

FIGURE 15–31. Asymmetric gluteal folds.

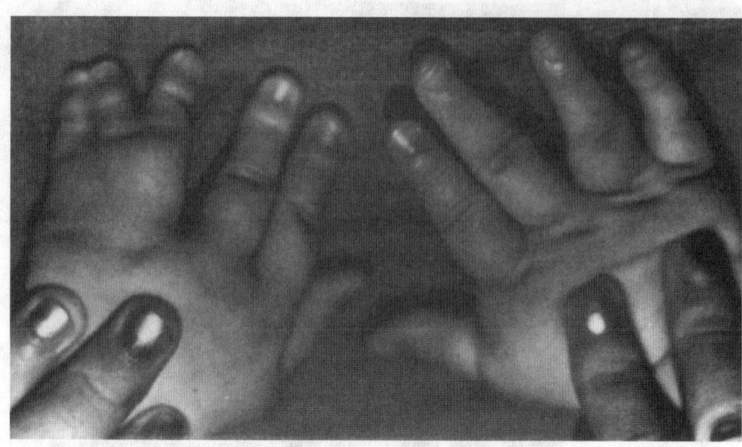

FIGURE 15–33. Polydactyly.

ment; evaluation of most cranial nerves; and evaluation of all developmental reflexes. Findings during the neurologic assessment are influenced by the gestational age and physical health of the newborn.

At rest, a newborn's posture is flexed, with extremities tight against the trunk. The neuromuscular portion of the gestational age assessment demonstrates the increasing muscle tone that the newborn develops as gestational age progresses. Scarf sign, popliteal angle, and heel-to-ear movements have less range of motion as gestational age increases. Leg and arm recoil also demonstrates how muscle tone normally becomes stronger as gestational age advances.

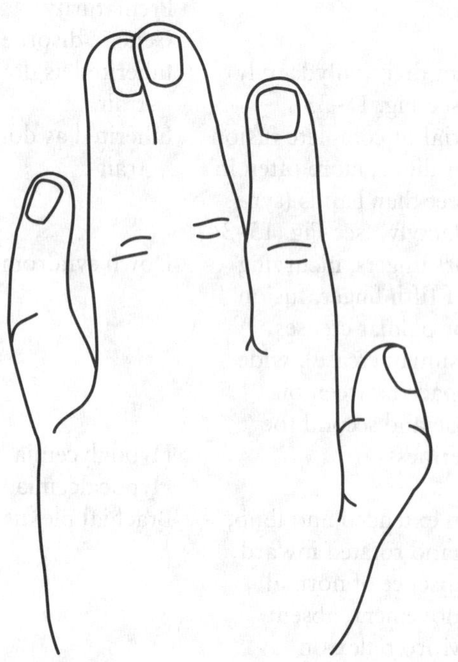

FIGURE 15–34. Syndactyly.

A healthy newborn's cry is strong and loud. Newborns cry for a variety of reasons. They cry in response to unpleasant environmental stimuli such as fatigue, hunger, cold or discomfort or because they want the attention of another person. Crying helps the parents develop parenting skills as they become more alert to interpreting their newborn's needs. Responding to a newborn cry helps facilitate attachment between parent and child and increases the newborn's feeling of security. They come to trust that there are people in their world who will respond to their needs (Pearson, 1999). A weak cry is associated with prematurity or illness; a high-pitched cry occurs with drug withdrawal, neurologic abnormalities, metabolic abnormalities, or meningitis.

All of the cranial nerves, with the exception of the olfactory nerve (CN I), should be routinely assessed in the newborn. The advent of UNHS programs has increased the sensitivity of evaluations of the acoustic nerve (CN VIII). Table 15–16 describes how to illicit a response to determine the integrity of each cranial nerve.

Reflexes are involuntary neuromuscular responses that provide protection from harm. In the newborn, reflexes reflect gestational age and can be altered by the experience of asphyxia (Pressler & Hepworth, 1997). Whether a specific reflex is present depends on the gestational age of the newborn. Newborns demonstrate two types of reflexes. The first type is protective in nature (ie, blink, cough, sneeze, and gag). The second type, which disappears during the first year of life, is a result of the neurologic immaturity of newborns. These reflexes are sometimes referred to as developmental or primitive reflexes. Developmental reflexes are all present at birth in the healthy term newborn. Appendix 15C describes how to elicit these reflexes, defines normal and abnormal responses, and explains at what age they disappear.

TABLE 15–16 ■ ASSESSING THE INTEGRITY OF CRANIAL NERVES

Cranial Nerve	Method of Assessment
CN I, olfactory	Not assessed in the neonate
CN II, optic	Newborn follows brightly colored object or face; blinks in response to light
CN III, oculomotor CN IV, trochlear CN VI, abducens	Pupils constrict equally in response to light; as newborn's head is moved to face one side or the other, eyes move in the opposite direction (dolls' eyes maneuver)
CN V, trigeminal	Presence of rooting and sucking reflexes; biting
CN VII, facial	Symmetry of facial movement while crying or smiling
CN VIII, acoustic	Positive Moro reflex or movement in the direction of sound; quiets to voice; hearing screening using brainstem auditory evoked response (BAER)
CN IX, glossopharyngeal CN X, vagus CN XII, hypoglossal	Coordination of suck and swallow; presence of gag reflex; tongue remains midline when mouth is open
CN XI, accessory	Head turns easily to either side; newborn attempts to move head back from side to midline; height of shoulders equal

SUMMARY

A formal assessment of all body systems is completed by the perinatal nurse soon after birth and repeated at intervals established by institutional protocol throughout the newborn's hospitalization. Informal assessments are ongoing and occur during caregiving activities. Performing the physical assessment provides a picture of how the newborn is adapting to extrauterine life. The development of keen physical assessment skills allows the perinatal nurse to detect subtle changes in the newborn's condition, identify or anticipate the development of problems, and intervene immediately to prevent or minimize these problems.

REFERENCES

American Academy of Pediatrics. (1995). Joint committee on infant hearing: 1994 position statement. *Pediatrics, 95*(1), 152–156.

American Academy of Pediatrics. (1999). Newborn and infant hearing loss: Detection and intervention. *Pediatrics, 103*(2), 527–530.

American Academy of Pediatrics & American College of Obstetricians and Gynecologists (AAP & ACOG). (1997). *Guidelines for perinatal care* (4th ed.). Washington, DC: Author.

Askin, D. F. (1997). *Acute respiratory care of the newborn.* Petaluma, CA: NICU INK.

Ballard, J. L., Khoury, J. C., Wedig, K., Wang, L., Ellers-Walsman, B. L., & Lipp, R. (1991). New Ballard Score, expanded to include extremely premature infants. *Journal of Pediatrics, 119*(3), 417–423.

Ballard, J. L., Novak, K. K., & Driver, M. (1979). A simplified score for assessment of fetal maturation of newly born infants. *Journal of Pediatrics, 95*(5, Pt. 1), 769–774.

Ballock, R. T., & Richards, B. S. (1997). Hip dysplasia: Early diagnosis makes a difference. *Contemporary Pediatrics, 14*(4), 108–117.

Bialik, V., Bialik, G. M., Blazer, S., Sujov, P., Wiener, F., & Berant, M. (1999). Developmental dysplasia of the hip: A new approach to incidence. *Pediatrics, 103*(1), 93–99.

Brown, T. J., Friedman, J., & Levy, M. L. (1998). The diagnosis and treatment of common birthmarks. *Clinics in Plastic Surgery, 25*(4), 509–525.

Cavaliere, T. A. (1996). Genitourinary Assessment. In E. P. Tappero & M. E. Honeyfield (Eds.), *Physical assessment of the newborn: A comprehensive approach to the art of physical examination* (pp. 103–116). Petaluma, CA: NICU INK.

Conner, G. K. (1996). Abdomen assessment. In E. P. Tappero & M. E. Honeyfield (Eds.), *Physical assessment of the newborn: A comprehensive approach to the art of physical examination* (pp. 81–90). Petaluma, CA: NICU INK.

Crawford, A. H., & Gabriel, K. R. (1987). Foot and ankle problems. *Orthopedic Clinics of North America, 18*(4), 649–666.

Darmstadt, G. L. (2000). The skin. In R. E. Behrman, R. M. Kliegman, & H. B. Jenson (Eds.), *Nelson's textbook of pediatrics* (16th ed., pp. 1965–2054). Philadelphia: W.B. Saunders.

Dubowitz, L. M. S., Dubowitz, V., & Goldberg, C. (1970). Clinical assessment of gestational age in the newborn infant. *Journal of Pediatrics, 77*(1), 1–10.

Donaldson, J. S., & Feinstein, K. A. (1997). Imaging of developmental dysplasia of the hip. *Pediatric Clinics of North America, 44*(3), 591–614.

Dodd, V. (1996). Gestational age assessment. *Neonatal Network, 15*(1), 27–36.

Elder, J. S. (2000). Urologic disorders in infants and children. In R. E. Behrman, R. M. Kliegman, & H. B. Jenson (Eds.), *Nelson's textbook of pediatrics* (16th ed., pp. 1619–1658). Philadelphia: W.B. Saunders.

Esterly, N. B. (1996). Cutaneous hemangiomas, vascular stains and malformations, and associated syndromes. *Current Problems in Pediatrics, 26*(1), 3–39.

Fernbach, S. A. (1998). Common orthopedic problems of the newborn. *Nursing Clinics of North America, 33*(4), 583–593.

Ferrer, F. A., & McKenna, P. H. (2000). Current approaches to the undescended testes. *Contemporary Pediatrics, 17*(1), 106–111.

French, L. M., & Dietz, F. R. (1999). Screening for developmental dysplasia of the hip. *American Family Physician, 60*(1), 177–184.

Gagliardi, L., Brambilla, C., Bruno, R., Martinelli, S., & Console, V. (1993). Biased assessment of gestational age at birth when obstetric gestation is known. *Archives of Disease in Childhood, 68*(1), 32–34.

Gallagher, P. G., Mahoney, M. J., & Gosche, J. R. (1999). Cystic hygroma in the fetus and newborn. *Seminars Perinatology, 23*(4), 341–356.

Glass, S. M. (1999). Routine care. In P. J. Thureen, J. Deacon, P. O'Neill, & J. Hernandez (Eds.), *Assessment and care of the well newborn* (pp. 188–196). Philadelphia: W.B. Saunders.

Green, M. (1998). Pediatric diagnosis: Interpretation of symptoms and signs in infants, children and adolescents, (6th ed.). Philadelphia: W. B. Saunders.

Hartley, A. H., & Rasmussen, J. E. (1990). Hemangiomas and spitz nevi. *Pediatric Review, 11*(9), 262–267.

Haslem, R. H. A. (2000). The nervous system. In R. E. Behrman, R. M. Kliegman, & H. B. Jenson (Eds.), *Nelson's textbook of pediatrics* (16th ed., pp. 1793–1867). Philadelphia: W. B. Saunders.

Hernandez, P. W., & Hernandez, J. A. (1999). Physical assessment of the newborn. In P. J. Thureen, J. Deacon, P. O'Neill, & J. Hernandez (Eds.), *Assessment and care of the well newborn* (pp. 114–164). Philadelphia: W.B. Saunders.

Hernandez, J. A., Zabloudil, C., & Hernandez, P. W. (1999). Adaptation to extrauterine life and management during transition. In P. J. Thureen, J. Deacon, P. O'Neill, & J. Hernandez (Eds.), *Assessment and care of the well newborn* (pp. 83–100). Philadelphia: W.B. Saunders.

Jackson, D., & Saunders, R. (1993). *Child health nursing*. Philadelphia: J.B. Lippincott.

Mason, J. A., & Herrmann, K. R. (1998). Universal infant hearing screening by automated auditory brainstem response measurement. *Pediatrics, 101*(2), 221–228.

Mehl, A. L., & Thomson, V. (1998). Newborn hearing screening: The great omission. *Pediatrics, 101*(1), 1–6.

Morelli, J. G. (1996). Hemangiomas and vascular malformations. *Pediatric Annals, 25*(2), 91–96.

Morrissy, R. T., & Weinstein, S. L. (1996). *Lovell and Winter's pediatric orthopaedics* (4th ed.). Philadelphia: Lippincott-Raven Publishers.

Pearson, J. (1999). Crying and calming: Important information and effective techniques to teach parents of full term newborns. *Mother-Baby Journal, 4*(5), 39–42.

Pressler, J. L., & Hepworth, J. T. (1997). Newborn neurologic screening using NBAS reflexes. *Neonatal Network, 16*(6), 33–46.

Rosenberg, N., Bialik, V., Norman, D., & Blazer, S. (1998). The importance of combined clinical and sonographic examination of instability of the neonatal hip. *International Orthopedics, 22*(3), 431–434.

Stoll, B. J., & Kliegman, R. M. (2000). Noninfectious disorders. In R. E. Behrman, R. M. Kliegman, & H. B. Jenson (Eds.), *Nelson's textbook of pediatrics* (16th ed., pp. 451–553). Philadelphia: W.B. Saunders.

Tachdjian, M. O. (1997). *Clinical pediatric orthopedics: The art of diagnosis and principles of management*. Stamford, CT: Appleton & Lange.

Ulshen, M. (2000). Clinical Manifestations of gastrointestinal disease. In R. E. Behrman, R. M. Kliegman, & H. B. Jenson (Eds.), *Nelson's textbook of pediatrics* (16th ed., pp. 1101–1107). Philadelphia: W.B. Saunders.

Versmold, H. T., Kitterman, J. A., Phibbs, R. H., Gregory, G. A., & Tooley, W. H. (1981). Aortic blood pressure during the first 12 hours of life in infants 610 to 4,220 grams. *Pediatrics, 67*(5), 703–713.

Witt, C. (1996). Skin assessment. In E. P. Tappero & M. E. Honeyfield (Eds.), *Physical assessment of the newborn: A comprehensive approach to the art of physical examination* (2nd ed., pp. 39–52). Petaluma, CA: NICU INK.

Witt, C. (1999). Neonatal Dermatology. In J. Deacon, & P. O'Neill (Eds.), *Core curriculum for neonatal intensive care nursing* (pp. 578–595). Philadelphia: W.B. Saunders.

Wong, D. L. (Ed.). (1998). *Whaley & Wong's nursing care of infants and children* (6th ed.). St Louis: Mosby–Year Book.

Yoshinaga-Itano, C. (1999). Benefits of early intervention for children with hearing loss. *Otolaryngology Clinics of North America, 32*(6), 1089–1102.

APPENDIX 15A

Characteristics of Infant State

Infant States	Body Activity	Eye Movements	Facial Movements	Breathing Pattern	Level of Response	Implications for Caregiving
Sleep States						
Deep sleep	Nearly still, except for occasional startle or twitch	None	Without facial movements, except for occasional sucking at regular intervals	Smooth and regular	Threshold to stimuli very high so that only very intense or disturbing stimuli will arouse infants	Caregivers trying to feed infants in deep sleep will probably find the experience frustrating. Infants will be unresponsive, even if caregivers use disturbing stimuli (flicking feet) to arouse infants. Infants may arouse only briefly and then become unresponsive as they return to deep sleep. If caregivers wait until infants move to a higher, more responsive state, feeding or caregiving will be much more pleasant.
Light sleep	Some body movements	Rapid eye movements (REM) Fluttering of eyes beneath closed eyelids	May smile and make brief fussy or crying sounds	Irregular	More responsive to internal and external stimuli. (When these stimuli occur, infants may remain in light sleep, return to deep sleep, or arouse to drowsy.)	Light sleep makes up the highest proportion of newborn sleep and usually precedes wakening. The brief fussy or crying sounds made during this state may make caregivers who are not aware that these sound occur normally think it is time for feeding, and they may try to feed infants before they are ready to eat.
Awake States						
Drowsy	Activity level variable, with mild startles interspersed from time to time; movement usually smooth	Eyes open and close occasionally, are heavy lidded with dull, glazed appearance	Some facial movements possible (Often there are none, and the face appears still.)	Irregular	React to sensory stimuli, although responses are delayed. (State change after stimulation is frequently noted.)	From the drowsy state, infants *may* return to sleep or awaken further. To facilitate waking, caregivers can provide something for infants to see, hear, or suck. This may arouse them to a quiet alert state, a more responsive state. Infants left alone without stimuli may return to a sleep state.

Quiet alert	Minimal	Brightening and widening of eyes	Face bright, shining, sparkling	Regular	Most attentive to environment, focusing attention on any stimuli that are present	Infants in quiet alert state provide much pleasure and positive feedback for caregivers. Providing something for infants to see, hear, or suck will often maintain this state. In the first few hours after birth, most newborns commonly experience a period of intense alertness before going into a long sleeping period.
Active alert	Much body activity; periods of fussiness possible	Eyes open with less brightening	Much facial movement; face not as bright as quiet alert state	Irregular	Increasingly sensitive to disturbing stimuli (hunger, fatigue, noise, excessive handling)	Caregivers may intervene at this stage to console and to bring infants to a lower state.
Crying	Increased motor activity, with color changes	Eyes tightly closed or open	Grimaces	More irregular	Extremely responsive to unpleasant external or internal stimuli.	Crying is the infants' communication signal. It is a response to unpleasant stimuli from the environment or from within infants (fatigue, hunger, discomfort). Crying tells us infants' limits have been reached. Sometimes infants can console themselves and return to lower states. At other times, they need help from caregivers.

From Pearson, J. (1999). Crying and calming: Important information and effective techniques to teach parents of full-term newborns. *Mother Baby Journal, 4*(5), 39–42.

APPENDIX 15B

Characteristics of the Ballard Gestation Age Assessment Tool

NEUROMUSCULAR MATURITY

Posture: Position the baby naturally assumes when lying quietly on his back. A very premature newborn lies with arms and legs extended or in whatever posture he is placed. As intrauterine development progresses, the fetus is capable of more and more flexion. At term, a newborn lies with his arms flexed to his chest, his hands fisted, and his legs flexed toward his abdomen.

Square window (wrist): Angle achieved when the newborn's palm is flexed toward his forearm. A preterm newborn's wrist exhibits poor flexion and makes a 90-degree angle with the arm. An extremely preterm newborn has no flexor tone and cannot achieve even 90-degree flexion. A term newborn's wrist can flex completely against the forearm.

Arm recoil: After first flexing the arms at the elbows against the chest, then fully extending and releasing them, term newborns resist extension and quickly return arms to the flexed position. Very preterm newborns do not resist extension and respond with weak and delayed flexion.

Popliteal angle: With the newborn supine and pelvis flat, flex his thigh to his abdomen and hold it there while extending his leg at the knee. The angle at the knee is estimated. The preterm newborn can achieve greater extension.

Scarf sign: While the newborn is supine, move his arm across his chest toward the opposite shoulder. A term newborn's elbow does not cross midline. It is possible to bring the preterm newborn's elbow much farther.

Heel to ear: Without holding the knee and thigh in place, move the newborn's foot as close to the ear as possible. A preterm newborn is able to get his foot closer to his head than a term baby.

PHYSICAL MATURITY

Skin: Assess for thickness, transparency, and texture. Preterm skin is smooth and thin with visible vessels. Extremely preterm skin is sticky and transparent. Term skin is thick, veins are difficult to see, and peeling may occur.

Lanugo: Fine hair seen over the back of premature newborns by 24 weeks' gestation. It begins to thin over the lower back first and disappears last over the shoulders.

Plantar creases: One or two creases over the pad of the foot at approximately 32 weeks' gestation. At 36 weeks, creases cover the anterior two thirds of the foot; at term, the whole foot. At very early gestations, the length from the tip of the great toe to the back of the heal is measured.

Breast tissue: Examined for visibility of nipple and areola and size of bud when grasped between thumb and forefinger. The very premature newborn does not have visible nipples or areolae. These become more defined and then raised by 34 weeks, with a small bud appearing at 36 weeks and growing to 5 to 10 mm by term.

Ear formation: Lack of cartilage in earlier gestation results in the ear folding easily and retaining this fold. As gestation progresses, soft cartilage provides increasing resistance to folding and increasing recoil. The pinnae are flat in very preterm newborns.

Adapted from Dodd, V. (1996). Gestational age assessment. *Neonatal Network, 15*(1), 27–36.

Incurving proceeds from the top down toward the lobes as gestation advances.

Genitalia: In males, rugae become visible at 28 weeks. By 36 weeks, the testes are in the upper scrotum, and rugae cover the anterior portion of the scrotum. At term, rugae cover the scrotum, and postterm, the testes are pendulous. In preterm females, the clitoris is prominent, and the labia minora are flat. By 36 weeks, the labia majora are larger, nearly covering the clitoris.

APPENDIX **15C**

Developmental Reflexes

Reflex	How Elicited	Normal Response	Abnormal Response	Duration of Reflex
Rooting and sucking	Touch cheek, lip, or corner of mouth with finger or nipple.	Newborn turns head in direction of stimulus, opens mouth, and begins to suck. In the term newborn, suck is coordinated and strong.	Weak or absent response seen with prematurity, neurologic deficit, or CNS depression from maternal drug ingestion.	Rooting disappears by 3 to 4 months; sucking disappears by 1 year
Swallowing	Place fluid on back of tongue.	Newborn swallows in coordination with sucking.	Gagging, coughing, or regurgitation of fluid; possibly associated with cyanosis secondary to prematurity, neurologic deficit, or injury.	Does not disappear
Extrusion	Touch tip of tongue with finger or nipple.	Newborn pushes tongue outward.	Continuous extrusion of tongue or repetitive tongue thrusting seen with CNS abnormalities or seizures.	Disappears by 6 months
Moro	Holding the newborn's head off the mattress slightly, let it drop quickly several inches into your hand.	Bilateral symmetric extension and abduction of all extremities, with thumb and forefinger forming characteristic "C," followed by adduction of extremities and return to relaxed flexion.	Asymmetric response seen with peripheral nerve injury (brachial plexus), fracture of clavicle or long bone of arm or leg, or birth trauma such as skull fracture.	Disappears by 6 months

Reflex	How Elicited	Normal Response	Abnormal Response	Duration of Reflex
Truck incurvature (Galant's reflex)	Use one hand to lift the prone newborn off a flat surface (ventral suspension). With a finger from the free hand, use some pressure to draw a line down the length of the back about an inch from the spinal column.	Newborn flexes pelvis toward the side stimulated.	Absence indicates spinal cord lesion or CNS depression.	Disappears by 4 months
Tonic neck (fencing)	Turn the newborn's head to one side when infant is resting in the supine position.	Extremities on the side to which the head is turned extends and opposite extremities flex. Response may be absent or incomplete immediately after birth.	Persistent response after 4 months may indicate neurologic injury.	Diminishes by 4 months
Startle	Expose the newborn to sudden movement or loud noise.	Newborn abducts and flexes all extremities and may begin to cry.	Absence of response may indicate neurologic deficit or deafness. Response may be absent or diminished during sleep.	Diminishes by 4 months
Crossed extension	Place the newborn in the supine position and extend one leg while stimulating the bottom of the foot.	Newborn's opposite leg flexes and extends rapidly as if trying to deflect stimulus to the other foot.	Weak or absent response is seen with peripheral nerve injury or fracture of a long bone.	Disappears by 6 months
Palmar grasp	Place a finger in the newborn's palm and apply slight pressure.	Newborn grasps finger; attempting to remove the finger causes newborn to tighten his grasp.	Weak or absent grasp in the presence of CNS deficit or nerve or muscle injury.	Does not disappear

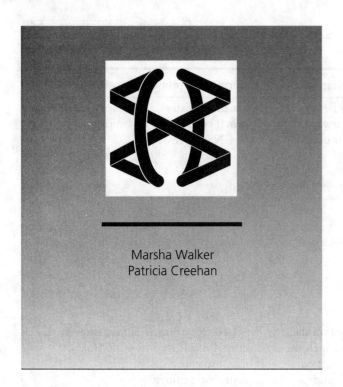

Marsha Walker
Patricia Creehan

CHAPTER 16

Newborn Nutrition

The decision about what to feed the newborn is frequently made long before giving birth. Many factors influence the decision, including education (Balcazar, Trier, & Cobas, 1995; Humphreys, Thompson, & Miner, 1998); age (Balcazar et al., 1995; Humphreys et al., 1998); previous experience (Humphreys et al., 1998); support from the husband, significant others (Tarkka, Paunonen, & Laippala, 1999; Trado & Hughes, 1996), or extended family (Littman, Mendendorp, & Goldfarb, 1994; Tarkka et al., 1999); prenatal breast-feeding education (Piper & Parks, 1996; Sciacca, Dube, Phipps, & Ratliff, 1995); and encouragement from peers (Schafer, Vogel, Viegas, & Hausafus, 1998; Tarkka et al., 1999) and professionals (Bentley et al., 1999; Patton, Beaman, Csar, & Lewinski, 1996; Trado & Hughes, 1996). The choice is not always based on all available information. The decision should not be a lifestyle choice but rather a health choice. However, a woman's choice of feeding method should be respected by healthcare providers.

This chapter offers information and guidelines for the perinatal nurse during the initiation and early days of lactation. The chapter emphasizes that breast-feeding is the ideal method of feeding the newborn and provides helpful information for the perinatal nurse working with families who choose to formula feed their newborn.

Human milk is a dynamic food, meeting the needs to construct an immune system, to grow and develop the brain, and to form attachments with other human beings. Research has produced compelling data about the advantages of breast-feeding for the mother and newborn. Exclusive use of formula is responsible for substantial expenditures of healthcare dollars during the first year of life for respiratory illness, otitis media, and gastrointestinal illness. Ball and Wright (1999) determined that, for 1,000 formula-fed babies, there was an excess of 2,033 office visits, more than 200 days of hospitalization, and more than 600 prescriptions compared with infants breast-fed for at least 3 months. Table 16–1 lists additional disadvantages associated with not breast-feeding.

INCIDENCE OF BREAST-FEEDING

Although breast-feeding rates have increased, the latest data suggest that only 64% of mothers breast-feed in the early postpartum period, 29% are still breast-feeding at 6 months of age, and 16% are breast-feeding at 1 year (United States Department of Health and Human Services [USDHHS], 2000). Given the importance of breast milk and breast-feeding to mothers, newborns, and the culture as a whole, experts in the United States have determined that increasing the rates and duration of breast-feeding continues to be a national health goal. The Healthy People 2010 target is that 75% of women will initiate breast-feeding, 50% of women will continue breast-feeding until 6 months of age, and 25% will be breast-feeding at 12 months of age (USDHHS, 2000). Display 16–1 identifies obstacles to meeting the Healthy People 2010 national goals.

A 1998 Ross Laboratory study determined that initiation of breast-feeding was most common among women who were Caucasian or Hispanic, older than 30 years of age, college educated, not enrolled in the Women, Infants, and Children (WIC) program, and living in the Mountain or Pacific regions of the United States. This

TABLE 16–1 ■ RISK OF SPECIFIC DISEASES WHEN NEWBORNS ARE BOTTLE-FED

Disease or Condition	Study	Result
Asthma	Oddy et al., 1999	27% increase in asthma by age 6 years 44% more likely to wheeze 74% more likely to have sleep disturbance from wheezing
Otitis media	Scariati, Grummer-Strawn, & Fein, 1997	70% increased risk
Diarrhea	Scariati et al., 1997	80% increased risk
Obesity	vonKries et al., 1999	Exclusive breast-feeding for 3–5 months reduced risk by 35%. Breast-feeding for 6–12 months reduced risk by 43%. Breast-feeding for >12 months reduced risk by 72%.
Diabetes	Mayer, Hannan, Gay, Lezotte, & Klingensmith, 1988	2–26% of type I diabetes attributable to not breast-feeding.
	Vaarala et al., 1999	Cow's milk is an environmental trigger of immunity to insulin in infancy.
Necrotizing enterocolitis (NEC)	Lucas & Cole, 1990	83% of NEC cases may be attributed to formula feeding
Cognitive development	Horwood & Furgusson, 1998	Up to an 8–10 point IQ deficit
	Greene, Lucas, Livingstone, Harland & Baker, 1995	Poorer academic performance in school

study determined that more than 80% of women living in Alaska, Colorado, Hawaii, Idaho, Montana, Oregon, Utah, and Washington breast-fed their newborns in the hospital. Breast-feeding was lowest among women who were African American, educated only through grade school, younger than 20 years of age, living in the eastern South Central region of the United States, and enrolled in the WIC program (Ross Products Division, 1998).

The American Academy of Pediatrics (AAP) confirms that, with few exceptions, human milk is preferred for all infants, including premature and sick newborns (AAP, 1997). The few contraindications to breast-feeding include galactosemia, human T-cell lymphotropic virus type (HTLV-1) infection, use of antimetabolites, therapeutic doses of radiopharmaceuticals, use of drugs of abuse, and human immunodeficiency virus (HIV) seropositivity of the mother.

PHYSIOLOGY OF MILK PRODUCTION

Several hormones are responsible for the dramatic breast changes that occur during pregnancy. Estrogen causes ductular sprouting, progesterone is responsible for lobular formation, and prolactin influences lobular and alveolar development. Prolactin stimulates receptors located on the surface of alveolar cells to initiate milk secretion. Prolactin is secreted from the anterior pituitary gland and stimulates production of colostrum, which appears in the third month of gestation. During this time, prolactin is involved in cell differentiation and the formation of lactocytes (ie, mammary secretory epithelial cells) that are capable of secreting milk components. Nipple growth is also related to blood levels of prolactin. By the second trimester, placental lactogen begins to stimulate the secretion of colostrum and is responsible for breast and areolar growth. The greatest breast growth usually occurs during the first 5 months of pregnancy. The increase in breast volume can range from 12 to 227 mL (Cox, Kent, Casey, Owens, & Hartmann, 1999). Some women, however, experience minimal breast enlargement during pregnancy—less than one cup size (Neifert, 1999). There is no relationship between breast growth during pregnancy and milk production at 1 month in mothers who breast-feed frequently (Cox et al., 1999). Human mammary glands have the ability to increase secretory tissue during lactation in response to increased demand for milk. Women who report little to no breast growth

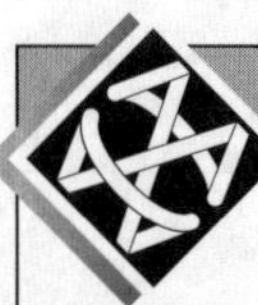

DISPLAY 16–1

Obstacles to Breast-feeding

Healthcare provider apathy, misinformation, and outdated clinical practices
Hospital policies
Inappropriate interventions and disruptions of breast-feeding
Lack of support and follow-up after discharge
Lack of broad cultural support
Lack of support in the workplace
Media portrayal of bottle-feeding as normal
Commercial pressures on mothers to bottle-feed or supplement with formula
- Formula club sign-up sheets in obstetric offices and clinics
- Prenatal formula starter kits
- Coupons for free formula
- Certificates for hospital discharge packs containing formula
- Cases of formula delivered to the homes of pregnant women
- Ads in parent magazines

Discounted formula available through the Internet

during pregnancy need more support to breast-feed frequently during the first 2 weeks of lactation, making sure that milk transfer is taking place (Cox et al., 1999).

Between 15 to 20 weeks' gestation, lactogenesis I occurs in most mothers (Cregan & Hartmann, 1999). This phase is the time when the breasts are capable of synthesizing the unique components of milk. Milk synthesis also requires insulin-induced cell division and the presence of cortisol. Lactogenesis II is defined as the onset of copious milk production 48 to 72 hours after the rapid drop in blood progesterone after delivery of the placenta (Lawrence & Lawrence, 1999). Viable placental fragments retained in the uterus can delay initiation of lactation until they are removed (Neifert, McDonough, & Neville, 1981). Copious milk production can also be delayed by 24 hours in mothers with type I diabetes mellitus (ie, insulin-dependent diabetes). A temporary imbalance may exist between the woman's need for insulin to regulate her own glucose levels and the amount required to contribute to the initiation of lactation (Arthur, Kent, & Hartmann, 1994; Neubauer et al., 1993). The type I diabetic mother should be encouraged to put the baby to breast 12 to 14 times during each 24 hours during the first 3 days to provide frequent, small doses of colostrum for glucose homeostasis in the infant and to stimulate milk production.

Although prolactin is necessary to maintain lactation, the concentration of blood prolactin does not regulate short-term or long-term rates of milk synthesis (Cox, Owens, & Hartmann, 1996). Prolactin levels are high during approximately the first 10 days postpartum and slowly decline over the next 6 months. Prolactin levels are also highest at night. It is thought that the frequent sucking acts as a stimulus to increase the binding capacity of prolactin receptor sites in the breast. This enhances tissue responsiveness, accounting for continued full milk production as prolactin concentrations decline over time.

Milk production closely matches the needs of the newborn. The degree of breast fullness at the end of each feeding influences the short-term rate of milk synthesis. The more efficiently the newborn nurses, the faster is the rate of milk synthesis and the higher its fat content (Daly, Owens, & Hartmann, 1993). The more milk left in the breast, the slower is the rate of milk synthesis. Leaving milk in the breasts for long periods can contribute to slower and lower amounts of milk production, a process referred to as the *feedback inhibitor of lactation* (Wilde, Addey, Boddy, & Peaker, 1995). This mechanism works independently such that each breast can have a different rate of milk synthesis depending on the frequency and degree of drainage on each side. There is also a decrease in the rate of milk synthesis overnight, because the interval between feedings during the night is probably the longest. Although some mothers with larger storage capacities in the breasts can accommodate longer durations between breast drainage (up to 8 to 9 hours) before milk synthesis is compromised, other mothers with smaller storage capacities could experience decreases in milk supplies sooner. Women with a large storage capacity may have greater flexibility in that their babies may not feed as often as an infant of a woman with a smaller storage capacity, even though they may be producing similar amounts of milk (Daly et al., 1993). Infants typically remove about 76% of the available milk at a feeding (Daly, Kent, Owens, & Hartmann, 1996).

Nipple stimulation prompts oxytocin to be released from the pituitary gland in a pulsatile manner numerous times during each feeding. The sensation that accompanies oxytocin's effect on breast tissue is referred to as the *let-down reflex* or the *milk ejection reflex.* Some mothers feel this as a heaviness or tingling sensation in the breast. Some mothers never feel the milk let down but observe milk leaking from the other breast or the newborn swallowing milk. Oxytocin causes the network of myoepithelial cells surrounding the alveoli to contract and expel milk into the larger ductules, making it available to the newborn. This increase in pressure inside the breast overcomes the resistance to the outflow of milk and creates a pressure gradient that allows the fluid inside the breast to move from an area of high pressure to an area of low pressure inside the newborn's mouth. Oxytocin also stimulates uterine contractions that control postpartum bleeding and promote involution. Mothers, especially multiparous women, feel these "after birth pains" during feedings for several days after the birth.

Oxytocin-producing neurons throughout the brain are thought to be associated with social behavior and attachment. In addition to being released in the maternal brain tissue, oxytocin is released into the newborn brain by means of milk transfer and is thought to modulate affiliative behavior between mother and newborn (Insel, 1997; Nelson & Panksepp, 1998). Touch, massage, and skin-to-skin contact stimulates oxytocin release. Separating mothers and newborns should be discouraged unless there is a medical indication (Uvnas-Moberg, 1997).

BIOSPECIFICITY OF HUMAN MILK

Human milk is a species-specific fluid. The composition is not static or uniform. Breast milk is designed to meet the needs of newborns to grow and develop a brain, protect the immature gut, be a substitute for an immature immune system, and assist in developing affiliative behavior. The composition of human milk changes over time. Colostrum (1 to 5 days postpartum) evolves to transitional milk (6 to 13 days postpartum) and then into mature milk (14 days and beyond). Milk composition also changes during feedings, during each 24 hours, and over the course of the entire lactation. Milk of preterm mothers differs from that of term mothers. In contrast, formula is an inert medium with none of the growth factors, enzymes, hormones, live cells, and other bioactive ingredients found in breast milk.

Colostrum is present in the breast from about 12 to 16 weeks of pregnancy. This first milk is thick and has a yellowish color the result of beta-carotene. Average energy value is about 18 kcal/ounce, compared with mature milk at 21 kcal/ounce (AAP, 1998). The volume of colostrum per feeding during the first 3 days postpartum ranges from 2 to 20 mL. Compared with mature milk, colostrum is higher in protein, sodium, chloride, potassium, and fat-soluble vitamins. It is rich in antioxidants, antibodies, interferon, fibronectin, and immunoglobulins, especially secretory IgA. Secretory IgA is antigen specific. When mothers come in contact with microbes, antibodies are synthesized in her milk, targeting pathogens in the newborn's immediate environment. These antibodies are passed to the newborn. Separating the mother and newborn interferes with this defense mechanism. Colostrum begins the establishment of normal bacterial flora in the newborn's gastrointestinal tract and exerts a laxative effect that begins elimination of meconium, decreasing the potential reabsorption of bilirubin.

Nutritional Components

Water

Human milk is composed of 87.5% water, in which all other components are dissolved, dispersed, or in suspension. Infants receiving adequate amounts of breast milk do not need additional water, even in hot, arid, or humid climates (Almroth, 1978).

Fat

Fat content of human milk ranges from 3.5% to 4.5% and contributes 50% of the calories. It varies during a feeding (rising at the end), increases over the first days of lactation, and shows diurnal rhythms. Total fat content is reduced in mothers who smoke (Vio, Salazar, & Infante, 1991) and increases when women nurse more frequently. The long-chain polyunsaturated fatty acids docosahexanoic acid and arachidonic acid contained in breast milk are found in the brain, retina, and central nervous system of newborn's and are necessary for the growth of these structures during the first year of life (Riordan, 1999). The absence of these fatty acids in formula is thought to contribute to differences in cognitive development (Anderson, Johnstone, & Remley, 1999).

Protein

Protein concentration is high in colostrum and settles to 0.8% to 1.0% in mature milk. The whey to casein ratio in human milk changes from 90:10 in the early milk, to 60:40 in mature milk, and 50:50 in late lactation (AAP, 1998). The whey protein that predominates in human milk is acidified in the stomach, forming soft curds that are easily digested and supply the infant with most of the nutrients in human milk. One of the components of the whey protein, lactoferrin, is important in the immunologic effects of human milk. The bacteriostatic effect of lactoferrin makes iron unavailable to pathogens that require the mineral (Riordan, 1999).

Carbohydrate

The principal carbohydrate in human milk is lactose. Lactose supports the colonization of the gut with microflora that increase the acidity of the intestine, decreasing growth of pathogens; ensures a supply of galactose and glucose, which are necessary for brain development; and enhances calcium absorption (Riordan, 1999).

Vitamins and Minerals

Breast milk contains all of the vitamins and minerals needed by most infants for about the first 6 months of life. After 6 months of exclusive breast-feeding, infants require an iron supplement (AAP, 1997). Mothers consuming a vegan diet with no dairy products may need supplemental vitamin B_{12} or an acceptable source in their diet. Breast-fed infants require about 30 minutes of exposure to sunlight per week if wearing only a diaper or 2 hours per week if fully clothed without a hat to maintain normal serum 25-OH-vitamin D levels (Specker, Valanis, Hertzberg, Edwards, & Tsang, 1985).

BREAST-FEEDING PROCESS

Preparation for Breast-feeding

Physical Preparation

There is no research supporting physical preparation of the breasts during pregnancy. Prenatal nipple rolling, application of creams, and expression of colostrum have not been shown to decrease pain or nipple trauma during the postpartum period. Use of methods to improve nipple erectility, such as Hoffman's exercises and breast shells, may decrease the incidence of breast-feeding (Alexander, Grant, & Campbell, 1992). Suggesting that a woman has an inferior nipple in need of correction may decrease her desire and motivation to successfully breast-feed, undermining the entire breast-feeding experience.

Prenatal Education

Women should be encouraged to attend prenatal breast-feeding classes. The current length of hospital stays puts pressure on the nurse, the mother, and the newborn to demonstrate effective breast-feeding before some mother–baby couples are ready. The fast learning pace in the inpatient setting and the mother's cognitive sluggishness for verbal instructions during the first 24 hours postpartum suggest that there could be a benefit in providing basic breast-feeding information before birth (Eidelman, Hoffman, & Kaitz, 1993.) Women report that their decision to breast-feed is influenced by biases of healthcare providers, parity, plans to return to work, and maternal confidence (Balcazar et al., 1995; O'Campo, Faden, Gielen, & Wang, 1992). Prenatal breast-feeding education programs increase the pregnant woman and her partner's knowledge about breast-feeding, increase the support women perceive from their partners around the decision to breast-feed, and increase breast-feeding rates and duration of breast-feeding (Hartley & O'Connor, 1996; Sciacca et al., 1995). In low-income populations, use of peer counselors has been shown to increase initiation, exclusivity, and duration of breast-feeding (Kistin, Abramson, & Dublin, 1994.)

Positioning

Women breast-feed successfully in many different positions. It is important for her to assume a relaxed, comfortable position with her back and arms well supported. If she is seated in a chair, placing a footstool beneath her feet decreases strain on her back and may discourages her from leaning forward over the baby. Some mothers benefit from a pillow on the lap or use one of the commercially available nursing pillows. These can be especially helpful when nursing twins. If the mother is lying on her side, place a pillow behind her back for support. Whatever position is used, instruct the mother to support her breast with her free hand, using four fingers underneath and the thumb on top of the breast in a "C hold" (Fig. 16–1).

Regardless of which position is used, the principles remain the same. The newborn and mother should be facing each other. The mother should not lean forward over the newborn but instead concentrate on bringing him toward her. The newborn should be loosely wrapped or not wrapped at all so the nurse and mother can clearly see the position. There is no need to be concerned about keeping the newborn warm because mother and baby generate body heat during breast-feeding. Skin-to-skin contact is useful for increasing a low temperature in a newborn during the transitional period. As the feeding progresses, if necessary, a light blanket may be placed over both for privacy.

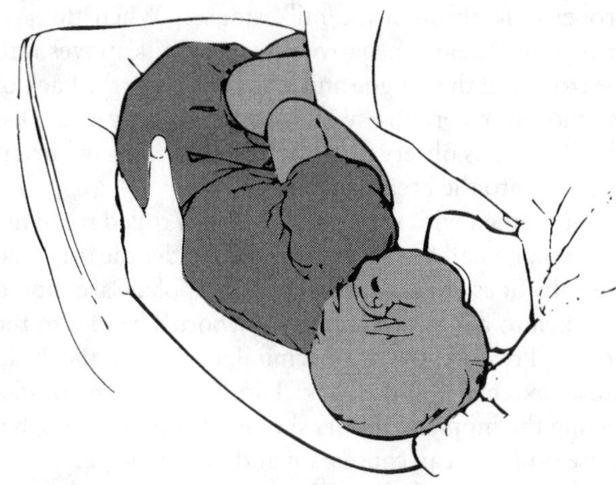

FIGURE 16–1. Cradle hold.

Cradle Hold

With the mother comfortably seated, the newborn is held in an sidelying position with their entire body completely facing the mother. Held on a slight incline, the newborn's lower arm is tucked around the outside of the breast. The newborn's body is in complete contact with the mother, with his legs wrapped around her waist. If the newborn is wrapped in a blanket, loosen it so his arms are free and he can move his legs. Avoid covering the infant's hands with the undershirt cuffs. The newborn's head rests on the mother's forearm, which along with her wrist and hands supports his back and bottom (see Fig. 16-1). Specially designed L-shaped pillows fit around the mother's waist and help to elevate and support her arm. Use of this pillow has been associated with increased length of breast-feeding at 2 weeks and 8 weeks (Humenick, Hill, & Hart, 1998). Regular bed pillows may also be used.

The cradle position can be modified by having the woman alter the position of her arms, using what is called the cross-cradle hold. This is a good position to use for preterm infants and infants with fractured clavicles. The newborn is placed in the same position as the cradle hold but held with the opposite arm such that the head is in the mother's hand and her forearm is supporting the back. This gives the mother much more control over positioning and, along with the clutch hold, may be easier to learn (Fig. 16–2).

Clutch Hold

The clutch position (ie, football hold) is useful for feeding preterm infants or twins and for mothers who have had a cesarean birth. The newborn is placed to the mother's side. Placing a pillow under the newborn raises him slightly and decreases the weight the mother needs to lift. The newborn's head is in her hand, and his feet are positioned toward her back. Care should be taken to ensure that the full weight of the breast does not rest on the newborn's chest (Fig. 16–3).

Sidelying

Sidelying position works well after a cesarean birth or if a woman has a very painful episiotomy. In this position, the newborn and mother are laying on their sides and facing each other. A small rolled blanket can be placed behind the newborn's back, or the mother can support him with her free arm (Fig. 16–4).

Supporting the Breast

Mothers are encouraged to support the breast in a C hold (see Fig. 16-1). The mother lifts her breast with her thumb on top and fingers below and against the chest wall. The thumb and fingers are away from the areola. This hold makes it easy for the mother to direct her nipple toward the center of the mouth during latch-on. Mothers are encouraged to use whichever hand is more comfortable. Pressure should not be applied to the breast with the thumb. The newborn's pug-shaped nose allows breathing through the grooves along the sides of the nares during breast-feeding, even when the nose is touching the breast. In all breast-feeding positions, pulling the newborn's

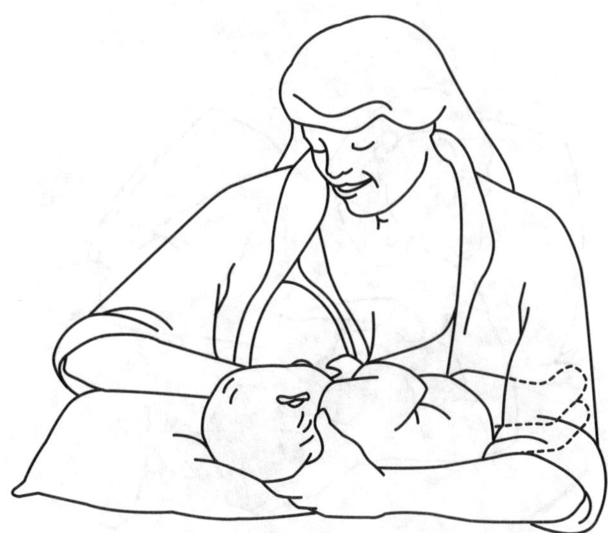

FIGURE 16–2. Modified cradle hold.

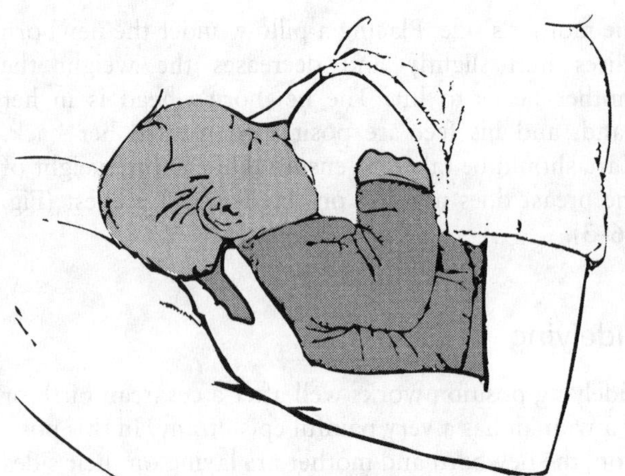

FIGURE 16–3. Clutch hold (football hold).

buttocks closer to the mother's body or gently lifting the breast causes the newborn's head to drop back slightly, providing room for breathing.

Latch-on

Latch-on is the process that the baby uses to attach to the breast. Proper attachment is necessary for pain-free and effective milk transfer. Once positioned comfortably, the mother moves the newborn's lips to the nipple. When the infant's mouth is wide open, she draws the newborn forward toward her. The lower lip and chin contact the breast first. The newborn should grasp the nipple and about 1 to 1.5 inches of the areola, pulling it as a unit forward and deep into his mouth. The tongue is cupped and forward over the lower gum. Peristaltic ripples from the anterior tongue to the posterior tongue propel milk through the milk sinuses. When the jaw lowers and creates negative pressure, milk moves into the trough of the tongue and is channeled to the back of the mouth, where the swallow reflex is triggered. Display 16–2 lists observations made when the newborn is latched onto the breast correctly.

For women with very large breasts, a rolled receiving blanket or small towel can be placed under the breast so the baby does not drag down on the nipple. Care should be taken to avoid pushing the newborn's head into the breast. Pressure on the occipital region of the head causes extension of the neck. Tilting, squeezing, or distorting the nipple or areola should also be avoided, because doing so can cause pain and skin damage.

If the mother feels a pinching or biting sensation while nursing, she should be instructed to pull down gently on the newborn's chin. This causes his mouth to open wider so that more of the areola goes in his mouth. If this does not work, have the mother insert her little finger into the side of the newborn's mouth to release the suction. She should begin again to achieve a better latch-on.

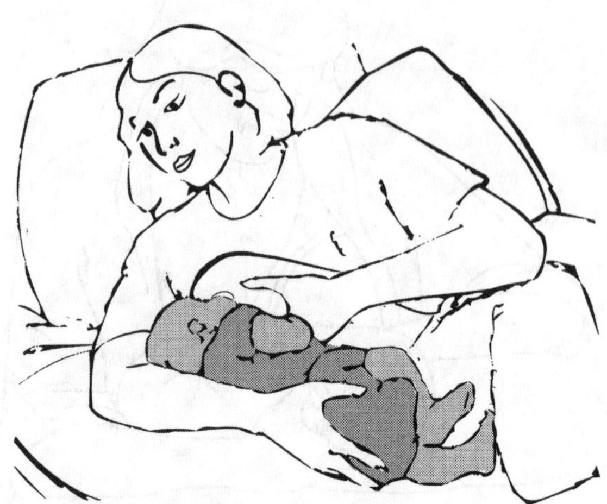

FIGURE 16–4. Side lying.

Milk Transfer

Milk transfer occurs when the newborn suckles effectively and the breast releases milk. Even though a newborn may suck at the breast for 15 minutes with

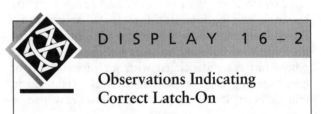

DISPLAY 16–2

Observations Indicating Correct Latch-On

- Lips are rolled outward.
- Clicking or smacking sounds are absent.
- Dimpled cheeks are absent.
- Muscles above and in front of the ear move.
- Both cheeks are equally close to the breast.
- Chin and nose are touching the breast.
- All of the nipple and part of the areola (at least 1 to 1.5 inches) is covered by the newborn's mouth.
- More of the areola is covered by the lower lip than the upper lip.
- Angle at the corner of the mouth is wide.
- When the lower lip is gently pulled away from the breast, the tongue is visible over the lower gum line.

his jaw moving up and down, it does not mean that there has been a transfer of milk. Display 16–3 lists the signs that are observed when milk transfer occurs.

BREAST-FEEDING MANAGEMENT

Getting Started

Breast-feeding should be initiated within an hour of birth. The newborn should be given the opportunity to seek and find the nipple. Nonsedated babies follow a predictable pattern of prefeeding behavior when held on the mother's chest immediately after birth that primes or imprints proper sucking mechanisms right from the start (Widstrom et al., 1987). Successful latch-on and suckling at this time greatly reduce sucking disorganization or dysfunction later on and contribute to increased breast-feeding duration (Righard & Alade, 1992). Sucking movements reach a peak 45 minutes after birth and decline until absent at 2 hours.

Analgesics given during labor have the potential for interfering with the early development of breast-feeding behavior, delaying the first breast-feeding, and negatively influencing breast-feeding long term. Newborn's whose mothers receive nalbuphine (Nubain) or butorphanol (Stadol) within an hour of birth or those whose mother's had no analgesia and who initiated breast-feeding within an hour of birth established effective breast-feeding significantly earlier than infants whose mothers had longer durations of analgesia and later initiation of breast-feeding (Crowell, Hill, & Humenick, 1994). Similar results were reported with use of alphaprodine (Nisentil) (Matthews, 1989). The perinatal nurse may be able to offset some of the side effects of labor medications by helping initiate breast-feeding early, keeping the mother and newborn together, and teaching the mother to put the newborn to breast when he demonstrates hunger cues (Walker, 1999).

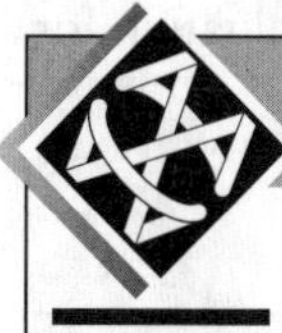

DISPLAY 16–3

Signs That Milk Transfer is Occurring

- Proper latch-on
- Vibration on the occipital region of the head
- Deep jaw excursion
- Mother verbalizes a drawing sensation on the breast
- Absence of clicking or smacking sounds indicating that the tongue has lost contact with the nipple and areola
- Drawing inward of the areolar margins
- Evidence of swallowing (ie, puff of air from the newborn's nose or audible swallows)
- Audible swallows (usually heard after onset of copious milk production)

Sustained Maternal Newborn Contact

Twenty-four hour rooming-in supports breast-feeding and is an integral component of family-centered maternity care. However, the practice of rooming-in needs to be flexible and its implementation respectful of the new mother. She may wish to move the newborn to the nursery in certain situations, such as fatigue or concern for newborn safety. Contact with the newborn enables a woman to recognize and respond to his needs and begin to develop confidence in her mothering role. Rooming-in provides opportunities for identifying hunger cues and to respond with a feeding (American College of Obstetricians and Gynecologists [ACOG], 2000). If the mother and newborn are together when the newborn demonstrates early hunger cues, she can begin feeding (Display 16–4). If the newborn is in a nursery, a healthcare provider witnesses the hunger cues and transports the newborn to the mother's room. During this delay, the newborn may become increasingly agitated, self-console, and return to sleep or become exhausted from crying and return to sleep. By the time the newborn reaches his

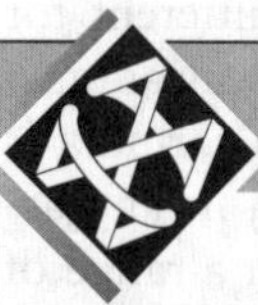

DISPLAY 16–4

Hunger Cues

- Rapid eye movements under the eyelids
- Sucking movements of the mouth and tongue
- Hand-to-mouth movements
- Body movements
- Small sounds
- Rooting
- Mouth opening in response to tactile stimulation
- Smacking of lips

mother, he is often sleeping or crying, and the optimal feeding opportunity is missed. Hunger cues can be observed for up to 30 minutes before the newborn begins a sustained cry for food. Feeding is most successful if initiated while the newborn is in a quiet, alert state. Crying is a late hunger cue, and it is often necessary to console the newborn before he will settle and feed well. Feeding before the newborn begins a sustained cry reduces stress and some of the accompanying undesirable physiologic side effects such as glycogen depletion, increased intracranial pressure, resumption of fetal circulation within the heart, disorganized sucking, and poor feeding. Extended contact with the newborn may facilitate a feeding pattern that includes clustered feedings (ie, 5 to 10 feedings over 2 to 3 hours, followed by a 4- to 5-hour deep sleep).

Frequency and Duration

Historically, fixed breast-feeding schedules were thought to be more scientific, safer because the stomach had to be emptied before allowing a refill, a way to prevent sore nipples, less disruptive for the family if the newborn was on a schedule, and more efficient on a maternity unit. Current understanding of this issue is that restricting breast-feeding in the early days after birth can increase the incidence of sore nipples, engorgement, and perceived need to supplement, and more women may discontinue breast-feeding by 6 weeks postpartum (Renfrew, Lang, Martin, & Woolridge, 2000). Breast-feeding patterns, however, vary widely between mother–baby pairs, over each 24-hour period, and during the course of the lactation. When no artificial time limits are placed on breast-feeding, the number of feedings during each 24 hours ranges from 8 to 14, depending on age, physiologic capacity of the stomach, ability of the newborn, and storage capacity of the breasts.

Frequency and duration of feedings is different for breast-fed and formula-fed newborns. The mean gastric half emptying time of breast milk and formula is quite different. Formula-fed infants have a mean gastric half emptying time of 65 minutes, with a range of 27 to 98 minutes; breast-fed infants have a mean gastric half emptying time of 47 minutes, with a range of 16 to 86 minutes (Van den Driessche, et al., 1999). A newborn consuming breast milk can be hungry 30 to 60 minutes after a feeding. Newborns who frequently nurse are not using their mother as a pacifier. They are learning to feed. The amount of colostrum available meets their current physiologic stomach capacity. Providing bottles of water or formula after nursing is not based on sound scientific principles. There is no evidence in the literature to support this practice.

The newborn feeds on the first breast until he is satiated. The newborn is finished when he comes off the breast by himself after swallowing for most of the feeding. If the mother is uncertain whether the newborn is satisfied, she can use alternate massage (ie, massage and compress the breast each time there is a pause between sucking bursts). When the newborn no longer sucks and swallows when she squeezes the breast, he is done on that side. The mother can then burp the newborn and offer the other breast. There are no time limits on the duration of feedings. In the first days after birth, some newborns nurse only from one breast at a feeding. The other side is offered at the next feeding, usually within 1 or 2 hours. Feeding frequently encourages an abundant milk supply, minimizes engorgement and sore nipples, enhances weight gain, reduces jaundice and hypoglycemia, and increases breast-feeding duration. Display 16–5 lists behavioral signs that indicate the newborn is satiated after feeding. Observing these cues provides new parents with positive feedback that increases their confidence.

Nursing Assessment

Breast-feeding assessments may be brief or comprehensive, depending on where in the perinatal period the mother is encountered and on whether she or the newborn is having problems. The assessment should include a physical evaluation of the breast, information about previous experiences with breast-feeding, knowledge level regarding the mechanics of breast-feeding, and an observation of at least one breast-feeding episode. The breast is evaluated for

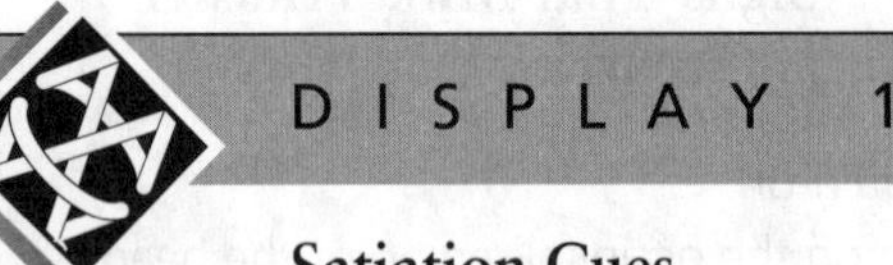

Satiation Cues

- Gradual decrease in number of sucks over course of feeding
- Pursed lips followed by pulling away from the breast and releasing the nipple
- Relaxed body
- Legs extended
- Absence of hunger cues
- Sleep
- Small amount of milk drools from mouth
- Contented state

protraction of the nipple. Approximately 10% of women have a truly inverted or nonprotractile nipple (Alexander et al., 1992). A truly inverted nipple is one that retracts or dimples when gentle tactile stimulation is applied. This condition is caused by the presence of embryologic tissue behind the nipple and areola (Lawrence & Lawrence, 1999). For most women, protraction of the nipple increases with breast-feeding and becomes more pronounced with subsequent pregnancies.

An initial assessment includes history of breast-feeding experience, problems with latch-on, sore nipples, engorgement, newborn weight gain, and amount and quality of social support. Knowing how long the mother exclusively breast-fed other children, when or if she introduced pacifiers and or bottles, how satisfied she was with the feeding experience, and how long she plans to breast-feed this newborn provides insight into the mother's style and potential problem areas. Without proper evaluation, nursing interventions may be inappropriate or inadequate.

Signs of Adequate Intake

Evaluating the newborn for adequate intake is based on elimination patterns, weight gain, condition of the mucous membranes, and behavioral observations. Table 16–2 outlines elimination patterns for the early days of life. If the number of wet diapers or bowel movements is below what is expected based on age, parents are instructed to notify their primary care provider. Wet diapers can be used to assesse hydration, and the number of bowel movements serves as a caloric assessment. Urine should be clear and pale yellow. Because urine contains an abundance of uric acid crystals during the first week of life, occasionally pink or rust-colored stain is apparent on the diaper. After the first week, presence of this pink stain is an indicator of insufficient intake. Superabsorbent diapers make it difficult for some parents to tell when the diaper is wet. Parents can place a soft, dry paper towel, tissue, or square of toilet paper inside the diaper with each change to more easily tell when the diaper is wet. Table 16–3 describes the estimated volume of urine output over the first 2 months of life. Stools change from meconium to transitional stools to yellow, seedy liquid. Yellow stool should be present by the end of the first week. Some infants stool as frequently as every feeding for the first 4 to 6 weeks.

Newborns regain their birth weight by 2 weeks of age and go on to gain 4 to 7 ounces each week or at least a pound per month. Most experts believe that newborns should not loose more than 7% of their birth weights (Lawrence & Lawrence, 1999). Physical signs that the newborn is sufficiently hydrated include mucous membranes that are moist and skin that doesn't remain tented when pinched. The newborn should also demonstrate a range of behaviors during the day, including being alert, acting hungry, being fussy, and acting satisfied after feeding.

Assessment Tools

Common methods of documenting breast-feeding interactions do not always provide useful information. Subjective words such as *well, fair,* and *poor* do not capture the data needed to assess adequate intake or effectively identify problem areas. Similarly, the phrase "breast-feeding well" does not capture information regarding latch-on, audible swallow, time frames, or satiation. Numerous breast-feeding assessment tools assist the perinatal nurse by providing consistent guidelines for evaluating individual feeding events, ensure continuity of care and communication between healthcare professionals, and provide a clear record in the chart of breast-feeding progress. One example of a breast-feeding assessment tool, the LATCH tool, is displayed in Table 16–4. Similar to an Apgar score, this tool assists the perinatal nurse to perform and document a thorough assessment and to identify areas where assistance

TABLE 16–2 ▪ ELIMINATION PATTERN DURING THE FIRST WEEK OF LIFE

Age (days)	Number of Wet Diapers	Number of Bowel Movements
1	1–2	1
2	2–3	2
3	3–4	3–4
4	4–5	3–4
5	4–5	3 or more
6	6–8	3 or more
7	8 or more	3 or more

TABLE 16–3 ■ ESTIMATED URINE VOLUME

Age (days)	Volume (mL)
1–2	15–60
3–10	50–300
11–60	250–450

and support are needed. A small amount of research supports the validity and reliability of breast-feeding assessment tools (Riordan & Koehn, 1997).

Supplemental Feedings

Supplemental feedings for term, healthy, breast-fed newborns are seldom necessary except for medical indications (AAP, 1997). Illnesses in the mother or newborn that may require supplementation include inborn errors of metabolism, very-low-birth-weight infants, preterm infants, and certain medications being taken by the mother. Use of supplements without a medical indication is associated with earlier cessation of breast-feeding (Chezem, Friesen, Montgomery, Fortman, & Clark, 1998). Placing formula or water bottles in the bassinet or at the bedside of a breast-feeding mother sends a negative message about her ability to successfully breast-feed.

Use of Pacifiers and Artificial Nipples

Artificial nipples and pacifiers are associated with incorrect sucking techniques at the breast (Righard, 1998), decreased total duration of breast-feeding (Aarts, Hornell, Kylberg, Hofvander, & Gebre-Medhin, 1999; Howard, et al., 1999; Righard & Alade, 1997; Victora, Behague, Barros, Olinto, & Weiderpass, 1997), and fewer feeds in 24 hours (Aarts, et al., 1999; Howard, et al., 1999; Victora, et al., 1997). Pacifier and bottle use are sometimes an indicator of breast-feeding difficulties. Mothers who request bottles or pacifiers may be doing so because they lack confidence in their ability to successfully breast-feed. These women may benefit from contact with a skilled perinatal nurse or lactation consultant to evaluate the situation.

TABLE 16–4 ■ LATCH: BREAST-FEEDING CHARTING SYSTEM

System Component	0	1	2
L Latch	Too sleepy or reluctant No latch achieved	Repeated attempts Hold nipple in mouth Stimulate to suck	Grasps breast Tongue down Lips flanged Rhythmic sucking
A Audible Swallowing	None	A few with stimulation	Spontaneous and intermittent <24 h old Spontaneous and frequent >24 h old
T Type of nipple	Inverted	Flat	Everted (after stimulation)
C Comfort (breast/nipple)	Engorged Cracked, bleeding, large blisters or bruises Severe discomfort	Filling Reddened small blisters or bruises Mild or moderate discomfort	Soft Nontender
H Hold (positioning)	Full assist (staff holds infant at breast)	Minimal assist (ie, place pillows for support, elevate head of bed) Teach one side; mother does other Staff holds and then mother takes over	No assist from staff Mother able to position and hold baby

From Jensen, D., Wallace, S., & Kelsey, P. (1994). LATCH: A breastfeeding charting system and documentation tool. *Journal of Obstetric Gynecologic, and Neonatal Nursing 23*, 27–32.

Hospital Discharge Packs

Many women in the United States come to the hospital expecting to receive some type of discharge "gift bag." The dilemma for perinatal nurses who support breast-feeding is that frequently these packs contain formula samples. Although research has not demonstrated that discharge packs with formula significantly decrease duration of breast-feeding (Bliss, Wilke, Acredolo, Berman, & Tebb, 1997; Dungy, Losch, Russell, Romitti, & Dusdieker, 1997), they do slightly increase the risk that parents will introduce formula during the first 6 weeks of life (Bliss, et al., 1997). Ideally, a discharge pack given to breast-feeding women does not contain formula samples but instead has products that support breast-feeding, such as a manual pump, chemical cold packs, and breast pads.

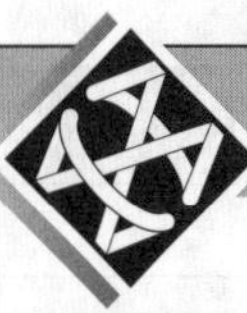

DISPLAY 16–6

Factors Contributing to a Reluctant Nurser

- Poor position at the breast
- Interruption in the organized sequence of prefeeding behaviors immediately after birth
- Use of medications during labor that may prolong the period of state disorganization
- Hypertonia (ie, jaw clenching, pursed lips, neck and back hyperextension, and tongue retraction or elevation)
- Infrequent feeds leading to an overly hungry newborn baby
- Excessive or prolonged crying resulting in behavioral disorganization
- Interference with imprinting on the breast from separation, artificial nipples, pacifiers, or nipple shields
- Excessive pressure on the occipital region of the baby's head from pushing the head forward into the breast
- Vigorous or deep suctioning or intubation causing swelling or pain in the mouth or throat
- Short or tight lingual frenulum

POTENTIAL BREAST-FEEDING PROBLEMS

Reluctant Nurser

Newborns are described as reluctant nursers when they latch-on only after many attempts, move their head from side to side without latching-on, fall asleep or aggressively push away from the breast and arch their back, have a preference for nursing only on one side, do not latch-on, or latch-on but feed ineffectively. Numerous factors can contribute to a newborn being reluctant to nurse (Display 16–6). Managing this situation requires that the nurse and parents be very patient and not give up on the newborn's ability to eventually latch-on correctly and nurse efficiently. Table 16–5 identifies interventions that the nurse can use to encourage the newborn who is reluctant to latch-on successfully.

Newborns should demonstrate at least one effective breast-feed before discharge. If the newborn has not latched-on at all by 24 hours, the mother should begin to express colostrum manually and feed with a syringe or cup. If the woman is unable to manually express colostrum, an electric or hand pump can be used as an alternative. These mothers should be referred to a lactation consultant for home follow-up and the primary care physician notified of the feeding difficulty.

Nipple Pain

Sore nipples are common during the early days of breast-feeding. Pain or tenderness may occur in the following situations:

- When the baby first latches on, but pain disappears during the feeding after the baby starts swallowing
- Periodically during the feeding
- Throughout an entire feeding

Physical findings include vertical or horizontal red or white lines on the breast; fissures, cracks, or bleeding from the nipple; and blisters or scabs on one or both nipples. Use of formula and pacifiers in the hospital have been associated with nipple pain at the time of discharge (Centuori et al., 1999). Display 16–7 outlines factors that contribute to nipple pain. Transient nipple pain usually peaks between the third and sixth days postpartum. Prolonged or severe soreness beyond the first week requires intervention.

Various interventions can be used by the perinatal nurse to assist a woman experiencing nipple pain continuously or intermittently with feedings (Table 16–6). None of the treatments for nipple pain, including lanolin (Brent, Rudy, Redd, Rudy, & Roth, 1998; Centuori et al., 1999; Pugh et al., 1996), breast shells (Brent et al., 1998), warm water compresses (Buchko et al., 1994; Pugh et al., 1998), expressed breast milk (Buchko et al., 1994; Pugh et al., 1998), air drying nipples (Buchko et al., 1994; Pugh et al., 1998), tea bags

TABLE 16–5 ■ RELUCTANT NURSER

Management	Rationale
Check positioning at the breast: Newborn completely facing mother with head, neck, and spine aligned Mouth directly in front of tip of nipple Newborn brought to breast and held close Mother does not lean forward, maneuver breast sideways, compress areola and insert it into the mouth, or tilt nipple up while attempting latch-on	Poor positioning increases the number of latch attempts needed before obtaining milk, which can frustrate the mother and baby. Incorrect position increases the chances that the newborn will not latch correctly, leading to sore nipples, engorgement, insufficient milk production, and slow weight gain.
Positioning depends on the newborn. Those who prefer the right side may need to be held in a football hold on the right breast and in a cradle or prone position for the left breast. Some babies do better when the mother is in a sidelying position. Breech babies may feed better sitting upright in the football hold. Babies with birth trauma, such as a cephalohematoma, may be more comfortable and feed better when held with the affected side up. Babies with a fractured clavicle may feed better in a football hold if the weight of the breast is kept off the chest or cradle hold with the affected side up.	Positioning in utero and events at birth may influence breast-feeding patterns. Several different positions need to be explored to find one that is satisfactory.
After birth, allow the newborn time to seek and find the nipple before removing him from his mother's chest.	This approach provides the opportunity for the prefeeding sequence of behaviors to occur, which increases the likelihood of proper attachment to the breasts.
Keep the mother and baby together. Place baby skin-to-skin on mother's chest. Instruct the mother to feed her baby on cue when he stirs, she sees rapid eye movements under the eyelids, she sees movements of the tongue and mouth, and the newborn exhibits hand-to-mouth movements or makes small sounds.	This approach reestablishes or repatterns the initial sucking sequence that may not have occurred immediately after birth. The mother can feel and see feeding cues and place him to the breast when he is most likely to latch-on.
For a newborn making rapid side-to-side head movements, touch the midline of the upper lip with a dropper of colostrum. Move him onto the breast as he follows the dropper to the nipple. When his mouth is wide open, place a few drops of water or colostrum on his tongue to elicit sucking and swallowing.	The dropper acts to provide external control and food incentives to attach and suck at the breast.
A newborn who arches can be placed in the football hold or with the mother lying on her side.	Positioning helps the newborn to relax and flex the back and hips to avoid arching and jaw clenching.
Provide latch and sucking incentives: A syringe placed in the side of the mouth can deliver a small amount of colostrum with each suck until the newborn demonstrates rhythmic suck and swallow at the breast. A syringe or soft clinic dropper can be used to elicit sucking.	These methods help prevent baby from pulling away from the breast before he latches on or swallows.

(continued)

TABLE 16–5 ■ RELUCTANT NURSER (continued)

Management	Rationale
Butterfly tubing attached to a 10-mL syringe and taped to the breast can provide these incentives as well as a supplement if needed.	
After crying hard for a while, the newborn may not be able to organize himself to feed. Allow him to suck on a finger or place the tubing on a finger and allow him to suck a little colostrum by finger feeding before putting him to the breast. If the newborn will not suck on a finger, place some colostrum in a medicine cup and have him sip from the cup until he calms down.	These interventions can calm the newborn and allow him to have a little food in his stomach so he is not so terrible hungry.
If the newborn does not open his mouth wide enough for painless latch-on or clenches his jaw while latching-on, hold the jaw between your thumb and index finger and move it gently a small amount from side to side.	This method helps inhibit jaw clenching.

(Buchko et al., 1994), and hydrogel moist wound dressings (Brent et al., 1998), has been shown to be more effective than any other. With this in mind, women would probably benefit from being instructed to use the easiest and most economic treatments, which include expressing colostrum or breast milk on nipples after feedings, letting the nipples air dry, or using warm, moist compresses to decrease discomfort. Colostrum and breast milk expressed on the nipple and areola have bacteriostatic qualities from the antibodies and antiinflammatory factors, which assist in the healing process (Brent et al., 1998; Pugh et al., 1996).

Candida albicans

If the mother complains of burning pain on the nipple or burning and shooting pains in the breast, a fungal infection (ie, thrush) may be present. This is usually caused by *Candida albicans*. Predisposing factors for mothers include

- Steroids (oral contraceptives, asthma medications)
- Broad-spectrum antibiotics
- Diabetes
- Obesity
- Poor endocrine function
- Infection in other family members or pets

Sources of *C. albicans* for newborns include

- Vaginal canal
- Artificial bottle nipples
- Pacifiers
- Antibiotic use
- Hands of the nurse or parent
- Mechanical irritant in the mouth (ie, disruption of oral mucosa from suctioning)

The mother may present with burning pain during or after feedings that does not improve with correct latch-on and positioning. She may have itching on the nipple or areola, with a pale or shiny spot on the areola and bright pink nipples. When *C. albicans* proliferates because of an upset in the balance of factors that normally keeps it in check, the usually noninvasive yeast can change to a fungus-like microbe that produces rhizoids. Rhizoids are long, rootlike structures able to pierce duct walls and release toxins or allergens into nearby tissues. This may be responsible for the burning sensation and shooting pains deep in the breast.

The newborn presents with white patches (ie, "crumbling curds") on the buccal mucosa, gums, or tongue that can travel to the hard and soft palate and down to the tonsils. It may also appear as pearly white or gray patches. If a patch is removed, a bright red base may be seen as a painfully eroded area. Most babies with thrush in the mouth also have the infection in the intestines and stools, which contributes to a *Candida*-caused diaper rash. Some newborn's mouths are colonized with *C. albicans*, but it is not clinically apparent. They may be fussy, have a poor appetite, breastfeed poorly, and experience general discomfort.

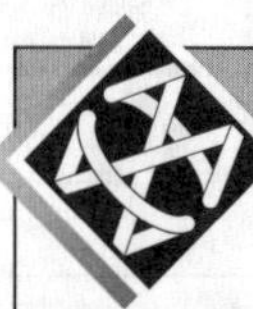

DISPLAY 16-7

Factors Contributing to Sore Nipples

- Transient pain while latching-on may occur from lack of a keratin layer on the nipple epithelium.
- Unrelieved negative pressure is present until the milk ejection reflex occurs and is relieved by the periodic swallowing of the baby.
- Manipulation of the nipple and areola such as squeezing it, tilting or pointing it up or down, or pushing it into the mouth
- Mother leaning over to "insert" the breast into the newborn's mouth
- Nipple and areola may not be in the mouth symmetrically or far enough
- Lips curled under rather than flared out
- Tongue behind lower gum and pinching or biting of the nipple
- Breast pushed sideways into the mouth rather than centered over where the nipple points naturally.
- Nipple confusion (ie, mouth configured for feeding on an artificial nipple or pacifier)
- Disorganized or dysfunctional sucking pattern
- Flat or retracted nipples
- Mouth not opened wide enough

The treatment depends on the location and severity of the infection. Treatment of the mother and newborn simultaneously is important, even if only one has clinical symptoms. Topical antifungals are used to treat skin *Candida.* Antifungal topical cream or lotion can be applied to the breast and nipple before and after each feeding. They can also be applied to the diaper area of the newborn and after breast-feeding to the newborn's mouth. Gentian violet in a weak aqueous solution of 0.5% to 1% can be directly applied to the nipple and areola and to the baby's mouth once each day for 3 to 7 days. The treatment for resistant or systemic candidiasis is oral fluconazole (200 to 400 mg), followed by 100 to 200 mg/day for 14 to 21 days (Hale, 1999; Hoover, 1999).

Jaundice

Early-onset jaundice appears after 24 hours of age, peaking on the third or fourth day of life, and steadily declines through the first month to normal levels. Clinical signs of hyperbilirubinemia are present in 50% to 60% of all newborns. Concentrations of unconjugated bilirubin can increase if production exceeds processing capabilities. Meconium is a reservoir for large amounts of unconjugated bilirubin that is reabsorbed into the circulation if there is a delay in eliminating the meconium. Failure to clear meconium quickly enhances enteric reabsorption and increases serum bilirubin levels. The laxative effect of colostrum promotes the rapid evacuation of meconium and reduces the unconjugated bilirubin available for reabsorption. Some hospital routines contribute to high bilirubin levels in breast-fed newborns. Systems that do not promote rooming-in decrease the number of feedings, as do scheduled feeds. Newborns given the most sugar water have the highest bilirubin levels (Kuhr & Paneth, 1982). Dextrose (5%) water has 6 calories per ounce, and colostrum has 18 calories per ounce. For every ounce of sugar water consumed, the newborn has a deficit in two thirds of the calories he needs to prevent intestinal reabsorption of bilirubin. Early exaggeration of physiologic jaundice can be reduced or eliminated by effective breast-feeding management that includes 8 to 12 feedings each 24 hours.

The technique of alternate breast massage has been used to increase milk supply when the newborn is sleepy or feeds inefficiently. When the mother notices that the newborn's rapid, shallow suckling movements decrease, she massages the base of her breast. She then alternates massaging the breast between periods of suckling.

The decision to begin phototherapy is complicated by the fact that the level of bilirubin that causes kernicterus is unknown and may differ from one newborn to another. After the first 48 hours of life, a healthy term newborn may not require phototherapy or interruption of breast-feeding until total serum bilirubin concentrations exceed 18 to 20 mg/dL. Management options when bilirubin levels go above 18 to 20 mg/dL include the following (Dixit & Gartner, 1999):

- Increasing the number of times during the day the newborn breast-feeds
- Use of alternate breast massage on each breast during feedings
- Pumping breast milk and giving it by cup as a supplement after nursing
- Phototherapy

In late-onset jaundice (ie, breast-milk jaundice), physiologic bilirubin levels decline at the end of the first week and then rise again, sometimes to much higher levels than originally. In rare situations, bilirubin levels may climb to 25 mg/dL or higher. Late-

TABLE 16–6. INTERVENTIONS FOR SORE NIPPLES

Management	Rationale
Suggest that the mother initiate the milk ejection reflex or express drops of colostrum before latch-on.	Colostrum or milk flow prevents traumatic sucking by causing swallowing at the start of the feeding.
Review and correct positioning:	
In the cradle hold, baby completely faces the mother and is held close with his legs, wrapped around the mother's waist.	Proper positioning and latch techniques prevent or alleviate many of the problems with sore nipples.
Four fingers are under the breast, and the thumb is on top, with all fingers off of the areola.	Proper positioning and latch-on can prevent or alleviate sore nipples.
The baby is brought to the breast with his mouth centered over where the nipple points.	Pushing the breast sideways to the newborn may cause vertical cracks on either side of the nipple.
Touch the lips to the nipple. When his mouth opens to its widest point, the newborn is drawn the rest of the way onto the breast.	Newborn must be brought close to the breast to facilitate enough of the areola begin drawn into the mouth rather than just the nipple tip.
If the mouth does not open wide enough or if the nipple feels pinched, the mother can use the side of her index finger under her breast to gently pull down on the chin. This also rolls out the lower lip. Some newborns who do not open wide enough may benefit from sucking on an adult's finger before feeds.	This technique helps draw into the mouth the portion of the breast needed to effect milk transfer without pain.
The mother can massage and compress the breast to initiate milk flow while waiting for the newborn to begin sucking. If the newborn pauses for long periods between sucking bursts, the mother can add the technique of alternate breast massage (ie, squeezing the breast when the newborn pauses.)	Milk flow regulates sucking and alleviates unrelieved negative pressure when the baby is not swallowing periodically. Alternate massage provides milk incentives to start the suck and swallow sequence.

(continued)

onset jaundice is thought to be caused by a component in the mother's milk that inhibits conjugation of bilirubin by the liver (Guthrie & Auerbach, 1999). Studies have demonstrated that there is a higher fat content in the milk of mothers whose newborns developed late-onset jaundice. If one infant develops late-onset jaundice, there is a high probability that subsequent infants born to the same mother will be affected. To determine whether a newborn has late-onset jaundice, a bilirubin level is assessed, and the mother is asked to formula feed for 24 hours, after which a second bilirubin level is determined. If the bilirubin level has begun to decrease a diagnosis of late-onset or breast-milk jaundice is made. No treatment is necessary for late-onset jaundice (Gartner, 1994).

Hypoglycemia

Hypoglycemia in a term newborn usually refers to a blood glucose level below 40 mg/dL. This is a common and usually transient occurrence in the immediate newborn period. Routine monitoring of blood glucose concentration in healthy term newborns is unnecessary. Conditions that increase the risk for hypoglycemia include being small for gestational age, being the smaller of two twins, being large for gestational age, having a low birth weight, being the infant of a diabetic mother, or having asphyxia, polycythemia, erythroblastosis fetalis, respiratory distress, and hypothermia. Hypoglycemia in breast-fed newborns can be prevented or greatly reduced by hospital policies that support breast-feeding:

TABLE 16–6. (continued)

Management	Rationale
Avoid extension of the baby's back or neck; align the head and trunk. The mother can use the football hold or prone position for a high-tone newborn.	Extension causes jaw clenching, with the tongue moving behind the lower gum.
The mother should avoid the tendency to depress the top of the breast or areola under the newborn's nose to create an airway. A properly positioned baby should have the tip of the nose touching the beast and can breathe without assistance. The mother should also avoid the scissors hold on the areola, which compresses it and flattens on inverted nipple.	The incorrect method pulls the nipple and areola out of the mouth and contributes to nipple sucking and blisters.
Feedings should occur on cue 8–12 times each 24 hours. Avoid trying to lengthen time intervals between feeds or feeding a bottle at night.	Feeding frequently avoids frantic, overly hungry pulling at the breast. Full, firm breasts make latch-on more difficult and painful.
Breast milk can be applied to the nipples after each feeding. Avoid creams, lotions, oils, and ointments unless medically indicated. Warm water compresses may also provide relief.	Some commercial preparations slow the healing process.
Avoid pacifiers, artificial nipples on bottles, and nipple shields. Use alternative devices for supplemental feeds if needed (eg, cup, syringe, dropper, feeding tube devices).	Some devices prevent incorrect patterning of mouth conformation. Artificial nipples do not elongate and compress like a human nipple. Their use weakens a baby's suck as the baby decreases sucking pressure to slow milk and regulate milk flow.

- Breast-feeding within an hour of birth
- Skin-to-skin contact between mother and newborn to prevent cold stress and use of glucose stores
- Breast-feeding 8 to 12 times per day
- Feeding in response to readiness cues, not on a schedule
- Not letting the newborn get to the point of crying (ie, crying rapidly depletes glycogen stores and can contribute to a steep decline in blood sugar levels)
- Pump or hand expressing colostrum into a spoon or cup for the newborn who is reluctant to suckle at the breast and feeding the newborn colostrum several times per hour until he able to feed effectively at the breast

Hypoglycemia that recurs or persists longer than 48 to 72 hours of age suggests an underlying medical condition and is not related to feeding. Documented hypoglycemia in an asymptomatic infant that does not respond to oral feeding or in a symptomatic infant usually necessitates intravenous glucose infusions. The mother should be encouraged to hand express or pump colostrum for oral feeds (by cup or spoon if the medical condition permits) to maintain a milk supply while the newborn is not nursing.

Engorgement

Lawrence and Lawrence (1999) describe engorgement of the breast in terms of three elements: congestion and vascularity, accumulation of milk, and edema caused by the swelling and obstruction of drainage of the lymphatic system. Engorgement can involve the areola, the body of the breast, or both areas. Areolar engorgement may be caused by distended lactiferous sinuses or reflect edema from large amounts of intravenous fluids infused during labor. Some amount of engorgement is normal. No engorgement is a sign of a problem that requires close follow-up. It may be related to retained placental fragments or minimal breast tissue growth during pregnancy. If areolar engorgement is caused by intravenous fluids, the areola may appear puffy and is responsive to cold-pack application. If distended with milk, the areola may envelop the nipple, and the whole unit is difficult for the baby to grasp. The mother should hand express some milk before putting the baby to breast to avoid tissue damage and pain.

Peripheral engorgement usually does not develop until 2 to 3 days after birth. Some swelling of the entire breast is normal, but if the breasts become hard, red, hot, shiny, and throb, physiologic engorgement has changed to pathologic engorgement. This can be extremely painful, and the mother needs to breast-feed very frequently using gentle, alternate massage. Hand expression may provide relief, and some women are made more comfortable by using ice packs, a bag of frozen peas wrapped around the breast, or application of chilled or room-temperature cabbage leaves. It is important to nurse even when engorged because prolonged milk stasis increases the risk of mastitis, is a major cause of insufficient milk, and contributes to sore nipples, poor latch-on, reduced milk transfer, and slow weight gain by the infant. Separating mothers and babies, especially at night, giving unnecessary supplements, skipping night feedings, and long intervals between feeds exacerbates the problem of engorgement. It is vital to maintain frequent and thorough drainage of the breasts at this time. Back pressure in the ducts can lead to atrophy of the milk secreting cells.

Plugged Duct and Mastitis

Small, tender breast lumps the size of a pea are sometimes encountered by breast-feeding mothers. Milk stasis or a component of the milk may contribute to this. Hot packs and massaging the lump while the baby is sucking helps move this blockage. Some women experience repeated plugging of ducts and describe fatty strings being expressed from the breast.

Continued milk stasis increases the risk for mastitis. Mastitis is an inflammatory condition of the breast that may or may not eventually or concurrently involve an infection. Display 16–8 describes symptoms of mastitis. When symptoms become severe, most clinicians treat with antibiotics. Although antibiotics treat the infection, they do not address the underlying cause of the mastitis. Antibiotic therapy must be accompanied by interventions to identify and correct the cause. Early identification of the cause and the use of appropriate interventions may halt the inflammatory process and prevent progression of an infection. Pain and inflammation at this point can be treated with a nonsteroidal antiinflammatory drug such as ibuprofen. If there is no improvement within 8 to 24 hours and the mother has obvious signs of a bacterial infection such as a discharge of pus from the nipple, continued fever, or a sudden spike of fever, she should contact her primary care provider immediately. Because *Staphylococcus aureus* is most commonly associated with breast infections, choices of antibiotics are generally penicillinase-resistant penicillins or cephalosporins that are effective against this organism. These antibiotics are safe, and the mother should continue breast-feeding frequently from the affected side.

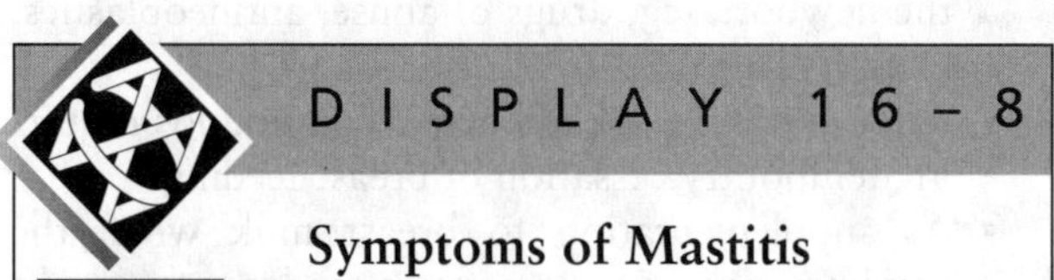

DISPLAY 16–8

Symptoms of Mastitis

- Fever >38°C (100.4°F)
- Flulike symptoms (eg, aching, chills)
- Pain or swelling at the site
- Red, hot, hard area that is often wedge shaped
- Red streaks extending from the lump toward the axilla

Insufficient Milk

Real or perceived insufficient milk supply is the most common reason for premature weaning. Qualitative research during the early postpartum period revealed that women become increasingly confident and empowered by breast-feeding or that their confidence progressively diminished as they expressed concerns about the adequacy of their breast milk. The perception of breast milk inadequacy was related to inability to quantify and visualize the amount of breast milk, anxiety about the adequacy of their own diet, inadequate and conflicting advice from healthcare professionals, and unmet needs for support and nurturing for themselves (Dykes & Williams, 1999).

A small percentage of women produce insufficient milk for anatomic or physiologic reasons. Psychologic, physiologic, and pathologic factors can lead to decreased production and ejection of milk (Biancuzzo, 2000). Psychological factors include stress, embarrassment, and pain, all of which may increase production of epinephrine, which causes blood vessels to constrict, and decrease oxytocin, which facilitates letdown. Physiologic factors include maternal illness, severe postpartum bleeding (Sheehan's syndrome), breast surgery (ie, reduction and augmentation), and conditions that interfere with the early, effective, and consistent stimulating of the breasts, such as restrictions on frequency and duration of feedings, more than 3 hours between feedings, skipping night feedings, and use of supplements. Pathologic factors that negatively affect milk production are related to endocrine problems. Women who do not develop breast tissue during pregnancy equal to an increase in at least one cup size are at risk for insufficient milk production. Perceived insufficient milk is often described by mothers when she experiences one or more of the following:

- Baby does not settle or fusses after a feeding.
- Baby wants to feed frequently (ie, growth spurt).
- Baby takes formula from a bottle directly after breast-feeding.
- Mother is unable to express much milk.
- Baby does not sleep through the night or is awake much of the day.
- Breasts are smaller and softer than they should be.
- Initial weight loss of baby after birth is a concern.

Strategies to handle real or perceived insufficient milk depend on the cause of the problem. Mismanagement of breast-feeding is the most common contributor to low milk production. This problem is usually revealed during a feeding history. Mothers should be breast-feeding 8 to 12 times each 24 hours with no supplements or pacifiers. A feeding observation is necessary to confirm whether the newborn is swallowing milk or simply engaging in nonnutritive sucking. Mothers should perform alternate massage and feed at closer intervals to increase milk production. Refer mothers to a lactation consultant for a thorough breast-feeding assessment and follow-up.

MEDICATIONS AND BREAST-FEEDING

Interruption of breast-feeding for women who are taking medications is usually an unnecessary and potentially damaging recommendation. Most medications have few side effects because the dose received by the newborn is usually less than 1% of the maternal dose and may be poorly bioavailable to the newborn. Antimetabolites and therapeutic doses of radiopharmaceuticals are examples of medications that are contraindicated. If a medication is necessary for only a short time, women can be assisted to pump and dispose of their milk until it is safe for the newborn to nurse. Ideally, newborns can be syringe or cup fed during this time. There are several excellent sources providing information on the safe use of medications for breast-feeding women (Display 16–9).

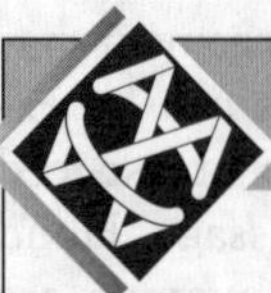

DISPLAY 16–9

References for Medications and Breast-feeding

Briggs, G. G., Freeman, R. K., & Yaffe, S. J. (1998). *Drugs in pregnancy and lactation.* (5th ed.) Baltimore: Williams & Wilkins.

Committee on Nutrition American Academy of Pediatrics. (1998). *Pediatric nutrition handbook* (4th ed.). Elk Grove Village, IL: Author.

Hale T. (1999). *Medications and mother milk* (8th ed.). Amarillo, TX: Pharmasoft Medical Publishing.

Lactation Fax Hotline, 24-hour fax-on-demand, registration required (806–356–9556)

Lactation Studies Center, Rochester, NY (716–275–0088)

Rocky Mountain Drug Consultation Center, Denver, CO (900–285–3784)

University of California at San Diego Drug Information Service, San Diego, CA (900–288–8273)

FORMULA FEEDING

Use of a commercially prepared, iron-fortified infant formula is another method of providing neonatal nutrition during the first year of life. Use of formula is indicated for newborns in the following situations (AAP, 1998):

- When their mother chooses not to breast-feed or not to breast-feed exclusively
- In the presence of maternal infections caused by organisms that may be transmitted through human milk
- If the newborn is diagnosed with an inborn error of metabolism causing intolerance to components of human milk, such as galactosemia or tyrosinemia
- When the mother has been exposed to foods, medications, or environmental agents that are excreted in human milk and may be harmful to the newborn (eg, drugs of abuse, antineoplastics, mercury, lead)
- After exposure to radioactive compounds requiring temporary cessation of breast-feeding
- As supplementation to breast milk when the newborn does not demonstrate adequate weight gain

Parents may benefit from an understanding that newborns fed formula have a greater risk of acute and chronic illness, allergies, and obesity. Parents with a family history of allergy or diabetes should be carefully counseled regarding the possible outcomes from the use of formula. Cow's milk; goat's milk; 1%, 2%, or fat-free milk; and evaporated milk are not recommended during the first year of life (AAP, 1998). These milk products do not contain adequate iron concentration, increase the renal solute load because of the amount of protein, sodium, potassium, and chloride, and may result in deficiencies in essential fatty acids, vitamin E, and zinc (AAP, 1998). Direct advertising of infant formulas to the public is a violation of the World Health Organization code and discouraged by the AAP. This important information should be provided to the woman in an objective manner. Some women may choose not to breast-feed. The purpose of the discussion is not to make them feel guilty about their choice.

Composition of Formula

Commercially prepared formula can never totally duplicate the hormones, immunologic agents, enzymes, and live cells found in human milk. In 1980, Congress passed the first Infant Formula Act, which was later revised in 1986. This legislation set minimum and maximum levels of certain nutrients and required that manufactures analyze all batches of formula and state on the labels the concentration of specific nutrients.

The concentrations of nutrients in formula varies slightly between manufacturers and are usually slightly higher in formula than breast milk to compensate for the possible lower bioavailability (AAP, 1998). Although formula companies may be able to provide a rationale for their individual differences, large, randomized clinical trials supporting their conclusions do not exist. Most formulas use cow's milk as the protein base. Because some newborns develop formula intolerance and some families are aware of existing milk intolerance, formula companies manufacture alternative formulas of special composition for newborns with gastrointestinal or metabolic disturbances.

Milk-Based Formula

Milk-based formula contains approximately 50% more protein than human milk. Concentrations of the two sources of protein, whey and casein, vary according to the manufacturer. During the processing of formula, the animal fat in cow's milk is removed and replaced with vegetable oils or a mixture of vegetable oil and animal fats. Using vegetable oil improves digestibility and absorption, eliminates cholesterol, increases the concentration of essential fatty acids, and reduces environmental pollutants (AAP, 1998). The major sources of carbohydrate in human milk and formula is lactose. The presence of lactose in the bowel is responsible for proliferation of acidophilic bacterial flora necessary to prevent the growth of pathogenic organisms. Most formulas are fortified with iron, minerals, and electrolytes such as calcium, phosphorus, magnesium, sodium, potassium, and chloride. Cow's milk is the source of most minerals and electrolytes, although some are added as inorganic salts.

Milk-based formulas are available for newborns with special needs. Newborns requiring a lower renal solute load, such as those with cardiovascular or renal disease, can use formulas containing low levels of minerals and electrolytes. Newborns with a lactose intolerance or a family history can be given a lactose-free formula in which glucose rather than lactose is the carbohydrate source. Because this formula contains very small amounts of lactose, it should not be given to newborns with galactosemia. There are also milk-based formulas in which the fat content has been lowered for newborns with fat malabsorption, bile duct obstruction, or severe cholestasis. Newborns who cannot digest protein (eg, cystic fibrosis, short gut syndrome, biliary atresia, cholestasis, and protracted diarrhea) or are severely allergic to cow's milk protein can receive formula in which the protein has been treated with heat and enzymes, decreasing the potential allergic response.

Soy Formulas

Soy formulas are used for newborns allergic to cow's milk proteins and by vegetarians. Although the major source of protein is soy, it is possible for a newborn allergic to cow's milk protein to also demonstrate an allergic reaction to soy protein. Soy formulas are also free of lactose and are recommended for newborns with lactase deficiency or galactosemia. The carbohydrate source in these formulas is sucrose.

Mechanics of Formula Feeding

The perinatal nurse should ensure that parents who choose to use commercially prepared formula have sufficient information and are doing so safely. Display 16–10 contains instructions for parents who choose to feed their newborns with formula. The primary healthcare provider can recommend the most appropriate formula. Formula is available as ready-to-feed, concentrated preparation to be diluted with water or as a powder to be mixed with water. Powdered mixes are more economical than ready-to-feed solutions, although it has been suggested that mixing water into the feeding may not always be done properly. In one trial, fewer than one half of the mothers mixed the feeding

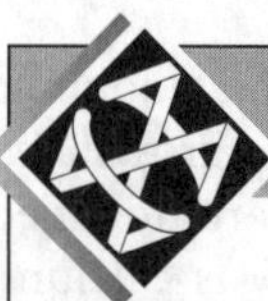

DISPLAY 16–10

Guidelines for Parents Using Formula

- Purchase cans that are not damaged. Check the expiration date, and wash the top of the can before opening.
- Wash bottles and artificial nipples in hot, soapy water or a dishwasher. Scrub bottles and nipples with a brush to loosen formula residue that adheres to crevices where bacteria may grow.
- Do not prop bottles or use products that hold a bottle in the newborn's mouth. This practice may contribute to ear infections, dental caries, choking, and aspiration.
- Newborns should be held during feedings.
- Formula does not need to be heated. It can be prepared and used at room temperature.
- Heating formula in a microwave oven can be dangerous and should be done very carefully. The microwave does not heat evenly, causing "hot spots" in the milk. The bottle should be shaken gently after heating so the temperature of the milk is evenly dispersed, and the temperature of the milk should be tested by sprinkling a few drops on the wrist.
- Once a can of formula has been opened or a bottle of powder formula mixed, it should be stored in the refrigerator and used within 48 hours.
- Formula remaining in a bottle after the newborn has drunk from it should be discarded, because it is an excellent medium for bacterial growth.

correctly, and 26% offered overly concentrated feedings, with the potential for serious consequence such as diarrhea (Lucas, Lockton, & Davies, 1992). Oral water intoxication can be the outcome of mixing too much water with the formula to stretch its availability or of offering water bottles to extend feeding times or to calm a fussy baby. These babies may present to the emergency room with seizures and apnea (Keating, Schears, & Dodge, 1991).

Standard commercially prepared formula contains 20 kcal/ounce and can be offered to newborns on demand. During the first 3 months of life, intake is approximately 150 to 200 mL/kg each day (AAP, 1998). This provides 100 to 135 kcal/kg per day. Weight gain should be approximately 25 to 30 g/day. Additional water is not necessary in the diet of a newborn.

Parents can begin feeding 0.5 ounce of formula at each feeding during the first 24 hours of life. During the next 24 hours, the feedings can be increased by 0.5-ounce increments, feeding the same volume for two to three feedings before increasing. Parents should not force the baby to finish the bottle and should feed on cue when the baby shows signs of hunger. The newborn should be burped after every 0.5 ounces or half-way through the feeding. The baby should be held at about a 45-degree angle, making sure to keep the nipple full of formula. After a can of formula has been opened, the contents should be stored in the refrigerator and used within 48 hours. Any formula remaining in the feeding bottle should be discarded, because it is an excellent medium for bacterial growth.

There is increasing evidence that feeding position may be responsible for increased incidence of otitis media in bottle-fed newborns (Tully, 1998). Supine feeding, positioning the newborn in a horizontal position, or propping the bottle for feeding has been associated with reflux of milk into the eustachian tubes. Researchers have identified a significant difference in the number of abnormal postfeeding tympanogram results when infants were fed in the supine position compared with those fed in the semi-upright position (Tully, Bar-Haim, & Bradley, 1995). Information such as this should be shared with parents choosing to bottle feed along with the following recommendations (Tully, 1998):

- Sit in a comfortable arm chair while feeding to reduce arm fatigue.
- Rest the newborn's head in the crook of the elbow, with his head facing the nipple (a position similar to the breast-feeding newborn).
- Avoid putting the newborn to bed with a bottle.
- Do not prop bottles.
- Keep the newborn upright after feeding for about 15 minutes before placing him in a supine position to sleep.

The perception of formula intolerance by parents and healthcare providers is usually related to symptoms of constipation, fussiness, abdominal cramps, and excessive spit-up or vomiting (Lloyd et al., 1999). In one study, the concentration of palm oil was reported to be responsible for perception of constipation. Using two different formulas to wean newborns from breast milk, the group receiving the formula containing palm oil had a decreased total number of stools, and they were firmer (Lloyd et al., 1999). Specific formula also influences the color of stools, making them more yellow and green, unlike breast-milk stools, which are usually brown.

LACTATION SUPPRESSION

In postpartum women who are not breast-feeding, milk leakage and breast pain begin 1 to 3 days postpartum, and engorgement begins between 1 to 4 days postpartum. Considerable pain may be experienced during this time. Various interventions have been suggested for many years to decrease milk leakage and pain associated with lactation suppression, but no interventions are supported by randomized, controlled clinical research. However, several interventions may make women more comfortable during this period:

- A well-fitting bra or sport bra worn 24 hours each day until the breasts are soft and nontender
- Cold packs applied to the breasts
- Mild over-the-counter analgesics taken according to manufacturers' recommendations
- Avoiding nipple or breast stimulation (although in extreme situations putting the baby to breast, hand expressing, or pumping a small amount of milk may provide relief)

Restricting fluids is neither necessary nor desirable. The breasts return to normal and tenderness decreases with 48 to 72 hours after engorgement occurs.

SUMMARY

The abundance of research on breast-feeding and human lactation clearly shows the importance of breast-feeding, the side effects of newborn formula use, and the evidence that many traditional newborn feeding practices have no scientific or physiologic validity. Parents and health professionals should be aware of this information. Healthcare professionals have an obligation to support changes in practice that have been shown to remove institutional barriers to breast-feeding. Clinical nurse specialists, educators, nurse managers, lactation consultants, hospital administrators, and physicians can take steps to see that breast-feeding is supported in their institution.

The Association of Women's Health, Obstetric and Neonatal Nurses (1999) supports breast-feeding as the optimal method of feeding and challenges its membership to foster environments that support breast-feeding. Display 16–11 identifies the responsibilities of nurses who care for women and newborns in the prenatal and postpartum periods. Many hospitals have chosen to model their policies and protocols after the Ten Steps to Successful Breast-feeding (Display 16–12) (Saadeh & Akre, 1996). This set of recommendations can facilitate successful breast-feeding by all women. In 1998, there were 17 hospitals and birthing centers in the United States and one in Canada that were designated "baby-friendly hospitals" (Davis, Okuboye, & Ferguson, 2000).

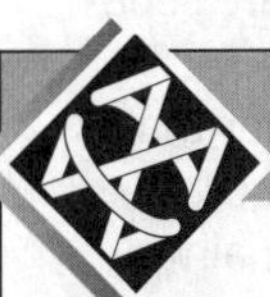

DISPLAY 16–11

Role of the Nurse in the Promotion of Breast-feeding

Attain knowledge about the benefits of breast-feeding. This should include anatomy and physiology of lactation, initiation of lactation, and management of common concerns and problems.

As part of preconception counseling, review the benefits of breast-feeding.

Provide breast-feeding education to all women during the prenatal period. This education should explore concerns, fears, and myths that may inhibit successful breast-feeding.

Work in collaboration with lactation specialists and other health care providers to optimize the breast-feeding experience for the mother and infant.

Integrate culturally appropriate and sensitive information into all breast-feeding education.

Ensure that breast-feeding is initiated in the immediate postpartum period whenever possible.

Promote nonseparation of mother and baby during the postpartum period.

Provide information about breast-feeding resources in the community at the time of hospital or birthing center discharge.

Use and conduct research related to breast-feeding.

From Association of Women's Health, Obstetric and Neonatal Nursing. (1999). *The role of the nurse in the promotion of breastfeeding.* Washington, DC: Author.

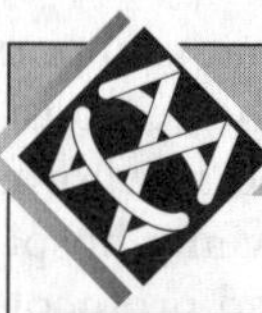

DISPLAY 16–12

Ten Steps to Successful Breast-feeding

1. Have a written breast-feeding policy that is routinely communicated to all healthcare staff.
2. Educate healthcare providers in skills necessary to implement this policy.
3. Inform all pregnant women about the benefits and management of breast-feeding.
4. Help mothers initiate breast-feeding within one-half hour of birth.
5. Show mothers how to breast-feed and how to maintain lactation even when they are separated from their newborns.
6. Give newborns no food or drink other than breast milk, unless medically indicated.
7. Allow mothers and newborns to remain together 24 hours each day.
8. Encourage breast-feeding on demand.
9. Give no artificial teats or pacifiers to breast-feeding newborns.
10. Foster the establishment of breast-feeding support groups, and refer mothers to them on discharge from the hospital or clinic.

From WHO/UNICEF Joint Statement. (1989). *Protecting and supporting breastfeeding: The special role of maternity services.* Geneva: World Health Organization.

The AAP (1998) recommends the introduction of solid foods for all infants between 4 and 6 months of age. Breast milk and formula should continue until the infant reaches 1 year of age. Ideally, the decision about the feeding method is a health decision. This choice has a significant effect on the health and development of the newborn, health of the mother, and cost of illness to the healthcare system. Breast-feeding saves millions of dollars each year by preventing disease. The perinatal nurse's interactions with families should reflect promotion, protection, and support of breast-feeding as the normal and natural way to feed a newborn.

REFERENCES

Aarts, C., Hornell, A., Kylberg, E., Hofvander, Y., & Gebre-Medhin, M. (1999). Breastfeeding patterns in relation to thumb sucking and pacifier use. *Pediatrics, 104*(4), E50.

Alexander, J. M., Grant, A. M., & Campbell, M. J. (1992). Randomized controlled trial of exercises for inverted and non-protractile nipples. *British Medical Journal, 304*(6833), 1030–1032.

Almroth, S., G. (1978). Water requirements of breastfed infants in a hot climate. *American Journal of Clinical Nutrition, 31*(7), 1154–1157.

American Academy of Pediatric Committee on Nutrition. (1998). *Pediatric nutrition handbook* (4th ed.). Elk Grove Village, IL: Author.

American Academy of Pediatrics Workgroup on Breastfeeding. (1997). Breastfeeding and the use of human milk. *Pediatrics, 100*(6), 1035–1039.

American College of Obstetricians and Gynecologists. (2000). *Breastfeeding: Maternal and infant aspects.* Washington, DC: Author.

Anderson, J. W., Johnstone, B. M., & Remley, D. T. (1999). Breastfeeding and cognitive development: A meta-analysis. *American Journal of Clinical Nutrition, 70*(4), 525–535.

Arthur, P. G., Kent, J. C., & Hartmann, P. E. (1994). Metabolites of lactose synthesis in milk from diabetic and non-diabetic women during Lactogenesis II. *Journal of Pediatric Gastroenterology and Nutrition, 19*(1), 100–108.

Association of Women's Health Obstetric and Neonatal Nursing. (1999). *The role of the nurse in the promotion of breastfeeding.* Washington, DC: Author.

Ball, T. M., & Wright, A. L. (1999). Health care costs of formula-feeding in the first year of life. *Pediatrics, 103*(4, Pt. 2), 870–876.

Balcazar, H., Trier, C. M., & Cobas, J. A. (1995). What predicts breastfeeding intention in Mexican-American and non-Hispanic white women: Evidence from a national survey. *Birth, 22*(2), 74–80.

Biancuzzo, M. (2000). Not enough milk: Reasons, rationale and remedies. Advance for Nurse Practitioners [On-line]. Available: www.advanceforNP.com.

Bliss, M. C., Wilkie, J., Acredolo, C., Berman, S., & Tebb, K. P. (1997). The effect of discharge pack formula and breast pumps on breastfeeding duration and choice of infant feeding method. *Birth, 24*(2), 90–97.

Bentley, M, E., Caulfield, L. E., Gross, S. M., Bronner, Y., Jensen, J., Kessler, L. A., & Paige, D. M. (1999). Sources of influence on intention to breastfeed among African-American women at entry to WIC. *Journal of Human Lactation, 15*(1), 27–34.

Brent, N., Rudy, S. J., Redd, B., Rudy, T. E., & Roth, L. A. (1998). Sore nipples in breastfeeding women: A clinical trial of wound dressings vs conventional care. *Archives in Pediatric Adolescent Medicine, 152*(11), 1077–1082.

Buchko, B. L., Pugh, L. C., Bishop, B. A., Chochran, J. F., Smith, L. R., & Lerew, D. J. (1994). Comfort measures in breastfeeding, primiparous women. *Journal of Obstetric Gynecologic and Neonatal Nursing, 23*(1), 46–52.

Centuori, S., Burmaz, T., Ronfani, L., Franiacomo, M., Quintero, S., Pavan, C., Davanzo, R., & Cattaneo, A. (1999). Nipple care, sore nipples, and breastfeeding: A randomized trial. *Journal of Human Lactation, 15*(2), 125–130.

Chezem, J., Friesen, C., Montgomery, P., Fortman, T., & Clark, H. (1998). Lactation duration: Influences of human milk replacements and formula samples on women planning postpartum employment. *Journal of Obstetric, Gynecologic, and Neonatal Nursing, 27*(6), 646–651.

Cox, D. B., Kent, J. C., Casey, T. M., Owens, R. A., & Hartmann, P. E. (1999). Breast growth and the urinary excretion of lactose during human pregnancy and early lactation: Endocrine relationships. *Experimental Physiology, 84*(2), 421–434.

Cox, D. B., Owens, R. A., & Hartmann, P. E. (1996). Blood and milk prolactin and the rate of milk synthesis in women. *Experimental Physiology, 81*(6), 1007–1020.

Cregan, M. D., & Hartmann, P. E. (1999). Computerized breast measurement from conception to weaning: Clinical implications. *Journal of Human Lactation, 15*(2), 89–96.

Crowell, M. K., Hill, P. D., & Humenick, S. S. (1994). Relationship between obstetric analgesia and time of effective breastfeeding. *Journal of Nurse-Midwifery, 39*(3), 150–155.

Daly, S. E. J., Owens, R. A., & Hartmann, P. E. (1993). The short-term synthesis and infant-regulated removal of milk in lactating women. *Experimental Physiology, 78*(2), 209–220.

Daly, S. E. J., Kent, J. C., Owens, R. A., & Hartmann, P. E. (1996). Frequency and degree of milk removal and the short-term control of human milk synthesis. *Experimental Physiology, 81*(5), 861–875.

Davis, L. J., Okuboye, S., & Ferguson, S. L. (2000). Healthy People 2010: Examining a decade of maternal and infant health. *AWHONN Lifelines, 4*(3), 26–33.

Dixit, R., & Gartner, L. M. (1999). The jaundiced newborn: Minimizing the risks. *Contemporary Pediatrics, 16*(4), 166–183.

Dungy, C. I., Losch, M. E., Russell, D., Romitti, P., & Dusdieker, L. B. (1997). Hospital infant formula discharge packages: Do they affect the duration of breastfeeding? *Archives in Pediatric Adolescent Medicine, 151*(7), 724–729.

Dykes, F., & Williams, C. (1999). Falling by the wayside: A phenomenological exploration of perceived breast milk inadequacy in lactating women. *Midwifery, 15*(4), 232–246.

Eidelman, A., Hoffman, N., & Kaitz, M. (1993). Cognitive deficits in women after childbirth. *Obstetrics and Gynecology, 81*(5, Pt. 1), 764–767.

Gartner, L. M. (1994). Neonatal jaundice. *Pediatric Review, 15*(11), 422–432.

Greene, L. C., Lucas, A., Livingstone, M. B., Harland, P. S., & Baker, B. A. (1995). Relationship between early diet and subsequent cognitive performance during adolescence. *Biochemical Society Transactions, 23*(2), 376S.

Guthrie, R. A., & Auerbach, K. G. (1999). Jaundice and the breastfeeding baby. In J. Riordan & K. G. Auerbach (Eds.), *Breastfeeding and human lactation* (2nd ed., pp. 375–391). Boston: Jones & Bartlett.

Hale, T. W. (1999). *Clinical therapy in breastfeeding patients.* Amarillo, TX: Pharmasoft Medical Publishing.

Hartley, B. M., & O'Connor, M. E. (1996). Evaluation of the "Best Start" Breast-feeding Education Program. *Archives of Pediatric and Adolescent Medicine, 150*(8), 868–871.

Hoover, K. (1999). Breast pain during lactation that resolved with fluconazole: Two case studies. *Journal of Human Lactation, 15*(2), 98–99.

Horwood, L. J., & Fergusson, D. M. (1998). Breastfeeding and later cognitive and academic outcomes. *Pediatrics, 101*(1), E9.

Howard, C. R., Howard, F. M., Lanphear, B., deBlieck, E. A., Eberly, S., & Lawrence, R. A. (1999). The effects of early pacifier use on breastfeeding duration. *Pediatrics, 103*(3), E33.

Humenick, S. S., Hill, P. D., & Hart, A. M. (1998). Evaluation of a pillow designed to promote breastfeeding. *The Journal of Perinatal Education, 7*(3), 25–31.

Humphreys, A. M., Thompson, N. J., & Miner, K. R. (1998). Intention to breastfeed in low-income pregnant women: The role of social support and previous experience. *Birth, 25*(3), 169–174.

Insel, T. R. (1997). A neurobiological basis of social attachment. *American Journal of Psychiatry, 154*(6), 726–735.

Jensen, D., Wallace, S., & Kelsay, P. (1994). LATCH: A breastfeeding charting system and documentation tool. *Journal of Obstetric, Gynecologic and Neonatal Nursing, 23*(1), 27–32.

Keating, J. P., Schears, G. J., & Dodge, P. R. (1991). Oral water intoxication in infants. *American Journal of Diseases in Children, 145*(9), 985–990.

Kistin, N., Abramson, R., & Dubin, P. (1994). Effect of peer counselors on breastfeeding initiation, exclusivity, and duration among low-income urban women. *Journal of Human Lactation, 10*(1), 11–15.

Kuhr, M., & Paneth, N. (1982). Feeding practices and early neonatal jaundice. *Journal of Pediatric Gastroenterology and Nutrition, 1*(4), 485–488.

Lawrence, R. A., & Lawrence, R. M. (1999). Breastfeeding: A guide for the medical profession (5th ed., pp. 255–258). St. Louis: Mosby.

Littman, H., Mendendorp, S. V., & Goldfarb, J. (1994). The decision to breastfeed: The importance of father's approval. *Clinical Pediatrics, 33*(4), 214–219.

Lloyd, B., Halter, R. J., Kuchan, M. J., Baggs, G. E., Ryan, A. S., & Masor, M. L. (1999). Formula tolerance in post breastfed and exclusively formula-fed infants. *Pediatrics, 103*(1), E7.

Lucas, A., & Cole, T. J. (1990). Breast milk and neonatal necrotizing enterocolitis. *Lancet, 336*(8730), 1519–1523.

Lucas, A., Lockton, S., & Davies, P. S. (1992). Randomized trial of a ready-to-feed compared with powdered formula. *Archives of Diseases of Children, 67*(7), 935–939.

Matthews, M. K. (1989). The relationship between maternal labor analgesia and delay in the initiation of breastfeeding in healthy neonates in the early neonatal period. *Midwifery, 5*(1), 3–10.

Mayer, E. J., Hamman, R. F., Gay, E., C., Lezotte, D. C., & Klingensmith, G. J. (1988). Reduced risk of IDDM among breastfed children. The Colorado IDDM Registry. *Diabetes, 37*(12), 1625–1632.

Neifert, M. R. (1999). Clinical aspects of lactation. Promoting breastfeeding. *Clinical Perinatology, 26*(2), 281–306.

Neifert, M. R., McDonough, S. L., & Neville, M. C. (1981). Failure of lactogenesis associated with placental retention. *American Journal of Obstetrics and Gynecology, 140*(4), 477–478.

Nelson, E. E., & Panksepp, J. (1998). Brain substrates of infant–mother attachment: Contributions of opioids, oxytocin, and norepinephrine. *Neuroscience and Biobehavioral Reviews, 22*(3), 437–452.

Neubauer, S. H., Ferris, A. M., Chase, C. G., Fanellim, J., Thompson, C. A., Lammi-Keefe, C. J., Clark, R. M., Jensen, R. G., Bendel, R. B., & Green, K. W. (1993). Delayed lactogenesis in women with insulin-dependent diabetes mellitus. *American Journal of Clinical Nutrition, 58*(1), 54–60.

O'Campo, P., Faden, R. R., Gielen, A. C., & Wang, M. C. (1992). Prenatal factors associated with breastfeeding duration: Recommendations for prenatal interventions. *Birth, 19*(4), 195–201.

Oddy, W. H., Holt, P. G., Sly, P. D., Read, A. W., Landau, L. I., Stanley, F. J., Kendall, G. E., & Burton, P. R. (1999). Association between breastfeeding and asthma in 6 year old children: Findings of a prospective birth cohort study. *British Medical Journal, 319*(7213), 815–819.

Patton, C. B., Beaman, M., Csar, N., & Lewinski, C. (1996). Nurses' attitudes and behaviors that promote breastfeeding. *Journal of Human Lactation, 12*(2), 111–115.

Piper, S., & Parks, P. L. (1996). Predicting the duration of lactation: Evidence from a national survey. *Birth, 23*(1), 7–12.

Pugh, L. C., Buchko, B. L., Bishop, B. A., Cochran, J. F., Smith, L. R., & Lerew, D. J. (1996). A comparison of topical agents to relieve nipple pain and enhance breastfeeding. *Birth, 23*(2), 88–93.

Renfrew, M. J., Lang, S., Martin, L., & Woolridge, M. W. (2000). Feeding schedules in hospitals for newborn infants. *Cochrane Database Systematic Review,* 2, CD000090.

Righard, L. (1998). Are breastfeeding problems related to incorrect breastfeeding technique and the use of pacifiers and bottles? *Birth, 25*(1), 40–44.

Righard, L., & Alade, M.. O. (1992). Sucking technique and its effects on success of breastfeeding. *Birth, 19*(4), 185–189.

Righard, L., & Alade, M. O. (1997). Breastfeeding and the use of pacifiers. *Birth, 24*(2), 116–120.

Riordan, J. (1999). The biological specificity of breastmilk. In J. Riordan & K. G. Auerbach (Eds.), *Breastfeeding and human lactation* (2nd ed., pp. 121–161). Boston: Jones & Bartlett.

Riordan, J. M., & Koehn, M. (1997). Reliability and validity testing of three breastfeeding assessment tools. *Journal of Obstetric Gynecologic and Neonatal Nursing, 26*(2), 181–187.

Ross Products Division. (1998). *Ross mother's survey.* Columbus, OH: Abbott Laboratories.

Saadeh, R., & Akre, J. (1996). Ten steps to successful breastfeeding: A summary of the rationale and scientific evidence. *Birth, 23*(3), 154–160.

Scariati, P. D., Grummer-Strawn, L. M., & Fein, S. B. (1997). A longitudinal analysis of infant morbidity and the extent of breastfeeding in the United States. *Pediatrics, 99*(6), E5.

Schafer, E., Vogel, M. K., Viegas, S., & Hausafus, C. (1998). Volunteer peer counselors increase breastfeeding duration among rural low-income women. *Birth, 25*(2), 101–106.

Sciacca, J. P., Dube, D. A., Phipps, B. L., & Ratliff, M. I. (1995). A breast feeding education and promotion program: Effects on knowledge, attitudes, and support for breast feeding. *Journal of Community Health, 20*(4), 473–490.

Specker, B. L., Valanis, B., Hertzberg, V., Edwards, N., & Tsang, R. C. (1985). Sunshine exposure and serum 25-hydroxyvitamin D concentrations in exclusively breastfed infants. *Journal of Pediatrics, 107*(3), 372–276.

Tarkka, A. T., Paunonen, M., & Laippala, P. (1999). Factors related to successful breast feeding by first time mothers when the child is 3 months old. *Journal of Advanced Nursing, 29*(1), 113–118.

Trado, M. G., & Hughes, R. B. (1996). A phenomenological study of breastfeeding WIC recipients in South Carolina. *Advanced Practice Nursing Quarterly, 2*(3), 31–41.

Tully, S. (1998). The right angle: Otitis media and infant feeding position. Advance for Nurse Practitioners [On-line]. Available: www.advanceforNP.com.

Tully, S. B., Bar-Haim, Y., & Bradley, R. L. (1995). Abnormal tympanography after supine bottle feeding. *Journal of Pediatrics, 126,* 105–111.

United States Department of Health and Human Services. (2000). *Healthy People 2010* (conference edition in two volumes). Washington, DC: Author.

Uvnas-Moberg, K. (1997). Physiological and endocrine effects of social contact. *Annals of the New York Academy of Sciences, 807*(1), 146–163.

Vaarala, O., Knip, M., Paronen, J., Hamalainen, A. M., Muona, P., Vaatainen, M., Ilonen, J., Simell, O., & Akerblom, H. K. (1999). Cow's milk formula feeding induces primary immunization to insulin in infants at genetic risk for type I diabetes. *Diabetes, 48*(7), 1389–1394.

Van den Driessche, M., Peeters, K., Marien, P., Ghoos, Y., Devlieger, H., & Veereman-Wauters, G., (1999). Gastric emptying in formula-fed and breast-fed infants measured with the C-octanoic acid breath test. *Journal of Pediatric Gastroenterology and Nutrition, 29*(1), 46–51.

Victora, C. G., Behague, D. P., Barros, F. C., Olinto, M. T., & Weiderpass, E. (1997). Pacifier use and short breastfeeding duration: Cause, consequence, or coincidence? *Pediatrics, 99*(3), 445–453.

Vio, F., Salazar, G., & Infante, C. (1991). Smoking during pregnancy and lactation: Its effects on breast milk volume. *American Journal of Clinical Nutrition, 54*(6), 1011–1016.

von Kries, R., Koletzko, B., Sauerwald, T., von Mutius, E., Barnert, D., Grunert, V., & von, Voss, H. (1999). Breast feeding and obesity: Cross sectional study. *British Medical Journal, 319*(7203), 147–150.

Walker, M. (1999). Epidurals and breastfeeding. *Birth, 26*(4), 275–276.

Wilde, C. J., Addey, C. V., Boddy, L. M., & Peaker, M. (1995). Autocrine regulation of milk secretion by a protein in milk. *Biochemical Journal, 305*(Pt. 1), 51–58.

Widstrom, A. M., Ransjo-Arvidsson, A. B., Christensson, K., Matthiesen, A. S., Winberg, J., & Uvnas-Moberg, K. (1987). Gastric suction in healthy newborn infants: Effects on circulation and developing feeding behavior. *Acta Paediatrica Scandinavica, 76*(4), 566–572.

WHO/UNICEF Joint Statement. (1989). *Protecting and supporting breastfeeding: The special role of maternity services.* Geneva: World Health Organization.

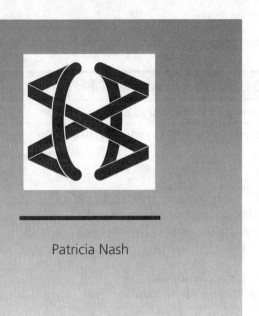

Patricia Nash

CHAPTER 17

Common Neonatal Complications

Most newborns with complications are identified and cared for in community hospitals or level II perinatal centers. Perinatal nurses must have a thorough understanding of pathophysiology and clinical signs of illness during the immediate newborn period. The length of stay limits the time to identify behavioral cues or subtle changes that could potentially compromise newborn well-being.

Common complications discussed in this chapter include respiratory distress, congenital heart lesions, hyperbilirubinemia, hypoglycemia, and sepsis. Neonatal abstinence syndrome is also included because of continuing data about chemical dependency among women during the childbearing years. The chapter concludes with a discussion of neonatal transport because, in some cases, the severity of the disease process necessitates transfer to a tertiary-care center.

RESPIRATORY DISTRESS

Respiratory distress is a major cause of neonatal morbidity and mortality despite significant technologic and pharmacologic advances during the past 30 years. Respiratory distress probably is the most common neonatal complication seen by the perinatal nurse and is a principal indication for neonatal transfer to tertiary-care units. Table 17–1 lists the perinatal events and associated respiratory diseases. The pathophysiology or causative factors of respiratory distress varies, but the result is decreased ability to exchange the oxygen and carbon dioxide necessary to ensure perfusion of well-oxygenated blood to vital organs and to remove metabolic waste products. Respiratory distress may be caused by obstruction or malformation, can develop as a consequence of acute lung injury, reflects prolonged transition to extrauterine life, and may occur in the presence of other medical or systemic problems. Five of the most common respiratory diseases occurring during the neonatal period are respiratory distress syndrome (RDS), meconium aspiration syndrome (MAS), pneumonia, transient tachypnea of the newborn (TTN), and persistent pulmonary hypertension of the newborn (PPHN).

Respiratory Distress Syndrome

RDS primarily occurs in preterm newborns. The incidence varies inversely with advancing gestational age. In the United States, 20,000 to 30,000 newborns each year develop RDS (Whitsett, Pryhuber, Rice, Warner, & Wert, 1999). The mortality rate for RDS is 32 deaths per 100,000 live births (March of Dimes, 1999). RDS is caused by insufficient amounts of surfactant or delayed or impaired surfactant synthesis. Surfactant decreases surface tension in the alveoli and functions as a stabilizer to prevent deflation during expiration. Without surfactant, atelectasis (ie, alveolar collapse) occurs, resulting in a series of events that progressively increase disease severity. These events include hypoxemia, hypercapnea, acidosis, pulmonary vasoconstriction, alveolar endothelial and epithelial damage, and subsequent protein-rich interstitial and alveolar edema. This cascade of events further decreases surfactant synthesis, storage, and release and worsens respiratory distress.

Meconium Aspiration Syndrome

Passage of meconium in utero is primarily seen in term or postterm gestations, is associated with chronic

TABLE 17–1 ■ CLINICAL CORRELATES OF PERINATAL HISTORY

History	Associated Respiratory Disease
Premature Birth	Respiratory distress syndrome (RDS)
Maternal diabetes	
Maternal hemorrhage	
Perinatal asphyxia	
Multiple gestation	RDS more common in second twin
Postmature Birth	Meconium aspiration syndrome
Nonreassuring fetal heart rate pattern	Persistent pulmonary hypertension
Meconium-stained amniotic fluid	
Perinatal asphyxia	
Oligohydramnios	Pulmonary hypoplasia
Polyhydramnios	Tracheoesophageal fistula with esophageal atresia
Choking on feedings	
Drooling	
Cesarean birth	Transient tachypnea
Prolonged rupture of fetal membranes	Pneumonia or sepsis
Maternal fever	
Traumatic delivery	Poor respiratory effort
Narcotics in labor	Poor respiratory effort

Adapted from Kenner, C., Brueggemeyer, A., & Gunderson, L.P. (1997). *Comprehensive Neonatal Nursing*. Philadelphia: W.B. Saunders.

or acute hypoxic events, and occurs in newborns younger than 36 weeks' gestation (Casey, 1999). Under normal intrauterine conditions, amniotic fluid does not enter the fetal lung. However, when the fetus experiences hypoxemia, gasping may result in aspiration of meconium-stained amniotic fluid. Approximately 13% of newborns are exposed to amniotic fluid stained by meconium; of these, 5% to 12% develop MAS (Wiswell et al., 2000). Passage of meconium in utero occurs as a physiologic maturational event, response to acute hypoxic events, and response to chronic intrauterine hypoxia (Klingner & Kruse, 1999). The amount and thickness of the meconium appear to directly affect the severity of respiratory distress. Once aspirated, meconium can obstruct large and small airways. Obstruction of the large or upper airways results in an acute hypoxic event postnatally. This may be prevented by suctioning the mouth, nasopharynx, oropharynx, and hypopharynx after the head is delivered and by suctioning the trachea by a laryngoscope immediately after birth. Meconium in the small or lower airways may result in obstruction of these airways or in an inflammatory response in the lung tissue. In the presence of meconium-stained fluid, suctioning on the perineum and intubation and suctioning the newborn immediately after birth may not prevent aspiration and aspiration pneumonia. Pneumonitis is an inflammatory response probably resulting from bile salts. Pneumonitis results in acute lung injury with protein-rich interstitial and alveolar edema. When meconium only partially obstructs the airway, a ball-valve effect results. Air enters the lower airways on inspiration but cannot escape on expiration. This causes overdistention of alveoli, leading to alveolar rupture and pulmonary air leaks. Pneumonitis and airway obstruction result in hypoxemia and acidosis, which cause increased pulmonary vascular resistance and subsequent PPHN (Casey, 1999). Figure 17–1 shows the pathogenesis of MAS.

Pneumonia

Pneumonia is acquired through vertical or horizontal transmission. Vertical transmission occurs in utero from the rupture of membranes for more than 24 hours, chorioamnionitis, intraamniotic infection, transplacental transmission of organisms, or aspiration of infected amniotic fluid or meconium. Horizontal transmission occurs in the nursery as pathogenic organisms are spread from hospital personnel, equipment, and parents. Horizontal transmission also includes secondary infections as a result of some other primary infection. Display 17–1 lists organisms that may cause pneumonia in the newborn. Pneumonia, like MAS, causes an inflammatory process, disrupting the normal barrier function of the pulmonary endothelium and epithelium, leading to abnormal protein permeability and edema of lung tissue.

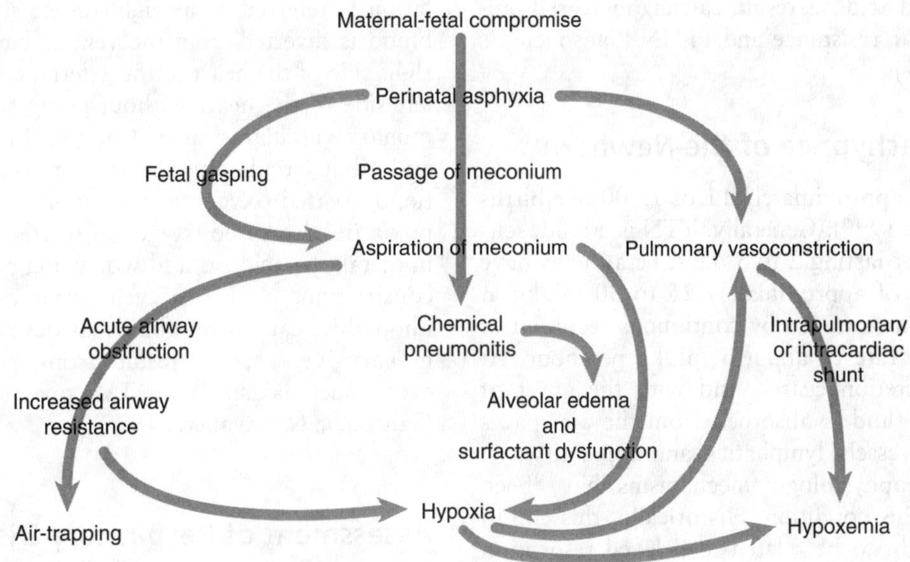

FIGURE 17–1. Pathogenesis of meconium aspiration syndrome.

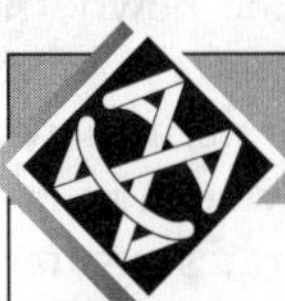

DISPLAY 17-1

Common Organisms Associated with Neonatal Pneumonia

TRANSPLACENTAL

Rubella
Cytomegalovirus
Herpes simplex virus
Adenovirus
Mumps virus
Toxoplasma gondii
Listeria monocytogenes
Mycobacterium tuberculosis
Treponema pallidum

AMNIOTIC FLUID

Cytomegalovirus
Herpes simplex virus
Enteroviruses
Genital mycoplasma
L. monocytogenes
Chlamydia trachomatis
M. tuberculosis
Group B Streptococcus (GBS)
Escherichia coli
Haemophilus influenzae (nontypeable)

AT DELIVERY

GBS
E. coli
Staphylococcus aureus
Klebsiella sp.
Other streptococci
H. influenzae (nontypeable)
Candida sp.
C. trachomatis

NOSOCOMIAL

S. aureus
Staphylococcus epidermidis
GBS
Klebsiella sp.
Enterobacter
Pseudomonas
Influenza viruses
Respiratory syncytial virus
Enteroviruses

From Hansen, T. N., Cooper, T. R., & Weisman, L. E. (Eds.). (1998). *Contemporary diagnosis and management of neonatal respiratory diseases* (2nd ed., p. 131). Newton, PA: Handbooks in Health Care.

Hypoxemia and acidosis result, causing increased pulmonary vascular resistance and PPHN (Sansoucie & Cavaliere, 1997).

Transient Tachypnea of the Newborn

TTN occurs in approximately 11 of 1,000 live births (Whitsett et al., 1999). Generally, TTN is a mild, self-limiting disorder lasting 2 to 5 days. Fetal lungs have a fluid volume of approximately 25 to 30 mL/kg at term, which is maintained by continuous secretion of lung fluid at a rate of about 5 mL/kg per hour. At birth, fluid secretion ceases, and with the onset of breathing, this fluid is absorbed from the air spaces through blood vessels, lymphatics, and upper airways.

Several pathophysiologic mechanisms have been suggested for this condition. Historically, this condition was thought to be related to delayed resorption of lung fluid by the pulmonary lymphatic system. Retained fluid causes bronchiolar collapse with air trapping or hyperinflation of the alveoli. Hypoxia (ie, decreased concentration of oxygen) results when poorly ventilated alveoli are perfused. Hypercarbia (ie, increased carbon dioxide) is caused by mechanical interference with alveolar ventilation by fluid. Decreased lung compliance results in tachypnea and increased energy needed to do the work of breathing. A second mechanism has to do with the fact that labor causes the active transport of chloride from plasma into the fetal lung fluid to cease. As the concentration of chloride becomes higher in the plasma, fetal lung fluid begins to be resorbed. Two thirds of the fetal lung fluid is absorbed before birth. Newborns without the benefit of labor and those born prematurely do not have the same amount of time to resorb lung fluid as those born after a normal course of labor (Speer & Hansen, 1998). Some authorities suggest that TTN could result from mild immaturity of the surfactant system. This idea is supported by lack of phosphatidylglycerol in amniotic fluid samples from newborns with TTN (Whitsett et al., 1999).

Persistent Pulmonary Hypertension of the Newborn

In fetal circulation, pulmonary blood vessels are constricted, causing most blood flow to bypass the lungs. This is appropriate for the fetus because the placenta rather than the fetal lung acts as the organ of gas exchange. PPHN is the result of a sustained elevation of the pulmonary vascular resistance (PVR) after birth, preventing transition to the normal extrauterine pattern of circulation. When the PVR remains elevated, blood bypasses the lungs by flowing through the foramen ovale or ductus arteriosus. This pattern of circulation is referred to as right-to-left shunting because blood is diverted from the venous circulation on the right side of the heart to the arterial circulation on the left side of the heart without going through the pulmonary vascular system. Chapter 14 compares fetal and adult circulations. Severe, prolonged hypoxemia (ie, decreased oxygen in the blood) progresses to hypoxia (ie, decreased oxygen in the tissues) and results in metabolic acidosis and worsening pulmonary vasoconstriction. A vicious cycle ensues. PPHN may be idiopathic, caused by abnormal development of pulmonary vessels, or result from pathophysiologic events such as asphyxia, MAS, pneumonia, and RDS (Sansoucie & Cavaliere, 1997).

Assessment of Respiratory Distress

Clinical signs of respiratory distress may be present at birth or occur at any time in the early neonatal period. These signs include tachypnea, grunting, retractions, nasal flaring, and cyanosis. Tachypnea is defined as a respiratory rate of more than 60 breaths/min. Tachypnea develops when the newborn attempts to improve ventilation. Because of the very compliant chest wall, especially in the preterm newborn, it is more energy efficient for the newborn to increase the respiratory rate, breathing at rates greater than 100 breaths/min for sustained periods, rather than increase the depth of respiration.

On expiration, a grunting sound is heard in newborns with respiratory distress. Grunting is the result of expired air passing through a partially closed glottis. The glottis closes in an effort to increase intrapulmonary pressure and to keep alveoli open. Keeping alveoli open during expiration is a compensatory response to decreased partial pressure of oxygen (PO_2). It allows more time for the passage of oxygen into the circulatory system. Grunting develops in an attempt to prevent atelectasis and to improve oxygenation and ventilation abnormalities.

Retractions are depressions observed between the ribs, above the sternum, or below the xiphoid process during inhalation. Retractions are the result of a very compliant chest wall and noncompliant lung. Compliance refers to the stiffness or distensibility of the chest wall and lung parenchyma. As the amount of negative intrathoracic pressure increases on inspiration, the rib cage expands until the soft tissue of the thorax and weak intercostal muscles are pulled inward toward the spine. The result is worsening atelectasis with marked oxygenation and ventilation abnormalities.

Nasal flaring occurs with respiratory distress as the newborn attempts to decrease airway resistance and increase the inflow of air. Nasal flaring may be seen immediately after birth, but beyond this period, it is considered abnormal (Askin, 1996).

Cyanosis results from inadequate oxygenation caused by atelectasis, poor lung compliance, and right-to-left shunting. Although the newborn's color is an indication of oxygenation, it is more appropriately monitored by using pulse oximetry or intermittently monitored by arterial or capillary blood gas determinations.

Interventions for Respiratory Distress

Care for newborns with respiratory distress focuses on oxygenation and ventilation, warmth, nourishment, and protection from harm. Adequate oxygenation and ventilation requires supportive mechanisms ranging from supplemental oxygen only to supplemental oxygen with mechanical ventilation. Pulse oximetry, arterial catheterization, and blood gas monitoring are methods for ensuring adequate gas exchange. In a preterm newborn, delivery of oxygen should be sufficient to maintain arterial oxygen tension at 50 to 80 mmHg, which corresponds to a pulse oximetry reading of approximately 90%. Because oxygen may be toxic to some tissue, care should be taken to avoid hypoxia. Hypoxia increases the risk of developing chronic lung disease and retinopathy of prematurity (Hey & Bell, 2000; Verklan, 1997). In a term newborn at risk for PPHN, oxygen delivery should be sufficient to maintain an arterial oxygen tension of more than 100 mmHg, and an oxygen saturation of 99% to 100%. Hypoxia must be avoided in term newborns because it is one of the most powerful stimuli for pulmonary vasoconstriction and the cycle of PPHN (Sansoucie & Cavaliere, 1997).

A neutral thermal environment is crucial in the care of a newborn with respiratory distress. Hypothermia or hyperthermia increase metabolic demands, leading to decreased oxygenation, metabolic acidosis, and worsening respiratory distress (Short, 1998). Newborns with respiratory distress are cared for under a radiant warmer or in an Isolette. Chapter 14 discusses thermoregulation.

Adequate nutrition frequently requires the administration of intravenous fluids during the early neonatal period. Care is taken to prevent hypoglycemia that may occur from respiratory distress and increased metabolic demands.

CONGENITAL HEART DISEASE

The cardiovascular system begins to develop in the third week of gestation and is fully functioning by the end of the eighth week. It is the first major organ system to function in the embryo. This fact may be one of the reasons why congenital heart disease (CHD) is so common, with an incidence of 8 per 1,000 live births (Paul, 1995; Witt, 1997). The cause of CHD cannot be ascribed to any single factor. Most cases are probably multifactorial, involving genetic predisposition and environmental factors. CHD can also be associated with chromosomal abnormalities and maternal–environmental factors, such as drug exposure or infection (Champawat & Torrence, 1996). Cardiac lesions are classified as cyanotic, acyanotic, or according to the hemodynamic characteristics related to pulmonary blood flow (Champawat & Torrence, 1996; Spilman & Furdon, 1998). Five of the most common cardiac lesions presenting in the early neonatal period include ventricular septal defect (VSD), tetralogy of Fallot (TET), patent ductus arteriosus (PDA), atrial septal defect (ASD), and transposition of the great arteries (TGA).

The assessment to exclude CHD includes the following:

- Close observation of cardiorespiratory status
- Palpation of peripheral pulses
- Blood pressures of the four extremities
- Chest radiograph to evaluate heart size and pulmonary vascularity
- Blood gas determinations to evaluate oxygenation and metabolic status
- Evaluation of response to oxygen

The newborn with CHD or persistence of a fetal shunt may present shortly after birth or within the first weeks of life with cyanosis or symptoms of congestive heart failure (CHF) (Paul, 1995). The newborn becomes cyanotic when gas exchange is impaired by pulmonary edema, blood flow to the lungs is restricted as a result of a structural abnormality, or blood flow is shunted away from the lungs (Furdon, 1997). In newborns with normal hemoglobin values, central cyanosis usually indicates an arterial hemoglobin saturation of less than 85% (Furdon, 1997). Several clinical signs indicate CHF:

- Tachypnea
- Respiratory distress
- Tachycardia
- Hepatomegaly
- Poor feeding

A murmur, if present, varies in quality and intensity, depending on the particular cardiac lesion present. Table 17–2 describes chest radiographic findings for each CHD.

If a VSD or ASD is present, allowing mixing of oxygenated and unoxygenated blood, only mild cyanosis

TABLE 17–2 ■ CONGENITAL HEART DEFECTS AND CHEST RADIOGRAPHY

Defect	Findings
Ventricular septal defects	Cardiomegaly and congestion (Wood, 1997)
Tetrology of Fallot	Pulmonary hypoperfusion and a boot-shaped heart (Paul, 1995)
Patent ductus arteriosus	Cardiomegaly and congestion (Wood, 1997)
Atrial septal defect	Cardiomegaly and congestion (Wood, 1997)
Transposition of the great arteries	Heart position described as an egg on a string (Paul, 1995; Witt, 1998)

occurs. If there is no intracardiac shunt, severe cyanosis is observed. With the exception of cyanosis, the physical examination is often otherwise unremarkable. In the newborn with a large VSD or ASD, signs of CHF develop over time as the PVR falls and the pulmonary blood flow increases. In newborns without an intracardiac shunt, severe hypoxemia and metabolic acidosis develop, followed by a rapid demise if emergency measures are not instituted.

Ventricular Septal Defect

Pathophysiology

Separation of the ventricles begins near the middle of the fourth week of gestation and is completed by the end of the seventh week (Witt, 1997). Incomplete division of the right and left ventricles results in a VSD. VSDs are classified by their anatomic location; perimembranous and muscular are the two most common types. A perimembranous VSD is located just below the aortic valve and accounts for 80% of all VSDs. A muscular VSD is located in the muscular septum. Between 75% and 80% of membranous and muscular VSDs close spontaneously. A VSD is considered an acyanotic lesion with increased pulmonary blood flow. The size and location of the defect, as well as the pulmonary-to-systemic vascular resistance ratio determine the degree of left-to-right shunt. The timing of the onset of symptoms is directly related to the normal fall in the PVR after birth (Wood, 1997).

Assessment

The onset of symptoms resulting from a VSD is related to the size of the defect and PVR. A newborn with a small defect may appear well and have few or no symptoms other than a harsh holosystolic murmur. The murmur develops as the PVR falls and is best heard over the left lower sternal border. A newborn with a large defect may present with symptoms of CHF at approximately 2 to 4 weeks of life. As with the smaller defects, the murmur is holosystolic and heard over the left lower sternal border. Preterm newborns with large VSDs present with symptoms sooner.

Tetralogy of Fallot

Pathophysiology

TET consists of a large perimembranous VSD, pulmonary stenosis, and aorta and right ventricle hypertrophy (Spilman & Furdon, 1998). This lesion is a result of disordered embryonic cardiac functioning. TET occurs during the embryonic stage of development, when some unknown factor influences functioning of the heart at the cellular level. This alteration in cellular function is partly responsible for determining development. Any transient change in work can alter cardiac tissue growth or distribution, causing this defect to occur (Witt, 1997). TET is generally considered a cyanotic lesion with decreased pulmonary blood flow, but the hemodynamics vary widely, depending on the severity of pulmonary stenosis, the size of the VSD, and the pulmonary and systemic vascular resistance. Newborns present with varying degrees of cyanosis at birth that worsens over the course of the first year of life (Spilman & Furdon, 1998).

Assessment

TET is the most common cyanotic heart disease seen in the first year of life. Newborns with TET present with cyanosis and symptoms of right-sided heart failure. The timing and degree of cyanosis depend on the severity of the pulmonary stenosis and may not be noticed until closure of the ductus arteriosus. In the case of pulmonary atresia and hypoplasia of the pulmonary arteries, marked cyanosis may be observed immediately after birth. The clinical signs of right-sided heart failure include hepatomegaly, tricuspid valve regurgitation, and a murmur best heard over the left lower sternal border.

Patent Ductus Arteriosus

Pathophysiology

The ductus arteriosus is a normal component of fetal circulation. The ductus arteriosus connects the pulmonary artery to the aorta, allowing blood to bypass the lungs. During fetal life the PVR is greater than the systemic vascular resistance. After birth, with spontaneous respiration, the arterial oxygen level increases, PVR decreases, and the ductus closes. If the ductus arteriosus does not close, blood begins to flow left to right as the PVR decreases. A PDA is an acyanotic lesion with increased pulmonary blood flow. It occurs much more commonly in preterm newborns, with the incidence inversely proportional to gestational age (Wood, 1997).

Assessment

The manifestation of PDA depends on the gestational age and the degree of lung disease. Preterm newborns generally develop signs associated with CHF at 3 to 7 days of life, but it can develop sooner in the smaller preterm newborn treated with surfactant. The development of clinical signs is related to the normal fall in the PVR. The classic murmur detected with a PDA is continuous and best heard over the left upper sternal border, radiating to the back.

Atrial Septal Defect

Pathophysiology

The separation of the atrium begins near the middle of the fourth week of gestation and is completed by the end of the sixth week, leaving the foramen ovale open between the two atria. An abnormality occurring during atrial separation can result in an ASD. An ASD is considered an acyanotic lesion with increased pulmonary blood flow. Approximately 10% of newborns with an ASD develop CHF as the PVR decreases (Wood, 1997).

Assessment

Newborns with an uncomplicated ASD are generally asymptomatic. However, about 10% present with signs of congestive failure, poor feeding, and poor growth. These symptoms develop as the PVR falls over the first few weeks of life. Associated with an ASD is a soft, systolic murmur best heard over the second intercostal space at the left upper sternal border.

Transposition of the Great Arteries

Pathophysiology

The truncus arteriosus begins to divide during the fifth week of gestation. As the cardiac tube folds, the vessel twists on itself and divides into two separate vessels. Transposition occurs because of a failure of the aorticopulmonary septum to grow in a spiral fashion, resulting in inappropriate migration of the vessels (Witt, 1997). The aorta arises from the right ventricle, and the pulmonary artery arises from the left ventricle, resulting in two parallel circulations. When these two arteries are transposed, unoxygenated blood returning from the body enters the right side of the heart and returns to the body, and oxygenated blood returning from the lung enters the left side of the heart and returns to the lungs. TGA is considered a cyanotic lesion with increased pulmonary blood flow. The degree of cyanosis depends on the amount of mixing of oxygenated and unoxygenated blood through the VSD (if present), patent foramen ovale, or PDA (Witt, 1998).

Assessment

The newborn with TGA presents with cyanosis, the degree of which depends on the presence or absence of other defects, such as a VSD or ASD. If a VSD or ASD is present, allowing mixing of oxygenated and unoxygenated blood, only mild cyanosis occurs. If there is no intracardiac shunt, severe cyanosis occurs. With the exception of cyanosis, the physical examination findings are often otherwise unremarkable. With a large VSD or ASD, signs of CHF develop over time as the PVR falls and the pulmonary blood flow increases. In the absence of an intracardiac shunt, severe hypoxemia and metabolic acidosis develop, followed by a rapid demise if emergency measures are not instituted.

Interventions for Congenital Heart Disease

Newborns with known or suspected CHD usually require transfer to a tertiary center for treatment and follow-up. The complete diagnostic workup and subsequent repair or palliative surgery are performed in centers with pediatric cardiac capabilities. Before transport, close observation and supportive care and treatment are warranted. Nursing care for newborns with known or suspected CHD includes the following:

- Cardiorespiratory monitoring
- Pulse oximetry
- Blood work, including blood gas determinations and ongoing assessment of color, perfusion, and degree of distress
- Maintaining a neutral thermal environment
- Intravenous hydration and nutrition
- Oxygen therapy, if appropriate, and mechanical ventilation, if required

Metabolic acidosis is treated with sodium bicarbonate, pulmonary edema with respiratory distress is treated with diuretics, and shock is treated with vasopressors and calcium gluconate. A lesion such as TGA without an intracardiac shunt is treated with prostaglandin E_1 to maintain patency of the ductus arteriosus until surgical correction takes place (Champawat & Torrence, 1997; Paul, 1995; Witt, 1998).

HYPOGLYCEMIA

Establishing the incidence of symptomatic and asymptomatic neonatal hypoglycemia is difficult because of lack of agreement among experts on the definition. One of the major difficulties associated with defining hypoglycemia is the lack of correlation between a given blood glucose level and clinical signs. Whether symptomatic or asymptomatic, hypoglycemia can be life threatening and can result in serious neurologic sequelae, such as brain injury, learning disabilities, and cerebral palsy (Brooks, 1997; Karp, Scardina, & Butler, 1995).

The generally accepted definition of hypoglycemia in the newborn is a blood glucose level less than 40 mg/dL (Ogata, 1999), although this may be changing. There is no evidence that the neonatal brain requires less glucose than that of an adult or is less sensitive to hypoglycemic injury. Some authorities have suggested that blood glucose levels should be maintained above 50 or 60 mg/dL (Schwartz, 1997; Stanley & Baker, 1999).

Pathophysiology

During fetal life, insulin is secreted by the fetal pancreas in response to glucose that readily crosses the placenta. At birth, the newborn's blood glucose level is approximately 70% to 80% that of the mother. After removal of placental circulation, the newborn must maintain glucose homeostasis. This requires initiation of various metabolic processes, including gluconeogenesis (ie, forming glucose from noncarbohydrate sources such as protein and fat) and glycogenolysis (ie, conversion of glycogen stores to glucose), as well as an intact regulatory mechanism and an adequate supply of substrate (Ogata, 1999). The cause of hypoglycemia is overuse of glucose, underproduction of glucose, or a combination of both. Table 17–3 shows clinical situations associated with overuse or underproduction of glucose.

Hypoglycemia develops at various hours of life, depending on cause. Transient symptomatic hypoglycemia usually occurs within the first 24 hours after birth but may not manifest until 72 hours or later. Symptomatic hypoglycemia, secondary to maternal or intrapartum causes, generally occurs during the first 2

TABLE 17–3 ■ ETIOLOGY OF NEONATAL HYPOGLYCEMIA

Condition	Causes
Increased use of glucose, hyperinsulinemia	Infant of a diabetic mother
	Islet cell hyperplasia
	Beckwith-Weidemann syndrome
	Insulin-producing tumors
	Maternal tocolytic therapy
	Hypothermia
	Malpositioned umbilical artery catheter
	Exchange transfusion
	Excessive maternal fluid administration in labor
	Rapid tapering of high glucose infusion
	Macrosomic infant
Decreased production or stores of glucose	Prematurity
	Small for gestational age
	Maternal starvation
Increased use and/or decreased production of glucose	Asphyxia
	Sepsis
	Shock
	Defects in carbohydrate or amino acid metabolism
	Endocrine deficiency
	Polycythemia

hours after birth. Hypoglycemia occurring after the first few hours after birth is most commonly caused by hyperinsulinemia, as in the infant of a diabetic mother (Stanley & Baker, 1999).

Assessment

Identification of those at risk for developing neonatal hypoglycemia facilitates planning and implementation of appropriate nursing care. This process begins with a review of maternal prenatal and intrapartum history for risk factors associated with neonatal hypoglycemia and a careful physical examination. Signs of hypoglycemia are nonspecific and not easily differentiated from many other common neonatal conditions (Display 17–2). Glucose values in normal term newborns fall after birth. Lowest levels are reached at 1 to 1.5 hours of age, after which they begin to rise.

Universal blood glucose screening before clinical signs develop is not recommended by the American Academy of Pediatrics (AAP, 1993). Selective screening of at-risk newborns is more appropriate and does not appear to decrease quality of care or result in adverse outcomes. Display 17–3 describes newborns at high risk for hypoglycemia who may benefit from routine screening.

Newborns at risk should be screened within 30 to 60 minutes after birth. Use of proper screening techniques is one of the most important nursing functions. Testing is performed using a bedside glucose oxidase stick method, such as the Chemstrip or a glucometer, approved by the U.S. Food and Drug Administration for use with newborns. Although glucose oxidase sticks are widely used, results depend on the hematocrit, blood source, and operator's skill (Halamek, Barron, & Stevenson, 1997). They have been shown to have considerable variance from actual blood glucose levels (AAP, 1993) and to lack reproducibility, especially for blood glucose levels less than 50 mg/dL (Halamek et al., 1997). One reason for variance is the source of the blood used for testing. Venous blood samples have blood glucose levels that are approximately 10% less than capillary or arterial specimens (Halamek et al., 1997). Another possible reason for variance and lack of reproducibility is improper storage or outdated shelf-life of test strips, which may result in inaccurate results. A third potential problem is contamination with isopropyl alcohol, which falsely elevates the results. To increase accuracy of blood glucose determination, isopropyl alcohol should be allowed to dry thoroughly before the skin is punctured, and the first drop of blood should be wiped away before a blood drop is placed on the test strip. It has also been recommended that color blindness testing be done on all staff who routinely perform glucose measurements read by eye and compared with a color chart (Brooks, 1997).

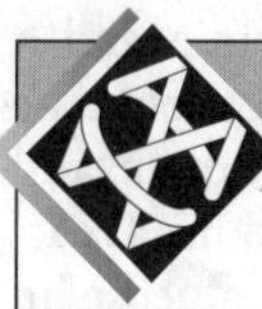

DISPLAY 17–3

Criteria for Routine Screening for Hypoglycemia

- Weight <2,500 g or >4,082 g
- Small for gestational age
- Large for gestational age
- <37 weeks' gestation
- Infants of diabetic mothers

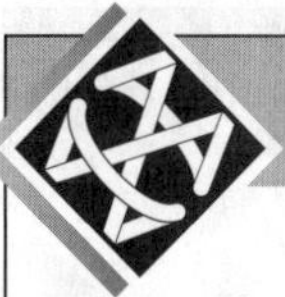

DISPLAY 17–2

Symptoms of Hypoglycemia

- Jitteriness, tremors
- Tachypnea, grunting
- Diaphoresis
- Cyanosis
- Lethargy
- Hypotonia
- Irritability
- Temperature instability
- Apnea
- Seizures, coma

Interventions

Newborns with asymptomatic hypoglycemia should be fed immediately and then retested. If results continue to be low (<40 mg/dL), they should be corroborated by laboratory determination and intravenous therapy started. The timing of laboratory measurements may also result in inaccurate values, because failure to determine the glucose level promptly after blood sampling results in red blood cell oxidation of glucose and produces falsely low values. Blood samples should be transported on ice and analyzed within 30 minutes (Stokowski, 1999). Newborns who have had a glucose level less than 40 mg/dL are at risk for subsequent episodes of hypoglycemia and should have bedside screening performed before feedings and when symptoms occur.

Newborns with symptomatic hypoglycemia and a low bedside blood glucose determination should be treated immediately and a blood sample drawn and sent to the laboratory for glucose evaluation. Treatment consists of an oral feeding of 5% glucose in water, formula, or breast-feeding if the newborn's condition is stable. Newborns who are unable to feed by nipple or those whose blood glucose levels do not respond to oral feedings are given a 200-mg/kg (2-mL/kg) bolus of 10% dextrose in water intravenously over 1 minute, followed by a continuous infusion, until the blood glucose level is stabilized. Correction of hypoglycemia should result in resolution of the symptoms. Intravenous administration is tapered off slowly, and the blood glucose level is monitored every 1 to 4 hours initially and then intermittently before feedings until stable. Newborns who experience persistent hypoglycemia may require an increased concentration of glucose, such as 12.5%, 15%, or 20%; dextrose solutions with concentrations greater than 12.5% require placement of a central line because of the risk of tissue extravasation. Other treatments for persistent or refractory hypoglycemia include glucagon, which promotes glycogenolysis and requires adequate stores, and corticosteroids, which induce gluconeogenic enzyme activity (Brooks, 1997).

The focus of nursing care in the perinatal unit is to prevent hypoglycemia when possible. Newborns should be fed within the first 2 hours of life. Care is taken to avoid cold stress and to recognize signs of respiratory distress and sepsis that can increase the newborn's risk for developing hypoglycemia.

HYPERBILIRUBINEMIA

Unconjugated or indirect hyperbilirubinemia resulting in clinical jaundice is detected in almost 50% of term and more than 75% of preterm newborns (Johnson & Bhutani, 1998). Unconjugated hyperbilirubinemia results from physiologic (Display 17–4) or pathologic causes (Display 17–5).

Pathophysiology

Bilirubin is produced from the breakdown of heme-containing proteins (Steffensrud, 1998). The major heme-containing protein is hemoglobin, which is the source of approximately 75% of the bilirubin produced. Heme is acted on by the enzyme heme oxygenase, releasing carbon monoxide and biliverdin. Biliverdin is then reduced to bilirubin through the activity of the enzyme biliverdin reductase (Steffensrud, 1998; Stevenson & Vreman, 1997). The degradation of every 1 g of hemoglobin produces 34 to 35 mg of bilirubin (Blackburn, 1995). Bilirubin, which is water insoluble, binds with albumin, a carrier protein, for transport to the liver. Bilirubin, but not albumin, diffuses into the liver cytoplasm, where it is transported to the endoplasmic reticulum for conjugation. Bilirubin combines with glucuronate with the help of glucuronyl transferase, the conjugating enzyme. Conjugated bilirubin is water soluble and excreted into bile and subsequently into the small intestine through the common bile duct. In the gut, conjugated bilirubin is excreted from the body or converted to unconjugated bilirubin by a gut enzyme (β-glucuronidase). If conversion to unconjugated bilirubin occurs, it is resorbed into the enterohepatic circulation (Blackburn, 1995).

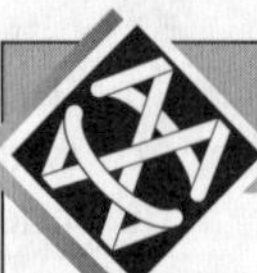

DISPLAY 17–4

Mechanisms Attributed to Physiologic Unconjugated Hyperbilirubinemia

- Increased bilirubin related to relative polycythemia and short (80–90 day) life span of fetal red blood cells
- Decreased uptake of bilirubin by the liver
- Decreased enzyme activity and ability to conjugate bilirubin
- Decreased ability to excrete bilirubin
- Breast-feeding

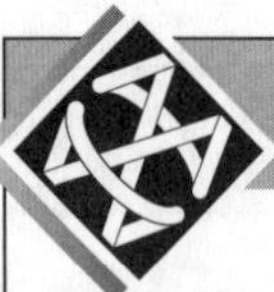

DISPLAY 17–5

Causes of Pathologic Unconjugated Hyperbilirubinemia

- Hemolytic disease of the newborn
- Bruising, hemorrhage
- Polycythemia
- Intestinal obstruction
- Metabolic conditions
- Prematurity
- Infection
- Respiratory distress

Excretion of conjugated bilirubin is facilitated by bacteria in the gut. Meconium contains large amounts of bilirubin, but excretion is inhibited in the newborn because of the sterility of the gut. Normal colonization of bacteria occurs over time and is facilitated by early and frequent feeding. Feeding introduces bacteria into the gut. Lack of bacterial flora allows conversion of conjugated bilirubin back to an unconjugated form. This, along with greater red cell mass per kilogram in the newborn than in the adult and a shortened red cell life span, sets the stage for development of physiologic unconjugated hyperbilirubinemia. Newborns produce twice as much bilirubin as adults (Rubaltelli, 1998; Stevenson & Vreman, 1997; Yao & Stevenson, 1995).

In a term newborn, physiologic unconjugated hyperbilirubinemia is characterized by a progressive increase in serum bilirubin to a peak of 5 to 8 mg/dL at 72 hours of age. Bilirubin levels slowly decline over the first 2 weeks of life to less than 1 mg/dL (Wheeler, 2000). Physiologic jaundice is considered exaggerated when bilirubin levels exceed 12 to 15 mg/dL in term newborns at 25 to 72 hours of life (AAP, 1994). In a preterm newborn, bilirubin continues to rise until the fifth postnatal day, reaching a peak of 10 to 15 mg/dL (Gartner & Lee, 1996).

Pathologic, unconjugated hyperbilirubinemia occurs in term and preterm newborns. Pathologic hyperbilirubinemia is most commonly associated with isoimmune hemolytic disease; blood group incompatibility results in an increased bilirubin load. Other causes include extravascular blood, polycythemia, intestinal obstruction, various metabolic conditions, prematurity, infection, and RDS (Blackburn, 1995). Table 17–4 lists maternal and newborn risk factors for hyperbilirubinemia.

Rising bilirubin levels engender concern that bilirubin encephalopathy (ie, kernicterus) may develop. Permanent damage to the central nervous system (CNS) results from deposition of unconjugated bilirubin in the brain, specifically in the basal ganglia, hippocampal cortex, subthalamic nuclei, and cerebellum (Blackburn, 1995). Clinical characteristics associated with kernicterus include poor Moro reflex, decreased tone, lethargy, poor feeding, high-pitched cry, opisthotonos, seizures, rigidity, and paralysis of upward gaze. There is no absolute level at which kernicterus occurs in all newborns. Gestational age, postnatal age, clinical condition, and the pathophysiologic process involved all play a part in determining what level of unconjugated bilirubin causes encephalopathy in a particular newborn (AAP, 1994). Kernicterus has been identified in newborns with bilirubin levels of 25 to 27 mg/dL (Yoa & Stevenson, 1995).

TABLE 17–4 ■ RISK FACTORS FOR HYPERBILIRUBINEMIA

Newborn	Maternal
Birth weight <1,500 g	Oxytocin
Preterm delivery	Forceps or vacuum delivery
Male sex	Diabetes
Hypothermia	East Asian heritage
Asphyxia	Native American heritage
Hypoalbuminemia	Pregnancy-induced hypertension
Sepsis	Family history of jaundice, liver disease, anemia, or splenectomy
Meningitis	Blood incompatibilities
Polycythemia (Hct >65%)	
Drugs that affect albumin binding	
Congenital hypothyroidism	
Bruising	
Poor feeding	
Inborn errors of metabolism	

Assessment

Clinical jaundice is apparent at serum bilirubin levels of 5 to 7 mg/dL (Gartner & Lee, 1996). Jaundice progresses in a caudal direction from head to the lower extremities. Visual recognition of jaundice is inaccurate and varies with the experience and level of training of the observer (Johnson & Bhutani, 1998).

A careful physical examination of any newborn presenting with jaundice aids in determining the cause of pathologic hyperbilirubinemia. The newborn should be examined for signs of prematurity, small size for gestational age, microcephaly, extravascular blood such as bruising and cephalhematoma, petechiae, and hepatosplenomegaly. In conjunction with the clinical examination, a number of laboratory tests may be done in the event of clinical jaundice (Display 17–6). When the diagnosis of hyperbilirubinemia is made, serum bilirubin levels should continue to be measured at least until they begin to decrease.

Interventions

In the late 1940s, exchange transfusion was the only available treatment for newborns with hyperbilirubinemia. In the mid-1950s, an observant nurse noticed that newborns exposed to sunlight had less clinical jaundice over exposed areas and decreased serum bilirubin levels. This observation led to the use of phototherapy, which remains the primary treat-

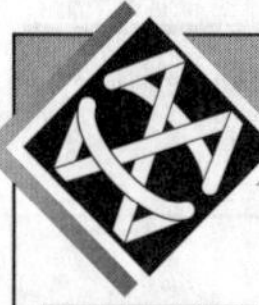

DISPLAY 17–6

Laboratory Tests to Evaluate the Cause of Jaundice

Total and direct bilirubin
Blood type
Coombs
Hematocrit
Peripheral smear for red blood cell morphology
Liver enzymes
Viral and/or bacterial cultures
pH
Serum albumin

ment for hyperbilirubinemia. In nearly all newborns, phototherapy decreases or blunts the rise in serum unconjugated bilirubin regardless of gestational age, race, or presence or absence of hemolysis. Phototherapy is used for treatment and prophylaxis of hyperbilirubinemia. No serious long-term side effects have been reported. Consensus does not exist in the literature or clinical practice about when phototherapy should be initiated or discontinued. Table 17–5 provides the recommendations from the AAP and Canadian Paediatric Society.

The goal of phototherapy is to decrease the level of unconjugated bilirubin. Phototherapy accomplishes this goal by means of

- Absorption of the light by bilirubin
- Photoconversion of bilirubin by photochemical reaction, restructuring the molecule
- Excretion of bilirubin through urine and bile (Blackburn, 1995)

The optimal light source is still under investigation; however, to be effective there must be illumination of an adequate area of exposed skin at a sufficiently short distance. Several types of phototherapy lamps are available: daylight white fluorescent, fluorescent green, special blue fluorescent, and quartz halogen (AAP, 1994). Because bilirubin absorbs visible light between 400 and 500 nm, any light source with irradiance in this range is effective. There is a known dose-response relationship between the light intensity and the rate of bilirubin decline. The standard recommended irradiance is 6 to 12 μW/cm^2 per nanometer. Irradiance should also be monitored using an irradiance meter; an ideal irradiance is 8 to 9 μW/cm^2 per nanometer. Bank lights, with a plexiglass shield placed closer than 36 cm from the newborn, should deliver adequate doses. Phototherapy can also be provided using a fiberoptic blanket that delivers irradiance of 15 to 20 μW/cm^2 per nanometer (McFadden, 1991). The newborn is placed naked under the phototherapy light and repositioned at least every 2 hours to ensure adequate light exposure to all areas. If a fiberoptic blanket is used, the blanket is wrapped around the newborn's trunk, and clothing is placed over the blanket. It is possible to provide "double" phototherapy by using two phototherapy lamps placed above and at an angle to the newborn or by placing the newborn on the fiberoptic blanket while a phototherapy lamp is above.

Although phototherapy has not been associated with any serious long-term effects, short-term side effects exist. The focus of nursing care is to prevent or minimize side effects. Newborns receiving phototherapy from phototherapy lamps are placed in an Isolette or under a radiant heat source, and axillary temperature is monitored at least every 2 hours to assess for hyperthermia. Hyperthermia can result in tachycardia and increased insensible water loss and dehydration. Loose stools are an unavoidable effect of phototherapy and can also result in increased insensible water loss and dehydration. Intake, output, and urine-specific gravity are measured accurately and documented. Meticulous skin care is necessary to prevent skin breakdown resulting from loose stools. A generalized macular rash frequently develops and resolves spontaneously when phototherapy is discontinued.

TABLE 17–5 ■ RECOMMENDATIONS FOR INITIATION OF PHOTOTHERAPY

Patient	American Academy of Pediatrics (1994)	Canadian Paediatric Society (1999)
Term infants 25–48 hours of age	Begin phototherapy when bilirubin levels are >15 mg/dL	Begin phototherapy when bilirubin levels are >10 mg/dL
Term infants 49–72 hours of age	Begin phototherapy when bilirubin levels are >18 mg/dL	Begin phototherapy when bilirubin levels are >15 mg/dL

From Wheeler, B. J. (2000). Kernicterus: Ancient history or ongoing threat? *Mother Baby Journal, 5*(2), 21–28.

The newborn's eyes are covered at all times while under phototherapy lamps to prevent retinal damage. An advantage of the fiberoptic blanket is that eye protection is unnecessary. Eye patches should be removed during feedings or at least every 4 hours to observe for drainage and to promote social stimulation and visual development. Corneal abrasions can result from eye patches that apply excessive pressure to the eyes (Blackburn, 1995). Although human studies have not shown irradiance effects on the developing gonads, animal studies have shown DNA strand breaks and chromatid exchanges and mutations. Diapers or small diaper-like devices are used as a shield for the testicles or ovaries (Blackburn, 1995).

Techniques are being investigated to predict which newborns will produce high levels of bilirubin and potentially be at risk for kernicterus, as well as methods that may replace traditional treatment with phototherapy. Knowing that carbon monoxide and biliverdin are produced in equal amounts has led researchers to investigate the possibility of noninvasive carbon monoxide monitoring. Identifying levels of carbon monoxide in blood and breath could be used as an index of heme degradation and help identify newborns at risk for exaggerated bilirubin production (Slusher et al., 1995). In 1980, it was discovered that certain metalloporphyrins (ie, family of compounds to which heme belongs) readily bind to heme oxygenase, inhibiting the enzyme's activity and resulting in decreased degradation of heme and bilirubin production. Tin-protoporphyrin and tin-mesoporphyrin are two such compounds that are potent inhibitors of heme oxygenase. These compounds are under investigation and may prove beneficial in the prevention of significant hyperbilirubinemia and associated neurologic sequelae (Steffensrud, 1998). Appendix 17A provides an algorithm for management of hyperbilirubinemia in the healthy term newborn.

NEONATAL SEPSIS

The incidence of neonatal sepsis is approximately 1 to 10 cases per 1,000 live births (Freij & McCracken, 1999; Schuchat et al., 2000). Variations in reported morbidity and mortality rates are related to methodologic factors such as healthcare institution practice, risk status of the population or community investigated, and clinical factors such as gestational age and birth weight (Table 17–6). Diagnosis of neonatal sepsis is based on clinical signs and evidence of a positive blood culture (Freij & McCracken, 1999). As technologic advances allow for the survival of progressively smaller preterm newborns, neonatal sepsis can potentially develop beyond the first month of life to 4 to 6 months of age (Witek-Janusek & Cusack, 1994).

TABLE 17–6 ■ NEONATAL SEPSIS—INCIDENCE AND MORTALITY RATES

Birth Weight	Incidence	Mortality Rate
>2,500 g	1 per 1,000	3%
1,000–2,500 g	4–9 per 10,000	30%
<1,000 g	26 per 1,000	90%

From Remington, J. S. & Klein, J. O. (Eds. (1995). *Infectious diseases of the fetus and newborn* (4th ed., pp. 835–890). Philadelphia: W. B. Saunders.

Pathophysiology

Many microorganisms are responsible for infection during the neonatal period (Display 17–7). The most common causative bacterial agents are group B β-hemolytic *Streptococcus* (GBS) and *Escherichia coli* (AAP, 1997b; Schuchat et al., 2000). Table 17–7 lists the common causative bacterial pathogens for neonatal sepsis. Infection occurs as a result of the following conditions:

- Intrauterine exposure by means of ascending infection from one or more of the endogenous flora of the cervix or vagina or, less commonly, by a transplacental route from maternal circulation

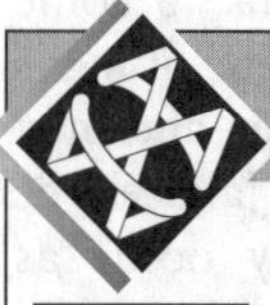

DISPLAY 17–7

Organisms Responsible for Neonatal Infection

Toxoplasms gondii
Rubella
Cytomegalovirus
Herpes
Human immunodeficiency virus
Treponema pallidum
Chlamydia trachomatis
Enterovirus
Other bacteria
Hepatitis B
Human papillomavirus

TABLE 17–7 ■ COMMON CAUSATIVE BACTERIAL PATHOGENS FOR NEONATAL SEPSIS

Early Onset	Late Onset
Common organisms	Coagulase-negative *Staphylococcus*
Group B *Streptococcus*	*Escherichia coli*
Escherichia coli	*Klebsiella* species
Haemophilus influenzae	*Enterobacter* species
Unusual organisms	*Candida* species
Staphylococcus aureus	*Malassezzia furfur*
Staphylococcus epidermidis	Other enteric organisms
Neisseria meningitidis	Group B *Streptococcus*
Streptococcus pneumoniae	Methicillin-resistant *Staphylococcus aureus*
Listeria monocytogenes	
Rare organisms	
Klebsiella pneumoniae	
Pseudomonas aeruginosa	
Enterobacter species	
Serratia marcescens	
Group A *Streptococcus*	
Group B *Streptococcus*	
Anaerobic species	

Remington, J. S., & Klein, J. O. (Eds.). (1995). *Infectious diseases of the fetus and newborn* (4th ed., pp. 835–890). Philadelphia: W.B. Saunders.

- Cutaneous transmission as the fetus passes through the birth canal
- Environmental contamination after the birth

Two patterns of development, early onset and late onset, are observed in neonatal sepsis. Early-onset sepsis occurs within 7 days of life. Frequently, inoculation occurred in utero. If symptoms are not present immediately after birth, most newborns become symptomatic within 12 hours. Development of signs in early-onset sepsis is generally very sudden and may rapidly progress to septic shock (Witek-Janusek & Cusack, 1994). Late-onset infection may occur as early as 1 week of age but more commonly after the first week of life. Late-onset infection usually results from exposure during the birth process or is the result of nosocomial transmission after birth from caregivers or invasive procedures. Because of immaturity of the newborn immune system and inability to localize infection, the most common clinical manifestations of sepsis are septicemia, pneumonia, and meningitis.

GBS acquired from the mother is the most common gram-positive organism causing sepsis in the newborn. Most of these infections could be prevented by use of prophylactic antimicrobials in at-risk women. The Centers for Disease Control and Prevention (CDC), AAP, and American College of Obstetricians and Gynecologists (ACOG) have recommended prevention and treatment strategies for mother and newborn. There are two maternal strategies: the risk-based approach and the screening-based approach. The risk-based approach is to treat all women with risk factors and labor at less than 37 weeks' gestation with intrapartum penicillin. The screening-based approach is to collect rectal and vaginal cultures for GBS at 35 to 37 weeks' gestation on all women. If the culture result is positive, the woman is treated during labor with penicillin. If the culture result is unknown during labor and risk factors are present, she is treated with intrapartum penicillin. If the culture result is negative, no treatment is indicated unless the mother has had a previous GBS-positive newborn (AAP, 1997a; ACOG, 1996; CDC, 1996; Schrag et al., 2000; Schuchat et al., 1996). Figures 17–2 and 17–3 show the CDC algorithm for addressing GBS.

Assessment

As with all neonatal complications, early identification of newborns at risk and prompt recognition of developing signs decreases morbidity and increases the chances of survival. Recognizing multiple risk factors is the first step in identifying newborns whose early days may be complicated by infection. Risk factors can be categorized as maternal, neonatal, and environmental.

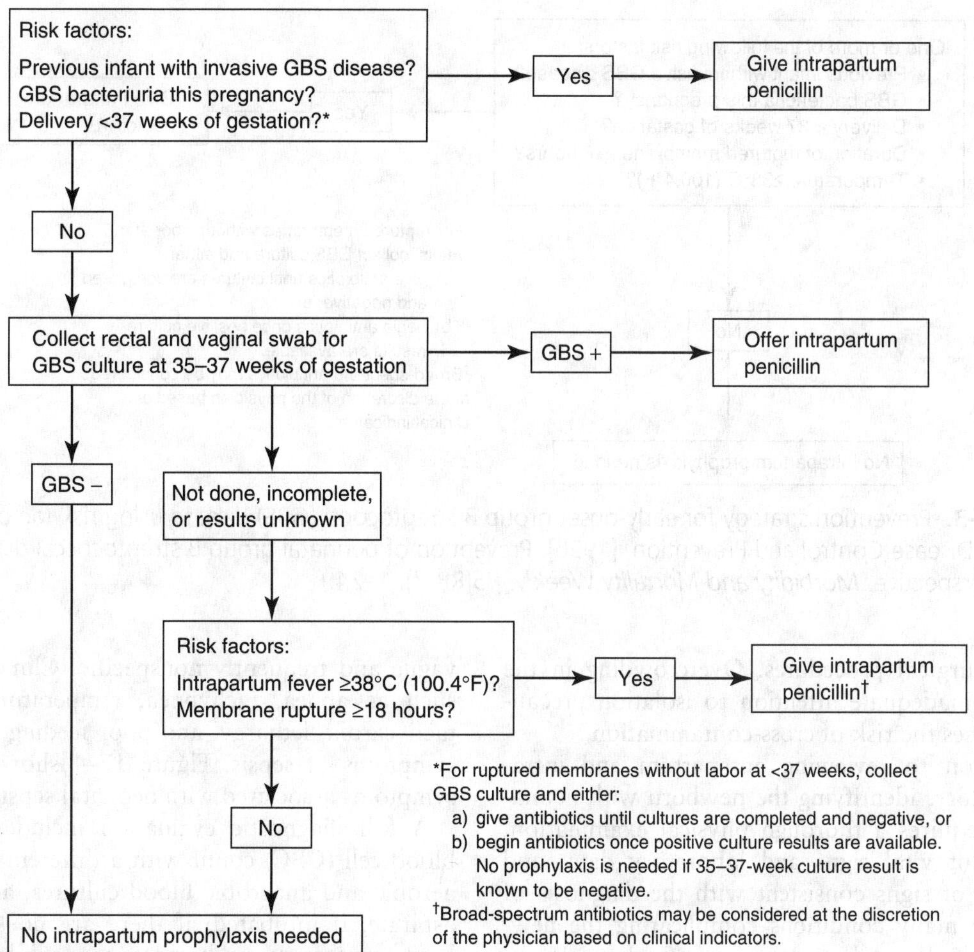

Risk factors:
Previous infant with invasive GBS disease?
GBS bacteriuria this pregnancy?
Delivery <37 weeks of gestation?*
Yes
Give intrapartum penicillin
No
Collect rectal and vaginal swab for GBS culture at 35–37 weeks of gestation
GBS +
Offer intrapartum penicillin
GBS –
Not done, incomplete, or results unknown
Risk factors:
Intrapartum fever ≥38°C (100.4°F)?
Membrane rupture ≥18 hours?
Yes
Give intrapartum penicillin†
No
No intrapartum prophylaxis needed
*For ruptured membranes without labor at <37 weeks, collect GBS culture and either:
a) give antibiotics until cultures are completed and negative, or
b) begin antibiotics once positive culture results are available.
No prophylaxis is needed if 35–37-week culture result is known to be negative.
†Broad-spectrum antibiotics may be considered at the discretion of the physician based on clinical indicators.

FIGURE 17–2. Prevention strategy for early-onset group B streptococci (GBS) disease using prenatal screening at 35 to 37 weeks. (From Centers for Disease Control and Prevention [1996]. Prevention of perinatal group B streptococcal disease: A public health perspective. *Morbidity and Mortality Weekly Report, 44*[RR-7], 1–24.)

A thorough review of antepartum and intrapartum history should specifically look for conditions that increase the risk of early-onset sepsis (Display 17–8). If the mother and newborn are cared for by different nurses, communication between healthcare team members is essential to ensure that maternal complications with potential impact on the newborn are not overlooked. The nurse caring for the mother during the postpartum period should notify the neonatal care provider if fever or other symptoms of infection develop.

The primary neonatal factors influencing development of sepsis are gestational age and birth weight. Gestational age and birth weight vary inversely with morbidity and mortality from sepsis. Preterm newborns may be exposed to the same organisms as term newborns, but their ability to fight infection is lessened. Other factors associated with increased risk of sepsis are resuscitation at birth and low Apgar scores. Congenital anomalies in which the skin or mucous membrane is not intact increase the risk of sepsis because a cutaneous port of entry is available for microorganisms. A history of a nonreassuring fetal heart rate pattern during labor, with or without meconium in the amniotic fluid, may identify fetuses at risk for infection. More male than female newborns develop sepsis, suggesting that the susceptibility may be sex linked (Witek-Janusek & Cusack, 1994).

The most obvious environmental risk for developing sepsis is admission to a newborn intensive care unit (NICU). Newborns in the NICU are compromised because of the original reason for admission along with being subjected to manipulation and invasive procedures that frequently puncture the skin, the first line of defense against infection. Environmental risks of nosocomial infection include use of equipment, indwelling catheters and chest tubes, inadequate handwashing or cleaning procedures, breaks in skin integrity, oxygen therapy and mechanical ventila-

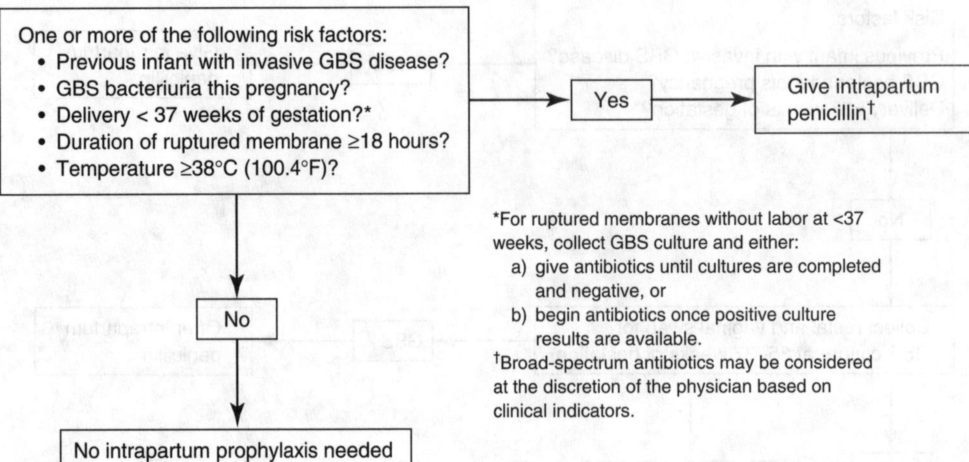
One or more of the following risk factors:
• Previous infant with invasive GBS disease?
• GBS bacteriuria this pregnancy?
• Delivery < 37 weeks of gestation?*
• Duration of ruptured membrane ≥18 hours?
• Temperature ≥38°C (100.4°F)?
Yes
Give intrapartum penicillin†
No
No intrapartum prophylaxis needed
*For ruptured membranes without labor at <37 weeks, collect GBS culture and either:
a) give antibiotics until cultures are completed and negative, or
b) begin antibiotics once positive culture results are available.
†Broad-spectrum antibiotics may be considered at the discretion of the physician based on clinical indicators.

FIGURE 17–3. Prevention strategy for early-onset group B streptococci (GBS) disease using risk factors. (From Centers for Disease Control and Prevention. [1996]. Prevention of perinatal group B streptococcal disease: A public health perspective. *Morbidity and Mortality Weekly, 45*[RR-7], 1–24.)

tion, and surgical procedures. Overcrowding in the nursery or inadequate attention to isolation precautions increases the risk of cross-contamination.

In addition to reviewing antepartum and intrapartum history, identifying the newborn with neonatal sepsis requires a thorough physical examination, evaluation of vital signs and laboratory data, and recognition of signs consistent with the diagnosis of sepsis. Like many conditions complicating the newborn period, the early signs of neonatal sepsis are vague and frequently nonspecific. Clinical indicators such as apnea, tachypnea, temperature instability, tachycardia, lethargy, and poor feeding may be early symptoms of sepsis. Figure 17–4 shows the clinical symptoms associated with neonatal sepsis.

A full diagnostic evaluation includes a complete blood cell (CBC) count with a differential cell count, aerobic and anaerobic blood cultures, and a tracheal aspirate, if intubated; if there are no CNS signs, a lumbar puncture can be postponed while awaiting the blood culture results (Gerdes, 1991). Anaerobic and aerobic blood cultures should be obtained before the initiation of antibiotic therapy from any newborn suspected of being septic. A positive blood culture is the only way to make a definitive diagnosis of bacterial sepsis. Superficial cultures from sites such as the nares, ear, throat, axillary, and umbilicus and cultures of gastric aspirate are rarely performed because they document colonization with a particular organism rather than bacteremia or sepsis. Other studies may include evaluation of acute phase reactants such as C-reactive protein. Acute-phase reactants increase in response to inflammation or tissue necrosis, theoretically providing a indicator of disease such as infection (Jaye & Waites, 1997).

DISPLAY 17–8

Maternal Factors Predisposing Newborns to Sepsis

- Preterm labor
- Premature rupture of the membranes
- Prolonged rupture of membranes
- Maternal sepsis
- Chorioamnionitis
- Intraamniotic infection
- Vaginal colonization with group B streptococci (GBS)
- Perineal colonization with *Escherichia coli*
- Prior birth of an infant with GBS
- Chemical dependency or substance abuse
- Urinary tract infection
- Foul-smelling amniotic fluid

Interventions

Many institutions have developed protocols for evaluations to exclude sepsis, including laboratory data and frequency of vital signs and clinical assessment. The CDC, AAP, and ACOG have also published certain recommendations for the management of a neonate born to a mother who received intrapartum antimicrobial prophylaxis for GBS. If there are signs of sepsis, the

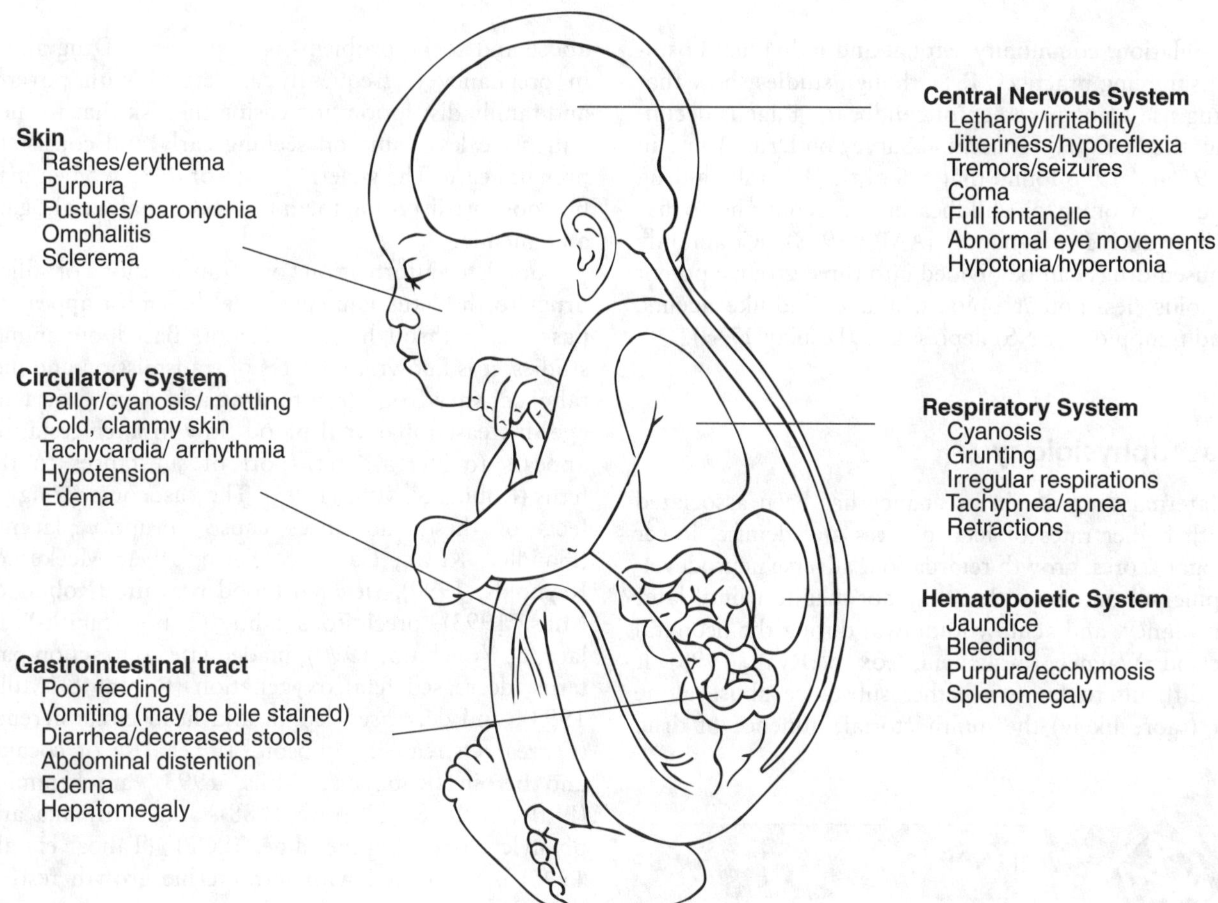

FIGURE 17–4. Clinical signs of neonatal sepsis. (From Wasserman, R. L. (1982.) Neonatal sepsis: The potential of granulocyte transfusion. *Hospital Practice, 17*(5), 98.)

newborn should receive a full diagnostic evaluation and antimicrobial therapy. If there are no signs of sepsis and the newborn is younger than 35 weeks' gestation, a CBC and blood culture should be obtained and the newborn observed for 48 hours or longer. If the newborn is 35 weeks' gestation or older and the mother received less than two doses of an antimicrobial agent, a CBC and blood culture should also be obtained and the newborn observed for 48 hours or longer. If the mother received two or more doses of an antimicrobial agent, no evaluation or therapy is required, although the newborn must still be observed for 48 hours or longer. This approach does not allow for early discharge (ACOG, 1996; Schuchat et al., 1996).

After the diagnostic evaluation has been completed, antimicrobial agents are initiated. For early-onset sepsis, ampicillin, a broad-spectrum antimicrobial that is bactericidal for gram-positive and gram-negative bacteria, is used in combination with an aminoglycoside such as gentamicin. The usual dosage of ampicillin is 50 to 100 mg/kg every 8 to 12 hours. When sepsis is complicated by meningitis, the dosage is increased to 100 to 200 mg/kg. The dose of gentamicin effective against *Pseudomonas*, *Klebsiella*, and *E. coli* has changed and depends on the gestational age and day of life. Treatment for sepsis continues for 7 to 10 days. If a diagnosis of meningitis is made, treatment may continue for 14 days. A spinal tap is usually done by day 10; if results remain positive, antimicrobials are continued for 21 days or until two sterile spinal fluid specimens are obtained. Antimicrobials are changed if results of blood cultures indicate a different medication would be more effective against the involved organism or less toxic to the newborn. After 48 to 72 hours, if the culture result is negative, antimicrobials may be discontinued (AAP, 1997b).

NEONATAL ABSTINENCE SYNDROME

Intrauterine exposure to illicit drugs may lead to neonatal intoxication or withdrawal. The incidence has been reported to be 3% to 50%, depending on the population, community setting, and individual hospital sampling practices. Even though studies show that drug use among women of childbearing age is declining, the National Household Survey on Drug Abuse in 1995 and 1996 found that 3% of the 4.1 million drug abusing women of childbearing age continue to use drugs during pregnancy (AAP, 1998). Commonly abused drugs can be divided into three groups: potent opioids, less-potent opioids, and opioid-like agents, and nonopioid (CNS) depressants (Display 17–9).

Pathophysiology

Maternal drug use in pregnancy has been associated with higher rates of fetal distress and demise, lower Apgar scores, growth retardation, adverse neurodevelopmental outcomes that may not manifest until later in infancy, and acute withdrawal during the neonatal period (Wagner, Katikaneni, Cox, & Ryan, 1998). It is difficult to know whether substance abuse alone or (more likely) the multifactorial influence of drug abuse and social problems is responsible. Drug abuse in pregnancy is frequently associated with poverty and family disruption, increasing the risk that women will place less value on seeking early and consistent prenatal care. The general health of these women may be poor, predisposing them to suboptimal weight gain and anemia.

Complete information on transmission of illicit drugs to the fetus is unavailable, but most appear to pass easily through the placenta. Based on animal studies, it is known that rates of transmission and metabolism vary from drug to drug and depend on fetal age. Increased maternal blood flow in later gestation appears to increase transport of substances to the fetus (Robins & Mills, 1993). The vasoconstricting effects of these substances cause abruptio placenta (Handler, Kistin, Davis, & Ferre, 1991; Meeker & Reynolds, 1990), elevated blood pressure (Robins & Mills, 1993), precipitous labor (Tabor, Smith-Wallace, & Yonekura, 1990), inadequate contraction patterns, decreased fetal oxygenation (Robins & Mills, 1993), and decreased length and head circumference (Ostrea, Ostrea, & Simpson, 1997). Use of cocaine and heroin (Robins & Mills, 1993), amphetamine (Little, Snell, & Gilstrap, 1988), and marijuana and phenylcyclohexyl piperidine (PCP) (Tabor et al., 1990) is associated with intrauterine growth restriction. Urogenital malformations are strongly associated with cocaine use in the first trimester (CDC, 1989). Cocaine is also thought to increase fetal vasoconstricting hormones, leading to increased blood pressure and an elevated heart rate (Woods, Plessinger, & Clark, 1987). These physiologic responses increase risk of cerebral ischemia and hemorrhagic lesions (Dixon & Bejar, 1989).

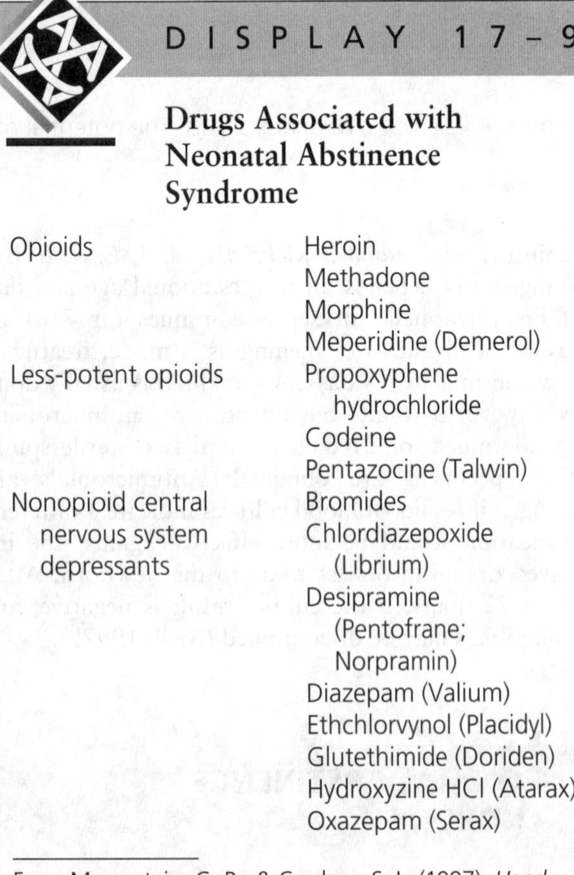

DISPLAY 17–9

Drugs Associated with Neonatal Abstinence Syndrome

Opioids	Heroin Methadone Morphine Meperidine (Demerol)
Less-potent opioids	Propoxyphene hydrochloride Codeine Pentazocine (Talwin)
Nonopioid central nervous system depressants	Bromides Chlordiazepoxide (Librium) Desipramine (Pentofrane; Norpramin) Diazepam (Valium) Ethchlorvynol (Placidyl) Glutethimide (Doriden) Hydroxyzine HCl (Atarax) Oxazepam (Serax)

From Merenstein, G. B., & Gardner, S. L. (1997). *Handbook of neonatal intensive care.* St. Louis: Mosby–Year Book. Copyright 1997 by Mosby–Year Book.

Assessment

Neonatal abstinence syndrome describes a range of symptoms the newborn experiences during withdrawal (Table 17–8). Although the most severe withdrawal symptoms are seen in the newborn exposed to opioids, symptoms can also occur after exposure to other drugs. Depending on the chemical agent the mother used, after several weeks or months, symptoms no longer represent withdrawal but instead represent the long-term effects of intrauterine drug exposure.

Clinical signs of opioid withdrawal usually begin 24 to 48 hours after birth, but they may not appear for as long as 10 days. Symptoms generally last for less than 2 weeks, but some infants show mild signs for up to 6 months (Botham, 1999). The severity of the abstinence syndrome depends on the drug or com-

TABLE 17–8 ■ SYMPTOMS OF NEONATAL ABSTINENCE SYNDROME

Site Affected	Symptoms
Central nervous system	Irritability and restlessness
	Shrill, high-pitched cry
	Tremors
	Hyperreflexia
	Altered sleep patterns
	Seizures
Gastrointestinal system	Vomiting
	Diarrhea
	Excessive sucking
	Poor feeding
Respiratory system	Tachypnea
	Stuffy nose
	Cyanosis
	Flaring
	Retractions
	Apnea
Autonomic nervous system	Yawning
	Sneezing
	Mottled skin
	Sweating
	Fever
Skin	Excoriations

bination of drugs used. The closer to the time of birth that the drugs are taken, the more severe the withdrawal symptoms (Weiner & Finnegan, 1998).

Methadone withdrawal is more severe than any other narcotic alone or cocaine alone (Robin & Mills, 1993). Approximately 75% of newborns with prenatal exposure to methadone develop withdrawal symptoms. Time of onset is variable. The newborn may have early withdrawal beginning at 24 to 48 hours or may have one or two types of late withdrawal, in which symptoms may appear shortly after birth, improve, and then reappear in 2 to 4 weeks, or there may be no symptoms until 2 to 3 weeks of age.

Heroin withdrawal begins within the first 2 weeks after birth, with an average onset at 72 hours. The duration of symptoms is 8 to 16 weeks or longer. There has been no correlation between the amount of maternal heroine abuse and severity of neonatal withdrawal (Flandermeyer, 1987). It is impossible to predict which newborns will develop severe symptoms of neonatal abstinence.

There is no clearly defined abstinence syndrome associated with in utero cocaine exposure (AAP, 1998). Several neurobehavioral abnormalities frequently occur after intrauterine cocaine exposure:

- Hypertonia
- Hyperactive startle reflex
- Irritability
- Tremulousness
- Tachypnea
- Loose stools
- State disorganization
- Poor feeding

These symptoms usually occur on day 2 or 3 and are more consistent with the cocaine effect itself, rather than withdrawal (AAP, 1998).

Preterm newborns are at lower risk for drug withdrawal, presumably because their CNS immaturity prevented damage from exposure to the drug or because of the decreased amount of time in utero when they were exposed to maternal substance abuse (AAP, 1998). It is more difficult to accurately assess the severity of abstinence in preterm newborns because the tools available were originally developed for use with term newborns. Many of the characteristics seen in neonatal drug withdrawal are common in preterm newborns, such as tremors, high-pitched cry, tachypnea, and poor feeding.

Interventions

Appropriate care of drug-exposed newborns begins with early identification and recognition of maternal drug abuse. Careful prenatal and postnatal maternal screening for substance abuse is essential. All women, regardless of racial or social background and perceived risk status, should be asked directly in a nonjudgmental manner about drug and alcohol use during pregnancy. Illicit drug use should be considered as potentially complicating all pregnancies. The level of suspicion should increase when the pregnant woman

- Has received no prenatal care
- Has a history of sexually transmitted diseases
- Insists on leaving the hospital shortly after birth
- Demonstrates signs of drug use such as needle marks and malnutrition
- Demands medication frequently and in large doses

Laws regulating toxicology screens without maternal consent vary from state to state, and the perinatal nurse should be aware of the laws in her state. When indicated, a maternal urine toxicology screen can be included as part of laboratory tests routinely ordered during the hospital admission process. If results are positive or not obtained, a urine toxicology screen or meconium assay is performed with a sample collected from the newborn's first void or stool (Ostrea et al., 1997). All newborns should be observed for signs of neonatal abstinence syndrome.

Many withdrawal symptoms can be successfully treated with basic supportive care (Display 17–10). These interventions increase the newborn's ability to regulate behavioral state, improve neuromotor control, and promote maternal newborn attachment. Minimal handling, swaddling, and a variety of positioning interventions have been used in an attempt to console and quiet the irritable, narcotic-withdrawing newborn. They can easily become overstimulated during the acute period of withdrawal (D'Apolito, 1999). Using a neonatal abstinence scoring system, narcotic-withdrawing newborns placed in a prone position demonstrated lower scores than narcotic-withdrawing newborns placed in other positions (Maichuk, Zahorodny, & Marshall, 1999).

Newborns who do not respond to symptomatic treatment alone may need medication. Ideally, the decision to begin medication is based on an objective assessment of symptoms such as the Neonatal Abstinence Scoring System (NASS) (Fig. 17–5). The newborn is assessed and scored every 2 hours for the first 48 hours and then every 8 hours while symptoms of withdrawal persist. Points are given for all behaviors or symptoms observed during the scoring interval. The newborn must be awake and calm to assess muscle tone, respirations, and Moro reflex. Observations should be made after feeding whenever possible, because hunger can mimic withdrawal. Temperature recorded on the scoring sheet should be obtained rectally, although an axillary temperature 2° F cooler may also indicate withdrawal. If the average of any three successive scores exceeds 8 points and is not reduced by nursing interventions, medications are initiated (Weiner & Finnegan, 1998). A simplified scoring system, the Neonatal Withdrawal Inventory (NWI), has been developed based on the NASS (Zahorodny et al., 1998).

A variety of medications are used to treat neonatal abstinence syndrome. The three most commonly used are diluted tincture of opium (DTO), paregoric, and phenobarbital; if opiate treatment is used, DTO is preferred over paregoric. Although these are the most commonly used medications in the treatment of neonatal withdrawal, liquid morphine and methadone are also available (AAP, 1998; Coghlan et al., 1999). Protocols for administration tapering and discontinuing these medications are available in the literature (D'Apolito & McRorie, 1996; Kandall, 1999). DTO controls all withdrawal symptoms, causes little impairment of the suck reflex, and contains few additives. Dosage is 0.05 mL/kg or 2 drops/kg every 4 to 6 hours; the dose may be increased by 2 drops every 4 hours until the desired effect is achieved. Side effects of DTO are sedation and constipation. Paregoric also contains opium (0.4%) and numerous additives. Dosage, tapering, and side effects are similar to DTO. Phenobarbital eases irritability, although it has little effect on relieving the gastrointestinal symptoms of withdrawal. Phenobarbital is given at a dose of 5 to 8 mg/kg per day in three divided doses, although some may require higher doses. Side effects of phenobarbital include sedation, poor suck reflex, and heightened sensitivity to pain.

Tapering and discontinuation of medications are best achieved using the NASS. After medication has been initiated, the newborn should be scored every 8 hours and reevaluated on a daily basis. If all scores are 8 or less, or the mean of any three successive scores is 7 or less, the dose should be maintained for 72 hours. If, after 72 hours, the scores are consistently 8 or less, or the mean of three successive scores is 7 or less, the dose should be decreased by 10%. This dose is maintained for 24 hours. If the mean score remains less than 8, the dose is decreased by 10% every 24 hours. When the dosage of DTO is 0.03 mg/kg per day or that of phenobarbital is 5 mg/kg per day or less, the medication is discontinued. After the medication has been discontinued, scoring continues until scores are 8 or less for 72 hours.

Because the symptoms of neonatal abstinence may not be completely resolved at the time of discharge, the parents need education to successfully care for the newborn. Parents should spend extended periods observing and interacting with their newborn in the presence of the nurse. These opportunities can be used by the nurse to observe parental interaction. Because drug-exposed newborns are discharged into an envi-

DISPLAY 17–10

Interventions to Support the Newborn Experiencing Withdrawal

Swaddling
Rocking
Decrease tactile stimulation
Dark room
Decrease environmental noise and stimulation
Water bed
Small, frequent feedings
Use of a pacifier

CENTRAL NERVOUS SYSTEM DISTURBANCES													
SIGNS AND SYMPTOMS	SCORE	AM						PM					
Excessive High-Pitched Cry	2												
Continuous High-Pitched Cry	3												
Sleeps <1 Hour After Feeding	3												
Sleeps <2 Hours After Feeding	2												
Sleeps <3 Hours After Feeding	1												
Hyperactive Moro Reflex	2												
Markedly Hyperactive Moro Reflex	3												
Mild Tremors Disturbed	1												
Moderate–Severe Tremors Disturbed	2												
Mild Tremors Undisturbed	1												
Moderate–Severe Tremors Undisturbed	4												
Increased Muscle Tone	2												
Excoloration (Specify Area):	1												
Myoclonic Jerks	3												
Generalized Convulsions	5												
METABOLIC/VASOMOTOR /RESPIRATORY DISTURBANCES													
Sweating													
Fever <101(99–100.8°F/37.2–38.2°C)	1												
Fever >101(38.2°C and Higher)	2												
Frequent Yawning (>3–4 times/interval)	1												
Mottling	1												
Nasal Stuffiness	1												
Sneezing (>3–4 times/interval)	1												
Nasal Flaring	2												
Respiratory Rate >60/Min.	1												
Respiratory Rate >60/Min. with Retractions	2												
GASTROINTESTINAL DISTURBANCES													
Excessive Sucking	1												
Poor Feeding	2												
Regurgitation	2												
Projectile Vomiting	3												
Loose Stools	2												
Watery Stools	3												
TOTAL SCORE													

FIGURE 17–5. Neonatal abstinence scoring system. (From Cloherty, J. P., & Stark, A. R. [1998]. *Manual of neonatal care* [4th ed., pp. 26–27]. Boston: Little, Brown.)

ronment where drug use may still be a factor, families are followed after discharge to ensure that growth and development is adequate and that parents are aware of and receive available community resources.

TRANSPORT AND RETURN TRANSPORT

Many conditions complicating the neonatal period do not begin with dramatic clinical symptoms. Experience and well-developed assessment skills allow perinatal nurses to recognize subtle changes and intervene before the newborn's condition worsens. Occasionally, the condition of the newborn and services available at a particular perinatal center necessitate transport to a level III NICU. The goal of neonatal transport is to bring a sick newborn to a tertiary-care center in stable condition. Stabilization is ongoing, beginning with the referring hospital through consultation with the tertiary center as needed until the arrival and eventual departure of the transport team. Stabilization takes many forms because of the diversity in the disease process and gestational age. Basic care needs of newborns requiring transport to a tertiary center include adequate oxygenation, prevention of hypothermia, prevention of hypoglycemia and conservation of energy, and maintenance of physiologic integrity. Appendix 17B offers an example of the documentation form used by a level III hospital during newborn transport.

After the newborn's condition is no longer critical, if an extended hospitalization is anticipated, the decision may be made to move the newborn back to the hospital in which he was born. This decision is made with input from neonatology staff at the level III center, the primary care provider who will care for the newborn in the level II hospital, nursing representatives of the level II institution, and the parents. The decision also is influenced by the parents' insurance carrier or managed care providers. Research on the impact of return transport has demonstrated inconsistent results. Several studies have shown that return transport of stable newborns to level II hospitals is safe and cost effective and that newborns demonstrate more consistent weight gains (Phibbs & Mortensen, 1992). These results were not, however, supported by later research (Pittard, Geddes, Ebeling, & Hulsey, 1993).

Return transport offers many advantages to family members of the high-risk newborn (Display 17–11). It can also be an extremely stressful process. It represents one more in a series of crises this family has experienced since the birth of their high-risk newborn (Klawitter, 1999). Maternal perceptions of the degree of stress caused by return transport are related to how well prepared they were by the level III hospital for transfer, how much the nursing care provided to their newborn differs between the two hospitals, and what medical problems their newborn develops after being transferred (Slattery, Flanagan, Cronenwett, Meade, & Chase, 1998). There is a negative correlation between the amount of stress mothers associated with the return transport and the quality of communication they had with healthcare providers at the receiving hospital. Women who perceived return transport of their newborn to be the most stressful reported the poorest experience of communicating with staff members (Flanagan, 1996).

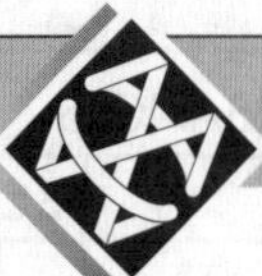

DISPLAY 17–11

Advantages of Return Transport to a Level II Nursery

- The newborn is usually closer to home, increasing the amount of time family members can spend with the newborn.
- Transport allows better use of beds in the level III intensive care unit.
- Cost of providing care in a level II hospital is generally less than in a level III institution.
- Ongoing communication is maintained between the level II and level III institutions.

To provide newborns with the best care possible, healthcare professionals within the referring hospital and between the referring hospital and tertiary center must communicate and work together as a team. The decision to transport back to the level II hospital first depends on whether the care needs of the newborn can be met at that institution. Communication between the level III and level II hospitals when a return transport is anticipated should begin several days before the actual transfer. This assists in preparing the parents, and the receiving hospital has time to anticipate staffing and equipment needs. Appendix 17C offers an example of a return transport care path used by the level III hospital. Using a formal documentation system provides the receiving hospital with information about the current condition of the newborn.

SUMMARY

Most newborns are born in level II hospitals. They are healthy at birth, develop no complications during the neonatal period, and are discharged to their homes with their mothers. A small minority of newborns are born with complications or develop complications immediately after birth. It is the newborn who develops complications that poses the challenge to the perinatal nurse. The nurse in a level II hospital must strive to identify in a timely fashion, care for appropriately, or stabilize the infant before transport to a level III facility and be prepared to accept the patient as a return transfer when he is no longer in need of intensive care.

REFERENCES

American Academy of Pediatrics. (1993). Routine evaluation of blood pressure, hematocrit and glucose in newborns. *Pediatrics, 92*(3), 474–476.

American Academy of Pediatrics. (1994). Practice parameter: Management of hyperbilirubinemia in the term newborn. *Pediatrics, 94*(4), 558–565.

American Academy of Pediatrics. (1997a). The 1997 AAP guidelines for prevention of early-onset group B streptococcal disease. *Pediatrics, 100*(3), 383–384.

American Academy of Pediatrics. (1997b). Summary of infectious diseases. In G. Peter (Ed.), *Red book: Report of the committee on infectious diseases* (24th ed., pp. 129–589). Elk Grove Village, IL: Author.

American Academy of Pediatrics Committee on Drugs. (1998). Neonatal drug withdrawal. *Pediatrics, 101*(6), 1079–1086.

American College of Obstetricians and Gynecologists (ACOG). (1996). Prevention of early-onset group B streptococcal disease in newborns. *American College of Obstetricians and Gynecologists Committee on Obstetric Practice, 173*, 1–8.

Askin, D. F. (1996). Chest and lung assessment. In E. P. Tappero & M. E. Honeyfield (Eds.), *Physical assessment of the newborn: A comprehensive approach to the art of physical examination* (pp. 67–76). Petaluma, CA: NICU INK.

Blackburn, S. (1995). Hyperbilirubinemia and neonatal jaundice. *Neonatal Network, 14*(7), 15–25.

Botham, S. (1999). Perinatal substance abuse. In J. Deacon & P. O'Neill (Eds.), *Core curriculum for neonatal intensive care nursing* (2nd ed., pp. 618–634). Philadelphia: W.B. Saunders.

Brooks, C. (1997). Neonatal hypoglycemia. *Neonatal Network, 16*(2), 15–21.

Canadian Paediatric Society. (1999). Approach to the management of hyperbilirubinemia in term newborn infants. *Paediatrics and Child Health, 4*(2), 161–164.

Casey, P. M. (1999). Respiratory distress. In J. Deacon & P. O'Neill (Eds.), *Core curriculum for neonatal intensive care nursing* (2nd ed., pp. 118–150). Philadelphia: W.B. Saunders.

Centers for Disease Control and Prevention (CDC). (1989). Urogenital anomalies in the offspring of women using cocaine during early pregnancy. *Morbidity and Mortality Weekly Report, 38*(31), 536, 541–542.

Centers for Disease Control and Prevention (CDC). (1996). Prevention of perinatal group B streptococcal disease: A public health perspective. *Morbidity and Mortality Weekly Report, 45*(R-7), 1–24.

Champawat, K. Y., & Torrence, C. R. (1996). Assessment and stabilization for transport of the infant with congenital heart disease. *Mother-Baby Journal, 1*(1), 33–38.

Coghlan, D., Milner, M., Clarke, T., Lambert, I., McDermott, C., McNally, M., Beckett, M., & Matthews, T. (1999). Neonatal abstinence syndrome. *Irish Medical Journal, 92*(1), 232–233.

D'Apolito, K. (1999). Comparison of a rocking bed and standard bed for decreasing withdrawal symptoms in drug-exposed infants. *American Journal of Maternal Child Nursing, 24*(3), 138–144.

D'Apolito, K. C., & McRorie, T. I. (1996). Pharmacologic management of neonatal abstinence syndrome. *Journal of Perinatal and Neonatal Nursing, 9*(4), 70–80.

Dixon, S. D., & Bejar, R. (1989). Echoencephalographic findings in neonates associated with maternal cocaine and methamphetamine use: Incidence and clinical correlates. *Journal of Pediatrics, 115*(5, Pt. 1), 770–778.

Flandermeyer, A. A. (1987). A comparison of the effects of heroin and cocaine abuse upon the neonate. *Neonatal Network, 6*(3), 42–48.

Freij, B. J., & McCracken, G. H. (1994). Acute infections. In G. B. Avery, M. A. Fletcher, & M. G. MacDonald (Eds.), *Neonatology: Pathophysiology and management of the newborn* (4th ed., pp. 1082–1116). Philadelphia: J.B. Lippincott.

Furdon, S. A. (1997). Recognizing congestive heart failure in the neonatal period. *Neonatal Network, 16*(7), 5–13.

Gartner, L. M., & Lee, K. S. (1996). Jaundice and liver disease. In A. A. Fanaroff & R. J. Martin (Eds.), *Neonatal-perinatal medicine diseases of the fetus and infant* (6th ed., pp. 1075–1117). St. Louis: Mosby–Year Book.

Gerdes, J. S. (1991). Clinicopathologic approach to the diagnosis of neonatal sepsis. *Clinics in Perinatology, 18*(2), 361–381.

Halamek, L. P., Benaron, D. A., & Stevenson, D. K. (1997). Neonatal hypoglycemia, part I: Background and definition. *Clinical Pediatrics, 36*(12), 675–680.

Handler, A., Kistin, N., Davis, F., & Ferre, C. (1991). Cocaine use during pregnancy: Perinatal outcomes. *American Journal of Epidemiology, 133*(8), 818–825.

Hansen, T. N., Cooper, T. R., & Weisman, L. E. (Eds.). (1998). *Contemporary diagnosis and management of neonatal respiratory diseases* (2nd ed., p. 31). Newton, PA: Handbooks of Health Care.

Hey, W. W., & Bell, E. F. (2000). Oxygen therapy, oxygen toxicity, and the STOP-ROP trial. *Pediatrics, 105*(2), 424–425.

Jaye, D. L., & Waites, K. B. (1997). Clinical applications of C-reactive protein in pediatrics. *Pediatric Infectious Disease Journal, 16*(8), 735–746.

Johnson, L., & Bhutani, V. K. (1998). Guidelines for management of the jaundiced term and near-term infant. *Clinics in Perinatology, 25*(3), 555–574.

Kandall, S. R. (1999). Treatment strategies for drug-exposed neonates. *Clinical Perinatology, 26*(1), 231–243.

Karp, T. B., Scardina, C., & Butler, L. A. (1995). Glucose metabolism in the neonate: The short and the sweet of it. *Neonatal Network, 14*(8), 17–23.

Klawitter, M. (1999). Back transport of the stable neonate: Easing the transition. *Mother-Baby Journal, 4*(3), 7–12.

Klingner, M. C. & Kruse, J. (1999). Meconium aspiration syndrome: Pathophysiology and prevention. *Journal of the American Board of Family Practice, 12*(6), 450–466.

Little, B. B., Snell, L. M., & Gilstrap, L. C. (1988). Methamphetamine abuse during pregnancy: Outcome and fetal effects. *Obstetrics and Gynecology, 72*(4), 541–544.

Maichuk, G. T., Zahorodny, W., & Marshall, R. (1999). Use of positioning to reduce the severity of neonatal narcotic withdrawal syndrome. *Journal of Perinatology, 19*(7), 510–513.

McFadden, E. A. (1991). The Wallaby phototherapy system: A new approach to phototherapy. *Journal of Pediatric Nursing, 6*(3), 206–208.

Meeker, J. E., & Reynolds, P. C. (1990). Fetal and newborn death associated with maternal cocaine use. *Journal of Analytical Toxicology, 14*(6), 379–382.

Merestein, G. B., & Gardner, S. L. (1997). *Handbook of neonatal intensive care.* St. Louis: Mosby–Year Book.

Ogata, E. S. (1999). Carbohydrate homeostasis. In G. B. Avery, M. A. Fletcher, & M. G. MacDonald (Eds.), *Neonatology: Pathophysiology and Management of the Newborn* (5th ed., pp. 1189–1230). Philadelphia: Lippincott, Williams & Wilkins.

Ostrea, E. M., Ostrea, A. R., & Simpson, P. M. (1997). Mortality within the first 2 years in infants exposed to cocaine, opiate or cannabinoid during gestation. *Pediatrics, 100*(1), 79–83.

Paul, D. E. (1995). Recognition, stabilization, and early management of infants with critical congenital heart disease presenting in the first days of life. *Neonatal Network, 14*(5), 13–20.

Phibbs, C., & Mortensen, L. (1992). Back transporting infants from neonatal intensive care units to community hospitals for recover care: Effect on total hospital charges. *Pediatrics, 90*(1), 22–26.

Pittard, W. B., Geddes, K. M., Ebeling, M., & Hulsey, T. C. (1993). Continuing evolution of regionalized perinatal care: Community hospital neonatal convalescent care. *Southern Medical Journal, 86*(8), 903–907.

Remington, J. S., & Klein, J. O. (Eds.). (1995). *Infectious diseases of the fetus and newborn* (4th ed., pp. 835–890). Philadelphia, W.B. Saunders.

Robins, L. N., & Mills, J. L. (1993). Effects of in utero exposure to street drugs. *American Journal of Public Health, 83*(Suppl.), 1–32.

Rubaltelli, F. (1998). Current drug treatment options in neonatal hyperbilirubinemia and the prevention of kernicterus. *Drugs, 56*(1), 23–30.

Sansoucie, D. A., & Cavaliere, T. A. (1997). Transition from fetal to extrauterine circulation. *Neonatal Network, 16*(2), 5–12.

Schrag, S. J., Zywicki, S., Farley, M. M., Reingold, A. L., Harrison, L. H., Lefkowitz, L. B., Hadler, J. L., Danila, R., Cieslak, P. R., & Schuchat, A. (2000). Group B streptococcal disease in the era of intrapartum antibiotic prophylaxis. *New England Journal of Medicine, 342*(1), 15–20.

Schuchat, A., Whitney, C., & Zangwill, K. (1996). Prevention of perinatal group B streptococcal disease: A public health perspective. *Morbidity & Mortality Weekly Report, 45*(RR-7), 1–21.

Schuchat, A., Zywicki, S. S., Dinsmoor, M. J., Mercer, B., Romaguera, J., O'Sullivan, M. J., Patel, D., Peters, M. T., Stoll, B., Levine, O. S., & the Prevention of Early-Onset Neonatal Sepsis Study Group. (2000). Risk factors and opportunities for prevention of early-onset neonatal sepsis: A multicenter case-control study. *Pediatrics, 105*(1), 21–26.

Schwartz, R. P. (1997). Neonatal hypoglycemia: how low is too low? *Journal of Pediatrics, 131*(2), 171–173.

Short, M. A. (1998). A comparison of temperatures in VLBW infants swaddled versus unswaddled in a double-walled incubator in skin control mode. *Neonatal Network, 17*(3), 25–31.

Slattery, M. J., Flanagan, V., Cronenwett, L. R., Meade, S. K., & Chase, N. S. (1998). Mothers' perceptions of the quality of their infants' back transfer. *Journal of Obstetrics, Gynecologic, and Neonatal Nursing, 27*(4), 394–401.

Slusher, T. M., Vreman, H. J., McLaren, D. W., Lewison, L. J., Brown, A., K., & Stevenson, D. K. (1995). Glucose-6-phosphate dehydrogenase deficiency and carboxyhemoglobin concentrations associated with bilirubin related morbidity and death in Nigerian infants. *Journal of Pediatrics, 126*(1), 102–108.

Speer, M. E., & Hansen, T. N. (1998). Transient tachypnea of the newborn. In T. N. Hansen, T. R. Cooper, & L. E. Weisman (Eds.), *Contemporary Diagnosis and Management of Neonatal Respiratory Diseases* (2nd ed., pp. 95–99). Newton, PA: Handbooks of Health Care.

Spilman, L. J., & Furdon, S. A. (1998). Recognition, understanding, and current management of cardiac lesions with decreased pulmonary blood flow. *Neonatal Network, 17*(4), 7–18.

Stanley, C. A., & Baker, L. (1999). The causes of neonatal hypoglycemia. *New England Journal of Medicine, 340*(15), 1200–1201.

Steffensrud, S. (1998). Tin-metalloporphyrins: An answer to neonatal jaundice? *Neonatal Network, 17*(5), 11–17.

Stevenson, D. K., & Vreman, H. J. (1997). Carbon monoxide and bilirubin production in neonates. *Pediatrics, 100*(2), 252–254.

Tabor, B. L., Smith-Wallace, T., & Yonekura, M. L. (1990). Perinatal outcome associated with PCP versus cocaine use. *American Journal of Drug and Alcohol Abuse, 16*(3–4), 337–348.

Verklan, M. T. (1997). Bronchopulmonary dysplasia: Its effects upon the heart and lung. *Neonatal Network, 16*(8), 5–12.

Wagner C. L., Katikaneni, L. D., Cox, T. H., & Ryan, R. M. (1998). The impact of prenatal drug exposure on the neonate. *Obstetric & Gynecology Clinics of North America, 25*(1), 169–194.

Weiner, S. M., & Finnegan, L. P. (1998). Drug withdrawal in the neonate. In B. B. Merenstein & S. L. Gardner (Eds.), *Handbook of neonatal intensive care* (4th ed.). St. Louis: Mosby.

Wheeler, B. J. (2000). Kernicterus: Ancient history or ongoing threat? *Mother-Baby Journal, 5*(2), 21–30.

Whitsett, J. A., Pryhuber, G. S., Rice, W. R., Warner, B. B., & Wert, S. E. (1999). Acute respiratory disorders. In G. B. Avery, M. A. Fletcher, & M. G. MacDonald (Eds.), *Neonatology, pathophysiology and management of the newborn* (4th ed., pp. 429–451). Philadelphia: J.B. Lippincott.

Wiswell, T. E., Gannon, C. M., Jacob, J., Goldsmith, L., Szyld, E., Weiss, K., Schutzman, D., Cleary, G. M., Filipov, P., Kurlat, I., Caballero, C. L., Abassi, S., Sprague, D., Oltorf, C., & Padula, M. (2000). Delivery room management of apparently vigorous meconium-stained neonates: Results of the multicenter international collaborative trial. *Pediatrics, 105*(1), 1–7.

Witek-Janusek, L., & Cusack, C. (1994). Neonatal sepsis: Confronting the challenge. *Critical Care Nursing Clinics of North America, 6*(2), 405–419.

Witt, C. (1997). Cardiac embryology. *Neonatal Network, 16*(1), 43–49.

Witt, C. (1998). Cyanotic heart lesions with increased pulmonary blood flow. *Neonatal Network, 17*(7), 7–16.

Wood, M. K. (1997). Acyanotic lesions with increased pulmonary blood flow. *Neonatal Network, 16*(3), 17–25.

Woods, J. R., Plessinger, M. A., & Clark, K. E. (1987). Effect of cocaine on uterine blood flow and fetal oxygenation. *Journal of the American Medical Association, 257*(7), 957–961.

Yao, T., & Stevenson, D. (1995). Advances in the diagnosis and treatment of neonatal hyperbilirubinemia. *Clinics in Perinatology, 22*(3), 741–758.

Zahorodny, W., Rom, C., Whitney, W., Giddens, S., Samuel, M., Maichuk, G., & Marshall, R. (1998). *Journal of Developmental and Behavioral Pediatrics, 19*(2), 89–93.

APPENDIX 17A

Algorithm for Management of Hyperbilirubinemia in the Healthy Term Infant

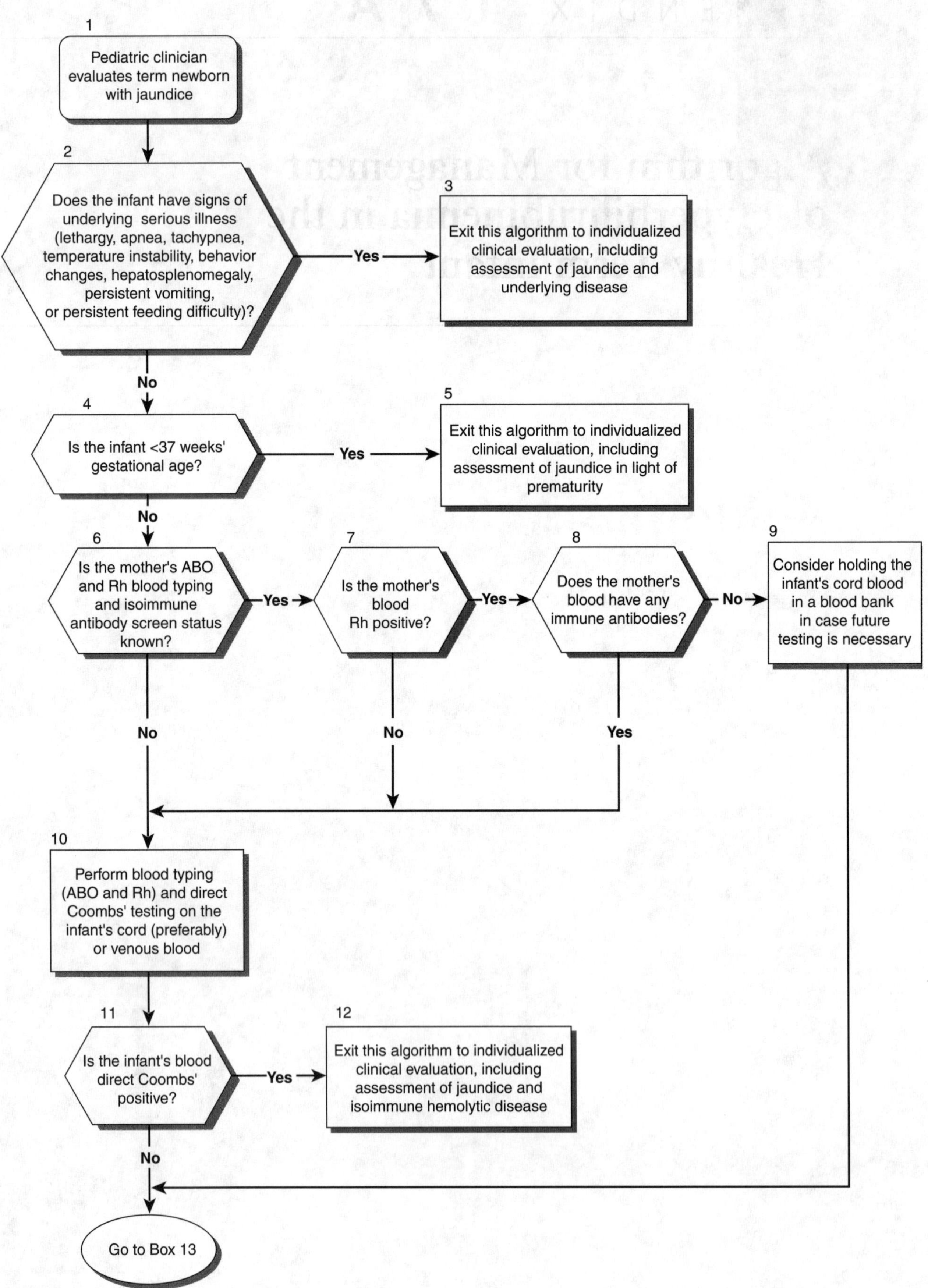
1
Pediatric clinician evaluates term newborn with jaundice
2
Does the infant have signs of underlying serious illness (lethargy, apnea, tachypnea, temperature instability, behavior changes, hepatosplenomegaly, persistent vomiting, or persistent feeding difficulty)?
Yes
3
Exit this algorithm to individualized clinical evaluation, including assessment of jaundice and underlying disease
No
4
Is the infant <37 weeks' gestational age?
Yes
5
Exit this algorithm to individualized clinical evaluation, including assessment of jaundice in light of prematurity
No
6
Is the mother's ABO and Rh blood typing and isoimmune antibody screen status known?
Yes
7
Is the mother's blood Rh positive?
Yes
8
Does the mother's blood have any immune antibodies?
No
9
Consider holding the infant's cord blood in a blood bank in case future testing is necessary
No
No
Yes
10
Perform blood typing (ABO and Rh) and direct Coombs' testing on the infant's cord (preferably) or venous blood
11
Is the infant's blood direct Coombs' positive?
Yes
12
Exit this algorithm to individualized clinical evaluation, including assessment of jaundice and isoimmune hemolytic disease
No
Go to Box 13

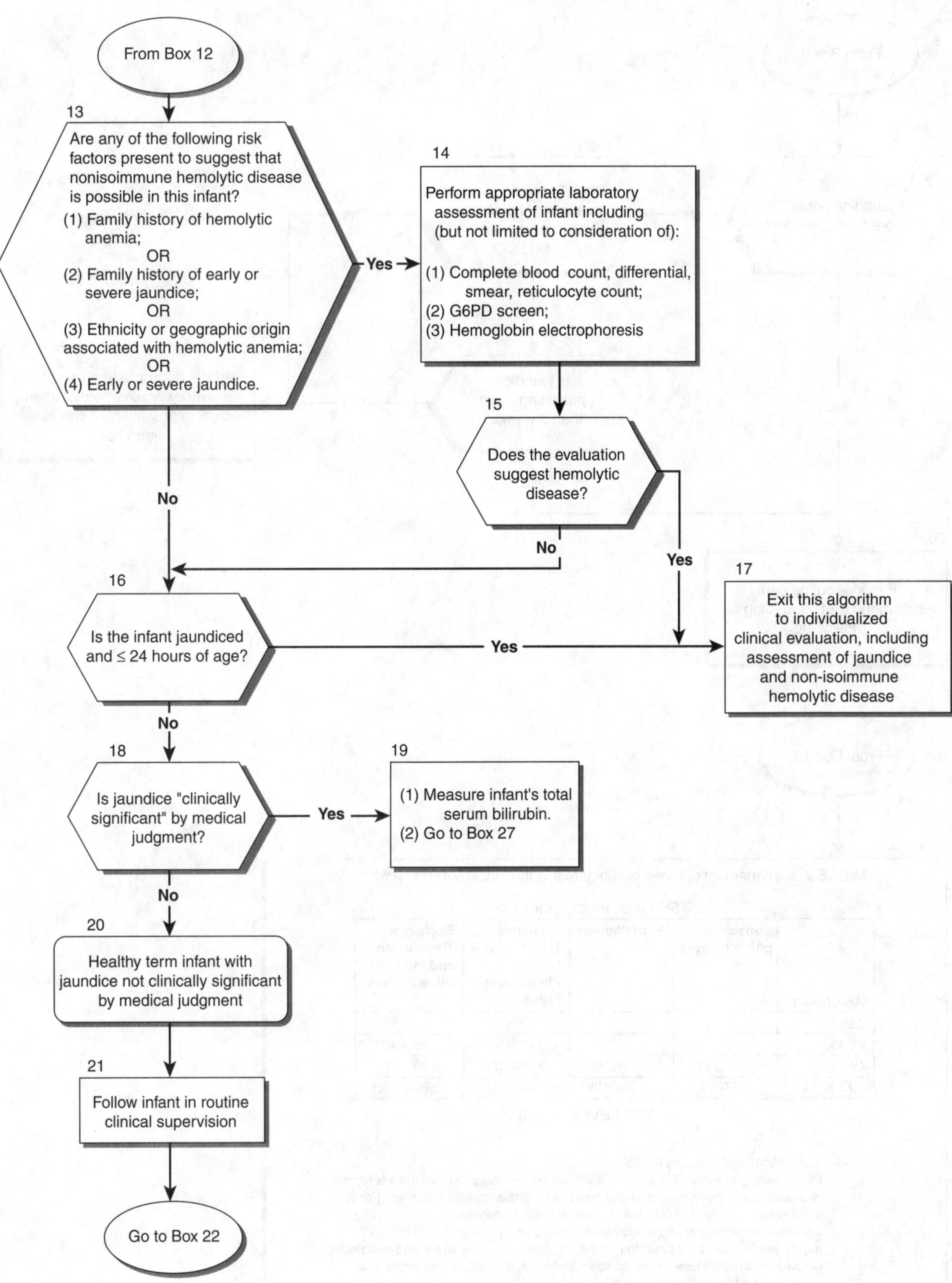
From Box 12
13
Are any of the following risk factors present to suggest that nonisoimmune hemolytic disease is possible in this infant?
(1) Family history of hemolytic anemia;
OR
(2) Family history of early or severe jaundice;
OR
(3) Ethnicity or geographic origin associated with hemolytic anemia;
OR
(4) Early or severe jaundice.
Yes
14
Perform appropriate laboratory assessment of infant including (but not limited to consideration of):
(1) Complete blood count, differential, smear, reticulocyte count;
(2) G6PD screen;
(3) Hemoglobin electrophoresis
15
Does the evaluation suggest hemolytic disease?
No
Yes
No
16
Is the infant jaundiced and ≤ 24 hours of age?
Yes
17
Exit this algorithm to individualized clinical evaluation, including assessment of jaundice and non-isoimmune hemolytic disease
No
18
Is jaundice "clinically significant" by medical judgment?
Yes
19
(1) Measure infant's total serum bilirubin.
(2) Go to Box 27
No
20
Healthy term infant with jaundice not clinically significant by medical judgment
21
Follow infant in routine clinical supervision
Go to Box 22

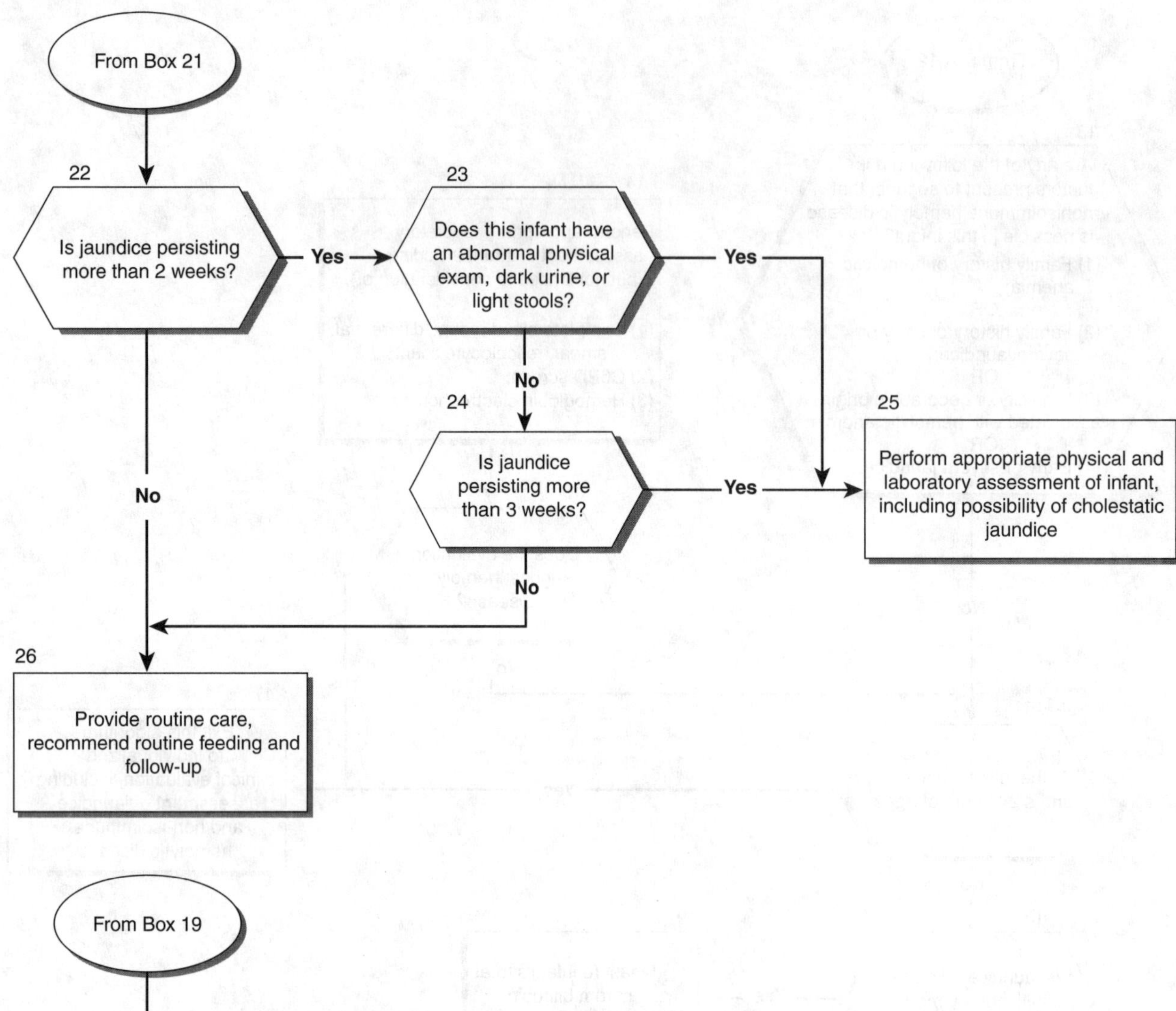

27

TABLE 2. Management of Hyperbilirubinemia in the Healthy Term Newborn*

TSB Level, mg/dL (μmol/L)

Age, hours	Consider phototherapy†	Phototherapy	Exchange Transfusion if Intensive Phototherapy Fails‡	Exchange Transfusion and Intensive Phototherapy
≤ 24	...	...	...	...
25-48	≥ 12(170)	≥ 15(260)	≥ 20(340)	≥ 25(430)
49-72	≥ 15(260)	≥ 18(310)	≥ 25(430)	≥ 30(510)
> 72	≥ 17(290)	≥ 20(340)	≥ 25(430)	≥ 30(510)

TSB LEVEL (mg/dL)[c]

* TSB indicates total serum bilirubin.

† Phototherapy at these TSB levels is a clinical option, meaning that the intervention is available and may be used *on the basis of individual clinical judgment.* For a more detailed description of phototherapy see the Appendix.

‡ Intensive phototherapy (Appendix) should produce a decline of TSB of 1 to 2 mg/dL within 4 to 6 hours and the TSB level should continue to fall and remain below the threshold level for exchange transfusion. If this does not occur, it is considered a failure of phototherapy.

§ Term infants who are clinically jaundiced at ≤24 hours old are not considered healthy and require further evaluation (see text).

APPENDIX **17B**

Loyola University Medical Center Perinatal Network: Acutely Ill Neonatal Transport Collaborative Carepath

COLLOBORATIVE CAREPATH: **ACUTELY ILL NEONATAL TRANSPORT**

Patient: ______ Date/Time of Birth: ______

Neonatologist/Pediatrician: ______ Infant Apgars: ______

Referring Obstetrician: ______ Gestational Age: ______

Referral Hospital Phone #: ______ Maternal Gravida/Parity: ______

Date: Time:	TRANSFER ACCEPTED (TIME) UNTIL TEAM ARRIVES	TEAM ARRIVAL (TIME________)	TEAM DEPARTURE (TIME________)	DISCHARGE OUTCOMES
Care Unit:	LEVEL II NURSERY			Safe transport
Consults/Physicians:	Neonatology/Pediatrician Written transfer order			Follow-up for return transport criteria
Tests: (Check all that were done)	_CBC _Blood Cultures _Blood Type/Coomb _Blood Gases _Glucose (serum) _Newborn Screen (PKU, etc.) _Mother's Maiden Name:______ _Mother's Social Security #:______ _Urine CIE _Urine Toxicology _Surface Cultures _CXR _X-ray post tube/line placement OTHER:______			Values available at time of transfer, except cultures
Treatment/ Procedures: (Check all that were done)	Resuscitation:_02 _Bag/Mask _Compressions _Medications _Intubation Tube size____ Cm at lip line____ _Surfactant Time________ Type________ _Umbilical Line _Chest Tube _Lumbar Puncture		Complete newborn identification verification	Infant stable for transport posttreatment intervention and identification
Activity:	Skin Care: Utilize pectin based barriers under any/all tape (ie., E.T., Umbilical lines, NG, etc.). Use of bowel bag (VI-drape) for abdominal defects.			Skin integrity will be maintained
Nutrition:	Intake: IV fluid______ Rate______ Enteric (type)______ Output: Urine: Mother desires: _Breast/ _Bottle Stool: Blood: Other:		TOTALS: Intake: Output	Promote optimal maintenance of hydration/nutrition

Medications: (Check or write meds given)	_EES _Vitamin K Antibiotics (Dosage/time): Ampicillin ________ Gentamicin ________ Other Meds: ______________		Medications ordered but not administered: ______________ ______________	Endorsement of medication plan
Assessment & Monitoring:	Evaluate: Skin color ________ Need for NG ________ Cardio/respiratory monitoring ___ V/S with dinamap B/P ________ Invasive B/P monitoring ______ Pulse oximetry ________ Anomalies/defects ________ Glucose screen (most recent level ________) time: ______			Stabilization for a safe transport
Expected Outcomes: (Check all that were done)	Items to prepare for transport: XEROX CHART: * _Baby Chart _Mother's delivery record _X-ray copies _Labelled cord blood _Mother's blood (pilot tubes) _Parent/Guardian available for consents _Referral Hospital "Release of Information" consent –Referral Hospital "procedure" consent(s) _Will fax unavailable items LUMC NICU FAX: 216-4125 Completion of appropriate consults; tests; procedures; skin care; nutritional evaluation; medication delivery; and assessment and monitoring	Referral center obtains transport consent. Transfer to Level III care initiated	Endorsements completed	Stabilization for safe transport
Psychosocial & Educational Needs: Patient & Family (Check all that were done)	_Reason for transport. _Chaplain notified. _Infant baptized, per parent request. _Polaroid picture taken and given to parent. _Parents see infant prior to departure.	Transport pack given to parents by transport team		Patient and family needs are met
Discharge Plan:		Transport team member signs for "receiving patient"	Document transfer. Discharge from computer. Complete neonatal transport log and nursery log. Complete charting, include: transport team arrival time, infant's condition on team's arrival and departure, and time of team departure with infant.	Safe transport and appropriate documentation completed

REFERRAL HOSPITAL R.N. (INITIALS) ______________(______) TRANSFER HOSPITAL R.N. (INITIALS) ______________(______)

REFERRAL HOSPITAL R.N. (INITIALS) ______________(______) TRANSFER HOSPITAL R.N. (INITIALS) ______________(______)

APPENDIX **17C**

Loyola University Medical Center Perinatal Network: Neonatal Return Collaborative Carepath

COLLABORATIVE CAREPATH: **NEONATAL RETURN TRANSPORT**

Patient: ______ Gestational age @ Birth: ______ DOL: ______ Date: ______

Birthweight: ______ Current Weight: ______ Diagnosis: ______ Current Condition: ______

Accepting Neonatologist/Pediatrician: ______ Referring Neonatologist: ______

Accepting Hospital: ______ Accepting Hospital Phone #: ______

Date: Time:	TRANSFER TIME AGREED UPON (TIME ______)	TIME TEAM ARRIVED AT LEVEL II (TIME____)	DISCHARGE OUTCOMES
Care Unit:	LEVEL III NURSERY	LEVEL II NURSERY	Safe Transport
Communication:	Nurse verifies consent for transfer. Nurse to Nurse report. Parent notification of tentative transfer time. Parent given Level II phone number.	Infant identification process completed	Return transport and infant identification safely completed
Tests: (Check all that are done)	_Newborn Screen (PKU, etc.) Date:______ _Hearing Screen Date:______ _Pass/ _Fail _Eye Exam Date:______ Follow-up: ______ _Last Hematocrit Date:______ Result: ______ _Drug Levels _Other pertinent Labs (ie, toxicology screen, blood cultures, blood gases, etc.) ______ ______		Values available and endorsed at time of transfer, except newborn screen
Treatment/ Procedures: (Check those applicable)	Environment: _Open Crib _Isolette (bed temperature______) _Warmer Respiratory Support: _None _02 % _NC____L flow _Hood _CPAP + _____ _Other: (Circumcision, etc.)______ ______		Infant stable for transport posttreatment intervention and identification
Medications: (list current medications)	MEDICATION DOSE ROUTE FREQUENCY LAST DOSE ______ If antibiotic, list day of treatment______/anticipated length of treatment______ _Immunization card provided to referral hospital		Endorsement of medication plan
Activity: (Check those applicable)	_Reflux precautions. _Kangaroo care. _Apnea and bradycardia status. _Other:______ ______		Outlined activities will be maintained

Nutrition:	Intake: IV fluid__________ Rate__________ IV lock in place, Last flushed:__________ Milk used:__________ Route: _CNG _Intermittent _ng _po/ng _po _ad lib Feeding amount:__________ Feeding frequency: q__________ Last feeding time:__________ Feeding issues: Emesis Reflux Residuals Other:__________ Breast: _Mom pumping _Attempted at breast _Breastfeeding well _Breastmilk supply brought with patient Output: Last Void:__________ Last Stool:__________ Problems:__________ Other:__________		Promote optimal maintenance of hydration/nutrition.
Assessment & Monitoring:	Head circumference:__________ Abdominal circumference:__________ Chest circumference:__________ Length:__________ V/S frequency:__________ Last V/S: T______ P______ R______ B/P ______ Pulse oximeter: _None _Continuous _Intermittent Pulse oximetry 0_2 Saturation range:________ to ________ Other:__________		Stabilization for a safe transport
Expected Outcomes:	Transfer Summary (history) prepared. _Brought with infant _To be faxed	Transfer Summary endorsed. Level II admission documentation initiated.	Hospitalization history endorsed for safe transition of care
Psychosocial & Educational Needs: Patient & Family (<u>Check those applicable</u>)	Parent contact history endorsed. Parent competencies achieved: _bath _temperature taking _diapering _feeding _CPR _Other: __________	Parent involvement and competencies endorsed to Level II. Personal belongings accepted by Level II.	Patient and family needs are met. Orientate parents to unit.
Discharge Plan:	Pediatrician identified__________ Neonatal Follow-up Clinic Appointment__________ Ophthalmology Follow-up Appointment__________ Other Follow-up needs:__________	Infant admitted to Level II for ongoing care and discharge planning	Safe transport and appropriate documentation completed

REFERRAL HOSPITAL R.N. (INITIALS) ____________________(________) TRANSFER HOSPITAL R.N. (INITIALS) ____________________(________)

REFERRAL HOSPITAL R.N. (INITIALS) ____________________(________) TRANSFER HOSPITAL R.N. (INITIALS) ____________________(________)

REFERRAL HOSPITAL M.D. ____________________

6/1 ccrt

PART 6

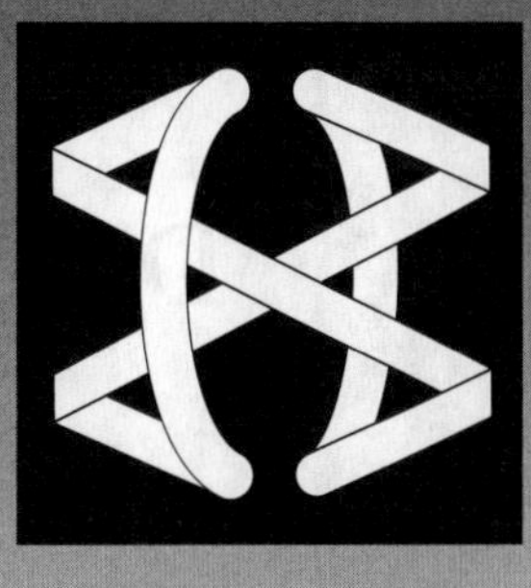

THE TRANSITION FROM HOSPITAL TO HOME

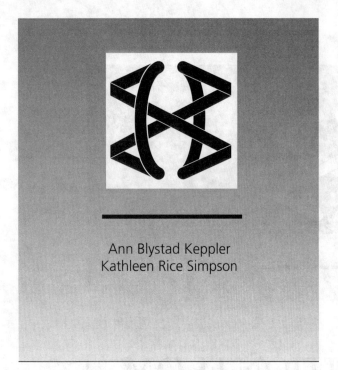

Ann Blystad Keppler
Kathleen Rice Simpson

CHAPTER 18

Discharge Planning

Almost 4 million babies are born every year in the United States in the approximately 6,000 hospitals that provide perinatal services (Ventura, Martin, Curtin, Mathews, & Park, 2000). The number of births in the United States increased by 2% in 1998, the first increase in the number of births since 1990 (Ventura et al., 2000). Childbirth is the most common reason for admission to hospitals in the United States (Agency for Health Care Policy and Research [AHCPR], 1999), but there are variations in the length of stay (LOS) for healthy women for vaginal and cesarean birth. These variations are based on maternal preferences, institutional policies, and health insurance coverage. During the past 20 years, there have been significant changes in LOS for childbirth. In 1980, the average LOS for vaginal birth was 3.2 days but had dropped to 1.7 days by 1995 (Curtin & Park, 1999). In 1998, the average LOS for vaginal birth increased to 2.1 days (AHCPR, 1999). The increase was related to state laws passed in 1995 and 1996 and the federal law (Newborns' and Mothers' Health Protection Act of 1996), which took effect in 1997 and 1998, requiring insurance companies to provide coverage for hospital stays of at least 2 days for vaginal births and of at least 4 days for cesarean births (Declercq, 1999).

According to the latest data from the *National Discharge Survey* of the National Center for Health Statistics (NCHS), the percentage of women hospitalized for 1 day or less for childbirth dropped from 37% in 1995 to 25% in 1997 (Kozak & Lawrence, 1999). Stays of 2 to 3 days for all births increased from 54% to 64% during this period. Women with vaginal births accounted for almost the entire decrease in stays of 1 day and the increase in stays of 2 to 3 days. The percentage of women who stayed longer than 4 days after cesarean birth also increased significantly (Kozak & Lawrence, 1999). The cost of an extra inpatient day per mother and baby is approximately $1,400 (Raube & Merrell, 1999).

Considerable controversy exists about whether an increase in LOS from 1 to 2 days after vaginal birth decreases the risk of neonatal readmission (Behram, Moschler, Sayegh, Garguillo, & Mann, 1998; Braveman, Egerter, Pearl, Marchi, & Miller, 1995; Danielsen, Castles, Damberg, & Gould, 2000; Lock & Ray, 1999; Maisels & Kring, 1998; Mandl, Brennan, Wise, Tronick, & Homer, 1997; Margolis, Gay, & Humphrey, 1998). Approximately 2% of newborns in the United States are readmitted during the first 2 weeks of life (Raube & Merrell, 1999). Even if an additional inpatient day prevented all neonatal readmissions, the cost of care for mothers and babies increases by 18% when mothers choose to stay 2 days instead of 1 day after vaginal birth (Raube & Merrell, 1999). Women discharged within 24 hours after childbirth without complications have clinical outcomes similar to women who in the past had longer lengths of stay (Beebe, Britton, Britton, Fan, & Jepson, 1996; Behram et al., 1998; Braveman et al., 1995; Grullon & Grimes, 1997; Grupp-Phelan, Taylor, Liu, & Davis, 1999; Kotagal et al., 1997; Kotagal, Atherton, Eschett, Schoettker, & Perlstein, 1999; Keppler & Roudebush, 1999; Lieu et al., 1998; Meikle, Lyons, Hulac, & Orleans, 1998; Welsh & Ludwig-Beymer, 1998).

The main outcomes related to LOS that have been studied are healthcare costs and maternal–newborn complications that require rehospitalization (Brumfield, 1998). Several researchers found that early discharge within 24 hours after vaginal birth was as safe as discharge after 48 hours or longer (Beck, 1991; Carty & Bradley, 1990; Hall & Carty, 1993; Welt, Cole, Meyers, Sholes, & Jelovsek, 1993). However, there are more factors related to the postpartum experience than risk of readmission to the hospital, safe care, and costs. Less attention has been given to patient and family satisfaction as an outcome variable in early discharge research. As evidenced by the grassroots consumer movement and subsequent state and federal legislation, many women prefer to have the option to stay in the hospital longer than 24 hours after they give birth.

CURRENT ISSUES

According to current trends, LOS for childbirth is now more realistically in line with the physical and psychosocial needs of the new mother and her family rather than the previous arbitrary mandates from health insurance companies in an effort to control costs. However, although LOS has increased, it is still relatively short in all settings (Martell, 2000). Discharge planning cannot be delayed until admission for childbirth. Women in active labor and women who have just given birth are not candidates for a discussion of learning needs or for typical classroom education about self-care or infant care. The woman's focus during the intrapartum period is on safe passage through labor and on a healthy childbirth experience. Rubin's (1961) classic research suggests that during the immediate postpartum period the new mother is not physically or emotionally ready to listen to extensive presentations of how to care for herself and her newborn. Postpartum women have transient deficits in cognition, particularly in memory function, the first day after giving birth (Eidelman, Hoffmann, & Kaitz, 1993). Women describe feeling confused and forgetful after childbirth. Fathers also have cognitive deficits, although to a lesser degree (Eidelman et al., 1993). New mothers recognize their infants by olfactory or tactile cues, senses that do not primarily require cognitive function (Eidelman & Kaitz, 1992; Kaitz, Lapidot, Bronner, & Eidelman, 1992). Traditional discharge planning that includes verbal transmission of information or instruction in child care techniques on the first postpartum day is poorly remembered (Eidelman et al., 1993). These findings underscore the importance of providing the family with appropriate written material they can review after discharge (Eidelman & Kaitz 1992; Eidelman et al., 1993). Priorities for most women in the first 24 hours postpartum are rest; time to touch, hold, and get to know their newborn; and an opportunity to review and discuss their labor and birth.

Childbearing is very different today from the experience nearly 50 years ago when Rubin began her research. Major changes include the availability of prenatal classes; women and families as active participants in all aspects of perinatal care; fathers, siblings, and other support persons present for labor and birth; epidural anesthesia or analgesia; open visiting; single-room maternity care; couplet care models; and shorter hospitalizations. However, despite the progress made toward a healthcare environment in which childbearing women have more participation and control, much of Rubin's work about the taking-in and taking-hold phases of the postpartum period remains valid.

The discharge planning process is ongoing during pregnancy, labor, and the postpartum period. Although education about maternal and infant care can occur during the inpatient stay, information should be offered during pregnancy and reinforced after discharge in many different settings, using a variety of teaching methods. The prenatal period provides a window of opportunity to prepare families for pregnancy and birth and to explain the postpartum and newborn periods (Booth, 1996; Cook & McIntire, 1995; Lieu et al., 1998; Martell, 2000; Owens, 1996; Trenam, 1995; Zwelling, 2000). Prenatal visits to the primary healthcare provider are an ideal time for the perinatal nurse to assess family learning needs and concerns and to offer information, support, and resources in a personalized way. Prenatal classes should provide education about pregnancy, health promotion, labor and birth, postpartum, maternal and infant care, and the transition to parenthood. Critical concepts can then be reviewed and reinforced during the postpartum stay.

Follow-up home visits or visits to outpatient clinics and offices offer the perinatal nurse another opportunity to assess knowledge, skills, and learning needs and to provide individualized education, support, and referrals (American Academy of Pediatrics [AAP], 1995; Britton, 1998; Brown & Johnson, 1998; Carpenter 1998; Jacobson, Brock, & Keppler, 1999; Keppler & Roudebush, 1999; Lieu et al., 2000). If home visits are not possible, follow-up phone calls after discharge provide the perinatal nurse an opportunity to clarify information and answer additional questions. Classes and support groups for new parents are another way for families to continue learning about maternal and infant care, parenting, and how to nurture the couple relationship.

Healthcare providers continue to struggle to find innovative ways to provide safe, cost-effective, comprehensive perinatal care in response to economic pressures. Although consumer pressures resulted in state and federal laws mandating minimal LOS coverage, costs remain a real issue for institutions and individual healthcare providers. Prenatal education in healthcare provider offices and in the classroom, combined with case management and written materials, effectively prepares women and their families for discharge (Jacobson et al., 1999; Keppler & Roudebush, 1999). Women feel more in control and express greater feelings of maternal confidence and competence when they have adequate knowledge about how to care for themselves and their newborns after discharge (Beger & Cook, 1998; Keppler & Roudebush, 1999; Lieu et al., 1998; Lieu et al., 2000). This chapter describes strategies for developing a comprehensive approach to discharge planning. Through the use of prenatal databases, prenatal classes, case-management models, clinical pathways, individualized assessment tools, postdischarge follow-up visits or phone calls, and a variety of creative and innovative teaching methods, perinatal nurses can ease the transition from hospital to home and ensure childbearing families have acquired enough information and skills to safely care for the mother and newborn.

PRENATAL PATIENT DATABASE

Early identification and entry into the system can facilitate prenatal preparation for hospitalization and postpartum discharge. Successful programs require communication among primary healthcare providers, prenatal educators, community resources, and the perinatal center. A simple, user-friendly system that incorporates demographic data, estimated date of birth, significant clinical history, family assessment and learning needs, participation in prenatal education programs, and a mechanism to communicate all pertinent information to the inpatient unit is critical. A computerized database is ideal, but traditional file systems in addition to communication in person or by phone, facsimile (fax), and email also work well. Healthcare providers at each institution can develop a prenatal patient database to meet specific needs. For example, when a woman registers her intent to give birth at the institution early in pregnancy, demographic and insurance data can be entered into the system. Primary healthcare providers and those in community prenatal clinics who refer women for inpatient care can be encouraged to send notification about women who have selected the institution for childbirth.

Some hospitals have developed Internet web sites where women can register for childbirth classes, seek prenatal care information, download patient education materials, and take a virtual tour of the facilities. Summaries of the educational and clinical backgrounds, services, office hours, and insurance plan participation of healthcare providers who have privileges at the institutions can offer valuable information to women who are in the process of selecting a healthcare provider and institution for birth. Links to offices of obstetricians, family practice physicians, and nurse midwives on staff can be helpful as well. Information about financial criteria for eligibility to participate in programs such as Medicaid and the Special Supplemental Feeding Program for Women, Infants, and Children (WIC) is useful to selected families. As more families of childbearing age gain access to the Internet, these web sites can meet the needs of patients and of the healthcare institutions.

Healthcare providers can provide mothers with a childbirth and parenting preparation book (or suggest one to be purchased) in early pregnancy, supply expectant families with information about the institution, and urge them to take a tour. Brochures describing all perinatal services available at the institution, including telephone numbers, are especially helpful and ideally should be available in the offices of all healthcare providers affiliated with the institution. Families should be informed about prenatal classes and encouraged to attend. Selected women and their families can be referred for case management, especially when the pregnancy or the social or economic situation is complex.

By the 36th week of pregnancy, a record of prenatal care should be sent by the primary healthcare provider to the perinatal institution (American Academy of Pediatrics & American College of Obstetricians and Gynecologists, 1997). This information can be added to the database. Specific, individualized care plans or guides developed by the case manager, social worker, or perinatal nurse for the woman's inpatient stay also should be added to the database. With this type of system, when the woman is admitted for childbirth, the perinatal nurse has valuable information about the current maternal–fetal health status, family learning needs, and education programs the family attended. The quality and quantity of prenatal data about the childbearing family enhances the perinatal nurse's ability to provide individualized care and teaching.

PRENATAL CLASSES

In the past, most prenatal classes consisted of a series lasting 6 to 8 weeks and focused primarily on preparation for labor and birth and, to a lesser extent, on pregnancy, infant care, and the transition to parenthood. For many working couples, making the time commitment to attend a series of six classes is often difficult. Factors such as perceived knowledge, support systems, transportation issues, work schedules, child care availability, and previous newborn and childbirth experience influence the decision to attend prenatal classes. Many institutions and perinatal educators have responded to consumer needs by streamlining content to decrease program length and offering alternatives such as weekend programs, flexible hours, and antepartum home visits.

Information about health promotion should be presented early in pregnancy to have the opportunity to make a difference in pregnancy outcomes. Early pregnancy classes may include several topics:

- Fetal growth and development
- Expected physical changes during pregnancy
- Normal discomforts of pregnancy
- Lifestyle modifications
- Nutrition
- Activity and exercise
- Effects of smoking cigarettes, drinking alcohol, and using illegal drugs
- Need to ask primary healthcare providers about use of over-the-counter medications and medications prescribed by other healthcare providers before use
- Warning signs of pregnancy complications, including a comprehensive discussion about preterm labor signs and symptoms and when to call their primary healthcare provider if these signs and symptoms should occur

Many hospitals have developed courses that cover early pregnancy content and have systems in place that prompt referral to these classes when women are seen for their first prenatal visit. Close partnerships with healthcare providers who are affiliated with the institution are essential to encourage women and their partners to attend classes that focus on early pregnancy health promotion.

Traditional prepared-childbirth classes are offered during the third trimester, when the mother and her partner are intent on learning about how to cope with labor pain and what to expect during labor and birth. Although the process of labor and birth is valuable content, information about parenthood and infant care is also important for expectant parents. Display 18–1 shows the course content for classes over 6 weeks that include prepared childbirth and infant care information. For couples unable to meet the 6-week time commitment, classes that meet less frequently can be designed. Options can include a 1-, 2-, or 3-week series covering critical content that is prioritized based on class time limitations. Display 18–2 lists sample curricula for prenatal classes based on a 1-, 2-, or 3-week series. Classes about parenting issues and infant care have been developed by many institutions. These classes are more commonly attended during pregnancy, but some institutions have been successful in offering these classes to new parents during evening hours and inviting them to bring their newborn.

Although there is a significant need for information to assist in preparing couples for labor and birth, pregnant women and their partners can benefit from a comprehensive educational program that includes preconception health promotion, healthy behaviors during the prenatal period, breast-feeding, the postpartum period, and infant care content. Display 18–3 provides the suggested course content from early pregnancy to the postpartum period. Prenatal education classes should be designed to meet the needs of the population served and based on the knowledge of what information and skills are useful and relevant to expectant parents at various stages of pregnancy. Classes should be made available to a variety of women, including teenagers, women who have previously given birth but desire a review class, women requesting private instruction, women who are hospitalized or on bed rest at home for much of their pregnancy, and women who speak a language other than English. Classes focusing on breast-feeding, sibling preparation, grandparents, car-seat safety, exercise during pregnancy, labor preparation for women who desire a vaginal birth after a previous cesarean birth (VBAC), and families expecting more than one baby complement the core curriculum.

A comprehensive educational program developed by parent and childbirth educators in partnership with healthcare providers, perinatal nurses, and parents is ideal. A curriculum designed using a team approach ensures that educators provide families with important information about pregnancy, childbirth, infant care, and the transition to parenthood. Parent and birth educators play a significant role in preparing families for the postpartum period. It is important that their work is valued and that there is ongoing communication between the educators and the perinatal unit staff, especially if the educators are not formally affiliated with the institution. Disappointments and unmet expectations for the labor, birth, and postpartum experience can be avoided if childbirth educators are fully familiar with the policies of the perinatal unit. In some institutions, educators are invited to attend staff meetings and retreats and are offered the opportunity to spend time on the unit with a labor nurse periodically to maintain an awareness of the daily realities of the childbirth experience and unit routines.

(text continues on page 618)

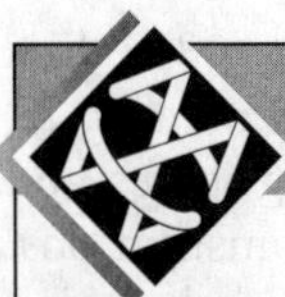

DISPLAY 18–1

Prepared Childbirth and Infant Care Class Curriculum Overview

Prepared Childbirth	*Infant Care*
Class I	
Introduction Discomforts of pregnancy Preterm labor Exercises Relaxation and breathing patterns Slow-paced breathing and progressive relaxation	Selecting a pediatrician Immunizations Childcare Babytime
Class II	
Preview of labor Relaxation and breathing patterns Favorite place, slow-paced, and bridged breathing Position changes for labor	Bathing video or bathing baby demonstration Changing or diapering Holding baby
Class III	
Birth video Goodybag Relaxation and breathing patterns Transition	Breast-feeding versus bottle-feeding video Burping Sleeping patterns Pacifiers
Class IV	
Labor, birth, and nursery tour Medical interventions	Newborn characteristics
Class V	
Labor rehearsal Review breathing and relaxation Emergency childbirth Cesarean birth video Medication, analgesia, anesthesia	Infant CPR Choking demonstration Illness and when to call pediatrician Parents as teachers video
Class VI	
Postpartum discussion Postpartum video Party	Safety video

Adapted from Harper, J. (1995). *Prenatal class content outline.* St. Louis: St. John's Mercy Medical Center.

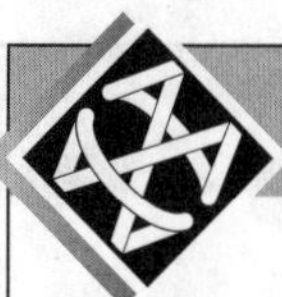

DISPLAY 18–2

Sample Curricula for Prenatal Classes

CLASS CONTENT: ONE 3-HOUR PRENATAL CLASS

Essentials to bring to the hospital
Early signs of labor and when to come to the hospital
What to expect during labor and birth
Formulating a birth plan
Anesthesia and analgesia options
Visiting policies
How to anticipate length of stay (LOS), third-party payer issues, precertification, deductibles, and copayments
Choosing a pediatrician
Warning signs of pregnancy complications, including preterm labor and preeclampsia
Maternal care issues: episiotomy care, normal lochia, afterpains, incision care, breast care, nutrition, rest, "baby blues"
Newborn care issues: umbilical cord care, circumcision care, breast-feeding, formula feeding, diapering, bathing, behavioral and satiation cues, crying, comforting, car seats, sleep positioning, and other safety issues
Videotapes and booklets to reinforce class content
Parent hotline number for additional questions
Community and institutional resources

CLASS CONTENT: TWO 3-HOUR PRENATAL CLASSES

Class I

Essentials to bring to the hospital
Formulating a birth plan
Early signs of labor, relaxation, and breathing techniques
When to come to the hospital
The admission process
Ambulation in early labor
Electronic fetal monitoring and intermittent auscultation
Labor induction and augmentation
Amniotomy
Active labor
Transition
Second stage of labor
Anesthesia and analgesia options, review of pain relief and comfort measures, nonpharmacologic and pharmacologic
The unanticipated cesarean birth
Visiting policies
How to anticipate LOS, third-party payer issues, precertification, deductibles, and copayments
Warning signs of pregnancy complications, including preterm labor and preeclampsia

Class II

Choosing a pediatrician
Maternal care issues: episiotomy care, normal lochia, afterpains, incision care, breast care, nutrition, rest, baby blues, sexuality issues, contraception, and family planning
Newborn care issues: umbilical cord care, circumcision care, breast-feeding, formula feeding, diapering, bathing, behavioral and satiation cues, sleep–awake state, crying, comforting, car seats, sleep positioning, other safety issues
Videotapes and booklets to reinforce class content
Parent hotline number for additional questions
Community and institutional resources

CLASS CONTENT: THREE 3-HOUR PRENATAL CLASSES

Class I

Brief overview of fetal development
Changes during pregnancy
Nutrition and lifestyle modification
Sexuality during pregnancy
Formulating a birth plan
Relaxation and breathing techniques
Childbirth options
Visiting policies
How to anticipate LOS, third-party payer issues, precertification, deductibles, and copayments
Choosing a pediatrician

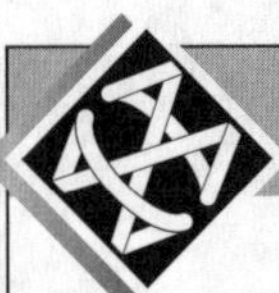

DISPLAY 18-2 (cont.)

Sample Curricula for Prenatal Classes

- Tour of perinatal unit
- Warning signs of pregnancy complications, including preterm labor and preeclampsia

Class II

- Essentials to bring to the hospital
- Early signs of labor and when to come to the hospital
- The admission process
- Ambulation in early labor
- Electronic fetal monitoring and intermittent auscultation
- Labor induction and augmentation
- Amniotomy
- Active labor
- Transition
- Second stage of labor
- Anesthesia and analgesia options, review of pain relief and comfort measures, nonpharmacologic and pharmacologic
- Reinforcement of relaxation and breathing techniques
- The unanticipated cesarean birth

Class III

- *Maternal care issues:* episiotomy care, normal lochia, afterpains, incision care, breast care, nutrition, rest, baby blues, sexuality issues, contraception and family planning
- *Newborn care issues:* umbilical cord care, circumcision care, breast-feeding, formula feeding, diapering, bathing, behavioral and satiation cues, sleep–awake state, crying and comforting, car seat, sleep positioning, other safety issues
- Videotapes and booklets to reinforce class content
- Parent hotline number for additional questions
- Community and institutional resources

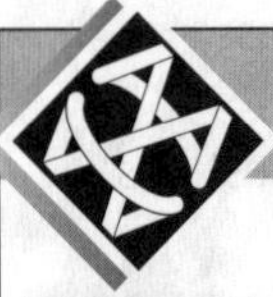

DISPLAY 18-3

Becoming Parents Course

The *Becoming Parents* course is designed to provide expectant families with the knowledge and skills needed to promote health during pregnancy and to prepare for childbirth and parenting. It reflects our philosophy that birth is one of life's most special events and that the role of family maternity education is to enhance the joy of this experience by providing families with support and education throughout the childbearing year in partnership with healthcare providers and hospital staff.

Celebrating Your Pregnancy—First Trimester

This informative and entertaining evening seminar focuses on how to grow a healthy baby and have a healthy pregnancy. You will learn about fetal growth and development, optimal lifestyle choices for pregnancy, workplace and environmental hazards to avoid, common changes in family relationships during pregnancy, how to be an informed healthcare consumer, and resources for education and support at Evergreen and in the community.
2-hour seminar

Growing the Baby of Your Dreams—Second Trimester

In the middle trimester, most families begin to imagine what their baby will look like and be like. You'll be amazed to discover the unique physical characteristics and capabilities of newborns and how able they are to respond to your love. We'll talk about what it means to be a parent and how becoming a parent affects your family relationships. You'll also learn about baby care and what supplies you'll need, and you will begin to master some of the labor coping skills such as relaxation and the first level of breathing. This series is also offered as *Christian Growing*

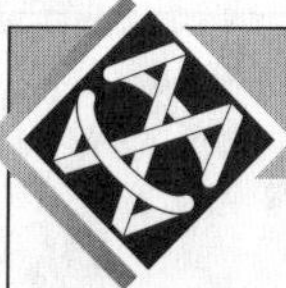

DISPLAY 18–3 (cont.)

Becoming Parents Course

Baby of Your Dreams, with time to discuss the spiritual aspects of pregnancy, birth, and parenting.
Two 2-hour classes or one 4-hour class, small group

Breast-feeding Basics—Second or Third Trimester
This class is recommended for all expectant families. You will learn about the health benefits of breast-feeding for mothers and infants, how to get off to a good start, how fathers, partners and family can support breast-feeding, and resources for support. A panel of families shares their breast-feeding experiences and valuable insights.
2-hour seminar

Breast-feeding and the 21st Century Family: Beyond the Basics—Second or Third Trimester (can be repeated after the birth)

Expectant mothers, fathers, partners, and family are encouraged to attend this class to learn about how breast-feeding fits into a busy lifestyle. You will learn how to express or pump breast milk, which pumps are best, how to store breast milk and for how long, and how to feed your baby when mother is away or at work. Tips for working mothers are provided. Breast-feeding Basics is a prerequisite.
2-hour seminar

Sneak Peek: A Look at Postpartum—Early Third Trimester
Take a peek at the realities of life with a newborn baby—the joys and the challenges. You will learn about physical recovery from birth and self-care to enhance healing and increase comfort. Also discussed are emotional and lifestyle changes to expect after delivery and resources to help you cope. A new-parent panel offers suggestions for a smooth transition to parenthood.
2-hour seminar

Birth Basics—Middle to Late Third Trimester

This class prepares you for childbirth. What to expect in labor and birth, how to develop an individual approach to birth, the partner's role in labor, breathing and relaxation techniques, methods of pain management, medical procedures, common variations in childbirth, and cesarean birth will be discussed. Included in this class is a tour of the Family Maternity Center. This series is also offered as Christian, Spanish-language, and Teen Birth Basics courses.
Four 2-hour classes or two 4-hour weekend classes, small group

OTHER CLASSES RELATED TO CHILDBIRTH AND EARLY PARENTING

During Pregnancy

- Vaginal Birth After Cesarean (VBAC)
- Labor and Birth Refresher
- Becoming Grandparents
- For Dads Only
- Sibling Preparation
- Car Safe Kids
- Maternity Fitness and Education
- Yoga for Pregnancy
- Family Maternity Center Tours

After Birth

- Parent–Baby Classes—a weekly class for parents and babies through the first year
- Yoga for New Moms
- Infant Massage
- Infant and Child CPR
- Early parenting seminars and series
  - Guiding Children's Behavior
  - Toddler Development
  - Parenting with Love and Logic
- Breast-feeding the Older Baby
- Starting Solids
- Infant Sleep and the Conflict with American Culture
- Young Moms Support Group
- This Is Not What I Expected—emotional support for new families in post partum

During Pregnancy or After

- IMET: Keys for Couples—a weekend seminar to strengthen couple relationships

In Special Circumstances

Private classes for childbirth preparation are available.

Adapted from Evergreen Hospital Medical Center. (1999).

EDUCATIONAL METHODS AND MATERIALS

Whether education is provided at the bedside, in a large auditorium, or in a small classroom, the teaching method must complement the information presented and must be appropriate for the learner. Skills such as comfort measures during labor, infant bathing, or cord care are most effectively taught by demonstration and return demonstration. Feelings and beliefs are best addressed individually or in a small group setting. Consideration should be given to personal learning styles and basic educational level and knowledge (Booth, 1995; Doak, Doak, & Root, 1985; Farrell, Bushnell, & Haag-Heitman, 1998; Freda, Damus, & Merkatz, 1999; O'Connor, 1997; Zwelling, 2000). Including parents as part of the prenatal education team enhances the likelihood that topics offered will be what parents want and need to know.

Written materials support and reinforce interactive learning. Books, pamphlets, brochures, and other handouts must have a consistent message and support the philosophy of the perinatal institution. There are several excellent resources in print, or the prenatal educators may develop their own educational materials. Selection or development of written materials should be based on the educational level of the population served and the financial resources available. The healthcare provider, educator, and representatives from the perinatal institution should collectively choose written materials and be familiar with the contents. Parents should be asked to evaluate the usefulness and helpfulness of the written materials. Providing families with standardized written materials can be a time-saving and cost-effective strategy. This approach provides a ready resource for parents at any time and potentially decreases the volume of calls to the perinatal center and to the primary healthcare provider. Written materials should be developed or chosen with consideration of the basic language level of the family and the language they speak. Families who do not speak English should be supplied with language-appropriate materials.

Some institutions use in-hospital television channels with programs on newborn bathing, cord and circumcision care, and breast-feeding and formula feeding. Purchased videos or those produced by the institution are another method of providing important information. The videos can be given as gifts, loaned to families, or purchased in the hospital gift shop. As with written materials, television instruction and videos need to be evaluated for consistent, correct information that is learner appropriate and reflects the philosophy of the perinatal institution.

FAMILY PREFERENCE PLAN

Involving women and their families in decisions about their perinatal care increases satisfaction and promotes a collaborative relationship between healthcare providers and families. A preference plan helps to individualize the family's care (Display 18–4). Women who are asked about care preferences feel their unique needs will be met by nurses and other healthcare providers. Advantages of methods that encourage women and their families to define their individual approach to birth, such as a birth plan or a list of family preferences, include validation of the family's knowledge of available labor and birth options and perinatal center policies. The family preference plan can be given to all pregnant women registered for birth or given to families during prenatal classes. The preference plan provides the healthcare provider with information about the family's special needs, concerns, and requests and allows the healthcare provider to have a meaningful discussion with the family members about their expectations. This discussion should occur during the pregnancy with the primary healthcare provider and with the perinatal nurse on admission to the unit for labor and birth.

Preference plans can be helpful in clarifying unit protocols and avoiding unmet expectations when women have plans for techniques or procedures that are not available on the unit. For example, the woman may have learned about the benefits of hydrotherapy in a Jacuzzi tub and wish to labor in the tub, but the unit may not have a Jacuzzi tub available; the woman may intend to use candles for aromatherapy although the unit may not allow burning candles for safety reasons; or the woman may plan to use a birthing ball during labor and the unit may not have birthing balls. If these limitations are known in advance of admission, alternative plans can be made. In the examples described previously, hydrotherapy can be provided in the shower, aromatherapy can be used with methods that do not include candles, and a birthing ball can be obtained on loan from a childbirth educator or purchased before admission.

The preference plan can be sent to the hospital with the prenatal care records or brought to the unit by the woman on admission for childbirth. Any system for recording childbirth preferences must ensure that the information is available to the nurses when the woman is admitted for labor and birth. The initial interaction during the admission process is used to develop rapport with the woman and her family and to get a sense of their expectations for their birth experience. Ideally, the amount of childbirth preparation

DISPLAY 18–4

Family Preference Plan

My name: ____________________ My doctor's name: ____________________

1. I would like to have these persons visit during labor:

   ____________________ ____________________

   ____________________ ____________________

2. My main support person is:
   Relationship: ____________________
3. For pain control/positioning during labor and birth, I would like to:
   ________ walk in room/halls
   ________ sit in recliner
   ________ use shower
   ________ use jacuzzi
   ________ use heat/cold/massage
   ________ listen to special music
   ________ use special focal point
   ________ use my own pillows
   ________ use squat bar
   ________ use foot pads on bed
4. I would like to have these persons present during birth:

   ____________________ ____________________

5. I have these religious requests:
   ________ birth blessing by chaplain
   ________ eucharist or communion
   ________ have visit by my own clergy
   ________ other: ____________________
   ________ none
6. After birth: I would like to:
   ________ place baby skin-to-skin
   ________ wrap baby in blanket before holding
   ________ breast-feed my baby
   ________ bathe my baby
   ________ have doctor circumcise my son
   ________ have pictures taken of my baby
   ________ keep baby in my room as long as he/she is stable
7. During my hospital stay, I would like to have my support person:
   ________ put baby skin-to-skin to him or her
   ________ assist with baby care
   ________ give the baby's first bath
   ________ spend the night in my room
   ________ take pictures of birth experience
8. I plan to attend, or have already attended, these classes/services during this pregnancy:
   ________ prenatal class
   ________ hospital OB tour
   ________ sibling class
   ________ exercise sessions
   ________ lamaze
9. Child care has been arranged for other dependent children:
   ________ during the hospital stay
   ________ after mom and baby go home
   ________ not applicable
   ________ other:

DISPLAY 18-4 (cont.)

Family Preference Plan

10. I plan to have my other child(ren) come to visit:
    ________ during labor
    ________ during birth
    ________ in the first 2-hour recovery time
    ________ after I arrive in my postpartum room
    ________ not at all
    ________ not applicable
11. After going home, these persons will help out for the first two days:
    ____
    ____
12. Additional ideas:
    ____
    ____
    ____
    ____
    ____

From Methodist Perinatal Center, Omaha, NE (1994).

and type of pain management anticipated during labor are topics covered during the admission assessment. A review of preferences for childbirth, including reinforcement of options that are available at the institution, works best to facilitate a positive experience. Although some labor nurses have negative feelings about written birth plans, a birth plan helps the nurse meet the couple's expectations and indicates the woman has given considerable thought to how she would like labor and birth to proceed. Every effort should be made to meet the expectations and wishes of the woman. The woman's desires for positioning, ambulation, and method of fetal assessment should be honored in ways that are consistent with safe care. If maternal or fetal status is such that the woman's wishes cannot be met within reason, a thorough discussion with adequate explanation of the rationale for the decision should occur. The woman should be allowed and encouraged to ask questions and be given appropriate answers. It may be necessary for the primary healthcare provider to talk to the woman in person or by telephone about her concerns. The nurse should acknowledge the woman's disappointment and assure her that every attempt to meet her expectations will be made if the clinical situation changes.

Arbitrary rules prohibiting more than one support person during labor and birth are contrary to the philosophy that the birth experience belongs to the woman and her family rather to those providing clinical care. Although healthcare providers are sometimes inclined to attempt to control this aspect of the birth process using various arguments for safety and convenience, when examined critically, these arguments have little scientific merit. Women should be able to choose who will be with them during this very special and unique life experience (Rouse & MacNeil, 2000). Family-centered care supports the concept that the "family" is defined by the childbearing woman. Families should be free to take still pictures and record video or audio tapes during labor and birth. Policies restricting cameras are in conflict with the philosophy that the birth experience should be, within reason, what the woman and her family desire. Concerns about safety, liability, privacy, and space limitations can be adequately addressed without restrictive policies about visitors and use of cameras during labor and birth if care providers are committed to meeting the needs of childbearing women and their support persons.

LEARNING-NEEDS ASSESSMENT

Learning-needs assessment tools assist nurses and families in identifying maternal learning needs and in documentation of the type and timing of prenatal education (Keppler & Roudebush, 1999; Memke, 1993).

A learning-needs assessment can be initiated at various times during the perinatal period, depending on when a woman has first contact with the hospital system. Opportunities include prenatal classes, prenatal visits, hospital tours, telephone contact with a case manager, during admission to the hospital, after birth, and at the mother–infant follow-up visit or contact.

Many families attending prenatal classes are first-time parents. A detailed assessment of individual learning needs discussed during the first prenatal class alerts prospective parents to information and skills they need to acquire by the time they are discharged from the hospital. The learning-needs assessment tool or the defined curriculum and supporting written materials document the information, the instruction provided, and the skills taught. When a formal learning-needs assessment tool is used during pregnancy, the tool is forwarded to the perinatal unit from the prenatal instructor to be stored with the woman's prenatal data. Display 18–5 is an example of a learning-needs assessment tool used after birth to assess the woman's knowledge of self-care and baby care, and it then becomes the discharge teaching record. Content marked with an asterisk is reviewed with all women before hospital discharge. Referencing specific content to written materials provides reinforcement and promotes use of materials as a reference for families and perinatal nurses.

For women who have not attended prenatal classes or completed a learning-needs assessment during a prenatal visit, the process begins on admission to the hospital. With the help of the labor nurse, families identify specific learning needs they want to address during the inpatient stay. Whether the needs assessment is completed before admission, during early labor, or after birth, the educational process begins as soon as possible for each family.

Primary responsibility for patient and family education varies with the institution. Patient education may be coordinated by the case manager, clinical nurse specialist, or perinatal educator; however, in any practice model, the perinatal staff nurse plays a key role. Critical concepts and essential information that families need have been identified. They are presented regardless of the family's past experience or self-assessment.

Maternal care includes the following concepts:

- Activity and rest
- Pain relief and comfort measures
- Care of the perineum and care of lacerations or episiotomy
- Breast care for breast-feeding women and lactation suppression for women who are formula feeding
- Postoperative cesarean birth instructions
- Expected emotional adaptations
- Signs of postpartum complications to report to the nurse in the hospital or to the healthcare provider after discharge

Newborn care care includes the following concepts:

- Newborn adaptation to extrauterine life: need to be held, need for thermoregulation, and need for comfort
- Newborn feeding cues
- Breast-feeding basics
- Formula-feeding basics
- Care of an infant who is spitting up or choking
- Use of the bulb syringe
- Umbilical cord care
- Circumcision care or care of the uncircumcised penis
- Position for sleep (ie, Back to Sleep campaign to reduce the risk of sudden infant death syndrome)
- Information about immunizations and newborn screening tests
- Signs of newborn complications to report to the nurse in the hospital or to the healthcare provider after discharge
- Safe use of car seats
- Appointment made for follow-up clinic or home visit offered by the hospital or community nursing agency
- When to schedule the first mother and newborn visits with their primary care provider

Written materials provided to the woman and her family should contain information about all critical concepts (Beger & Cook, 1998; Keppler & Roudebush, 1999; Lieu et al., 1998).

Before discharge, knowledge and skills about self-care and infant care are validated. Validation can be accomplished by discussion with the new mother during which understanding is verbalized or by demonstration of critical skills such as feeding, sleeping position, or umbilical cord care. No one method of validation is superior; nurses in each institution can develop a system with enough flexibility to meet the needs of the population served. Validation ensures that women who indicate that they need no additional information are truly prepared and knowledgeable. The goal is for all women to verbalize understanding or demonstrate skills related to all critical concepts. Women with special needs who have not demonstrated knowledge of critical concepts or have not acquired the skills to care for themselves or their infants are referred for follow-up support and care. Referrals are made to the clinical nurse specialist, lactation consultant, social worker, dietitian, or home care agency.

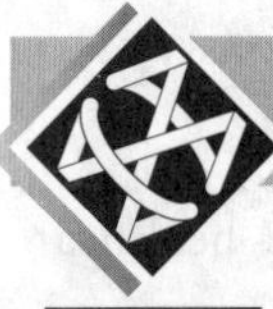

DISPLAY 18-5

Mother–Baby Discharge Record

I know this already	Doesn't apply to me	I need to know more	Please go through the following list and check whether you understand each topic or need to know more. Please read ...*For Moms and Babies* booklet given to you **after** the birth of your baby.		Booklet page #	NURSES MUST INITIAL Mother & family reviewed/ demonstrated
			POSTPARTUM			
			Activity – how much is OK		11	*
			Care of perineum and episiotomy		7,8	*
			Postoperative C-section instructions		9	*
			Signs of postpartum complications		11	*
			Changes in vaginal bleeding, return of my period		7	
			Comfort measures for afterpains, constipation and hemorrhoids		7,9	
			Postpartum "baby blues," depression, hormonal changes		10	
			Postpartum exercises for the first weeks		11	
			How to minimize milk production if I'm not nursing		8	
			BABY CARE			
			What to do if baby is choking or gagging		14	*
			How to do skin care/cord care		14	*
			How to take care of the circumcision or genital area	Type: Bell/Gomco	13	*
			How to know if my baby is sick and what to do		21	
			What is jaundice and how to detect it		15	
			Use and cleaning of bulb syringe		14,15	*
			How and when to burp baby		17	
			How to position baby after feeding		17	*
			How to complete and obtain a birth certificate		20,21	
			BREAST-FEEDING			
			I attended Breastfeeding class/watched Breast-feeding video	☐ YES ☐ NO		
			How to position baby for feeding		23	*
			How to get baby to latch onto my nipple properly		23	*
			Removal of baby from my nipple		24	*
			What is the supply and demand concept		23,24	*
			When does breast milk come in		25	
			Implications of supplementing for breast-feeding mothers		24	
			Prevention and comfort measures for sore nipples		24	
			Prevention and comfort measures for engorgement		25	
			How to express milk by hand/breast pump		25	
			BOTTLE FEEDING			
			How and when to feed my baby a bottle		16	*
			Reasons for NOT propping bottles		17	
			What formula should my baby drink		16	
			State Law requires use of infant car seat. I have a baby/infant car seat and know how to use it.	☐ YES ☐ NO		

Discharge weight _____ lb _____ oz
Medications:
Mother: None   Prescriptions: ____________
Baby: None   Prescriptions: ____________
Discharge Instructions: ____________

Follow-up doctor's appointment:
Mother: Date: ____________
Baby: Date: ____________
Please call your doctor if you have any questions or concerns.

My discharge instructions have been explained to me and I have received a copy.

Signature: ____________

Person receiving infant: ____________

Postpartum
Discharge Nurse: ____________ Date: ________ Time: ________

Nursery Nurse: ____________ Date: ________

White–Mother's Record; **Canary**–Baby's Record; **Pink**–Mother

MOTHER-BABY DISCHARGE RECORD

St. John's Mercy Medical Center/St. Louis, MO

Form 583 (11/93)

PKU (Repeat) Instructions (if necessary): By state law your baby must be tested for these metabolic diseases. Bring your baby to the admitting lab on 2L (next to the escalators) within 3-5 days after discharge. No appointment is necessary. You may come Monday through Friday and Saturday morning. There will be no additional charge. Call 569-6814 for specific hours.

Metabolic Screen (PKU/Thyroid/Galactosemia)
Date: ________ Time: ________ Repeat needed: ☐ YES ☐ NO
(If yes - see instructions above.)

Nurses Signature(s) and Initials	

PATIENT IDENTIFICATION

Follow-up contacts to ensure that the critical concepts have been learned and to verify the woman can safely care for her infant and herself can occur at a follow-up clinic or home visit, during a phone assessment, through involvement in support groups and community programs, or at healthcare provider office visits. Assessment of maternal knowledge and skills is documented on the clinical pathway, discharge teaching record, or other appropriate medical record form.

CASE MANAGEMENT

Case management is an excellent way to enhance the quality of perinatal services. In a case-management model, the case manager interacts with the expectant woman and her family over the continuum of perinatal care from entry into the system through the postpartum period, including follow-up visits after discharge. The case manager coordinates a case load of families in collaboration with the nursing staff, physicians, midwives, and other healthcare professionals. An obvious advantage of this approach is that there is one person with comprehensive knowledge of each family and responsibility to ensure all important and special needs are addressed. Coordination and collaboration enhance continuity of care, promote cost-effective use of resources, ensure expected maternal–newborn outcomes occur in a timely manner, and improve family, healthcare provider, and nurse satisfaction. As the case manager follows the woman and her family during pregnancy, potential risk factors and educational needs are identified, and the adequacy of family and community support system is assessed. The case manager can then make appropriate referrals and develop a care plan or guide for the antepartum, intrapartum, and postpartum periods. Display 18–6 shows a sample case management record.

The case manager uses a variety of opportunities to identify and contact pregnant women in the system during the prenatal period. Ideally, the case manager initially contacts women after a referral is received from the healthcare provider's office, insurance company, public health nurse, or prenatal educator. The first contact is usually made by telephone, although some institutions report success by sending newly pregnant women information about prenatal classes and inviting them to take tours of the perinatal center. The woman then contacts the case manager at her convenience. Method and type of initial contact are based on the population served.

Women are encouraged to attend prenatal classes during which learning needs and risks are identified. For women who are unable to attend prenatal classes, assessment can be accomplished through alternative methods. For example, a prenatal visit with the case manager can be arranged to coincide with a prenatal office appointment. Women who present to the hospital without prenatal care or who are emergently transferred from another facility are managed from the time they arrive or when contact is made for tertiary care referral. When the woman's clinical situation is complicated by maternal or infant health problems or difficult emotional and social circumstances, the case manager may meet with the mother or with the entire family.

During the inpatient stay, the case manager and primary nurse work in collaboration. The primary nurse reviews the learning-needs assessment and patient care plan completed during the prenatal period. Discussion with the woman can determine whether the data are still accurate or if there are new needs or areas of concern. A new mother and father may not have confidence in their ability to care for the newborn despite participation in prenatal classes, presentation of maternal–newborn care content, and satisfactory demonstration of expected skills such as umbilical cord care, diapering, feeding, and holding the newborn. Maternal confidence affects family discharge needs. It is also important to identify and address concerns that the mother and family feel are important, even though data may not have been identified by the primary nurse or case manager as significant. Common issues that can inhibit confidence are perceived feeding difficulties, inability to soothe the crying newborn, prior parenting experience, limited financial resources, and past physical or emotional problems.

The medical record is reviewed for indications of preexisting physical and psychosocial conditions. If complicating factors with the potential for affecting the discharge needs of the mother or newborn are identified, the case manager is notified. The family's knowledge and current use of institutional and community resources are evaluated. Possession of supplies and equipment in the home that are necessary to provide safe care for the newborn is determined.

Based on the learning-needs assessment form, the case manager or primary nurse initiates or reinforces maternal–newborn teaching. As the case manager completes the teaching process or makes referrals, there is communication with the primary nurse. Appropriate referrals to institutional and community resources are made. Examples of inpatient referrals are to the clinical nurse specialist, lactation consultant, nutritionist, nurse midwife, nurse practitioner, physician, or social worker. Outpatient referral can be made to community services such as home healthcare agencies, parent support groups, WIC services, breast-feeding support

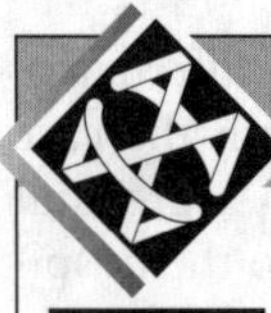

DISPLAY 18–6

Evergreen Hospital Medical Center
Family Maternity Center
Prenatal Care Management Guide Worksheet

Name ______________________ Age ____ EDB _____ Physician/Midwife ______________

Husband/Partner ______________________ Phone H ______________________ W ______________________

Full term pregnancies ____ Preterm births _____ Miscarriages _____ TAB ____ Live Children _____ Losses _____

Pregnancy History:

Past notable pregnancy/birth/postpartum experiences (eg, past C/Birth, poor experience, fast labor, PIH, preterm birth, hemorrhage, etc.)

Any current pregnancy complications? (eg, hypertension, anemia, low platelets, expecting twins/triplets, needle phobia, latex allergy, dietary needs such as allergies, vegan)

Current medications:

Social history (eg, insurance, home support, list people with whom she lives, community support such as WIC, PHN, Healthystart program, plans to relinquish baby and has chosen adoptive family, counseling, possibility of abuse or domestic violence, and additional needs identified)

Emotional well-being (eg, past history of mood disorders, seeing a counselor, medications, past or current history of sexual abuse, physical abuse or rape)

Education needs (eg, Becoming Parents Course, has read books and written materials and identified education needs)

Special needs or requests for labor and birth (eg, support persons, doula, pain management plan, desires to be a "no information patient," what the family needs from their nurse, consultations during inpatient stay)

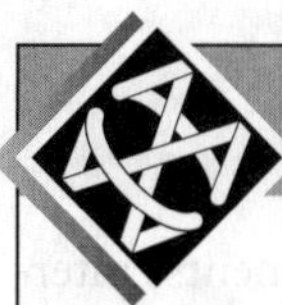

DISPLAY 18–6 (cont.)

Evergreen Hospital Medical Center
Family Maternity Center
Prenatal Care Management Guide Worksheet

For Baby (eg, physician chosen for baby, feeding method, concerns about feeding, requests oral vitamin K, delayed eye prophylaxis, will decline certain procedures, infant has known medical condition requiring neonatology presence at birth or transfer to another center)

For Postpartum (eg, needs referral to lactation consultant, social services, bereavement service, community resources and support groups, additional classes)

Use this worksheet during prenatal telephone or in-person contact to develop a plan of care for the inpatient stay and time following discharge. Care guide to be attached to prenatal record: White copy is chart copy and purple copy to physician or midwife. Additional copies to Breast-feeding Center, Postpartum Care Center, Special Care Nursery, Social Service, Infant's physician, Dietary, etc., as appropriate.

Evergreen Hospital Medical Center 1999. Used with permission.

groups, and community health clinics. The case manager may also coordinate services that include follow-up telephone calls or postpartum home visits.

ROLE OF THE STAFF NURSE

Not all perinatal centers have developed case-management positions or have nurses in advanced-practice roles. Staff nurses plan, coordinate, and participate in successful discharge planning programs. Ideally, prenatal educators have a partnership with unit-based nurses. However, in many institutions, resources for prenatal education are limited, and perinatal staff nurses also teach prenatal classes. In some cases, the staff nurse fills the roles of prenatal educator, case manager, and inpatient care provider. Benefits of this approach include presentation of realistic expectations of what will happen during hospitalization by someone providing direct patient care and a heightened awareness of consumer desires and concerns related to the childbearing experience.

In many institutions, staff nurse committees develop clinical pathways, care plans, individualized maternal–newborn learning-needs assessment tools, and prepare patient educational materials. The staff nurse has the most interaction with the woman and her family during the postpartum hospitalization. Ultimately, responsibility for ensuring women and their families have the necessary information and skills related to maternal–newborn care rests with the nurse at the bedside.

Opportunities for teaching occur during all aspects of clinical care. Assessment of the perineum, laceration, or episiotomy can include instructions about perineal care, suggestions to increase comfort, characteristics of normal lochia, and issues related to sexual activity. While checking the fundus, the nurse can discuss involution and afterbirth pains. The initial newborn bath given in the mother's room provides an excellent opportunity to teach the family about newborn physical characteristics, sleep and awake states, ways to comfort a crying infant, and infant sensory and behavioral capabilities. A discussion about newborn sleep and awake states can lead to suggestions for ensuring adequate maternal rest after discharge. While assisting the new mother with breast-feeding, the nurse can provide information about infant feeding cues, position, and latch-on; normal feeding patterns; and resources for help after discharge. While helping mothers who are formula feeding, information about formula preparation, care of feeding equipment, how to hold the baby, and how to suppress lactation can be offered. If family members are present, involving them in discussions promotes family–newborn attachment and encourages their participation with newborn care at home.

Ideally, the staff nurse has sufficient time before discharge to review critical areas of maternal–newborn education and to help mothers and families acquire the skills needed for maternal and newborn care. The nurse documents that essential education was provided to mothers and families on the mother's and infant's institutional clinical pathway or discharge teaching forms. Mothers and their partners have cognitive deficits in the first day after birth. They learn by experiencing and doing, and they forget detailed, scripted verbal information (Beger & Cook, 1998; Eidelman et al., 1993; Farrell et al., 1998). The method of teaching used during inpatient education must be developed to meet the learning needs of the new mother and her partner (Eidelman et al., 1993). Written materials that highlight essential information serve as a resource for families after they are home. Perinatal staff nurses, breast-feeding consultants, and postpartum and home visit nurses continue to play an important role in answering patient questions after discharge. Some institutions have "warm lines" with designated staff to triage calls from new mothers and refer them to appropriate healthcare providers. Other institutions routinely refer calls about newborn care to nurses in the newborn nursery. If this is the practice, it is important to keep a log of the calls, the patient's name, the primary healthcare provider, questions asked, advice given, and referrals. A system in place to notify the primary healthcare provider about their patients' questions and the resolutions is ideal. Because of liability issues, some institutions have discontinued giving advice to new parents over the phone and have initiated policies that direct parents to call their primary healthcare provider for all questions and concerns after discharge. If the call involves an obvious emergency, parents can be told to bring the baby to the emergency department instead of waiting to contact and receive a call back from their primary healthcare provider.

The inpatient perinatal nurse influences successful transition from hospital to home by assessing individual learning needs, giving accurate information, encouraging independence in self-care and newborn care, and promoting confidence in the mothering and parenting role. A positive experience during childbirth and in the immediate postpartum period sets the stage for continued adaptation to parenthood at home.

CARE PATHS

Care paths are used to ensure that assessments, interventions, and appropriate outcomes are accomplished within a limited time. The ability to look at care in distinct time frames across the perinatal continuum increases the possibility that mothers and their families receive essential education and support from early pregnancy through the postpartum period. The inpatient stay is short; therefore, much of the education families need for postpartum and newborn care must begin prenatally and continue throughout the impatient stay rather than being delayed until immediately before discharge. Care paths are used as a prospective overview of the entire childbearing process, beginning during the prenatal period and continuing through postpartum follow-up visits or phone calls and including ongoing evaluation of program effectiveness and patient satisfaction.

Care paths provide a timeline for assessments, interventions, teaching, and evaluation for further follow-up. Appendix 18A provides a series of care paths designed for expectant parents that begin at 12 weeks of pregnancy and continue until the infant is 12 months old. Parents can use the pathways to anticipate and plan for specific phases of the pregnancy, labor, birth, and the postpartum period. Common diagnostic tests and procedures, medications, assessments, activity, diet, and discharge planning tips are listed. Suggestions for classes appropriate for each phase of the continuum from pregnancy to postpartum are included. A copy of the family care path should be given to all families as part of their written materials. Providing families with a copy of the care path ensures that they know what to expect during all aspects of pregnancy, labor, birth, and the postpartum period. A care path written in understandable language promotes collaboration between families and the perinatal healthcare team. Women and families have a concise resource describing the healthcare provider's thoughtful plan for their care. They can be reassured that their educational and healthcare needs will be met in an individualized way during the course of their pregnancy, labor, birth, and postpartum period.

Care paths are also used in the inpatient setting to assist healthcare providers in planning clinical aspects of care and education. Frequency of maternal–newborn assessments and common interventions are outlined. Care path time frames are adjusted based on the method of birth and expected LOS. It is important to allow for flexibility as needed according specific maternal–newborn needs and unplanned complications. Some maternal and newborn complications occur with enough frequency that specific care paths or clinical algorithms may be developed to guide consistent and safe care, such as for preterm labor and postpartum care of the woman who gave birth preterm after a period of antepartum bed rest, hypertensive disorders of pregnancy, and newborn hyperbilirubinemia. In addition to clinical aspects of care, critical maternal–newborn educational content to be discussed with all families before discharge is listed and the appropriate time for discussion indicated. Teaching may be completed before the scheduled time frame; it should not occur later than the scheduled time unless a special plan to address the content is made and documented in the medical record along with a notation about why the teaching was not completed.

Care paths provide an organized approach to meeting clinical care and teaching goals in specific time frames, but other methods can be equally successful in streamlining perinatal services and accomplishing desired patient care and educational outcomes. Use of routine antepartum, intrapartum, and postpartum orders; traditional nursing care plans; and maternal–newborn teaching checklists can ensure that all women are provided similar clinical care and educational opportunities in the inpatient setting. Essential components of all types of plans for care are flexibility and the ability to individualize care based on the specific needs of the woman and newborn (Joint Commission on Accreditation of Healthcare Organizations, 2000).

POSTDISCHARGE FOLLOW-UP

In response to the current LOS, many perinatal centers offer postdischarge follow-up home or clinic visits or telephone calls. The AAP's *Committee on the Fetus and Newborn* (1995) recommends that in-person follow-up by a knowledgeable clinician occurs within 48 hours of discharge after a maternity stay of 48 hours or less. The optimal time for assessing mothers and their infants is between 3 and 4 days after birth when infections, poor infant feeding, excessive weight loss, jaundice, and other problems become evident (Jacobson et al., 1999; Keppler & Roudebush, 1999; Maisels & Kring, 1997).

In-person follow-up visits afford the perinatal nurse an opportunity to carefully assess maternal and infant well-being and provide the family with continuing education and support (Gagnon et al., 1997). In some institutions, the primary staff nurse may see the family for the follow-up visit. The family may return to the hospital and be seen in a room set aside for outpatient follow-up visits, or the primary nurse may make a follow-up visit at the family's home. In other institutions, the volume of visits is large enough to require a separate nursing staff for follow-up visits (Britton, 1998; Brown & Johnson, 1998; Carpenter, 1998; Frank-Hanssen, Hanson, & Anderson, 1999; Jacobson et al., 1999; Keppler & Roudebush, 1999; Lieu et al., 1998; Lieu et al., 2000; Olds et al., 1999).

Medical complications identified during the visit are immediately referred to the primary healthcare provider. Other issues or concerns are addressed during the visit or referred to an appropriate resource. A record of assessments, including pertinent information such as maternal and infant vital signs, infant weight, hyperbilirubinemia, patient concerns, and referrals made, is sent or faxed to the healthcare provider on the day of the visit (AAP, 1995).

When in-person follow-up visits are not offered, a postdischarge phone call gives families another opportunity to ask questions and receive important information and referrals. The perinatal nurse, using a standardized assessment tool, asks the family about infant feeding and elimination patterns, cord care, infant appearance and behavior, maternal comfort, lochia flow, perineal care, breast care, and maternal emotional well-being (Display 18–7). The nurse asks the mother if she has any concerns about herself or her infant and reminds the mother about specific situations that would warrant a telephone call to the healthcare provider. The nurse refers the mother to the written materials provided by the institution for further information.

Ideally, all women should receive a visit or telephone call after discharge from the hospital. If resources are limited, the following criteria define circumstances for which postdischarge follow-up is essential:

- LOS less than 24 hours after a vaginal birth
- LOS less than 48 hours after a cesarean birth
- Limited or no prenatal care
- Infant feeding problems identified during hospital stay
- Infant gestational age of less than 37 weeks
- Risk factors for developing hyperbilirubinemia
- Health conditions putting mother or infant at risk for complications
- Lack of adequate support system
- Women who express or show they feel overwhelmed, very anxious, or depressed
- Discharge evaluation indicating the need for further teaching

The nurse providing postdischarge follow-up should have access to essential patient information, including maternal age, health history, delivery infor-

DISPLAY 18–7

Early Discharge Follow-Up Telephone Call Report

Mother: Age ________ G/P ________ Vag Birth ________ C/Birth ________

Marital status: S M W Discharge date: ________

Baby: Sex: M F Gestational age: ________

Newborn birth weight ________ Discharge weight ________

Breast ________ Formula ________ Person making call: ________

BABY CARE	NO CONCERNS	PROBLEM IDENTIFIED	SUGGESTION MADE
Circumcision assessment			
Cord assessment			
Jaundice			
Changes in Newborn:			
Behavior			
Feeding			
Temperature			
Breast-feeding:			
# wet diapers			
# & character of stools			
latch-on/positioning			
Frequency of feeding/24 hours			
Breast & nipple assessment:			
Sore nipples			
Cracked nipples			
Breast fullness			
Suck/swallow assessment			
Other concerns			
Formula Feeding:			
# wet diapers			
# & characteristics of stools			
Ounces/feedings			
Frequency of feedings			
Skin appearance			
Sleep patterns			
Ability to care for newborn			

MATERNAL CARES	NO CONCERNS	PROBLEM IDENTIFIED	SUGGESTION MADE
Lochia			
Episiotomy			
Incision			
Discomforts:			
Breast			
Perineal			
Incisional			

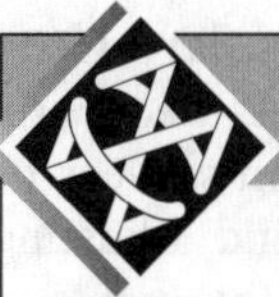

DISPLAY 18–7 (cont.)

Early Discharge Follow-Up Telephone Call Report

MATERNAL CARES	NO CONCERNS	PROBLEM IDENTIFIED	SUGGESTION MADE
Cramping			
Calf/leg tenderness			
Hemorrhoids			
Voiding:			
Frequency			
Dysuria			
Bowel Movement			
Emotional:			
Weepy			
Fatigue			
Sadness			
Onset of feelings			
Adequate rest:			
Taking naps			
Sleeps well when baby sleeps			
Other			
Ability to care for self			

REFERRALS	DATE	PROBLEM IDENTIFIED	SUGGESTION MADE
Lactation Consultant			
Social Services			
Physician			
Clinical Specialist			
Home Health Care			
WIC			
Other			

From Methodist Perinatal Center, Omaha, NE (1994)

mation, newborn assessment, infant weight, method of infant feeding, and name of the infant's and mother's healthcare provider. The nurse's assessment is documented and maintained as part of the permanent medical record. Periodic review of accumulated assessment forms provide the institution with important data to be able to identify common concerns and outcomes. Data can be used to revise and strengthen patient educational programs and patient care provided as part of discharge planning.

PROGRAM EVALUATION

An essential first step in program evaluation is identification of goals and expected outcomes. Primary outcome criteria include family knowledge about maternal–newborn care, ability to identify support persons and community resources, and familiarity with signs and symptoms of complications that warrant a call to the primary healthcare provider. Criteria met at discharge and in the immediate postpartum period should be included in the evaluation process. Quantitative and qualitative approaches to data collection are useful.

Quantitative evaluation may be concurrent or retrospective review of medical record data, tracking readmissions, or keeping a log of parent's phone calls to the nursery or maternity unit (Edmonson, Stoddard, & Owens, 1997; Keppler & Roudebush, 1999; Soskolne, Schumacher, Fyack, Young, & Schork, 1996; Welsh & Ludwig-Beymer, 1998). Care path variance data provides information about maternal–newborn teaching and care completed within suggested time frames during the inpatient stay. Primary healthcare providers can participate in data collection by tracking phone calls, commonly asked questions, and nonroutine office visits. Data collected from postdischarge follow-up assessment tools can be used to identify topics of maternal and newborn care that suggest perinatal education was effective and identify areas for improvement. Results of individual follow-up contacts can be compared with learning-needs assessments completed before discharge. If data analysis suggest specific topics should be covered in more depth in the inpatient setting, staff nurses can make appropriate revisions in their teaching strategies.

Qualitative methods of evaluation such as patient interviews, focus groups, written surveys, and letters or phone calls from parents who have used programs and services are additional valuable sources of data (Beger & Cook, 1996; Handler et al., 1996, 1998; Walker, Watters, Nadon, Graham, & Niday, 1999; Zwelling, 2000). Women and their families frequently identify important issues not addressed on surveys or evaluation tools. Tracking data trends and adjusting discharge plans accordingly leads to improvements in the system. For example, if analysis of the parents' phone call log indicates many calls about a particular issue such as cord care, parent teaching plans can be redesigned to include comprehensive coverage of that topic (Lane et al., 1999; Lieu et al., 1998). Childbearing family surveys may suggest a need to offer more flexibility in class schedules. Prenatal class evaluations provide information about class content and teaching methods that parents found useful (Beger & Cook, 1996; Fishbein & Burggraf, 1998). Prenatal classes can be revised based on consistent themes in participant feedback.

An additional benefit of soliciting patient feedback about services provided is the ability to share with perinatal educators and staff nurses positive remarks about their individual contributions. Women often take time to write lengthy comments about their prenatal educator and the nurses who cared for them during the inpatient stay or during the outpatient home or clinic visit. Although perinatal nurses often feel rushed to accomplish all there is to do in the limited time available, it is gratifying to know nurses can still make a positive difference. Conversely, a complaint or criticism offered by the mother or her family about a staff member, the educational program, or the hospital stay is always valuable. Complaints can increase the nurse's understanding of how the family perceived their interactions with the nurse and the care provided. With this insight, the nurse has the opportunity to make improvements in clinical or interpersonal skills. Complaints also provide the institution with an opportunity to change or revise existing programs to meet consumer expectations. A well-designed postpartum discharge-planning program can be cost-effective if unnecessary calls and return visits to the healthcare provider or institution are decreased and readmissions to the hospital are decreased or remain stable (Bragg, Rosenn, Khoury, Miodovnik, & Siddiqi, 1997; Keppler & Roudebush, 1999; Lee, Perlman, Ballantyne, Elliot, & To, 1995, Lieu et al., 1998; Marbella, Chetty, & Layde, 1998; Soskolne et al., 1996; Welsh & Ludwig-Beymer, 1998). However, to demonstrate a change in readmissions or a decrease in unnecessary calls and return visits, a systematic method of data collection and analysis must be in place. As healthcare dollars become more scarce, increased sophistication in linking clinical and financial positive outcomes to perinatal educational and discharge planning programs will be critical.

SUMMARY

Criteria for postpartum LOS continue to provide challenges for perinatal nurses. Traditional approaches to prenatal educational and discharge planning are obsolete. Opportunities for teaching in the inpatient setting are limited. Innovative educational programs that begin in early pregnancy and continue after discharge are essential to meet the needs of today's childbearing families. Qualitative and quantitative data about program effectiveness are a critical component of discharge planning.

REFERENCES

Agency for Healthcare Policy and Research. (1999). *Hospital inpatient statistics*. Silver Springs, MD: AHCPR Publications Clearinghouse.

American Academy of Pediatrics (AAP) Committee on the Fetus and Newborn. (1995). Hospital stay for healthy newborns. *Pediatrics, 96*(4, Pt. 1), 788–790.

American Academy of Pediatrics & American College of Obstetricians and Gynecologists. (1997). *Guidelines for perinatal care* (4th ed.). Elk Grove Village, IL: Author.

Beck, C. T. (1991). Early postpartum discharge programs in the United States: A literature review and critique. *Women and Health, 17*(1), 125–138.

Beebe, S. A., Britton, J. R., Britton, H. L., Fan, P., & Jepson, B. (1996). Neonatal mortality and length of newborn hospital stay. *Pediatrics, 98*(2, Pt. 1), 231–235.

Beger, D., & Cook, C. A. (1998). Postpartum teaching priorities: The viewpoints of nurses and mothers. *Journal of Obstetric, Gynecologic, and Neonatal Nursing, 27*(2), 161–168.

Behram, S., Moschler, E. F., Sayegh, S. K., Garguillo, F. P., & Mann, W. J. (1998). Implementation of early discharges after uncomplicated vaginal deliveries: Maternal and infant complications. *Southern Medical Journal, 91*(6), 541–545.

Booth, T. (1995). *Family-centered education. The process of teaching birth*. Minneapolis: International Childbirth Educators Association.

Booth, T. (1996). Redesigning your classes to meet today's challenges. *International Journal of Childbirth Education, 11*(2), 24–25.

Bragg, E. J., Rosenn, B. M., Khoury, J. C., Miodovnik, M., & Siddiqi, T. A. (1997). The effect of early discharge after vaginal delivery on neonatal readmission rates. *Obstetrics and Gynecology, 89*(6), 930–933.

Braveman, P., Egerter, S., Pearl, M., Marchi, K., & Miller, C. (1995). Problems associated with early discharge of newborns and mothers: A critical review of the literature. *Pediatrics, 96*(4, Pt. 1), 716–726.

Braveman, P., Kessel, W., Egerter, S., & Richmond, J. (1997). Early discharge and evidence-based practice: Good science and good judgment. *Journal of the American Medical Association, 278*(4), 334–336.

Britton, J. R. (1998). Postpartum early hospital discharge and follow-up practices in Canada and the United States. *Birth, 25*(3), 161–168.

Brown, S. G., & Johnson, B. T. (1998). Enhancing early discharge with home follow-up: Pilot project. *Journal of Obstetric, Gynecologic, and Neonatal Nursing, 27*(1), 33–38.

Brumfield, C. G. (1998). Early postpartum discharge. *Clinical Obstetrics and Gynecology, 41*(3), 611–625.

Carpenter, J. A. (1998). Shortening the short stay. *AWHONN Lifelines, 2*(1), 28–34.

Carty, E. M., & Bradley, C. F. (1990). A randomized controlled evaluation of early postpartum hospital discharge. *Birth, 17*(4), 199–204.

Cook, S., & McIntire F. (1995). Meaningful postpartum advice can make a difference. *International Journal of Childbirth Education, 10*(3), 32–34.

Curtin, S. C., & Park, M. M. (1999). Trends in the attendant, place and timing of births, and in the use of obstetric interventions: United States, 1989–97. *National Vital Statistics Reports, 47*(27), 1–12.

Danielsen, B., Castles, A. G., Damberg, C. L., & Gould, J. B. (2000). Newborn discharge timing and readmissions: California, 1992–1995. *Pediatrics, 106*(1), 31–39.

Declercq, E. (1999). Making US maternal and child health policy: from "early discharge" to "drive through deliveries" to a national law. *Maternal Child Health Journal, 3*(1), 5–17.

Doak, C. C., Doak, L. G., & Root, J. H. (1985). Teaching patients with low literacy skills. *Journal of Reading, 12*, 639–646.

Edmonson, M. B., Stoddard, J. J., & Owens, L. M. (1997). Hospital readmission with feeding-related problems after early postpartum discharge of normal newborns. *Journal of the American Medical Association, 278*(4), 299–303.

Eidelman, A. I., Hoffmann, N. W., & Kaitz M. (1993). Cognitive deficits in women after childbirth. *Obstetrics and Gynecology, 81*(5, Pt. 1), 764–767.

Eidelman, A. I., & Kaitz, M. (1992). Olfactory recognition: A genetic or learned capacity? *Journal of Developmental Behavior and Pediatrics, 13*(2), 126–127.

Farrell, M., Bushnell, D. D., & Haag-Heitman, B. (1998). Theory and practice for teaching the childbearing couple. *Journal of Obstetric, Gynecologic, and Neonatal Nursing, 27*(6), 613–618.

Fishbein, E. G., & Burggraf, E. (1998). Early postpartum discharge: How are mothers managing? *Journal of Obstetric, Gynecologic, and Neonatal Nursing, 27*(2), 142–148.

Frank-Hanssen, M. A., Hanson, K. S., & Anderson M. A. (1999). Postpartum home visits: Infant outcomes. *Journal of Community Health Nursing, 16*(1), 17–28.

Freda, M. C., Damus, K., & Merkatz, I. R. (1999). Evaluation of the readability of ACOG patient education pamphlets. *Obstetrics and Gynecology, 93*(5), 771–774.

Gagnon, A. J., Edgar, L., Kramer, M. S., Papageorgiou, A., Waghorn, K., & Klein, M. C. (1997). A randomized trial of a program of early postpartum discharge with nurse visitation. *American Journal of Obstetrics and Gynecology, 176*(1, Pt. 1), 205–211.

Grullon, K. E., & Grimes, D. A. (1997). The safety of early pospartum discharge: A review and critique. *Obstetrics and Gynecology, 90*(5), 860–865.

Grupp-Phelan, J., Taylor, J. A., Liu, L. L., & Davis, R. L. (1999). Early newborn hospital discharge and readmission for mild and severe jaundice. *Archives of Pediatric and Adolescent Medicine, 153*(12), 1283–1288.

Hall, W. A., & Carty, E. M. (1993). Managing the early discharge experience: Taking control. *Journal of Advanced Nursing, 18*(4), 574–582.

Handler, A., Raube, K., Kelley, M. A., & Giachello, A. (1996). Women's satisfaction with prenatal care settings: A focus group study. *Birth, 23*(1), 31–37.

Handler A., Rosenberg, D., Raube, K., & Kelley, M. A. (1998). Health care characteristics associated with women's satisfaction with prenatal care. *Medical Care, 36*(5), 679–694.

Jacobson, B. B., Brock, K. A., & Keppler, A. B. (1999). The Post Birth Partnership: Washington State's comprehensive approach to improve follow-up care. *Journal of Perinatal and Neonatal Nursing, 13*(1), 43–52.

Kaitz, M., Lapidot, P., Bronner, R., & Eidelman, A. I. (1992). Parturient women can recognize their infants by touch. *Developmental Psychology,* (28), 35–39.

Keppler, A. B., & Roudebush, J. L. (1999). Postpartum follow-up care in a hospital-based clinic: An update on an expanded program. *Journal of Perinatal and Neonatal Nursing, 13*(1), 1–14.

Kotagal, U. R., Atherton, H. D., Bragg, E., Lippert, C., Donovan, E. F., & Perlstein, P. H. (1997). Use of hospital-based services in the first three months of life: Impact of an early discharge program. *Journal of Pediatrics, 130*(2), 250–256.

Kotagal, U. R., Atherton, H. D., Eschett, R., Schoettker, P. J., & Perlstein, P. H. (1999). Safety of early discharge for Medicaid newborns. *Journal of the American Medical Association, 282*(12), 1150–1156.

Kozak, L. J., & Lawrence, L. (1999). National hospital discharge survey: Annual summary, 1997. *Vital and Health Statistics, Series 13: Data from the National Health Survey, 144,* i–iv, 1–46.

Lane, D. A., Kauls, L. S., Ickovics, J. R., Naftolin, F., & Feinstein, A. R. (1999). Early postpartum discharges. Impact on distress and outpatient problems. *Archives of Family Medicine, 8*(3), 237–242.

Lee, K. S., Perlman, M., Ballantyne, M., Elliot, I., & To, T. (1995). Association between duration of neonatal hospital stay and readmission rate. *Journal of Pediatrics, 127,* 758–766.

Lieu, T. A., Wikler, C., Capra, A. M., Martin, K. E., Escobar, G. J., & Braveman, P. A. (1998). Clinical outcomes and maternal perceptions of an updated model of perinatal care. *Pediatrics, 102*(6), 1437–1444.

Lieu, T. A., Braveman, P. A., Escobar, G. J., Fischer, A. F., Jensvold, N. G., & Capra, A. M. (2000). A randomized comparison of home and clinic follow-up visits after early postpartum hospital discharge. *Pediatrics, 105*(5), 1058–1065.

Lock, M., & Ray, J. G. (1999). Higher neonatal morbidity after routine early hospital discharge: Are we sending newborns home too early? *Canadian Medical Association Journal, 161*(3), 249–253.

Maisels, M. J., & Kring, E. (1997). Early discharge from the newborn nursery—effect on scheduling of follow-up visits by pediatricians. *Pediatrics, 100*(1), 72–74.

Maisels, M. J., & Kring, E. (1998). Length of stay, jaundice, and hospital readmission. *Pediatrics, 101*(6), 995–998.

Mandl, K. D., Brennan, T. A., Wise, P. H., Tronick, E. Z., & Homer, C. J. (1997). Maternal and infant health: Effects of moderate reductions in postpartum length of stay. *Archives of Pediatric and Adolescent Medicine, 151*(9), 915–921.

Marbella, A. M., Chetty, V. K., & Layde, P. M. (1998). Neonatal hospital lengths of stay, readmissions, and charges. *Pediatrics, 101*(1), 32–36.

Margolis, L. H., Gay, K., & Humphrey, A. D. (1998). The role of state maternal and child health programs in the issue of newborn discharge. *Maternal and Child Health Journal, 21*(1), 45–54.

Martell, L. K. (2000). The hospital and the postpartum experience: A historical analysis. *Journal of Obstetric, Gynecologic, and Neonatal Nursing, 29*(1), 65–72.

Meikle, S. F., Lyons, E., Hulac, P., & Orleans, M. (1998). Rehospitalizations and outpatient contacts of mothers and neonates after hospital discharge after vaginal delivery. *American Journal of Obstetrics and Gynecology, 179*(1), 166–171.

Memke, K. L. (1993). Linking patient education with discharge planning. In B. E. Giloth (Ed.), *Managing hospital-based patient education* (pp. 153–164). Chicago: American Hospital Publishing.

Olds, D. L., Henderson, C. R., Kitzman, H. J., Eckenrode, J. J., Cole, R. E., & Tatelbaum, R. C. (1999). Prenatal and infancy home visitation by nurses: Recent findings. *Future Child, 9*(1), 44–65, 190–191.

O'Connor, J. (1997). I taught; why didn't they learn? (Using teaching methods to reach both sides of the brain). *International Journal of Childbirth Education, 12*(1), 5–10.

Owens, C. W. (1996). Incorporating parenting information into childbirth classes. *International Journal of Childbirth Education, 11*(1), 14–15.

Raube, K., & Merrell, K. (1999). Maternal minimum-stay legislation: Cost and policy implications. *American Journal of Public Health, 89*(6), 922–923.

Rouse, C. L., & MacNeil, J. (2000). Should there be policies to restrict visitors during labor and birth? *MCN American Journal of Maternal Child Nursing, 25*(1), 8–9.

Rubin, R. (1961). Puerperal change. *Nursing Outlook,* 11, 828–831.

Soskolne, E. I., Schumacher, R., Fyack, C,. Young, M. L., & Schork, A. (1996). The effect of early discharge and other factors on readmission rates of newborns. *Archives of Pediatric and Adolescent Medicine, 150*(4), 373–379.

Trenam, G. (1995). The first few days postpartum: Preparing families for the adjustment. *International Journal of Childbirth Education, 10*(3), 35–36.

Ventura, S. J., Martin, J. A., Curtin, S. C., Mathews, T. J., & Park, M. M. (2000). Births: Final data for 1998. *National Vital Statistics Report, 48*(3), 1–100.

Walker, C. R., Watters, N., Nadon, C., Graham, K., & Niday, P. (1999). Discharge of mothers and babies from hospital after birth of a healthy full-term infant: Developing criteria through a community-wide consensus process. *Canadian Journal of Public Health, 90*(5), 313–315.

Welsh, C., & Ludwig-Beymer, P. (1998). Shortened lengths of stay: Ensuring continuity of care for mothers and babies. *Lippincott's Primary Care Practitioner, 2*(3), 284–291.

Welt, S. I., Cole, J. S., Myers, M. S., Sholes, D. M., & Jelovsek, F. R. (1993). Feasibility of postpartum rapid hospital discharge: A study from a community hospital population. *American Journal of Perinatology, 10*(5), 384–387.

Zwelling, E. (2000). Trendsetter: Celeste Phillips, the mother of family-centered maternity care. *Journal of Obstetric, Gynecologic, and Neonatal Nursing, 29*(1), 90–94.

APPENDIX 18A

Pregnancy, Having a Baby, and Parenting Pathway

The Pathways

The pathways on the following pages are like a roadmap to help you anticipate how pregnancy, birth, and the post birth period generally progress. We hope this helps you to participate in your care and plan for your own experience.

Consultations	Diagnostic Tests	Procedures	Medications	Assessments	Activity	Diet	Hospital Discharge Planning	Teaching and Learning
Pregnancy: 12–32 Weeks								
If needed, you may be referred to a dietitian to talk about your nutritional needs. You may be referred to the Maternal–Fetal Medicine Department at the hospital for tests if needed or consultation with the genetic counselor. You may be referred to the hospital social worker who can link you to community and hospital resources. You may be referred to the Clinical Nurse Specialist for Care Planing.	Early in your pregnancy, laboratory tests will be done to get baseline information. An alpha-fetoprotein or triple screen may be ordered to check fetal well-being. Sometimes, a glucose tolerance test is ordered to see if you have elevated blood sugar.	Your physician or midwife may have you get an ultrasound to check the size of your baby or to answer other questions. Sometimes, an amniocentesis is ordered along with the ultrasound to check fetal well-being and maturity.	You will be taking prenatal vitamins. You need to avoid smoking, alcohol, and recreational drugs. Do not take *any* medications (prescribed or over-the-counter) that are not approved by your physician or midwife first.	The office staff will assess your health needs and your baseline weight, pulse, blood pressure, and other physical signs. You will have a pelvic examination. Your baby's heart rate will be assessed.	Your physician or midwife will discuss exercise and activity with you. In general, there will probably be no need to restrict your activities.	Your book, *Pregnancy, Childbirth, and the Newborn (PCN)*, will help you make sure you are eating healthy foods.	You will select your baby's physician. You will begin to make plans for your support needs, for baby equipment and supplies, and help at home after the birth of your baby. **Cesarean birth:** You will want to plan for additional household help.	You begin your *Becoming Parents Course* by taking classes at the hospital such as "Celebrating Your Pregnancy" and "Maternity Fitness." In the second trimester, you will take "Growing the Baby of Your Dreams, Breastfeeding Basics, and Breastfeeding and the 21st Century Family." Call *(425) 899-3000* to register. If you wish to arrange private instruction, call *(425) 899-2658*. You may have your questions answered at each pregnancy visit, in your prenatal classes,or by calling The Evergreen Health Line: *(425) 899-3000*.
Pregnancy: 32–40 Weeks								
If needed, you may be referred to a dietitian to talk about nutritional needs. You may be referred to Maternal–Fetal Medicine Department at the hospital for tests and	Laboratory tests may be ordered. You can count your baby's movements by using the "Fetal Movement Count" in the Pregnancy and Birth section in your *Maternity*	A nonstress test (NST) is sometimes ordered by the physician or midwife to check fetal well-being. An ultrasound or an amniocentesis may be ordered to check	You continue taking your vitamins and iron supplements if prescribed by your physician or midwife.	You begin to have frequent office visits, and your physical well-being and the baby's will be assessed frequently. You may have a pelvic examination as you	You may need to change your activity level when you are excessively tired or uncomfortable (listen to your body). If you are still working, pace yourself and	You will want to drink plenty of fluids. You may find it more comfort able to eat several small meals rather than three large meals.	You will complete the forms in the *Maternity Patient Information Guide* ("Your Hospital Stay" section), including "Evergreen Babies on Line,"	Sneak Peek Birth Basics VBAC Seminar Labor and Birth Refresher Grandparents Siblings Dads Only Maternity Fitness Yoga for Pregnancy

consultations. Physical therapy may be ordered for extreme back pain or other pregnancy related concerns. If you have any concerns about your hospitalization or special needs during your labor and birth, you can arrange a care conference by calling *(425) 899-3602*.	*Patient Information Guide*. If you think your baby is moving less often, be sure to count fetal movements and talk with your physician or midwife.	fetal well-being and maturity. After your 36th week of pregnancy, come to the Family Maternity Center's Information Desk in the Center's lobby between 7:00 AM and 9:00 PM, Monday through Friday, or 7:00 AM to 5:00 PM, Saturday and Sunday, to sign consent forms for your care during hospitalization. At other times, you may come to the Maternity Center's communication front desk near the floral donor recognition wall.		get close to your due date.	take rest breaks when you feel tired.		First Foto, and the Birth Certificate information. You will purchase a car seat.	
Latent Phase of Labor You will want to call the following and notify them your labor has begun *before coming to the hospital:* 1. Call your physician or midwife if you have been asked to do so. 2. Call the Family Maternity Center Charge Nurse *(425) 899-3500*.	You can count your baby's fetal movements at home. See "Fetal Movement Count" in the "Pregnancy and Birth" section of *The Maternity Patient Information Guide.*	An ultrasound can be done to confirm your baby's position (head down or breech).	You should not take any medications unless your physician or midwife has told you to do so.	You can time your contractions from the beginning of one to the beginning of the next. You can keep a record for an hour or so. Call the Family Maternity Center at *(425) 899-3500* before coming into the hospital so that we are ready for you when you arrive.	Refer to the chart on page 162 of the *PCN*. This chart will outline appropriate activities for this stage of your labor (latent phase).	If you feel like eating and drinking liquids, go ahead; light meals and fluids are important for energy later in labor.	If you have children at home, finalize arrangements for their care while you are away. Place your newborn's car seat into the car so it is ready to bring the baby home. Make sure that you have packed clothing and diapers for the baby's homecoming.	Review and finalize your birth plan. You have a chance to ask questions of your physician or midwife and the charge nurse or your labor nurse.

(continued)

Consultations	Diagnostic Tests	Procedures	Medications	Assessments	Activity	Diet	Hospital Discharge Planning	Teaching and Learning
3. Call your husband or partner and doula or support person. *Labor induction and cesarean birth:* If your cesarean birth or induction is scheduled and you go into labor, call your physician or midwife and the Family Maternity Center *(425) 899-3500.* *DO NOT EAT OR DRINK IF YOU ANTICIPATE A CESAREAN BIRTH.* An anesthesiologist will consult with you before your cesarean section.	If your membranes have ruptured or you think they have, you may be tested for the presence of amniotic fluid in the vagina in your physician's or midwife's office or in the hospital.						If you are planning to formula feed, make sure that you have formula at home (refer to the "Infant Feeding" section of your *Maternity Patient Information Guide.* Read *Formula Feeding Basics* and talk with your baby's healthcare provider for guidance).	
Labor and Birth Your physician or midwife has left directions about your care in labor, and your nurse will manage your labor according to their plan. The physician or midwife will be in contact with your nurse and notified of your progress in labor. Your midwife may spend a lot of time with you during your labor.	A test to determine if your water has "broken" may be performed. Your urine will be checked for protein and glucose.	An episiotomy occasionally is done at delivery time if needed (see page 154 in *PCN*). A vacuum extractor or forceps may be used to assist in the birth if needed. Refer to pages 183–188 in *PCN* for other procedures. *Cesarean birth:* You will have a urinary catheter placed in your bladder	Refer to pages 212–213 in the PCN. *Cesarean birth:* You will receive anesthesia (see page 189 in *PCN*). This will be an epidural or a spinal. You will also receive epidural medication to provide pain relief for the first several hours after birth. You will be given a medication by mouth that decreases stomach	Your heart rate, respirations, blood pressure, and temperature will be monitored periodically. An electronic fetal monitor will be used to assess the well-being of your baby and strength of your contractions. Vaginal examinations will be done periodically to check the progress of your labor.	Refer to pages 144–145 and pages 163–164 in *PCN.* You will be encouraged to walk, move about, and explore the Family Maternity Center while you are in labor. You may find the Jacuzzi very soothing as your labor progresses. Refer to the chart on pages 163–164 in *PCN* for sug-	You may eat and drink according to your physician's or midwife's orders.	The expected time that you will be going home will be determined by your physician or midwife and your nurse will talk with you about getting ready to go home. The usual length of stay after a vaginal birth is about 24 hours and 2 to 3 days after a cesarean. The length of stay may be longer if you have a medical	Identification bands will be placed on the baby and on you and your partner. Your nurse will talk to you about the security of your baby while you are in the hospital. In the first hours after birth, your nurse will give your baby his/her first bath, show you how to diaper your baby, and show how to soothe a fussy baby.

If it is determined that your baby will require any special care at birth or shortly after birth, a special care nursery nurse, pediatrician, or neonatologist will be called to attend the delivery of your baby. If you choose to have an epidural, an anesthesiologist will be called at the right time in labor. *Cesarean birth:* An anesthesiologist will consult with you.		after you have received your anesthesia.	acid. An antibiotic may be added to your intravenous (IV) line. *IV line:* You will have an IV if you are going to have an epidural; otherwise, only if ordered by your physician or midwife. You will receive antibiotics by IV if you are positive for group B Streptoccus. *Cesarean birth:* An IV line will be started.	*Cesarean birth:* You will have a heart monitor, and blood pressure monitor, and the oxygen level in your blood will be checked.	gestions for activity and partner role.		need to stay longer; for example, you have a fever or need for continued IV medication.	
After Delivery: 0–2 Hours								
Your baby's physician will be notified that your baby has arrived. A pediatrician or neonatologist may be called to come and see the baby if special care is required. A Special Care Nursery registered nurse may examine your baby and provide care.	Blood may be drawn from you, if needed, for blood typing and the Rh factor if indicated. Blood may be drawn from your baby's heel if there is concern about your baby's blood sugar level. Blood may be drawn from the baby if there is a concern about jaundice or infection.	Your nurse will cover you with a warmed blanket, which will feel wonderful after the hard work of labor. Ice packs will be placed on your perineum to reduce swelling and discomfort.	Pitocin may be added to your IV line or given by injection to prevent excessive uterine bleeding (nursing your baby has the same effect). Your Self-Administration Medication (SAM) kit will be given and explained to you. This kit contains mild pain relievers and medication to soften bowel movements (stool softener).	*Mom:* Your physical vital signs, including pulse and blood pressure, will be monitored frequently. The firmness of the uterus will be felt through your abdomen (when the uterine muscle is firmly contracted you are less likely to bleed heavily). You will be encouraged to empty your bladder, and your nurse will assist you to the bathroom.	You will be given food if you are hungry and something to drink if you are thirsty. Many mothers are very hungry after a vaginal birth.	Whatever you want!! Your nurse will provide you with a meal soon after birth. In addition, you have a refrigerator in your room, and a microwave is available if you wish to have your favorite foods brought from home. There are no foods you need to avoid if you are breast-feeding.	You will begin to discuss your going-home arrangements with your nurse and family.	Your nurse will review with you your copy of the *Evergreen Mother and Baby Care* book. Your nurse will teach you • How to relieve any perineal discomfort • How to minimize lightheadedness while getting out of bed • About your medications • About proper latch and position for breastfeeding • How to formula feed • Normal newborn characteristics • How to keep the baby warm

(continued)

Consultations	Diagnostic Tests	Procedures	Medications	Assessments	Activity	Diet	Hospital Discharge Planning	Teaching and Learning
			Your baby will receive an injection of vitamin K; erythromycin eye ointment will be placed in the baby's eyes (see page 242 in PCN); and the hepatitis B vaccination given. *IV line:* Your IV will be continued if it is necessary.	If you had an epidural, the catheter taped to your back will be removed. *Cesarean birth:* The feeling will gradually return to the lower half of your body. This will be monitored by your nurse. *Baby:* Your baby will be given an Apgar score test (see page 158 in *PCN*. Your baby will be weighed and measured for length. The baby's physical signs, including heart and respiratory rate and temperature, will be accessed.	The first hours after your baby's birth are magical—at this time babies are more alert, responsive, and ready to feed than they will be for the next several hours. You will want to take this opportunity to begin nursing your baby. Your nurse will be available to help you if you need it. If you plan to formula feed your baby, you will take advantage of the same opportunity to offer your baby his/her first bottle. Your nurse will be available to help you with this. If you have had an epidural, you will be encouraged to move your toes and feet as feeling returns. You will be encouraged to move about and to take a shower when you are ready.	If you had a cesarean, your physician or midwife will order an appropriate diet for you after surgery.		• How to diaper • Security for your baby You will have many chances to ask questions, because your nurse will be caring only for you during the recovery time after birth.

After Delivery: 2 Hours–Going Home

You will be seen by your physician or midwife

Your baby's physician will examine your baby.

You will be seen by a lactation consultant (a registered nurse with special expertise in assisting nursing mothers and babies) if needed or as you request.

Because you will need less intense nursing care, you will have a postpartum nurse and her assistant who will care for you and 4 to 5 other mothers and babies.

Blood will be drawn from your baby's heel for newborn screening tests (see Newborn Care section of *Mother and Baby Care* book). Blood may also be taken from your baby's heel to check the blood sugar, check for jaundice or for infection.

If you choose to do so, your baby boy will be circumcised.

Cesarean birth: Your urinary catheter will be removed.

If your incision has been closed with staples, they will be removed, and Steri-Strip tapes will be applied.

You may take medication for discomfort from your *SAM* kit. You will also be taking stool softener.

Rhogam and the mumps, measles, and rubella (MMR) immunization will be given to you if indicated.

IV line: Your IV will be removed.

Cesarean birth: If you had a cesarean, you will begin to take Percoset or Vicodin by mouth for pain. Your nurse will provide you with pain medication. Be sure to call her if you are in pain.

The nurse will be constantly but quietly assessing the baby's overall status during the next 20 hours.

Your nurse will examine your breasts and assess your uterus and bladder. The nurse will also check your vaginal discharge (lochia) and check your blood pressure and vital signs.

The baby will have vital signs assessed, a full physical examination, and an assessment of feeding and elimination patterns.

Let how you feel guide your activity.

To get the rest you need and to take advantage of your nursing care, you may wish to limit your visitors. Some families have found that too many visitors who stay too long keep them from having private time and cause them to feel fatigued. Let your nurse know if you wish to limit visitors.

Baby and family pictures can be taken for "Evergreen Babies On-Line" and First Foto takes baby pictures.

Your baby will enjoy her/his first bath in your room in our special bathing sinks. You or a family member may bathe the baby or help the nurse to bathe your baby. This is a good time to take pictures.

Many women experience a decrease in appetite, but other women are hungry.

Let your body guide you; eat if you are hungry, and drink if you are thirsty.

Your nurse, in consultation with your physician or midwife, will let you know when you can expect to go home. You will want to complete your birth certificate and the First Foto information.

Your nurse will make your Postpartum Care Center appointment. You will be seen there when your baby is 2 to 4 days old. The nurse will make a referral to the Breastfeeding Center for a follow-up appointment if you are having breast-feeding challenges and review when to see your physician or midwife and your baby's physician after discharge.

You and your family are encouraged to attend the "Baby Care and Feeding" class while in the hospital.

Your nurse will show you how to nurse your baby lying down so that you can rest and feed your baby at the same time.

You will learn about how your baby shows he/she is ready to feed, how often and how long to feed, and how to know if the baby is getting enough.

If you are formula feeding, you will learn how to mix the formula, how much and how often to feed, and what formulas are recommended.

Your nurse will talk to you about how many wet diapers and bowel movements to expect. (Refer to the Newborn Care Infant Feeding section in *Mother and Baby Care* book.)

Your nurse will show you how to care for the umbilical cord, skin, circumcision, and how to take the baby's temperature.

(continued)

Consultations	Diagnostic Tests	Procedures	Medications	Assessments	Activity	Diet	Hospital Discharge Planning	Teaching and Learning
					Cesarean birth: You will be assisted to get out of bed and walk. Your activity will gradually increase as you are able.			You will be shown how to put your baby into his/her car seat. Your nurse will discuss postpartum warning signs to report to your physician or midwife. (See Warning Signs for Mother and Infant in *Mother and Baby Care* book.)
After Birth: 1–14 Days								
When your baby is 2 to 4 days of age, you will return to the *Postpartum Care Center: (425) 899-3602.* You will return to the baby's physician at 8 to 14 days. You can call the Breast-feeding Center if you are having difficulty feeding: *(425) 899-3494.*	A second newborn screening test occurs at 7 to 14 days of age. This test is done in your baby's healthcare provider's office or at the hospital. Check with your baby's physician to determine where the test will be done. (See Screening Tests in the *Mother and Baby Care* book). Your baby may have a blood test for jaundice.	Baby boys may have their circumcision done as an outpatient. The cord clamp may be removed at the *Postpartum Care Center* visit if it was not removed in the hospital.	You may continue taking medication from your SAM kit as needed. You may receive Rhogam or MMR at your *Postpartum Care Center* visit if this was not done in the hospital. *Cesarean birth:* You may take oral pain medication as needed. Your pain medication may cause constipation—be sure to takeyour stool softener and eat high-fiber foods.	Your own and your baby's physical well-being will be checked at your visit at the *Postpartum Care Center.* You will have your perineum and incision checked, given suggestions to increase your comfort, and be assisted with infant feeding. Your baby will be weighed, checked for jaundice, and have vital signs assessed and cord checked. Any specific concerns you have about yourself or your infant will be addressed. If a medical problem is detected, your physician	Although you may feel quite fit, do *not* overdo activity!!! Don't do anything that increases your bleeding, makes you tired, or causes you pain. Your joints are still at risk for injury, so avoid any jerky exercises. As long as you do not feel overly tired, light-headed, and are not taking any narcotic pain medications, you may drive. Avoid heavy lifting. Brisk walking is fine, and you may wish to refer to *PCN* page 230 and the Postpartum Exercise section in the	Eat the nutritious foods you enjoy. It is common to have a decrease in appetite for several weeks after giving birth. Refer to diet and weight loss in the *Mother and Baby Care* book.		Use your *Baby Mother and Care* book to provide you with information about common baby- and mother-care concerns. Postpartum Warning Signs for mother and infant to be reported to your healthcare providers are listed in the boxes on the last page. Resources for help are listed in your *Mother and Baby Care* book under Resource Phone List. For breast-feeding information, call *(425) 899-3494.* You are encouraged to go to the Parent–Baby Classes, an educational support group for new parents. (See Parent–Baby Classes in your

				or midwife or your baby's physician will be contacted.	*Mother and Baby Care* book.) *Cesarean birth:* You will appreciate additional help in your home at this time. You have had surgery. Give yourself time to heal and for your endurance to return.			*Mother and Baby Care* book.) Call *(425) 899-3000,* to register. You may return to the hospital for the Baby Care and Feeding Class if you were unable to attend earlier. Call *(425) 899-3500* for times. *Cesarean birth:* Discuss with your physician or midwife the events that led to the decision to deliver your baby by cesarean. Most causes are nonrepeating, and it is likely that if you choose to have another baby, you will be encouraged to deliver vaginally (see *PCN,* page 194).
After Birth: 14 Days–1 Year								
You may call the *Breast-feeding Center* anytime you have questions about nursing your baby: *(425) 899-3494.* You may call the *Postpartum Care Center* with any concerns about postpartum adjustment: *(425) 899-3602.*		Your physician or midwife will discuss the best time for you to resume having Pap tests. See the Newborn Care Immunization section in your *Mother and Baby Care* book.	Continue your prenatal vitamins or multivitamins.		You will gradually return to all normal activities.	Eat the nutritious foods you enjoy. Refer to diet and weight loss in the *Mother and Baby Care* book.		You can continue with parent–baby classes until your baby is 1 year old. Also offered are • This is Not What I Expected—Emotional Care for New Families; call *(425) 899-3602* for information. • Support Group for Young Moms • Yoga for the New Mom (continued)

Consultations	Diagnostic Tests	Procedures	Medications	Assessments	Activity	Diet	Hospital Discharge Planning	Teaching and Learning
Your baby will be seen regularly by his/her physician during the first year. You will be seen by your midwife or physician 4–6 weeks after birth. Family planning options will be discussed at that time.								• Breast-feeding the Older Baby • Starting Solids • IMET: Keys for Couples

From Evergreen Hospital Medical Center.

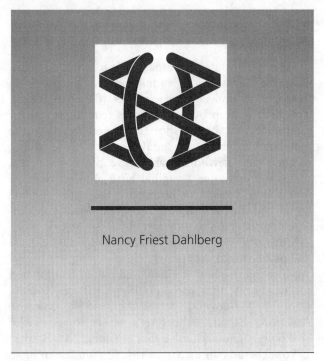

Nancy Friest Dahlberg

CHAPTER 19

Postpartum Home Care

A critical component of comprehensive perinatal nursing care during the postpartum period is a well-designed, universally accessible home follow-up program for childbearing women and their families. Despite recent increases in the inpatient length of stay (LOS) for childbirth, the time in the hospital remains relatively short for mothers to recover from the labor and birth process and to assimilate the knowledge they need to care for themselves and their newborn after discharge. Fundamental changes in reimbursement for perinatal care, a continued emphasis on appropriate inpatient LOS, cost-reduction strategies, consumer demand for increased participation in the childbirth experience, and favorable outcomes for women and newborns who receive postpartum home care are factors that have influenced the availability of these services. Unfortunately, some third-party payers eliminated coverage for postpartum home care when state and federal legislation established minimum coverage for LOS after childbirth, limiting availability and access to home care for some women. Despite limited reimbursement, all women can benefit from participation in a comprehensive postpartum follow-up program.

REVIEW OF THE LITERATURE

Decreasing LOS for childbirth is not a new phenomenon. As early as 1943, there were reports in the literature about efforts to discharge women 2 to 5 days postpartum with home care follow-up services instead of the then traditional 10-day stay (Guerriero, 1943). During the 1960s, early discharge programs were instituted in response to maternity hospital bed shortages (Hellman, Kohl, & Palmer, 1962). During the 1970s and 1980s, similar programs were developed at the request of patients and families; however, not until the 1990s did the practice become widespread. Norr and Nacion (1987) reviewed all postpartum early discharge programs published between 1960 and 1985 and concluded that discharge less 48 hours after birth has generally been safe for mothers and infants. Beck's (1991) review of early discharge programs in the United States provided similar results concerning the favorable statistics on maternal and infant morbidity.

Several randomized studies comparing early postpartum discharge and follow-up home visits have been published (Armstrong, Fraser, Dadds, & Morris, 1999; Brooten et al., 1994, 1996; Carty & Bradley, 1990; Gagnon et al., 1997; Lieu et al., 2000; Olds, Henderson, Tatelbaum, & Chamberlin, 1986; Waldenstrom, 1987; Yanover, Jones, & Miller, 1976). In an early study, Yanover and colleagues (1976) found that discharge as early as 12 hours after birth, when combined with home visits by a perinatal nurse practitioner, was safe, economically feasible, and well accepted by childbearing women. Women's choice in staying in the hospital or going home early had an influence on patient satisfaction with the postpartum experience in Waldenstrom's (1989) qualitative study. In families randomized to the early-discharge group, 92% of women and 83% of men reported positive experiences. Men in the early-discharge group were also more involved in changing, bathing, and holding the newborn (Waldenstrom, 1988). In another study (Carty & Bradley, 1990), postpartum women were randomly assigned to three discharge times: 12 to 24 hours, 25 to 48 hours, and 4 days. Based on LOS, women received one to five home visits by a perinatal nurse during the first 10 days postpartum. Results indicated low maternal and neonatal morbidity for all groups. Breast-feeding success at 1 month and satisfaction with nursing care was significantly higher for early-discharge groups. Women with a 4-day LOS scored higher on measures of depression and lower on scores of confidence in the mothering role than did the early-discharge groups.

Norr, Nacion, and Abramson (1989) studied the impact of early discharge with home follow-up visits for low-income women and their infants. In this study, women who were discharged less than 48 hours after birth with their newborns reported higher maternal satisfaction and less maternal concerns than the control group. No differences in maternal–newborn morbidity were found for traditional versus shorter LOS. Newborns receiving home visits after hospital discharge were less likely to require hospital readmission or outpatient care (Braveman et al., 1996; Meikle, Lyons, Hulac, & Orleans, 1998). Brown and Johnson (1998) evaluated the cost savings of decreased hospital LOS and home follow-up services provided by perinatal nurses. They found that women and newborns who participated in an early discharge program that included home visits had 10 times less nonroutine healthcare expenditures in the 6 weeks after birth compared with the group who received standard care (Brown & Johnson, 1998). However, not all researchers found that early discharge resulted in cost savings. A study comparing mothers who stayed 1 night with those who stayed 2 nights found that a 1-night LOS was associated with more distress and more pediatric problems and greater use of outpatient services than a 2-night LOS (Lane, Kauls, Ickovics, Naftolin, & Feinstein, 1999).

In the mid-1990s, a "very early discharge" (<24 hours after uncomplicated vaginal birth) became a norm in some parts of the United States (Brumfield, 1998). There was a strong national response to this trend. Women and their families felt postpartum hospital stays were too short. The public outcry against healthcare insurance company practices to reduce costs and provide less services in general and against "drive-through deliveries" specifically led to federal and state legislation mandating coverage for minimal postpartum LOS (Declercq & Simmes, 1997). The Newborns and Mothers Health Protection Act of 1996, effective January 1, 1998, ensures that the third-party payer must reimburse the hospital for a minimum of 48 hours after an uncomplicated vaginal birth and for 96 hours after an uncomplicated cesarean birth (Declercq, 1999). This care is under the direction of a physician and with the consent of the mother.

Twenty-six states have passed legislation strengthening the federal law by adding a home care provision to maternity and newborn services (Bateman, 1998). This home care provision requires reimbursement for one home visit after a shorter hospital stay than the mandated hours of hospital care. In these states, mothers and newborns who leave the hospital less than 48 hours after a vaginal birth and less than 96 hours after a cesarean birth have the option of one home visit. Before hospital discharge, primary healthcare providers are required to discuss appropriate follow-up with each mother based on individual clinical and psychosocial situations.

Most studies show no increased risk of readmission for newborns after early discharge (Bragg, Rosenn, Khoury, Miodovnik, & Siddiqi, 1997; Kotagal, Atherton, Eshett, Schoettker, & Perlstein, 1999; Soskolne, Schumacher, Fyock, Young, & Schork, 1996). There is an increased risk of jaundice in newborns who are discharged less than 24 hours after birth, but there is no evidence that an additional inpatient day can prevent readmission for jaundice and subsequent complications (Grupp-Phelan, Taylor, Liu, & Davis 1999; Lock & Ray 1999). Maisles and Kring (1998) found a LOS less than 72 hours significantly increased the risk of readmission for newborn jaundice. Based on their findings, Maisles and Kring (1998) recommend that the American Academy of Pediatrics (AAP) guidelines for follow-up observation of newborns who are discharged less than 48 hours after birth be extended to newborns who are discharged less than 72 hours after birth. In a study of almost 48,000 newborns in Washington state during 1989 and 1990, researchers found that discharge before 30 hours of life was associated with a significantly increased risk of infant mortality (Malkin, Garber, Broder, & Keeler, 2000). These investigators suggested that infants discharged early were more likely to die within 1 year of birth of cardiac problems, infection, and sudden infant death syndrome (SIDS) than infants discharged after 30 hours of life, but it is unclear how an extra day in the hospital or a postpartum home visit would have decreased risk of death for the infants who died within the first year.

Evidence suggests that there are long-term benefits of postpartum home care when services are provided until the infant is 2 years old (Olds et al., 1994, 1997, 1999). Results showed that home visits by nurses have enduring effects on certain aspects of prenatal caregiving, safety of the home, and children's use of the healthcare system (Olds et al., 1994). A 20-year study found that the use of nurses as home visitors was a key factor in successful outcomes (Olds et al., 1999). According to Olds and coworkers (1999), at a minimum, home visit programs should be targeted to the neediest populations. In the studies of Olds and colleagues (1994, 1997, 1999), postpartum home visits by registered nurses until the infant was 2 years old were associated with reduced rates of childhood injuries and ingestions that may be related to child abuse and neglect, an increased interval between pregnancies, a decrease in the number of subsequent pregnancies, and an increased likelihood that the mother would reenter the workforce. Additional positive outcomes were a reduction in the use of welfare, child abuse and neglect, and criminal behavior on the part of low-income, unmarried mothers for up to 15 years after the birth of the first child (Olds et al., 1997, 1999). Although results of the studies by Olds and coworkers are encouraging, few programs provide home visits covering the infant's first 2 years of life.

Published studies about early discharge for mothers and newborns have limited generalizability because of differences in hospital LOS, criteria for discharge, and inconsistencies in definition of the term *early*, type of care providers, and the number of follow-up visits (Armstrong et al., 1999; Braveman et al., 1996; Britton, 1998; Brooten et al., 1994; Brown & Johnson, 1998; Brumfield et al., 1996; Carty & Bradley, 1990; Drummond, Boucher, Chisholm, Geraci, & Kay, 1984; Frank-Hanssen, Hanson, & Anderson, 1999; Gazmararian & Solomon, 1997; Jones, 1997; Kotagal et al., 1999; Lieu et al., 2000; Olds, Henderson, Tatelbaum, & Chamberlin, 1986; Yanover et al., 1976). Although limitations of available published studies exist, all investigators cite the need for comprehensive follow-up perinatal care for women and newborns after discharge. More data are needed on what constitutes a quality home care follow-up program, including types of service most beneficial for selected populations (Braveman, Egerter, Pearl, Marchi, & Miller, 1995).

The American Academy of Pediatrics and The American College of Obstetricians and Gynecologists (AAP & ACOG, 1997) have established guidelines for LOS and follow-up care for mothers and newborns. A home visit or telephone call within 48 hours of discharge is recommended for mothers who go home less than 48 hours after vaginal birth or less than 96 hours after cesarean birth (AAP & ACOG, 1997). An examination by an experienced healthcare provider within 48 hours after discharge is recommended for newborns who go home less than 48 hours after vaginal birth (AAP & ACOG, 1997).

Although consensus in the literature and in practice does not exist concerning the number of visits and type of service that should be provided, there is enough evidence to support the benefits of postpartum home care follow-up for childbearing women and families. The perinatal nurse can ease the transition from hospital to home by providing comprehensive assessments and appropriate interventions and by coordinating referrals to other healthcare resources as necessary (Simpson, 1996).

The Association of Women's Health, Obstetric and Neonatal Nurses (AWHONN, 1994, 1998) has developed standards and guidelines for the nursing care of women and newborns in the home setting. The American Nurses Association (ANA) addressed the need for home visits after a shortened hospital stay in their 1995 position statement *Home Care for Mother, Infant, and Family Following Birth*. They recommend a reasonable hospital LOS for childbirth, followed by a postpartum home visit for low-risk mothers and newborns based on identified needs. For mothers and newborns at risk for poor health and development, 1 year of periodic home visits is recommended. According to the ANA (1995), postpartum home visits by a registered nurse should be a national standard of care and include the following:

- Provide early identification of complications, preventing costly rehospitalization
- Bridge the gap between hospital discharge and the first follow-up visit with primary healthcare providers
- Promote efficient use of existing healthcare resources
- Provide care in the most appropriate environment considering the recovery needs of the mother, adaptation of the newborn, and developmental tasks of the family

Key recommendations included in the ANA's (1995) position statement are listed in Display 19–1.

MODELS OF SERVICES

Healthcare providers at each perinatal center should develop strategies to meet the needs of the mothers and newborns after postpartum discharge. As part of discharge planning, options should be identified within the community for ongoing care needed for mothers and newborns discharged less than 48 hours after vaginal birth and less than 96 hours after cesarean birth. Perinatal home care follow-up services can be developed based on nursing resources, institutional goals, third-party payer influence, and home care agency availability in the community (Dahlberg & Koloroutis, 1994). Hospital-based programs, freestanding agencies, public health departments, and hospital acute care postpartum nurses providing fol-

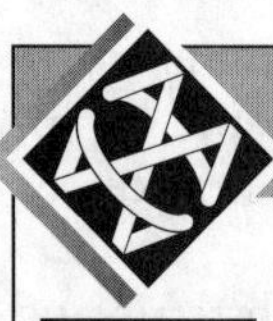

DISPLAY 19–1

Key Recommendations from the American Nurses Association 1995 Position Statement on Home Care for Mother, Infant, and Family After Birth

The American Nurses Association supports

- The rights of new mothers, newborns, and new families to have their healthcare needs addressed
- Recognition of postpartum nursing as an essential component of maternity care
- Access by families to perinatal nursing care provided by registered nurses in the hospital and at home
- Redefinition and clarification of the roles of the inpatient postpartum nurse, the postpartum home care nurse, and the perinatal home care nurse
- Maternity programs that include, based on the individual assessment of mother and infant needs, a reasonable hospitalization and provision of postpartum home nursing care as a national standard of care
- Reimbursement for perinatal and postpartum home nursing by registered nurses that is adequate and recognizes the mother and infant as separate patients
- Availability of nursing services in the home for all high-risk pregnant women and newborns and through the first year of life for infants at risk for poor health and development
- Nursing care beyond the immediate postpartum period as a necessary component to the continuing health of women, infants, and families

low-up home visits are some of the home care services available.

Individual state home care licensure rules and regulations guide the type of program options available when a home care program structure is being considered. The governing body, home care rules, and regulations may also require physician orders and direct communication with the perinatal nurse for home care services. Participating physicians must be aware of the scope of services available in the home and the medical indications for home care. Close communication and collaboration with physician colleagues promote the appropriate use of services and increase the likelihood that services ordered will be covered by the patient's healthcare insurance company.

The goal of home care services is to provide an opportunity for mothers, newborns, and their families to receive technical, psychological, and therapeutic support for their individual needs after they leave the hospital (AWHONN, 1998). Home care services bridge the interests of families, healthcare providers, third-party payers, and community resources; coordinate efforts; minimize duplication; and fill gaps in the healthcare system (Dahlberg & Koloroutis, 1994). There are regional variations in who pays for and who provides postpartum home care services. In some areas of the country, state and local health departments provide home care services. In other areas, these services are provided by hospitals or private home care agencies. Although there are differences in the methods of reimbursement and provision of home care, telephone contact and one to two home visits usually are included (Simpson, 1996).

Ideally, during a postpartum home visit, the perinatal nurse conducts a thorough physical, psychosocial, and learning-needs assessment of the mother and newborn, provides appropriate nursing interventions, communicates and coordinates care with the primary healthcare provider, and makes referrals to other community resources as necessary (Frank-Hanssen et al., 1999). Nursing assessments, interventions, and referrals contribute to effective care management, positive maternal–newborn outcomes, and, for selected populations, may result in cost savings. Most postpartum home visit programs involve one to two visits for healthy mothers and newborns. Additional visits may be ordered as needed based on the individual clinical situation.

ESSENTIAL COMPONENTS OF QUALITY PERINATAL HOME CARE SERVICES

Discharge Criteria

Successful outcomes depend on a commitment from healthcare providers to offer comprehensive discharge planning, thorough patient and family assessment, education, and support with coordination of institutional and community resources (Dahlberg & Koloroutis, 1994). The birth plan and postpartum care, including the expected LOS for uncomplicated vaginal births, should be discussed with women and support persons during prenatal clinic visits and educational classes. The childbearing family can then have realistic expectations, know their options, and make appropriate plans. It is essential that home visits remain a covered service for private and government insurance, because very early or early discharges are an option and choice for many women and their newborns (AAP & ACOG, 1997; ANA, 1995; Welt, Cole, Myers, Sholes, & Jelovsek, 1993).

There are established guidelines and suggested criteria for discharging childbearing women in less than 48 hours after a vaginal birth and less than 96 hours after a cesarean birth (AAP & ACOG, 1997) (Display 19–2). The guidelines for nursing practice, health education, and counseling developed by AWHONN (1994) can be used to develop protocols for postpartum home care. Careful screening is essential to avoid sending women and newborns that are at risk for complications home too soon. Plans that include patient and family education and assessment of support-person availability are also important.

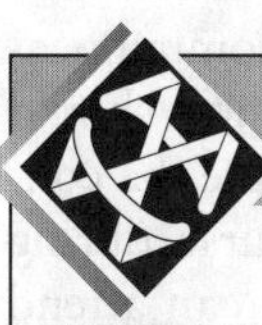

DISPLAY 19–2

Suggested Criteria for Discharge in Less Than 48 Hours for a Vaginal Birth and Less Than 96 Hours for a Cesarean Birth

- The mother had an uncomplicated birth after a normal antepartum and postpartum course
- Pertinent laboratory data are within normal limits for both mother and newborn
- The newborn is stable and able to maintain thermal homeostasis, has urinated and passed one stool, and demonstrates feeding abilities
- Arrangements are made for postpartum follow-up care for mother and newborn
- Mother is ready to care for herself and the newborn
- Newborn has no evidence of jaundice
- Family members or other support persons are available to the mother for the first few days after discharge
- The mother is aware of possible complication and has been instructed to notify the appropriate practitioner, as necessary
- The institution has in place mechanisms to address patient's questions that arise after discharge

From American Academy of Pediatrics & American College of Obstetricians and Gynecologists. (1997). Guidelines for perinatal care (4th ed.). Elk Grove Village, IL: Author.

Healthcare providers may find it helpful to use checklists or similar evaluation tools to assess mothers' readiness for discharge (see Chapter 18). Learning-needs assessment and physical assessment can be combined on a single form or documented separately. Some institutions use a single documentation tool for mother and baby, whereas others maintain two medical records. Clinical pathways are also excellent tools for determining patient and family status at discharge, because expected goals and outcomes are evaluated and appropriate nursing interventions can be initiated before sending the mother and infant home.

Before discharge, the primary healthcare provider and the mother–baby nurse should discuss current needs and appropriate follow-up care with each family. If the mother chooses early discharge, the primary healthcare provider probably will recommend that the mother and newborn be examined within 48 hours after they go home (AAP & ACOG, 1997). The primary healthcare provider or the mother may prefer to have a nurse provide this care in the home rather than returning to an outpatient office or clinic.

Appropriate and Timely Referral

To initiate the referral process, it is essential that the discharging facility communicate with the home care provider so the family experiences coordinated care and a seamless transition to home (Dahlberg & Koloroutis, 1994). This communication can occur through a written referral or verbal report. The home care agency needs to have current and complete information to provide appropriate care to the mother, newborn, and family. Referral information should include the mother's and newborn's histories and the plan of care, including physician orders, infant feeding assessment, and individual nursing care needs of the mother and newborn. This process is essentially a report from the hospital nursing staff to the home care nursing staff, ensuring continuity of care and capitalizing on care already given.

Efforts to decrease duplication of services have resulted in the hospital and home care agency cooperating to determine the best process for the exchange of information to assist in the discharge and transition to home. Appendix 19A has an example of a referral form for home care. In some programs, home care nurses use selected portions of inpatient medical records of the mother and newborn rather than transferring information onto a referral form. The AWHONN (1994, 1998) standards and guidelines for professional nursing home care practice for mothers and newborns are helpful in designing a comprehensive perinatal home care program.

Although the number of nursing visits, telephone calls, and additional services offered vary with each perinatal home care agency, a basic program is described in Display 19–3. When the discharge plan of care includes a referral to home care for follow-up services, the inpatient nurse facilitates the referral as part of the plan of care for the mother, newborn, and family. After receiving the referral, the home care nurse reviews the information and determines whether the referral is appropriate for their agency. If there are reasons the agency cannot provide care to this mother and newborn (eg, geographic limitations, health insurance plan participation, clinical status, required interventions), the home care nurse notifies the hospital and primary care provider and assists in identifying the appropriate home care agency.

On first day home, the family receives a call from the home care nurse for an assessment. This is a structured telephone assessment, reviewing maternal and newborn health issues and addressing any areas of concern the mother and her family may be having at this time (Appendix 19B). Through the telephone interview, the nurse and mother can determine the need for a home visit. If the nurse and mother agree that mother and newborn are doing well and do not have any identified medical problems or concerns, they may decide a home visit is not needed. If however, the nurse identifies clinical situations that warrant a home visit, it can be arranged at a mutually agreeable day and time. If urgent clinical issues are identified during the initial telephone call, the home visit may be scheduled for that day. Occasionally, it may not be possible to schedule a home visit on the day of the telephone assessment, even when the nurse has identified urgent clinical issues. In this case, the mother should be given the option of another resource and encouraged to seek resolution of the clinical problem. For example, a clinic or office visit or visit to a lactation consultant should be scheduled to address the urgent issue until the nurse can see the mother and baby in the home. Based on the clinical urgency of the situation, the primary healthcare provider may need to be notified.

For healthy mothers and babies, the home visit occurs on the day after the telephone assessment, which is within 48 hours of discharge. Occasionally, the visit is earlier or later, based on the individual needs of the family. State legislation may also stipulate the time frame of the home visit. The mother has the right to decline a home visit, and the nurse can assist the mother in making a follow-up plan with the appropriate resource as indicated.

It is important to have resources when communication barriers exist. Each home care agency should have interpreter services available to translate the conversation between the woman and the nurse during the telephone assessment call. Interpreters can attend the home visit with the nurse to provide ongoing translation throughout the home care services. Family members who speak English and who are willing to act as translators can also be helpful. There are services available to allow hearing-impaired mothers to participate in the telephone assessment. The agency can arrange for a person who knows sign language to accompany the nurse during the home visit if appropriate.

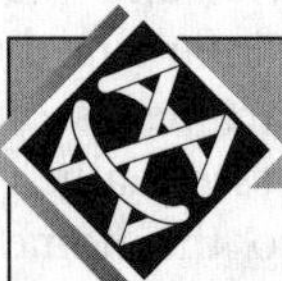

DISPLAY 19–3

Suggested Prenatal Home Care Services

- Referral to home care on the day of hospital discharge
- Structured phone call to the mother on the day after hospital discharge that screens for maternal and newborn complications
- Day of home visit scheduled
- Home visit(s) completed and ongoing plan of care determined
- Follow-up phone calls as indicated and discharge from home care when ongoing plan of care is established, resources are identified, and referrals are completed as needed

Plan of Care

The home care nurse reviews the information obtained during the telephone interview and develops a plan of care. The plan of care is based on established agency protocols and adapted to meet the individual needs of the woman and newborn. The perinatal home care nurse uses knowledge of physical, psychosocial, and learning needs of new mothers to promote a healthy postpartum experience (AWHONN, 1998). Assessments, teaching, support, and interventions as needed comprise a comprehensive plan of care for the new mother and newborn.

The first few days at home can be challenging and stressful, even when the childbirth experience has been wonderful and the newborn eagerly anticipated. The process of integrating a new baby into the household coincides with major changes and adjustments in the lives of parents. If adequate social support systems (eg, grandparents, family members, friends, doulas, child care, housekeeping services) are not available, new parents may be overwhelmed with the needs of the newborn. The new mother must cope with fatigue, discomfort, changes in body image, and possible frustration as she tries to learn her newborn's patterns and ways of communicating. Fatigue is frequently reported by new mothers in the first few days at home with their newborns and can have a cumulative effect on physical discomforts, mood swings, and changes in relationships inherent in the physical and emotional transition to motherhood (Ruchala & Halstead, 1994).

The goal of home care services is to safely and effectively care for the mother and newborn in their home after a hospital birth. This includes a physical assessment of the mother and newborn to identify complications and subsequent medical interventions; an infant feeding assessment (ie, breast-feeding or bottle feeding); addressing any issues of concerns about mothers own health or self-care, the health of the newborn, and newborn care; and reinforcing education already provided from prenatal education, clinic, birthing, and postpartum care. The home care nurse must be knowledgeable about the educational materials provided to the patients from the clinic or hospital to ensure the instructions given by the home care nurse are consistent. The nurse needs to be aware of hospital and community resources available to the family. It is often during the home visit that the family is ready to learn about ongoing educational programs and available resources. Support persons and family members are invited to participate in the home visit if the mother desires. Subsequent home visits are based on the individual needs identified (AWHONN, 1994, 1998; AWHONN & Johnson & Johnson, 1996).

Adjustment and coping with the stress of a newborn varies with each family. During the first few days postpartum, women have a need to describe the labor and birth process (Rubin, 1961). The home care nurse can ask the mother about her childbirth experience, which assists in fulfilling a developmental task in the transition to motherhood and can be the first opening to successful nurse–patient communication. Nursing assessments and interventions occur concurrently. During the assessment of physical status, learning needs, and psychological adaptation to parenting, the nurse has the opportunity to reinforce earlier teaching, answer questions and concerns, and refer to appropriate community resources as needed. Each new mother has unique abilities and learning needs. A collaborative approach is more successful than a lecture approach in promoting maternal confidence in parenting skills (Hall & Carty, 1993). The home care nurse can establish mutually acceptable goals with the mother for the home visit time. The home care program protocols, primary healthcare provider's orders, clinical situation, and intent of the home visit also guide and direct the home visit.

NURSING ASSESSMENTS

The home care nurse should be prepared to address the following maternal–newborn topics. Not all of the listed topics are covered during a home care visit, but they may be included in the care provided during home visits based on the assessment and individual needs of the mother and newborn (AAP & ACOG, 1997; AWHONN, 1994, 1998; AWHONN & Johnson & Johnson, 1996).

Physical Assessment

Maternal physical assessments include the following (not in order of importance):

- Review of antepartum, intrapartum, and immediate postpartum events
- Vital signs (eg, temperature, blood pressure, pulse, respirations)
- Breasts and nipple condition
- Fundal height and location
- Lochia: color, consistency, and amount
- Perineum
- Episiotomy
- Abdominal incision
- Edema
- Pain or discomfort level
- Elimination patterns: voiding and bowel movements
- Nutritional status
- Sleeping patterns
- Emotional assessment, postpartum blues or depression
- Activity level
- Sexuality issues
- Self-care ability
- Social support system available
- Cultural and religious norms and practices regarding postpartum recovery

Newborn physical assessments include the following (not in order of importance):

- Vital signs (eg, temperature, pulse, respirations)
- Fontanelles
- Color
- Evaluation for presence of neonatal jaundice
- Condition of skin

- Umbilical cord
- Circumcision
- Reflexes: suck, grasp, and Moro
- Nutritional status: feeding patterns
- Elimination patterns: voiding and stooling
- Activity, sleep–wake cycles

Learning-Needs Assessment

Maternal Topics

Maternal learning-needs topics include the following:

- Pericare
- Incision or episiotomy care
- Breast care
- Diet and fluid intake
- Sexuality
- Contraception
- Potential complications
- When to call perinatal nurse, nurse midwife, or obstetrician
- When to return for postpartum office visit
- Pain management and what medications are safe during breast-feeding
- Domestic violence assessment
- Cultural groups within the community
- Body image changes
- Activity level and when to return to normal activity
- Rest requirements
- Normal baby blues versus postpartum depression or psychosis

Newborn Topics

Physical care topics for the newborn include the following:

- Skin care and bathing
- Umbilical cord care
- Circumcision and care of the uncircumcised penis
- Normal hormonal influence, vaginal discharge, and breast enlargement
- Diapering and rash treatment
- Newborn positioning: side and back versus prone
- Use of bulb syringe for suctioning secretions
- Temperature assessment
- Comforting techniques
- Normal growth and development
- Maternal–newborn attachment
- Sibling behaviors
- Safety issues, including car seats, pets, and toys
- Infant cardiopulmonary resuscitation
- Potential complications
- When to call perinatal nurse, pediatric nurse practitioner, or pediatrician
- When to return for first newborn office visit

Bottle-feeding topics include the following:

- Amount, type, and frequency
- Adequacy of intake
- Positioning
- Burping
- Resources available to answer bottle feeding questions and provide support

Breast-feeding topics include the following:

- Adequate milk supply, engorgement
- Demand feeding and frequency
- Positioning
- Latching-on
- Let-down
- Burping
- Support bra
- Nipple care
- Strategies to assess breast-feeding adequacy
- Strategies to cope with sore nipples
- Importance of rest and increased diet and fluid intake
- Resources available to answer breast-feeding questions and provide support
- Availability of certified lactation nurse consultant for phone consultation or visit
- Use of a breast-feeding assessment tool (Matthews, 1993; Schlomer, Kemmerer, & Twiss, 1999)

Newborn behaviors and cues include the following:

- Crying
- Sleep–wake pattern
- Individual temperaments
- Response to parenting and reciprocal cues

Psychosocial Assessment

A psychosocial assessment includes the following topics:

- Maternal–newborn attachment process
- Emotional response to parenting
- Perceptions of childbirth experience
- Family interactions
- Coping and adaptation abilities
- Maternal role assumption
- Body image adjustment
- Identification of support persons
- Social, economic, and cultural factors
- Knowledge of community resources

Environmental Assessment

An environmental assessment includes the following topics:

- Obvious safety issues
- Adequate heat and temperature control
- Telephone availability
- Infant crib, pets, and toys
- Equipment, such as a thermometer

NURSING INTERVENTIONS

Perinatal nursing interventions during home visits are directed toward reinforcing earlier instructions, providing assistance with self-care, promoting health education, providing emotional support, validating childbirth experiences, and emphasizing support and referral resources available in the community (AWHONN, 1994, 1998). Additional services that may be provided on an as-needed basis are staple removal for abdominal incisions, wound care, obtaining samples for laboratory testing (eg, newborn screen and bilirubin determination, maternal hemoglobin and hematocrit determinations), and initiating and monitoring newborn phototherapy.

An assessment of the home environment is incorporated in the home visit. A safety checklist is a valuable tool to ensure that all aspects of safety are addressed. The nurse can assist the family in obtaining community resources available to address conditions such as health hazards (eg, poor sanitation, infestation) and physical hazards (eg, broken windows, lack of heat, poor lighting, other unsafe housing conditions) or financial needs.

Nursing interventions are based on the needs of the individual mother, newborn, and family. The unique difference in nursing practice in the home is that the nurse is practicing alone, and critical thinking and communication skills are crucial to safe and effective care. When the home care nurse determines that the clinical findings are outside of normal limits, the family is informed, and the primary healthcare provider is contacted to determine the most appropriate follow-up care needed. The plan may include additional nursing visits, clinic visits, or ongoing reporting to the physician. Some situations may require immediate attention and require a trip to the emergency department or urgent care center.

At each home visit, the home care nurse determines the need for ongoing care and referrals. If there are clinical issues requiring further home visits, the home care nurse contacts the primary care provider, establishes the plan of care, obtains needed orders, and then obtains authorization from the funding source for further visits. The home care nurse may determine that the needs of the family may be met through other members of the healthcare team such as social services, lactation consultants, and support groups. After the home care nurse has completed the home visits needed and made appropriate referrals, the nurse can follow-up through phone calls to validate the plan identified is working for this family. If the plan has not been successful, the nurse determines the reason and facilitates changes in the plan of care to better meet their needs. When the needs of the family are met or a plan is in place to meet those needs, the mother and newborn can be discharged from home care services. At discharge, the home care nurse reviews with the mother the plan and timing of clinic appointments for herself and the newborn.

OUTCOME MONITORING AND QUALITY CARE

Documentation of nursing assessments, interventions, evaluations, and the discharge summary must be as meticulous and complete during perinatal home visits as during inpatient care (AWHONN, 1998). Each perinatal home care program should have established standards for medical record documentation. It is also important to record summaries of nurse–patient phone consultations. Examples of documentation tools (eg, Postpartum Home Care Referral, Postpartum Assessment Phone Call, Maternal Assessment Note and Care Plan, Infant Assessment Note and Care Plan) are presented in Appendices 19A through 19D. If complications arise, nursing interventions, physician orders, and follow-through actions are included. A copy of documentation tools about the home visit should be provided to the primary care provider to be included in the maternal–newborn medical record.

The clinical findings of a perinatal home care program should be reviewed and included in the quality management of the agency. Data should be collected about maternal–newborn complications, including those that require additional home visits, an unscheduled visit to the office or clinic of the primary healthcare provider, and readmissions to the hospital. Early postpartum discharge followed by home visits has not been found to result in an increase risk of newborn or maternal readmission to the hospital for healthy mothers and babies. Occasionally, a clinical situation may result in a newborn or maternal readmission. Factors associated with newborn readmission after an early discharge are breast-feeding, vaginal birth with a LOS less than 72 hours, neonatal jaundice, gestational age less than 37 weeks, or discharge weight less than 3 kg (Egerter, Braveman, & Marchi, 1998; Soskolne et al., 1996). Factors associated with maternal readmission are cesarean birth, operative vaginal birth, and wound infections (Lydon-Rochelle, Holt, Martin, & Easterling, 2000). Ability to track readmission rates related to maternal and newborn complications, as well as the treatment and resolution of complications that do not require readmission, is essential in the evaluation of nursing care provided and in planning future care strategies. Display 19–4 lists the suggested categories to include in a comprehensive morbidity database that are helpful in evaluating outcomes related to perinatal home care services.

Home phototherapy has allowed some newborns to remain home and receive treatment for hyperbilirubinemia. Additional nursing visits are arranged on a daily basis to initiate home phototherapy and monitor the newborn's improvement. The home care nurse can identify maternal infections and facilitate consultation with the healthcare provider and the appropriate treatment obtained. Other complications may necessitate a return visit to the healthcare provider's office. Any interventions performed at home instead of the hospital are cost-effective and are more convenient for the mother and family.

In addition to morbidity and cost data, maternal satisfaction with perinatal home care services is also an important quality indicator. An example of a patient satisfaction tool is provided in Appendix 19E. There is evidence to support a high level of maternal satisfaction with postpartum home visits (Armstrong et al., 1999; Brooten et al., 1994; Carty & Bradley, 1990; Drummond, Boucher, Chisholm, Geraci, & Kay, 1994; Gazmararian & Solomon, 1997; Jones, 1997). Patient and family feedback obtained through satisfaction surveys can assist the program in process improvements. The data also help the nurses understand how their home visits support the mother and newborn during the first days home. At the time of the home visit, surveys can be given to the mother with a postage-paid envelope for her to mail at her convenience. When the surveys are received in the office, the home care nurse and program leadership team can review the individual surveys and summaries. Survey data provides useful feedback about quality of service. The following are examples of mothers' responses:

- "The part of the home visit that was most valuable to me was answering all my questions and having the examination for myself and my baby."
- "Just having the nurse available for the questions you don't remember to ask while in the hospital was great."
- "It's nice to have a nurse come out a few days later. There are always more questions when you get home. I didn't have a home care nurse with my first baby—I'm glad I did this time."

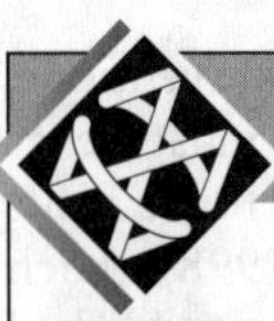

DISPLAY 19–4

Suggested Categories for Morbidity Statistics Database

All readmissions

Maternal complications
- Infections: incision, episiotomy, breast, urinary tract, endometrium
- Vaginal bleeding
- Anemia
- Fever
- Gastrointestinal
- Inadequate maternal–newborn attachment
- Clinical depression
- Social support deficit
- Abuse or battering
- Unsafe or inadequate environment

Newborn complications
- Jaundice
- Dehydration
- Feeding instabilities
- Failure to thrive or inadequate weight gain
- Infections: cord stump, circumcision, eyes, thrush
- Unsafe or inadequate environment
- Abuse

NURSE PROVIDERS OF PERINATAL HOME CARE

Orientation and Education

AWHONN (1994) has published guidelines for didactic content and clinical skill verification for professional nurse providers of perinatal home care services that are useful in planning a comprehensive orientation program. A thorough knowledge of normal postpartum and newborn care, potential complications, and appropriate nursing interventions is essential for the perinatal nurse providing care in the home. Inpatient mother–newborn care is an ideal way to gain this level of expertise. Practice in the home setting requires a high degree of autonomy and independence. It is also important for nurses to remember that they are guests in the home and that the goal is to facilitate the family's ability to cope using their own resources.

Nursing responsibilities during home care for women and newborns have been outlined by AWHONN (1998) and may include the following actions:

- Planning for comprehensive home health services, 24 hours each day and 7 days each week, for the woman, newborn, and family
- Acting as a coordinator in communicating a plan of care between the woman and the primary healthcare provider
- Acting as a liaison with ancillary healthcare providers
- Developing and supervising a written plan of care for the homemaker or home health aide
- Acting as the patient's advocate by promoting informed decision-making about care
- Orienting, supervising, and evaluating individuals on the home health team as appropriate

A didactic course covering the content outline suggested in the AWHONN (1994) guidelines provides basic knowledge needed for home care practice. A clinical practicum with an experienced preceptor is an essential part of a comprehensive orientation to perinatal home care nursing (Simpson & Creehan, 1998). Evaluation and documentation of core competencies through clinical skill verification and knowledge base assessment should be as thorough as those provided in the inpatient setting. Requirements for continuing education are also desirable to maintain excellence in practice. Criteria have been suggested for employment:

- Registered professional nurse status
- Three years' perinatal nursing experience
- Successful completion of orientation and ongoing support and mentoring available for 6 months to 1 year
- Seven to 15 contact hours of continuing education in perinatal nursing per year

Annual performance evaluations are based on patient satisfaction data; accurate, complete, and timely documentation; and consistent, appropriate nursing interventions and follow-up; and peer review, self-assessment, and manager review.

Personal Safety

A final issue unique to nursing practice in the home setting is that of personal safety. Each agency should have in place policies to address various situations that could compromise the safety of the nurse in the community. There should be a system to locate the nurse if necessary and a reliable method for communication between the agency and nurse. Beepers and cellular telephones are ideal ways to ensure rapid communication and the ability to call for help in unanticipated dangerous situations. The office must have the address and phone numbers of the patients the nurse is visiting each day. The agency or institution should have a check-in policy; nurses should report changes in their schedules and check in at the completion of their assignments so that they are accounted for at the end of the day. Orientation should include directions regarding the immediate actions the nurse should take when encountering potentially unsafe situations such as abusive others in the home, weapons, illegal drugs, and hazardous pets. Self-defense techniques should be addressed along with situations to avoid, such as groups of people in doorways or corners leading to the home. If traveling by car, preventive maintenance and adequate fuel are important to avoid being stranded. A heightened awareness of personal safety and common sense are the best approaches to decrease the likelihood of involvement in a potentially dangerous situation.

SUMMARY

Research has suggested that an early hospital discharge is safe and effective for appropriately screened women and newborns. There appears to be a high level of satisfaction with early discharge when followed by perinatal home care nursing services. Data related to the financial benefits are also encouraging. As healthcare services are increasingly scrutinized for quality and cost-effectiveness, programs such as perinatal home care, with positive clinical outcomes, high levels of patient satisfaction, and cost reduction potential will continue. During the past decade, the traditional role of the postpartum nurse has evolved to include care in the home. More research is needed about the types of follow-up services after hospital discharge and related outcomes. Perinatal nurses are challenged to expand their practice into the community to meet the needs of childbearing women and families. Perinatal nurses have the opportunity to improve outcomes and enhance the childbirth experience by providing quality nursing care in the home setting.

REFERENCES

American Academy of Pediatrics & American College of Obstetricians and Gynecologists (AAP & ACOG). (1997). *Guidelines for perinatal care* (4th ed.). Elk Grove Village, IL: Author.

American Nurses Association (ANA). (1995). *Home care for mother, infant, and family following birth* (Position Statement). Washington, DC: Author.

Armstrong, K. L., Fraser, J. A., Dadds, M. R., & Morris, J. (1999). A randomized controlled trial of nurse home visiting to vulnerable families with newborns. *Journal of Paediatric and Child Health, 35*(3), 237–244.

Association of Women's Health, Obstetric and Neonatal Nurses (AWHONN). (1994). *Didactic content and clinical skills verification for professional nurse providers of perinatal homecare.* Washington, DC: Author.

Association of Women's Health, Obstetric and Neonatal Nurses (AWHONN). (1998). *Standards and guidelines for professional nursing practice in the care of women and newborns* (5th ed). Washington, DC: Author.

Association of Women's Health, Obstetric and Neonatal Nurses & Johnson & Johnson Consumer Products. (1996). *Compendium of postpartum care.* Washington, DC: Author.

Bateman, S. (1998). A fourth trimester with home care. *Caring, 17*(5), 18–20.

Beck, C. T. (1991). Early postpartum discharge programs in the United States: A literature review and critique. *Women and Health, 17*(1), 125–138.

Bragg, E. J., Rosenn, B. M., Khoury, J. C., Miodovnik, M., & Siddiqi, T. A. (1997). The effect of early discharge after vaginal delivery on neonatal readmission rates. *Obstetrics and Gynecology, 89*(6), 930–933.

Braveman, P., Egerter, S., Pearl, M., Marchi, K., & Miller, C. (1995). Problems associated with early discharge of newborns and mothers: A critical review of the literature. *Pediatrics, 96*(4, Pt. 1), 716–726.

Braveman, P., Miller, C., Egerter, S., Bennett, T., English, P., Katz, P., & Showstack, J. (1996). Health service use among low-risk newborns after early discharge with and without nurse home visiting. *Journal of the American Board of Family Practice, 9*(4), 254–260.

Britton, J. R. (1998). Postpartum early hospital discharge and follow-up practices in Canada and the United States. *Birth, 25*(3), 161–168.

Brooten, D., Roncoli, M., Finkler, S., Arnold, L., Cohen, A., & Mennuti, M. (1994). A randomized trial of early hospital discharge and home follow-up of women having cesarean birth. *Obstetrics and Gynecology, 84*(5), 832–838.

Brooten, D., Knapp, H., Borucki, L., Jacobsen, B., Finkler, S., Arnold, L., & Mennuti, M. (1996). Early discharge and home care after unplanned cesarean birth: Nursing care time. *Journal of Obstetric, Gynecologic, and Neonatal Nursing, 25*(7), 595–600.

Brown, S. G., & Johnson B. T. (1998). Enhancing early discharge with home follow-up: A pilot project. *Journal of Obstetric, Gynecologic, and Neonatal Nursing, 27*(1), 33–38.

Brumfield, C. G. (1998). Early postpartum discharge. *Clinical Obstetrics and Gynecology, 41*(3), 611–625.

Brumfield, C. G., Nelson, K. G., Stotser, D., Yarbaugh, D., Patterson, P., & Sprayberry, N. K. (1996). 24 Hour mother-infant discharge with a follow-up home health visit: Results in a selected Medicaid population. *Obstetrics and Gynecology, 88*(4, Pt. 1), 544–548.

Carty, E. M., & Bradley, C. F. (1990). A randomized, controlled evaluation of early postpartum hospital discharge. *Birth, 17*(4), 199–204.

Dahlberg, N. L., & Koloroutis, M. (1994). Hospital-based perinatal homecare program. *Journal of Obstetric, Gynecologic, and Neonatal Nursing, 23*(8), 682–686.

Declercq, E. (1999). Making US maternal and child health policy: From "early discharge" to "drive through deliveries" to a national law. *Maternal-Child Health Journal, 3*(1), 5–17.

Declercq, E., & Simmes, D. (1997). The politics of "drive through deliveries": Putting early postpartum discharges on the legislative agenda. *The Milbank Quarterly, 75*(2), 175–203.

Drummond, R. C., Boucher, J. D., Chisholm, D., Geraci, R. C., & Kay, S. (1994). Mother care: Cost effective program in maternal-infant care. *Home Healthcare Nurse, 2*(5), 41–43.

Egerter, S. A., Braveman, P. A., & Marchi, K. S. (1998). Follow-up of newborns and their mothers after early hospital discharge. *Clinics in Perinatology, 25*(2), 471–481.

Frank-Hanssen, M., Hanson, K. S., & Anderson, M. A. (1999). Postpartum home visits: Infant outcomes. *Journal of Community Health Nursing, 16*(1), 17–28.

Gagnon, A. J., Edgar, L., Kramer, M. S., Papageorgiou, A., Waghorn, K., & Klein, M. C. (1997). A randomized trial of a program of early postpartum discharge with nurse visitation. *American Journal of Obstetrics and Gynecology, 176*(1, Pt. 1), 205–211.

Gazmararian, J. A., & Solomon, F. M. (1997). Receipt of home health care after early discharge: Results from a national managed care organization. *Maternal-Child Health Journal, 1*(3), 151–156.

Grupp-Phelan, J., Taylor, J. A., Liu, L. L., & Davis, R. L. (1999). Early newborn hospital discharge and readmission for mild and severe jaundice. *Archives of Pediatric and Adolescent Medicine, 153*(12), 1283–1288.

Guerriero, W. (1943). A maternal welfare program for New Orleans. *American Journal of Obstetrics and Gynecology, 46*, 312–313.

Hall, W. A., & Carty, E. M. (1993). Managing the early discharge experience: Taking control. *Journal of Advanced Nursing, 18*(4), 574–582.

Hellman, L., Kohl, S., & Palmer, J. (1962). Early hospital discharge in obstetrics. *Lancet, 1* (4), 227–232.

Jones, P. M. (1997). Patient satisfaction with home care after early postpartum hospital discharge. *Home Care Provider, 2*(5), 235–243.

Kotagal, U. R., Atherton, H. D., Eshett, R., Schoettker, P. J., & Perlstein, P. H. (1999). Safety of early discharge for Medicaid newborns. *Journal of the American Medical Association, 282*(12), 1150–1156.

Lane, D. A., Kauls, L. S., Ickovics, J. R., Naftolin, F., & Feinstein, A. R. (1999). Early postpartum discharges. Impact on distress and outpatient problems. *Archives of Family Medicine, 8*(3), 237–242.

Lieu, T. A., Braveman, P. A., Escobar, G. J., Fischer, A. F., Jensvold, N. G., & Capra, A. M. (2000). A randomized comparison of home and clinic follow-up visits after early postpartum hospital discharge. *Pediatrics, 105*(5), 1058–1065.

Lock, M., & Ray, J. G. (1999). Higher neonatal morbidity after routine early hospital discharge: Are we sending newborns home too early? *Canadian Medical Association Journal, 161*(3), 249–253.

Lydon-Rochelle, M., Holt, V. L., Martin, D. P., & Easterling, T. R. (2000). Association between method of delivery and maternal rehospitalization. *Journal of the American Medical Association, 283*(18), 2411–2416.

Maisels, M. J., & Kring, E. (1998). Length of stay, jaundice, and hospital readmission. *Pediatrics, 101*(6), 995–998.

Malkin, J. D., Garber, S., Broder, M. S., & Keeler, E. (2000). Infant mortality and early postpartum discharge. *Obstetrics and Gynecology, 96*(2), 183–188.

Matthews, M. K. (1993). Assessments and suggested interventions to assist newborn breastfeeding behavior. *Journal of Human Lactation, 9*(4), 243–248.

Meikle, S. F., Lyons, E., Hulac, P., & Orleans, M. (1998). Rehospitalizations and outpatient contacts of mothers and neonates after hospital discharge after vaginal delivery. *American Journal of Obstetrics and Gynecology, 179*(1), 166–171.

Norr, K. F., & Nacion, K. (1987). Outcomes of postpartum early discharge, 1960–1986: A comparative review. *Birth, 14*(3), 135–141.

Norr, K. F., Nacion, K. W., & Abramson, R. (1989). Early discharge with home follow-up: Impact on low-income mothers and infants. *Journal of Obstetric, Gynecologic, and Neonatal Nursing, 18*(2), 133–141.

Olds, D. L., Eckenrode, J., Henderson, C. R.. Jr., Kitzman, H., Powers, J., Cole, R., Sidora, K., Morris, P., Pettit, L. M., & Luckey, D. (1997). Long-term effects of home visitation on maternal life course and child abuse and neglect: Fifteen-year follow-up of a randomized trial. *Journal of the American Medical Association, 278*(8), 637–643.

Olds, D. L., Henderson, C. R., Jr., & Kitzman, H. J. (1994). Does prenatal and infancy nurse home visitation have enduring effects on qualities of parental caregiving and child health at 25 to 50 months of life? *Pediatrics, 93*(1), 89–98.

Olds, D. L., Henderson, C. R., Jr., Kitzman, H. J., Eckenrode, J. J., Cole, R. E., & Tatelbaum, R. C. (1999). Prenatal and infancy home visitation by nurses: Recent findings. *Future Child, 9*(1), 44–65, 190–191.

Olds, D. L., Henderson, C. R., Jr., Tatelbaum, R., & Chamberlin, R. (1986). Improving the delivery of prenatal care and outcomes of pregnancy: A randomized trial of nurse home visitation. *Pediatrics, 77*(1), 16–28.

Rubin, R. (1961). Puerperal change. *Nursing Outlook, 9*, 753–755.

Ruchala, P. L., & Halstead, L. (1994). The postpartum experience of low-risk women: A time of adjustment and change. *Maternal-Child Nursing Journal, 22*(3), 83–89.

Schlomer, J. A, Kemmerer, J, & Twiss, J. J. (1999). Evaluating the association of two breastfeeding assessment tools with breastfeeding problems and breastfeeding satisfaction. *Journal of Human Lactation, 15* (1), 35–39.

Soskolne, E. I., Schumacher, R., Fyock, C., Young, M. L., & Schork, A. (1996). The effect of early discharge and other factors on readmission rates of newborns. *Archives of Pediatric and Adolescent Medicine, 150*(4), 373–379.

Simpson, K. R. (1996). *Easing the transition from hospital to home: Postpartum discharge planning and homecare services* (Nursing Module). White Plains, NY: March of Dimes Birth Defects Foundation.

Simpson, K. R., & Creehan, P. A (Eds.). (1998). *AWHONN's Competence validation for perinatal providers: Orientation, continuing education and evaluation.* Philadelphia: Lippincott.

Waldenstrom, U. (1987). Early discharge with domiciliary visits and hospital care: Parents' experiences of two modes of postpartum care. *Scandinavian Journal of Caring Sciences, 1*(2), 51–58.

Waldenstrom, U. (1988). Early and late discharge after hospital birth: Father's involvement in infant care. *Early Human Development, 17*(1), 19–28.

Waldenstrom, U. (1989). Early discharge as voluntary and involuntary alternatives to a longer postpartum stay in hospital: Effects on mothers' experiences and breast feeding. *Midwifery, 5*,(4), 189–196.

Welt, S. I., Cole, J. S., Myers, M. S., Sholes, D. M., & Jelovsek, F. R. (1993). Feasibility of postpartum rapid discharge: A study from a community hospital population. *American Journal of Perinatology, 10*(5), 384–387.

Yanover, M. J., Jones, D., & Miller, M. D. (1976). Perinatal care of low-risk mothers and infants: Early discharge with homecare. *New England Journal of Medicine, 294*(13), 702–705.

APPENDIX **19A**

Home Care Assessment Form

Minnesota OB Homecare
Phone: 612-863-4478
Fax: 612-863-4568

UNITED HOSPITAL
POSTPARTUM HOME CARE REFERRAL

Mother's Name: ____________________________

Address/Phone where mother will be staying:

Address: ____________________________

City: ____________________________

Phone #(____) ____________________________

☐ **Address & Phone Verified**

Language Spoken: ☐ English ☐ Other: __________

Understands English: ☐ Well ☐ Poor

☐ Mother Needs Interpreter ☐ Hearing Impaired

Who interpreted in hospital: ______________

Phone: (____) ______________

Mom's MD/Midwife: (Full Name) ______________

Phone #: (____) ______________

Next Appt: ______________

MOTHER:

Gravida ____ T ____ P ____ A ____ L ____

Marital Status: S M W D Sep

Normal Maternal Exam: ☐ Yes ☐ No (explain below)

☐ Vaginal Birth ☐ C/Birth

Epis/Incision: ______________

Meds: ______________

Allergies: ______________

☐ Needs Large BP Cuff

OTHER ISSUES:

Diabetic: ______________

Hgb pp, if abnormal: ______________

Psycho/Social Issues:

☐ Parent/Child Interaction ☐ Limited Support System

☐ Mental Health Status ☐ Drug Use/Dependency

☐ Previous Losses ☐ Hx of Domestic Violence

☐ Other: ______________

Husband/Significant Other: ______________

Baby's Name: ______________ ☐ M ☐ F

Delivery Data/Time: __________ @ __________

Mother's Discharge Date/Time: __________ @ __________

Baby's MD (Full Name): ______________

Phone #: (____) ______________

Next Appt: ______________

BABY:

Gestation: __________ weeks ☐ Fetal Loss

Birth Weight: __________ Discharge wt: __________

Apgars: 1 __________ 5 __________

Feedings: ☐ Breast ☐ Bottle ☐ Both

Feeding Issues: ______________

____

Normal Infant Exam: ☐ Yes ☐ No (explain below)

Circumcised: ☐ Yes ☐ No

Additional Order:

☐ Home care to draw newborn screen
**Must send lab-slip home with family.

____

ADDITIONAL COMMENTS or
ABNORMAL FINDINGS FOR MOTHER OR BABY:

____

____

____

____

____

____

____

____

Mom aware of referral: ☐ Yes ☐ No

REFERRAL COMPLETED BY: ______________

☐ ***Faxed to Minnesota OB Homecare @ 613-863-4568:*** ☐ ***Facesheet*** ☐ ***Referral***

☐ ***Faxed to PHN*** ______________ ***County:*** ☐ ***Facesheet*** ☐ ***Referral***

Currently being seen by PHN: ☐ Yes ☐ No

APPENDIX **19B**

Telephone Assessment Form

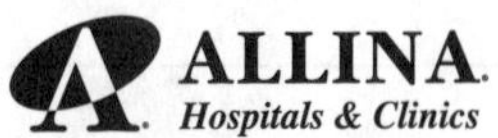

POSTPARTUM ASSESSMENT PHONE CALL

OB HOMECARE

MOTHER'S NAME	SSN	MD	D/C DATE
INFANT NAME	ID#	MD	DOB / D/C DATE
☐ MALE ☐ FEMALE	☐ PRIMIP ☐ MULTIP	☐ VAG ☐ C/BIRTH	BIRTH WT / D/C WT

QUESTION	RESPONSE	EDUC PROV
1) ARE YOU FEELING AS WELL AS YOU THOUGHT YOU WOULD NOW THAT YOU ARE HOME?	☐ YES ☐ NO	
2) IF NO: WHAT ARE YOU EXPERIENCING THAT IS DIFFERENT OR CHALLENGING FOR YOU?	☐ PAIN ☐ BLEEDING ☐ FATIGUE ☐ OVERWHELMED	
3) HOW OFTEN IS BABY EATING?	☐ Q1–2H ☐ Q2–3H ☐ Q3–4H	
4) BREAST-FEEDING / LATCH ASSESSMENT:		

	0	1	2
L LATCH	• Too sleepy or reluctant • No latch achieved	• Repeated attempts • Hold nipple in mouth • Stimulate to suck	• Grasps breast • Tongue down • Lips flanged • Rhythmical sucking
A AUDIBLE SWALLOWING	• None	• A few with stimulation	• Spontaneous and intermittent <24° • Spontaneous and frequent
T TYPE OF NIPPLE	• Inverted	• Flat	• Everted (after stimulation)
C COMFORT	• Engorged • Cracked, bleeding, large blisters or bruises • Severe discomfort	• Filling • Reddened/small blisters or bruises • Mild/moderate discomfort	• Soft • Nontender
H HOLD (Positioning)	• Full assist (staff holds)	• Minimal assist (ie, pillows, ↑HOB) • Teach one side, mom does other • Staff holds →mom takes over	• No assist from staff • Mom able to position/hold baby

TOTAL SCORE:_______/10

☐ pumping & bottling
☐ advised on cup feeding / dropper feeding
☐ patient is seeing lactation consultant
☐ patient to call lactation consultant for appt.
☐ OBHC RN advised lactation consultant of breast-feeding issue

QUESTION	RESPONSE	EDUC PROV
(5-6) BOTTLE FEEDING: 5) HOW MUCH FORMULA IS TAKEN AT EACH FEEDING?	☐ 1oz ☐ 2oz ☐ 3oz	
6) ANY PROBLEMS WITH FEEDING?	☐ YES ☐ NO	
7) HOW MANY WET DIAPERS HAS BABY HAD IN LAST 24 HRS? (4–6 IF > 3 DAYS OLD)	☐ 1–2 ☐ 3–4 ☐ 5–6 ☐ >6	
8) WHAT COLOR WAS YOUR BABY'S LAST STOOL?	☐ NO STOOLS ☐ TRANSITIONAL ☐ MECONIUM ☐ MUSTARD	
9) DOES BABY APPEAR JAUNDICED? (OPTIONAL)	☐ NO ☐ YES: DESCRIBE:	
10) DO YOU HAVE A CLINIC APPT FOR BABY?	☐ YES ☐ NO	
11) IF YOU HAVE A PROBLEM, DO YOU KNOW THE RESOURCES AVAILABLE TO YOU?	☐ YES ☐ NO ☐ B:PBB ☐ CLINIC ☐ 911	

NURSE'S SIGNATURE ______________________ **DATE / TIME** ________ @ ________

Message left: 1) date/time: ________ @ ________ ☐ on answering machine ☐ with person ____________
2) date/time: ________ @ ________ ☐ on answering machine ☐ with person ____________
3) date/time: ________ @ ________ ☐ on answering machine ☐ with person ____________

VISIT SCHEDULED: Date: ________

NO VISIT; REASON:
☐ Medical criteria not met
☐ Planned phone call only
☐ No call back from patient
☐ Unable to locate patient
☐ Mother declined, follow-up in clinic
☐ Referral to PHN: ____________
☐ Other ____________

COMMENTS: ______________________________

APPENDIX **19C**

Maternal Assessment Form

ALLINA Hospitals & Clinics

OB HOMECARE

MATERNAL ASSESSMENT NOTE AND CARE PLAN

MEDICAL RECORD NUMBER (SSN) ☐☐☐-☐☐-☐☐☐☐ TIME IN ☐☐☐☐

DATE ☐☐☐☐☐☐ TIME OUT ☐☐☐☐

CLIENT NAME:			
BILLABLE: ○ YES ○ NO			
ACTIVITY ID ● RNV620	BRANCH ● 62		
PHYSICIAN NAME:	PHONE:	DELIVERY DATE:	HOSP DISCHARGE DATE:
PHYSICIAN PLEASE NOTE:			

EXPECTED OUTCOME:
* Client will verbalize/demonstrate knowledge of postpartum self care and care for newborn
* Client will demonstrate knowledge of breast and/or bottle-feeding techniques and methods for problem solving.

TPR: ________________

B/P: ____________

CURRENT MEDICATION

☐ None ☐ PNV (1, po, qd) ☐ Ibuprofen (600 mg, po, q6hprn)
☐ Stool softener (1–2, po, qd) ☐ Other ________________

ALLERGIES

☐ None ☐ ________________

	WNL	Educ Prov	Exceptions
PROGNOSIS Good / excellent			
RESPIRATORY Quiet, regular, nonlabored			
BREASTS Nipples intact; nontender, nonengorged			
UTERUS Fundus firm, at or below umbilicus; non-tender; lochia not excessive; no foul odor			
CARDIOVASCULAR Pulse regular, no calf tenderness; No edema or <+2 (+1 slight, +2 indentation 10–15 sec.) (+3 deep indent, +4 marked deep indent)			
PERINEUM / INCISION Intact, no s/s of infection; Hemorrhoids without problems			
ELIMINATION Voiding & stooling w/o difficulty			

	WNL	Educ Prov	Exceptions
NUTRITION Good appetite; adequate food/fluids			
SLEEP / REST / ACTIVITY Sleeps when baby sleeps; up as tolerated; no functional limitations			
PARENT / INFANT ATTACHMENT Demos positive interaction w/baby			
PSYCHOSOCIAL / MENTAL STATUS Alert & oriented; actively participates at visit; asking appropriate questions			
SUPPORT SYSTEM Support system involved; has respite support			
SAFETY Aware of s/s of complications; verbalizes emergency plan (ie, clinic ph#, poison control, 911, etc)			
FAMILY RESOURCES Family, hospital, community parenting groups, etc.			

WE FIND MOST FREQUENTLY ASKED QUESTIONS OF MOMS HOME FROM THE HOSPITAL ARE:

1) DO YOU KNOW HOW / WHEN TO TAKE YOUR PAIN MEDS? ☐ Yes ☐ No ________________
DO YOU HAVE QUESTIONS ABOUT SIDE EFFECTS? ☐ Yes ☐ No ________________

2) DO YOU KNOW WHEN TO RESUME NORMAL ACTIVITIES? SEXUAL RELATIONS? ☐ Yes ☐ No ________________

3) DO YOU HAVE THE INFO NEEDED TO CARE FOR YOURSELF & YOUR BABY? ☐ Yes ☐ No ________________
IF NOT, HOW CAN I HELP? OR: WHAT CAN I DO FOR YOU?

CONFERENCE WITH: ☐ PHYSICIAN ☐ VISIT NOTE FAXED TO MD OFFICE ☐ SENT TO MD W/PT ☐ INSURANCE ☐ NONE ☐ OTHER ________

PLAN OF CARE:

☐ Has the B:PBB Resource Book
☐ Call MD with questions or concerns;
• Routine clinic visit scheduled: ☐ Yes ☐ No
☐ Discharged at home visit OR ☐ Follow-up call by visiting nurse

DISCHARGE DATE:

____

☐ See next visit for discharge date

(SELF CARE, GOALS MET)

DV SCREEN:

\+ – ?

Resources given:

Y N

____

____

170103 (12/99)

Nurse's Signature ________________________________

APPENDIX 19D

Infant Assessment Form

ALLINA
Hospitals & Clinics

OB HOMECARE

INFANT ASSESSMENT NOTE AND CARE PLAN

MEDICAL RECORD NUMBER ☐☐☐☐☐☐ TIME IN ☐☐ ☐☐

DATE ☐☐ ☐☐ ☐☐ TIME OUT ☐☐ ☐☐

CLIENT NAME:		
BILLABLE: ○ YES ○ NO		
ACTIVITY ID ○ BPV620 ○ RNV620	**BRANCH** ● 62	
PHYSICIAN NAME:	**PHONE:**	**MOTHER'S NAME:**
DOB:	**HOSPITAL DISCHARGE DATE:**	**DAYS OLD AT VISIT:**
PHYSICIAN PLEASE NOTE:		

TPR: ________ **WEIGHT:** Birth: ____________ D/C: ____________ **Today:** ____________ (☐ ≥10% wt loss)

FEEDING: ☐ Breast ☐ Bottle

BREAST-FEEDING: ● Nursing Q _____ hrs **SCORE** ________/10

LATCH	0	1	2	EDUC
LATCH	• Too sleepy or reluctant • No latch achieved	• Repeated attempts • Hold nipple in mouth • Stimulate to suck	• Grasps breast • Tongue down • Lips flanged • Rhythmical sucking	
AUDIBLE SWALLOWING	• None	• A few with stimulation	• Spontaneous and intermittent <24° • Spontaneous and frequent	
TYPE OF NIPPLE	• Inverted	• Flat	• Everted (after stimulation)	
COMFORT	• Engorged • Cracked, bleeding, large blisters or bruises • Severe discomfort	• Filling • Reddened/small blisters or bruises • Mild/moderate discomfort	• Soft • Nontender	
HOLD (Positioning)	• Full assist (staff holds)	• Minimal assist (ie, pillows, ↑HOB) • Teach one side, mom does other • Staff holds →mom takes over	• No assist from staff • Mom able to position/hold baby	

BOTTLE FEEDING:	WNL	Educ
• eating every ________ hours • amount taken: __________ oz		
• Recognizes proper bottle position		
• Knowledge of formula preparation		

ELIMINATION:

URINARY: Amt wet diapers /24 hrs: ______

BOWEL: Stools /24 hrs: ______

☐ meconium ☐ transitional ☐ mustard

	WNL	Educ Prov	Exceptions
SKIN / MUCOSA Warm, dry, intact, no bruises, no abrasions, eyes clear			
CARDIOVASCULAR A/P 120-160, regular, pink			
RESPIRATORY RR 30-60, quiet, nonlabored			
G/U ASSESS Normal appearance of gender/function, no s/s of infection, circ healing			

	WNL	Educ Prov	Exceptions
NEURO Alert, active periods, responds to stimuli, good muscle tone			
MUSCULOSKELETAL Extremities symmetrical, MAE, flat fontanelles			
JAUNDICE None, face only			
SAFETY Parents aware of s/s of illness; verbalizes emergency plan (ie, 911, poison control); safe environment, has car seat			
PARENT/INFANT ATTACHMENT Positive interaction w/baby demo'd			

LABS:

☐ Newborn Screen Drawn

☐ Bili drawn: Time to lab: ________ RESULTS: ______________

MEDICATION: ☐ None ☐ ________________________________

EXPECTED OUTCOMES:

- Family will verbalize/demonstrate knowledge of care for newborn
- Family will receive education & support in areas of interest & concern

CONFERENCE WITH: ☐ Physician ☐ Physician via copy w/mother ☐ Visit Note FAXED To MD Office ☐ Insurance ☐ None ☐ Other __________

PLAN OF CARE:

☐ Family has the B:PBB Resource Book

☐ Family to call MD/clinic with questions or concerns; • Routine clinic visit scheduled: ☐ Yes ☐ No

DISCHARGE DATE: __________

☐ See next visit for discharge date

(FAMILY CARE, GOALS MET)

170104 (12/99)

Nurse's Signature ________________________________

APPENDIX **19E**

Patient Satisfaction Form

CASE#				
OFFICE USE ONLY				

Minnesota OB Homecare

O Antepartum O Postpartum

Month

Hospital	O ANW O UNITED O MERCY O UNITY O BUFFALO O ST. FRANCES
	O DISTRICT MEMORIAL O REGINA O OTHER ALLINA O NON-ALLINA

PLEASE FILL IN THE BUBBLES BY USING BLACK PEN

Thinking about your experience with us, how would you rate the following:	Poor	Fair	Good	Very Good	Excellent
1. Your overall home care experience.	O	O	O	O	O
2. How clearly we gave instructions.	O	O	O	O	O
3. The support given to you by the nurses.	O	O	O	O	O
4. The opportunity given to you by the nurses.	O	O	O	O	O
5. The nurse's ability to answer questions.	O	O	O	O	O
6. Your relationship with the nurse.	O	O	O	O	O
7. The scheduling of your visit.	O	O	O	O	O
8. How do your family members rate the home care visit?	O	O	O	O	O
9. Would you recommend our service to others?		O Yes	O No		

10. What did you find most valuable?

____

____

11. Do you have any suggestions for improvements?

____

____

12. Would you like a follow-up call regarding your comments? O Yes O No

Name: ______________________________

Daytime Phone Number: ________________________

Please return via the enclosed postage paid envelope.
THANK YOU!

APPENDIX A

Item Bank Questions and Answer Key

QUESTIONS

Chapter 1

Multiple Choice

1. One explanation for the United States consistently ranking unfavorably with other developed countries in perinatal care outcomes is that
   a. environmental hazards are greater in the United States.
   b. healthcare dollars are not evenly distributed across populations.
   c. pregnant women in the United States experience more stress than women in other countries.

2. The most common reason for admission of women to the hospital in the United States is
   a. cardiac disease.
   b. childbirth.
   c. hysterectomy.

3. Administrative costs are greatest in hospitals that are
   a. for-profit.
   b. government-owned.
   c. not-for-profit.

4. Healthcare costs are funded
   a. almost equally by private and government sources.
   b. primarily from government sources.
   c. primarily from private sources.

5. An indicator used to evaluate the state of healthcare in developed and underdeveloped countries is the rate of
   a. birth.
   b. death.
   c. infant mortality.

6. The age group most likely to be without health insurance is
   a. children 4–10 years.
   b. elderly 65–80 years.
   c. young adults 18–24 years.

7. The trend for hospital length of stay for childbirth over the last 3 years has been
   a. downward.
   b. fluctuating.
   c. upward.

8. Cost-containment strategies are based on data regarding
   a. clinical outcomes.
   b. financial bottom line.
   c. patient satisfaction.

9. Cost-consciousness strategies are based on data regarding
   a. evidence and clinical outcomes.
   b. physician satisfaction.
   c. predetermined financial targets.

10. Much of contemporary perinatal practice is based on
    a. past practice.
    b. patient satisfaction data.
    c. research evidence.

11. Providing perinatal care based on the premise that birth is a natural process requiring minimal selected interventions will result in care that is
    a. high quality, high cost.
    b. high quality, low cost.
    c. low quality, high cost.

12. Outcome monitoring for nursing practice was started by
    a. Florence Nightingale.
    b. Health Care Financing Agency (HCFA).
    c. Joint Commission on Accreditation of Healthcare Organizations (JCAHO).

13. A perinatal outcome measure sensitive for nursing care is

a. birth care satisfaction.
b. cost per unit of service.
c. length of stay.

14. Professional registered nurses commonly account for what portion of the total hospital workforce?
a. one-third
b. one-half
c. two-thirds

15. Nursing school enrollment over the past 5 years has
a. decreased.
b. increased.
c. remained constant.

16. The average age of registered nurses in the United States is
a. 32.
b. 38.
c. 44.

Fill in the Blank

17. Overall patient satisfaction with hospitalization is usually determined by the patient's perception of the quality of ______ he or she received.
18. Perinatal practice committees function best when they are jointly chaired by a ______ and a ______.
19. The accreditation body for hospitals is the ______.
20. The national professional association for perinatal nurses is ______.

Chapter 2

Multiple Choice

1. The estimated number of births in U.S. hospitals each day is
a. 7,000.
b. 9,000.
c. 11,000.

2. The organization that publishes the Standards and Guidelines for Professional Nursing Practice in the Care of Women and Newborns is the
a. American Nurses Association.
b. Association of Women's Health, Obstetric and Neonatal Nursing.
c. National Perinatal Association.

3. The percentage of nurses in the United States who are male is
a. 4%.
b. 6%.
c. 8%.

4. The percentage of nurses in the United States who are baccalaureate prepared is
a. 41%.
b. 51%.
c. 61%.

5. Nursing licensure in the United States is governed by
a. federal law.
b. professional association regulations.
c. state nurse practice acts.

6. The legal basis empowering the government to protect the public's health, safety and welfare is
a. certification.
b. licensure.
c. registration.

7. By which of the following nationally recognized processes can a nurse demonstrate qualification and special knowledge in a defined area of nursing practice?
a. certification
b. competence validation
c. licensure

8. To establish professional negligence, the most difficult entity for the claimant to prove is
a. breach of duty.
b. causation.
c. damages.

9. Professional nursing liability is most commonly increased by the absence of
a. adequate medical record documentation.
b. annual competency validation.
c. current unit policies and procedures.

10. An incident-management program will
a. include "near misses" with potential for adverse outcomes.
b. identify and discipline those at fault.
c. increase institutional and nursing liability.

11. Nurse/physician difference of opinion about patient management should be
a. considered unprofessional behavior.
b. discussed with the patient's family.
c. focused on the issue in question.

12. Despite repeated requests to a physician to come to the bedside to evaluate a deteriorating maternal condition, the physician has failed to respond. The nurse appropriately
a. consults with another physician in the unit.
b. institutes the unit chain of command.
c. provides the intervention indicated.

13. A criterion by which the quality of a certification organization can be evaluated is a
    a. high pass rate on certification examinations.
    b. minimum of requirements for being tested.
    c. psychometrically sound test process.
14. A characteristic of an unsafe perinatal unit is
    a. frequent use of the chain of command.
    b. nurse–physician difference of opinion.
    c. presence of peer review processes.
15. A characteristic of a safe perinatal unit is
    a. hierarchical professional relationships.
    b. policies supported by local standards.
    c. the clearly stated purpose of safety first.

Fill in the Blank

16. Intrapartum nursing is unique among the nursing specialties because the nurse–patient ratio for care of laboring women is a minimum of ______.
17. In the United States, nurse practice acts are the responsibility of legal entities called ______.
18. One of the most significant barriers to advancing the professional and economic status of nursing today is ______.
19. To prove professional negligence, the following must be established:
    1) ______
    2) ______
    3) ______
    4) ______
20. When the professional registered nurse (RN) delegates a selected nursing task to an unlicensed assistive personnel (UAP), the RN is responsible for determining if
    1) ______
    2) ______
21. Failure to exercise reasonable care is termed ______.
22. Malpractice is defined as ______.
23. Communication between patients and healthcare providers can be protective against ______.
24. The majority of obstetric lawsuits result from five commonly recurring clinical problems, which are
    1) ______
    2) ______
    3) ______
    4) ______
    5) ______
25. Over time, successful institutions continually redefine risk in the context of accidents that do not occur, and the process termed the ______ occurs, which leads to mistakes.
26. The reason organizations continue to use unsafe practices and systems is ______.
27. Most clinical errors that occur in perinatal care do not result in maternal–fetal injury because ______.
28. During clinical emergencies, the timing of medical record documentation is often ______.
29. The practice of duplicate documentation on the fetal monitoring strip and the medical record is ______ and contributes to ______.
30. A serious adverse event is defined by the Joint Commission on Accreditation of Healthcare Organization (JCAHO) as a ______.
31. Staffing ratios for perinatal units have been developed by
    1) ______
    2) ______
    3) ______
32. The recommended nurse-to-patient ratio during oxytocin administration is ______.
33. The recommended nurse-to-patient ratio for patients in the second stage of labor is ______.
34. The federal law that prevents patient "dumping" and defines requirements for care of patients who present to the hospital under emergency circumstances is ______.
35. The three obligations that must be met under the Emergency Medical Treatment and Active Labor Act (EMTALA) law are to
    1) ______
    2) ______
    3) ______
36. According to the EMTALA law, a pregnant woman who is having contractions is considered to have a(n) ______.
37. Notifying the charge nurse when the staff nurse remains concerned about a physician's plan of care, after appropriate attempts to resolve the issues, is an example of implementing the ______.
38. Frequent and regular use of the chain of command for resolving clinical conflicts indicates ______ and leads to ______.
39. All perinatal nurses engaged in the practice of nursing should be insured for ______.
40. Institutional liability policies cover nurses for acts that are ______.
41. Institutional liability policies may not cover nurses for acts that are ______.

Chapter 3

Fill in the Blank

1. List six factors that inhibit teamwork between nurses and physicians.
    1) ______
    2) ______
    3) ______

4) ______
5) ______
6) ______
2. List five characteristics of a successful team.
1) ______
2) ______
3) ______
4) ______
5) ______
3. The doctor–nurse game is communication that results in ______.
4. The ultimate advantage to perinatal teamwork is a(n) ______ approach to perinatal care, which leads to ______ and decreased ______.
5. Teams achieve better performance than ______.

Chapter 4

Multiple Choice

1. A 25-year-old Vietnamese woman admitted to the birthing unit requests that her husband stay in the waiting area until after she gives birth. The appropriate response is based on the nurse's knowledge that
   a. all husbands should be present during labor and birth.
   b. the husband may fear his response to his wife giving birth.
   c. the woman's request should be honored.

2. Wang Din Wah, a Laotian mother who is 24 hours postpartum, rejects the nurse's instructions to bring the newborn back to the clinic by the seventh day of life for a phenylketonuria (PKU) test. Wang's reasons for this refusal are most likely based on
   a. her lack of recognition of appropriate health-care for the baby.
   b. the baby's early care being provided largely by the maternal grandmother.
   c. the first month after birth being considered a time for confinement and rest.

3. Berta Wolf Creek is 4 hours postpartum and requests permission to take her placenta home with her. Appropriate instruction by the nurse would include
   a. keeping the placenta in a leakproof container.
   b. requiring disposal of the placenta by internment (burial).
   c. keeping the placenta frozen until burial.

4. Maria Ochoa, a 23-year-old Filipino American, is 18 weeks pregnant. After receiving a prescription for prenatal vitamins, she tells the nurse that her mother has warned her to take only herbal medication during pregnancy. The nurse appropriately
   a. advises Maria that the pills are only vitamins and not considered medication.
   b. assesses the significance of Maria's mother's advice.
   c. reminds her that the vitamins were ordered by the nurse-midwife.

5. The percentage of the U.S. population who are African American or black is nearly
   a. 6%.
   b. 13%.
   c. 20%.

6. An African-American/black woman who, because she believes she should not swallow her saliva and carries a spit cup with her during pregnancy, is most likely from
   a. Barbados.
   b. Haiti.
   c. West Indies.

7. A major cultural group of childbearing women at increased risk for alcoholism, heart disease, cirrhosis of the liver, and diabetes mellitus is the population of women who are
   a. African American/black.
   b. American Indian/Alaskan native.
   c. Asian American/Pacific Islanders.

8. According to the hot/cold theory, pregnancy is thought to be which kind of a condition?
   a. cold
   b. hot
   c. lukewarm

9. Match the sacred day of worship with the religious group.

a. Sunday ______	1. Jewish or Seventh-Day Adventists
b. sunset Friday to sunset Saturday ______	2. Most Christians
c. sunset Thursday to sunset Friday ______	3. Muslims

10. Ethnocentrism is the belief that
   a. cultural values are major determiners of one's behavior.
   b. every cultural group has a core or center of common beliefs.
   c. values and practices of one's own culture are superior.

11. A woman whose discharge plan includes her mother-in-law caring for her and her newborn during the postpartum period by tradition is most likely culturally including
    a. Korean.
    b. Laotian.
    c. Tongan.

12. What percentage of nurses come from racial or ethnic minority backgrounds?
    a. 9%
    b. 13%
    c. 17%

13. Goals each nurse can set to increase cultural competence while caring for culturally diverse childbearing women and their families are described as
    a. culturally driven.
    b. externally based.
    c. self-generated.

Fill in the Blank

14. Identify at least three strategies useful to increase the cultural competence of the nurse.
    1) ______
    2) ______
    3) ______

Chapter 5

Multiple Choice

1. By 32 weeks of gestation in a normal pregnancy, blood volume increases by approximately
   a. 1000 mL.
   b. 1300 mL.
   c. 1600 mL.

2. During pregnancy, the position for optimum maternal cardiac output is
   a. lateral.
   b. semi-Fowler's.
   c. supine.

3. During labor, maternal cardiac output
   a. decreases slightly.
   b. increases progressively.
   c. remains the same.

4. An intravenous fluid bolus is given before epidural anesthesia to prevent
   a. hypotension.
   b. renal hypoperfusion.
   c. sympathetic blockade.

5. Normally during pregnancy, maternal sitting and standing systolic blood pressure readings
   a. decrease, then increase.
   b. increase progressively.
   c. remain unchanged.

6. The volume of the maternal autotransfusion immediately after birth is
   a. 600 mL.
   b. 800 mL.
   c. 1000 mL.

7. The normal range for maternal PaO_2 levels in late pregnancy is
   a. 94–98 mm Hg.
   b. 99–103 mm Hg.
   c. 104–108 mm Hg.

8. The slight increase in pH that occurs during pregnancy is due to
   a. decrease in hemoglobin and hematocrit.
   b. increase in renal excretion of bicarbonate.
   c. increase in ventilatory rate.

9. During pregnancy, serum urea and creatine levels
   a. decrease.
   b. increase.
   c. remain constant.

10. Heartburn is common during pregnancy due to
    a. decreased gastric motility.
    b. increased secretion of hydrochloric acid.
    c. relaxation of the esophageal sphincter.

11. A physical finding that may occur during pregnancy in response to normal cardiovascular changes is
    a. decreased heart rate.
    b. dependent edema.
    c. elevated blood pressure.

12. The average blood loss during vaginal birth is
    a. 300–400 mL.
    b. 500–600 mL.
    c. 700–800 mL.

13. The average blood loss during cesarean birth is
    a. 600 mL.
    b. 800 mL.
    c. 1000 mL.

14. During pregnancy, cardiac output increases approximately
    a. 10%–25%.
    b. 30%–50%.
    c. 60%–75%.

15. Cardiac output is greatest during which period of the birth process?
   a. first stage, active phase
   b. immediately after birth
   c. second stage

16. A cardiovascular parameter which normally decreases during pregnancy is
   a. heart rate.
   b. stroke volume.
   c. systemic vascular resistance.

17. An expected white cell count during early postpartum is
   a. 8,000–10,000 mm^3.
   b. 13,000–15,000 mm^3.
   c. 20,000–22,000 mm^3.

18. Which of the following coagulation factors does not increase during pregnancy?
   a. fibrin
   b. platelets
   c. fibrinogen

19. Which of the following increases during pregnancy?
   a. colloid oncotic pressure
   b. glomerular filtration rate
   c. serum creatinine levels

20. By term, blood flow to the uterus is approximately
   a. 200 mL/min.
   b. 500 mL/min.
   c. 800 mL/min.

21. During pregnancy, the pigmented line in the skin that traverses the abdomen longitudinally from the sternum to the symphysis is called the
   a. linea nigra.
   b. spider nevus.
   c. striae gravidarum.

22. Which of the following is a change occurring in the respiratory system during pregnancy?
   a. oxygen consumption increases 15%–20%
   b. respiratory rate decreases 5%
   c. tidal volume decreases 30%–40%

23. A finding that can be considered a normal finding during pregnancy is
   a. glycosuria.
   b. hematuria.
   c. proteinuria.

24. The respiratory system parameter that decreases during pregnancy is the
   a. functional residual capacity.
   b. minute ventilation.
   c. tidal volume.

25. A clotting factor that decreases during pregnancy is/are
   a. coagulation factors XI, XIII.
   b. fibrin.
   c. plasma fibrinogen.

Fill in the Blank

26. The increase in cardiac output and decrease in heart rate following delivery are due to ______.
27. The greater increase in plasma volume than in red cell volume results in a state called ______.
28. The hypercoagulability state of pregnancy is due to ______ and ______.
29. During pregnancy, maternal oxygen consumption ______.
30. The primary determinant of volume hemostasis is ______.
31. The renal clearance of many substances is increased during pregnancy due to the ______.
32. Normal stretching of the skin and hormonal changes during gestation may produce "stretch marks" that are called ______.
33. The hormone released from the anterior pituitary that is responsible for initiating lactation is ______.
34. The hormone crucial in maintaining the endometrium and therefore the pregnancy is ______.
35. Management of the pregnant woman with diabetes requires blood glucose values rather than urine glucose values because ______.
36. The ______ is the system which undergoes the most profound changes during pregnancy.
37. After childbirth, the contracted uterus shunts blood from the uterine vessels into the systemic circulation causing a(n) ______ of approximately 1000 mL.
38. Increases in plasma volume and red cell mass result in an increase in ______ during pregnancy.
39. Cardiac output progressively decreases and returns to nonpregnant levels by ______.
40. The ______ accommodates one third of the additional blood volume at term.
41. The hormone ______ produces relaxation of smooth muscle and vasodilation.
42. Blood pressure reaches its lowest point in the ______ trimester.
43. During pregnancy, the woman becomes resistant to the pressor effects of ______.
44. Pregnancy is considered a ______ state due to the increases of several essential coagulation factors.

45. The pregnant woman is at increased risk for venous thrombus formation due to _______ and _______.
46. _______ are lipid substances that affect smooth muscle contractility, play an important role in the mechanism of labor, and are potent vasodilators.
47. Irregularly shaped brown blotches on the face are known as _______, or the "mask of pregnancy."
48. The bluish discoloration of the cervix occurring during pregnancy is known as _______ sign.

Chapter 6

Multiple Choice

1. The developmental task of the first trimester is
   a. identification of the maternal role.
   b. movement from conflict and ambivalence to acceptance.
   c. resolution of the approach–avoidance conflict related to childbirth and loss of control.

2. A necessary element for the development of a therapeutic relationship with a perinatal client is
   a. establishment of healthy, clear boundaries between the woman and the nurse.
   b. kind and sympathetic judgments to guide the woman toward an appropriate maternal role.
   c. sharing of relevant personal information that demonstrates the empathy of the perinatal nurse.

3. The changes and transitions affecting the mind, body, and soul during pregnancy are best defined using a
   a. holistic model.
   b. physiologic model.
   c. psychosocial model.

4. A major issue during the third trimester is
   a. the physical changes of pregnancy.
   b. fetal well-being.
   c. ambivalence about the maternal role.

5. Symptoms of postpartum depression include
   a. agitation and anger.
   b. anxiety and irritability.
   c. hallucinations and delusions.

6. When the length of postpartum hospitalization is short, discharge planning should include
   a. a brief psychiatric assessment to rule out potential for postpartum psychosis.
   b. directing the new mother to look up the telephone numbers of postpartum resources.
   c. identifying with the new mother and her partner/key support people.

7. Reva Rubin suggests that during the postpartum period it is helpful for the new mother to
   a. accept constructive criticism from the nurse so that she can learn to correctly care for her infant.
   b. be encouraged to focus on the infant's needs exclusively so that she can provide care following discharge.
   c. put meaning into the childbirth experience by verbalizing her reality.

8. The estimated percentage of new mothers who experience "baby blues" is
   a. 30%–40%.
   b. 50%–60%.
   c. 70%–80%.

9. Discharge teaching for the new mother and family includes information that labile moods should stabilize and organization and confidence should increase by
   a. 4 weeks.
   b. 8 weeks.
   c. 12 weeks.

Fill in the Blank

10. Ten elements of a comprehensive psychosocial assessment include
    1) _______
    2) _______
    3) _______
    4) _______
    5) _______
    6) _______
    7) _______
    8) _______
    9) _______
    10) _______
11. Participants included in the psychosocial assessment are _______, _______, and _______.
12. The data obtained during a psychosocial assessment are used to develop _______, _______, and _______.
13. There is a strong correlation between mood and anxiety disorders before pregnancy and _______.
14. A critical aspect of holistic care planning for the perinatal client involves coordination of _______.
15. During the second trimester, women are increasingly vulnerable to _______.
16. When conducting a psychosocial assessment, it is important to determine the _______, _______, and _______ of mood or emotional disturbances.

17. Most women do not seek help with depressive disorders following birth because ______.
18. Maternal role attainment is a process that develops over approximately ______ months.
19. The mother is better able to meet the needs of her infant when ______.

Chapter 7

Multiple Choice

1. Over the past 40 years, the incidence of preterm birth in the United States has
   a. declined.
   b. increased.
   c. remained the same.

2. An appropriate recommendation for weight gain for an underweight pregnant woman would be
   a. 20 lbs.
   b. 25 lbs.
   c. 30 lbs.

3. Delayed entry into prenatal care is associated with physical violence in
   a. older women of higher socioeconomic status.
   b. older women of lower socioeconomic status.
   c. younger women of higher socioeconomic status.

4. The time during pregnancy when blood pressure is lowest in the normotensive woman is the
   a. first trimester.
   b. second trimester.
   c. third trimester.

5. The time when measurement of fundal height in centimeters should correlate with gestational age is
   a. after 20 weeks' gestation.
   b. near term.
   c. before 20 weeks' gestation.

6. Planning culturally specific care includes
   a. making sure that a translator is available when requested.
   b. noting patterns of decision making in the family.
   c. using a translator at each visit.

7. A nonreactive nonstress test at 39 weeks' gestation is an indication for
   a. expedited delivery.
   b. further testing.
   c. reassurance about fetal status.

8. Health promotion and education to improve pregnancy outcome in the next generation should begin when
   a. children are in elementary school.
   b. pregnancy occurs in the peer group.
   c. teens are sexually active.

9. An appropriate gestational age for a glucose screening test is at
   a. 23 weeks' gestation.
   b. 26 weeks' gestation.
   c. 29 weeks' gestation.

10. Risk assessment for all women during the initial prenatal visit should include
    a. complete health history.
    b. triple screen.
    c. ultrasound for fetal anomalies.

11. Which of the following women would be at risk for nutritional problems during pregnancy?
    a. advanced maternal age.
    b. cigarette smoker.
    c. Gravida III, Term I, Preterm 0, Abortion I, Living Child I.

12. An effect of cigarette smoking during pregnancy is increased incidence of
    a. low-birth weight and prematurity.
    b. neonatal TTNB (transient tachypnea).
    c. pregnancy-induced hypertension.

13. Maternal serum alpha-fetoprotein specifically screens for
    a. heart defects.
    b. neural tube defects.
    c. placental defects.

14. If both parents are affected by sickle cell disease, the risk of their children being affected by sickle cell disease is
    a. 25%.
    b. 50%.
    c. 100%.

15. A primary method of fetal surveillance during pregnancy is
    a. fetal kick counts.
    b. nonstress testing.
    c. ultrasonography.

16. The most significant food shortages for low-income women occur
    a. at the end of the month when federal/local resources diminish.
    b. before Women, Infants, and Children (WIC) eligibility is determined.
    c. postpartum, when fatigue prevents appointments with WIC.

17. A key component of preterm birth prevention education is
    a. discussing the hospital admission criteria.
    b. empowering the woman to act on her own instincts and self-knowledge.
    c. involving the significant other in the teaching.

Fill in the Blank

18. The monitoring of fetal activity by "kick counts" is initiated at ______ weeks' gestation.
19. It is recommended that every woman have an initial serology and gonorrhea culture (GC), and that the tests be repeated at ______ weeks.
20. The recommended weight gain for an obese woman during pregnancy is ______.
21. Approximately ______ % of human malformations are caused by genetic factors alone.
22. A ______ is an agent that causes congenital malformations.
23. A biophysical profile summative score of ______ or greater is considered a sign of fetal well-being.
24. Male and female genitalia are recognizable by ______ weeks of gestation.
25. Tay-Sachs disease is a recessive disorder common in families of ______ ancestry.
26. The anticoagulant drug ______ is a known teratogen.
27. A ______ contraction stress test is reassuring.
28. Amniocentesis for genetic evaluation is usually done between ______ and ______ weeks' gestation.
29. The three basic components of prenatal care are
    1) ______
    2) ______
    3) ______
30. Moderate physical activity during an uncomplicated pregnancy maintains ______ and ______ fitness.
31. Diagnosis of gestational diabetes mellitus is made when a glucose tolerance test result has ______.
32. Maternal serum alpha-fetoprotein testing is offered between ______ and ______ weeks' gestation.
33. A healthy fetus usually has ______ perceivable movements in one hour.
34. The five parameters assessed in the biophysical profile are
    1) ______
    2) ______
    3) ______
    4) ______
    5) ______

Chapter 8

Hypertensive Disorders

Multiple Choice

1. A diagnosis of severe preeclampsia is consistent with a 24-hour urine showing protein excretion of
    a. 1.0 g/L.
    b. 3.0 g/L.
    c. 5.0 g/L.
2. An indication of impending magnesium sulfate toxicity in the patient being treated for preeclampsia is the absence of
    a. deep tendon reflexes.
    b. fetal movement.
    c. urine output.
3. The therapeutic range of serum magnesium during magnesium sulfate therapy to prevent eclamptic seizures is
    a. 1–4 mg/dL.
    b. 5–8 mg/dL.
    c. 9–12 mg/dL.
4. The first priority in the care of a patient during an eclamptic seizure is to
    a. administer an anticonvulsant agent.
    b. ensure a patent airway.
    c. establish IV access.
5. Diagnosis of preeclampsia requires the presence of hypertension and
    a. edema.
    b. headaches.
    c. proteinuria.
6. Severe preeclampsia can be diagnosed in the presence of
    a. excretion of 4500 gms protein in a 24-hour urine collection.
    b. serial diastolic blood pressures of at least 110 mm Hg.
    c. serum blood urea nitrogen (BUN) of 10 with a serum creatinine of 1.0.

Fill in the Blank

7. ______ disorders of pregnancy are the most common medical complication of pregnancy.
8. A diastolic blood pressure of ______ mm Hg on two occasions of at least 6 hours apart is necessary for diagnosis of severe preeclampsia.
9. The blood pressure should be recorded with the pregnant woman in the ______ position.

10. ______ is the drug of choice to prevent seizure activity in the patient with preeclampsia.
11. Maternal morbidity from hypertension in pregnancy results from
    1) ______
    2) ______
    3) ______
    4) ______
12. The goals of antihypertensive therapy in the woman with preeclampsia are to ______ and to ______.
13. Laboratory markers for HELLP syndrome are ______, ______, and ______.
14. A leading cause of maternal morbidity following an eclamptic seizure is ______.

Bleeding

Multiple Choice

1. Invasion of the trophoblastic cells into the uterine myometrium is termed placenta
   a. accreta.
   b. increta.
   c. percreta.

2. Prostaglandin $F_2\alpha$ (Hemabate) is most likely to fail to control hemorrhage in women with
   a. chorioamnionitis.
   b. multiple gestation.
   c. previous cesarean section.

3. Painless, bright red vaginal bleeding at 28 weeks' gestation is most likely due to
   a. abruptio placentae.
   b. placenta previa.
   c. uterine rupture.

4. A clinical finding with a dehiscence of a uterine scar during a trial of labor after cesarean birth (TOLAC) is
   a. cessation of uterine contractions.
   b. Fetal heart rate (FHR) with variable decelerations.
   c. sudden decrease of intrauterine pressure.

5. The initial drug of choice for excessive bleeding in the immediate postpartum period is
   a. Methergine IM.
   b. oxytocin IV infusion.
   c. prostaglandin 15-MF_{2a} suppository.

Fill in the Blank

6. Vasa previa is the result of a ______ insertion of the cord.
7. For the fetus to maintain adequate oxygenation, the maternal oxygen saturation must be at least ______%.
8. ______ is a late sign of hypovolemia in the woman experiencing bleeding during pregnancy.
9. Obstetric factors predisposing a woman to disseminated intravascular coagulation are
    1) ______
    2) ______
    3) ______
    4) ______
    5) ______
    6) ______
    7) ______

Preterm Labor and Birth

Multiple Choice

1. Which of the following is not a common symptom of preterm labor?
   a. headache
   b. menstrual-like cramps
   c. pelvic pressure

2. The risk factor most predictive of preterm labor is prior
   a. low-birth-weight baby.
   b. preterm birth.
   c. preterm labor.

3. When considering nursing care of the woman in preterm labor, which of the following is true?
   a. Maternal transport to a high-risk center has improved outcome over neontal transport to a special care nursery.
   b. The effect of antenatal glucocorticoid treatment is immediate.
   c. Tocolysis has great effectiveness in delaying preterm birth by 7 days.

4. A drug that is used for tocolysis but is not classified as a beta-mimetic is
   a. Procardia.
   b. ritodrine.
   c. terbutaline.

5. To accurately be called preterm, an infant must be
   a. born at gestational age <37 weeks.
   b. <10th percentile in weight.
   c. small for gestational age.

6. The best method for teaching pregnant women about the symptoms of preterm labor is
   a. asking about symptoms at each prenatal visit.
   b. computer-aided instruction.
   c. providing pamphlets to read.

7. When beginning IV hydration for a woman with preterm contractions, the nurse should remember that
   a. IV fluids should be administered with the expectation for tocolysis with a beta-mimetic.
   b. preterm labor contractions usually diminish within one hour of initiation of IV hydration.
   c. the first liter of IV fluid should be administered within the first hour of the admission.
8. Antenatal glucocorticoid administration for acceleration of fetal lung maturation is appropriate
   a. for all women who could deliver preterm.
   b. in two doses given 24 hours apart.
   c. once a week from the time of the first preterm symptoms until delivery.
9. Bed rest has been shown by research to
   a. allow the pregnant woman to gain appropriate amounts of weight.
   b. cause bone demineralization.
   c. inhibit preterm labor contractions.
10. Smoking increases the risk of preterm birth by
    a. 20%.
    b. 30%.
    c. 40%.

Fill in the Blank

11. The rate of preterm birth in the United States is currently ______%.
12. During the past several decades, rates of preterm birth have ______.
13. We now know that the term "Braxton-Hicks contractions" should be ______ from prenatal care teaching.

Diabetes

Multiple Choice

1. An indication to initiate insulin in a pregnant woman with gestational diabetes is
   a. fasting blood suger (FBS): >95 mg/dL on two or more occasions.
   b. FBS: normal but 2 hour; postprandial: >100 mg/dL.
   c. FBS: >105 mg/dL and 2-hour postprandial: >120 mg/dL.
2. Hypoglycemia is defined as a plasma blood glucose of
   a. 70 mg/dL.
   b. 80 mg/dL.
   c. 90 mg/dL.
3. To assist in controlling blood glucose, the recommendation for pregnant women with well-controlled diabetes is to exercise
   a. daily for less than 30 minutes.
   b. every other day for 45 minutes.
   c. three times a week for 20 minutes.
4. Women with a history of gestational diabetes with a normal postpartum follow-up test should be tested for overt diabetes
   a. annually.
   b. every 3 years.
   c. before a subsequent pregnancy.
5. Blood glucose values from reflectance meters are
   a. comparable to laboratory values.
   b. 14% above laboratory plasma values.
   c. 14% below laboratory plasma values.
6. The preferred non-nutritive sweetener to use during pregnancy is
   a. aspartame.
   b. saccharin.
   c. sucrose.
7. Preterm labor in women with diabetic ketoacidosis should be treated with
   a. hydration.
   b. magnesium sulfate.
   c. terbutaline.
8. Diagnostic testing for gestational diabetes includes 3-hour FBS evaluation after administation of
   a. 28 jelly beans.
   b. 50 gram glucose solution.
   c. 100 gram glucose solution.
9. Insulin dosage during periods of nausea and vomiting in pregnant women should be
   a. administered with no adjustment.
   b. based on a sliding scale.
   c. withheld until nausea is resolved.
10. Weekly nonstress testing should be initiated in women with vascular disease beginning at the gestational age of
    a. 28 weeks.
    b. 30 weeks.
    c. 32 weeks.

Fill in the Blank

11. ______ diabetes results due to an autoimmune reaction directed at the pancreas following an environmental trigger.

12. Metabolic changes in the first half of pregnancy characterized by fat storage is called the ______ phase.
13. List five diabetogenic hormones of pregnancy.
    1) ______
    2) ______
    3) ______
    4) ______
    5) ______
14. ______ insulin is recommended for use during pregnancy because of the decreased risk of transmitting anti-insulin antibodies to the fetus.
15. Four specific symptoms of hyperglycemia are
    1) ______
    2) ______
    3) ______
    4) ______

Cardiac Disease

Multiple Choice

1. The incidence of congenital cardiac disease is
   a. 1:100 live births.
   b. 1:500 live births.
   c. 1:1000 live births.

2. Maternal outcomes in pregnancies of women with Marfan's syndrome are related to
   a. cardiac dysrhythmias.
   b. degree of aortic root dilation.
   c. hypervolemia of pregnancy.

3. Coronary artery disease in pregnancy is rare due to
   a. hormonal protection against atherosclerosis.
   b. maternal production of relaxin.
   c. progesterone-mediated vasodilation.

4. The incidence of myocardial infarction during pregnancy is
   a. 1:1000.
   b. 1:10,000.
   c. 1:100,000.

5. Peripartum cardiomyopathy is categorized as
   a. dilated cardiomyopathy.
   b. hypertrophic cardiomyopathy.
   c. restrictive cardiomyopathy.

6. A pregnant woman with New York Heart Association (NYHA) class II cardiac disease is symptomatic with
   a. bed rest.
   b. mild exertion.
   c. moderate exertion.

7. The drug of choice to treat epidural analgesia-related hypotension for a pregnant woman with a cardiac disorder would be
   a. dopamine.
   b. ephedrine.
   c. phenylephrine.

8. The time during labor when the greatest cardiac stress occurs is
   a. immediately after the end of the third stage.
   b. late first stage (transition).
   c. second stage with descent.

9. The release of catecholamines, which occurs with stimulation of the sympathetic nervous system,
   a. has no effect on uteroplacental perfusion.
   b. increases uteroplacental perfusion.
   c. limits uteroplacental perfusion.

10. An initial sign of inadequate cerebral perfusion is
    a. low pulse oximeter readings.
    b. restlessness.
    c. unequal pupil dilation.

Fill in the Blank

11. ______ regulate the distribution of extracellular fluid.
12. Mitral and aortic stenosis are examples of cardiac diseases caused by ______.
13. Severe consequences from myocardial infarction are ______ in pregnancy.
14. Current risk counseling for pregnant women with cardiac disease is based upon the ______ and the ______.
15. The NYHA classification system for cardiac disease categorizes patients by ______.

Pulmonary Complications

Multiple Choice

1. During pregnancy, predicted values of peak expiratory flow rates are
   a. decreased.
   b. increased.
   c. unchanged.

2. The mainstay of asthma therapy is
   a. beta-2 agonists.
   b. corticosteroids.
   c. immunotherapy.

3. Moderate–severe asthma is apparent when respiratory rate is greater than
   a. 20/minute.

b. 30/minute.
c. 40/minute.

4. During an exacerbation of asthma, there is
   a. decreased functional residual capacity.
   b. increased expiratory airflow.
   c. increased peripheral vascular resistance.

5. A breath sound rarely auscultated in asthmatics is
   a. rales.
   b. rhonchi.
   c. wheezes.

6. The most commonly seen pneumonia of pregnancy is
   a. aspiration.
   b. bacterial.
   c. viral.

7. The major factor predisposing pregnant women to severe pneumonia is
   a. altered maternal immune status.
   b. diminished maternal ventilatory reserve.
   c. increased capillary permeability.

8. When aspiration pneumonia occurs during pregnancy, it is most commonly a result of
   a. bronchitis.
   b. eclampsia.
   c. smoking.

9. Initial arterial blood gases in the pregnant woman with pneumonia usually reflect significant
   a. acidosis.
   b. hypercapnia.
   c. hypoxia.

10. Hypoxia should be suspected when a pregnant woman is noted to have
   a. hypotension.
   b. increased urine output.
   c. restlessness.

Fill in the Blank

11. Exacerbations of asthma will occur during the intrapartum period _______ % of the time.
12. Oxygen saturation of greater than _______ % by pulse oximetry is vital for a pregnant woman with pneumonia.
13. Following delivery, _______ % of women will return to the prepregnancy status of their asthma.
14. A lifestyle risk factor that may increase a woman's risk of acquiring pneumonia during pregnancy is _______.
15. The most common bacterial pathogen in pneumonia during pregnancy is _______.
16. The maternal position that best supports maximum oxygenation is _______.
17. Common inhalation irritants for many asthmatics are _______.
18. Markers for potentially fatal asthma are _______.
19. Maternal complications of pneumonia during pregnancy are _______.
20. During pregnancy, _______% of women with asthma will experience worsening of their symptoms.

Multiple Gestation

Multiple Choice

1. The placental configuration most likely to require a cesarean birth is
   a. diamniotic–dichorionic.
   b. monochorionic–diamniotic.
   c. monochorionic–monoamniotic.

2. Dizygotic twinning occurs when
   a. the fertilized egg divides into two or more zygotes.
   b. two identical unfertilized eggs are fertilized by two sperm.
   c. two or more eggs are fertilized separately.

3. Monozygotic twinning occurs
   a. as a random event.
   b. as a result of ovulation induction.
   c. when two eggs are fertilized simultaneously.

4. The major cause of morbidity in triplets is
   a. cord entanglement.
   b. prematurity.
   c. traumatic delivery.

5. The type of twinning associated with a higher rate of congenital anomalies is
   a. dizygotic twinning.
   b. intermediary twinning.
   c. monozygotic twinning.

6. Vaginal delivery can be anticipated when the presentation of twin fetuses is
   a. baby A breech–baby B breech.
   b. baby A breech–baby B vertex.
   c. baby A vertex–baby B vertex.

True or False

7. Although rare, each dizygotic twin could have a different chromosomal disorder.

Chapter 9

Multiple Choice

1. According to AWHONN and the American College of Obstetricians and Gynecologists (ACOG), in the absence of risk factors, FHR should be assessed during second stage labor every
   a. 5 minutes.
   b. 15 minutes.
   c. 30 minutes.

2. An appropriate lubricant to use for vaginal examinations during labor is
   a. povidone–iodine gel.
   b. sterile water.
   c. water-soluble jelly.

3. According to the American Society of Anesthesiologists (ASA) Guidelines For Obstetrical Care, an elective cesarean could be done when the woman has been NPO for at least
   a. 4 hours.
   b. 5 hours.
   c. 6 hours.

4. An involuntary urge to push is most likely a sign of
   a. low fetal station.
   b. occiput posterior fetal position.
   c. transition.

5. An appropriate solution to use for amnioinfusion is
   a. 5% dextrose in lactated Ringer's solution (D5/LR).
   b. 5% dextrose in water (D5W).
   c. lactated Ringer's solution..

6. An increased risk for shoulder dystocia is associated with
   a. maternal diabetes.
   b. post-date pregnancy.
   c. trial of labor after cesarean (TOLAC).

7. The primary factor that would allow second stage labor to continue beyond 2 hours is that
   a. epidural anesthesia is in place with level <T10.
   b. FHR is reassuring as the presenting part descends.
   c. maternal pushing efforts result in progress.

8. Using the Zavanelli maneuver to resolve shoulder dystocia involves
   a. assisting the woman to a knee–chest position.
   b. elevating the fetal head back through the vagina.
   c. sweeping an arm to deliver the posterior shoulder.

9. ACOG defines uterine hyperstimulation as
   a. contraction duration of >60 seconds.
   b. contraction frequency q 2–3 minutes.
   c. contractions >5 in 10 minutes.

10. A high probability of successful induction of labor is associated with a Bishop score of
    a. >4.
    b. >6.
    c. >8.

11. Appropriate treatment of hyperstimulation after dinoprostone administration is
    a. IV bolus of D5W.
    b. terbutaline 0.25 mg SQ.
    c. vaginal irrigation with normal saline.

12. In the absence of complications, immediate postpartum maternal vital signs should be assessed every
    a. 5 minutes for 30 minutes.
    b. 15 minutes for 1 hour.
    c. 30 minutes for 2 hours.

13. ACOG recommends a dosing interval for misoprostol of every
    a. 1–2 hours.
    b. 3–6 hours.
    c. 6–12 hours.

14. The most common reason for hospital readmission following operative birth is
    a. endometritis.
    b. hemorrhage.
    c. wound infection.

15. Vacuum extractor cup placement on the fetal head should not exceed
    a. 5 minutes.
    b. 10–15 minutes.
    c. 20–30 minutes.

16. Anesthesia personnel are required to remain with a postanesthesia care unit (PACU) patient until the
    a. monitoring equipment has been applied.
    b. PACU nurse accepts responsibility for the patient.
    c. patient is alert and oriented.

17. The normal length of the pregravid cervix is
    a. 2.5–3 cm.
    b. 3.5–4 cm.
    c. 4.5–5 cm.

18. True labor is characterized by
    a. effacement and/or dilation of the cervix.
    b. painful uterine contractions.
    c. suprapubic discomfort at regular intervals.

19. One liter of D5/LR provides
    a. 100 calories.
    b. 225 calories.
    c. 500 calories.

20. Facilitating a family-centered birth experience involves
    a. allowing immediate family members to participate.
    b. providing a waiting area for siblings.
    c. supporting family as defined by the childbearing woman.

Fill in the Blank

21. Diastolic blood pressure measurements taken from an automatic blood pressure device are typically ______ than diastolic measurements utilizing a stethoscope and a mercury cuff.

22. The enzyme oxytocinase facilitates plasma clearance of oxytocin via the maternal ______ and ______.

23. During the second stage of labor, an alternative to squatting that provides the same benefits is ______.

24. Bearing down efforts accompanied by prolonged breath-holding typifies ______ pushing, which has associated negative maternal and fetal ______ effects.

25. AWHONN's second stage labor nursing management protocol for a woman with epidural anesthesia encourages rest until the occurrence of ______.

26. The McRoberts maneuver is used to facilitate birth when there is an occurrence of ______, and requires the nurse to assist the woman to ______ her legs at the ______ and at the ______.

27. Adverse outcomes associated with episiotomy include
    1) ______
    2) ______
    3) ______

28. Measures to aid perineal stretching and aid in the goal to avoid episiotomy include
    1) ______
    2) ______
    3) ______

29. Women who have a support person with them in labor have been found to have
    1) ______
    2) ______
    3) ______

30. Before the use of a cervical ripening or labor induction agent, the following should be assessed:
    1) ______
    2) ______
    3) ______

31. Risks associated with stripping of membranes include
    1) ______
    2) ______
    3) ______

32. An interval of ______ hours is recommended between the final dose of dinoprostone and oxytocin administration.

33. Nursing documentation following amniotomy should include:
    1) ______
    2) ______
    3) ______

34. A ______ degree laceration extends into the rectal lumen.

35. The maternal landmarks that must be identified to determine fetal stations are the ______.

36. With a physician or certifed nurse midwife (CNM) order, nurses with appropriate training may administer the cervical ripening agents ______ and ______.

37. ______ is a contraindication for the use of misprostol and Cervidil.

38. A nursing measure to use before forcep application to help prevent maternal trauma is ______.

39. The recommendations for use of the vacuum extractor device state that the pressure should not exceed ______ mm Hg.

40. Requirements for post-anesthesia recovery care include availability of
    1) ______
    2) ______
    3) ______
    4) ______
    5) ______
    6) ______
    7) ______

41. According to ACOG, selection criteria for women who are candidates for vaginal birth after cesarean (VBAC) include
    1) ______
    2) ______
    3) ______
    4) ______
    5) ______

42. ______ is a sign of impending uterine rupture in women experiencing a trial of labor after prior cesarean delivery.

43. Four maternal factors proposed as being responsible for initiation of labor are
    1) ______
    2) ______
    3) ______
    4) ______

44. If any of the following findings are present in a pregnant woman, the perinatal provider should be notified promptly.
    1) ______
    2) ______
    3) ______
    4) ______
    5) ______
    6) ______

45. The Bishop score evaluates these five parameters.
    1) ______
    2) ______
    3) ______
    4) ______
    5) ______

46. Unnecessary interventions during labor increase the risk of ______.

47. Informed consent for VBAC correctly includes discussion about
    1) ______
    2) ______
    3) ______

Chapter 10

Multiple Choice

1. When auscultation is used for fetal assessment during labor for a low-risk woman, the FHR should be auscultated in the first stage of labor every
   a. 5 minutes.
   b. 15 minutes.
   c. 30 minutes.

2. For a low-risk woman in the second stage of labor, the FHR should be auscultated every
   a. 5 minutes.
   b. 10 minutes.
   c. 15 minutes.

3. The normal FHR baseline
   a. decreases during labor.
   b. fluctuates during labor.
   c. increases during labor.

4. Bradycardia in the second stage of labor following a previously normal tracing may be caused by fetal
   a. hypoxemia.
   b. rotation.
   c. vagal stimulation.

5. A likely cause of fetal tachycardia with moderate variability is
   a. fetal hypoxemia.
   b. maternal fever.
   c. vagal stimulation.

6. Loss of FHR variability can result from
   a. fetal scalp stimulation.
   b. medication administration.
   c. vaginal examination.

7. The primary goal in treatment for late decelerations is to
   a. correct cord compression.
   b. improve maternal oxygenation.
   c. maximize uteroplacental blood flow.

8. The most frequently observed type of FHR deceleration is
   a. early.
   b. late.
   c. variable.

9. Amnioinfusion may be useful in alleviating decelerations that are
   a. early.
   b. late.
   c. variable.

10. Findings indicative of progressive fetal hypoxemia are
    a. late decelerations, moderate variability, and stable baseline rate.
    b. prolonged decelerations recovering to baseline and moderate variability.
    c. rising baseline rate and absent variability.

11. Fetal metabolic acidemia is indicated by an arterial cord gas pH of 7.18 and a base deficit of
    a. 3.

b. 6.
c. 12.

12. Fetal bradycardia can result during
a. sleep state.
b. umbilical vein compression.
c. vagal stimulation.

13. While caring for a 235-lb laboring woman who is HIV seropositive, the external FHR tracing is difficult to obtain. An appropriate nursing action would be to
a. apply a fetal scalp electrode.
b. auscultate for presence of FHR variability.
c. notify the attending midwife or physician.

14. FHR decelerations that are benign and do not require intervention are
a. early.
b. late.
c. variable.

15. FHR decelerations that result from decreased uteroplacental blood flow are
a. early.
b. late.
c. variable.

16. FHR decelerations that result from umbilical cord compression are
a. early.
b. late.
c. variable.

17. Brief accelerations of the FHR that precede and/or follow variable decelerations are called
a. overshoots.
b. shoulders.
c. uniform accelerations.

18. A FHR pattern likely to develop with severe fetal anemia is
a. lambda.
b. saltatory.
c. sinusoidal.

19. A work-up for maternal systemic lupus erythematosus would likely be ordered in the presence of fetal
a. complete heart block.
b. premature ventricular contractions.
c. supraventricular tachycardia.

Fill in the Blank

20. Late decelerations are characterized by decelerations of the FHR that begin at the ______ of the contraction, do not return to the basel
until ______ the contraction ends, and o
with every contraction.

21. Variable decelerations are characterized by decelerations that have ______ timing in relation to the contractions, but always have a(n) ______ change in rate.

22. Early decelerations are characterized by a drop in FHR that begins at the ______ of a contraction and recovers to the ______ by the end of the contraction. Early decelerations are ______ and do not require intervention.

23. Nursing interventions for late decelerations include ______ the oxytocin if it is infusing.

24. Reassuring FHR tracings have an absence of decelerations and may show accelerations and/or ______ variability as recorded by a fetal scalp electrode.

25. Whenever a very unusual FHR pattern occurs that cannot be easily characterized, the possibility of a fetus with ______ should be considered.

26. Most fetal dysrhythmias are not life-threatening, except for ______, which may lead to fetal congestive heart failure.

27. Decreased baseline variability may be caused by multiple factors including ______, ______, and ______.

28. In the presence of variable decelerations, progressive hypoxemia may be characterized by an increasing ______, loss of ______, and the presence of ______ following the deceleration.

29. Late decelerations associated with acute conditions may be caused by uterine ______.

30. If the FHR tracing does not revert to a reassuring tracing following interventions for late decelerations, adminstration of ______ to stop or decrease uterine activity may be indicated.

31. Uterine resting tone and the intensity of contractions are measured in mm Hg only when a/an ______ is being used.

32. A sinusoidal pattern may develop in the Rh sensitized fetus or the fetus who is ______.

33. In the presence of maternal and/or fetal risk factors, auscultation of the fetal rate should occur every ______ minutes in the active phase of the

and every ______ minutes in labor.

variability is defined as

decelerations can best be accomplished by ______.

36. In the presence of late or variable decelerations, two parameters that reassure the nurse of adequate fetal oxygenation are ______ and ______.

37. Evidence shows that when an electronic fetal monitoring tracing is interpreted as nonreassuring or indicative of fetal stress, a well-oxygenated newborn is delivered at least ______% of the time.

38. In the presence of FHR accelerations greater than 15 bpm above baseline and lasting more than 15 seconds, the fetal condition is comparable to the fetal blood gas pH of at least ______ and is considered ______.

39. To correctly interpret a baseline FHR as tachycardic or bradycardic, the rate must persist for a minimum of ______ minutes.

40. In assessing fetal well-being, the most important characteristic of the FHR is ______.

41. Nursing interventions to maximize uteroplacental blood flow include
   1) ______
   2) ______
   3) ______
   4) ______
   5) ______

42. The normal FHR baseline range is ______ bpm to ______ bpm.

43. The normal range for fetal oxygen saturation ($FSpO_2$) is between ______ and ______.

44. A trend in fetal oxygen saturation ($FSpO_2$) data that would be nonreassuring is ______.

Chapter 11

Multiple Choice

1. Pain during the first stage of labor is caused by
   a. cervical and lower uterine segment stretching and traction on ovaries, fallopian tubes, and uterine ligaments.
   b. pressure on the urethra, bladder, and rectum by the descending fetal presenting part.
   c. uterine muscle hypoxia, lactic acid accumulation, and distention of the pelvic floor muscles.

2. The release of maternal catecholamines during labor results in
   a. FHR baseline tachycardia.
   b. increased metabolic rate and oxygen consumption.
   c. uterine hypoperfusion and decreased blood flow to the placenta.

3. Effleurage is defined as
   a. a form of visualization.
   b. firm pressure on specific pressure points.
   c. light massage over any area of the body.

4. The purpose for administration of medications such as promethazine hydrochloride (Phenergan), hydroxyzine hydrochloride (Vistaril), and propriomazine (Largon) during early labor is to
   a. decrease pain of contractions.
   b. potentiate effects of narcotics.
   c. provide sedation and relieve anxiety.

5. The epidural catheter for labor pain management is generally placed between the
   a. 2nd and 3rd lumbar vertebrae.
   b. 3rd and 4th lumbar vertebrae.
   c. 4th and 5th lumbar vertebrae.

6. Symptoms of an intravascular injection of a local anesthetic agent include
   a. light-headedness and bradycardia.
   b. numbness of the tongue and decreased blood pressure.
   c. tachycardia and tinnitus.

7. Continued use of one breathing technique during labor may provide insufficient stimulation or distraction to interfere with pain perception. This phenomena is referred to as
   a. habituation.
   b. repetition.
   c. monotony.

8. A medication commonly given to women who are experiencing prolonged latent labor to produce a period of sleep is
   a. butorphanol (Stadol).
   b. pentobarbital (Nembutal).
   c. promethazine hydrochloride (Phenergan).

9. Neonatal respiratory depression could result from the maternal administration of IV opioids if birth occurs within
   a. 1 hour or after 4 hours following administration.
   b. 2–3 hours of administration.

c. 12 hours of administration.

10. The advantage of using nalbuphine (Nubain) to relieve pain associated with labor is
    a. less effect on frequency and duration of contractions.
    b. less respiratory depression.
    c. short onset of action and longer duration of action.

11. The initial intervention to suggest for a woman experiencing pain on one side during a continuous epidural infusion is to
    a. maintain the woman in a lateral position, off the painful side.
    b. request that an anesthesiologist reevaluate the woman.
    c. turn the woman toward the side with pain.

12. Ephedrine is used to correct which side effect of epidural anesthesia/analgesia?
    a. hypotension
    b. nausea and vomiting
    c. pruritus

13. A medication given to reverse the symptom of a distended bladder during a continuous epidural infusion is
    a. bupivacaine.
    b. epinephrine.
    c. naloxone.

14. Research has demonstrated that continuous support by a doula during labor
    a. decreases the stress male partners felt during labor in their role as "coach".
    b. decreases use of analgesia, oxytocin, and forceps; decreases incidence of cesarean sections; and significantly shortens labor.
    c. has less impact on a woman's perception of her labor than continuous support by a registered nurse.

15. Touch/massage is thought to decrease or interrupt the pain of labor by
    a. activating large myelinated nerve fibers.
    b. activating the same type of nerve fibers that would transmit sensations of pain from the uterus.
    c. interrupting the "habituation" that occurs when labor is prolonged.

16. When pruritus occurs in the presence of an opioid in the epidural infusion, the nurse can correctly tell the patient that this symptom will most likely subside in about
    a. 15 minutes.
    b. 45 minutes.
    c. 1–2 hours.

17. Advantages of combined spinal epidural technique are
    a. decreased hypotension, decreased motor blockade, increased maternal satisfaction.
    b. decreased hypotension, faster onset of pain relief, decreased pruritis.
    c. faster onset of pain relief, decreased motor blockade, increased maternal satisfaction.

18. Maintaining a horizontal position in labor promotes
    a. descent of the presenting part.
    b. increased perception of pain.
    c. maternal oxygenation and comfort.

19. Women with a fetus in an occiput posterior position commonly are more comfortable
    a. in knee–chest position.
    b. side-lying with pillows behind their back and between their knees.
    c. sitting in a chair with their feet on a stool.

Fill in the Blank

20. ______ pressure equalizes the pressure exerted on all parts of the body.

21. The advantages of bupivacaine (Marcaine) over lidocaine (Xylocaine) and chloroprocaine (Nesacaine) for use in epidural analgesia/anesthesia is less ______ and fewer ______.

22. A major limitation for recommendation of all nonpharmacologic methods of pain relief in labor is the lack of large ______.

Questions 23–27 relate to the following statement: Using the Gate Control Theory, explain how each nonpharmacologic pain management strategy (23–27) interrupts the transmission of painful stimuli (options a–c).

23. ______ hydrotherapy

24. ______ focal point

25. ______ breathing techniques

26. ______ labor support

27. ______ relaxation
    a. measures to reduce painful stimuli
    b. methods that activate peripheral sensory receptors and inhibit pain awareness
    c. cognitive techniques that reduce a woman's negative psychological reaction to pain

Questions 28–33 relate to the following statement: Complications associated with epidural anesthesia (28–33) are related to the use and amount of which type of medication (a or b)?

28. _______ hypotension

29. _______ late decelerations

30. _______ neonatal hyperthermia

31. _______ persistent occiput posterior

32. _______ urinary retention

33. _______ pruritus
   a. local anesthesia
   b. narcotic

34. Imagery is also known as _______.

35. Following administration of an opioid during early labor, frequency and duration of contractions and FHR variability may _______.

36. To decrease transfer of medication to the fetus, IV push narcotics should be given (circle the correct answer) before/after/during uterine contractions.

37. Medications such as Nubain and Stadol are categorized as _______.

38. Respiratory depression following epidural anesthesia with a combination of narcotic and local anesthetic is most likely related to the _______.

39. A fluid bolus should be administered before the initiation of regional analgesia/anesthesia to decrease the potential for maternal _______.

40. Auditory and visual stimulation serve as a _______ during labor, decreasing the perception of painful stimuli.

Chapter 12

Multiple Choice

1. A normal hemodynamic/hematologic change occurring during the immediate postpartum period is
   a. decreased white blood cell count.
   b. elevated blood pressure.
   c. increased cardiac output.

2. During the postpartum period, normal respiratory and acid–base changes include
   a. decreased base excess.
   b. hypercapnia.
   c. increased PCO_2.

3. Postpartum teaching about sexual activity includes the information that
   a. interest in sexual activity may increase due to hormonal changes.
   b. lubricants will not be needed due to increased vaginal mucus.
   c. sexual intercourse should be avoided until vaginal bleeding has ceased.

4. A normal physiologic finding during the immediate postpartum period is
   a. dizziness when sitting up from a reclining position.
   b. saturation of the peripad every 15 minutes.
   c. urinary output of 25 mL/hour.

5. An appropriate nursing intervention for postpartum hemorrhage is
   a. bimanual pressure.
   b. bladder catheterization.
   c. continuous fundal massage.

6. On the second postpartum/postoperative day following her cesarean delivery, a woman exhibits hypotension, dyspnea, hemoptysis, and abdominal/chest pain. The nurse recognizes these as signs and symptoms of
   a. endometritis.
   b. pulmonary embolism.
   c. sepsis.

7. Normal metabolic changes during the postpartum period include increased levels of
   a. blood glucose.
   b. plasma renin and angiotensin II.
   c. prolactin.

8. The most significant factor influencing a woman's successful transition to motherhood is
   a. emotional support and physical involvement in child care by a significant other.
   b. regular attendance at parent support group meetings.
   c. resumption of a positive and satisfying sexual relationship with her partner.

9. Postpartum endometritis is
   a. associated with internal monitoring, amnioinfusion, prolonged labor, and prolonged rupture of membranes.
   b. effectively treated with a single dose of ampicillin or cephalosporin.
   c. less frequent following cesarean birth due to sterile technique used during surgery.

10. Disruptions in the integrity of the anal sphincter, third-degree tears, and sphincter weakness are
    a. associated with increased incidence of incontinence of flatus/stool.
    b. prevented through the judicious use of operative delivery.
    c. problems freely discussed by women with their healthcare providers.

11. The nurse can positively affect a new mother's self-concept and mothering abilities by encouraging
    a. establishment of a feeding schedule that the mother finds satisfying.
    b. supportive family and friends to participate in learning opportunities and infant care during hospitalization.
    c. the mother to provide as much of the infant care as possible.

12. Appropriate fundal massage for postpartum uterine atony involves using
    a. continuous two-handed pressure on the uterus until bleeding stops.
    b. firm one-handed pressure on the fundus until clots are expressed.
    c. two hands and the force needed to effect uterine contraction.

13. Stress incontinence during the postpartum period is more likely to be associated with the techniques used to manage which stage of labor?
    a. first
    b. second
    c. third

14. No more than 800 mL of urine should be removed during postpartum catheterization to minimize the potential for
    a. bladder spasm.
    b. hypertension.
    c. hypotension.

15. The most effective prevention of endometritis is use of
    a. early pericare.
    b. handwashing.
    c. intrapartum antibiotics.

16. The most likely cause of a decline in sexual interest/activity during the postpartum period is
    a. bleeding from the vagina.
    b. fatigue.
    c. vaginal dryness.

17. Postpartum hemorrhage is associated with administration of
    a. dicloxacillin.
    b. methadone.
    c. terbutaline.

18. Peak cardiac output after birth occurs at
    a. 1–5 minutes.
    b. 10–15 minutes.
    c. 30 minutes.

19. A normal hematologic change during the postpartum period is a/an
    a. drop in hematocrit between days 2 and 4.
    b. increase in the sedimentation rate.
    c. leukocytosis of 25–30,000/µL.

20. Nutritional counseling for women who breastfeed should include increasing caloric intake by
    a. 300 calories.
    b. 400 calories.
    c. 500 calories.

Fill in the Blank

21. To increase venous return during postpartum hemorrhage, the woman should be positioned with _______.

22. A white blood cell count of 28,000/mm^3 on postpartum day 2 would be considered _______.

23. Vital signs within normal limits do not rule out hypovolemic shock in a woman who has experienced a postpartum hemorrhage because alterations in vital signs do not occur until _______.

24. _______ is an assessment technique for identification of deep vein thrombosis.

25. When a postpartum woman displays dyspnea and chest pain, the nurse most appropriately suspects _______.

26. The first blood pressure response to hypovolemia would be decreased _______.

27. Counseling regarding contraceptive methods must include information about the _______, _______, and _______.

28. Symptoms of postpartum blues include
    1) _______
    2) _______
    3) _______
    4) _______
    5) _______

29. During the initial postpartum period, the nurse should assess _______, _______, and _______

every 15 minutes for at least 1 hour or more often if indicated.

30. Typically, postpartum blues occur at ______ days postpartum and continue for no more than a few days.

31. The normal postpartum physiologic diuresis begins within ______ hours of delivery and continues up to ______ days.

32. The acronym BUBBLERS, used to organize postpartum assessment, stands for
    1) ______
    2) ______
    3) ______
    4) ______
    5) ______
    6) ______
    7) ______
    8) ______

33. For each 500 cc of blood loss, the hematocrit will decrease ______% and the hemoglobin will decrease ______ g/dL.

34. Assessment findings suggesting the development of mastitis include
    1) ______
    2) ______
    3) ______
    4) ______

35. Essential topics to be discussed during postpartum teaching are
    1) ______
    2) ______
    3) ______
    4) ______

36. A major factor affecting emotional adjustment during the postpartum period in low-risk women is ______.

37. The first hour after birth is the time of greatest risk for postpartum hemorrhage because ______.

38. Symptoms indicating the development of postpartum preeclampsia are
    1) ______
    2) ______
    3) ______

39. It is important that the nurse has the drug ______ readily available when patients are receiving heparin therapy for thrombophlebitis.

40. Symptoms of impending postpartum eclamptic seizure are
    1) ______
    2) ______
    3) ______
    4) ______
    5) ______

Chapter 13

Multiple Choice

1. Miscarriage occurs in what percentage of pregnancies?
   a. 15%
   b. 20%
   c. 25%

2. Tim and Ann have experienced the death of their 2-day-old son, Tyler, from meconium aspiration. During this acute phase of grief, the nurse would expect a grief response of
   a. acceptance.
   b. guilt.
   c. denial.

3. The nurse provides parents with special mementos and pictures of their deceased newborn to make the experience more real. This should be helpful based on the acute grief response of
   a. anger.
   b. inability to maintain organized patterns of activity.
   c. preoccupation with the deceased.

4. When asked, "Why did this happen?", the nurse's best response is to
   a. listen and provide comfort.
   b. offer explanations.
   c. reflect the question.

5. When parents decide that they do not want to take home the photographs of their infant, the nurse most appropriately
   a. discards the photos.
   b. files the photos for future retrieval.
   c. packs the pictures with their belongings.

Fill in the Blank

6. Losses can be divided into four types.
   1) ______
   2) ______
   3) ______
   4) ______

7. ______ grief describes grief experienced by the parents before the expected death of a child.

8. Parents may experience _______ grief when their child has a deformity because they are continually reminded that the child is not "perfect".

9. Bereaved parents can take pleasure in the memories of their child who has died through _______ grief, which brings gentle sadness in remembering.

10. Participating in a(n) _______ provides parents with the emotional support of others who have experienced a similar loss.

11. The nurse should preserve special mementos for the parents such as _______, _______, and _______.

12. An appropriate response to a bereaved family during acute grief, when the family is irritable or angry, would be to _______.

13. When a mother expresses thoughts about having caused the death of her baby, the nurse should reassure her that _______.

14. A(n) _______ support group is one where bereaved parents can enter and leave at will.

15. Repressing feelings after caring for a family who has experienced a loss may cause the nurse to feel _______, _______, and _______.

16. When nurses experience overload in caring for bereaved families, they may be helped by talking with skilled members of the _______ to process their feelings.

17. Novice nurses who want to work with bereaved families can gain experience by
    1) _______
    2) _______
    3) _______

Chapter 14

Multiple Choice

1. The newborn's metabolism of brown fat occurs
   a. immediately after birth.
   b. in response to cold stress.
   c. when oxygen saturation is below 90.

2. A 10-minute Apgar is assigned when the
   a. 1-minute Apgar is less than 8.
   b. 5-minute Apgar is less than 7.
   c. newborn has required resuscitation.

3. During the first week of life, newborns are at risk for bleeding because
   a. milk intake is inadequate to supply vitamin K requirements.
   b. several clotting factors are being under-produced by the spleen.
   c. the liver is immature and not yet producing several clotting factors.

4. According to the American Academy of Pediatrics, vitamin K should be administered
   a. after the infant is weighed and measured.
   b. after 2 hours of life.
   c. within 1 hour of birth.

5. After administration of eye prophylaxis, excess erythromycin ophthalmic ointment is correctly
   a. left in place until absorbed.
   b. removed using sterile water.
   c. wiped away after 1 minute.

6. According to research, there is an association between shorter separation time and umbilical cord care using
   a. alcohol.
   b. sterile water.
   c. triple antibiotic dye.

7. The key to infant abduction prevention is a
   a. carefully obtained set of newborn footprints.
   b. state of the art electronic infant abduction alert.
   c. systematic infant safety program.

8. Vitamin K is produced by the newborn as
   a. a normal compensatory mechanism whenever bleeding occurs.
   b. a response to the parenteral administration of vitamin K.
   c. the gastrointestinal tract becomes colonized with bacteria following initiation of feeding.

9. As part of the algorithm for performing neonatal resuscitation, medications are administered when the
   a. code team physician orders them.
   b. heart rate is below 60 after PPV with 100% oxygen.
   c. heart rate is 60–80 and not increasing.

10. Initiation of respirations is triggered in the brain by decreased concentration of
    a. carbon dioxide.
    b. oxygen.
    c. surfactant.

11. Fetal pulmonary vascular resistance is
    a. equal to neonatal.
    b. higher than neonatal.
    c. lower than neonatal.

12. In the fetus, most blood is shunted away from the lungs through the
    a. ductus arteriosus.
    b. ductus venosus.
    c. foramen ovale.

13. Clamping the umbilical cord at birth causes
    a. decreased blood pressure and decreased systemic vascular resistance.
    b. increased blood pressure and decreased systemic vascular resistance.
    c. increased blood pressure and increased systemic vascular resistance.

14. The major factor contributing to closure of the ductus arteriosus is sensitivity to
    a. decreasing arterial carbon dioxide concentration.
    b. decreasing left ventricular pressure.
    c. increasing arterial oxygen concentration.

15. In a healthy newborn, the ductus arteriosus will have closed or will be closing by
    a. 1–6 hours of life.
    b. 12–24 hours of life.
    c. 48–72 hours of life.

16. The premature infant is more susceptible to evaporative heat loss because of
    a. decreased body surface area.
    b. decreased muscle tone.
    c. increased permeability of skin.

17. Hemorrhagic disease of the newborn is prevented by administration of
    a. vitamin A.
    b. vitamin D.
    c. vitamin K.

18. To protect newborns from infection with hepatitis B virus, all newborns
    a. born to mothers with unknown HBsAg status should receive one dose of vaccine within 12 hours of birth.
    b. should be screened for HBsAg within 12 hours of birth.
    c. should receive the first dose of hepatitis vaccine within 12 hours of birth.

19. Intrauterine infection should be suspected when the newborn has elevated
    a. IgA.
    b. IgG.
    c. IgM.

20. An infant born to a group B streptococcus positive mother who did not receive antibiotics during labor is at risk for
    a. hyperbilirubinemia.
    b. hypoglycemia.
    c. pneumonia.

Fill in the Blank

The following nursing interventions support the newborn's transition to extrauterine life by interrupting what mechanism of heat loss (a–d)?

21. ______ dry newborn thoroughly, remove wet linen

22. ______ when necessary use humidified, warmed oxygen

23. ______ place cover between newborn and metal scale

24. ______ preheat radiant warmer
    a. evaporation
    b. convection
    c. conduction
    d. radiation

25. Maternal intrauterine transmission of ______ antibodies protects the newborn from bacterial and viral infections for which the mother has already produced antibodies.

26. The action that best protects newborns from infection is ______.

27. A 2000 g infant should receive ______ mg of vitamin K.

28. Erythromycin ophthalmic ointment protects newborns from the organisms ______ and ______.

29. Immediately following birth, in the absence of spontaneous respirations, a nurse begins giving the newborn positive pressure ventilation. The second nurse should ______.

30. Respiratory adaptations during the transition to extrauterine life are dependant on ______, ______, and ______ stimuli to the brain.

31. In utero, oxygenated blood flows from the placenta to the fetus through the ______.

32. During fetal life, the placenta is an organ of ______ vascular resistance.

33. The vessels in the umbilical cord are two ______ and one ______.

34. The four main mechanisms of heat loss in the neonate are ______, ______, ______, and ______.

35. Nonshivering thermogenesis generates heat in the newborn through _______.

36. Hypothermia in the neonate increases _______ consumption.

37. The action of surfactant is to _______ in the alveoli.

38. In neonatal resuscitation, chest compressions should be initiated if the heart rate is below _______ bpm.

39. Women who are positive for group B streptococcal infection should be treated with _______ during labor.

40. Postpartum practices that increase breast-feeding duration include _______ and _______.

Chapter 15

Multiple Choice

1. In a newborn with hypospadias, the urinary meatus is located on the
   a. anterior surface of the glans.
   b. posterior surface of the glans.
   c. tip of the glans.

2. A nevus simplex "stork bite"
   a. is usually elevated, rough, and dark red.
   b. most often appears on the neck, forehead, and eyelids.
   c. will not blanch with pressure.

3. Tears are usually absent in a baby until the age of
   a. 2–4 weeks.
   b. 2–3 months.
   c. 4–6 months.

4. Newborn femoral pulses would characteristically be decreased or absent in
   a. congenital heart abnormalities.
   b. hip dysplasia.
   c. sepsis.

5. A persistent newborn heart rate of less than 100 beats per minute is consistent with
   a. congenital heart block.
   b. congestive heart failure.
   c. vagal stimulation.

6. Using the Silverman Index to assess a newborn's respiratory effort, a score of zero indicates
   a. moderate respiratory distress.
   b. no respiratory distress.
   c. severe respiratory distress.

7. In the neonate, blood pressure in the lower extremities is usually
   a. higher than in the upper extremities.
   b. lower than in the upper extremities.
   c. no different than in the upper extremities.

8. The normal umbilical cord contains
   a. one artery and one vein.
   b. two arteries and one vein.
   c. two veins and one artery.

9. Jaundice within the first 24 hours of life may be related to
   a. asphyxia.
   b. cardiac disease.
   c. sepsis.

10. Edema over the presenting part of a newborn's head that feels spongy and resolves within a few days of life is characteristic of
    a. caput succedaneum.
    b. cephalhematoma.
    c. trauma during birth.

11. A gestational age assessment indicating the greatest degree of physical maturity is
    a. labia majora covering clitoris and labia minora.
    b. labia majora large and labia minora small.
    c. prominent clitoris and enlarging labia minora.

12. Newborn jaundice appears initially on the
    a. head and face.
    b. trunk and extremities.
    c. sclera.

13. To measure fontanelles accurately, a ruler or measuring tape is placed
    a. across the widest diameter.
    b. diagonally from bone to bone.
    c. from suture line to suture line.

14. A crossed-eyed appearance in a newborn is called
    a. hypertelorism.
    b. nystagmus.
    c. strabismus.

15. Bowel sounds are expected to be present in the newborn
    a. after passage of first meconium stool.
    b. immediately after birth.
    c. within 1 hour of birth.

16. A prominent xiphoid process identified during a newborn physical assessment is
    a. a normal finding.
    b. associated with intrauterine growth retardation.

c. indicative of respiratory distress.

17. The most common finding in assessment of the newborn's skin is a
a. hemangioma.
b. Mongolian spot.
c. nevus simplex.

18. Permanent eye color is present by the age of
a. 2 months.
b. 4 months.
c. 6 months.

19. In a newborn, the skin lesion that has discrete borders and does not blanch to pressure or lighten with age is a
a. hemangioma.
b. Mongolian spot.
c. port wine stain.

20. The presence of the red reflex in the newborn indicates
a. congenital cataracts.
b. intact cornea and lens.
c. weak eye musculature.

21. Umbilical hernias are more commonly seen in newborns who are
a. African American.
b. Native American.
b. South East Asian.

22. Screening programs evaluating newborns at high risk for hearing loss will potentially miss what percentage of newborns with hearing loss?
a. 25%
b. 50%
c. 75%

23. The most common abnormal neck finding in newborns is
a. cystic hygroma.
b. torticollis.
c. webbing.

24. The Moro reflex should disappear by the age of
a. 2 months.
b. 4 months.
c. 6 months.

25. A genitourinary finding in a gestational age assessment of a newborn male at 36 weeks' gestation is
a. rugae becoming visible.
b. pendulous scrotum.
c. testes in the upper scrotum.

26. During the first few days of life, the percentage of newborns with developmental hip dysplasia that is identified during physical assessment is
a. 40%.
b. 60%.
c. 80%.

27. A scrotal mass which does not transilluminate is a/an
a. hydrocele.
b. inguinal hernia.
c. testis.

Fill in the Blank

28. When examining the clavicles, _______ is felt by the examiner if there is a fracture present.

29. At birth, newborns are covered with an odorless, white, cheesy substance called _______.

30. Epstein's pearls are composed of _______ cells.

31. Popping sensations (similar to indenting a ping-pong ball) felt when when palpating the parietal or occipital bones of a newborn are called _______.

32. The anterior fontanelle normally closes at about _______ months.

33. The posterior fontanelle normally closes at about _______ months.

34. Apnea refers to pauses in respirations which last _______ seconds or longer.

35. Newborns can see an object clearly when the object is _______ inches away.

36. _______ describes the inability to completely retract the foreskin of the penis.

37. _______ is an asymmetric neck deformity in which the head is noted to be pulled toward the effected side, with the chin pointing toward the opposite shoulder, due to injury to the _______ muscle.

38. Acrocyanosis is the result of _______ and tends to worsen if the newborn becomes chilled.

39. _______ is a compensatory mechanism that decreases upper airway resistance, allowing more air to enter the nasal passages.

40. Newborn _______ are involuntary protective neuromuscular responses.

Chapter 16

Multiple Choice

1. A woman who presents with a history of minimal increase in breast tissue during pregnancy should be informed that
   a. the amount of breast tissue influences milk production.
   b. breast growth during pregnancy does not influence milk production.
   c. breast tissue will increase as she nurses.

2. The onset of milk production in a postpartum woman is triggered by the
   a. periodic stimulation of oxytocin.
   b. rapid rise in prolactin.
   c. sudden decrease in progesterone.

3. A pregnant woman who asks what she should do to prepare her nipples for breast-feeding is correctly informed that nipple exercises
   a. do little to prevent nipple soreness.
   b. improve nipple erectility.
   c. reduce the incidence of engorgement.

4. Frequent breast-feeding during the first 24 hours postpartum increases newborn
   a. immunity.
   b. sleep cycles.
   c. weight gain.

5. Breast engorgement in the breast-feeding mother is minimized by
   a. avoiding unnecessary nipple stimulation.
   b. nursing without time limits.
   c. pumping after nursing.

6. As maternal prolactin levels decline over time, what is responsible for continued milk production?
   a. newborn sucking
   b. maternal ingestion of adequate fluids
   c. return of normal estrogen levels

7. During a home visit to a 4-day-old breast-feeding newborn, the nurse observes jaundice. Which of the following interventions should be suggested to the mother?
   a. increasing the frequency of breast-feeding
   b. supplementing breast-feeds with water
   c. temporarily pumping and discarding her breast milk

8. A newborn is reported to have breast-fed very well during the first hour after birth. The baby is now 12 hours old and has not had a second successful feeding. The nurse should
   a. advise the mother to give water every 2-3 hours.
   b. review newborn sleep cycles and hunger cues.
   c. teach the mother to pump her breasts.

9. A woman calls the hospital asking what she should do for her 10-day-old breast-feeding newborn who wants to nurse "all the time." The nurse should recommend that the mother
   a. continue breast-feeding based on the newborn's cues.
   b. offer formula if the newborn is still hungry after breast-feeding.
   c. use other comforting techniques to space feedings at least 2 hours apart.

10. A bottle-feeding mother asks if she should give her baby water. The nurse should instruct her to
    a. add a little extra water to the formula on hot days.
    b. feed the newborn properly mixed formula.
    c. give the newborn water between feedings if fussy.

11. The hormone responsible for milk ejection is
    a. oxytocin.
    b. progesterone.
    c. prolactin.

12. The mother can encourage the newborn to open his mouth wider while nursing by
    a. applying a small amount of downward pressure on the newborn's chin.
    b. guiding the newborn's head toward the breast.
    c. leaning forward toward the newborn.

13. Compared to mature milk, colostrum is higher in
    a. fat.
    b. IgG.
    c. protein.

14. As human milk matures, the concentration of immunoglobins and proteins
    a. decreases.
    b. increases.
    c. remains the same.

15. A mother holds her breast with her thumb on top and fingers below; she is using the hold called
    a. "C".
    b. circle.
    c. cup.

16. Formula-feeding is recommended for newborns with
    a. galactosemia.
    b. jaundice.
    c. thalassemia.

17. After opening a can or bottle of formula, the contents should be used within
    a. 24 hours.
    b. 48 hours.
    c. 72 hours.

18. The most economic formula preparation is
    a. concentrate.
    b. powder.
    c. ready-to-feed.

19. Methods to increase comfort while suppressing lactation include
    a. applying heat to the breast.
    b. limiting fluid intake for 48 hours.
    c. wearing a firm-fitting bra.

Fill in the Blank

20. Healthy People 2010 target for percentage of women breast-feeding at discharge is _______.

21. Colostrum's yellow color is due to its high _______ level.

22. A hard, tender area in the breast of a breast-feeding woman should be treated with _______ and _______.

23. When the breast-feeding baby is correctly latched onto the mother's breast, the tongue covers the _______.

24. Hunger cues can be observed for _______ minutes before the newborn begins sustained crying.

25. General guidelines for newborn weight gain during the first few weeks of life are regaining birth weight by _______ weeks and gaining _______ ounces a week or at least _______ pounds a month.

26. Current thinking is that newborns will lose _______% of their birth weight in their first few days of life.

27. The easiest, most economic treatments for nipple pain are _______.

28. Alternate breast massage is used to _______.

29. Instructions for alternate breast massage are to _______.

30. Feeding the infant in the _______ position may decrease the risk of otitis media.

Chapter 17

Multiple Choice

1. Transient tachypnea develops more often in the newborn who is born
    a. by cesarean section.
    b. after a prolonged first stage of labor.
    c. small for gestational age.

2. In a newborn, tachypnea is defined as a respiratory rate greater than
    a. 40/minute.
    b. 60/minute.
    c. 80/minute.

3. A cardiac lesion considered to be cyanotic is
    a. ASD.
    b. PDA.
    c. TGA.

4. A cardiac lesion which results in decreased pulmonary blood flow is
    a. ASD.
    b. TET.
    c. PDA.

5. A medication used to maintain patency of the ductus arteriosus is
    a. caffeine.
    b. indomethacin.
    c. prostaglandin E_1.

6. Hypoglycemia in the infant born to an insulin-dependent diabetic mother, occurs after birth between
    a. 1–3 hours.
    b. 5–7 hours.
    c. 8–10 hours.

7. One etiology of hypoglycemia is decreased production of glucose, which should be suspected in the newborn who is
    a. cold-stressed.
    b. the infant of a diabetic mother.
    c. small for gestational age.

8. Clinical jaundice is first apparent at serum bilirubin levels of
    a. 1–3 mg/dL.
    b. 5–7 mg/dL.
    c. 9–11 mg/dL.

9. In a full-term newborn, physiologic hyperbilirubinemia is characterized by a progressive increase in serum bilirubin that peaks at
    a. 24 hours.
    b. 48 hours.

c. 72 hours.

10. Gastrointestinal symptoms associated with neonatal abstinence syndrome include
    a. constipation.
    b. diarrhea.
    c. flatulance.

11. Which drug, when used alone, is responsible for the most severe withdrawal symptoms in the newborn?
    a. cocaine
    b. heroin
    c. methadone

12. When ruling out sepsis in the newborn, the broad-spectrum antimicrobial agents most commonly initiated after cultures have been obtained are
    a. ampicillin/cephalosporin.
    b. ampicillin/gentamicin.
    c. penicillin/gentamicin.

13. IV antibiotic treatment for neonatal sepsis should continue for
    a. 3–5 days.
    b. 7–10 days.
    c. 12–14 days.

14. Hypothermia can cause
    a. decreased metabolic demand.
    b. hypoglycemia.
    c. metabolic alkalosis.

15. A sign of hypoglycemia in the newborn is
    a. decreased skin turgor.
    b. increased appetite.
    c. temperature instability.

16. An indication to screen for hypoglycemia is an infant who is
    a. a second twin weighing 3000 grams.
    b. born at 38 weeks' gestation.
    c. small for gestational age.

17. In the newborn, physiologic hyperbilirubinemia is characterized by a progressive increase in serum bilirubin to a peak of
    a. 5 mg/dL at 72 hours of age.
    b. 8 mg/dL at 72 hours of age.
    c. 10 mg/dL at 48 hours of age.

18. Infants undergoing phototherapy should have axillary temperatures monitored at least every
    a. 30 minutes.
    b. 1 hour.
    c. 2 hours.

19. Infants born to cocaine-addicted mothers frequently exhibit
    a. constipation.
    b. feeding difficulties.
    c. lethargy.

20. Which of the following interventions is useful to support an infant experiencing abstinence syndrome?
    a. massage
    b. music
    c. rocking

21. The diagnosis of neonatal sepsis is made in the presence of a positive culture of
    a. blood.
    b. both blood and urine.
    c. urine.

Fill in the Blank

22. Surfactant _______ surface tension in the alveoli and functions as a stabilizer to prevent collapse during expiration.

23. When meconium only partially obstructs the airway, a _______ effect results where air enters the lower airways on inspiration but cannot _______ on expiration.

24. The _______ is the first major organ system to function in the embryo.

25. A ventricular septal defect (VSD) is considered to be a(n) _______ lesion with _______ pulmonary blood flow.

26. The three pathophysiologic findings in tetrology of Fallot are
    1) _______
    2) _______
    3) _______

27. The incidence of the congenital heart defect, _______, is inversely proportional to gestational age.

28. An atrial septal defect (ASD) is considered to be a(n) _______ lesion with _______ pulmonary blood flow.

29. With transposition of the great arteries in two _______ circulations; the degree of cyanosis present depends upon the amount of mixing through the _______, if present, _______ or _______.

30. Glucose homeostasis requires the initiation of various metabolic processes including _______

forming glucose from noncarbohydrate sources and _______, conversion of glycogen stores to glucose.

31. As bilirubin levels rise, there is concern that bilirubin encephalopathy, also known as _______, will develop.

32. In nearly all newborns, phototherapy decreases or blunts the rise in serum _______ bilirubin regardless of gestational age, race, or presence or absence of hemolysis.

33. A variety of medications are used to treat neonatal abstinence syndrome. The three most commonly used are _______, _______, and _______.

34. _______ is the one common side effect of all of the medications used to treat neonatal abstinence.

35. The two bacterial agents most commonly associated with neonatal sepsis are _______ and _______.

36. The primary neonatal factors influencing the development of sepsis are _______ and _______.

37. Once sepsis has been diagnosed, antibiotic therapy must continue for _______ days.

38. Intrapartum administration of prophylactic antibiotics has proven to be beneficial in preventing _______.

39. Heroin withdrawal in a newborn may last _______ weeks.

40. Skin care is important during phototherapy because the infant often has _______.

41. An infant born to a mother who received tocolytic therapy would be prone to _______.

42. Tachypnea is defined as a respiration rate of _______ breaths per minute.

43. To prevent meconium aspiration syndrome, the mouth and pharynx may be suctioned _______ the head is delivered.

44. Narcotics used to manage labor pain may result in _______ respiratory effort in the newborn.

45. The mortality rate associated with neonatal sepsis increases as birth weight _______.

Chapter 18

Multiple Choice

1. Discharge planning begins
   a. during the prenatal period.
   b. in the immediate postpartum period.
   c. when the mother is admitted for labor.

2. The woman's focus during the intrapartum period is
   a. bonding with her newborn.
   b. opportunity to review her labor after the birth.
   c. safe passage through her labor and birth.

3. Encouraging postpartum parents to complete a learning needs assessment
   a. avoids duplication of teaching done during prenatal care.
   b. decreases the amount of time the nurse will spend teaching.
   c. helps parents recognize information needed before discharge.

4. According to the American Academy of Pediatrics, postpartum follow-up contacts are ideally made
   a. at a scheduled 2-week well baby visit.
   b. by the primary perinatal nurse by phone contact.
   c. in person in the home or outpatient clinic.

5. The primary reason to give a copy of the family clinical pathway to childbearing women and their families is to
   a. explain prenatal care as they enter the system.
   b. facilitate care during the inpatient stay.
   c. promote collaboration between women and their primary care providers.

6. The increase in the quality and quantity of prenatal data about the childbearing family provided by a database results in
   a. effective use of available nursing staff.
   b. enhanced individualized care and teaching.
   c. optimal use of economic resources.

7. Prenatal class curriculum is ideally developed by prenatal educators
   a. after consultation with the medical staff.
   b. following the advice of professional associations.
   c. in partnership with healthcare providers and parents.

8. The development of effective teaching methods and materials include consideration of

a. reading and comprehension levels of the expectant family.
b. staff preferences for class materials and schedules.
c. use of large group presentations to maximize use of resources.

9. A family preference plan
   a. assists in avoiding the development of maternal complications.
   b. formulates most realistically at admission for labor.
   c. involves women and their families in decisions about their care.

10. The optimal time for case managers to become involved with the expectant woman and her family is
    a. during the intrapartum period by referral from the perinatal nurse.
    b. from entry into the system through the postpartum period.
    c. when the woman meets the definition of being at high risk for problems.

11. The essential first step in program evaluation is
    a. identifying goals and expected outcomes.
    b. reviewing patient satisfaction surveys.
    c. trending data from prenatal class evaluations.

Fill in the Blank

12. Postpartum women have transient deficits in cognition, particularly in memory function the _______ day following birth.

13. Discharge planning that relies on verbal transmission of information or instruction in childcare techniques on the first postpartum day will be _______.

14. The discharge planning process begins _______.

15. Opportunities to identify learning needs of women and their families include:
    a. _______
    b. _______
    c. _______
    d. _______

16. In any practice model for prenatal and birth education, the following people play a key role in designing curriculum that includes postpartum education:
    a. _______
    b. _______
    c. _______
    d. _______

17. No matter where perinatal instruction is given, the teaching method must _______ and _______.

18. Skills such as comfort measures for labor or postpartum perineal care are most effectively taught by _______

19. Written materials given to women and their families must
    a. _______
    b. _______
    c. _______

20. A family preference plan encourages women and their families to define _______.

21. A family preference plan helps the perinatal nurse _______.

22. List three critical concepts that must be addressed in maternal postpartum care.
    a. _______
    b. _______
    c. _______

23. List three critical concepts that must be addressed in newborn care.
    a. _______
    b. _______
    c. _______

24. Before discharge, knowledge and skills about self- and infant care are validated. Validation can be accomplished by _______.

25. Adequacy of maternal knowledge and skills is documented on _______.

26. When the case manager is able to coordinate care effectively in the perinatal period, the following outcomes are achieved:
    a. _______
    b. _______
    c. _______
    d. _______

27. The hospital-based perinatal nurse influences successful transition from hospital to home by
    a. _______
    b. _______
    c. _______
    d. _______

Chapter 19

True or False

1. State legislation for maternity length of stay is consistent across the United States.
2. Care coordination between the hospital and home care agency is of key importance to provide continuity of care to the mother and newborn.
3. Nursing interventions are based on the needs of the individual mother, newborn, and family.
4. There is no evidence to support early discharge as a safe practice.
5. Early discharge is a new concept in obstetrics for mothers and newborns.
6. The goal of home care services is to safely and effectively care for the mother and newborn in their home following a hospital birth.
7. AWHONN and the ANA support the practice of nursing in the home for mothers and newborns.
8. Personal safety for the home care nurse is not of concern because these families want the home care nurse to come and support them and check on their baby.

Multiple Choice

9. The primary reason for neonatal readmission after early discharge is
   a. hyperbilirubinemia.
   b. sepsis.
   c. weight loss.
10. Studies about early discharge for mothers and newborns have limited application to the general population because
    a. discharge criteria are not consistent.
    b. "early" has various definitions.
    c. the studies are not published.

Fill in the Blank

11. Early discharge criteria include
    1) ______
    2) ______
    3) ______
    4) ______
12. The nursing role in home care is
    1) ______
    2) ______
    3) ______
    4) ______
13. List 4 components of a postpartum maternal assessment in the home.
    1) ______
    2) ______
    3) ______
    4) ______
14. List 4 components of a newborn assessment in the home following an early discharge.
    1) ______
    2) ______
    3) ______
    4) ______

ANSWER KEY

Chapter 1

1. b
2. b
3. a
4. a
5. c
6. c
7. c
8. b
9. a
10. a
11. b
12. a
13. a
14. c
15. a
16. c
17. care
18. physician, nurse
19. Joint Commission on Accreditation of Healthcare Organizations (JCAHO)
20. Association of Women's Health, Obstetric and Neonatal Nurses (AWHONN)

Chapter 2

1. c
2. b
3. a
4. a
5. c
6. b
7. a
8. b
9. a
10. a
11. c
12. b
13. c
14. a
15. c
16. 1:2
17. state legislatures
18. the lack of a four-year college degree in nursing as a criterion for entry into practice
19. duty, breach of duty, damages (injury), causation (proximate cause)
20. the task is suitable for delegation, the UAP is competent to perform the task
21. negligence
22. negligence by a professional
23. lawsuits/litigation/"suits"
24. 1) inability to recognize and/or appropriately respond to both antepartum and intrapartum fetal compromise
    2) inability to effect a timely cesarean birth (30 minutes from decision to incision when indicated by maternal or fetal condition)
    3) inability to appropriately resuscitate a depressed infant
    4) inappropriate use of oxytocin or misoprostol leading to uterine hyperstimulation, uterine rupture, fetal compromise and/or death
    5) inappropriate use of forceps/vacuum/fundal pressure leading to maternal/fetal trauma and/or preventable shoulder dystocia
25. normalization of deviance
26. they get away with it, nothing "bad" happens
27. most mothers and babies are healthy
28. retrospective
29. outdated, error
30. sentinel event
31. AWHONN, ACOG, AAP
32. 1:2
33. 1:1
34. the Emergency Medical Treatment and Labor Act (EMTALA)
35. 1) provide a medical screening exam for every patient
    2) provide stabilization and treatment for every patient with an emergency medical condition
    3) transfer according to the guidelines outlined in the statute
36. emergency medical condition
37. chain of command
38. ongoing problems with nurse/physician communication; deterioration in nurse/physician relationships
39. liabilities to third parties arising out of their professional practice
40. within the scope of employment
41. criminal

Chapter 3

1. 1) gender issues
   2) traditional roles of physicians and nurses
   3) institutional policies and organizational structures
   4) methods and amount of financial compensation
   5) wide disparity in level of educational preparation
   6) licensure and professional accountability
2. 1) consensus (agreeing to agree)
   2) mutual accountability
   3) organizational discipline
   4) clearly defined tasks
   5) clearly defined time frames

3. getting the doctor to order an intervention, medication, or laboratory test and have it look like his/her idea rather than that of the nurse.
4. evidence-based, maternal–fetal safety, likelihood of adverse outcomes.
5. individuals

Chapter 4

1. c
2. a
3. a
4. b
5. b
6. b
7. c
8. b
9. a-2, b-1, c-3
10. c
11. a
12. b
13. c
14. Enhance communication skills, develop linguistic skills, determine who the family decision-makers are, understand that agreement may not indicate comprehension, utilize nonverbal communication, use appropriate names and titles, and use culturally appropriate teaching techniques.

Chapter 5

1. c
2. a
3. b
4. a
5. c
6. c
7. c
8. c
9. a
10. c
11. b
12. b
13. c
14. b
15. b
16. c
17. c
18. b
19. b
20. b
21. a
22. a
23. a
24. a
25. a
26. autotransfusion of approximately 1000 mL at birth
27. physiologic anemia of pregnancy
28. increased levels of coagulation factors, placental fibrinolysis factors
29. increases
30. renal sodium
31. increased glomerular filtration rate
32. striae gravidarum
33. prolactin
34. progesterone
35. glycosuria is normal during pregnancy
36. cardiovascular
37. autotransfusion
38. blood volume
39. 6 weeks' postpartum
40. uterus
41. progesterone
42. second
43. angiotensin II
44. hypercoagulable
45. coagulation change, venous stasis
46. prostaglandins
47. melasma
48. Chadwick's sign

Chapter 6

1. b
2. a
3. a
4. b
5. b
6. c
7. c
8. c
9. a
10. 1) family and social history
    2) psychiatric history
    3) mental status
    4) self-concept/self-esteem
    5) support systems
    6) stressors
    7) coping strategies
    8) spirituality
    9) neurovegetative signs
    10) knowledge of the pregnancy experience
11. pregnant woman, family, nurse
12. nursing diagnoses, care plans, and strategies for nursing care delivery
13. exacerbation or recurrence in the postpartum period
14. the multidisciplinary team providing care for the woman and her family
15. emotional nuances in relationships with family and professionals
16. frequency, duration, and intensity
17. they believe it is a normal reaction secondary to the stress of becoming a mother
18. 10
19. her own physical and psychological needs have been met

Chapter 7

1. b
2. c
3. a
4. b
5. a
6. b
7. b
8. a
9. b
10. a
11. b
12. a
13. b
14. c
15. a
16. a
17. b
18. 28
19. 36
20. 15 lbs
21. 10
22. teratogen
23. 8
24. 12
25. Jewish
26. Coumadin

27. negative
28. 15, 20
29. 1) early and continuing risk assessment
    2) health promotion
    3) medical and psychosocial intervention
30. cardiorespiratory, muscular
31. two or more abnormally elevated values
32. 15, 20
33. 10
34. 1) fetal tone
    2) fetal reflex movement
    3) fetal breathing
    4) amniotic fluid volume
    5) nonstress test

Chapter 8

Hypertensive Disorders

1. c
2. a
3. b
4. b
5. c
6. b
7. hypertensive
8. 110
9. semi-Fowler's
10. magnesium sulfate
11. 1) abruptio placentae
    2) disseminated intravascular coagulation
    3) hepatic failure
    4) acute renal failure
12. prevent maternal cerebral vascular accident; maintain uteroplacental perfusion
13. hemolysis; elevated liver enzymes; low platelets
14. aspiration

Bleeding

1. b
2. a
3. b
4. b
5. b
6. velamentous
7. 95
8. hypotension
9. 1) abruptio placentae
    2) hemorrhage
    3) preeclampsia
    4) amniotic fluid embolism
    5) sepsis
    6) cardiopulmonary arrest
    7) massive transfusion therapy
    8) saline termination of pregnancy
    9) dead fetus syndrome

Preterm Labor and Birth

1. a
2. b
3. a
4. b
5. a
6. a
7. a
8. b
9. b
10. c
11. 1.6
12. increased
13. eliminated

Diabetes

1. c
2. a
3. c
4. b
5. c
6. a
7. b
8. c
9. a
10. a
11. type 1
12. anabolic
13. 1) prolactin
    2) estrogen
    3) progesterone
    4) human placental lactogen
    5) cortisol
14. human
15. 1) polyuria
    2) polyphagia
    3) polydipsia
    4) blurred vision

Cardiac Disease

1. a
2. b
3. a
4. b
5. a
6. c
7. c
8. a
9. c
10. b
11. capillaries
12. rheumatic fever
13. rare
14. type of cardiac disorder, the secondary complications
15. functional ability

Pulmonary Complications

1. c
2. b
3. b
4. c
5. a
6. b
7. b
8. b
9. b
10. c
11. 10
12. 95
13. 75
14. illicit drug use, cigarette smoking, alcohol abuse, chronic illness
15. *streptococcus pneumoniae*
16. high Fowler's
17. pollens, molds, dust mites, animal dander, cockroach antigens, air pollutants, strong odors, food additives, tobacco smoke
18. systemic steroid therapy >4 wks; three visits for asthma recently; history of multiple hospitalizations for asthma; history of hypoxic seizure, hypoxic syncope, or intubation; history of admission to ICU for asthma
19. preterm labor, empyema, bacteremia, pneumothorax, atrial fibrillation, respiratory failure
20. 33

Multiple Gestation

1. c
2. c
3. a
4. b
5. c
6. c
7. true

Chapter 9

1. b
2. c
3. c
4. a
5. c
6. a
7. b
8. b
9. c
10. c
11. b
12. b
13. b
14. c
15. c
16. b
17. b
18. a
19. b
20. c
21. lower
22. kidneys, liver
23. sitting on the toilet
24. closed glottis, hemodynamic
25. spontaneous bearing-down efforts (urge to push)
26. shoulder dystocia, flex, knee, hip
27. blood loss, infection, pain, third and fourth degree laceration, delayed healing, sexual dysfunction, scarring.
28. 1) open glottis—gentle pushing
    2) spontaneous rather than directed pushing
    3) upright position in second stage
29. 1) fewer perinatal complications
    2) shorter labors
    3) fewer Neonatal Intensive Care Unit (NICU) admissions
30. 1) maternal status
    2) fetal well-being
    3) cervical status
31. bleeding, infection, rupture of membranes, umbilical cord prolapse
32. 6–12 hours
33. color and amount of fluid, FHR before procedure, fetal response to procedure
34. fourth
35. ischial spines
36. misoprostol, Cervidil
37. prior cesarean birth or uterine scar
38. emptying the maternal bladder
39. 500–600
40. 1) oxygen delivery system
    2) continuous and intermittent suction
    3) blood pressure monitoring equipment
    4) ECG monitoring equipment
    5) pulse oximeter
    6) adjustable lighting
    7) means to assure patient privacy
41. 1) one or two prior low transverse cesarean births
    2) clinically adequate pelvis
    3) no prior uterine surgery or rupture
    4) physician immediately available and capable of performing emergent cesarean birth
    5) surgical team and anesthesia personnel available for emergent cesarean birth
42. pain at the prior incision site
43. 1) stretching of uterine muscles
    2) pressure on the cervix
    3) endogenous oxytocin
    4) change in estrogen:progesterone ratio
44. 1) vaginal bleeding
    2) acute abdominal pain
    3) temperature of 100.4°F or higher
    4) preterm labor
    5) premature preterm rupture of membranes
    6) hypertension
45. 1) dilation
    2) effacement
    3) station
    4) consistency
    5) position
46. iatrogenic injuries to the mother and/or fetus
47. 1) risks
    2) benefits
    3) alternative approaches

Chapter 10

1. c
2. c
3. b
4. c
5. b
6. b
7. c
8. c
9. c
10. c
11. c
12. c
13. c
14. a
15. b
16. c
17. b
18. c
19. a
20. peak, after
21. variable, abrupt
22. beginning, baseline rate benign
23. decreasing or discontinuing
24. moderate
25. congenital anomalies
26. supraventricular tachycardia
27. three of the following:

    medications
    prematurity
    fetal sleep

fetal dysrhythmia
anesthetic agents
cardiac anomaly
28. baseline rate, variability, overshoots
29. hyperstimulation
30. tocolytics
31. intrauterine pressure catheter
32. anemic
33. 15,
5
34. 6–25
35. changing maternal position
36. variability, normal baseline rate
37. 50
38. 7.20, reassuring
39. 10
40. variability
41. 1) increasing IV fluids
    2) maintaining lateral maternal position
    3) administering O_2 by mask
    4) decreasing or discontinuing oxytocin
    5) delaying the next dose of Prepidil, Cervidil, or Cytotec
42. 110, 160
43. 30%, 70%
44. less than 30% between contractions

Chapter 11

1. a
2. c
3. c
4. c
5. c
6. c
7. a
8. b
9. a
10. b
11. c
12. a
13. c
14. b
15. a
16. b
17. c
18. b
19. a
20. hydrostatic
21. motor blockade, neonatal neurobehavioral effects
22. randomized controlled clinical trials
23. a
24. b
25. b
26. c
27. c
28. a
29. a
30. a
31. a
32. b
33. b
34. daydreaming
35. decrease
36. during
37. opioids/narcotics or agonist/antagonists
38. narcotic
39. hypotension
40. distraction

Chapter 12

1. c
2. c
3. c
4. a
5. b
6. b
7. b
8. a
9. a
10. a
11. b
12. c
13. b
14. c
15. b
16. b
17. c
18. b
19. c
20. c
21. legs elevated 20 degrees to 30 degrees.
22. nonpathologic leukocytosis.
23. a loss of 15–20% of the total blood volume.
24. measurement of the affected leg circumference or Homans' sign
25. pulmonary embolism
26. pulse pressure to 30 mm Hg or less
27. advantages, disadvantages, prevention of sexually transmitted diseases
28. 1) insomnia
    2) weepiness
    3) anxiety
    4) irritability
    5) poor concentration
29. vital signs, lochia, uterine tone/position
30. 3–6
31. 12, 5
32. 1) breast
    2) uterus
    3) bladder
    4) bowel
    5) lochia
    6) episiotomy/incision
    7) emotional response
    8) Homans' sign
33. 2–4, 1–1.5
34. 1) fever and chills
    2) localized tenderness
    3) palpable, hard, reddened mass
    4) tachycardia
35. 1) pelvic floor exercises
    2) postpartum exercise
    3) sexuality
    4) contraception
36. fatigue
37. large venous areas are exposed after placental expulsion
38. 1) blood pressure of 140/90
    2) headache
    3) decreased urine output
39. protamine sulfate
40. 1) severe persistent headache
    2) scotomata
    3) blurred vision
    4) photophobia
    5) epigastric or right upper quadrant pain

Chapter 13

1. b
2. a
3. c
4. a
5. b
6. 1) loss of significant other
   2) loss of some aspect of self

   3) loss through stages of growth and development
   4) loss of external objects
7. anticipatory
8. chronic
9. bittersweet
10. support group
11. footprints, name bands, lock of hair
12. listen
13. her feelings are normal
14. ongoing
15. out of control, tearful, self-focused
16. multidisciplinary team
17. 1) reading books on grief
    2) attending conferences
    3) working with an appropriate role model

Chapter 14

1. b
2. b
3. c
4. c
5. c
6. b
7. c
8. b
9. b
10. b
11. b
12. a
13. c
14. c
15. c
16. c
17. c
18. a
19. c
20. c
21. a
22. b
23. c
24. c
25. IgG
26. handwashing
27. 1
28. chlamydia and gonococcus
29. evaluate the heart rate
30. chemical, mechanical, sensory
31. umbilical vein
32. low
33. arteries, vein
34. evaporation, convection, conduction, and radiation
35. brown fat
36. oxygen
37. lower surface tension
38. 60
39. antibiotics
40. early suckling, uninterrupted contact between mother and newborn

Chapter 15

1. b
2. b
3. c
4. b
5. a
6. b
7. a
8. b
9. c
10. a
11. a
12. a
13. b
14. c
15. a
16. a
17. c
18. c
19. c
20. b
21. a
22. b
23. a
24. c
25. c
26. b
27. b
28. crepitus
29. vernix
30. epithelial
31. craniotabes
32. 18
33. 2–4
34. 20
35. 8–10
36. phimosis
37. torticollis; sternocleidomastoid
38. vasomotor instability
39. flaring
40. reflexes

Chapter 16

1. b
2. c
3. a
4. c
5. b
6. a
7. a
8. b
9. a
10. b
11. a
12. a
13. c
14. a
15. a
16. a
17. a
18. b
19. c
20. 75%
21. beta-carotene
22. warm compresses, frequent feedings
23. lower gum
24. 30 minutes
25. 2, 4–7, 1
26. 7
27. colostrum or breast milk on nipples after feeding; letting nipples air dry; warm, moist compresses
28. increase milk supply
29. massage the base of the breast when the infant stops sucking; alternate massaging of the breast between periods of sucking
30. semi-upright

Chapter 17

1. a
2. b
3. c
4. b
5. c
6. a
7. c
8. b
9. c
10. b
11. c
12. b
13. b
14. b
15. c
16. c
17. b
18. c
19. b
20. c
21. a
22. decreases
23. ball–valve, escape
24. cardiovascular system

25. acyanotic, increased
26. 1) VSD
    2) pulmonary stenosis
    3) aorta and right ventricular hypertrophy
27. PDA
28. acyanotic, increased
29. parallel, VSD, PDA, patent foramen, ovale (PFO)
30. gluconeogenesis glycolysis
31. kernicterus
32. unconjugated or indirect
33. dilute tincture of opium (DTO), paregoric, phenobarbital
34. sedation
35. group B β-hemolytic *Streptococcus*, *E-coli*
36. gestational age birth weight
37. 7–10
38. early onset group B strep sepsis
39. 8–16 weeks
40. loose stools
41. hypoglycemia
42. >60
43. once
44. poor
45. decreases

Chapter 18

1. a
2. c
3. c
4. c
5. c
6. b
7. c
8. a
9. c
10. b
11. a
12. first
13. poorly remembered
14. during the prenatal period
15. prenatal classes, prenatal visits to primary care providers, case managers, intrapartum stay, postdischarge follow-up visits and contacts
16. parent and birth educators, healthcare providers, perinatal nurses, the woman and her family
17. complement the information presented; must be appropriate for the learner
18. demonstration and return demonstration
19. have a consistent message, support the philosophy of the institution, support and reinforce interactive learning
20. their individual approach to birth
21. individualize the family's care
22. Three of the following:
    activity and rest
    pain relief and comfort measures
    care of the perineum
    breast care for breast-feeding women and lactation suppression for formula-feeding women
    postoperative cesarean birth instructions
    expected emotional adaptations
    signs of postpartum complications to report to the nurse or healthcare provider after discharge
23. Three of the following:
    newborn adaptation to extrauterine life
    feeding cues
    breast-feeding basics
    formula-feeding basics
    care of an infant who spits up or chokes
    umbilical cord care
    circumcision care and care of the uncircumcised penis
    position for sleep
    information about immunizations and newborn screening tests
    signs of newborn complications to report to the nurse or to the healthcare provider after discharge
    safe use of car seats
24. discussion with the new mother during which understanding is verbalized or by demonstration of critical skills such as feeding or cord care
25. the clinical pathway, discharge teaching form, or other appropriate document in the patient chart
26. continuity of care is enhanced, cost-effective use of resources is promoted, expected maternal and infant outcomes are ensured and occur in a timely manner, and family, healthcare provider and nurse satisfaction are improved
27. assessing individual learning needs, giving accurate information, encouraging independence in self- and newborn care, and promoting confidence in the mothering and parenting role

Chapter 19

1. False
2. True

3. True
4. False
5. False
6. True
7. True
8. False
9. a
10. a
11. 1) mother had uncomplicated pregnancy, birth, and postpartum course
    2) newborn has stable vital signs
    3) no evidence of newborn jaundice
    4) mother ready to care for self and newborn
12. 1) thorough physical assessment of mother and newborn
    2) psychosocial and learning needs assessment
    3) communication and coordination of care with healthcare team
    4) referrals as appropriate
13. Suggested answers:
    vital signs
    breasts and nipple condition
    incision—episiotomy or cesarean birth incision
    elimination patterns
    emotional assessment
    support system assessment
14. Suggested answers:
    vital signs
    color, including jaundice
    skin condition
    eating patterns
    elimination—wet diapers and stools: color and frequency
    circumcision, if appropriate
    activity

INDEX

Note: Page numbers follwed by *f* indicate figures; those followed by *t* indicate tables; those followed by *d* indicate displays.

Abdomen, of newborn, 504, 530–532, 532*f*, 533*t*, 534*f*
Abdominal circumference, 513, 514*f*, 530
Abdominal fetal guidance, with twins, 267, 267*d*
Abduction, of newborns, 506, 506*t*
ABNS (American Board of Nursing Specialties), 25
Abortion(s), spontaneous, 478–479. *See also* Perinatal death
  in multiple gestation, 260–261, 262d
ABR (auditory brainstem response), 522
Abruptio placentae, 193–195, 194*f*
  clinical manifestations of, 194–195
  diagnosis of, 195
  fetal and neonatal complications of, 497*t*
  incidence of, 191
  management of, 195
  with multiple gestation, 264
  in preeclampsia, 182*t*, 187
  recurrent, 194
  risk factors for, 194, 194*d*
  terminal bradycardia with, 393, 394*t*
  and uterine rupture, 356–357
Abscess, breast, 460
Absent variability, in fetal heart rate, 380*t*, 395, 395*t*, 400*t*
Abstinence syndrome, neonatal, 591–596
  assessment of, 592–593, 593*t*, 594, 595*f*
  incidence of, 591–592
  interventions for, 593–596, 594*d*
  pathophysiology of, 592, 592*d*
  symptoms of, 592–593, 593*t*
Abuse
  maternal trauma due to, 206
  in prenatal risk assessment, 136, 166
Acardia, 261
Accelerated starvation, 222
Accelerations, of fetal heart rate, 380*t*, 390–391, 390*f*
Accessory nerve, assessment of, 541*t*
Accountability
  mutual, 56, 59
  of nurses, 29–31
    vs. physicians, 57–58
Accreditation, of healthcare organizations, 11–13
ACE (angiotensin-converting enzyme) inhibitors, teratogenic effects of, 148*t*
Acid–base changes, postpartum, 451
Acidemia, fetal
  bradycardia and, 393, 393*t*
  fetal heart rate patterns with, 404–405, 404*t*
  tachycardia and, 392, 392*t*
Acidosis, 379
ACLS (advanced cardiac life support) care, 354*d*
Acoustic nerve, assessment of, 541*t*
Acquired immunodeficiency syndrome (AIDS). *See* Human immunodeficiency virus (HIV)
Active alert state, of newborn, 545
Active management of labor (AMOL), 345–346
Activity(ies)
  with cardiac disease, 296
  with multiple gestation, 266
  postpartum, 475
Activity restriction
  for preeclampsia, 185
  for preterm labor and birth, 214
Acute perinatal twin transfusion (AperiTTS), 263
Acyclovir, for varicella pneumonia, 252
Adaptation, 115–123
  assessment of, 115–116, 116*d*
  collaborative care and referral for, 116–117
  during labor and birth, 120–121, 121*d*
  in postpartum period, 121–123, 122*d*
  during pregnancy, 117–120, 117*d*, 118*d*, 120*d*
Administrative costs, 3
Admission assessment, 302–303, 306*d*, 367–368
Adoption, relinquishment for, 479
Adrenal glands, during pregnancy, 109
Advanced cardiac life support (ACLS) care, 354*d*
Advanced practice nurses (APNs), 23, 129
Adverse outcomes, 32–35, 35*d*, 36*d*, 37, 40–41
AFI (amniotic fluid index), 154
AFP (alpha-fetoprotein), 142, 146*t*
  with diabetes, 230*t*
  with multiple gestation, 257, 258
African Americans, 73–76, 75*f*
  comparative statistical data on, 74*t*
  core values of, 75
  cultural beliefs and practices of, 75–76
  pregnancy-induced hypertension in, 173, 174, 174*t*, 175
  preterm labor and delivery in, 74*t*, 209
Afterload, 237*d*
  with maternal cardiac disease, 242, 242*t*
AGA (appropriate for gestational age), 514
Age
  gestational
    appropriate for, 514
    assessment of, 513–514, 515*f*, 546–547
    large for, 514
    and sepsis, 589
    small for, 514
  maternal, 133
    and pregnancy-induced hypertension, 174–175, 175*t*
Agonist, 237*d*
AIDS. *See* Human immunodeficiency virus (HIV)
Alanine aminotransferase (ALT, SGPT), during pregnancy, 106, 106*t*
Alaskan natives, 74*t*, 75*f*, 76
Albumin, during pregnancy, 106, 106*t*
Alcohol use
  cultural differences in, 82
  fetal and neonatal complications due to, 495*t*
  history of, 162
  in prenatal risk assessment, 135–136, 161–163
  teratogenic effects of, 148*t*
Aldosterone
  in preeclampsia, 180*t*
  during pregnancy, 104
Alert states, of newborn, 545
Aleutians, 74*t*, 75*f*, 76
Alfentanil (Alfenta), for labor pain, 434
Alkaline phosphatase, during pregnancy, 106, 106*t*
Allergen immunotherapy, for asthma, 248
All-fours maneuver, 326
Alpha-fetoprotein (AFP), 142, 146*t*
  with diabetes, 230*t*
  with multiple gestation, 257, 258
ALT (alanine aminotransferase), during pregnancy, 106, 106*t*
Alternate breast massage, 564, 565*t*
Alveoli, maturation of, 496
Ambulation, during labor, 314, 316*f*, 425*t*
American Board of Nursing Specialties (ABNS), 25
American Indians, 74*t*, 75*f*, 76
  pregnancy-induced hypertension in, 174*t*
American Nurses' Credentialing Center (ANCC), 23, 24
Amino acid excretion, during pregnancy, 105, 105*t*
Aminopterin, teratogenic effects of, 148*t*
Amniocentesis, 142, 146*t*
  with diabetes, 230*t*
  with multiple gestation, 265
Amnioinfusion, 349–350
  for nonreassuring fetal heart rate, 392
Amnionitis, 497*t*
Amniotic fluid index (AFI), 154
Amniotic membranes. *See* Membranes
Amniotomy, 342
AMOL (active management of labor), 345–346
Ampicillin
  for group B streptococcal infection, 591
  for pneumonia, 252, 253*t*
ANA Code of Ethics, 29
Analgesia
  and breast-feeding, 557
  complications of, 497*t*
  epidural. *See* Epidural anesthesia and analgesia
  intrathecal, 438
  for labor pain, 432–433, 433*t*, 434*t*
  regional. *See* Regional anesthesia and analgesia
Anal sphincter damage, 452–453
ANCC (American Nurses' Credentialing Center), 23, 24
Androgens, teratogenic effects of, 148*t*
Anemia
  and fetal and neonatal complications, 495*t*
  with multiple gestation, 258
  physiologic, of pregnancy, 99
Anesthesia
  complications of, 497*t*
  epidural. *See* Epidural anesthesia and analgesia
  intrathecal, 438
  local, 434
  maternal deaths related to, 312
  with multiple gestation, 270
  postoperative recovery from, 453
    with cesarean section, 351–353, 352*d*, 353*f*, 354*d*, 355*d*, 375
  regional. *See* Regional analgesia and anesthesia
Anger, in acute grief work, 481*t*
Angiotensin
  in postpartum period, 448
  in preeclampsia, 180*t*
  during pregnancy, 104
Angiotensin-converting enzyme (ACE) inhibitors, teratogenic effects of, 148*t*
Angiotensinogen, during pregnancy, 104
Ankyloglossia, 524
Antagonist, 237*d*

Antenatal care. *See* Prenatal care
Antepartum risk assessment. *See* Prenatal risk assessment
Antiarrhythmic medications, for maternal cardiac disease, 242
Antibiotic prophylaxis, for bacterial endocarditis, 243
Antibiotic therapy, for pneumonia, 252–253, 253*t*
Anticipatory grief, 479, 480
Anticipatory stage, in transition to parenthood, 468
Antidiuretic hormone, 109
Antidumping law, 42–44
Antihistamines, for asthma, 248
Antihypertensive therapy, for preeclampsia, 185, 189
Antiinflammatory therapy, for asthma, 248
Antimicrobial therapy, for pneumonia, 252–253
Anus, of newborn, 530
Anxiety, during labor and birth, 328
Anxiety disorders
  history of, 116–117
  with multiple gestation, 257
  postpartum, 123
AperiTTS (acute perinatal twin transfusion), 263
Apgar score, 503
Apnea, in newborn, 527, 528*t*
APNs (advanced practice nurses), 23, 129
Appropriate for gestational age (AGA), 514
Apresoline (hydralazine hydrochloride), for preeclampsia, 189
Areola
  engorgement of, 566
  during pregnancy, 111, 551
Arm(s), of newborn, 535
Arm recoil, 546
Arterial blood gases, in asthma, 246
Arteries, 238
Arteriovenous anastomoses, in multiple gestations, 255, 262
Artery-to-artery anastomoses, in multiple gestations, 262
Ascites, 533*t*
ASD (atrial septal defect), 580*t*, 581
Asian Americans, 75*f*, 76–78
  comparative statistical data on, 74*t*
  core values of, 77
  cultural beliefs and practices of, 77–78
  dermal practices of, 82
  pregnancy-induced hypertension in, 173–174, 174*t*
Aspartate aminotransferase (AST, SGOT), during pregnancy, 106, 106*t*
Asphyxia, 379
Aspiration pneumonia, 251, 253
Assessment
  admission, 302–303, 306*d*, 367–368
  cultural, 84*d*, 137–138
  vs. data collection, 30
  fetal. *See* Fetal assessment
  of newborn. *See* Newborn(s), assessment of
  prenatal risk. *See* Prenatal risk assessment
AST (aspartate aminotransferase), during pregnancy, 106, 106*t*
Asthma, 244–249
  acute exacerbations of, 249
  antepartum care for, 249
  bottle-feeding and, 551*t*
  clinical manifestations of, 245, 246, 246*d*
  defined, 244
  environmental control for, 247
  inpatient management of, 249
  labor and birth with, 249
  laboratory findings in, 246
  nursing assessment of, 245–246, 245*d*, 246*d*
  nursing interventions for, 246–247
  ongoing maternal and fetal assessment with, 247
  pathophysiology of, 244–245
  patient education on, 246–247
  pharmacologic therapy for, 242–249
  potentially fatal, 245–246, 245*d*
  significance and incidence of, 244
  triggers for, 244, 245*t*, 247
Atrial septal defect (ASD), 580*t*, 581
Atrioventricular heart block, bradycardia due to, 394
Attachment, family–newborn, 329, 508
  with cesarean birth, 353–354, 355*f*, 356*f*
Attention focusing, for labor pain, 431
Attitudes, cultural differences in, 72*d*
Audit, of medical records, 27, 28*d*
Auditory brainstem response (ABR), 522
Auditory techniques, for labor pain, 424*t*, 431–432
Augmentation of labor, 345
  contraindications for, 332*d*
  criteria for, 332*d*
  defined, 329–330
  incidence of, 330
  indications for, 332*d*
  staffing during, 346
Auscultation, intermittent, of fetal heart rate, 304–308, 379, 383, 384*d*, 385*d*
Autonomic nervous system, 238, 239*d*
  in fetal heart rate, 387, 388*d*
Autonomic neuropathy, with diabetes, 221
Autotransfusion, postpartum, 450
Awake states, of newborn, 544–545

"Baby blues," 122, 468
Baccalaureate degree, 26, 57
Back, of newborn, 539, 539*f*, 539*t*
Bacterial endocarditis, antibiotic prophylaxis for, 243
Bacterial pneumonia, 251
Bacteriuria, postpartum, 460–461
Balanced Budget Act, 4
Ballard Maturational Score (BMS), 514, 515*f*, 546–547
Balloon catheters, for cervical ripening, 335–336
Barbiturates, for labor pain, 432
Barlow maneuver, 537, 537*f*
Baroreceptors, in fetal heart rate, 388, 388*d*
Barrier methods, 466–467
Baseline fetal heart rate, 380*t*, 390
  alterations in, 392–394, 392*t*, 393*t*, 394*f*
Bathtub, laboring in, 427–428, 429*t*
B cells, during pregnancy, 111, 111*t*
Bearing down, 314–322, 319*f*, 320*d*–321*d*
Becker muscular dystrophy, carrier frequency for, 145*d*
Becoming parents course, 616*d*–617*d*
Bed rest
  effects of, 464
  during labor, 425
  postpartum recovery after, 464
  for preeclampsia, 185
  for preterm labor and birth, 214
Behavioral characteristics, with substance abuse, 162
Behavior factors, in prenatal risk assessment, 132*d*, 133–137, 137*d*
Belief system, cultural differences in, 72*d*
Benchmarking, 11
Bereavement
  nursing assessment of, 485
  nursing interventions for, 486–487, 487*t*–489*t*
  nursing management of, 481*t*, 485–490
  ontologic perspective of, 485
  sociologic perspective on, 483–484
  spiritual perspective of, 484–485
  stages of, 476, 477*d*
  support groups for, 485, 486*d*, 490
Best Practice Network, 11
Beta-adrenergic agents, for preterm labor and birth, 216*d*, 217*d*, 218
Betamethasone, for preterm labor and birth, 219
Beta-mimetics
  for preterm labor and birth, 216*d*, 217*d*, 218
  tocolytic therapy with, 373
β_2 agonists, for asthma, 247–248
Bigeminy, fetal, 401
Bilirubin. *See also* Jaundice
  metabolism of, 584
Bilirubin encephalopathy, 585
Biliverdin, 584
Biochemical evaluation, prenatal, 139*d*, 140–141, 141*t*, 142
Biochemical markers, for preterm labor and delivery, 144–147, 209–210
Biochemical tests, for multiple gestation, 256–257
Biophysical profile (BPP), 154
  with multiple gestation, 266
Birth
  adaptations during, 120–121, 121*d*
  breech. *See* Breech birth
  care paths for, 636–637
  cesarean. *See* Cesarean birth
  complications of, 497*t*
  documentation of, 304, 370–375
  emotional support during, 328–329
  episiotomy during, 326–328
  facilitation of, 301–302
  forceps-assisted, 346, 347–348, 347*t*
    complications of, 347–348, 497*t*
  fundal pressure during, 322–323, 322*f*
  with multiple gestation
    environment for, 266–268, 267*d*
    method of, 268–270, 268*f*, 269*d*, 270*d*
  operative vaginal, 346–349, 347*t*
  perineum care during, 326–328, 328*d*
  positions for, 313–314, 316*f*–318*f*, 320*d*
  precipitous, 497*t*
  pushing during, 314–322, 319*f*, 320*d*–321*d*
  with shoulder dystocia, 323–326, 323*f*, 324*f*, 327*d*
  vacuum devices during, 348–349
Birth ball, 314, 316*f*
Birth canal, lacerations of, 199
Birthing ball, 314, 316*f*
Birthing room
  procedures performed on newborn in, 506–508, 506*t*, 507*d*
  resuscitation in, 502, 502*d*, 503*f*
Birth outcome, prenatal care and, 129–130
Birth plan, 618–620, 619*d*–620*d*
Birth rate, 125
Birth weight, 513
  low. *See* Low-birth-weight (LBW) infants
Bishop pelvic scoring system, 333–334, 334*t*
Bittersweet grief, 483
Blacks. *See* African Americans
Bladder
  in postpartum period, 449
  during pregnancy, 103
Bladder exstrophy, 533*t*
Bleeding
  intracranial, with vacuum extraction, 348
  with multiple gestation, 264
  postpartum. *See* Postpartum hemorrhage
  during pregnancy, 190–206
    due to abnormal placental implantation, 195–196, 196*f*
    due to abruptio placentae, 193–195, 194*d*, 194*f*
    hemorrhagic and hypovolemic shock due to, 205–206, 205*d*
    home care management of, 203, 293–294
    inpatient management of, 203–206
    nursing assessment of, 200–203, 202*d*, 203*t*
    nursing interventions for, 203–206
    due to placenta previa, 192–193, 192*d*, 193*f*
    significance and incidence of, 190–191
    due to trauma, 206
    due to uterine rupture, 197–198, 197*d*
    due to vasa previa, 196–197, 197*d*
Bleeding time, in preeclampsia, 180*t*
Blink reflex, 520
Blood chemistry, for hypertension during pregnancy, 188*d*
Blood flow
  distribution of, during pregnancy, 100
  through heart, 237–238, 238*f*
Blood gases
  arterial, in asthma, 246
  umbilical cord, 408–409, 409*t*

Blood pressure (BP)
with antepartum bleeding, 201–202
and fetal heart rate, 388*d,* 389*d*
during labor, 308–309
with multiple gestation, 259*t*
of newborn, 529–530, 530*f,* 531*t*
postpartum, 448–449, 453–454, 457
in preeclampsia, 180*t,* 184*d,* 186–187
during pregnancy, 100, 140
Blood sugar levels. *See* Glucose, plasma
Blood transfusion
for antepartum bleeding, 202, 203*t,* 204
for hypovolemic shock, 205, 205*d*
Blood urea nitrogen (BUN)
in postpartum period, 449
in preeclampsia, 180*t*
during pregnancy, 104*t*
Blood volume
in preeclampsia, 179, 180*t*
during pregnancy, 98–99, 98*t*
"Blueberry muffin" spots, in newborn, 518*t*
BMS (Ballard Maturational Score), 514, 515*f,* 546–547
Body changes, during second trimester, 118–119
Bonding, of multiples, 273
Bottle feeding, 551*d,* 568–571, 570*d,* 650
Bowel movements, of newborn, 559, 559*t*
Bowel sounds, of newborn, 530–531, 532
BP. *See* Blood pressure (BP)
BPP (biophysical profile), 154
with multiple gestation, 266
Brachial cleft cyst, 527*t*
Brachial plexus palsy, 539*t*
Brachial sinus, 527*t*
Bradycardia
fetal, 380*t,* 393–394, 393*t,* 394*f,* 403
in newborn, 531*t*
terminal, 393, 394*t*
Braxton-Hicks contractions, 212
Breach of duty, 31–32
Breast(s)
engorgement of, 566–567
of newborn, 526, 528*f,* 546
in postpartum period, 474
during pregnancy, 111, 551–552
Breast abscess, 460
Breast-feeding, 550–568, 571–572
advantages of, 550, 551*t*
analgesics and, 557
after cesarean birth, 555, 556*f*
choice of, 550
contraindications to, 551
cultural differences in, 74*t*
with diabetes, 233, 234, 552
engorgement with, 566–567
frequency and duration of, 558, 558*d*
home care assessment, 650
hospital discharge packs and, 561
hunger cues for, 557–558, 557*d*
hypoglycemia and, 565–566
incidence of, 550–551
initiation of, 557
insufficient milk with, 567–568
jaundice and, 564–565
latch-on in, 556, 556*d*
management of, 557–561
mastitis with, 460, 567, 567*d*
maternal-newborn contact and, 508, 557–558, 557*d,* 562*t*
medications and, 568, 568*d*
milk transfer during, 556–557, 557*d*
of multiples, 273, 273*f,* 554, 555
nipple pain with, 561–564, 564*d,* 565*t*–566*t*
nursing assessment of, 558–560, 559*t,* 560*t*
obstacles to, 552*d*
physiology of milk production in, 551–553
plugged duct with, 567
positioning for, 554–555, 555*f,* 556*f*
with reluctant nurser, 562*t*
with sore nipples, 565*t*–566*t*
potential problems in, 561–568
prenatal education for, 157, 554, 617*d*
preparation for, 554
process of, 554–557
of reluctant nurser, 561, 561*d,* 562*t*–563*t*
role of nurse in promotion of, 571–572, 571*d,* 572*d*
satiation cues for, 558, 558*d*
signs of adequate intake with, 559, 559*t,* 560*t*
supplemental feedings with, 560
supporting breast during, 554, 555–556, 555*f*
use of pacifiers and artificial nipples with, 560
Breast massage, alternate, 564, 565*t*
Breast milk
biospecificity of, 553–554
insufficient, 567–568
Breast-milk jaundice, 564–565
Breathing
by newborn, 494–497, 504, 526–528, 528*t*
patterned, for labor pain, 431
Breech birth
breast-feeding after, 562*t*
complications of, 497*t*
forceps-assisted, 347
positional deformities in newborn due to, 535, 535*f*
with twins, 269, 270*d*
Brethine. *See* Terbutaline (Brethine)
Bronchodilators, for asthma, 247–248
Brow presentation, complications of, 497*t*
Bruising, in newborn, 516
Brushfield spots, 521*t*
Bulk flow, 237
BUN. *See* Blood urea nitrogen (BUN)
Bupivacaine, epidural anesthesia with, 434
Butorphanol (Stadol), for labor pain, 433, 434*t*

Café au lait spots, in newborn, 518*t*
Calcaneovalgus foot, 538, 539*f*
Calcium channel blockers, for preterm labor and birth, 216*d,* 217*d,* 218
Calcium intake, during pregnancy, 110
Caloric intake, during pregnancy, 107
Cambodians, 78
Candida albicans, sore nipples due to, 563–564
Capillaries, 238
Captopril, teratogenic effects of, 148*t*
Caput succedaneum, 518, 519*f*
Carbamazepine, teratogenic effects of, 148*t*
Carbohydrate
in breast milk, 554
in formula, 569
Carbon dioxide levels, during pregnancy, 102
Carbon dioxide transfer, maternal-fetal, 385–387, 386*f,* 387*d*
Cardiac disease
congenital, 579–582, 580*t*
carrier frequency for, 145*d*
labor and birth with, 243
during pregnancy, 235–255
activity with, 296
clinical management of, 242–243, 242*t,* 243*t*
diet for, 296
fetal and neonatal complications with, 495*t*
heparin therapy for, 295, 296
home care management of, 295–296
nursing assessment of, 240–242, 241*d*
physiology and terminology related to, 237–238, 237*d,* 238*f,* 239*d*
risk factor assessment and counseling for, 239–240, 240*d,* 241*t*
significance and incidence of, 235–237, 236*t,* 237*d*
signs and symptoms of, 241*d*
Cardiac output
defined, 237*d*
with epidural anesthesia, 99
during labor and birth, 99, 100*t*
with maternal cardiac disease, 242, 242*t*
peripartum, 243, 243*t*
postpartum, 450
in preeclampsia, 179, 180*t,* 181*t*
during pregnancy, 98*t,* 99
Cardiomyopathy, 235
Cardiovascular disease. *See* Cardiac disease
Cardiovascular system
anatomy of, 237–238, 238*f*
bulk flow in, 237
function of, 237
homeostasis of, 238
innervation of, 238, 239*d*
of newborn, 497–499, 498*f,* 504, 528–530
in postpartum period, 450, 475
during pregnancy, 98–101, 98*t,* 100*t,* 101*t*
vessels in, 238
Care
quality of. *See* Quality of care
standards of, 7–8, 8*d,* 31–32, 35–37
Care paths, 626–627, 633–642
Care plan, for home care services, 648–649
Carpal tunnel syndrome, postpartum, 450
Carrier frequencies, 145*d*
Carrier screening, 146*t*
Case management, 623–625, 624*d*–625*d*
prenatal, 154–157
Caucasians, 75*f,* 80
comparative statistical data on, 74*t*
pregnancy-induced hypertension in, 174*t*
Causation, 31, 32
Cavernous hemangiomas, 516, 516*f*
Cellular immunity, during pregnancy, 111*t*
Central nervous system (CNS), with maternal cardiac disease, 241
Central nervous system (CNS) depressants, neonatal withdrawal from, 592*d*
Central nervous system (CNS) disorders, and fetal and neonatal complications, 495*t*
Cephalohematoma, 519*f,* 519*t*
breast-feeding with, 562*t*
with vacuum extraction, 348
Cephalopelvic disproportion, 345
Cephalosporin, for pneumonia, 252, 253*t*
Cerebral disturbances, in preeclampsia, 184*d*
Cerebral palsy, fetal heart rate monitoring and, 411, 412*d*
Ceremonial and ritual system, cultural differences in, 72*d*
Certification
of healthcare organizations, 11–13
of nurses, 23–25, 24*d,* 25*d*
Certified nurse midwives (CNMs), 129
Cervical dilation, 298, 301, 302*f,* 304*t*–305*t*
Cervical incompetence, fetal and neonatal complications with, 495*t*
Cervical length assessment, for preterm labor and birth, 210
Cervical ripening, 334–341
criteria for, 331*d*
defined, 329
indications for, 331*d*
informed consent for, 332–333, 377
mechanical methods of, 334–336
nurse's role in, 333
pharmacologic methods of, 97, 336–341, 338*d*–339*d*
protocols and policies for, 333, 333*d*
risk-benefit analysis of, 332–333
staffing during, 346
Cervical status, assessment of, 333–334, 334*t*
Cervidil, for cervical ripening, 336, 337–340, 338*d*
Cervix
during multiple gestation, 260*t*
postpartum, 447
during pregnancy, 110
Cesarean birth, 350–358
attachment to newborn with, 353–354, 355*f,* 356*f*
for bradycardia, 394
breast-feeding after, 555, 556*f*
complications of, 350
incidence of, 350
indications for, 350
induction of labor and, 350
intraoperative care for, 351*d*–352*d*
joint educational programs on, 64–65
with multiple gestation, 269–270, 270*d*
postanesthesia recovery care for, 351–353, 352*d,* 353*f,* 354*d,* 355*d*
postpartum care after, 463–464, 474
preoperative care for, 351*d*

Cesarean birth, (*continued*)
for shoulder dystocia, 326
standards and guidelines for, 351–353
for uterine rupture, 393
vaginal birth after, 354–358
benefits of, 356
candidates for, 356
contraindications to, 356
costs of, 357
incidence of, 350
with multiple gestation, 270
nursing care for, 357
predicting success of, 357
risks of, 357
uterine rupture with, 355–358
Chadwick's sign, 110
Chain of command, 45, 46*f*
Charting by exception, 39
CHD (congenital heart disease), 579–582, 580*t*
carrier frequency for, 145*d*
Chemical dependency, in prenatal risk assessment, 135–136, 161–163
Chemoreceptors, in fetal heart rate, 387–388, 388*d*
Chest, of newborn, 525–528, 527*t*, 528*f*, 528*t*
Chest circumference, 513, 514*f*, 525
CHF (congestive heart failure)
maternal, 495*t*
neonatal, 579
Childbirth. *See* Birth
Childbirth education, 157, 612–613, 614*d*–617*d*
Childbirth preparation
class curriculum for, 614*d*
and labor pain, 422–423, 423*f*
Chinese Americans, pregnancy-induced hypertension in, 174*t*
Chlamydia pneumoniae, 251, 253*t*
Chloasma, 109
Chloroprocaine (Nesacaine), epidural anesthesia with, 434
Cholera, prenatal immunization for, 169
Cholesterol, serum, during pregnancy, 106
Chorioamnionic membranes. *See* Membranes
Chorionic villus sampling (CVS), 143, 146
with multiple gestation, 265
Chronotrope, 237*d*
Church of Jesus Christ of Latter-Day Saints, 81, 81*t*
Cigarette smoking
and fetal and neonatal complications, 495*t*
history of, 162
and preeclampsia, 176
in prenatal risk assessment, 135
and preterm labor and birth, 209, 213–214
Circulation
fetal, 497–498, 498*f*
neonatal, 498–499
Circumcision
female, 80–81, 94
male, 81, 533–534
Circumoral cyanosis, 515, 526*t*
Classes, prenatal, 157, 612–613, 614*d*–617*d*
Clavicle, fractured, 504, 535
breast-feeding with, 562*t*
Cleft lip/palate, 524, 525*f*, 526*t*
carrier frequency for, 145*d*
Clinical indicator, 37
Clinical nurse specialists (CNSs), 129
Clinical practice bulletins, 31–32
Clinical protocols, 37–38
Clitoris, 532, 533
Closed-glottis pushing, 314–315, 403, 404*f*
Clotting factors
in preeclampsia, 180*t*, 181*t*
during pregnancy, 101, 101*t*
Clubfoot, 538, 538*f*, 539*f*
Clutch hold, 555, 556*f*
CNMs (certified nurse midwives), 129
CNS. *See* Central nervous system (CNS)
CNSs (clinical nurse specialists), 129
Coaches, fathers as, 421
Coagulation factors
in preeclampsia, 180*t*, 181*t*
during pregnancy, 101, 101*t*
Coagulation profile, for hypertension during pregnancy, 188*d*
Co-bedding, of premature multiples, 272
Cocaine, teratogenic effects of, 149*t*
Cocaine withdrawal, 593
Code of Ethics, 29
Cognitive development, bottle feeding and, 551*t*, 553
Cognitive techniques, for labor pain, 424*t*, 430–431
Cold, for labor pain, 427–428, 427*t*, 429*t*
Cold stress, in newborn, 500, 501*f*, 501*t*
Colloid(s), in preeclampsia, 184–185
Colloid oncotic pressure, during pregnancy, 98*t*
Colloid osmotic pressure, in preeclampsia, 181*t*
Coloboma, 521*t*
Colostrum, 111, 551, 553
Combined spinal epidural (CSE), 436–437
Comfort measures, during labor, 419*d*
"Common cause" variation, 51–52
Communication
cultural assessment of, 138
culturally competent, 83, 84–86, 85*d*
within multicultural health care team, 89*d*
nonverbal, 86
in teamwork, 55–56, 60*d*, 61–62
Compensation, of nurses *vs.* physicians, 56
Competence, on team, 61
Competence validation, 26–27, 28*d*
Complete blood count, for hypertension during pregnancy, 188*d*
Condoms, 466–467
Conductive heat loss, 500, 501*t*
Conferences, 28
Confidentiality, of patient records, 15
Conflict resolution, 44–45, 46*f*
Congenital dislocation of the hip, 535–538, 536*d*, 536*f*, 537*f*, 539, 539*f*
Congenital heart disease (CHD), 579–582, 580*t*
carrier frequency for, 145*d*
Congestive heart failure (CHF)
maternal, 495*t*
neonatal, 579
Conjoined twins, 262
Consensus, 58–59, 60*d*, 62–63
Consent, informed, 16*d*
for induction of labor, 332–333, 377
Constipation
with formula feeding, 570–571
postpartum, 452
during pregnancy, 106
Continuing education, 27–29
Continuous subcutaneous insulin infusion (CSII), 229
Contraception, postpartum, 466–467
Contraction(s)
coupling of, 381, 382*f*
duration of, 304*t*–305*t*, 310, 380
frequency of, 310, 380, 381
in hyperstimulation, 381, 382*f*
intensity of, 304*t*–305*t*, 310, 380
normal, 381, 382*f*
physiology of, 298–300
tripling of, 381
Contraction stress test (CST), 153–154
with multiple gestation, 265
Convection heat loss, 500, 501*t*
Coping mechanisms, with substance abuse, 162
Copper T380, 467
Cord compression, decelerations due to, 399*t*, 403
Cordocentesis, 144
Core performance measures, 12
Corkscrew maneuver, 325
Coronary artery disease, 235
Corticosteroids, for asthma, 248
Corticotropin-releasing hormone, during pregnancy, 109
Cortisol
in onset of labor, 299*d*
during pregnancy, 109
Cost(s), healthcare, 2–4
Cost containment, *vs.* cost consciousness, 4–5
Coumarin derivatives, teratogenic effects of, 148*t*
Counseling, prenatal, 155–157, 156*d*
Counterpressure, for low-back pain, 427, 427*f*
Couplet care, 453
Coupling, of contractions, 381, 382*f*
Cow's milk formula, 569
Crackles, 527
Cradle hold, 555, 555*f*
Cranial nerves, assessment of, 540, 541*t*
Craniosynostosis, 518
Craniotabes, 518
Crash symptoms, 162
Creatinine, serum, in preeclampsia, 180*t*, 184*d*
Creatinine clearance
in preeclampsia, 180*t*
during pregnancy, 104*t*
Creation, loss of, 477
Cromolyn, for asthma, 248
Crossed extension reflex, 549
Cruising phase, of labor, 421–422, 422*d*
Crying, in newborn, 496, 540, 545
and breast-feeding, 557–558, 563*t*
Cryoprecipitate, for antepartum bleeding, 202, 203*t*
Cryptorchidism, 534
CSE (combined spinal epidural), 436–437
CSII (continuous subcutaneous insulin infusion), 229
CST (contraction stress test), 153–154
with multiple gestation, 265
Cubans, pregnancy-induced hypertension in, 174*t*
Cultural assessment, 84*d*, 137–138
Cultural competence
characteristics of, 82–83, 83*d*
institutional factors in, 88, 88*d*
process of, 70, 71*f*
strategies fostering, 89*d*
Cultural difference. *See also* Racial differences
Cultural differences
in childbearing and meaning of birth, 72–73
examples of, 68
in experiences of pain, 73
in gender roles, 72–73, 72*d*
in genetic disorders, 145*d*
importance of, 68–69
nursing education on, 88
in practices associated with childbearing, 73
in prenatal care, 74*t*, 127
Cultural frameworks, 69–71, 69*f*–71*f*, 72*d*
Cultural groups, 73–82
African Americans (blacks), 73–76, 74*t*, 75*f*
American Indians and Alaskan Natives, 74*t*, 75*f*, 76
Asian Americans and Pacific Islanders, 74*t*, 75*f*, 76–78
biologic and physiologic variations between, 81–82
comparative statistics for, 73, 74*t*, 75*f*
deeply religious women, 81, 81*t*
Hispanics and Latinos, 74*t*, 75*f*, 78–80
immigrants and refugees, 80
nontraditional, 80–82
ritually circumcised women, 80–81
whites (Caucasians), 74*t*, 75*f*, 80
Cultural imposition, 82
Cultural practices, 72*d*, 86–88, 87*t*
Culture
defined, 68
domains of, 70
influence on pregnancy, childbirth, and parenting of, 72*d*
integration into nursing care of
barriers to, 82–83
long-term strategies for, 88–89, 88*d*, 89*d*
techniques for, 84–88, 84*d*–86*d*, 87*t*
Culture care resources, 94
Culture care theory, 69, 69*f*
"Cupping," 82
Curanderismo, 79
Cutaneous techniques, for labor pain, 424*t*, 425–430
Cutis marmorata, in newborn, 516
CVS (chorionic villus sampling), 143, 146
with multiple gestation, 265

Cyanosis
circumoral, 515, 526*t*
in newborn, 514–515, 518*t*, 531*t*, 579
Cyst
brachial cleft, 527*t*
thyroglossal duct, 527*t*
Cystic fibrosis
carrier frequency for, 145*d*
carrier screening for, 146*t*
Cystic hygroma, 525, 527*f*
Cystitis, postpartum, 461
Cystocele, 452
Cytomegalovirus, teratogenic effects of, 150*t*
Cytotec (misoprostol)
for cervical ripening, 338*d*–339*d*, 340–341
for induction of labor, 345

Damages, 31, 32
Danazol, teratogenic effects of, 148*t*
Dancing, during labor, 425*t*
Dangling position, during labor, 426*t*
Database, prenatal patient, 612
Data collection, *vs.* assessment, 30
DBP (diastolic blood pressure), during pregnancy, 100
DDH (developmental dysplasia of the hip), 535–538, 536*d*, 536*f*, 537*f*, 539, 539*f*
Death, perinatal. *See* Perinatal death
Decelerations
early, 380*t*, 396, 397*f*, 399*t*
late, 380*t*, 396, 397*f*, 398*f*, 399*t*
prolonged, 380*t*, 397*f*, 398–399, 399*t*
variable, 380*t*, 396–398, 397*f*, 399*t*, 402–403
Decision-making, cultural difference in, 85
Decongestants, for asthma, 249
Deep sleep state, of newborn, 544
Deep tendon reflexes (DTRs), in preeclampsia, 187
Delayed pushing, 321–322
"Delegate up," 57
Delegation, to unlicensed assistive personnel, 30–31
Delivery. *See* Birth
Demerol (meperidine), for labor pain, 433, 434*t*
Demographic factors, in prenatal risk assessment, 132*d*, 133
Denial, in bereavement, 477*d*
Depo-Provera, 466
Depression
with multiple gestation, 257
postpartum, 123, 468
predisposing factors for, 137*d*
Developmental dysplasia of the hip (DDH), 535–538, 536*d*, 536*f*, 537*f*, 539, 539*f*
Developmental reflexes, 540, 548–549
Deviance, normalization of, 34–35
Dexamethasone, for preterm labor and birth, 219
Diabetes mellitus
bottle-feeding and, 551*t*
breast-feeding with, 233, 234, 552
cultural differences in, 82
gestational
ambulatory and home care management of, 225–230, 294–295
classification of, 221
clinical manifestations of, 224–225
defined, 107, 221
development of overt diabetes after, 234–235, 234*d*
diabetic ketoacidosis due to, 221, 222, 224–225, 231, 232*t*
diagnosis of, 224, 224*t*
exercise therapy for, 226, 227*d*
fetal assessment for, 230, 230*t*
incidence of, 107
inpatient management of, 231
insulin therapy for, 229
intrapartum management of, 231–233, 233*d*
metabolic monitoring for, 227–228, 227*d*
with multiple gestation, 258
nursing assessments and interventions for, 225
nutrition therapy for, 226
pathophysiology of, 222–223
patient education for, 225–226, 226*d*
pharmacologic therapy for, 229
postpartum management of, 234–235, 448
screening for, 107–108, 141, 223–224, 223*d*
significance and incidence of, 219–221
perinatal morbidity with, 220–221
pregestational, 219–235
ambulatory and home care management of, 225–230, 294–295
clinical manifestations of, 224–225
diabetic ketoacidosis due to, 222, 224–225, 231, 232*t*
elective delivery with, 230*t*, 233
exercise therapy for, 226, 227*d*
fetal and neonatal complications with, 495*t*
fetal assessment for, 230, 230*t*
inpatient management of, 231
insulin therapy for, 108, 228–229, 228*d*, 229*d*
intrapartum management of, 231–233, 233*d*
metabolic monitoring for, 227–228, 227*d*
nursing assessments and interventions for, 225
nutrition therapy for, 226
pathophysiology of, 222–223
patient education for, 225, 225*d*
pharmacologic therapy for, 228–229, 228*d*, 229*d*
postpartum management of, 233–234, 448
sick day management for, 228–229, 229*d*, 295
significance and incidence of, 219–221
type 1, 221
type 2, 221–222
shoulder dystocia with, 324
Diabetic ketoacidosis (DKA), during pregnancy, 108, 221, 222, 224–225, 231, 232*t*
Diabetogenic state, of pregnancy, 107, 222
Diagnosis, nursing, 30
Diamniotic twins, 254*t*, 255
Diaphragm, contraceptive, 467
Diarrhea, bottle-feeding and, 551*t*
Diastasis, of rectus muscles, 451
Diastolic blood pressure (DBP), during pregnancy, 100
DIC (disseminated intravascular coagulation), risk factors for, 204, 204*d*
Dichorionic twins, 254*t*, 255
Diet. *See also* Nutrition
for cardiac disease, 296
cultural assessment of, 138
for diabetes, 226
of newborn. *See* Breast-feeding; Formula feeding
postpartum, 453, 475
and preeclampsia, 176
in prenatal risk assessment, 134–135, 134*d*, 135*d*
and preterm labor and birth, 214, 294
religious prohibitions on, 81*t*
Diethylstilbestrol, teratogenic effects of, 149*t*
Dilantin (phenytoin)
for preeclampsia, 188–189
teratogenic effects of, 149*t*
Dilapan, 335
Dilated cardiomyopathy, 235
Diluted tincture of opium (DTO), for neonatal abstinence syndrome, 594
Dinoprostone
for cervical ripening, 336–340, 338*d*
for postpartum hemorrhage, 200*t*
Diphtheria, prenatal immunization for, 170
Disagreements, in teamwork, 60*d*
Discharge
early, 3–4, 10, 14, 610–611
criteria for, 646–647, 647*d*
guidelines for, 645
and home care services, 643–644
follow-up after, 611, 627–630, 628*d*–629*d*
Discharge planning, 610–642
current issues in, 611–612
evaluation of, 630
referral for home care services in, 647–648, 648*d*, 657
role of staff nurse in, 625–626
Discharge record, 622*d*
Disintegration, in bereavement, 477*d*
Dislocation, of hip, congenital, 535–538, 536*d*, 536*f*, 537*f*, 539, 539*f*
Disseminated intravascular coagulation (DIC), risk factors for, 204, 204*d*
Distraction, for labor pain, 431
Diuresis, postpartum, 449
Diuretics, in preeclampsia, 184–185
Dizygotic (DZ) twins, 254, 254*t*, 255*d*, 256
DKA (diabetic ketoacidosis), during pregnancy, 108, 221, 222, 224–225, 231, 232*t*
Documentation
of labor and birth, 304, 370–375
legal aspects of, 32, 38–40
of shoulder dystocia, 326, 327*d*
Dolls' eyes maneuver, 541*t*
Domestic violence
maternal trauma due to, 206
in prenatal risk assessment, 136, 166
Doppler ultrasonography
of fetal heart rate, 381, 383, 383*f*, 384*d*
of multiple gestation, 265
Double-marker screening, 142, 146*t*
Doulas, 422
Downsizing, 9–10
Down syndrome
biochemical screening for, 142, 146*t*
eyes in, 521*t*
fingers in, 539*t*
neck in, 527*t*
Dream(s)
loss of, 477
during second trimester, 119
during third trimester, 120
Dromotrope, 237*d*
Drooling, 526*t*
Drowsy state, of newborn, 544
Drug abuse
fetal and neonatal complications with, 495*t*
history of, 163
in prenatal risk assessment, 135–136, 161–163
Drug-induced sinusoidal fetal heart rate pattern, 400
Drug withdrawal, neonatal. *See* Abstinence syndrome, neonatal
DTO (diluted tincture of opium), for neonatal abstinence syndrome, 594
DTRs (deep tendon reflexes), in preeclampsia, 187
Dubowitz Scoring System, 514
Duchenne muscular dystrophy, carrier frequency for, 145*d*
Ductus arteriosus, 499
patent, 580*t*, 581
Ductus venosus, 498
"Dumping," 42–44
Duty, 31
breach of, 31–32
Dyspnea, during pregnancy, 102
Dysrhythmias, fetal, 401–402, 402*f*
Dystocia, 345
DZ (dizygotic) twins, 254, 254*t*, 255*d*, 256

Ear(s), of newborn, 504, 521–523, 523*t*
appearance and structure of, 521, 522*f*, 523*t*
and gestational age, 546–547
and hearing, 521–523, 522*d*, 523*d*, 523*t*
position of, 521, 521*f*, 523*t*
Ear canal, 521
Early decelerations, 380*t*, 396, 397*f*, 399*t*
Early discharge, 3–4, 10, 14, 610–611
criteria for, 646–647, 647*d*
guidelines for, 645
and home care services, 643–644
Ecchymosis, in newborn, 516

ECG (electrocardiogram)
for antepartum bleeding, 203
with maternal cardiac disease, 240–241
Eclampsia, 178, 189–190
postpartum, 450
Economics, of healthcare, 2–4
Ectopic pregnancy, 479–480
Edema
in newborn, *518t*
under scalp, 518, *519f*
in pregnancy-induced hypertension, 180–183, 187
Education. *See also* Patient education
childbirth, 157, 612–613, *614d–617d*
continuing, 27–29
culturally appropriate material for, 86, *86d*
joint programs for physicians and nurses, 63–65
maternal, 133
of nurses *vs.* physicians, 56–57
for perinatal home care, 652–653
prenatal, 155–157, *156d*
on breast-feeding, 554
preparatory, 25–26
Effleurage, for labor pain, 429, *430f*
EFM. *See* Electronic fetal monitoring (EFM)
Elective delivery, with diabetes, *230t*, 233
Electrocardiogram (ECG)
for antepartum bleeding, 203
with maternal cardiac disease, 240–241
Electrolyte(s)
for diabetic ketoacidosis, 231, *232t*
postpartum, 449
during pregnancy, 103–104
Electronic fetal monitoring (EFM), 378–405
audit of, *28d*
and cerebral palsy, 411, *412d*
during contraction stress test, 153–154
decision tree for, *413f*
for diabetic ketoacidosis, 231, *232t*
vs. Doppler ultrasound, 381, 383, *383f*, *384d*
efficacy of, 411
via fetal scalp electrode, 381–383
historical perspectives on, 378–379
vs. intermittent auscultation, 383, *384d*, *385d*
joint educations programs on, 63–64
during labor, 303, *306d–307d*, 310, 411–412, *412d*
with multiple gestation, *259t*
nomenclature for, 64
during nonstress test, 153
during oxytocin induction or augmentation, *307d*
patient education about, 409
physiologic basis for, 383–388
sources of artifact or error in, 382, *384t*
specificity, sensitivity, and reliability of, 411–412
strip review of, 63–64
techniques of, 380–383
after trauma, 206
and uterine activity, 380–381, *382f*
Elimination
by newborn, 559, *559t*, *560t*
postpartum, 475
Emergency medical condition (EMC), 43–44
Emergency Medical Treatment and Labor Act (EMTALA), 42–44
Emotion(s)
during first trimester, 117–118
during labor and birth, 120–121
during postpartum period, 121–122, 475
during second trimester, 118–119
during third trimester, 119–120
Emotional support, during labor and birth, 328–329, 419, *419d*
Employment, maternal, 133, 136
EMTALA (Emergency Medical Treatment and Labor Act), 42–44
Enalapril, teratogenic effects of, *148t*
Encephalopathy, bilirubin, 585
Endocrine system, during pregnancy, 108–109
Endometritis, postpartum, 458–459
Endomyometritis, postpartum, 458
Endomyoparametritis, postpartum, 458
Endothelial dysfunction, in preeclampsia, 180–183, *181t*
Engorgement, *566–567*
Enterocele, 452
Environmental assessment
postpartum, 651
prenatal, *132d*, 133–137, *137d*
Environmental control, for asthma, 247
EOAE (evoked otoacoustic emissions), 522
Ephedrine, for maternal cardiac disease, 242
Epicanthal folds, 520, *521t*
Epidural anesthesia and analgesia, 434–438
advantages of, *436d*
with asthma, 249
cardiac output with, 99
combined spinal, 436–437
complications of, 437–438, *438t*
contraindications to, *435d*
historical development of, 434–435
maternal-fetal assessment with, 309
with multiple gestation, 270
nursing care for, *440t–442t*
standard, 436, *437f*
walking, 437, *437d*
Episiotomy, 326–328, 452, 454
Epispadias, *535t*
Epistaxis, during pregnancy, 102
Epstein's pearls, 524
Ergonovine maleate, for postpartum hemorrhage, 457
Errors, 32–35, *35d*, *36d*, 37, 40–41
Erythema toxicum, 517
Erythromycin, for pneumonia, 252, *253t*
Erythromycin ointment, for newborn, 508
Escherichia coli, pneumonia due to, 251
Eskimos, *74t*, *75f*, 76
Esophagus, during pregnancy, 105
Estriol
during pregnancy, 97, 144
and preterm labor and birth, 144–147, 210
screening for, 142, 144–147, *146t*
Estrogen
in lactation, 551
in onset of labor, *299d*
during pregnancy, 96–97
Ethical considerations, with multiple gestation, 266
Ethics, 29–30
Ethiopians, 76
Ethnic differences. *See* Cultural differences; Racial differences
Ethnocentrism, 82
Ethnocultural considerations, 70, *71f*
Etretinate, teratogenic effects of, *150t*
Evaluation, in nursing process, 30
Evaporative heat loss, 500, *501t*
Evidence-based practice, 5–7, *5d*, *7d*
"Evil eye," 79
Evoked otoacoustic emissions (EOAE), 522
Exercise(s)
for diabetes, 226, *227d*
pelvic-floor, 465
postpartum, 465
in prenatal risk assessment, 136
Expectations, by patient, 13–14
Expiratory reserve volume, during pregnancy, 102, *102t*
External relations, of team, *60d*
External version, with twins, 267, *267d*
Extremities, of newborn, 504–506
Extrusion reflex, 548
Eye(s)
of newborn, 504, 520, *521t*
sunset, *521t*
Eye contact, cultural difference in, 86
Eye movement, 520
Eye prophylaxis, for newborn, 508
Eyesight, 520

Face presentation, complications of, *497t*
Facial nerve
assessment of, *541t*
paralysis of, *524f*
Failure to progress, 345
False labor, *301d*
Family
cultural assessment of, 138
with multiple gestation, 257, 271–272
Family-centered care, 301–302, 620
Family history
of pregnancy-induced hypertension, 177
in prenatal risk assessment, 133
of substance abuse, 163
Family-newborn attachment, 329, 508
with cesarean birth, 353–354, *355f*, *356f*
Family nurse practitioners (FNPs), 129
Family preference plan, 618–620, *619d–620d*
Fasting, during labor, 312–313
Fasting plasma glucose (FPG), 224, *227t*, 234, *234t*
Fat
in breast milk, 553
in formula, 569
Fatigue, postpartum, 449–450, 468
Fat metabolism, during pregnancy, 108
FBS (fetal blood sampling), 144, *146t*, 406
Fear-tension-pain cycle, 423, *423f*
Feedback inhibitor of lactation, 552
Feeding, adaptive and maladaptive behaviors for, *469d*
Feet, of newborn, 535, 538, *538f*, *538t*, *539f*
Femoral pulses, of newborn, 504, 529, *531t*
Fencing reflex, 549
Fentanyl (Sublimaze), for labor pain, 434, *434t*
Ferguson reflex, 299, *299d*, 314
Fertility program
multiple gestation due to, 258
spontaneous abortion with, 260–261
Fetal acidemia
bradycardia and, 393, *393t*
fetal heart rate patterns with, 404–405, *404t*
tachycardia and, 392, *392t*
Fetal activity, assessment of. *See* Fetal movement counting (FMC)
Fetal alcohol syndrome, *148t*
Fetal assessment, 140, 147–154, *153d*
with asthma, 247
during labor, 378–414
fetal blood sampling for, 406
of fetal heart rate. *See* Fetal heart rate (FHR) monitoring
fetal oxygen saturation monitoring for, 406–408, *407f*, *408f*
fetal scalp stimulation for, 405, *405f*
historical perspectives on, 378–379
of umbilical cord blood gases, 408–409, *409t*
with maternal cardiac disease, 242
with maternal diabetes, 230, *230t*
Fetal blood sampling (FBS), 144, *146t*, 406
Fetal complications
intrapartum risk factors and, *497t*
maternal risk factors and, *495t*
of multiple gestation, 261–263, *263d*
recurrent, *496d*
Fetal compromise, in preeclampsia, *182t*, 187
Fetal death, 479. *See also* Perinatal death
in preeclampsia, *182t*
Fetal development, 147, *152d*
Fetal distress, 379
Fetal fibronectin (fFN), 144
and induction of labor, 334
and preterm labor and birth, 209–210
Fetal head position, 309–310
Fetal heart rate (FHR)
accelerations of, *380t*, 390–391, *390f*
in antepartum bleeding, 202
baseline, *380t*, 390
alterations in, 392–394, *392t*, *393t*, *394f*
characteristics of normal, 390–391, *390f*
decelerations of
early, *380t*, 396, *397f*, *399t*
late, *380t*, 396, *397f*, *398f*, *399t*
prolonged, *380t*, *397f*, 398–399, *399t*
variable, *380t*, 396–398, *397f*, *399t*, 402–403

documentation of, 39
maternal oxygen status and, 385
medical record audit of, 28*d*
nursing assessment of, 409–410, 410*d*
periodic and episodic changes in, 395–399, 397*f*, 399*t*
physiology of, 387–388, 387*f*, 388*d*–389*d*
in preeclampsia, 187
during pushing, 315
uterine, placental, and umbilical blood flow and, 385–387, 386*f*, 387*d*
variability in, 380*t*, 390
absent, 380*t*, 395, 395*t*, 400*t*
alterations in, 394–395, 395*t*
baseline, 390
long-term, 390
marked, 380*t*, 395
minimal, 380*t*, 395, 395*t*, 400*t*
moderate, 380*t*, 394–395, 400*t*
short-term, 390
Fetal heart rate (FHR) monitoring, 378–405
audit of, 28*d*
and cerebral palsy, 411, 412*d*
during contraction stress test, 153–154
decision tree for, 413*f*
for diabetic ketoacidosis, 231, 232*t*
via Doppler ultrasound, 381, 383, 383*f*, 384*d*
efficacy of, 411
via fetal scalp electrode, 381–383, 384*t*
historical perspectives on, 378–379
via intermittent auscultation, 379, 383, 384*d*, 385*d*
joint educations programs on, 63–64
during labor, 303, 306*d*–307*d*, 310, 411–412, 412*d*
with multiple gestation, 259*t*
nomenclature for, 64
during nonstress test, 153
during oxytocin induction or augmentation, 307*d*
patient education about, 409
physiologic basis for, 383–388
sources of artifact or error in, 382, 384*t*
specificity, sensitivity, and reliability of, 411–412
strip review of, 63–64
techniques of, 380–383
after trauma, 206
and uterine activity, 380–381, 382*f*
Fetal heart rate (FHR) patterns, 392–405
assessment of evolution of, 402–405, 403*f*, 404*f*, 404*t*
bradycardia, 380*t*, 393–394, 393*t*, 394*f*, 403
communication with primary providers about, 410–411
prior to death, 403–405, 404*t*
definitions of terms for, 379–380, 380*t*
documentation of, 410, 410*d*
dysrhythmias, 401–402, 402*f*
and fetal acidemia, 404–405, 404*t*
joint educational programs on, 63–64
management of variant, 400*t*
nonreassuring, 379
evolution of, 402–405, 403*f*
interventions for, 391–392
overshoots, 402
saltatory, 400–401
shoulders, 402
sinusoidal, 399–400, 401*f*
tachycardia, 389*t*, 392–393, 392*t*
unusual, 399–402, 401*f*, 402*f*
Fetal hydrops, and preeclampsia, 178
Fetal hypoxemia, 387*f*, 388
Fetal loss, in multiple gestation, 260–261, 262*d*
Fetal macrosomia, due to gestational diabetes mellitus, 220
Fetal malposition, and fetal and neonatal complications, 495*t*
Fetal monitoring. *See* Electronic fetal monitoring (EFM)
Fetal movement counting (FMC), 152–153
with diabetes, 230, 230*t*
with multiple gestation, 265
Fetal oxygen saturation ($FSpO_2$), 406–408, 407*f*, 408*f*
Fetal presentation
abnormal, fetal and neonatal complications of, 497*t*
Leopold maneuver for, 311*f*, 497*t*
with multiple gestation, 267*d*, 268–270, 268*f*, 269*d*, 270*d*
Fetal scalp electrode (FSE), 310, 381–383, 384*t*
Fetal scalp stimulation, 405, 405*f*
Fetal surveillance, 147–154
assessment of fetal activity in, 152–153
with asthma, 247
basic, 140
biophysical profile in, 154
contraction stress test in, 153–154
indications for, 153*d*
with maternal diabetes, 230, 230*t*
with multiple gestation, 264–266
nonstress test in, 153
Fetoscope, 379, 383, 384*d*, 385*d*
Fetus-in-fetus, 261
Fetus papyraceus, 255, 261
fFN (fetal fibronectin), 144
and induction of labor, 334
and preterm labor and birth, 209–210
Fibrin, during pregnancy, 101*t*
Fibrinogen
in preeclampsia, 180*t*
during pregnancy, 101*t*
Fibrinolysis, during pregnancy, 101
Fibronectin, fetal, 144
and induction of labor, 334
and preterm labor and birth, 209–210
Filipinos, 78
pregnancy-induced hypertension in, 174*t*
Fingers, of newborn, 539*t*, 540*t*
First trimester
adaptations during, 117–118, 117*d*
hypoglycemia in, 222
prenatal education in, 156*d*
Flow sheet(s), 39, 40
labor, 370–375
Fluconazole, for *Candida,* 564
Fluid and electrolyte balance
postpartum, 449
during pregnancy, 103–104
Fluid needs, postpartum, 453
Fluid replacement
for antepartum bleeding, 202, 203*t*, 204
for hypovolemic shock, 205, 205*d*
Fluid resuscitation
for abruptio placentae, 195
for diabetic ketoacidosis, 231, 232*t*
FNPs (family nurse practitioners), 129
Focus groups, 14
Focusing, for labor pain, 431
Folic acid antagonists, teratogenic effects of, 148*t*
Follow-up, postdischarge, 611, 627–630, 628*d*–629*d*
Fontanelles, 310, 518, 519*t*, 520*f*
Football hold, 555, 556*f*
Foramen ovale, 498
Forceps-assisted birth, 346, 347–348, 347*t*
complications of, 347–348, 497*t*
Foreskin, of newborn, 533–534
Formal stage, in transition to parenthood, 468
Formula feeding, 551*d*, 568–571, 570*d*, 650
FPG (fasting plasma glucose), 224, 227*t*, 234, 234*t*
Fragile X syndrome, carrier screening for, 146*t*
Fraternal twins, 254, 254*t*, 255*d*, 256
Fresh-frozen plasma, for antepartum bleeding, 202, 203*t*
Fresh whole blood, for antepartum bleeding, 202, 203*t*
Friedman curve, 300
FSE (fetal scalp electrode), 310, 381–383, 384*t*
$FSpO_2$ (fetal oxygen saturation), 406–408, 407*f*, 408*f*
Functional residual capacity, during pregnancy, 102, 102*t*
Fundal height, 140
with multiple gestation, 256, 260*t*
Fundal massage, postpartum, 453*f*, 454, 456, 457
Fundal pressure, 322–323, 322*f*
with shoulder dystocia, 325

GAI (General Acculturation Index) scale, 70–71
Galant's reflex, 549
Gallbladder, during pregnancy, 106
Gap junctions, and labor, 299
Gas exchange, during pregnancy, 102
Gaskin maneuver, 326
Gas pains, postpartum, 455
Gastric reflux, during pregnancy, 105
Gastrointestinal system
postpartum, 452
during pregnancy, 105–106, 106*t*
Gastroparesis, diabetic, 221
Gastropathy, diabetic, 221
Gastroschisis, 533*t*
Gate-control theory, 424
GBS (group B streptococcal) infection
maternal, 495*t*
neonatal, 508–510, 509*f*, 510*f*, 588, 589*f*, 590*f*
GDM. *See* Gestational diabetes mellitus (GDM)
Gender roles
cultural differences in, 72–73, 72*d*
and teamwork, 54–55
General Acculturation Index (GAI) scale, 70–71
Genetic basis, for preeclampsia, 177
Genetic counseling, for multiple gestation, 261
Genetic disorders, prenatal risk assessment for, 142, 143*d*, 144*f*, 145*d*, 146*t*
Genital mutilation, 80–81, 94
Genitourinary system, of newborn, 506, 532–534, 534*f*, 535*t*, 547
Gentamicin, for group B streptococcal infection, 591
Gentian violet, for *Candida,* 564
Gestational age
appropriate for, 514
assessment of, 513–514, 515*f*, 546–547
large for, 514
and sepsis, 589
small for, 514
Gestational diabetes mellitus (GDM), 219–235
ambulatory and home care management of, 225–230, 294–295
classification of, 221
clinical manifestations of, 224–225
defined, 107, 221
development of overt diabetes after, 234–235, 234*d*
diabetic ketoacidosis due to, 221, 222, 224–225, 231, 232*t*
diagnosis of, 224, 224*t*
exercise therapy for, 226, 227*d*
fetal assessment for, 230, 230*t*
incidence of, 107
inpatient management of, 231
insulin therapy for, 229
intrapartum management of, 231–233, 233*d*
metabolic monitoring for, 227–228, 227*d*
with multiple gestation, 258
nursing assessments and interventions for, 225
nutrition therapy for, 226
pathophysiology of, 222–223
patient education for, 225–226, 226*d*
pharmacologic therapy for, 229
postpartum management of, 234–235, 448
screening for, 107–108, 141, 223–224, 223*d*
significance and incidence of, 219–221
Getting phase, of labor, 422*d*
Globulins, during pregnancy, 106*t*
Glomerular filtration rate (GFR)
in preeclampsia, 180*t*
during pregnancy, 103
Glomerulonephritis, fetal and neonatal complications with, 495*t*
Glossopharyngeal nerve, assessment of, 541*t*
Glucocorticoid administration, for preterm labor and birth, 219

Glucose
administration during labor, 313
plasma
fasting, 224, 227*t*, 234, 234*t*
impaired, 234, 234*t*
during labor, 231
monitoring of, 227
postpartum, 448
postprandial, 227, 227*t*
preprandial, 227*t*
values for, 224, 227–228, 227*t*
in urine, during pregnancy, 104–105, 104*t*
Glucose challenge test, 139*d*
Glucose metabolism, during pregnancy, 107–108
Glucose Screening Test (GST), 141
Glucose tolerance, impaired, 234, 234*t*
Glucose tolerance test, oral, 141, 233–234, 234*t*
Gluteal folds, asymmetrical, 539, 539*f*
Glycemic goals, for pregnancy, 227, 227*t*
Glycosuria, during pregnancy, 104–105
Goals, of perinatal team, 60–61, 60*d*
Graduate degree, 23
Gravidity, and preeclampsia, 177
Gray color, of newborn, 518*t*
Grief
acute, 480, 481*t*
anticipatory, 479, 480
behaviors caused by, 481*t*
bittersweet, 483
chronic, 482, 482*d*
duration of, 483
psychological perspective on, 480–483
resolution of, 482–483
shadow, 483
types of, 480–482, 482*d*
Group B streptococcal (GBS) infection
maternal, 495*t*
neonatal, 508–510, 509*f*, 510*f*, 588, 589*f*, 590*f*
Grunting, by newborn, 526, 527*t*, 578
GST (Glucose Screening Test), 141
Guidelines, practice, 31–32, 35–37
Guilt, in acute grief work, 481*t*

Haemophilus influenzae, pneumonia due to, 251, 252, 253*t*
Hair
of newborn, 518–520, 519*t*
during pregnancy, 109
Haitian women, 75
Half-identical twinning, 254, 255
Hands, of newborn, 535
Hands-and-knees position, during labor, 314, 317*f*, 426*t*
Hard palate, cleft, 524, 525*f*, 526*t*
Hawaiians, pregnancy-induced hypertension in, 174*t*
HBV (hepatitis B virus)
newborn immunization for, 510–511
prenatal immunization for, 169, 171
HCFA (Health Care Financing Administration), 12
hCG (human chorionic gonadotropin)
during pregnancy, 96
screening for, 142, 146*t*
Head, of newborn, 504, 517–520, 518*f*–520*f*, 519*t*
Headaches
postpartum, 450
during pregnancy, 109
Head circumference, 513, 514*f*, 517, 519*t*
Head compression, decelerations due to, 399*t*, 403
Head position, fetal, 309–310
Health beliefs and practices, cultural assessment of, 138
Healthcare costs, 2–4
Healthcare environment, and labor pain, 423
Health Care Financing Administration (HCFA), 12
Healthcare organizations, accreditation and certification of, 11–13
Health insurance, 3
Health promotion, prenatal, 157–158
Hearing loss, 521–523, 522*d*, 523*d*, 523*t*
Heart
auscultatory areas of, 529, 529*f*
blood flow through, 237–238, 238*f*
during pregnancy, 98
Heart block, fetal, 394, 401
Heart disease. *See also* Cardiac disease
congenital, 579–582, 580*t*
carrier frequency for, 145*d*
Heart failure, congestive
maternal, 495*t*
neonatal, 579
Heart murmur
in newborn, 529, 529*d*, 531*t*
during pregnancy, 98
Heart rate
fetal. *See* Fetal heart rate (FHR)
of newborn, 529
during pregnancy, 98, 98*t*
with cardiac disease, 242
Heart sounds
in newborn, 529, 531*t*
during pregnancy, 98
Heat, for labor pain, 427–428, 427*t*, 429*t*
Heat loss, mechanisms of, 500, 501*t*
Heat production, in newborn, 499–500
Heave, 529
Heel to ear, 546
HELLP syndrome, 178, 189
Hemangiomas, 516, 516*f*
Hematocrit
with multiple gestation, 260*t*
postpartum, 450
during pregnancy, 100
Hematologic changes
postpartum, 450–451
during pregnancy, 100–101
Hematoma, subgaleal, with vacuum extraction, 348
Heme, 584
Hemodynamic changes, postpartum, 450
Hemodynamic monitoring, with maternal cardiac disease, 241
Hemoglobin electrophoresis, 142
Hemoglobin levels
with multiple gestation, 258, 260*t*
postpartum, 450
during pregnancy, 100
Hemoglobinopathies
carrier screening for, 146*t*
fetal and neonatal complications with, 495*t*
Hemolysis, in preeclampsia, 182*t*
Hemophilia, carrier frequency for, 145*d*
Hemorrhage. *See* Bleeding
postpartum. *See* Postpartum hemorrhage
Hemorrhagic shock, 205–206
Hemorrhoids
postpartum, 452
during pregnancy, 106
Heparin
antenatal, 295, 296
during labor and birth, 243
for pulmonary embolism, 463
for thrombophlebitis, 462
Hepatic dysfunction, in preeclampsia, 181*t*–182*t*, 184*d*
Hepatic rupture, in preeclampsia, 181*t*–182*t*
Hepatitis, fetal and neonatal complications with, 495*t*
Hepatitis A, prenatal immunization for, 172
Hepatitis B virus (HBV)
newborn immunization for, 510–511
prenatal immunization for, 169, 171
Herbs, prenatal use of, 135
Hernia(s)
inguinal, 532, 532*f*, 535*t*
postpartum, 452
umbilical, 530, 532*f*
Heroin withdrawal, 593
High-reliability organizations, 34
Hinduism, 81*t*
Hip, developmental dysplasia of, 504–506, 535–538, 536*d*, 536*f*, 537*f*
Hispanics, 75*f*, 78–80
comparative statistical data on, 74*t*
core values of, 79
cultural beliefs and practices of, 79–80
pregnancy-induced hypertension in, 174*t*
HIV. *See* Human immunodeficiency virus (HIV)
Holding-out phase, of labor, 421, 422*d*
Homans sign, 455, 462
Home care management
of antepartum bleeding, 203, 293–294
of diabetes, 225–230, 294–295
of multiple gestation, 266
postpartum, 643–665
benefits of, 644–645
discharge criteria and, 646–647, 647*d*
early discharge and, 643–644
environmental assessment in, 651
essential components of, 646–649, 647*d*, 648*d*
interpreter for, 648
learning-needs assessment in, 650
maternal assessment in, 649, 650, 661
models of, 645–646
newborn assessment in, 649–650, 663
nurse providers of, 652–653
nursing assessments in, 649–651, 656–663
nursing interventions in, 651
orientation and education for, 652–653
outcome monitoring and quality care with, 651–652, 652*d*, 665
personal safety in, 653
physical assessment in, 649–650
plan of care for, 648–649
psychosocial assessment in, 650
recommendations on, 645, 646*d*
referral for, 647–648, 648*d*, 657
review of literature on, 643–645
schedule for, 648
telephone assessment for, 659
of preeclampsia, 183, 292–293
of preterm labor and birth, 214–215, 215*d*, 294
Home uterine activity monitoring (HUAM), 214–215
H_1-receptor antagonists, for labor pain, 432
Hospital discharge packs, 561
Hospitalization. *See* Inpatient management
Host defense, during pregnancy, 111–112, 111*t*
hPL (human placental lactogen), during pregnancy, 96
Human chorionic gonadotropin (hCG)
during pregnancy, 96
screening for, 142, 146*t*
Human chorionic somatomammotropin, during pregnancy, 96
Human immunodeficiency virus (HIV)
fetal and neonatal complications of, 495*t*
fetal heart rate monitoring with, 383
prenatal screening for, 141
Human placental lactogen (hPL), during pregnancy, 96
Humoral immunity, during pregnancy, 111*t*
Hunger cues, and breast-feeding, 557–558, 557*d*
Husband, labor support by, 421–422, 422*d*
Hydatiform mole, and preeclampsia, 178
Hydralazine hydrochloride (Apresoline), for preeclampsia, 189
Hydration, intravenous. *See* Intravenous (IV) fluids
Hydrocele, 534, 535*t*
Hydronephrosis, physiologic, of pregnancy, 103
Hydrotherapy, during labor, 427–428, 429*t*
Hydroureter, of pregnancy, 103
Hydroxyzine hydrochloride (Vistaril), for labor pain, 432
Hygiene, postpartum, 475
Hygroma, cystic, 525, 527*f*
Hygroscopic dilators, synthetic, 335
Hymen, imperforate, 533, 534*f*
Hymenal tag, 533
Hyperbilirubinemia. *See* Jaundice
Hyperemesis gravidarum, 105
Hyperglycemia, during pregnancy, 107, 222–223

Hyperinsulinemia
  fetal, 223
  during pregnancy, 107, 222
Hypermagnesemia, 373
Hyperpigmentation, during pregnancy, 109
Hyperreflexia, in preeclampsia, 182*t*
Hyperstimulation, uterine, 381, 382*f*
  with Cervidil, 338*d*, 340
  defined, 330, 381
  with misoprostol, 339*d*, 340, 341
  with oxytocin, 344
  with Prepidil, 337, 338*d*
Hypertelorism, 520
Hypertension
  cultural differences in, 82
  persistent pulmonary, of newborn, 499, 578
  in pregnancy, 173–190
    activity restriction for, 185
    by age, 174–175, 175*t*
    antepartum management of, 185, 186*t*
    chronic, 175*t*, 177–178
      fetal and neonatal complications with, 495*t*
    cigarette smoking and, 176
    clinical manifestations of, 179–183
    colloids for, 184–185
    complications of, 184*d*
    defined, 179
    with diabetes, 221
    differential diagnosis of, 183
    diuretics for, 184–185
    eclampsia, 178, 189–190
    expedition of birth for, 186*t*
    family history of, 177
    fetal hydrops and, 178
    genetic basis for, 177
    gestational age at first prenatal visit and, 177
    gravidity and parity and, 177
    HELLP syndrome, 178, 189
    home care management of, 183, 292–293
    hydatiform mole and, 178
    incidence of, 173–174, 174*t*, 175*t*
    inpatient management of, 183–184
    laboratory tests for, 187–188, 188*d*
    mild *vs.* severe, 183, 184*d*
    morbidity and mortality from, 174
    with multiple gestation, 178, 263–264
    nursing assessment and interventions for, 183–189
    nutrition and, 176
    ongoing assessment for, 185–187
    pathophysiology of, 178–179, 180*t*–182*t*, 183*f*
    pharmacologic therapies for, 188–189
    postpartum management of, 189
    preeclampsia, 178–179, 183–189
    pregnancy complications and, 178
    by race, 173–174, 174*t*, 175
    risk factors for, 174–178, 176*d*
    socioeconomic status and, 175–176
    transient, 178
    urinary tract infection and, 178
  pregnancy-induced, 178, 179–183
    defined, 178
    family history of, 177
    fetal and neonatal complications of, 495*t*
    significance and incidence of, 173–174, 174*t*, 175*t*
Hyperthyroidism, during pregnancy, 108
Hypnotics, for labor pain, 432
Hypocalcemia, in infant of diabetic mother, 220
Hypoglycemia
  clinical manifestations of, 225, 583*d*
  defined, 225
  with diabetes, 221
  in first trimester, 222
  in infant of diabetic mother, 220
  during labor, 233, 233*d*
  neonatal, 565–566, 582–584, 582*t*, 583*d*
Hypoglycemic agents, oral, 228
Hypokalemia, due to diabetic ketoacidosis, 231
Hypomagnesemia, in infant of diabetic mother, 220
Hypospadias, 535*t*
Hypotelorism, 520
Hypotension, orthostatic, postpartum, 449
Hypothermia, in newborn, 500, 501*f*, 501*t*
Hypothyroidism, during pregnancy, 108
Hypovolemic shock
  postpartum, 457
  during pregnancy, 205, 205*d*
Hypoxemia, fetal, 387*f*, 388
Hypoxia
  acute intrapartum, 411, 412*d*
  in preeclampsia, 182*t*

Ice packs
  for labor pain, 428
  for perineal edema, 454
Identical twins, 254–255, 254*t*, 256
Identification, of newborn, 506–508, 506*t*, 507*d*
Idiopathic thrombocytopenic purpura (ITP), fetal and neonatal complications with, 495*t*
IFG (impaired fasting glucose), 234, 234*t*
Igs. *See* Immunoglobulins (Igs)
IGT (impaired glucose tolerance), 234, 234*t*
IISW (intradermal injections of sterile water), for labor pain, 429–430, 430*f*
Ileus, postpartum, 452
Illicit drugs
  fetal and neonatal complications with, 495*t*
  history of, 163
  in prenatal risk assessment, 135–136, 161–163
Imagery, for labor pain, 430–431
Immigrants, 80
Immune system
  breast milk and, 553
  of newborn, 500–502
Immunity, during pregnancy, 111–112, 111*t*
Immunization
  newborn, for hepatitis B virus, 510–511
  during pregnancy, 168–172
Immunoglobulins (Igs)
  in breast milk, 553
  in newborn, 501
  during pregnancy, 111, 111*t*
Immunotherapy, for asthma, 248
Impaired fasting glucose (IFG), 234, 234*t*
Impaired glucose tolerance (IGT), 234, 234*t*
Implementation, in nursing process, 30
Incident management, 40–41
Incontinence
  anal, 452–453
  stress, 449
Indemnification and contribution, 46
Individuation, of multiples, 273
Indomethacin, for preterm labor and birth, 216*d*, 217*d*, 218–219
Induction of labor
  with asthma, 249
  cervical status and, 333–334, 334*t*
  and cesarean birth, 350
  contraindications for, 332*d*
  criteria for, 331*d*
  defined, 329, 330
  fetal fibronectin as marker for success of, 334
  incidence of, 330
  indications for, 330–331, 331*d*
  informed consent for, 332–333, 377
  mechanical methods of, 341–342
  nurse's role in, 333
  pharmacologic methods of, 343–345
  protocols and policies for, 333, 333*d*
  risk-benefit analysis of, 330, 332–333
  staffing during, 346
Infant care, classes in, 614*d*, 617*d*
Infant mortality, 126, 126*d*
  cultural differences in, 74*t*
  with multiple gestation, 253–254
  with preterm birth, 207, 208
Infection(s)
  intraamniotic, fetal and neonatal complications with, 495*t*
  neonatal, 587–591
    assessment of, 588–590
    clinical signs of, 590, 591*f*
    diagnosis of, 590
    early-onset, 588, 588*t*
    of eye, 508
    group B beta-hemolytic streptococcal, 508–510, 509*f*, 510*f*, 588, 589*f*, 590*f*
    immune system and, 501–502
    incidence and mortality rates for, 587, 587*t*
    interventions for, 590–591
    late-onset, 588, 588*t*
    pathophysiology of, 587–588, 587*d*, 588*t*, 589*f*
    risk factors for, 588–590, 590*d*
  postpartum (puerperal), 458–461
  during pregnancy, 111
  preterm labor and birth due to, 211
  urinary tract
    postpartum, 460–461
    and preeclampsia, 178
    during pregnancy, 103
  wound, 459
Infertility, 479, 480*d*
Influenza, pneumonia due to, 251
Influenza vaccine
  for asthma, 249
  prenatal, 169
Informality, in teamwork, 60*d*
Informal stage, in transition to parenthood, 468
Informed consent, 16*d*
  for induction of labor, 332–333, 377
Inguinal hernia, 532, 532*f*, 535*t*
Inheritance patterns, 142, 143*d*, 144*f*
Injury, in legal sense, 31, 32
Inotrope, 237*d*, 242–243
Inpatient management
  of antepartum bleeding, 203–206
  of asthma, 249
  of diabetes, 231
  of multiple gestation, 266
  of preeclampsia, 183–184
Inspiratory reserve volume, during pregnancy, 102, 102*t*
Institutional politics, and teamwork, 56
Insulin pump, 229
Insulin resistance, during pregnancy, 107, 222
Insulin therapy
  for diabetic ketoacidosis, 231, 232*t*
  during labor, 231–233
  postpartum, 233, 448
  during pregnancy, 108, 228–229, 228*d*, 229*d*
Insurance, 3
  professional liability, 45–47
Integument. *See* Skin
Intercostal muscles, of newborn, 496–497
Intermediary twinning, 254, 255
Intermittent auscultation, of fetal heart rate, 304–308, 379, 383, 384*d*, 385*d*
Internal version, with twins, 267, 267*d*
Interpreter(s), 83, 138
  for home care services, 648
Intestines, during pregnancy, 105–106
Intraamniotic infection, fetal and neonatal complications with, 495*t*
Intracranial hemorrhage, with vacuum extraction, 348
Intracranial pressure, of newborn, 519*t*
Intradermal injections of sterile water (IISW), for labor pain, 429–430, 430*f*
Intrapartum management
  of diabetes, 231–233, 233*d*
  of multiple gestation, 266–270
Intrapartum risk factors, fetal and neonatal complications with, 497*t*
Intrathecal analgesia and anesthesia, 438
Intrauterine devices (IUDs), 467
Intrauterine fetal death (IUFD), in preeclampsia, 182*t*
Intrauterine growth restriction (IUGR)
  with diabetes mellitus, 220
  with multiple gestation, 254
  with preeclampsia, 182*t*, 184*d*
  with preterm birth, 208
Intrauterine pressure catheter (IUPC), 310, 380, 381

Intravenous (IV) fluids
during labor, 313
for nonreassuring fetal heart rate, 391
in preeclampsia, 184–185
for preterm labor and birth, 215
In utero resuscitation, 391
Inverted nipples, 558–559
Iris, 520, 521*t*
Iron deficiency, postpartum, 451
Iron requirements, during pregnancy, 100
Irritability, in acute grief work, 481*t*
Ischial spines, 309
Islamic women, 81, 81*t*
Isotretinoin, teratogenic effects of, 150*t*
ITP (idiopathic thrombocytopenic purpura), fetal and neonatal complications with, 495*t*
IUDs (intrauterine devices), 467
IUFD (intrauterine fetal death), in preeclampsia, 182*t*
IUGR, Intrauterine growth restriction (IUGR)
IUPC (intrauterine pressure catheter), 310, 380, 381
IV fluids. *See* Intravenous (IV) fluids

Japanese Americans, pregnancy-induced hypertension in, 174*t*
Jaundice, 584–587
algorithm for management of, 600–602
assessment of, 585, 586*d*
breast-milk, 564–565
clinical manifestations of, 515–516, 585
early-onset, 564
etiology of, 518*t*, 584*d*
incidence of, 515
in infant of diabetic mother, 220
late-onset, 564–565
pathologic, 584*d*, 585
pathophysiology of, 584–585
phototherapy for, 564, 585–587, 586*t*
home, 652
physiologic, 584*d*, 585
risk factors for, 585*t*
with vacuum extraction, 348
Jews, Orthodox, 81, 81*t*
Joint(s), during pregnancy, 110
Joint Commission on Accreditation of Healthcare Organizations (JCAHO), 11–13
Joint educational programs, for physicians and nurses, 63–65
Journal clubs, 27–28
Judaism, 81, 81*t*

Kanamycin, teratogenic effects of, 149*t*
Kegel exercises, 465
Kernicterus, 585
Ketoacidosis, diabetic, during pregnancy, 108, 221, 222, 224–225, 231, 232*t*
Ketones, in urine, 227
Kidney function. *See* Renal function
Kinship system, cultural differences in, 72*d*
Klebsiella pneumoniae, pneumonia due to, 251
Kneeling, during labor, 314, 317*f*, 426*t*
Knowledge and belief system, cultural differences in, 72*d*
Koreans, 78

Labetalol, for preeclampsia, 189
Labia majora, 532, 533
Labia minora, 532
Labor, 298–350
active management of, 345–346
adaptations during, 120–121, 121*d*
admission assessment for, 302–303, 306*d*, 367–368
amnioinfusion during, 349–350
augmentation of, 345
contraindications for, 332*d*
criteria for, 332*d*
defined, 329–330
incidence of, 330
indications for, 332*d*
staffing during, 346
cardiac output during, 99, 100*t*
care paths for, 635–637
cervical ripening for, 334–341
criteria for, 331*d*
defined, 329
indications for, 331*d*
informed consent for, 332–333, 377
mechanical methods of, 334–336
nurse's role in, 333
pharmacologic methods of, 336–341, 338*d*–339*d*
protocols and policies for, 333, 333*d*
risk-benefit analysis of, 332–333
staffing during, 346
clinical interventions during, 329–350
documentation of, 304, 370–375
duration of, 300–301, 302*f*, 304*t*–305*d*
emotional support during, 328–329
facilitation of, 301–302
false *vs.* true, 300, 301*d*
fetal assessment during, 378–414
historical perspectives on, 378–379
fetal blood sampling during, 406
fetal heart rate monitoring during, 303, 306*d*–307*d*, 310, 411–412, 412*d*
fetal oxygen saturation monitoring during, 406–408, 407*f*, 408*f*
fetal scalp stimulation during, 405, 405*f*
flow sheet for, 370–375
fundal pressure during, 322–323, 322*f*
induction of
cervical status and, 333–334, 334*t*
and cesarean birth, 350
contraindications for, 332*d*
criteria for, 331*d*
defined, 329, 330
fetal fibronectin as marker for success of, 334
incidence of, 330
indications for, 330–331, 331*d*
informed consent for, 332–333, 377
mechanical methods of, 341–342
nurse's role in, 333
pharmacologic methods of, 343–345
protocols and policies for, 333, 333*d*
risk-benefit analysis of, 330, 332–333
staffing during, 346
intravenous fluids and oral intake during, 312–313
Leopold maneuvers during, 310, 311*f*
maternal-fetal status during, 302–309, 306*d*–308*d*
nursing assessments during, 302–310
onset of, 298–300, 299*d*
fetal fibronectin as marker for, 334
positions for, 313–314, 316*f*–318*f*, 320*d*
premonitory signs of, 300
stage(s) of, 301, 304*t*–305*t*
active, 301, 304*t*
first, 301, 304*t*–305*t*
latent, 301, 304*t*
second, 305*t*, 314–322, 319*f*, 320*d*–321*d*
third, 305*t*
transition, 301, 305*t*
umbilical cord gases during, 408–409, 409*t*
uterine activity assessment during, 310
vaginal examinations during, 309–310
vital signs during, 306*d*, 308–309
Laboratory tests, prenatal, 139*d*, 140–141, 141*t*, 142
with multiple gestation, 258, 260*t*
Labor-delivery-recovery postpartum rooms (LDRPs), 14
Laboring down, 321–322
Labor pain, 417–442
analgesics for, 432–433, 433*t*, 434*t*
attention focusing and distraction for, 431
auditory or visual techniques for, 424*t*, 431–432
childbirth preparation and, 422–423, 423*f*
cognitive techniques for, 424*t*, 430–431
counterpressure for, 427, 427*f*
cultural differences in experience of, 73
cutaneous techniques for, 424*t*, 425–430
cyclic nature of, 423, 423*f*
descriptions of, 418, 418*t*
effleurage for, 429, 430*f*
epidural anesthesia and analgesia for, 434–438
advantages of, 436*d*
with asthma, 249
cardiac output with, 99
combined spinal, 436–437
complications of, 437–438, 438*t*
contraindications to, 435*d*
historical development of, 434–435
maternal-fetal assessment with, 309
with multiple gestation, 270
nursing care for, 440*t*–442*t*
standard, 436, 437*f*
walking, 437, 437*d*
gate-control theory of, 424
healthcare environment and, 423
heat and cold for, 427–428, 427*t*, 429*t*
imagery for, 430–431
intradermal injections of sterile water for, 429–430, 430*f*
intrathecal analgesia and anesthesia for, 438
labor support and, 419–422, 419*d*, 420*d*, 422*d*
local anesthetic for, 434
music for, 431–432
nonpharmacologic management of, 423–432, 424*t*
pain tolerance and, 423
paracervical block for, 439
parenteral opioids for, 432–433, 433*t*, 434*t*
patterned breathing for, 431
pharmacologic management of, 432–442
physiologic basis for, 417–418
physiologic responses to, 418
positioning and movement for, 425–427, 425*t*–426*t*
psychosocial factors influencing, 418–423
pudendal block for, 434, 435*f*
regional anesthesia and analgesia for, 434–442
delayed pushing with, 321–322
maternal and fetal assessment with, 307*d*–308*d*, 440*d*
nursing guidelines for, 438–439, 440*d*
nursing interventions with, 438–439, 440*d*, 440*t*–442*t*
and position for labor and birth, 314
relaxation for, 430, 431*d*
saddle block for, 439–442
sedatives and hypnotics for, 432
touch and massage for, 428
Labor Progress Chart, audit of, 28*d*
Labor support, 419–422, 419*d*, 420*d*, 422*d*
Lacerations, of birth canal, 199
Lactation. *See also* Breast-feeding
feedback inhibitor of, 552
Lactation suppression, 571
Lactocytes, 551
Lactoferrin, 553–554
Lactogen, placental, 551
Lactogenesis, 552–553
Lactose, 554, 569
Lactose-free formula, 569
Lactose intolerance, cultural differences in, 82
La manita de azabache, 79
Lamicel, 335
Laminaria tents, 334–335
Language, second, 85
Language barrier, 83, 138
Language line services, 94
Lanugo, 517, 546
Large for gestational age (LGA), 514
Large intestine, during pregnancy, 105–106
Largon (propiomazine), for labor pain, 432
Latch-on, 556, 556*d*
LATCH tool, 559–560, 560*t*
Late decelerations, 380*t*, 396, 397*f*, 398*f*, 399*t*
Latinos, 75*f*, 78–80
comparative statistical data on, 74*t*
core values of, 79
cultural beliefs and practices of, 79–80
pregnancy-induced hypertension in, 174*t*

LBW infants. *See* Low-birth-weight (LBW) infants
LDRPs (labor-delivery-recovery postpartum rooms), 14
Lead, teratogenic effects of, 149*t*
Leadership, of team, 60*d*, 61
Learning-needs assessment, 620–623, 622*d*, 650
Leg(s), of newborn, 535, 535*f*
Legal issues, 29–47
  conflict resolution, 44–45, 46*f*
  documentation, 32, 38–40
  duty, 31
    breach of, 31–32
  Emergency Medical Treatment and Labor Act, 42–44
  errors, 32–35, 35*d*, 36*d*, 37, 40–41
  incident management, 40–41
  injury and legal causation, 32, 33*d*
  institutional policies and procedures, 37–38
  nursing accountability and responsibility, 29–31
  professional liability, 31–32, 33*d*
  professional liability insurance, 45–47
  risk management, 32–35, 35*d*, 36*d*
  risk modification, 37
  staffing, 41–42, 42*t*
  standards of care and practice guidelines, 32, 33*d*, 35–37
  working with unlicensed assistive personnel, 30–31
Legionella pneumophila, pneumonia due to, 251, 253*t*
Length of stay (LOS), 3–4, 10, 14, 610–611
  guidelines for, 645
  and home care services, 643–644
Leopold maneuvers, 310, 311*f*
Let-down reflex, 552–553
Letting-go phase, in transition to parenthood, 469
Leukocytes
  in newborn, 501
  during pregnancy, 101, 111, 111*t*
Leukocytosis, postpartum, 451
LGA (large for gestational age), 514
Liability, professional, 31–32, 33*d*
Liability insurance, professional, 45–47
Licensure, of nurses, 22–23
  vs. physicians, 57–58
Lidocaine (Xylocaine), epidural anesthesia with, 434
Lifestyle factors, in prenatal risk assessment, 132*d*, 133–137, 137*d*
Lifestyle modification, for preterm labor and birth, 212–214
Ligaments, during pregnancy, 110
Light sleep state, of newborn, 544
Linea nigra, 109
Lip(s)
  assessment of, 526*t*
  cleft, 524, 525*f*, 526*t*
Lipids, serum, during pregnancy, 106*t*
Lispro, 229
Listening, in teamwork, 60*d*
Lithium, teratogenic effects of, 149*t*
Liver function
  of newborn, 531
  in postpartum period, 451
  in preeclampsia, 181*t*–182*t*, 184*d*
  during pregnancy, 106, 106*t*
Local anesthetic, for labor pain, 434
  epidural, 434–438, 438*t*
Lochia, 447, 448*t*, 474
  with multiple gestation, 259*t*
LOS (length of stay), 3–4, 10, 14, 610–611
  guidelines for, 645
  and home care services, 643–644
Loss
  causes of, 478–480
  perceptions of, 477–478
  phenomenology of, 476–480
  types of, 476–477, 478*t*
Low-back pain, during labor, 417
  counterpressure for, 427, 427*f*
  intradermal injections of sterile water for, 429–430, 430*f*
Low-birth-weight (LBW) infants
  cultural differences in, 74*t*
  defined, 207–208
  incidence of, 207
  mortality rate for, 208
  sepsis in, 589
Low-lying placenta, 192, 193*f*
Lung(s), of newborn, 494–497, 525–528, 527*t*, 528*f*, 528*t*
Lunge, during labor, 425*t*
Lung volume, during pregnancy, 101–102, 102*t*
Lupus, cultural differences in, 82
Lymphatic system, 238
Lymphocytes, in newborn, 501

Macrosomia
  due to gestational diabetes mellitus, 220
  shoulder dystocia with, 324
Macules, in newborn, 518*t*
Magnesium sulfate ($MgSO_4$)
  complications of, 497*t*
  for preeclampsia, 188, 189, 373
  for preterm labor and birth, 216*d*, 217*d*, 218
  tocolytic therapy with, 373
Male children, cultural preferences for, 87
Malpractice, 31–35, 33*d*, 35*d*, 36*d*
Managed care
  emergency treatment with, 43
  healthcare costs with, 2–3, 4
Manual extraction, complications of, 497*t*
Manual version, complications of, 497*t*
MAP. *See* Mean arterial pressure (MAP)
Marfan syndrome, 235
Marital status, 133
Marked variability, in fetal heart rate, 380*t*, 395
MAS (meconium aspiration syndrome), 575–576, 577*f*
  amnioinfusion for, 349–350
Mask of pregnancy, 109
Massage
  for labor pain, 428
  postpartum uterine, 454, 454*f*, 456, 457
Mastitis, 460, 567, 567*d*
MAST suit, for antepartum bleeding, 204–205
Maternal age, 133
  and pregnancy-induced hypertension, 174–175, 175*t*
Maternal assessment, in home care, 649, 650, 661
Maternal care, learning-needs assessment for, 621, 622*d*
Maternal complications
  fetal and neonatal complications with, 495*t*
  of multiple gestation, 263–264, 264*d*
Maternal education, 133
Maternal employment, 133, 136
Maternal-fetal oxygen transfer, 385–387, 386*f*, 387*d*
Maternal-fetal status, during labor, 302–309, 306*d*–308*d*
Maternal mortality, 126–127
  anesthesia-related, 312
  due to bleeding, 190
  cultural differences in, 74*t*
  pregnancy-related, 127
Maternal-newborn attachment, 508
  with cesarean birth, 353–354
Maternal-newborn contact, and breast-feeding, 508, 557–558, 557*d*, 562*t*
Maternal physical assessment, in postpartum home care, 649
Maternal role attainment, 468–469
Maternal serum alpha-fetoprotein (MSAFP), 142, 146*t*
  with diabetes, 230*t*
  with multiple gestation, 257, 258
Maternal transfer, 274–276, 275*d*
Maternity Center Association (MCA), 15–16, 16*d*
McRoberts maneuver, 324*f*, 325
Mean arterial pressure (MAP)
  postpartum, 457
  during pregnancy, 140
  in pregnancy-induced hypertension, 179
Measles
  pneumonia due to, 252
  prenatal immunization for, 168, 172
Measurements, of newborn, 513, 514*f*
Meconium
  assessment of, 533*t*
  and jaundice, 564
Meconium aspiration syndrome (MAS), 575–576, 577*f*
  amnioinfusion for, 349–350
Meconium-stained fluid, fetal and neonatal complications of, 497*t*, 504
Medicaid, 3, 4, 12
Medical antishock trousers (MAST suit), for antepartum bleeding, 204–205
Medical history
  in prenatal risk assessment, 131*d*, 132–133
  with substance abuse, 161
Medical record(s), 38–40
  audit of, 27, 28*d*
  confidentiality of, 15
Medical screening examination (MSE), legal issues with, 43
Medicare, 3, 4, 12
Medications
  and breast-feeding, 568, 568*d*
  history of, 163
Melasma, 109
Membranes
  rupture of
    premature, 497*t*
      with multiple gestation, 264
    prolonged, 497*t*
  stripping of
    for cervical ripening, 336
    for induction of labor, 341–342
Men, historical roles of, 54–55
Meningitis, 591
Menstruation
  pseudo-, 533
  return of, 447–448
Mental status, postpartum, 475
Meperidine (Demerol), for labor pain, 433, 434*t*
Mercury, teratogenic effects of, 149*t*
Metabolic changes
  postpartum, 448–449
  during pregnancy, 107–108, 107*t*
Metabolic monitoring, for diabetes, 227–228, 227*t*
Metatarsus adductus, 538, 538*f*, 538*t*
Methadone withdrawal, 593
Methotrexate, teratogenic effects of, 148*t*
Methylergonovine maleate, for postpartum hemorrhage, 199–200, 200*t*, 457
Methyl-prostaglandin $F_{2\alpha}$, for postpartum hemorrhage, 200, 200*t*, 457
Mexican Americans, 75*f*, 78–80
  comparative statistical data on, 74*t*
  core values of, 79
  cultural beliefs and practices of, 79–80
  pregnancy-induced hypertension in, 174*t*
  religious beliefs of, 81
$MgSO_4$. *See* Magnesium sulfate ($MgSO_4$)
Micrognathia, 525*t*
Milia, 517
Milk-based formula, 569
Milk ejection reflex, 552–553
Milk transfer, during breast-feeding, 556–557, 557*d*
Minerals, in breast milk, 554
Minimal variability, in fetal heart rate, 380*t*, 395, 395*t*, 400*t*
Minute ventilation, during pregnancy, 102, 102*t*
Mirror twinning, 255
Miscarriage, 478–479. *See also* Perinatal death
Misoprostol (Cytotec)
  for cervical ripening, 338*d*–339*d*, 340–341
  for induction of labor, 345
Mission, of perinatal team, 60–61, 60*d*
Mistakes, 32–35, 35*d*, 36*d*, 37, 40–41

Moderate variability, in fetal heart rate, 380*t*, 394–395, 400*t*
Mohel, 81
Molar pregnancy, and preeclampsia, 178
Molding, 517, 518*f*
Mongolian slant, of palpebral fissures, 520, 521*t*
Mongolian spots, 82, 517, 517*f*
Monitrices, 422
Monoamniotic twins, 254*t*, 255
Monochorionic twins, 254*t*, 255
Monovular-dispermic twinning, 254, 255
Monozygotic (MZ) twins, 254–255, 254*t*, 256
Montgomery's follicles, 111
Mood disorders, 116–117
Moral and value system, cultural differences in, 72*d*
Moraxella catarrhalis, pneumonia due to, 251, 253*t*
Mormonism, 81, 81*t*
Moro reflex, 523*t*, 548
Morphine, for labor pain, 433, 434*t*
Mother. *See also* Maternal
  readmission of, 652
Mother-baby discharge record, 622*d*
Mottling, in newborn, 516
Mourning, 484
Mouth, of newborn, 504, 524, 524*f*, 525*f*, 526*t*
Movement, for labor pain, 425–427, 425*t*–426*t*
MSAFP (maternal serum alpha-fetoprotein), 142, 146*t*
  with diabetes, 230*t*
  with multiple gestation, 257, 258
MSE (medical screening examination), legal issues with, 43
Mucous membranes, of newborn, 524, 526*t*, 559
Mucous plug, 110
Multicultural health care team, 89*d*
Multidisciplinary practice committee, 6–7, 62–63
Multiple gestation, 253–274
  anemia with, 258
  anesthesia with, 270
  antepartum management of, 257–266, 259*t*–260*t*
  biochemical tests for, 256–257
  birth environment for, 266–268, 267*d*
  bonding and individualization with, 273
  breast-feeding with, 273, 273*f*, 554, 555
  cervical examinations with, 258
  clinical assessment of, 256
  complications of
    antepartum, 260–266
    fetal and newborn, 261–263, 263*d*, 495*t*
    maternal, 263–264, 264*d*
    postpartum, 271
    undiagnosed, 497*t*
  ethical considerations with, 266
  family adjustments to, 257, 271–272
  due to fertility program, 258
  fetal loss with, 260–261, 262*d*
  fetal presentation and method of birth for, 267*d*, 268–270, 268*f*, 269*d*, 270*d*
  fetal surveillance with, 264–266
  follow-up pediatric care and neonatal assessment with, 273
  genetic counseling for, 261
  grief over death in, 274
  higher-order, 270–271
  history of, 254
  home care for, 266
  hospital management of, 266
  identification of, 256–257
  incidence of, 253–254
  intrapartum management of, 266–270
  medical history of, 256
  neonatal intensive care for, 254, 272
  nutritional needs with, 258–260
  physiology of, 254–256, 254*t*, 255*d*
  preeclampsia with, 178
  prenatal education with, 257
  preterm birth with, 207
  psychological aspects of, 257, 258
  resources and support organizations for, 258, 274
  screening for, 256
  separation at discharge with, 272
  significance of, 253–254
  specialized clinics for, 258
  ultrasonography of, 256
  undiagnosed, complications of, 497*t*
  well baby care for, 272
Mumps, prenatal immunization for, 168
Murmur
  in newborn, 529, 529*d*, 531*t*
  during pregnancy, 98
Muscular dystrophy, carrier frequency for, 145*d*
Musculoskeletal system
  of newborn, 505–506, 534–539, 539*t*
  during pregnancy, 110
Music, for labor pain, 431–432
Muslims, 81, 81*t*
Mutual accountability, 56, 59
Mycoplasma pneumoniae, 251, 253*t*
Myocarditis, 235
Myometrium, during labor, 298, 299–300
MZ (monozygotic) twins, 254–255, 254*t*, 256

Nails
  of newborn, 535
  during pregnancy, 109
Nalbuphine (Nubain), for labor pain, 433, 434*t*
Naloxone hydrochloride (Narcan), 433
Narcotics
  for labor pain
    epidural, 434–435, 438*t*
    intrathecal, 438
    parenteral, 432–433, 433*t*, 434*t*
  neonatal withdrawal from, 592–593, 592*d*
Narrative notes, 39, 40
Nasal flaring, 523, 526, 527*t*, 578–579
Nasal stuffiness, during pregnancy, 102
NASS (Neonatal Abstinence Scoring System), 594, 595*f*
National Commission for Certifying Agencies (NCCA), 25
National Council of State Boards Licensing Exam (NCLEX), 23
National Council of State Boards of Nursing (NCSBN), 23
Native Americans, 74*t*, 75*f*, 76
  pregnancy-induced hypertension in, 174*t*
Natural family planning, 467
Natural killer cells, during pregnancy, 111, 111*t*
Nausea, during pregnancy, 105
NCCA (National Commission for Certifying Agencies), 25
NCLEX (National Council of State Boards Licensing Exam), 23
NCSBN (National Council of State Boards of Nursing), 23
Near misses, 37
Neck, of newborn, 504, 524–525, 525*f*, 525*t*
Necrotizing enterocolitis (NEC), bottle-feeding and, 551*t*
Necrotizing fasciitis, postpartum, 459–460
Nedocromil, for asthma, 248
Negligence, 45
Nembutal (pentobarbital), for labor pain, 432
Neonatal Abstinence Scoring System (NASS), 594, 595*f*
Neonatal intensive care unit (NICU)
  and infections, 589–590
  for multiples, 254, 272
Neonatal mortality
  cultural differences in, 74*t*
  preterm delivery and, 126, 126*d*
Neonate. *See* Newborn(s)
Nephropathy, diabetic, 221
Nesacaine (chloroprocaine), epidural anesthesia with, 434
Neural tube defects (NTDs)
  carrier frequency for, 145*d*
  screening for, 146*t*
Neurologic assessment, of newborn, 506, 539–540, 541*t*, 548–549
Neurologic changes
  in postpartum period, 449–450
  during pregnancy, 109
Neuromuscular maturity, of newborn, 546
Neuropathy, diabetic, 221
Nevus flammeus, 516
Nevus simplex, 516–517
Nevus vasculosus, 516
Newborn(s)
  abdomen of, 504, 530–532, 532*f*, 533*t*, 534*f*
  abduction of, 506, 506*t*
  abstinence syndrome in, 591–596
    assessment of, 592–593, 593*t*, 594, 595*f*
    incidence of, 591–592
    interventions for, 593–596, 594*d*
    pathophysiology of, 592, 592*d*
    symptoms of, 592–593, 593*t*
  adaptation to extrauterine life by, 494–511
  Apgar score of, 503
  assessment of, 308*d*, 513–549
    equipment for, 513
    of gestational age, 513–514, 515*f*, 546–547
    in home care, 649–650
    initial, 502–506, 505*f*
    for multiples, 273
    sequence for, 513
    skills used in, 513
    of state, 513, 544–545
  attachment with family of, 508
  back of, 539, 539*f*, 539*t*
  breasts of, 526, 528*f*, 546
  cardiovascular system of, 497–499, 498*f*, 504
  care of
    classes on, 614*d*, 617*d*
    home care assessment for, 650
    learning-needs assessment for, 621, 622*d*
  chest and lungs of, 494–497, 525–528, 527*t*, 528*f*, 528*t*
  circulation of, 498–499
  complications in, 575–608
    intrapartum risk factors and, 497*t*
    maternal risk factors and, 494, 495*t*
    with multiple gestation, 261–263, 263*d*
    recurrent, 496*d*
  congenital heart disease in, 579–582, 580*t*
  crying in, 496, 545
  death of, 479. *See also* Perinatal death
  developmental dysplasia of hip in, 535–538, 536*d*, 536*f*, 537*f*, 539, 539*f*
  developmental reflexes of, 540, 548–549
  ears of, 504, 521–523, 523*t*
    appearance and structure of, 521, 522*f*, 523*t*
    and gestational age, 546–547
    and hearing, 521–523, 522*d*, 523*d*, 523*t*
    position of, 521, 521*f*, 523*t*
  elimination pattern of, 559, 559*t*, 560*t*
  eyes of, 504, 508, 520, 521*t*
  feet of, 535, 538, 538*f*, 538*t*, 539*f*
  fingers and toes of, 539*t*, 540*t*
  genitourinary system of, 506, 532–534, 534*f*, 535*t*, 547
  head of, 504, 517–520, 518*f*–520*f*, 519*t*
  hepatitis B vaccine for, 510–511
  hypoglycemia in, 565–566, 582–584, 582*t*, 583*d*
  identification of, 506–508, 506*t*, 507*d*
  immune system adaptation in, 500–502
  infections in, 587–591
    assessment of, 588–590
    clinical signs of, 590, 591*f*
    diagnosis of, 590
    early-onset, 588, 588*t*
    of eye, 508
    group B beta-hemolytic streptococcal, 508–510, 509*f*, 510*f*, 588, 589*f*, 590*f*
    immune system and, 501–502
    incidence and mortality rates for, 587, 587*t*
    interventions for, 590–591
    late-onset, 588, 588*t*
    pathophysiology of, 587–588, 587*d*, 588*t*, 589*f*
    risk factors for, 588–590, 590*d*
  jaundice in, 584–587
    algorithm for management of, 600–602
    assessment of, 585, 586*d*
    breast-milk, 564–565

clinical manifestations of, *515–516*
early-onset, 564
etiology of, *518t, 584d*
incidence of, 515
in infant of diabetic mother, 220
late-onset, *564–565*
pathologic, *584d,* 585
pathophysiology of, 584–585
phototherapy for, 564, 585–587, *586t*
physiologic, *584d,* 585
risk factors for, *585t*
with vacuum extraction, 348
"less than perfect," 479
measurement of, 513, *514f*
meconium aspiration syndrome in, 575–576, *577f*
mouth of, 504, 524, *524f, 525f, 526t*
musculoskeletal system of, 504–506, 534–539, *539t*
neck of, 504, 524–525, *525f, 525t*
neurologic system of, 506, 539–540, *541t,* 548–549
nose of, 523–524, *523t*
nutrition of. *See* Breast-feeding; Formula feeding
persistent pulmonary hypertension of, 499, 578
physiologic changes in, 494–502
pneumonia in, 528–530, 576–578, *577t*
readmission of, 651–652
respiratory distress in, 527, *528t,* 575–579, *576t*
respiratory system of, 494–497, 504
resuscitation of, 502, *502d, 503f*
joint education programs on, 64
safety of, 506–508, *506t, 507d*
skin of, 504, 514–517, *518t*
color of, 514–516
erythema toxicum of, 517
and gestational age, 546
hemangiomas of, 516, *516f*
milia on, 517
Mongolian spots on, 517, *517f*
nevus simplex of, 516–517
port wine stain of, 516
texture of, 517
turgor of, 517
stabilization of, 502
thermoregulation in, 499–500, *501f, 501t*
transient tachypnea of, 578
transport and return transport of, 596, *596d,* 603–608
umbilical cord care for, 508
vitamin K for, 508
weight gain of, 559
Newborn rash, 517
New York Heart Association functional classification system, 239–240, *240t*
Nicardipine, for preterm labor and birth, 218
Nicotine. *See* Cigarette smoking
Nicotine replacement products, 214
NICU (neonatal intensive care unit)
and infections, 589–590
for multiples, 254, 272
Nifedipine (Procardia), for preterm labor and birth, *216d, 217d,* 218
Nightingale, Florence, 21
Nipple(s)
artificial, 560
inverted, 558–559
during pregnancy, 111, 551
sore, 561–564, *564d, 565t–566t*
supernumerary, 526
Nonreassuring fetal heart rate, 379
evolution of, 402–405, *403f*
interventions for, 391–392
Nonshivering thermogenesis, 499
Nonstress test (NST), 153
with diabetes, *230t*
with multiple gestation, 264–265
Nonverbal communication, 86
Normalization of deviance, 34–35
Normative behavior, cultural differences in, *72d*
Noropin (ropivacaine), epidural anesthesia with, 434
Norplant, 466
Nose, of newborn, 523–524, *523t*
NTDs (neural tube defects)
carrier frequency for, *145d*
screening for, *146t*
Nubain (nalbuphine), for labor pain, 433, *434t*
Nurse(s)
certification of, 23–25, *24d, 25d*
competence validation of, 26–27, *28d*
continuing education of, 27–29
educational preparation of, 25–26
licensure of, 22–23
traditional roles of, 55–56
Nurse practice acts, 23
Nurse-sensitive outcomes, 8–9
Nurse-to-patient ratios, 41–42, *42t*
Nursing. *See* Breast-feeding
Nursing assessments
during labor, 302–310
in postpartum home care, 649–651, 656–663
Nursing conferences, 28
Nursing diagnosis, 30
Nursing practice, perinatal, 22
Nursing research, culturally sensitive, 88–89
Nursing shortage, 16–18
Nutrition. *See also* Diet
in breast milk, 553–554
in formula, 569
during labor, 312–313
with multiple gestation, 258–260
of newborn. *See* Breast-feeding; Formula feeding
postpartum, 452, 475
and preeclampsia, 176
during pregnancy, 107
in prenatal risk assessment, 134–135, *134d, 135d*
and preterm labor and birth, 214, 294
Nutritional assessment and counseling, prenatal, 155
Nutrition therapy, for diabetes, 226
Nystagmus, 520

OAE (otoacoustic emissions), 522
Obesity
bottle feeding and, *551t*
cultural differences in, 82
fetal and neonatal complications with, *495t*
during pregnancy, 107
Obsessive-compulsive disorder (OCD), postpartum, 123
Obstetric history
in prenatal risk assessment, *131d,* 132–133
with substance abuse, 161
Obstetric status, in prenatal risk assessment, *131d,* 138
OCT (oxytocin challenge test), 153–154
Oculomotor nerve, assessment of, *541t*
Office of Inspector General (OIG), 12
OGTT (oral glucose tolerance test), 141, 233–234, *234t*
Olfactory cravings, 135
Oligohydramnios
fetal and neonatal complications of, *497t*
in preeclampsia, *182t*
Oliguria, in preeclampsia, *184d*
Omphalitis, *533t*
Omphalocele, *533t*
Omphalomesenteric duct, *533t*
Open-glottis pushing, 319–321, 403
Opioids
for labor pain
epidural, 434–435, *438t*
intrathecal, 438
parenteral, 432–433, *433t, 434t*
neonatal withdrawal from, 592–593, *592d*
Opium, diluted tincture of, for neonatal abstinence syndrome, 594
Optic nerve, assessment of, *541t*
Oral contraceptives, 466
Oral glucose tolerance test (OGTT), 141, 233–234, *234t*
Oral hypoglycemic agents, 228
Oral intake, during labor, 312–313
Organizational discipline, 59
Organizational structure, and teamwork, 56
Organization-focused outcomes, 9
Organization of Teratology Information Services, 134
Orthodox Jews, 81, *81t*
Orthostatic hypotension, postpartum, 449
Ortolani maneuver, 536, *536f*
Otitis media, bottle-feeding and, *551t,* 570
Otoacoustic emissions (OAE), 522
Outcome(s)
accreditation and certification of healthcare organizations and, 11–13
effect of downsizing, re-engineering, and decreased resources on, 9–10
monitoring of, 8–13
nurse-sensitive, 8–9
organization-focused, 9
patient-focused, 9
provider-focused, 9
realistic goals for, 10–11
Ovarian function
postpartum, 447–448
during pregnancy, 110
Overshoot, 402
Over-the-counter medications, history of, 163
OxiFirst, 406–408, *407f, 408f*
Oxygen administration
for diabetic ketoacidosis, 231, *232t*
for newborn, 579
for nonreassuring fetal heart rate, 391
for pneumonia, 252
Oxygen consumption, during pregnancy, 102
"Oxygen debt," postpartum, 451
Oxygen saturation
with antepartum bleeding, 202–203
fetal, 406–408, *407f, 408f*
with oxytocin induction, 344
Oxygen status, maternal, and fetal heart rate, 385
Oxygen transfer, maternal-fetal, 385–387, *386f, 387d*
Oxytocin, 109
audit of, *28d*
for augmentation of labor, 345
complications of, *497t*
for induction of labor, *339d,* 343–344
after cervical ripening with misoprostol, 341
during labor, 299–300, *299d*
in lactation, 552–553
for postpartum hemorrhage, 199, *200t,* 457
Oxytocin challenge test (OCT), 153–154

Pacific Islanders, *74t, 75f,* 76–78
pregnancy-induced hypertension in, 173–174, *174t*
Pacifiers, 560
Packed red blood cells, for antepartum bleeding, 202, *203t*
$PaCO_2$
postpartum, 451
during pregnancy, 102, *102t*
PACs (premature atrial contractions), fetal, 401
PACU. *See* Postanesthesia care unit (PACU)
Pain
labor. *See* Labor pain
nipple, 561–564, *564d, 565t–566t*
postpartum, 454–455
Pain tolerance, 423
Palate, cleft, 524, *525f, 526t*
Pallor, in newborn, *518t*
Palmar erythema, during pregnancy, 109
Palmar grasp reflex, 549
Palm oil, in formula, and constipation, 570–571
Palpebral fissures, Mongolian slant of, 520, *521t*
Pancreas, during pregnancy, 107–108
Panic disorder, postpartum, 123

PaO_2
postpartum, 451
during pregnancy, 102, 102*t*
Paracervical block, 439
Paramethadione, teratogenic effects of, 150*t*
Parasympathetic nervous system, 238, 239*d*
in fetal heart rate, 387, 388*d*
Parathyroid glands, during pregnancy, 108
Parathyroid hormone (PTH), during pregnancy, 108
Paregoric, for neonatal abstinence syndrome, 594
Parenthood, transition to, 468–470, 469*d*–470*d*
Parenting pathway, 626–627, 633–642
Parenting style, cultural assessment of, 138
Paresthesia, during pregnancy, 109
Parity
and labor progression, 300–301, 302*f*
and preeclampsia, 177
Participation, in teamwork, 60, 60*d*
Partner, labor support by, 421–422, 422*d*
Patent ductus arteriosus (PDA), 580*t*, 581
Patient assessment, *vs.* data collection, 30
Patient database, prenatal, 612
Patient education
on asthma, 246–247
on breast-feeding, 157, 554, 617*d*
on childbirth preparation, 157, 612–613, 614*d*–617*d*
culturally appropriate material for, 86, 86*d*
on diabetes, 225–226, 225*d*, 226*d*
on fetal heart rate monitoring, 409
on insulin therapy, 228–229, 228*d*, 229*d*
learning-needs assessment for, 620–623, 622*d*
methods and materials for, 618
on multiple gestation, 257
postpartum, 464–467
prenatal, 155–157, 156*d*
role of staff nurse in, 625–626
Patient-focused outcomes, 9
Patient records. *See* Medical record(s)
Patient rights, 15–16, 16*d*
Patient satisfaction, 13–14
with home care services, 652, 665
Patterned breathing, for labor pain, 431
PDA (patent ductus arteriosus), 580*t*, 581
Pediatric care, for multiples, 273
Pelvic floor, postpartum, 447, 474
Pelvic-floor exercises, 465
Penis, of newborn, 533, 535*t*
Pentobarbital (Nembutal), for labor pain, 432
Percutaneous umbilical blood sampling (PUBS), 144, 146*t*
Perinatal death, 476–491
bereavement with
nursing assessment of, 485
nursing interventions for, 486–487, 487*t*–489*t*
nursing management of, 481*t*, 485–490
ontologic perspective on, 485
sociologic perspective on, 483–484
spiritual perspective on, 484–485
stages of, 476, 477*d*
support groups for, 485, 486*d*, 490
grief over
acute, 480, 481*t*
anticipatory, 479, 480
behaviors caused by, 481*t*
chronic, 482, 482*d*
duration of, 483
psychological perspective on, 480–483
resolution of, 482–483
types of, 480–482, 482*d*
healing the healer in, 490
loss in, 476–480
causes of, 478–480
perceptions of, 477–478
types of, 476–477, 478*t*
mourning over, 484
of multiples, 274
rites of passage for, 483–484
Perinatal home care services. *See* Home care management, postpartum
Perinatal nursing practice, 22
Perinatal practice committee, 6–7
Perineal care
during birth, 326–328, 328*d*
postpartum, 455
Perineal edema, ice pack for, 454
Perineal hygiene, during vaginal examinations, 310
Perineal lacerations, 326–327, 328*d*
Perineal massage, 327–328
Perineal nerve damage, during pushing, 315
Perineum, postpartum, 447, 474
Peripheral pulses, of newborn, 529, 531*t*
Peripheral vascular resistance, in preeclampsia, 180*t*, 181*t*
Persistent pulmonary hypertension of the newborn (PPHN), 499, 578
Personal stage, in transition to parenthood, 468
Personnel issues, 16–18
Petechiae, in newborn, 516, 518*t*
PGE (prostaglandin E), for postpartum hemorrhage, 200*t*
PGE_1 (prostaglandin E_1)
for cervical ripening, 338*d*–339*d*, 340–341
for induction of labor, 345
PGE_2 (prostaglandin E_2), for cervical ripening, 97, 336–340, 338*d*
$PGF_{2\alpha}$ (prostaglandin $F_{2\alpha}$), for postpartum hemorrhage, 200, 200*t*, 457
pH, during pregnancy, 102*t*
Phenergan (promethazine hydrochloride), for labor pain, 432
Phenobarbital, for neonatal abstinence syndrome, 594
Phenylephrine, for maternal cardiac disease, 242
Phenytoin (Dilantin)
for preeclampsia, 188–189
teratogenic effects of, 149*t*
Philosophy
of care, 62, 63*d*
unit, 6
Phimosis, 534
Phototherapy, 564, 585–587, 586*t*
home, 652
Physical activity, in prenatal risk assessment, 136
Physical appearance, with substance abuse, 162
Physical assessment
of newborn. *See* Newborn(s), assessment of
in postpartum home care, 649–650
in prenatal risk assessment, 138
Physical maturity, of newborn, 546–547
Physical status, postpartum, 455–456
Physician(s), traditional roles of, 55–56
Physician–nurse relationship, factors affecting, 54–58, 54*d*
Physiologic anemia of pregnancy, 99
Physiologic intervention, 391
Physiologic positions, during labor, 316*f*
PI (pulsatility index), 265
Pica, 75, 135
PIH. *See* Pregnancy-induced hypertension (PIH)
Pillows, during labor, 427
Pilonidal dimple, 539, 539*f*
Pinna, 521
Pituitary glands, during pregnancy, 108–109
Placenta
abnormal adherence of, 191, 195–196, 196*f*
cultural differences in disposal of, 72
in immune system, 111–112
and lactogenesis, 552
low-lying, 192, 193*f*
premature separation of. *See* Abruptio placentae
Placenta accreta, 191, 196, 196*f*
Placenta increta, 196, 196*f*
Placental abruption. *See* Abruptio placentae
Placental blood flow, 110
and fetal heart rate, 385–387, 386*f*, 387*d*
Placental insufficiency, fetal and neonatal complications of, 497*t*
Placental lactogen, 551
Placental migration, 192
Placental site, postpartum, 447
Placenta percreta, 196, 196*f*
Placenta previa, 192–193
clinical manifestations of, 192
defined, 192
diagnosis of, 192–193
factors associated with, 192, 192*d*
fetal and neonatal complications of, 497*t*
incidence of, 190–191
management of, 193
with multiple gestation, 264
partial, 192, 193*f*
total, 192, 193*f*
Placentation, in multiple gestations, 255–256
Plague, prenatal immunization for, 169
Plan of care, for home care services, 648–649
Plantar creases, 546
Plasma, fresh-frozen, for antepartum bleeding, 202, 203*t*
Plasma volume
postpartum, 450
in preeclampsia, 179, 180*t*
during pregnancy, 98*t*, 99
Platelet concentrate, for antepartum bleeding, 202, 203*t*
Platelet counts
in preeclampsia, 180*t*, 184*d*
during pregnancy, 101, 101*t*
Platelet dysfunction, in preeclampsia, 182*t*
Plethora, in newborn, 518*t*
Plugged duct, 567
PMI (point of maximal impulse), 528–529
Pneumococcus, prenatal immunization for, 170
Pneumocystis carinii pneumonia, 253*t*
Pneumonia
in newborn, 528–530, 576–578, 577*t*
in pregnancy, 249–253
aspiration, 251, 253
bacterial, 251
causes of, 250, 250*d*
clinical manifestations of, 251–252
defined, 250
nursing assessment of, 252
nursing interventions for, 252
pathophysiology of, 250–251
pharmacologic therapy for, 252–253, 253*t*
significance and incidence of, 249–250
varicella, 250, 251–253
viral, 251–252
Pneumonitis, in meconium aspiration syndrome, 576, 577*f*
Point of maximal impulse (PMI), 528–529
Polar body twinning, 254, 255
Policies, institutional, 37–38
Poliomyelitis, prenatal immunization for, 168
Polycythemia, due to diabetes, 220
Polydactyly, 539*t*, 540*t*
Polyhydramnios
fetal and neonatal complications of, 497*t*
with multiple gestation, 264
in twin-to-twin transfusion syndrome, 262–263
Popliteal angle, 546
Port wine stain, 516
Positioning
for antepartum bleeding, 202
for breast-feeding, 554–555, 555*f*, 556*f*
with reluctant nurser, 562*t*
with sore nipples, 565*t*, 566*t*
and cardiac output, 99
for formula feeding, 570
for labor and birth, 313–314, 316*f*–318*f*, 320*d*
and episiotomy, 327
for labor pain, 425–427, 425*t*–426*t*
for nonreassuring fetal heart rate, 391
Postanesthesia care unit (PACU)
discharge from, 353, 353*f*, 375
equipment in, 355*d*
standards for care in, 351–353, 352*d*, 354*d*
Postdischarge follow-up, 611, 627–630, 628*d*–629*d*
Postpartum depression (PPD), 123, 468
predisposing factors for, 137*d*
Postpartum hemorrhage, 198–200, 456–458
causes of, 191, 199, 199*d*, 452*d*
defined, 198, 456
early, 199, 452*d*, 456
hematologic changes due to, 450–451

incidence of, 191, 456
late, 199, 452*d*
management of, 199–200, 200*t*, 201*f*, 456*d*, 457–458
with multiple gestation, 271
risk factors for, 456–457
due to uterine inversion, 198, 198*d*
Postpartum period, 446–475
acid–base changes in, 451
activity in, 475
adaptations during, 121–123, 122*d*
anal sphincter damage in, 452–453
anatomic and physiologic changes during, 446–453
with antepartum bed rest, 464
anxiety disorders in, 123
bladder in, 449
breasts in, 474
cardiovascular system in, 450, 475
care paths for, 637–642
cervix in, 447
after cesarean birth, 463–464, 474
complications during, 456–463
clinical signs and symptoms of, 464*d*
with multiple gestation, 271
contraception in, 466–467
daily assessments and interventions for, 474–475
depression in, 123, 468
predisposing factors for, 137*d*
diabetes management in, 233–235, 234*d*
education in, 464–467
elimination in, 475
emotional status in, 475
exercise in, 465
fatigue in, 449–450, 468
fluid balance and electrolytes in, 449, 453
follow-up in, 611, 627–630, 628*d*–629*d*
gastrointestinal changes in, 452
hematologic changes in, 450–451
hemodynamic changes in, 450
hemorrhage during. *See* Postpartum hemorrhage
hernias in, 452
home care services in, 643–665
benefits of, 644–645
discharge criteria and, 646–647, 647*d*
early discharge and, 643–644
environmental assessment in, 651
essential components of, 646–649, 647*d*, 648*d*
interpreter for, 648
learning-needs assessment in, 650
maternal assessment in, 649, 650, 661
models of, 645–646
newborn assessment in, 649–650, 663
nurse providers of, 652–653
nursing assessments in, 649–651, 656–663
nursing interventions in, 651
orientation and education for, 652–653
outcome monitoring and quality care with, 651–652, 652*d*, 665
personal safety in, 653
physical assessment in, 649–650
plan of care for, 648–649
psychosocial assessment in, 650
recommendations on, 645, 646*d*
referral for, 647–648, 648*d*, 657
review of literature on, 643–645
schedule for, 648
telephone assessment for, 659
hygiene in, 475
immediate, 453–454, 454*f*
infections in, 458–461
kidneys in, 449
learning-needs assessment in, 464–465
liver changes in, 451
lochia in, 447, 448*t*, 474
maternal-fetal assessment during, 308*d*
mental status in, 475
metabolic changes in, 448–449
muscles in, 451
neurologic changes in, 449–450
nursing care in, 453–456
nutritional needs in, 453, 475
observation in, 375
ovarian function in, 447–448
pain management in, 454–455
pelvic-floor exercises in, 465
pelvic floor (perineum) in, 447, 474
physical status in, 455–456
placental site in, 447
psychosis in, 123
psychosocial status in, 455
recovery from anesthesia during, 351–353, 352*d*, 353*f*, 354*d*, 355*d*, 375
respiratory changes in, 451
sexuality in, 465–466, 465*d*
skin in, 451, 474
stress incontinence in, 449
stressors in, 468
thrombophlebitis and thromboembolism in, 461–463
transition to parenthood in, 468–470, 469*d*–470*d*
uterine involution in, 446–447, 447*d*, 474
vagina in, 447
weight changes in, 451
Posture, of newborn, 540, 546
Potassium, serum, during pregnancy, 103–104
PPD (postpartum depression), 123, 468
predisposing factors for, 137*d*
PPHN (persistent pulmonary hypertension of the newborn), 499, 578
PPROM (preterm premature rupture of the membranes), with multiple gestation, 264
Practice bulletins, 31–32
Practice changes, 63
Practice committee, multidisciplinary, 6–7, 62–63
Practice guidelines, 31–32, 35–37
Preauricular sinus, 521, 522*f*, 523*t*
Preauricular skin tags, 521, 522*f*, 523*t*
Precipitous birth, complications of, 497*t*
Precordium, of newborn, 528, 531*t*
Preeclampsia
activity restriction for, 185
by age, 174–175, 175*t*
antepartum management of, 185, 186*t*
chronic hypertension and, 177–178
cigarette smoking and, 176
clinical manifestations of, 179–183
colloids in, 184–185
complications of, 184*d*
defined, 178
differential diagnosis of, 183
diuretics in, 184–185
expedition of birth for, 186*t*
family history of, 177
fetal hydrops and, 178
genetic basis for, 177
gestational age at first prenatal visit and, 177
gravidity and parity and, 177
home care management of, 183, 292–293
hydatiform mole and, 178
incidence of, 173–174, 174*t*, 175*t*
inpatient management of, 183–184
laboratory tests for, 187–188, 188*d*
on labor flow sheet, 373
mild *vs.* severe, 183, 184*d*
morbidity and mortality from, 174
with multiple gestation, 178, 263–264
nursing assessment and interventions for, 183–189
nutrition and, 176
ongoing assessment for, 185–187
pathophysiology of, 178–179, 180*t*–182*t*, 183*f*
pharmacologic therapies for, 188–189
postpartum management of, 189
pregnancy complications and, 178
by race, 173–174, 174*t*, 175
risk factors for, 174–178, 176*d*
socioeconomic status and, 175–176
urinary tract infection and, 178
Preference plan, 618–620, 619*d*–620*d*
Pregnancy
adaptations during, 117–120, 117*d*, 118*d*, 120*d*
bleeding during, 190–206
due to abnormal placental implantation, 195–196, 196*f*
due to abruptio placentae, 193–195, 194*d*, 194*f*
hemorrhagic and hypovolemic shock due to, 205–206, 205*d*
home care management of, 203, 293–294
inpatient management of, 203–206
nursing assessment of, 200–203, 202*d*, 203*t*
nursing interventions for, 203–206
due to placenta previa, 192–193, 192*d*, 193*f*
significance and incidence of, 190–191
due to uterine rupture, 197–198, 197*d*
due to vasa previa, 196–197, 197*d*
cardiac disease during, 235–255
activity with, 296
clinical management of, 242–243, 242*t*, 243*t*
diet for, 296
heparin therapy for, 295, 296
home care management of, 295–296
nursing assessment of, 240–242, 241*d*
physiology and terminology related to, 237–238, 237*d*, 238*f*, 239*d*
risk factor assessment and counseling for, 239–240, 240*d*, 241*t*
significance and incidence of, 235–237, 236*t*, 237*d*
cardiovascular system during, 98–101, 98*t*, 100*t*, 101*t*
care paths for, 634–635
diabetes during, 219–235
ambulatory and home care management of, 225–230, 294–295
classification of, 221
clinical manifestations of, 224–225
diabetic ketoacidosis due to, 222, 224–225, 231, 232*t*
elective delivery with, 230*t*, 233
exercise therapy for, 226, 227*d*
fetal assessment for, 230, 230*t*
inpatient management of, 231
insulin therapy for, 108, 228–229, 228*d*, 229*d*
intrapartum management of, 231–233, 233*d*
metabolic monitoring for, 227–228, 227*d*
nursing assessments and interventions for, 225
nutrition therapy for, 226
pathophysiology of, 222–223
patient education for, 225, 225*d*
pharmacologic therapy for, 228–229, 228*d*, 229*d*
postpartum management of, 233–234
screening for, 107–108, 141, 223–224, 223*d*
sick day management for, 228–229, 229*d*, 295
significance and incidence of, 219–221
type 1, 221
type 2, 221–222
diabetogenic state of, 107, 222
ectopic, 479–480
endocrine system during, 108–109
gastrointestinal system during, 105–106, 106*t*
hospital admission during, 303, 306*d*
host defense and immunity during, 111–112, 111*t*
hypertension in, 173–190
activity restriction for, 185
by age, 174–175, 175*t*
antepartum management of, 185, 186*t*
chronic, 175*t*, 177–178
cigarette smoking and, 176
clinical manifestations of, 179–183
colloids in, 184–185
complications of, 184*d*
defined, 179
with diabetes, 221

Pregnancy (*continued*)
hypertension in (*continued*)
differential diagnosis of, 183
diuretics in, 184–185
eclampsia, 178, 189–190
expedition of birth for, 186*t*
family history of, 177
fetal hydrops and, 178
genetic basis for, 177
gestational age at first prenatal visit and, 177
gravidity and parity and, 177
HELLP syndrome, 178, 189
home care management of, 183, 292–293
hydatiform mole and, 178
incidence of, 173–174, 174*t*, 175*t*
inpatient management of, 183–184
laboratory tests for, 187–188, 188*d*
mild *vs.* severe, 183, 184*d*
morbidity and mortality from, 174
with multiple gestation, 178, 263–264
nursing assessment and interventions for, 183–189
nutrition and, 176
ongoing assessment for, 185–187
pathophysiology of, 178–179, 180*t*–182*t*, 183*f*
pharmacologic therapies for, 188–189
postpartum management of, 189
preeclampsia, 178–179, 183–189
pregnancy complications and, 178
pregnancy-induced, 178, 179–183
by race, 173–174, 174*t*, 175
risk factors for, 174–178, 176*d*
socioeconomic status and, 175–176
transient, 178
urinary tract infection and, 178
immunization during, 168–172
integumentary system during, 109
mask of, 109
metabolic changes during, 107–108, 107*t*
musculoskeletal system during, 110
neurologic system during, 109
physiologic anemia of, 99
physiologic hydronephrosis and hydroureter of, 103
prolonged, and fetal and neonatal complications, 495*t*
pulmonary complications of, 243–253
asthma, 244–249, 245*d*, 245*t*, 246*d*
pneumonia, 249–253, 250*d*, 253*t*
renal system during, 103–105, 104*t*, 105*t*
reproductive hormonal changes during, 96–98
reproductive system during, 110–111
respiratory system during, 101–102, 102*t*
trauma during, 206
Pregnancy and Related Conditions performance set, 12
Pregnancy-associated maternal death, 127
Pregnancy-induced hypertension (PIH), 178, 179–183. *See also* Pregnancy, hypertension in
defined, 178
family history of, 177
fetal and neonatal complications of, 495*t*
significance and incidence of, 173–174, 174*t*, 175*t*
Pregnancy mortality rate, 127
Pregnancy mortality ratio, 127
Pregnancy-related maternal death, 127
Pregnancy status
in prenatal risk assessment, 131*d*, 138
with substance abuse, 161
Preload, 237*d*
with maternal cardiac disease, 242, 242*t*
Premature atrial contractions (PACs), fetal, 401
Premature rupture of membranes, 497*t*
with multiple gestation, 264
Premature ventricular contractions (PVCs), fetal, 401
Prematurity. *See* Preterm labor and birth
Prenatal care
access to, 127–129
adequate, 129–130
for asthma, 249
biochemical evaluation in, 139*d*, 140–141, 141*t*, 142
and birth outcome, 129–130
case management in, 154–157
cultural differences in, 74*t*, 127
decision to seek, 128
education and counseling in, 155–157, 156*d*
on breast-feeding, 554
health promotion in, 157–158
initial visit in, 130–138, 139*d*
late, 127, 129–130
and preeclampsia, 177
for multiple gestation, 257–266, 259*t*–260*t*
nursing interventions in, 154
nutrition in, 155
ongoing, 138–147, 139*d*–140*d*
for preeclampsia, 185, 186*t*
schedule of, 130, 139*d*–140*d*
with multiple gestation, 258
selection of provider for, 128–129
social services in, 155
social trends affecting, 126
Prenatal classes, 157, 612–613, 614*d*–617*d*
Prenatal diagnosis, 142–147, 146*t*
alpha-fetoprotein in, 142, 146*t*
amniocentesis for, 142, 146*t*
biochemical markers for, 144–147
carrier screening in, 146*t*
chorionic villus sampling for, 143, 146*t*
double and triple marker screening in, 142, 146*t*
fetal blood sampling for, 144, 146*t*
indications for, 142, 145*d*
ultrasonography for, 143–144
Prenatal patient database, 612
Prenatal risk assessment, 130–147, 131*d*–132*d*
abuse in, 136, 166
alpha-fetoprotein in, 142, 146*t*
amniocentesis in, 142, 146*t*
biochemical evaluation in, 139*d*, 140–141, 141*t*, 142
biochemical markers in, 144–147
biophysical profile in, 154
blood pressure in, 140
carrier screening in, 146*t*
chorionic villus sampling in, 143, 146*t*
cigarette smoking in, 135
contraction stress test in, 153–154
cultural factors in, 137–138
current obstetric status in, 131*d*, 138
demographic factors in, 132*d*, 133
double and triple marker screening in, 142, 146*t*
fetal activity in, 152–153
fetal blood sampling in, 144, 146*t*
fetal development in, 147, 152*d*
fetal surveillance in, 140, 147–154, 153*d*
for genetic disorders, 142, 143*d*, 144*f*, 145*d*, 146*t*
initial prenatal visit in, 130–138, 139*d*
lifestyle factors in, 132*d*, 133–137, 137*d*
medical and obstetric history in, 131*d*, 132–133
nonstress test in, 153
nutrition in, 134–135, 134*d*, 135*d*
ongoing prenatal care in, 138–147, 139*d*–140*d*
physical activity in, 136
physical examination in, 138
prenatal diagnostic evaluation in, 142–147, 145*d*, 146*t*
psychosocial factors in, 132*d*, 133, 136–137, 137*d*
stress in, 136
substance abuse in, 135–136, 161–163
for teratogens, 147, 148*t*–151*t*
ultrasonography in, 143–144
weight gain in, 135, 135*d*
Prepared childbirth
class curriculum for, 614*d*
and labor pain, 422–423, 423*f*
Prepidil, for cervical ripening, 336, 337, 338*d*
Prepuce, 533–534
Prescription medications, history of, 163
Presentation
abnormal, fetal and neonatal complications of, 497*t*
Leopold maneuver for, 311*f*, 497*t*
with multiple gestation, 267*d*, 268–270, 268*f*, 269*d*, 270*d*
Preterm labor and birth, 207–219
bed rest for, 214
beta-mimetics for, 216*d*, 217*d*, 218
biochemical markers for, 144–147, 209–210
cervical length assessment for, 210
clinical manifestations and nursing assessment of, 211
costs of, 207
cultural differences in, 74*t*
definitions for, 207–208
due to diabetic ketoacidosis, 231
diet and, 214, 294
drug withdrawal with, 593
glucocorticoid administration for, 219
history of, 208–209
home care management of, 214–215, 215*d*, 294
home uterine activity monitoring for, 214–215
incidence of, 207
indomethacin for, 216*d*, 217*d*, 218–219
infant mortality with, 207, 208
due to infection, 211
intravenous hydration for, 215
lifestyle modification for, 212–214
magnesium sulfate for, 216*d*, 217*d*, 218
with multiple gestations, 207
and neonatal mortality, 126, 126*d*
nifedipine for, 216*d*, 217*d*, 218
pathophysiology and causes of, 210–211
patient education for, 211–212
in preeclampsia, 182*t*
prevention of, 211–219
racial differences in, 209
risk factors for, 208–210, 208*d*
screening for, 209–210
signs and symptoms of, 211–212
smoking cessation for, 213–214
tocolytic therapy for, 215–219, 216*d*, 217*d*
weight gain and, 214
Preterm premature rupture of the membranes (PPROM), with multiple gestation, 264
Privacy, right to, 15
Procardia (nifedipine), for preterm labor and birth, 216*d*, 217*d*, 218
Procedures, institutional, 37–38
Professional issues, 22–29
certification, 23–25, 24*d*, 25*d*
competence validation, 26–27, 28*d*
continuing education, 27–29
educational preparation, 25–26
licensure, 22–23
perinatal nursing practice, 22
Professional liability, 31–32, 33*d*
Professional liability insurance, 45–47
Professional organizations, 7–8, 8*d*
Professional standards, 7–8, 8*d*
Progestasert, 467
Progesterone
in lactation, 551
in onset of labor, 299, 299*d*
during pregnancy, 97
Program evaluation, 630
Projections, 116
Prolactin
in lactation, 551, 552
in postpartum period, 448
during pregnancy, 97–98
Prolonged decelerations, 380*t*, 397*f*, 398–399, 399*t*
Prolonged pregnancy, fetal and neonatal complications with, 495*t*
Prolonged rupture of membranes, 497*t*
Promethazine hydrochloride (Phenergan), for labor pain, 432
Propiomazine (Largon), for labor pain, 432
Prostaglandin(s)
during labor, 97

in onset of labor, 299, 299*d*
during pregnancy, 97
Prostaglandin E (PGE), for postpartum hemorrhage, 200*t*
Prostaglandin E_1 (PGE_1)
for cervical ripening, 338*d*–339*d*, 340–341
for induction of labor, 345
Prostaglandin E_2 (PGE_2), for cervical ripening, 97, 336–340, 338*d*
Prostaglandin $F_{2\_}$ ($PGF_{2\_}$), for postpartum hemorrhage, 200, 200*t*, 457
Prostaglandin inhibitors, for preterm labor and birth, 216*d*, 217*d*, 218–219
Protein
in breast milk, 553–554
in formula, 569
Proteinuria
in postpartum period, 449
in preeclampsia, 179–180, 181*t*, 184*d*, 187
during pregnancy, 105
Prothrombin time, during pregnancy, 101*t*, 106*t*
Protocols, institutional, 37–38
Provider-focused outcomes, 9
Proximate cause, 31, 32, 51
Prune belly syndrome, 533*t*, 534*f*
Pseudoephedrine, for asthma, 249
Pseudomenstruation, 533
Pseudosinusoidal fetal heart rate pattern, 400
Psyche, impact on childbirth of, 328–329
Psychological aspects, of multiple gestation, 257, 258
Psychosis, postpartum, 123
Psychosocial adaptation, 115–123
assessment of, 115–116, 116*d*
collaborative care and referral for, 116–117
during labor and birth, 120–121, 121*d*
in postpartum period, 121–123, 122*d*, 455
during pregnancy, 117–120, 117*d*, 118*d*, 120*d*
Psychosocial assessment
in postpartum home care, 650
in prenatal risk assessment, 132*d*, 133, 136–137, 137*d*
Psychosocial history, with substance abuse, 161–162
PTH (parathyroid hormone), during pregnancy, 108
PUBS (percutaneous umbilical blood sampling), 144, 146*t*
Pudendal block, 434, 435*f*
Puerperal infections, 458–461
Puerto Ricans, pregnancy-induced hypertension in, 174*t*
Pulmonary blood flow, in newborn, 496
Pulmonary complications, of pregnancy, 243–253
asthma, 244–249, 245*d*, 245*t*, 246*d*
pneumonia, 249–253, 250*d*, 253*t*
Pulmonary embolism, postpartum, 461–463
Pulmonary vascular resistance (PVR)
of fetus *vs.* newborn, 496, 498, 499, 578
during pregnancy, 100
Pulsatility index (PI), 265
Pulse(s)
with multiple gestation, 259*t*
of newborn, 504, 529, 531*t*
postpartum, 450, 453–454
Pulse oximetry, fetal, 406–408, 407*f*, 408*f*
Pupils, 520, 521*t*, 541*t*
Purpose statements, unit, 6
Purpura
idiopathic thrombocytopenic, fetal and neonatal complications with, 495*t*
in newborn, 518*t*
Pushing, 314–322, 319*f*, 320*d*–321*d*
and fetal heart rate, 403, 404*f*
Pustules, in newborn, 518*t*
PVCs (premature ventricular contractions), fetal, 401
PVR (pulmonary vascular resistance)
of fetus *vs.* newborn, 496, 498, 499, 578
during pregnancy, 100
Pyelonephritis, postpartum, 461

Quality of care, 2–18
accreditation and certification of healthcare organizations in, 11–13
benchmarking in, 11
cost containment *vs.* cost consciousness in, 4–5
downsizing, re-engineering, and decreased resources in, 9–10
economics and, 2–4
evidence-based practice and, 5–7, 5*d*, 7*d*
outcome monitoring in, 8–13
patient rights in, 15–16, 16*d*
patient satisfaction in, 13–14
personnel issues in, 16–18
regulatory agencies and professional standards in, 7–8, 8*d*
service excellence in, 13–16
Quality of service, 8
Quiet alert state, of newborn, 545

Rabies, prenatal immunization for, 169, 171
Racial differences. *See also* Cultural differences
in multiple gestation, 254
in pregnancy-induced hypertension, 173–174, 174*t*, 175
in preterm labor and birth, 209
Radiation, teratogenic effects of, 151*t*
Radiation heat loss, 500, 501*t*
Rales, 527
Rash, newborn, 517
RBC(s) (red blood cells), packed, for antepartum bleeding, 202, 203*t*
RBC (red blood cell) volume, during pregnancy, 98*t*, 99, 100
RDS (respiratory distress syndrome), 575
in infant of diabetic mother, 220–221
Readmission, 651–652
Reality vaginal pouch, 467
Rebolus, 439
Recertification, 24–25
Records, medical. *See* Medical record(s)
Rectocele, 452
Rectus muscles, diastasis of, 451
Recumbency, for labor and birth, 313, 314
Red blood cell(s) (RBCs), packed, for antepartum bleeding, 202, 203*t*
Red blood cell (RBC) volume, during pregnancy, 98*t*, 99, 100
Red cell mass, in preeclampsia, 180*t*
Red reflex, 520
Re-engineering, 9–10
Referral, for home care services, 647–648, 648*d*, 657
Reflectance meter, 227
Reflexes, developmental, 540, 548–549
Refugees, 80
Regional anesthesia and analgesia, 434–442
delayed pushing with, 321–322
epidural, 434–438
intrathecal, 438
by local infiltration, 434
maternal and fetal assessment with, 307*d*–308*d*, 440*d*
nursing guidelines for, 438–439, 440*d*
nursing interventions with, 438–439, 440*d*, 440*t*–442*t*
paracervical block for, 439
and position for labor and birth, 314
by pudendal block, 434, 435*f*
by saddle block, 439–442
Registered nurse, labor support by, 419–421, 420*d*
Regulatory agencies, 7–8
Rehydration, for diabetic ketoacidosis, 231, 232*t*
Reintegration, in bereavement, 477*d*
Relaxation, for labor pain, 430, 431*d*
Relaxin, during pregnancy, 97
Religious influences, cultural assessment of, 138
Religious women, deeply, 81, 81*t*
Relinquishment, for adoption, 479
Reluctant nurser, 561, 561*d*, 562*t*–563*t*
Renal clearance, during pregnancy, 103, 104*t*
Renal failure, due to antepartum bleeding, 204
Renal function
with maternal cardiac disease, 241
of newborn, 531, 532*f*
in postpartum period, 449
in preeclampsia, 180*t*, 181*t*
during pregnancy, 103–105, 104*t*, 105*t*
Renal insufficiency, fetal and neonatal complications of, 495*t*
Renal plasma flow (RPF)
in preeclampsia, 180*t*
during pregnancy, 103
Renin
in postpartum period, 448
during pregnancy, 104, 109
Renin-angiotensin-aldosterone system, in preeclampsia, 180*t*
Reproductive hormonal changes, during pregnancy, 96–98
Reproductive system, during pregnancy, 110–111
Residual volume, during pregnancy, 101–102, 102*t*
Resistance index (RI), 265
Resources
decreased, 9–10
for multiple gestation, 258, 274
Respiration, with multiple gestation, 259*t*
Respiratory complications, of pregnancy, 243–253
asthma, 244–249, 245*d*, 245*t*, 246*d*
pneumonia, 249–253, 250*d*, 253*t*
Respiratory distress, in newborn, 527, 528*t*, 575–579, 576*t*
Respiratory distress syndrome (RDS), 575
in infant of diabetic mother, 220–221
Respiratory rate
of newborn, 525
during pregnancy, 102*t*
Respiratory system
with maternal cardiac disease, 241
of newborn, 494–497, 504, 525–528, 527*t*, 528*f*, 528*t*
postpartum, 451
during pregnancy, 101–102, 102*t*
Responsibility, 29–31
Resting, adaptive and maladaptive behaviors for, 469*d*
Restraint, 15
Restructuring, 9–10
Resuscitation
fluid
for abruption placentae, 195
for diabetic ketoacidosis, 231, 232*t*
neonatal, 502, 502*d*, 503*f*
joint educational programs on, 64
in utero, 391
Retinoids, teratogenic effects of, 150*t*
Retinopathy, diabetic, 221
Retractile testes, 534
Retractions, 526, 527*t*, 578
Return transport, of newborn, 596, 596*d*, 607–608
Rhizoids, 563
Rh negative factor, cultural differences in, 82
Rh sensitization, and fetal and neonatal complications, 495*t*
RI (resistance index), 265
Rights
exercise of, 15
notice of, 15
of patient, 15–16, 16*d*
Risk assessment, prenatal. *See* Prenatal risk assessment
Risk management, 32–35, 35*d*, 36*d*
Risk modification, 37
Rites of passage, for perinatal death, 483–484
Ritodrine hydrochloride (Yutopar), for preterm labor and birth, 216*d*, 217*d*, 218
Rituals, cultural differences in, 72*d*, 138
Rocking, during labor, 317*f*
Roles
gender, 54–55
of physicians and nurses, 55–56
on team, 60*d*

Rooming-in, and breast-feeding, 557–558
Root cause analysis, 41, 50–52
Rooting reflex, 548
Ropivacaine (Naropin), epidural anesthesia with, 434
RPF (renal plasma flow)
in preeclampsia, 180*t*
during pregnancy, 103
Rubella
prenatal immunization for, 168
teratogenic effects of, 150*t*
Rubeola, pneumonia due to, 252

Saddle block, 439–442
Safety
legal aspects of, 32–35, 35*d*, 36*d*
of newborn, 506–508, 506*t*, 507*d*
in postpartum home care, 651, 653
right to, 15
Salivary estriol, 144–147, 210
Saltatory fetal heart rate pattern, 400–401
Samoans, 78
Satiation cues, for breast-feeding, 558, 558*d*
Satisfaction, of patient, 13–14
with home care services, 652, 665
SBP (systolic blood pressure), during pregnancy, 100
Scalp electrode, fetal, 310, 381–383, 384*t*
Scalp stimulation, fetal, 405, 405*f*
Scaphoid, 533*t*
Scarf sign, 546
Schwartz-Dixon maneuver, 32
Sclera, 520, 521*t*
Scrotum, of newborn, 534, 535*t*
S/D (systolic/diastolic) ratio, 265
Seclusion, 15
Secobarbital sodium (Seconal), for labor pain, 432
Second trimester
adaptations during, 118–119, 118*d*
blood pressure during, 100
cardiac output during, 99
prenatal education in, 156*d*
Sedatives, for labor pain, 432
Seizure(s), in eclampsia, 185, 189–190
Seizure disorders, fetal and neonatal complications of, 495*t*
Self-assessment, of team, 59–65, 60*d*
Self-perception, adaptive and maladaptive, 470*d*
Semisitting position, during labor, 318*f*
Sentinel event(s), 40–41
root cause analysis in response to, 41, 50–52
Sepsis. *See* Infection(s)
Septic pelvic thrombophlebitis, 463
Septic shock, 459
Service, quality of, 8
Service excellence, 13–16
Seventh Day Adventism, 81, 81*t*
Sexual abuse, 328–329
Sexuality, postpartum, 465–466, 465*d*
Sexually transmitted diseases, and fetal and neonatal complications, 495*t*
SGA (small for gestational age), 514
SGOT (aspartate aminotransferase), during pregnancy, 106, 106*t*
SGPT (alanine aminotransferase), during pregnancy, 106, 106*t*
Shadow grief, 483
Shock
in bereavement, 477*d*
hemorrhagic, 205–206
hypovolemic
postpartum, 457
during pregnancy, 205, 205*d*
septic, 459
Short staffing, 16–18
Shoulder(s), in fetal heart rate monitoring, 402
Shoulder dystocia
complications of, 497*t*
diagnosis of, 324–325
documentation of, 326, 327*d*
interventions for, 323, 323*f*, 324*f*, 325–326
joint educational programs on, 64
labor and birth with, 323–326, 323*f*, 324*f*, 327*d*
risk factors for, 324
Shower, during labor, 427–428, 429*t*
Siblings
attachment by, 329, 354, 356*f*
present at birth, 329
Sick day management, for diabetes, 228–229, 229*d*, 295
Sickle cell disease
carrier frequency for, 145*d*
cultural differences in, 82
and fetal and neonatal complications, 495*t*
screening for, 142, 143*d*, 144*f*
Sidelying position
for breast-feeding, 555, 556*f*
during labor, 316*f*, 318*f*, 426*t*
Significant other, labor support by, 421–422, 422*d*
Silverman-Anderson Index, 526, 527*t*
Sinus, preauricular, 521, 522*f*, 523*t*
Sinusoidal fetal heart rate pattern, 399–400, 401*f*
Sitting, during labor, 314, 317*f*, 425*t*–426*t*
Skills checklists, 26–27
Skin
of newborn, 504, 514–517, 518*t*
color of, 514–516
erythema toxicum of, 517
and gestational age, 546
hemangiomas of, 516, 516*f*
milia on, 517
Mongolian spots on, 517, 517*f*
nevus simplex of, 516–517
port wine stain of, 516
texture of, 517
turgor of, 517
in postpartum period, 451, 474
during pregnancy, 109
Skin tags, preauricular, 521, 522*f*, 523*t*
Skin-to-skin contact, 500
Skull, of newborn, 519*t*
Sleep states, of newborn, 544
Slow dancing, during labor, 425*t*
Small for gestational age (SGA), 514
Small intestine, during pregnancy, 105–106
Smegma, 534
Smoking. *See* Cigarette smoking
Smoking cessation, 213–214
Social network, for bereavement, 483–484
Social services, prenatal, 155
Social trends, and birth rate, 126
Sociocultural system, 70, 71*f*
Socioeconomic status
and preeclampsia, 175–176
in prenatal risk assessment, 132*d*, 133
Sodium, serum, during pregnancy, 103–104
Soft palate, cleft, 524, 525*f*, 526*t*
Somatic distress, in acute grief work, 481*t*
Sonography. *See* Ultrasonography
Sore nipples, 561–564, 564*d*, 565*t*–566*t*
Sorrow, chronic, 482, 482*d*
Soy formulas, 569
Spanish, perinatal teaching materials in, 94
"Special cause" variation, 51–52
Speciality nurse, 23, 24
Spermicides, 467
Spider nevi, during pregnancy, 109
Spiral arteries, in preeclampsia, 182*t*, 187
Spiritual beliefs, and bereavement, 484–485
Spleen, of newborn, 531
Spontaneous abortion, 478–479. *See also* Perinatal death
in multiple gestation, 260–261, 262*d*
Square window, 546
Squatting, during labor, 313–314, 318*f*, 426*t*
Stabilization, of newborn, 502
Stadol (butorphanol), for labor pain, 433, 434*t*
Staffing, 41–42, 42*t*
Staff nurse, in discharge planning, 625–626
Standards, of care, 7–8, 8*d*, 31–32, 35–37
Standards and Guidelines for Professional Nursing Practice in the Care of Women and Newborns, 29
Standards of Clinical Nursing Practice, 29
Standing, during labor, 425*t*
Staphylococcus aureus, pneumonia due to, 251
Startle reflex, 549
Starvation, accelerated, 222
State, of newborn, 513, 544–545
State boards of nursing, 23
Station, 309
Stereotypical generalization, 86
Sterile water, intradermal injections of, for labor pain, 429–430, 430*f*
Sterilization, 467
Stillbirth, 479. *See also* Perinatal death
Stimulation, adaptive and maladaptive behaviors for, 469*d*
Stomach, during pregnancy, 105
Stool, of newborn, 559, 559*t*
Stork bite, 516–517
Strabismus, 520
Strawberry hemangioma, 516
Streptococcal infection
maternal, 495*t*
neonatal, 508–510, 509*f*, 510*f*, 588, 589*f*
Streptococcus pneumoniae, 251, 252, 253*t*
Streptomycin, teratogenic effects of, 149*t*
Stress
and postpartum depression, 137*d*
in prenatal risk assessment, 136
and teamwork, 59
Stress incontinence, postpartum, 449
Stressor, postpartum, 468
Stress test, 153–154
in multiple gestation, 265
Stretch marks, 109, 451
Striae gravidarum, 109, 451
Stripping of the membranes
for cervical ripening, 336
for induction of labor, 341–342
Stroke volume
defined, 237*d*
in preeclampsia, 181*t*
during pregnancy, 98*t*, 99
"Stuck twin" syndrome, 262
Style diversity, in team, 60*d*
Subgaleal hematoma, with vacuum extraction, 348
Sublimaze (fentanyl), for labor pain, 434, 434*t*
Substance abuse
fetal and neonatal complications with, 495*t*
history of, 163
in prenatal risk assessment, 135–136, 161–163
Sucking, evaluation of, 526*t*
Sucking blisters, 524
Sucking reflex, 548
Sufentanil (Sufenta), for labor pain, 434
Sugar water, and jaundice, 564
Sunrise Model, 69, 69*f*
Sunset eyes, 521*t*
Supernumerary nipples, 526
Supervision, 30
Supine position, for labor and birth, 313, 314
Supplemental feedings, 560
Support groups, for bereavement, 485, 486*d*, 490
Support organizations, for multiple gestation, 258, 274
Support person, 301, 329, 620
Suprapubic pressure, for shoulder dystocia, 323*f*, 325
Supraventricular tachycardia (SVT), fetal, 401
Surfactant, 496
Surrendering phase, of labor, 422*d*
Suture lines, 310, 518, 520*f*
SVR (systemic vascular resistance), during pregnancy, 98*t*, 100
Swallowing reflex, 548
Sweeping the membranes. *See* Stripping of the membranes
Sympathetic nervous system, 238, 239*d*
in fetal heart rate, 387, 388*d*
Symphysiotomy, 326
Syndactyly, 539*t*, 540*t*
Synthetic hygroscopic dilators, 335
Syphilis, teratogenic effects of, 150*t*

Systemic vascular resistance (SVR), during pregnancy, 98t, 100
Systolic blood pressure (SBP), during pregnancy, 100
Systolic/diastolic (S/D) ratio, 265
Systolic murmur, during pregnancy, 98

T_3 (triiodothyronine), during pregnancy, 108
T_4 (thyroxine), during pregnancy, 108
Tachycardia
  fetal, 389t, 392–393, 392t
    supraventricular, 401
  in newborn, 531t
Tachypnea, in newborn, 526, 528t
  transient, 578
Tactylon, 467
Taking-hold phase, in transition to parenthood, 468–469
Taking-in phase, in transition to parenthood, 468
Talipes calcaneovalgus, 538, 539f
Tap, 529
Tay-Sachs disease
  carrier frequency for, 145d
  cultural differences in, 82
  screening for, 142, 146t
T cells, during pregnancy, 111, 111t
Team(s) and teamwork, 53–66
  advantages of, 53–54
  barriers to, 54–58, 54d
  challenges and opportunities with, 65
  characteristics of, 59–65, 60d
  communication in, 55–56, 60d, 61–62
  consensus in, 58–59, 60d, 62–63
  defined, 58–59
  disagreements in, 60d
  external relations of, 60d
  informality in, 60d
  joint educational programs in, 63–65
  leadership of, 60d, 61
  listening in, 60d
  mission, vision, or goals of, 60–61, 60d
  multicultural, 89d
  mutual accountability in, 56, 59
  organizational discipline in, 59
  participation in, 60, 60d
  potential benefits of, 65–66
  professional competence and capabilities in, 61
  roles and work assignments with, 60d
  self-assessment of, 59–65, 60d
  stress and, 59
  style diversity in, 60d
  trends conducive to, 58
Teammates, fathers as, 421
Tears, 520
Teeth, 524
Telephone assessment form, for home care services, 659
Temperature, with multiple gestation, 259t
Temperature regulation, in newborn, 499–500, 501f, 501t
Teratogens, 145d, 147, 148t–151t
Teratology Information Services, 134
Terbutaline (Brethine)
  for asthma, 247–248
  for hyperstimulation of uterine activity, 337, 340, 341
  for preterm labor and birth, 216d, 217d, 218
Terminal bradycardia, 393, 394t
Testes, of newborn, 534, 535t
Testicular torsion, 535t
Testosterone, during pregnancy, 109
Testosterone derivatives, teratogenic effects of, 148t
Tetanus, prenatal immunization for, 170, 171
Tetracycline, teratogenic effects of, 149t
Tetralogy of Fallot (TET), 580–581, 580t
TGA (transposition of the great arteries), 580t, 581
Thalassemia
  cultural differences in, 82
  screening for, 142
Thalidomide, teratogenic effects of, 149t
Thecal cells, during pregnancy, 110
Thermal environment, for newborn, 579
Thermogenesis, nonshivering, 499
Thermoregulation, in newborn, 499–500, 501f, 501t
Third trimester
  adaptations during, 119–120, 120d
  prenatal education in, 156d
Thrill, 529
Thrombocytopenia, in preeclampsia, 182t, 184d
Thrombocytopenic purpura, idiopathic, fetal and neonatal complications with, 495t
Thromboembolism
  postpartum, 461–463
  prophylaxis for, 243
Thrombophlebitis, postpartum, 461–463
Thrush, sore nipples due to, 563–564
Thyroglossal duct cyst, 527t
Thyroid disease, fetal and neonatal complications with, 495t
Thyroid gland
  of newborn, 525, 527t
  in postpartum period, 448
  during pregnancy, 108
Thyroid hormone, during pregnancy, 108
Thyroxine (T_4), during pregnancy, 108
Tidal volume, during pregnancy, 102, 102t
Tincture of opium, for neonatal abstinence syndrome, 594
Tobacco use. *See* Cigarette smoking
Tocodynamometer, 310, 381
Tocolytic therapy, 215–219, 216d, 217d
  on labor flow sheet, 373
Toes, of newborn, 539t, 540t
Tongue, of newborn, 524, 526t
Tongue tie, 524
Tonic neck reflex, 549
TORCH infections, fetal and neonatal complications of, 495t
Torticollis, 524
Total lung volume, during pregnancy, 101, 102t
Touch, for labor pain, 428
Toxoplasmosis, teratogenic effects of, 151t
Training. *See* Education
Transcultural Assessment Model, 69, 70f
Transcultural Nursing Model, 69, 70f
Transfer
  to another hospital or home, 43–44
  maternal, 274–276, 275d
  neonatal, 596, 596d, 603–608
Transference, 116
Transfusion
  for antepartum bleeding, 202, 203t, 204
  for hypovolemic shock, 205, 205d
  twin-to-twin, 255, 261, 262–263, 263d
Transient tachypnea of newborn (TTN), 578
Transport
  to another hospital or home, 43–44
  maternal, 274–276, 275d
  neonatal, 596, 596d, 603–608
Transposition of the great arteries (TGA), 580t, 581
Transverse lie, complications of, 497t
TRAP (twin reversed arterial perfusion), 263
Trauma, during pregnancy, 206
Treponema pallidum, teratogenic effects of, 150t
Trigeminal nerve, assessment of, 541t
Triggers, for asthma, 244, 245t, 247
Triiodothyronine (T_3), during pregnancy, 108
Trimethadione, teratogenic effects of, 150t
Trimethoprim/sulfamethoxazole, for pneumonia, 252, 253t
Triple-marker screening, 142, 146t
Triplets. *See* Multiple gestation
Tripling, of contractions, 381
Trisomy 18, screening for, 146t
Trophoblast, immune system of, 112
Trunk incurvature, 549
TTN (transient tachypnea of newborn), 578
TTS (twin-to-twin transfusion syndrome), 255, 261, 262–263, 263d
Tubal ligation, 467
Tuberculosis, cultural differences in, 82
Turner syndrome, neck in, 527t4
Twin(s). *See* Multiple gestation
Twin embolization syndrome, 261
Twin reversed arterial perfusion (TRAP), 263
Twin-to-twin transfusion syndrome (TTS), 255, 261, 262–263, 263d
Tympanic membrane, 521
Typhoid, prenatal immunization for, 170

UAPs (unlicensed assistive personnel), working with, 30–31
Ultrasonography, 143–144
  with diabetes, 230t
  Doppler
    of fetal heart rate, 381, 383, 383f, 384d
    of multiple gestation, 265
  of multiple gestation, 256, 260t, 265–266
Umbilical blood flow, and fetal heart rate, 385–387, 386f, 387d
Umbilical blood sampling, percutaneous, 144, 146t
Umbilical cord
  assessment of, 504, 530, 533t
  care for, 508
  cultural differences in care of, 72
  knot in, 497t
  prolapsed, 497t
  rupture or tearing of, 497t
  velamentous insertion of, 497t
Umbilical cord blood gases, 408–409, 409t
Umbilical hernia, 530, 532f
Undescended testes, 534, 535t
Unit philosophy, 6
Unlicensed assistive personnel (UAPs), working with, 30–31
Urachus, patent, 533t
Urea, during pregnancy, 104t
Uric acid
  in preeclampsia, 180t
  during pregnancy, 104t
Urinary bladder
  in postpartum period, 449
  during pregnancy, 103
Urinary meatus, 532–533, 535t
Urinary tract infections (UTIs)
  fetal and neonatal complications with, 495t
  postpartum, 460–461
  and preeclampsia, 178
  during pregnancy, 103
Urination
  by newborn, 535t
  in postpartum period, 449
Urine, ketones in, 227
Urine color, of newborn, 559
Urine output
  in antepartum bleeding, 203, 204
  of newborn, 559, 559t, 560t
  postpartum, 449
Urine tests, for hypertension during pregnancy, 188d
Uterine activity
  and fetal heart rate, 380–381, 382f
  hyperstimulation of. *See* Uterine hyperstimulation
  during labor, 307d, 310
  monitoring of, 214–215
    with diabetic ketoacidosis, 231, 232t
    with multiple gestation, 259t
  reduction of, for nonreassuring fetal heart rate, 391
Uterine atony, postpartum hemorrhage due to, 199
Uterine blood flow, and fetal heart rate, 385–387, 386f, 387d
Uterine contractions
  coupling of, 381, 382f
  duration of, 304t–305t, 310, 380
  frequency of, 310, 380, 381
  in hyperstimulation, 381, 382f
  intensity of, 304t–305t, 310, 380
  normal, 381, 382f
  physiology of, 298–300
  tripling of, 381

Uterine dehiscence, 197, 198
with VBAC, 355
Uterine hyperstimulation, 330, 381, 382*f*
with Cervidil, 338*d*, 340
defined, 330, 381
with misoprostol, 339*d*, 340, 341
with oxytocin, 344
with Prepidil, 337, 338*d*
Uterine inversion, 191, 198, 198*d*, 454
Uterine involution, 446–447, 447*d*, 474
Uterine malformation, fetal and neonatal complications with, 495*t*
Uterine massage, postpartum, 454, 454*f*, 456, 457
Uterine prolapse, 452, 454
Uterine resting tone, 380–381
Uterine rupture
abruptio placentae and, 356–357
clinical manifestations of, 197–198
diagnosis of, 198
factors associated with, 197, 197*d*
incidence of, 191
management of, 198, 357–358
with misoprostol, 340
neonatal morbidity with, 357
terminal bradycardia with, 393, 394*t*
with VBAC, 191, 355–358
Uterine vascular resistance, during pregnancy, 100
Utero-placental insufficiency, late decelerations due to, 399*t*
Uterus, during pregnancy, 110
UTIs. *See* Urinary tract infections (UTIs)
Uvula, 524, 525*t*

Vaccination
newborn, for hepatitis B virus, 510–511
during pregnancy, 168–172
Vacuum extraction, 346, 348–349
complications of, 347, 348, 349, 497*t*
Vagina
postpartum, 447
during pregnancy, 110
Vaginal birth
of triplets, 270, 271*d*
of twins, 267, 267*d*, 268–269, 269*d*
Vaginal birth after cesarean (VBAC), 354–358
benefits of, 356
candidates for, 356
contraindications to, 356
costs of, 357
incidence of, 350
with multiple gestation, 270
nursing care for, 357
predicting success of, 357
risks of, 357
uterine rupture with, 355–358
Vaginal discharge, in newborn, 533
Vaginal examinations, during labor, 309–310
Vaginal pouch, 467
Vagus nerve, in fetal heart rate, 387, 388*d*
Validation, in learning-needs assessment, 621
Valium, for seizures, 185
Valproic acid, teratogenic effects of, 150*t*
Valsalva maneuver, 315
Value system, cultural differences in, 72*d*
Valvular stenosis, 235
Vanishing twin syndrome, 255, 261, 262*d*
Variability, in fetal heart rate, 380*t*, 390
absent, 380*t*, 395, 395*t*, 400*t*
alterations in, 394–395, 395*t*
baseline, 390
long-term, 390
marked, 380*t*, 395
minimal, 380*t*, 395, 395*t*, 400*t*
moderate, 380*t*, 394–395, 400*t*
short-term, 390
Variable decelerations, 380*t*, 396–398, 397*f*, 399*t*, 402–403
Varicella
of newborn, 252–253
prenatal immunization for, 171, 252
teratogenic effects of, 151*t*
Varicella pneumonia, 250, 251–253
Varicella-zoster immune globulin (VZIG), 252, 254
Vasa previa, 191, 196–197, 197*d*, 497*t*
Vascular resistance
of fetus *vs.* newborn, 496, 498, 499, 578
during pregnancy
in preeclampsia, 180*t*, 181*t*
pulmonary, 100
systemic, 98*t*, 100
uterine, 100
Vascular system, 238
Vasoactive substances, altered response to, in preeclampsia, 181*t*
Vasoconstriction, in preeclampsia, 179
Vasopressin, 109
Vasospasms, in preeclampsia, 179, 180–183, 187
VBAC. *See* Vaginal birth after cesarean (VBAC)
Veins, 238
Vein-to-vein anastomoses, in multiple gestations, 262
Velamentous insertion, of umbilical cord, 497*t*
Ventilation, during pregnancy, 102
Ventricular septal defect (VSD), 580, 580*t*
Vernix, 518*t*
Very-low-birth-weight (VLBW) infants
incidence of, 207
mortality rate for, 208
Videos, on infant care, 618
Vietnamese, 78
Viral pneumonia, 251–252
Vision
of newborn, 520
of perinatal team, 60–61, 60*d*
in preeclampsia, 184*d*
Vistaril (hydroxyzine hydrochloride), for labor pain, 432
Visual techniques, for labor pain, 424*t*, 431
Vital capacity, during pregnancy, 102, 102*t*
Vital signs
with antepartum bleeding, 201–202
during labor and birth, 306*d*, 308–309
with multiple gestation, 259*t*
Vitamin(s)
in breast milk, 554
prenatal, 135
Vitamin A, teratogenic effects of, 150*t*
Vitamin K, for newborn, 508
VLBW (very-low-birth-weight) infants
incidence of, 207
mortality rate for, 208
Volume depletion, in preeclampsia, 179
Vomiting, during pregnancy, 105
VSD (ventricular septal defect), 580, 580*t*
VZIG (varicella-zoster immune globulin), 252, 254

Waiting phase, of labor, 422*d*
Walking
with epidural analgesia, 437, 437*d*
during labor, 314, 316*f*, 425*t*
Warfarin, teratogenic effects of, 148*t*
"Warm lines," 626
Water immersion, during labor, 427–428, 429*t*
WBC (white blood cell) count, during pregnancy, 101
Weight
birth, 513
low. *See* Low-birth-weight (LBW) infants
maternal, and fetal and neonatal complications, 495*t*
Weight gain
of newborn, 559
during pregnancy, 107, 107*t*
with multiple gestation, 258–260
in prenatal risk assessment, 135, 135*d*
and preterm labor and birth, 214
Weight loss, postpartum, 451
Well baby care, for multiples, 272
West Indians, 76
WHCNPs (women's healthcare nurse practitioners), 129
Whirlpool tub, during labor, 427–428, 429*t*
White(s), 75*f*, 80
comparative statistical data on, 74*t*
pregnancy-induced hypertension in, 174*t*
White blood cell (WBC) count, during pregnancy, 101
WHO (World Health Organization), 16
Whole blood, fresh, for antepartum bleeding, 202, 203*t*
Withdrawal
neonatal, 591–596
assessment of, 592–593, 593*t*, 594, 595*f*
incidence of, 591–592
interventions for, 593–596, 594*d*
pathophysiology of, 592, 592*d*
symptoms of, 592–593, 593*t*
symptoms of, 162
Witnesses, fathers as, 421
Women, historical roles of, 54–55
Women's healthcare nurse practitioners (WHCNPs), 129
Woods corkscrew maneuver, 325
Work assignments, on team, 60*d*
Workshops, 28
World Health Organization (WHO), 16
Wound infections, postpartum, 459
Written materials, on infant care, 618

Xiphoid process, 525
Xiphoid retractions, 526, 527*t*
Xylocaine (lidocaine), epidural anesthesia with, 434

Yellow fever, prenatal immunization for, 168
Yin/yang polarity, 77
Yutopar (ritodrine hydrochloride), for preterm labor and birth, 216*d*, 217*d*, 218

Zavanelli maneuver, 326
Zygosity, 254–255, 254*t*, 256